IMMUNE HEMOLYTIC ANEMIAS

IMMUNE HEMOLYTIC ANEMIAS

SECOND EDITION

LAWRENCE D. PETZ, M.D.
Emeritus Professor of Pathology and Laboratory Medicine
University of California
Los Angeles, California

Chief Medical Officer
StemCyte
Arcadia, California

GEORGE GARRATTY, Ph.D., FRCPath.
Scientific Director
American Red Cross Blood Services
Southern California Region

Clinical Professor of Pathology and Laboratory Medicine
University of California
Los Angeles, California

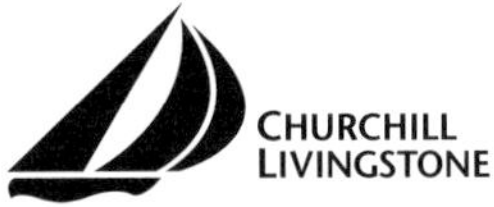

An Imprint of Elsevier

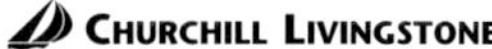
CHURCHILL LIVINGSTONE
An Imprint of Elsevier
The Curtis Center
Independence Square West
Philadelphia, Pennsylvania 19106

Notice

Medicine is an ever-changing field. Standard safety precautions must be followed, but as new research and clinical experience broaden our knowledge, changes in treatment and drug therapy may become necessary or appropriate. Readers are advised to check the most current product information provided by the manufacturer of each drug to be administered to verify the recommended dose, the method and duration of administration, and contraindications. It is the responsibility of the treating physician, relying on experience and knowledge of the patient, to determine dosages and the best treatment for each individual patient. Neither the Publisher nor the editor assumes any liability for any injury and/or damage to persons or property arising from this publication.

The Publisher

Library of Congress Cataloging-in-Publication Data

Petz, Lawrence D.
Immune hemolytic anemias / Lawrence D. Petz, George Garratty.—2nd ed.
p. ; cm.
Rev. ed. of: Acquired immune hemolytic anemias. 1980.
Includes bibliographical references.
ISBN 0-443-08559-5
1. Hemolytic anemia, Autoimmune. I. Garratty, George. II. Petz, Lawrence D. Acquired immune hemolytic anemias. III. Title.
[DNLM: 1. Anemia, Hemolytic, Autoimmune. WH 170 P513i 2004]
RC641.7.H4P47 2004
616.1'52—dc21

2003043767

Printed in United States of America

Last digit is the print number: 9 8 7 6 5 4 3 2 1

Preface to the Second Edition

We thought we might have set a record for the longest time between editions of a book, since the first edition of this book, entitled *Acquired Immune Hemolytic Anemias*, was published 24 years ago. However, our mentor, Professor Sir John Dacie, published the third edition of *Autoimmune Haemolytic Anaemias* (Volume 3 of *The Haemolytic Anemias*) in 1992, just 30 years after the publication of the previous edition of that volume!

We have been flattered during these long years by a number of physicians, immunohematologists, and blood bankers who insist that they still use the first edition and have continued to press us for the second. As with the first edition, this book is intended primarily as a useful source of information for those who care for patients who have immune hemolytic anemias, that is, clinicians with patient care responsibility and blood bank professionals, including physicians and technical staff. However, this purpose cannot be properly served without an adequately detailed scientific background, and we have endeavored to supply this. We have attempted to be rather comprehensive, but we do not intend this book to be only a reference volume and have therefore included practical aspects of the evaluation and management of patients with hemolysis.

Patients with immune hemolytic anemias are sufficiently common as to constitute an important problem, but, on the other hand, they are sufficiently unusual that it is difficult for many individuals outside of referral centers to acquire adequate experience to feel at ease in managing the multitude of problems such patients may present. We earnestly hope that sharing our experiences through the medium of this book will be of value to others who confront such problems less commonly.

During the years between editions of this text, medical disciplines that were rather early in their developmental stages, such as hematopoietic cell and solid organ transplantation, have emerged to be major components of health care and have contributed to the emergence of entirely new causes of immune hemolysis. Also, new "generations" of drugs have been developed, one of the consequences of which is an expansion of the causes of drug-induced immune hemolytic anemias. Molecular biology and DNA technology have evolved to become a part of our everyday scientific lives and are being utilized in hematology as in all other disciplines. We have attempted to bring our first edition up to date while not ignoring important earlier contributions. We have added chapters on Historical Concepts of Immune Hemolytic Anemias, Hemolytic Disease of the Fetus and Newborn, Immune Hemolysis Associated with Transplantation, and Hemolytic Transfusion Reactions.

As we emphasized in the preface to the first edition, one of the important aspects of diagnosis and management of patients with immune hemolytic anemias is that the care of such patients depends on a knowledge of some aspects of both clinical and laboratory medicine. Although this is true throughout clinical medicine, a problem of particular magnitude is created by the need for clinicians to be able to interpret such unusual laboratory tests as the direct antiglobulin test with monospecific antiglobulin sera and the specificity and thermal range of allo- and autoantibodies. Similarly, laboratory personnel should be able to assist clinicians in the interpretation of important data, as when transfusion is indicated for a patient whose serum reacts with all RBCs in compatibility tests. Accordingly, one of the primary purposes of this book is to present both the clinical and laboratory aspects of immune hemolytic anemias in a single volume. We strongly feel that neither laboratory personnel (including physicians) nor clinicians can optimally contribute to the care of patients with immune hemolytic anemias without a firm understanding of both aspects of the subject.

Lawrence D. Petz
George Garratty

Preface to the First Edition

This book is intended to be a useful source of information for those who care for patients who have immune hemolytic anemias, i.e., clinicians with primary responsibility for patient management, physicians concerned with laboratory medicine, including blood bank directors, and the technical staff of such laboratories. It is not intended as an encyclopedic review or as a "tour de force" exposition of facts that are of interest primarily to those with extensive background and a highly specialized interest in the field.

Patients with immune hemolytic anemias are sufficiently common as to constitute an important problem but, on the other hand, are sufficiently unusual that it is difficult for many individuals outside of referral centers to acquire adequate experience to feel at ease in managing the multitude of problems such patients may present. We have had a special interest in these disorders and we earnestly hope that sharing our experiences through the medium of this book will be of value to others who confront such problems less commonly. We include previously unpublished data concerning our experiences with various phases of the diagnosis and management of more than 300 patients, as well as a review of relevant information available in the medical literature.

Although the primary purpose of this book is, therefore, to be a source of information that will be of value in management of patients, this purpose cannot be adequately served merely by a superficial exposition of "practical" facts, and we do not intend this book to be a manual of patient care. We trust that the interested reader would demand an adequately detailed scientific background to make meaningful the recommended laboratory procedures and their clinical interpretation. For example, the knowledge that the direct antiglobulin (Coombs') test performed on red cells from patients with cold agglutinin syndrome is invariably positive using anit-C3d antiglobulin serum and invariably negative using anti-IgG antiglobulin serum is of some clinical value (Ch. 6). When such information is augmented by an understanding of pertinent aspects of the serum complement system (Ch. 3) and the mechanisms of immune hemolysis (Ch. 4), one then has a basis for understanding such facts and their clinical significance.

Writing this book presents a unique problem. That is, one of the important aspects of diagnosis and management of patients with immune hemolytic anemias is that the care of such patients depends upon a knowledge of some aspects of both clinical and laboratory medicine. Although this is true throughout medicine, a problem of unusual magnitude is created by the fact that most clinicians have very little exposure to immunohematology. Results of direct antiglobulin tests with monospecific antiglobulin sera and the characterization of serum antibody specificity and thermal range is information that is difficult or impossible for most practicing physicians to utilize. This problem is augmented by the fact that laboratory personnel are faced with difficult technical tasks, and, in the very best of hands, uncertainties may remain. For example, in regard to blood transfusion (Ch. 10), what is the probability of not detecting a red cell alloantibody in the serum of a patient with autoimmune hemolytic anemia when the serum reacts with all donor cells tested, and what is the risk of transfusion of blood that is incompatible because of the presence of an autoantibody? One of the prime purposes of this book, and one of the more difficult tasks we faced in writing it, is to present both the laboratory and clinical aspects of immune hemolytic anemias in a single volume in a manner that is understandable by those in both fields. Neither laboratory personnel (including physicians) nor clinicians can optimally contribute to the care of patients with immune hemolytic anemias without an understanding of both aspects of the subject. Therefore, it is our firm opinion that, with few exceptions (e.g., some sections concerning technical details which may justifiably be ignored by clinicians, and some aspects of therapy which may not be essential knowledge for technologists), the information herein is important to those in both clinical and laboratory medicine for proper management of patients with immune hemolytic anemias.

Lawrence D. Petz
George Garratty

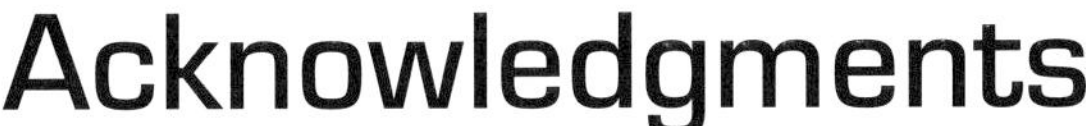

Acknowledgments

As indicated in the first edition, we are both indebted to Professor Sir John Dacie for the privilege of working in his laboratory at the Royal Postgraduate Medical School and Hammersmith Hospital in London. His teachings served as a foundation for our work and, moreover, we have attempted to emulate his dedication and precision in scientific investigation.

Grateful acknowledgment is also due to the numerous physicians and technologists who were kind enough to refer interesting and challenging clinical and laboratory problems to us. Without this continued support it would have been impossible to acquire the experience and data necessary to compile this volume. In addition, we appreciate the collaboration of our colleagues at the City of Hope Medical Center, Duarte, California, and the University of California Los Angeles Medical Center (Dr. Petz) and American Red Cross Blood Services, Southern California Region (Dr. Garratty).

We would especially like to thank some extraordinary medical technologists who were not just a "pair of hands" in the laboratory but were innovative contributors to the design and results of our studies: Donald Branch (now the proud possessor of a PhD); Alana (Loni) Calhoun, Patricia Arndt, Regina Leger, Sandra Nance, and Nina Postoway. Their relevant roles were obvious from our publications mentioned throughout the book. Dr. Garratty would especially like to thank Ann Tunick, his administrative assistant (since 1978), who typed multiple error-free drafts of material, found and formatted references, and dealt imperturbably with all problems that arose. Without her help Dr. Garratty's contributions would never have appeared in this book!

Both of us would like to acknowledge the tremendous support of our wives (Thelma Petz and Eileen Garratty), who put up with our working every weekend and many evenings without too many grumbles!

Contents

CHAPTER 1

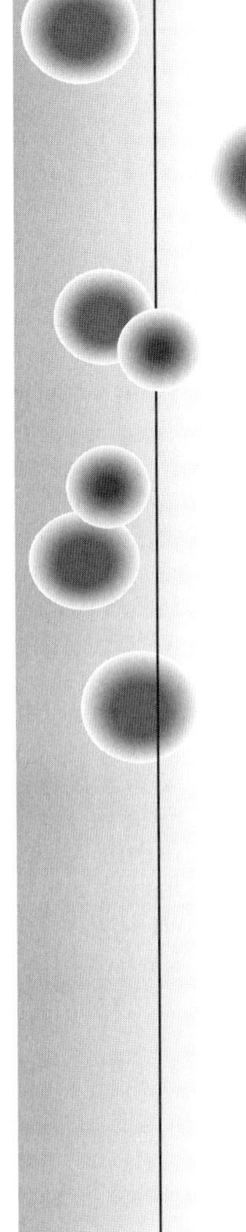

Historical Concepts of Immune Hemolytic Anemias

Immune hemolysis is a shortening of red blood cell (RBC) survival due, directly or indirectly, to antibodies. These antibodies may be autoantibodies or alloantibodies. This chapter will deal mainly with historical aspects of autoimmune hemolytic anemia (AIHA), followed by a brief discussion of historical aspects of hemolytic transfusion reactions.

AIHA is an acquired immunologic disease in which the patient's RBCs are selectively attacked and destroyed (hemolysed) by autoantibodies produced by the patient's own immune system. Shortened RBC survival is frequently associated with the presence of a reticulocytosis, spherocytes in the peripheral blood film, autoantibodies in the patient's serum, and occasionally splenomegaly, hemoglobinemia, and hemoglobinuria. Although these facts are common knowledge now, it was not always so. Reviewing how these concepts developed over the centuries by observation and clinical and laboratory experimentation is both fascinating and instructive.

It is evident that concepts that collectively led to our present understanding of AIHA required knowledge of the existence of RBCs, understanding the possibility of anemia without blood loss, distinguishing hemoglobinuria from hematuria, understanding the mechanism by which hemoglobinuria occurs, recognizing the process of agglutination, understanding the distinction between congenital and acquired disorders, understanding that premature destruction of RBCs can cause anemia and jaundice, recognizing spherocytes and abnormal osmotic fragility of RBCs and determining their significance in patients with hemolysis, recognizing reticulocytes, determining that serum antibodies may cause destruction of foreign cells and also autologous cells, developing means to measure RBC survival, developing diagnostic assays for antibodies, refuting the concept of *horror autotoxicus*, and understanding the role of the spleen and splenectomy.

The discoveries that led to the development of our knowledge about these concepts are herein reviewed in the approximate order in which the relevant observations were made. Here, then, is how our knowledge of AIHA came to be. The development of this short review was aided significantly by previous reviews on various aspects of hemolysis and AIHA.[1-9]

THE LESSONS OF HISTORY

Everyone who studies the stories of discovery in what has come to be called the field of hematology will recognize the early gropings in the midst of profound ignorance and the difficulties that confronted the investigators. We have gained an understanding of biology that could hardly have been dreamed of only a short time ago, let alone at the time of the first tentative forays into the unknown. Moreover, understanding has been crowned by tangible benefits for humanity. It is worthwhile to consider how such great progress comes about and why. How is knowledge achieved, and what can we learn from the process by which important discoveries were made?[10]

The first lesson to be learned of history is that the path of progress is anything but straight. The course of research has been likened to the flow of a stream that ultimately becomes a rushing torrent whose importance is obvious. This certainly has been the history of research in hematology.

It certainly does not follow that, because a concept is plausible and is in accord with the understanding of the time, it is necessarily correct. The following pages provide many examples of misinterpretations resulting from such an assumption. Furthermore, because they have been plausible, such views often have endured and have stood in the way of acceptance of observations and interpretations that proved to be the correct ones.

Discovery begins with an observation or the posing of a question. But observation is not as simple as it sounds. Indeed, many look but few see. It is the exceptional person who recognizes the unusual event or manifestation. Still fewer pursue it to new understanding. Many may ask questions but few have the imagination, the energy, and the overpowering drive to persist in the search for an answer, especially when this must be done in the face of difficulties and failures and even despite scorn from their peers.

Imagination and industry alone, however, have not sufficed. Means have had to be devised to explore the questions that were posed. When these were provided, it is impressive to see what the introduction of a new technique made possible for an area of inquiry. A simple example, described later, is the introduction of the antiglobulin test, which very rapidly led to a much clearer distinction between immune and nonimmune hemolytic anemias.

Progress depends on the contributions of many. Moreover, scientific discipline has benefited from developments in other fields, progress in one field spurring another, and vice versa. As knowledge has grown, it has become impossible for a single human being to encompass the whole, and the discovery and growth of understanding have become more and more dependent on interchange among scientific disciplines.

Still another aspect of the progress of understanding is worth noting. It is not generally appreciated how often curiosity concerning an observation made at the bedside by clinicians has led to far-reaching investigations. An example is the observation of hemoglobinuria, which led to the understanding of destruction of RBCs and to the early delineation of certain clinical syndromes (e.g., paroxysmal cold hemoglobinuria [PCH], paroxysmal nocturnal hemoglobinuria [PNH], and march hemoglobinuria) characterized by hemoglobin in the urine.

Investigators have not always been farseeing and logical, moving steadily and directly to their goal, nor did they fail to make mistakes. Indeed, incorrect theories have hampered the advance of knowledge, especially when these theories were widely disseminated and were pronounced by eminent authorities. A number of such examples appear in the following pages.

It follows that authorities must be humble and novices skeptical.

EARLIEST DESCRIPTIONS OF POSSIBLE ACQUIRED HEMOLYTIC ANEMIA

The first written description of what may have been an acquired hemolytic anemia, albeit not of an immune nature, was Galen's description in 150 AD of a person bitten by a viper whose "skin turned the color of a ripe leek."[1,4,11] Galen's understanding of physiology was such that he implicated the spleen as leading to the skin discoloration, an association of the spleen and hemolysis that was not confirmed until the late nineteenth century.[1]

PCH may have been described as early as 1529 by Johannes Actuarius, a court physician in Constantinople. In his work, *De Urinis*, Acturarius described a condition in which the urine is "azure & livid as well as black" in patients being of melancholic humor and complaining of loss of strength, after an exposure to cold.[4] Further mention of PCH seems, however, to be absent for nearly 300 years, until the latter half of the nineteenth century.

EARLY EXPERIMENTAL INVESTIGATION OF BLOOD

Description of Red Blood Cells. The development of the scientific method led to the seminal discoveries of the circulation of blood by Harvey in the early sixteenth century and the cardinal experiments with transfusion of blood by Lower in England and Denis in Paris in the mid-seventeenth century. Despite this interest in blood, the discovery of the RBCs had to await the appearance of the microscope around 1650. The first observation of an RBC was likely made by Malpighi in 1661, when he described the circulation of RBCs in the capillaries, and this was followed in 1663 by Swammerdan's description of minute globules in the blood of a frog. A decade later, human RBCs were described in detail by van Leeuwenhoek (Fig. 1-1),[12] who also established their size at about $\frac{1}{3000}$ of an inch by comparing an RBC with a grain of sand of known size.

John Huxham, in 1770, described the changing shapes of degenerating RBCs and, importantly, recognized that such cells were the origin of hemoglobin.[4]

Anemia without Blood Loss. In 1843, Andral (Fig. 1-2) described a spontaneous anemia, which arises without any prior blood loss.[13] He quantified red blood globules in healthy patients and reported

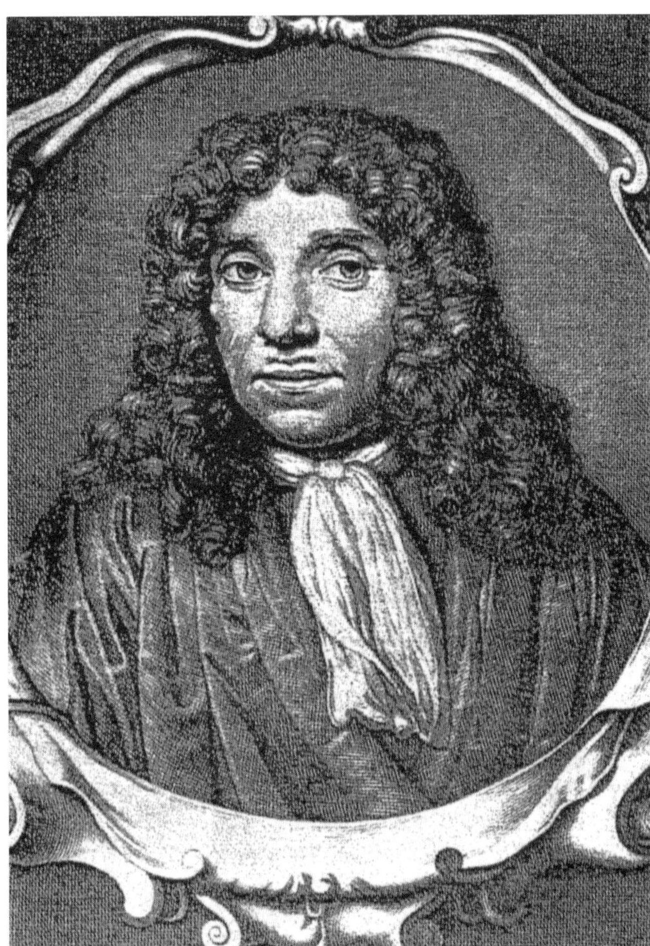

FIGURE 1-1. Antonj van Leeuwenhoek (1632–1723). (From Wintrobe MM: Milestones on the path of progess. In: Wintrobe MM (ed): Blood, Pure and Eloquent. New York: McGraw-Hill Book Company, 1980:1–31.)

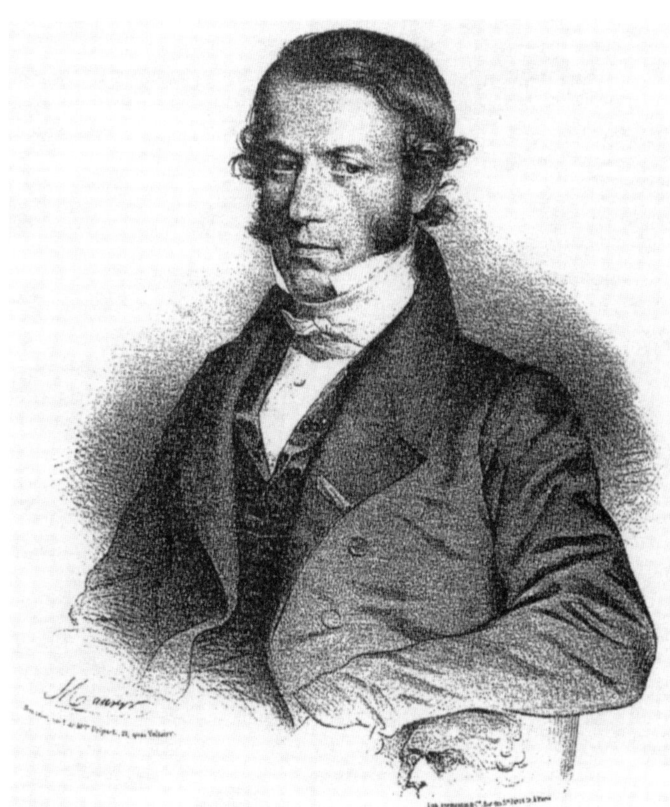

FIGURE 1-2. Gabriel Andral (1797–1876). (From Wintrobe MM: Milestones on the path of progress. In: Wintrobe MM (ed): Blood, Pure and Eloquent. New York: McGraw-Hill Book Company, 1980:1–31.)

16 early case of anemia. Although he provided no other information concerning the patients' condition, what is important in relation to hemolytic anemia is the observation of anemia without prior blood loss.

Hemoglobinuria. Vogel, in 1853,[14] stated that the matter in the urine is the same as that in the blood and suggested that the matter in the urine consists of a "decomposition of blood discs." He suggested that the degree of blood decomposition can readily be ascertained by the degree of coloration in the urine, and he indicated a connection between fevers, colored urine, decomposition of blood discs, and anemia. This represents one of the early examples of the association between a decreased RBC count and the term *anemia.* It also represents early evidence suggesting that anemia may be secondary to infections.

RED BLOOD CELL AGGLUTINATION

The description of the phenomenon of RBC agglutination and its development as a tool in elucidating blood groups took place in the last 30 years of the nineteenth century in Germany and Austria, and were reviewed in depth in 2002 by Hughes-Jones and Gardner.[15] The discoveries were largely the work of three people: Adolf Creite, a medical student in Göttingen, Germany; Leonard Landois, Director of the Physiological Institute at the University of Greifswald, Germany; and Karl Landsteiner, working in the Pathological Anatomy Institute in Vienna, Austria.[15]

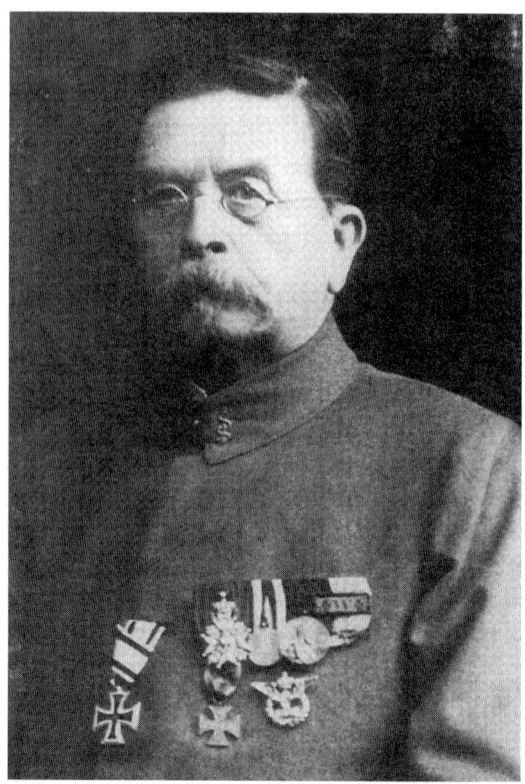

FIGURE 1-3. Adolf Creite, about 1920. (From Hughes-Jones NC, Gardner B: Red cell agglutination: The first description by Creite (1869) and further observations made by Landois (1875) and Landsteiner (1901). Br J Haematol 2002;119:889–893.)

Adolph Creite. Creite's (Fig. 1-3) almost unknown contribution was published in 1869 under the title "Investigations concerning the properties of serum proteins following intravenous injection."[16] His work is quite remarkable in that it showed that serum proteins had the property of both "dissolving" and bringing about "clustering" of red cells, that is, *lysis* and *agglutination* in present-day terms, anticipating the discovery of antibodies by a quarter of a century.

Creite injected sera from calf, pig, dog, sheep, cat, chicken, duck, and goat into rabbits. The first three had little or no effect on the recipient, but the sera of the latter five almost always resulted in the appearance of "blood-stained urine," general malaise, and death of the animal. He noted that the urine was free of intact RBCs. He concluded that serum contains agents that are able to dissolve red cells "directly." He performed additional experiments in which he removed protein from the serum before its injection and observed that "all of the urine samples examined until the evening of the following day are normal." Accordingly, he concluded that the most likely active ingredients were serum proteins, but added, "However, I cannot say how they function."

He also performed in vitro experiments and provided a remarkably clear account of what is probably the first description of agglutination. He reported, "If you add blood serum from any of the animals with which I have carried out my experiments to a drop of fresh rabbit blood, then you observe under the microscope that in the regions where the foreign serum mixes with the rabbit red cells, the cells suddenly flow together in a peculiar way forming different shaped drop-like clusters with irregular branches. I believed that I had found an explanation for the appearance of blood in the urine, as it was possible that some blood cells had dissolved completely."

Leonard Landois. RBC agglutination and lysis were put on an even firmer basis by Landois, who published an extensive monograph on the subject of transfusion,[17] which included a section describing his in vitro experiments. In his experiments, Landois was successful in demonstrating both lysis and agglutination. (It should be noted that the terms *lysis* and *agglutination* were not in use until the end of the nineteenth century. For *lysis*, both Creite and Landois used a German word meaning "dissolve"; for agglutination, words translatable as "accumulation," "ball formation," or "sticky clumps" were used.) Landois also distinguished *agglutination* from *rouleaux*, for which he used the term, "like rolls of coins."

Landois added 4 to 5 mL of clear serum into a test tube and then added fresh defibrinated blood. He incubated the mixture at 37°C to 38°C or at room temperature and observed the initiation of the RBC lysis.

"Sooner or later the mixture becomes completely clear and transparent and the cells are no longer visible. I observe the whole process of the lysis and the changes in red cell shape under the microscope." Commenting on another experiment on the mixing of cells and serum, Landois described the changes in shape of RBCs and added, "The cells develop the ability to stick to neighboring cells" and "form larger or smaller clumps."

Karl Landsteiner. At the turn of the century, there was a considerable amount of disagreement and confusion about the occurrence and significance of agglutination in both health and disease.[15] It was at this point that Landsteiner (Fig. 1-4) entered the field.[17a,b] The first suggestion of the existence of serum agglutinins and red cell antigens within what would finally be known as the ABO blood group system is to be found as a footnote in a publication by Landsteiner in 1900.[18] In it he states, "The serum of healthy individuals not only have an agglutinating effect on animal red cells but also on human red cells from different individuals. It remains to be decided whether this phenomenon is due to individual differences or to the influence of injuries or bacterial infection." In a detailed paper in 1901, he reported that he obtained sera and red cells from 29 different people, including himself and four medical colleagues, to study agglutination reactions. The reason that Landsteiner was successful in elucidating the mechanism underlying intraspecies agglutination where others had failed arose from the nature of Landsteiner's experimental design. He used all of the sera against all of the samples of RBCs, using "checkerboard" blocks of five or six different sera and RBCs in 144 combinations. He found that certain sera would agglutinate the RBCs of certain other people. This discovery of isoagglutination became the basis of human blood-group classification, which would subsequently be found to have relevance for autoantibody specificity in AIHA.

In his characteristically brief but data-filled paper of 1901,[19] Landsteiner further noted and pointed out that the blood isoagglutinins retained their activity after drying and redissolving. Also, he observed agglutination with serum extracted after 14 days from blood dried on a cloth. "The reaction may be suited to establish the identity or more correctly the non-identity of a blood specimen." This predicted the value of Landsteiner's discovery to forensic medicine in the future. The closing statement in his paper was, "Finally, it might be mentioned that the reported observations may assist in the explanation of various consequences of therapeutical blood transfusions." In three pages, Landsteiner compressed knowledge that would fill thousands of pages in the future.[20]

On November 8, 1930, Karl Landsteiner was awarded the Nobel Prize (Fig. 1-5). The lecture given by Landsteiner at the conferment of his Noble Prize was based on the "differences in the blood of human individuals." More than a century later, his theories about isoantigens are accepted and are a fundamental part of the theoretical basis of immunology, tissue transplantation, forensic medicine, and population genetics.[21,22]

FIRST DESCRIPTION OF HEMOLYTIC ANEMIA

The concept that premature destruction of RBCs might lead to a disease state and jaundice was first suggested in 1871 by Vanlair and Masius.[1,23] These observers described a patient with anemia and marked splenomegaly without hepatomegaly. The patient suffered acute attacks of left upper quadrant pain and jaundice without acholia, and passed reddish brown urine. Morphologic evidence of an RBC abnormality was suggested by finding spherical dwarf cells in the peripheral blood that they called *microcytes.* The authors postulated that clinical jaundice could result from two different mechanisms: "mechanically by reabsorption or liver induced" and "paradoxical icterus." The latter group included the "blood induced icterus," where excessive amounts of colorant material is released from the blood cells and followed by the formation of bile which is deposited in the tissues. More explicitly, they stated that "there are at least a certain number of non-mechanical types of icterus which are caused by the exaggerated destruction of red cells and the transformation to bilirubin of released hematin." This concept was essentially correct, but little attention was paid to this remarkable publication and, for almost 30 years, hepatic disease, jaundice, and hemolytic anemia became hopelessly intertwined.[1]

THE DISTINCTION BETWEEN CONGENITAL AND ACQUIRED HEMOLYTIC ANEMIAS

At the turn of the twentieth century, Hayem[24] (Fig. 1-6) and Minkowski[25] showed that the jaundice associated with hemolytic anemia was distinct from that of hepatic diseases. Hayem made the distinction between congenital and acquired hemolytic anemias, whereas Minkowski described only a hereditary condition. Hayem has repeatedly been said to be the first to describe acquired hemolytic anemia, although he did not name it that, but, instead, coined the term *chronic infectious splenomegalic icterus.*[24] Minkowski is credited with the first clear recognition of icterus due to hemolytic anemia (*chronic hereditary acholuric icterus*) separate from obstructive jaundice; he associated the anemia with urobilinuria and splenomegaly and postulated that RBC destruction was attributable to lesions in the spleen.[25]

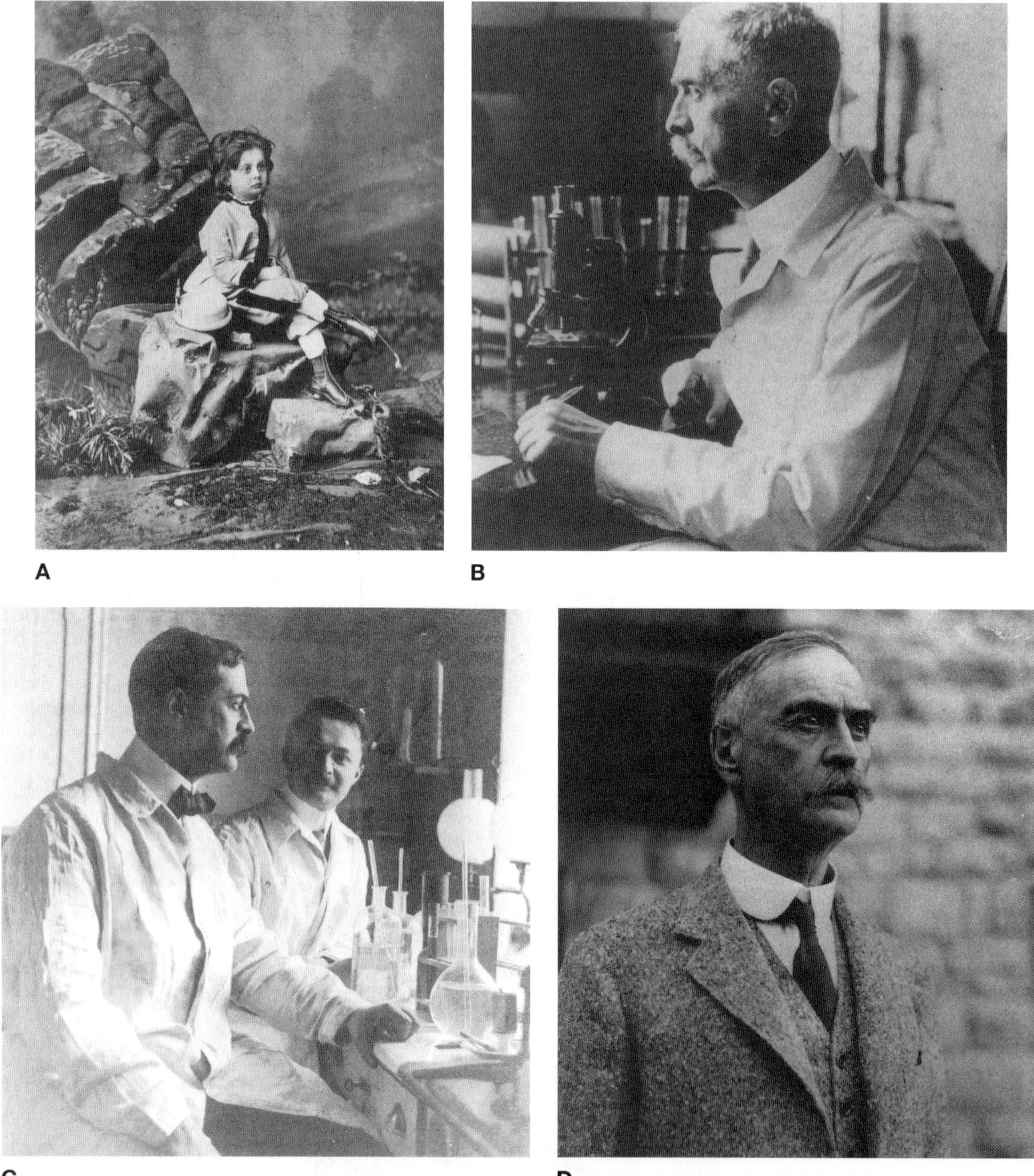

FIGURE 1-4. Karl Landsteiner at various times in his life. (*A*) Landsteiner at about the age of 5 (c. 1873), posing in a Husara riding costume on the photographer's papier-maché rocks. (*B*) Photograph of Landsteiner probably taken at the Institute for Pathological Anatomy, where he worked from 1897 to 1907. (*C*) Landsteiner and his coworker, Emil Prášek from Belgrade, December 1913. The two worked together on the chemical manipulation of the specificity of serum albumin. (*D*) Landsteiner at about the time he left Europe for the United States. (From Mazumbar MH: Species and Specificity. An Interpretation of the History of Immunology. Cambridge, UK: Cambridge University Press, 1995.)

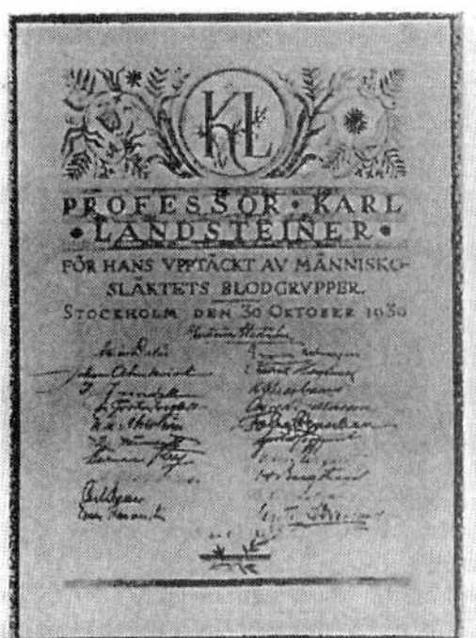

PROFESSOR · KARL
· LANDSTEINER ·
FÖR HANS VPPTÄCKT AV MÄNNISKO-
SLÄKTETS BLODGRVPPER.
STOCKHOLM DEN 30 OKTOBER 1930

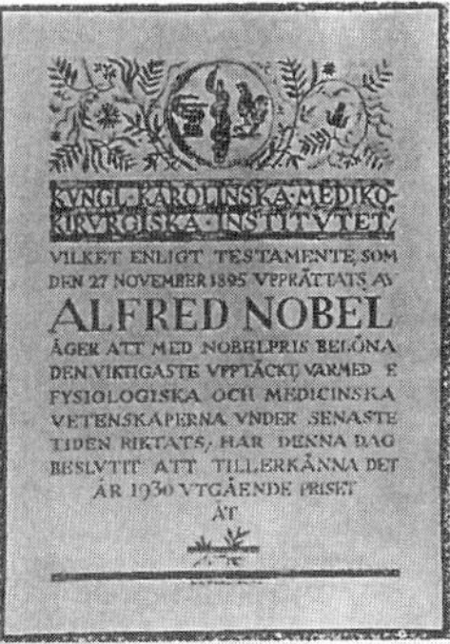

KVNGL · KAROLINSKA · MEDIKO-
KIRVRGISKA · INSTITVTET
VILKET ENLIGT TESTAMENTE SOM
DEN 27 NOVEMBER 1895 VPPRÄTTATS AV
ALFRED NOBEL
ÄGER ATT MED NOBELPRIS BELÖNA
DEN VIKTIGASTE VPPTÄCKT, VARMED E
FYSIOLOGISKA OCH MEDICINSKA
VETENSKAPERNA VNDER SENASTE
TIDEN RIKTATS, HAR DENNA DAG
BESLVTIT ATT TILLERKÄNNA DET
ÅR 1930 VTGÅENDE PRISET
ÅT

FIGURE 1-5. The Noble Prize certificate for Karl Landsteiner in 1930. (From Tagarelli A, Piro A, Lagonia P, Tagarelli G: Karl Landsteiner: A hundred years later. Transplantation 2001;72:3–7.)

DESCRIPTION OF SPHEROCYTES AND ANALYSIS OF THEIR SIGNIFICANCE

Vanlair and Masius[23] described the case of a young woman who developed icterus, recurrent attacks of left upper quadrant abdominal pain, and splenomegaly shortly after giving birth. The patient's mother and sister were also icteric, and the sister's spleen was enlarged. The most remarkable aspect of this paper lies in their description of the blood findings. Although they made no mention of anemia and had no concept of hemolysis as a pathological process, they unmistakably described RBCs that we now recognize as spherocytes with remarkable clarity (Fig. 1-7). The authors noted that some of the RBCs, which they called microcytes, were smaller than normal RBCs, 3 to 4 μm in diameter, spherical in shape, and the contours were completely smooth. They concluded, "The jaundice of our patient appears to be a peculiar type of icterus. The fact that the patient's mother and sister had a slight jaundice and that the sister had an enlarged spleen may indicate that this condition is one disease entity."

Naegli is often credited with first use of the term *spherocyte*. However, according to Crosby[26] (Fig. 1-8), two British army officers, Christophers and Bentley, were the first. They were assigned to India to study

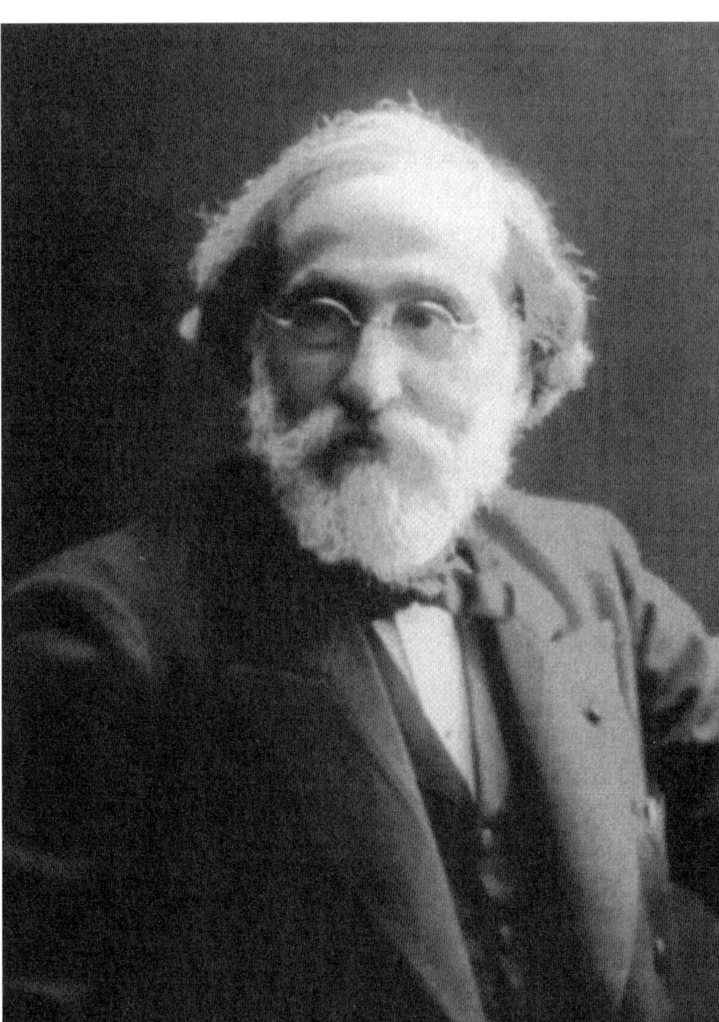

FIGURE 1-6. Georges Hayem. (From Packman CH: The spherocytic haemolytic anaemias. Br J Haematol 2001;112:888–899.)

blackwater fever and made very careful descriptions of spherocytes in a monograph published in 1909. Naegli also proposed that the spherocyte was pathognomonic of congenital hemolytic icterus, an observation that constricted thinking about hemolytic icterus for the next 15 or 20 years. In fact, many authorities began to doubt the existence of an acquired type of hemolytic icterus, regarding the disease as a variation on the congenital form.

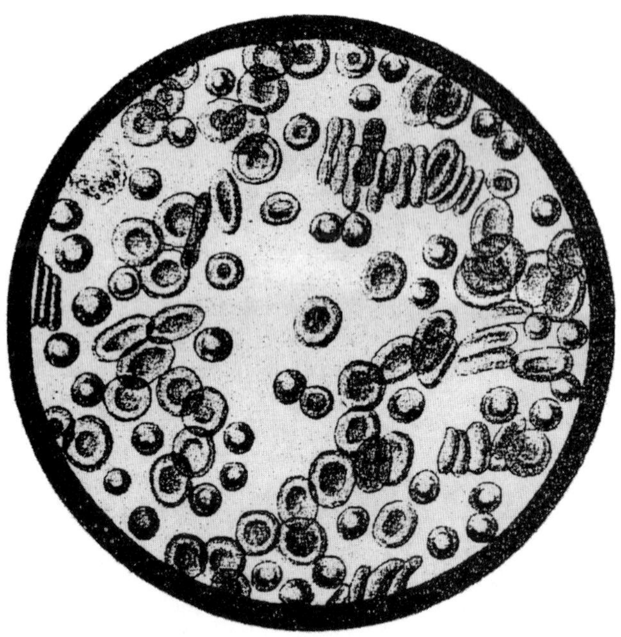

I

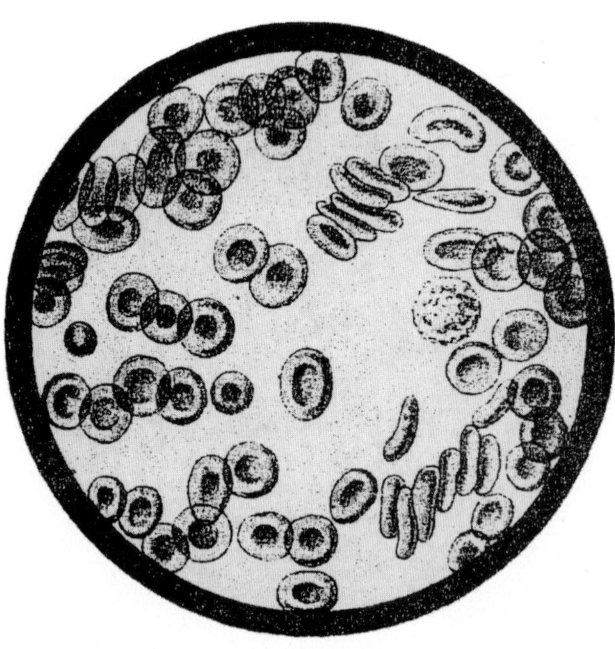

II

FIGURE 1-7. A reproduction of part of the tinted lithograph illustrating the paper by Vanlair and Masius (1871) entitled *De la microcythémie*. I is a drawing of the patient's blood. II is a drawing of control normal blood. (From Dacie JV: The life span of the red blood cell and circumstances of its premature death. In: Wintrobe MM (ed): Blood, Pure and Eloquent. New York: McGraw-Hill Book Company, 1980:211–255.)

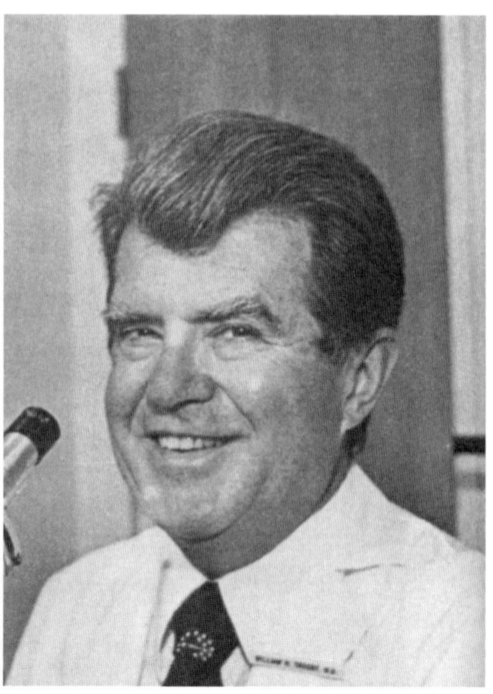

FIGURE 1-8. William H. Crosby. (From Wintrobe MM: Blood, Pure and Eloquent. New York: McGraw-Hill Book Company, 1980:XVIII. Reproduced with permission of The McGraw-Hill Companies.)

OSMOTIC FRAGILITY OF RED BLOOD CELLS

During the first decade of the twentieth century, a number of significant studies of the osmotic fragility of RBCs were conducted. Chaufford[27] (Fig. 1-9) noted that RBCs of several patients, but not those of normal subjects, were hemolysed by hypotonic saline. He developed an osmotic fragility test, in which RBCs were placed in a series of tubes containing successively decreasing concentrations of saline. The osmotic fragility was expressed as the concentration of saline at which hemolysis began and at which hemolysis was complete (Fig. 1-10). Chauffard recognized that the liver was not at fault and that the disorder was a result of hemolysis. He wrote, "Perhaps after this clinical and hematologic inquiry, the cause of the hemolytic theory could be considered as won." This observation finally enabled physicians to distinguish hepatic and hemolytic jaundice, as Ribbierre had recently (in 1903) demonstrated that the cells from patients with hepatic jaundice are resistant to osmotic stress.[7]

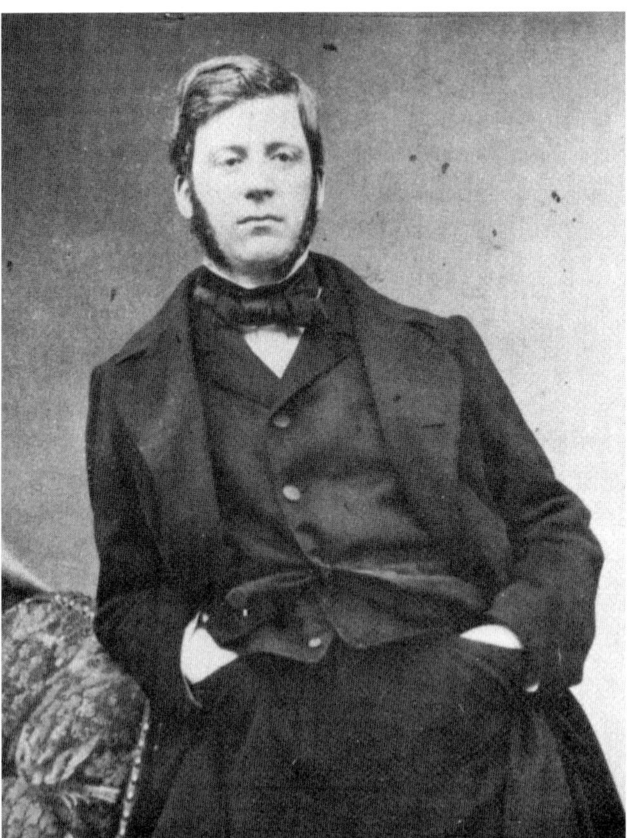

FIGURE 1-9. Anatole Chauffard (1855–1932). (From Dacie JV: The life span of the red blood cell and circumstances of its premature death. In: Wintrobe MM (ed): Blood, Pure and Eloquent. New York: McGraw-Hill Book Company, 1980:211–255.)

Of course, Chauffard and coworkers[27] had discovered the in vitro pathophysiological expression of the spherical microcytes described by Vanlair and Massius[23] almost 40 years earlier. However, they were probably unaware of the work of these early investigators and they certainly made no association between microcytic spherical cells and increased osmotic fragility. That correlation was noted much later by Haden.[28]

RETICULOCYTES

About 1 year after his description of increased osmotic fragility in congenital hemolytic icterus, Chauffard and Fiessinger[29] and Chauffard[30] stained RBCs from patients with hemolytic icterus with Pappenheim's[31] (Fig. 1-11) solution and noted large numbers of cells containing a peculiar basophilic granulation or reticulum, which they called "granular degeneration." Ehrlich had first described this special staining method in 1881[7] and noted increased numbers of reticular cells in anemic patients. Vaughan,[32] in 1903, noted these granular cells constituted about 1% of the RBCs in normal subjects. Chauffard had hoped to explain the anatomical lesion that underlay the increased fragility of the RBCs. What he actually discovered, or rediscovered, was the reticulocytosis that is now a hallmark of hemolytic anemia. Chauffard's drawing[30] of a blood smear stained with Pappenheim stain from a patient with familial hemolytic icterus is shown in Figure 1-12.

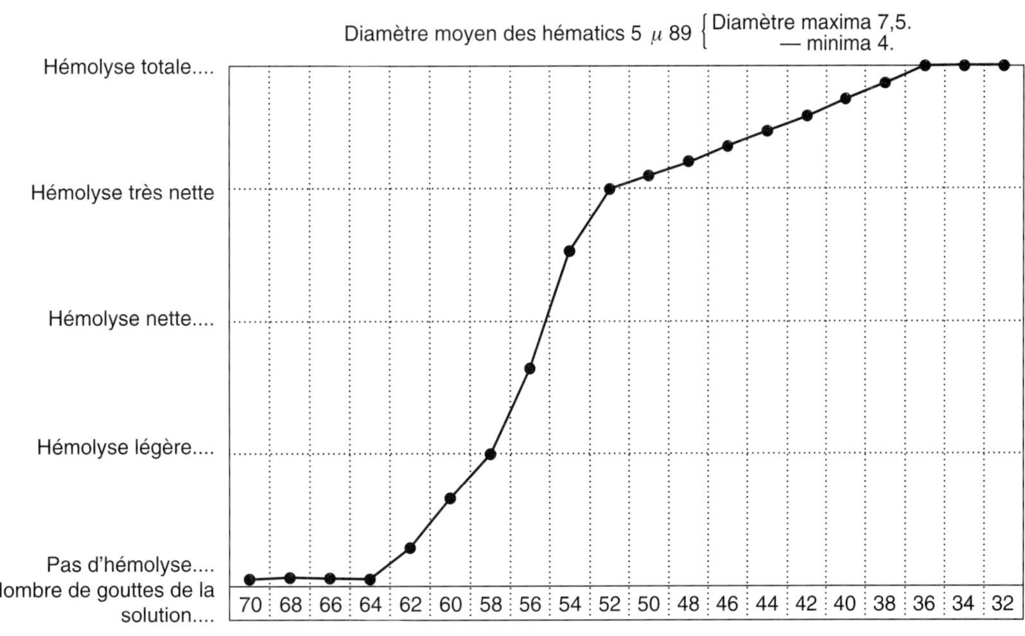

FIGURE 1-10. The figure illustrates the "precocious and prolonged" lysis in hypotonic saline of the red cells of a patient suffering from ictère congénital de l'adulte (hereditary spherocytosis). (From Dacie JV: The life span of the red blood cell and circumstances of its premature death. In: Wintrobe MM (ed): Blood, Pure and Eloquent. New York: McGraw-Hill Book Company, 1980:211–255.)

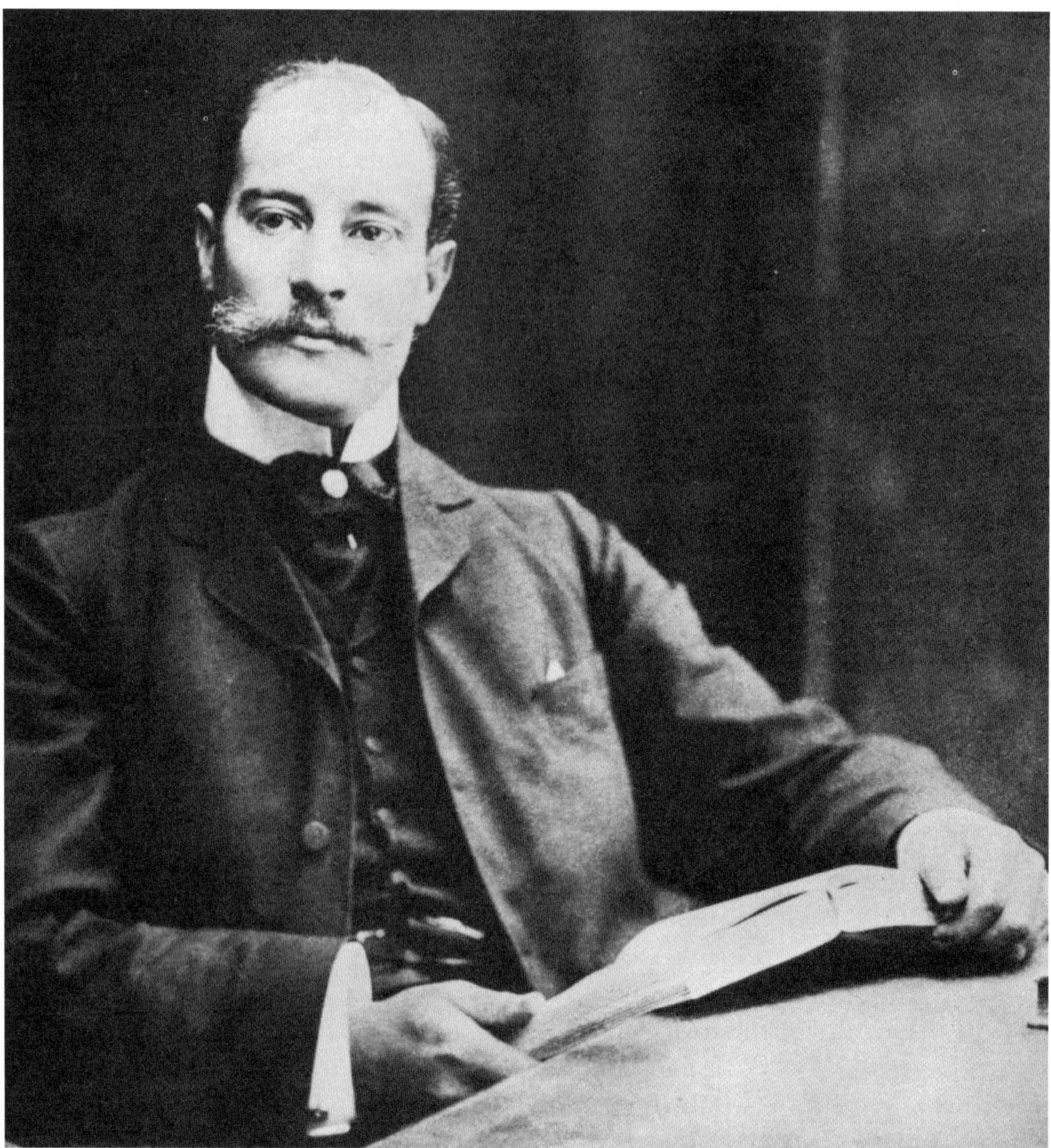

FIGURE 1-11. Artur Pappenheim (1870–1916). (From Lajtha LG: The common ancestral cell. In: Wintrobe MM (ed): Blood, Pure and Eloquent. McGraw-Hill Book Company, 1980:81–95. Reproduced with permission of The McGraw-Hill Companies.)

THE CONCEPTS OF IMMUNE HEMOLYSIS AND *HORROR AUTOTOXICUS*

In an impressive series of studies commencing in 1899,[33] Paul Ehrlich (Fig. 1-13) and Julius Morgenroth sought to identify the constituents and to define the mechanisms involved in the phenomenon of immune hemolysis, which Jules Bordet had only recently described.[34] Such studies involved the immunization of animals with foreign RBCs, a procedure resulting in an immune serum whose thermostable antibody would collaborate with a thermolabile substance (variously termed *complement, alexin,* or *cytase*) to cause the specific destruction in vitro of the erythrocyte species used for immunization.[8] During the course of these studies, Ehrlich and Morgenroth attempted repeatedly to induce the animal to form hemolytic antibodies to its own cells. These attempts to elicit the formation of *auto*antibodies were uniformly unsuccessful, and, at best, they were only able to produce antibodies able to agglutinate or to hemolyse the RBCs of certain other members of the same species.

Ehrlich had postulated, in his landmark paper of 1897, that antibody formation was part of the normal

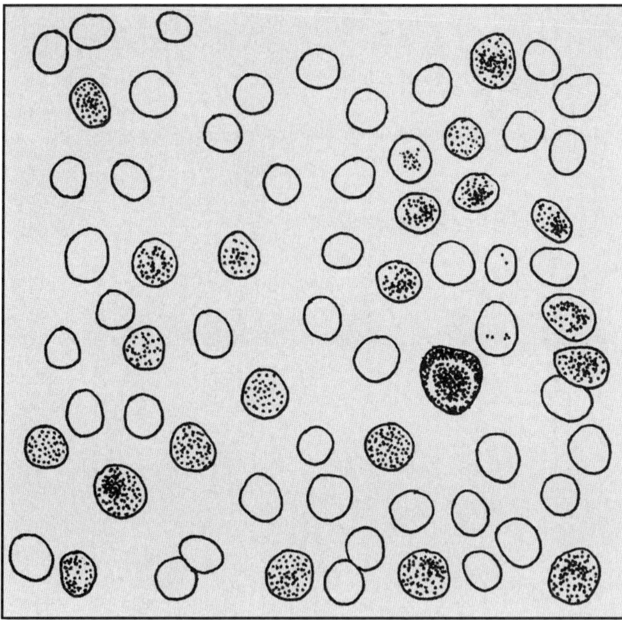

FIGURE 1-12. Drawing of a blood smear (Pappenheim stain) as seen by Chauffard (1908). The granular appearing cells are reticulocytes from a patient with familial haemolytic icterus. (From Packman CH: The spherocytic haemolytic anaemias. Br J Haematol 2001; 112:888–899.)

physiological process of cellular digestion and so might theoretically be stimulated by autochthonous as well as by foreign substances.[8] Nevertheless, he pointed out, "It would be dysteleologic in the highest degree, if under these circumstances self-poisons of the parenchyma—autotoxins—were formed."[35,35a] Thus, "we might be justified in speaking of a *horror autotoxicus* of the organism."[36]

THE FIRST DESCRIPTION OF AN AUTOIMMUNE HEMOLYTIC ANEMIA

The first AIHA in which clinical and diagnostic laboratory findings were clearly described is PCH.[37] This appears, at first, to be surprising because PCH is the least common type of AIHA. Its early recognition is due to the fact that hemoglobinuria is a striking symptom, a fact that also explains the early recognition of march hemoglobinuria and PNH. It is also true that PCH was much more common than it is at present because a majority of cases recorded in the early medical literature were associated with late stage syphilis or congenital syphilis. In the early 1900s, over 90% of patients with chronic PCH had a positive test for syphilis and approximately 30% showed clinical evidence of the disease.[38] With the effective treatment of syphilis and the virtual elimination of the congenital form, "classic" syphilitic PCH is now an extremely rare disorder, as is chronic PCH. It was in patients with the chronic form of PCH that exposure to cold resulted in a paroxysm of hemoglobinuria.[39,40]

In the latter part of the nineteenth century, there were a number of reports of PCH. Dressler[41] is generally credited with being the first (in 1854) to give a clear description. His patient was a 10-year-old boy who may have had congenital syphilis. After exposure to cold, he passed red urine that gradually paled to clear to a natural color. Microscopic examination of the urine showed "dirty brown pigment" but no blood corpuscles. PCH, however, seems also likely to have been the diagnosis in the patient described by Elliotson in *The Lancet* in 1832[3,42] who had heart disease and cold "fits" and passed bloody urine "whenever the east wind blew."

Subsequently, several excellent clinical accounts were published during the 1860s.[3] The authors realized that exposure to cold precipitated that attacks and that the urine contained blood pigment, but no blood cells. Wiltshire[43] described an infant, perhaps the youngest such patient ever recorded, who passed bloody urine, free from RBCs in the sediment, when the "weather was particularly inclement."

The term *hemoglobinuria* seems to have been used first by Secchi in 1872, but it is not clear whether the patient he described had PCH.[44]

In 1879, Stephen Mackenzie, at the London Hospital, elaborated on the pathophysiology of PCH.[45] He described a young boy who had a sallow complexion and yellow eyes and whose urine was black. The microscopic examination and spectroscopic analysis of the urine showed it contained abundant hemoglobin but no RBCs. He suggested that the discolored urine was due to blood solution or disintegration (hemolysis) and stated that it must take place in some part of the organism. He believed that the hemolysis occurred in the "genito-urinary apparatus," most probably the kidney.

Kuessner, in 1879, made the important observation that serum obtained by "cupping" a patient during an attack of hemoglobinuria was tinged red.[46] This probably was the first direct evidence derived from observations in humans that indicated that the hemoglobin in the urine was being derived from hemoglobin liberated in the plasma, rather than being, in some mysterious way, of renal origin. Indeed, Mackenzie modified his previous theory of erythrocyte destruction, suggesting that the role of the kidney is in fact passive, and that the corpuscle solution, or hemolysis, occurs in the vasculature.[47]

EARLY DIAGNOSTIC TESTS FOR PAROXYSMAL COLD HEMOGLOBINURIA

Although there were many clinical descriptions of PCH in the nineteenth-century medical literature documenting the relationship of acute attacks to exposure to cold and the fact that the urine contained blood pigment but no blood corpuscles, the pathophysiology was not understood.

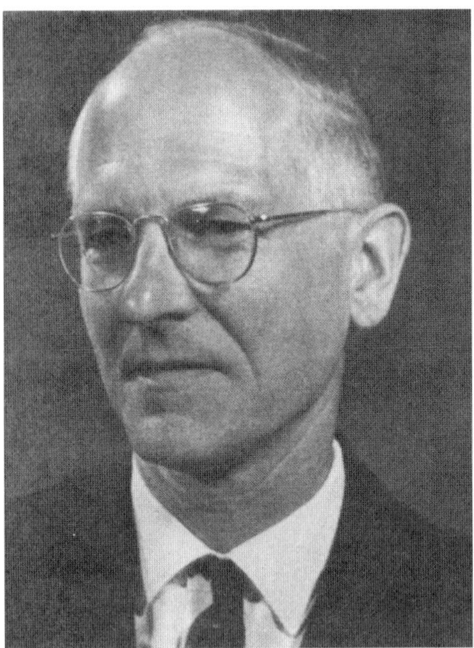

FIGURE 1-24. Professor Sir John Dacie laid the foundation for the investigation of hemolytic anemias. His persistence and experimental approach enabled him to demonstrate the vast complexity of the factors involved in the anemias due to hemolysis, and for this he has justifiably been considered a pioneer.[81a] He was also responsible for training many hematologists from numerous countries, including the present authors. (From Wintrobe MM: Blood, Pure and Eloquent. New York: McGraw-Hill Book Company, 1980:XVIII. Reproduced with permission of The McGraw-Hill Companies.)

body to serum globulin, i.e., an antiglobulin. All the necessary thinking had been done!"

Coombs obtained some "very crude [rabbit] antihuman globulin serum" from a coworker and the "very first experimental protocols with Race and Mourant showed quite clearly that the procedure was going to work." They absorbed the antiglobulin serum (AGS) with human group AB Rh-positive RBCs and then incubated Rh-positive RBCs in sera known to contain incomplete Rh antibodies. The sensitized cells agglutinated in the antiglobulin serum and the appropriate controls were negative. The first account of what we now call the indirect antiglobulin test was published by Coombs, Mourant, and Race in 1945.[88] The authors were bold enough to state, "This test may have useful applications in detecting fine degrees of sensitization in other antigen-antibody systems. . . ." This has turned out to be an understatement, for quite apart from the tests on red cells and bacteria covering all the isotypes of antibody, an antiglobulin step or stage is a regular component in very many immunoassay procedures.[85]

A more substantial paper[89] was published in the same year in the *British Journal of Experimental Pathology*, and just as the printer's page proofs were on the point of dispatch back to the publisher, Mourant came across a paper in the German literature from 1908 by Carlo Moreschi[90] (Fig. 1-28) that described enhancement of red cell agglutination with an "antiserum to serum." An acknowledgment was added to the proofs as an addendum. Coombs states, "The lesson is that one should never refer to a discovery or a test as being new."[84]

Coombs, Mourant, and Race next went on to demonstrate RBC sensitization in babies with hemolytic disease of the newborn using the direct antiglobulin test (DAT).[91] Cord RBCs from patients agglutinated when exposed to the antihuman antiglobulin reagent, but cells from healthy babies did not agglutinate.

One of the positive tests they observed in newborns appeared at first to be a false positive since there were no Rh antibodies in the mother's serum. However, Race went on to demonstrate the test was a true positive but that it was not caused by an Rh antibody. The mother's name was Kell, and this was the start of Race's research on the Kell blood group system.

In 1947, Coombs and Mourant[92] demonstrated that the component in AGS that reacted with RBCs coated with Rh antibody was in all probability an anti-gamma globulin. They showed that the addition of a small amount of gamma globulin to the antiglobulin serum rendered it incapable of agglutinating cells coated with Rh antibody, whereas the addition of alpha globulin or beta globulin had only a slight effect, which could be ascribed to contamination with traces of gamma globlulin.

An interesting phenomenon observed by Dacie[93] was that the addition of gamma globulin to AGS produced a reagent that could discriminate between the RBCs of individual patients with AIHA. Thus, although in many instances the positive antiglobulin reaction was abolished by adding the gamma globulin, this was not true in all cases. It seemed clear that in those cases in which the reaction was inhibited, the autoantibody on the cell was itself a gamma globulin, but that when the reaction was not affected, the material on the RBC surface could not be gamma globulin. The "nongamma protein" was eventually shown to consist of components of complement fixed to the cell as a result of antibody-antigen interaction.[93,94]

Use of the Antiglobulin Test to Distinguish Immune from Nonimmune Acquired Hemolytic Anemias. At the time of the discovery of the antiglobulin test, there was great difficulty in distinguishing hemolytic anemia that was familial from that which was acquired. The only laboratory test available was the measurement of osmotic fragility, which was abnormal in familial hemolytic icterus (now called *hereditary spherocytosis*). However, Dameshek and Schwartz[74] pointed out that spherocytes causing increased osmotic fragility could develop in cases that were clearly acquired hemolytic anemia.

Barbara Dodd described the fact that she and Kathleen Boorman, who were working at the South London Transfusion Centre with the director, John Loutit, who was already an authority in the field of anemias, were in a privileged position.[95] They had visited Cambridge, where Race revealed to them the secrets of the antiglobulin test before it had appeared in print. Dodd states that, "I shall never forget the gleam

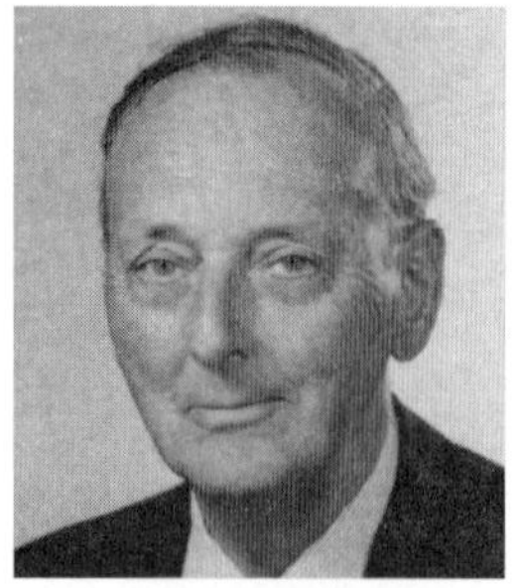

A

FIGURE 1-25. (*A*) Patrick Mollison. (*B*) A 1947 photograph taken at the Lister Institute in London showing, from left to right: Louis K. Diamond whose research clarified the pathogenesis of hemolytic disease of the fetus and newborn as well as the optimal management of that disorder; Patrick L. Mollison, a pioneer in the field of blood transfusion and editor of ten editions of the famous text, *Blood Transfusion in Clinical Medicine*; Robert R. Race, an eminent immunohematologist who, along with his long-time collaborator, Ruth Sanger, made innumerable contributions to the field of RBC genetics and serology; and Sir Ronald A. Fisher, a famous geneticist/biostatistician who, together with Race, devised a classification of the Rh blood group system that is still used. (Courtesy of Professor P. L. Mollison.)

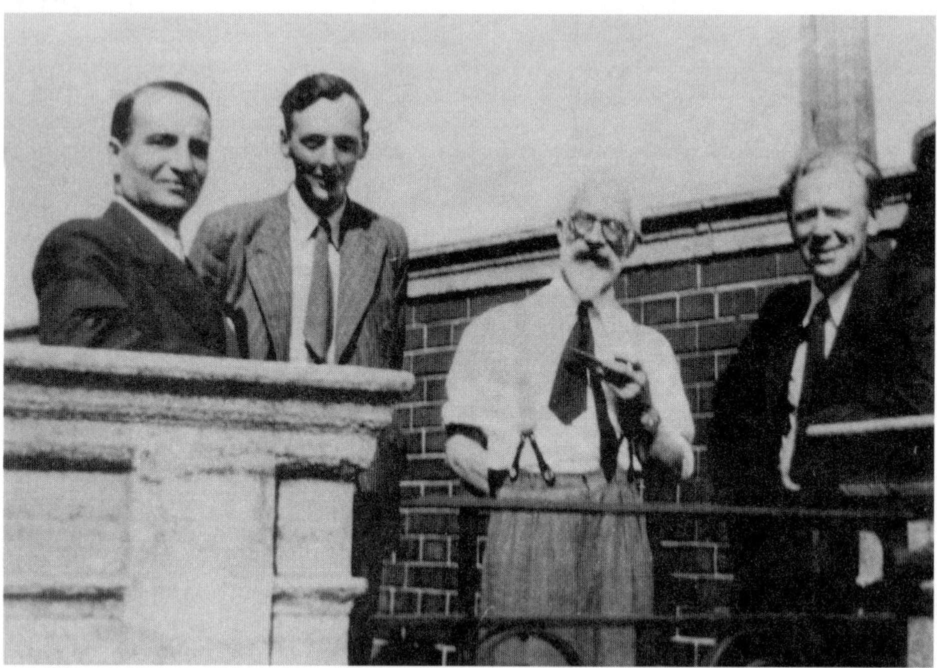

B

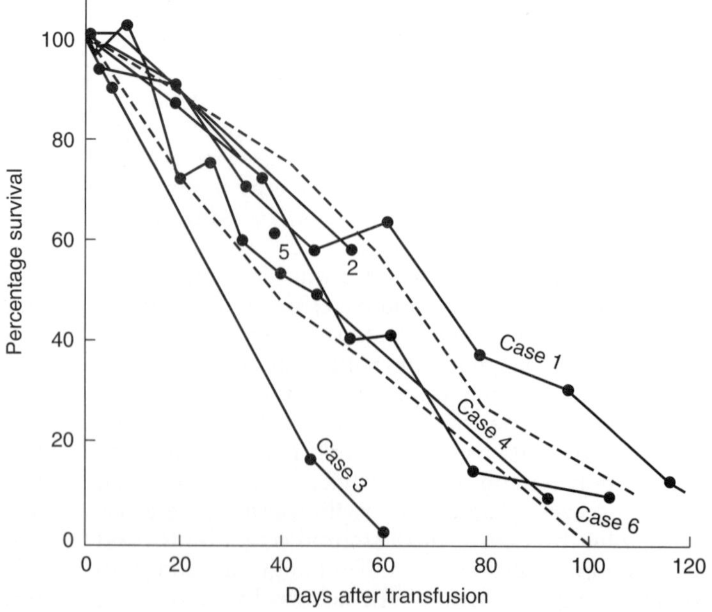

FIGURE 1-26. Dacie and Mollison, using the Ashby technique, were the first to demonstrate that normal RBCs survive normally in patients with familial hemolytic anemia. The figure shows survival of RBCs from normal donors after transfusion to six patients with familial hemolytic anemia. Case 3 was an Rh-negative patient who was later found to have developed an alloantibody to Rh, accounting for the shortened survival of transfused Rh-positive RBC. Although not shown in the figure, survival in cases 2 and 5 was followed to completion and found to exceed 100 days in each case. The dotted lines indicate the limits of survival in a group of normal recipients (Mollison, unpublished observations). (From Dacie JV, Mollison PL: Survival of normal erythrocytes after transfusion to patients with familial haemolytic anaemia (acholuric jaundice). The Lancet, volume i, May 1, 1943, pp 550–552.)

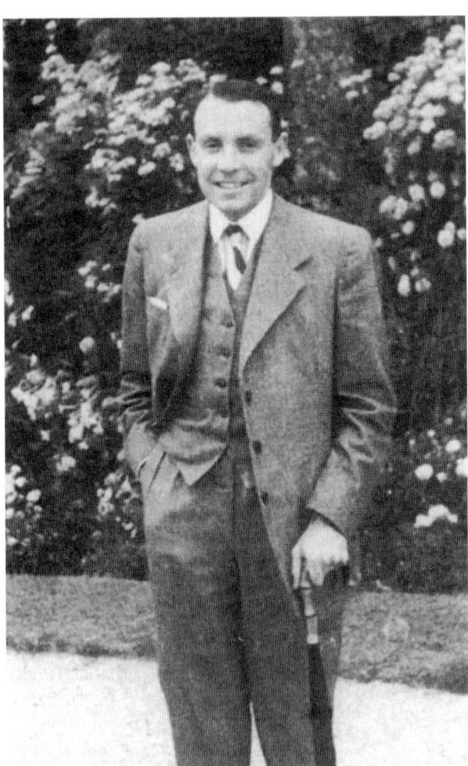

FIGURE 1-27. Robin R. A. Coombs. (Photograph by Lawrence E. Young M.D., Fellows' Garden, Kings College, Cambridge University, 1950. From Packman CH: The spherocytic haemolytic anaemias. Br J Haematol 2001;112:888–899.)

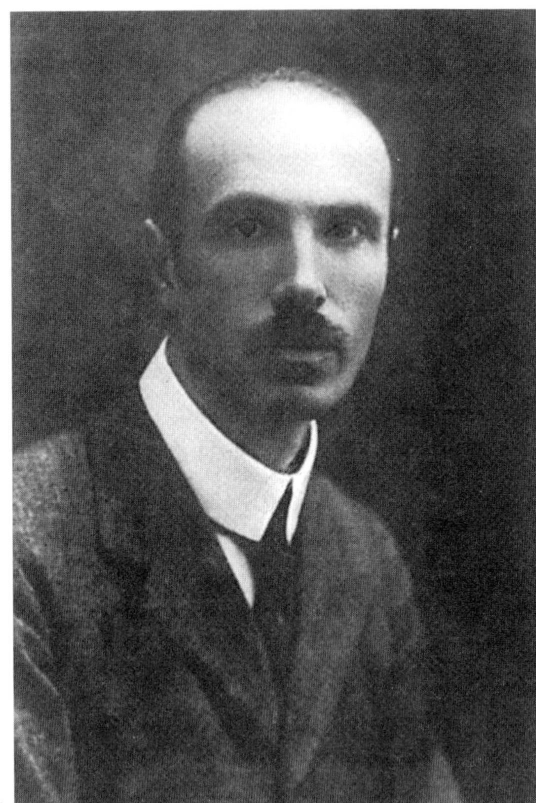

FIGURE 1-28. A photographic portrait of Carlo Moreschi. (From Coombs RR: Historical note: Past, present and future of the antiglobulin test. Vox Sang 1998;74:67–73.)

in his eye when we returned from Cambridge with a description of the new test!" They quickly collected the RBCs of 17 patients with familial hemolytic anemia and 5 others with hemolytic anemia of the acquired type. "It was enormously exciting then, but no surprise now, to find that the 5 patients having acquired type had positive DATs, whereas the 17 familials were negative." They concluded (correctly) that the agglutination tests "will discriminate the congenital from the acquired form [of hemolytic icterus], and that it indicates that the acquired form is due to a process of immunization, whereas the congenital form is not." Thus, not only had they found a test that would distinguish between the familial and acquired forms of hemolytic anemia, but they had also demonstrated a difference in their etiology.

A Note about Carlo Moreschi. Carlo Moreschi was deep in immunological research at Pavia at the turn of the twentieth century. He published two particularly interesting papers[90,96] describing enhancement of agglutination with antiserum to serum (i.e., with antiglobulin) (Table 1-1). However, incomplete antibodies were unknown at the time and general acceptance or use of this procedure never resulted. Dr. Coombs paid tribute to Moreschi and his researches in a lecture to the Italian Association of Medical Analysts and Pathologists entitled "Moreschi and Some Recent Developments in Agglutination." There seemed to be little interest in the agglutination or in Moreschi himself. However, 6 months after the lecture was published in the Italian medical journal *l'Informatore Medico*,[97] Dr. Coombs received a letter from Dr. Pietro de Ruggieri, who was a steroid chemist in Milan and who was a nephew of Carlo Moreschi. He was delighted with the reference to his long-since-dead uncle.

THE CONCEPT OF AUTOIMMUNE HEMOLYTIC ANEMIA

In 1951, Young and associates[98] were the first to coin the term *autoimmune hemolytic anemia*. It was theorized that the production of an autoantibody was the result of a breakdown in the "regulatory contrivances," thus leading to autoimmunization. However, the concept that a patient could produce autoantibodies was vigorously resisted by some. Witebsky,[99] in particular, was reluctant to draw the conclusion that the RBC coating material demonstrated by the antiglobuin test was a true autoantibody. He considered it unproved that the RBC could be involved in autoimmunization, with the implied breaking of the principle of horror autotoxicus. This reluctance to accept the autoimmune nature of antiglobulin test–positive hemolytic anemias led to the use for a time of the noncommittal term "antiglobulin-positive hemolytic anemia."[100]

TABLE 1-1. TRANSLATED FROM MORESCHI (1908), DEMONSTRATING THE PRINCIPLE OF THE ANTI-GLOBULIN (COOMBS) REACTION

Rabbit RBCs	Goat Immune Serum or Goat Normal Serum	Rabbit Precipitating Serum	Agglutination with	
			Immune Serum	Normal Serum
1 mL	0.005 mL	0.0001 mL	0	0
1 mL	0.005 mL	0.005 mL	Scant	0
1 mL	0.005 mL	0.001 mL	Marked	0
1 mL	0.005 mL	0.005 mL	Very marked	0
1 mL	0.005 mL	0.01 mL	Very marked	0
1 mL	0.005 mL	0.05 mL	Very marked	0
1 mL	0.005 mL	0.1 mL	Very marked	0
1 mL	–	0.1 mL	0	0
1 mL	0.01 mL	–	0	0
2 hr room temperature	Cells centrifuged and washed with normal saline	2 hr room temperature		

Rabbit RBCs were incubated with goat immune serum, washed, and incubated with rabbit antibody to goat serum (precipitating serum). The RBCs agglutinated in a dose-dependent manner. The controls, lacking either goat immune serum or rabbit precipitating serum, showed no agglutination.
Reproduced with modification from Packman CH: The spherocytic haemolytic anaemias. British Journal of Haematology 112:888–899.

Through the extensive writings and teaching of such eminent physicians as Dameshek, the concept of an autoimmune etiology for some types of acquired hemolytic anemias gradually obtained general recognition and application.[1]

RADIOACTIVE CHROMIUM (^{51}CR) AND DF^{32}P

The first studies using ^{51}Cr were reported by Gray and Sterling[101] in 1950 from Boston. They found that the labeled RBCs lost radioactivity at a rate more rapid than could be predicted from the known normal life span of dog RBCs and, consequently, did not recognize the potential usefulness of the method in determining long-term RBC survival.[102] Later, Ebaugh and coworkers[103] labeled normal blood with ^{51}Cr and transfused it into normal human volunteers. Subsequently, the amount of radioactivity per milliliter of RBCs was quantitated and a simultaneous evaluation was made of the RBC survival by the Ashby differential agglutination technique. They found that the two curves reached extinction point at the same time. Calculations of the two curves were consistent with the hypothesis that chromium was leaking from the RBCs in an exponential fashion with a mean half-life of 77 ± 12 days. Correcting for this leakage, the curve for the two techniques approximated that determined by the straight-line Ashby differential agglutination survival curve.[103]

The value of the isotope as a harmless label of RBCs was soon confirmed in many centers throughout the world, and because the ^{51}Cr could be used to label patients' own RBCs and to study their survival in their own circulation, as well as to label transfused blood, Ashby's elegant but laborious technique, with its inherent limitations and technical difficulties soon became obsolete.

^{51}Cr is still widely used in studies of RBC life span and in the measurement or blood volume, although it is not an ideal label because of the elution of the label from the RBCs. The nearest rival to ^{51}Cr is DF^{32}P, which was first reported in 1954 to be a potentially a satisfactory label for RBCs.[104] The DF^{32}P technique has the advantage over ^{51}Cr in that once attached to the RBCs, it is not eluted.

The elimination curve of normal RBCs in a healthy recipient, as demonstrated by the Ashby method or by the use of DF^{32}P, is virtually a straight line, and this is consistent with the concept of gradually increasing senescence rather than of random elimination in which the cells would be destroyed indiscriminately regardless of age. Indeed, the analysis of survival curves has contributed most significantly to the understanding of the pathogenesis of increased hemolysis.[3]

COLD AGGLUTININ SYNDROME (CAS)

Cold agglutinins were initially demonstrated by Landsteiner in animal blood in 1903[105] and in human blood by Mino in 1924,[106] but their significance in human disease was not accurately appreciated until several decades later. The first determination of titers in an acute postpneumonic cold agglutinin disease was made by Clough and Richter in 1918.[107] A recognition of the relationship between cold agglutinins, hemolytic anemia, Raynaud's phenomenon, and hemoglobinuria began to emerge with the case reports of Iwai and Mei-Sai in 1925 and 1926.[108,109] Their first patient was a 36-year-old Chinese man giving a 6-year

*As mentioned in Chapter 2, describing the skin manifestations in cold agglutinin syndrome as Raynaud's phenomena is, strictly speaking, incorrect.[110] Raynaud's disease, the consequence of vasoconstriction, leads in sequence of three phenomena: First, the affected part becomes white and perhaps numb; then it becomes swollen, stiff and livid; and finally, when the vasoconstriction passes off, the part becomes red due to reactive hyperemia. In CAS the changes, which preferably are termed *acrocyanosis*, or literally "blue extremity," differ from those of Raynaud's disease in the absence of an initial white phase because there is no history of Raynaud's disease.* His serum contained a cold agglutinin that reacted to a titer of 1,000 at 0°C and reacted up to 30°C against normal RBCs as well as those of the patient. They demonstrated that the circulation of the patient's blood through fine tubes was impeded when the blood was cooled to 5°C and suggested that the Raynaud's phenomenon might be related to mechanical obstruction by autoagglutinated RBCs. In their second patient, a woman aged 78, they showed that cooling of the fingers was associated with breaking of the column of blood in the capillaries of the nail bed. However, in neither case did the authors describe hemoglobinuria or anemia.

Druitt,[113] writing from Madras in 1873, described in detail the history of a doctor, aged 51 years, who over a period of at least 6 years had experienced attacks of numbness of the feet and a purplish blue discoloration of the hands on exposure to cold. These attacks might be followed by the passage of "hematinuria." The patient obtained relief from his symptoms when he went to live in a warm climate (India). Druitt believed that the nervous system and the blood were involved and suggested that the blood was undergoing "a hemolysis, a decomposition or necrosis of the blood globules."

Roth, in 1935, reported a 59-year-old man who suffered from Raynaud's phenomenon affecting his hands, feet, and nose when exposed to mild degrees of cold.[114] More severe chilling produced hemoglobinuria. The author noted that the patient's blood underwent rapid autoagglutination after withdrawal, which was reversed by warming.

In the same year, Ernstene and Gardner[115] reported a 38-year-old man who had attacks of hemoglobinuria and Raynaud's phenomenon on exposure to cold. Autoagglutination of his blood was noted at room temperature, red blood cell counts were difficult to perform, the cold agglutinin titer was 1280, and he was anemic with a hemoglobin of 10.5 g/dL.

Despite these early reports, CAS did not receive wide recognition and the pathogenetic role of cold agglutinins was not well accepted. Indeed, as late as 1943, Stats and Wasserman[116] published a review in which they stated that in the great majority of cases cold hemagglutination was innocuous, although "in some cases" of hemolytic anemia, PCH, Raynaud's syndrome, and peripheral gangrene, the cold hemagglutination is of pathogenetic significance. Accurate descriptions of the syndrome and features that distinguished it from other forms of AIHA appeared during the 1950s.[117]

The hemolytic activity of serum of patients with cold agglutinin disease had not been well recognized because the pH of blood rapidly rises to pH 8 and higher in vitro following the loss of CO_2, and the antibodies do not cause optimal lysis at alkaline pH. Dacie[118] demonstrated the presence of cold hemolysins in sera containing cold agglutinins by adding a trace of hydrochloric acid to produce a slightly acid pH value. However, he still used the two-step temperature arrangement in the classic Donath-Landsteiner test. In 1953 Schubothe pointed out that hemolysis caused by the cold agglutinins does not have a bithermic mode of action but takes place monothermically.[119,120] He introduced the term *cold hemagglutinin disease* to separate the disorder from other acquired hemolytic anemias.

In the 1950s it ultimately became apparent that there existed an obscure and rather unusual syndrome, which affected almost exclusively elderly subjects, that was characterized by mild to moderate hemolytic anemia and by the presence in the patient's serum of cold agglutinins at high titers, so that massive and rapid autoagglutination took place if their blood, after withdrawal, was allowed to cool to room temperature. In cold weather the patients suffered from what was often described as Raynaud's phenomenon, affecting the fingers, toes, and earlobes, and sometimes this led to local gangrene. Hemoglobinuria, too, often developed in cold weather. This is the condition we now refer to as cold CAS.

Discovery of Blood Group Specificity of Pathologic Cold Agglutinins. Early studies of the specificity of the cold agglutinin in patients with CAS demonstrated no blood group specificity. Mino[121] is usually quoted as having introduced the concept of the "nonspecific" nature of cold agglutinins; he concluded that all human RBCs shared a common receptor and that no distinction could be made with regard to reactivity between cells of different ABO groups. However, Wiener and his coworkers[122] reported in 1956 that they had tested a serum derived from a patient with CAS against 22,964 blood samples! Five samples only, as well as the patient's own RBCs, were not agglutinated at room temperature. The insensitive RBCs were designated "i" or "I-negative," and the serum was said to contain "anti-I" ("I" for individuality). Thus started the unraveling of the complex Ii blood group system (see Chapter 6). By far the most common type of high-titer cold antibody reacts with the I antigen, a small minority with the i antigen, and a few antibodies react with antigens other than I and i (see Chapter 7).

The Physical Nature of Cold Agglutinins. The antibodies also have been studied by physical means. First, the use of the ultracentrifuge showed that in sera containing large amounts of a cold autoantibody, this would separate as a high-density protein and might also be visualized as a distinct sharp peak in the beta-gamma region on simple paper electrophoresis.[123] Subsequently, when methods of immunoelectrophoresis became available, it was clearly shown that not only were these protein peaks composed of macroglobulin (IgM) but that they were also monoclonal. In that respect CAS is analogous to Waldenström's macroglobulinemia in that the basis of both disorders is

vasoconstriction, and in that the blue cyanotic phase is more intense; the affected part may in fact become deep purple. There is, too, no final hyperemic phase. Marshal et al.[111] and Hillestad[112] showed that the blood flow reactions to chilling are quite distinct from those in Raynaud's disease proper. No evidence of an abnormal vascular response could be obtained. Both processes can, however, lead to local gangrene.

the formation by the patient of large amounts of an IgM paraprotein.

Subsequently, numerous case reports and detailed reviews of clinical findings, laboratory features, serologic and immunochemical characterization of the antibodies, and the pathogenesis of CAS have been published (see Chapter 3).

MORE RECENT EVENTS

The investigators who, in the early days, contributed to our understanding of AIHA as we know it today were clinicians in the true sense of the word. They studied at the bedside and in clinical laboratories, using their minds, hands, eyes, and ears; their most sophisticated instrument was a microscope. Information transmittal and retrieval were rudimentary at best; if the journals were available, the language was more probably foreign to the reader than not, either French, German, or English. They made errors, but they also identified and corrected them, so as to lay a foundation for the more sophisticated studies that were to come.

The second half of the twentieth century brought important new insights into the diagnosis, pathogenesis, and management of AIHA. Important advances occurred concerning the roles of RBC structure and biochemistry, the specificity of autoantibodies and their molecular structure, the molecular nature and reaction mechanism of serum complement, the concept of drug-induced immune hemolytic anemias including drug-induced AIHA, mechanisms of hemolysis, RBC structure, and its genetic regulation. Future years will undoubtedly bring new understandings of pathogenesis at the molecular and genetic level, and new means of treatment, possibly involving the sciences of stem cell transplantation and gene replacement therapy.

HISTORICAL NOTES REGARDING HEMOLYTIC TRANSFUSION REACTIONS

The fascinating history of blood transfusion has been reviewed in a number of publications[124-127] and, among descriptions of the early attempts at transfusion therapy, are dramatic accounts of hemolytic transfusion reactions. This is to be expected because transfusions were carried out long before there was knowledge of blood groups or current good manufacturing practices.

The Early History of Blood as a Therapeutic Measure. Blood, in one form or another, was mentioned as a possible therapeutic measure throughout ancient times. The Egyptians were said to advocate blood baths for purposes of recuperation and rejuvenation. As late as the fifteenth century, blood was recommended to remedy a variety of ailments, such as lunacy, fits, palsy, melancholia, and bad disposition, but not for blood loss or anemia, as would have seemed more logical.

There is an apocryphal story that when Pope Innocent VIII was on his deathbed in 1492, a last desperate attempt at his survival was made on the recommendation of an unknown physician. He received the blood of three youths supposedly via transfusion, although more likely as a draught. The fact is that shortly thereafter he passed on, to Heaven, doubtlessly. The prescribing physician wisely and quickly disappeared—in which direction is not recorded.[125]

Early Suggestions for Transfusions. Up to the seventeenth century, blood must have been given only by mouth. Direct transfusion into the circulation had to await the discovery that there was a circulation. The beginnings of transfusion therapy date from the mid-seventeenth century following Harvey's momentous discovery of the circulation of the blood. He announced in a monumental treatise, *De Motu Cordis*, that blood circulated within the body in a closed system, maintained by the heart acting as a pump, and that the blood was sent to the limbs through the arteries and returned through the veins, whose valves did not oppose its course that way. This stimulated actual experimentation with injections into the bloodstream.[125]

FIRST RECORD OF TRANSFUSIONS

The first well-documented transfusions were carried out by two widely separated investigators, one English, the other French. Because both individual and national priorities were at stake, considerable controversy was engendered and numerous publications resulted as to who should be accredited with doing the first transfusion.[128-131]

In England, a young physiologist and physician, Richard Lower (Fig. 1-29), of Oxford, participated in experiments of injecting opiates, emetics, and other medicines into the veins of living animals. As he stated in letters then and in a book published later, this stimulated ideas about injecting large quantities of blood from different animals. In February 1665, he developed the needed surgical skill and performed his first successful transfusion, from the cervical artery of one dog into the jugular vein of another, previously almost agonally exsanguinated. The recipient animal was promptly restored to a healthy active state. There was no untoward reaction, for dogs do not have natural isoagglutinins, although they do vary in blood group antigens. Lower's experiments were recorded in the *Journal des Savants* of January 31, 1667.[124]

THE FIRST RECORDS OF HEMOLYTIC TRANSFUSION REACTIONS

In France, a philosopher-mathematician and physician, Jean-Baptiste Denis (Fig. 1-30), performed the first transfusion of a human on June 15, 1667. His patient was a boy of 15, a sufferer from a prolonged febrile illness and profound lethargy. He had been subjected

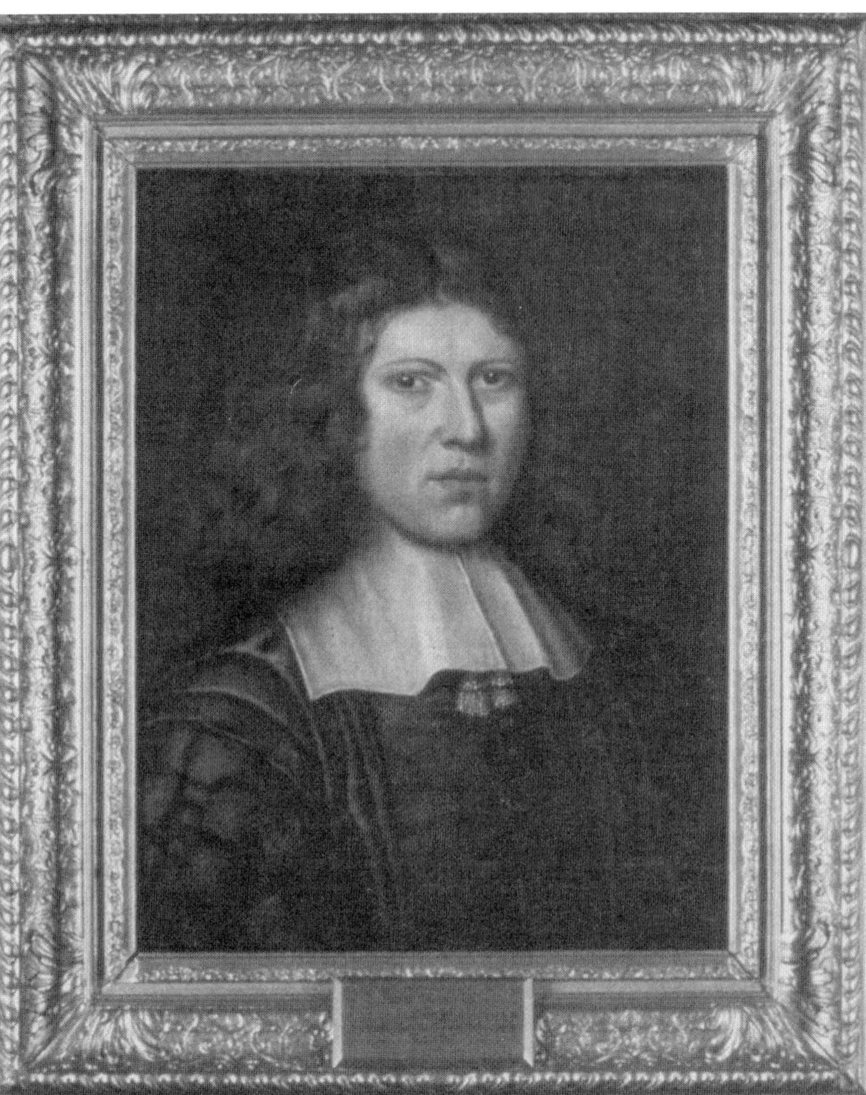

FIGURE 1-29. Richard Lower (1631–1691). Oil painting by Jacob Huysmans. (From Moore P: Blood and Justice. Chichester, England: John Wiley & Sons Ltd., 2003.)

to, and had somehow managed to survive, 20 phlebotomies. Denis succeeded in transfusing him with about 9 ounces of sheep's blood and actually "cured" him of his ailment. Encouraged by this success, Denis tried his good fortune again. This time he used a healthy paid volunteer who received 20 ounces of sheep's blood without recorded difficulties except for feeling "very great heat" along the vein in his arm and later voiding "black urine." Although the black urine strongly suggests a hemolytic transfusion reaction, he was otherwise asymptomatic and was so little disturbed that he proceeded to butcher the sheep and then went off on a drinking bout with companions.[125]

A third subject, a Swedish nobleman already moribund, did not fare so well and died soon after an attempted transfusion.

Next Denis treated a man who had episodes of violent maniacal behavior. The transfusion was on December 19, 1667, with 5 or 6 ounces of blood from the femoral artery of a "gentle calf," which "might dampen his spirits." The patient seemed to improve. A few days later the procedure was repeated. This time, there developed all the signs now recognized as typical of a severe hemolytic transfusion reaction. Denis's description can be considered a medical classic[132]:

> As soon as the blood began to enter into his veins, he felt the heat along his arm and under his armpits. His pulse rose and soon after we observed a plentiful sweat over all his face. His pulse varied extremely at this instant and he complained of great pains in his kidneys, and that he was not well in his stomach, and that he was ready to choke unless given his liberty. He was made to lie down and fell asleep, and slept all night without awakening until morning. When he awakened he made a great glass full of urine, of a color as black as if it had been mixed with the soot of chimneys.[124]

Denis recounted that the following morning the subject also manifested hemoglobinuria and had epistaxis. However, by the third day his urine cleared, and he improved his mental status and returned to his wife. Denis attributed the color of the urine to a "black

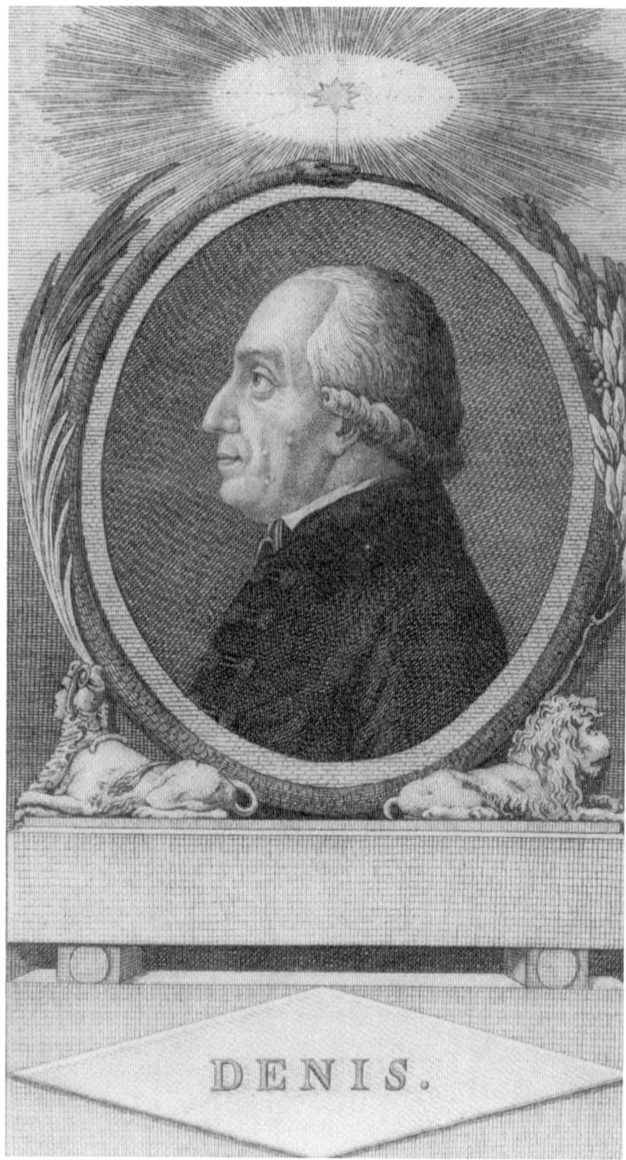

FIGURE 1-30. Jean-Baptiste Denis (From Moore P; Blood and Justice. Chichester, England: John Wiley & Sons Ltd., 2003.)

choler" that had been retained in the body and had sent vapors to the brain that caused the subject's mental disturbance.[132] Several months later the patient again became violent and irrational and his wife insisted on yet another transfusion. Denis attempted this but without success because the man was violent and would not cooperate. He died the following night.

By this time, Lower had also initiated transfusion in humans. On November 23, 1667, he and his skilled associate Edmund King performed their first human transfusion before The Royal Society. The patient was a 22-year-old member of the clergy who was "somewhat unbalanced, whose brain was considered a little too warm." It was hoped that the operation would alter his character. Accordingly, he was bled from his antecubital vein for 6 or 7 ounces and then he was connected via silver tubes and quills to a sheep's carotid artery. It was surmised that during 2 minutes, 9 to 10 ounces of blood were so transferred. The patient afterward "found himself very well" and 6 days later gave the society a talk in Latin telling how much better he felt. Nowhere was any comment recorded about the effect of the transfusion on the patient's temperament or his "too warm brain."[125]

NATIONAL AND INTERNATIONAL CONTROVERSY

In an action that presages modern medicine, the wife of the patient who was transfused by Denis sued him, charging that the transfusion had killed her husband.[124,125,127] Considerable furor was raised among Parisian physicians, but at the trial the defense was successful in proving that the man had been poisoned with arsenic by his wife. Although Denis was thus exonerated, the Paris Society of Physicians declared itself against such experiments and persuaded the criminal court in Paris on April 17, 1668, to forbid further transfusions without approval from the Faculty of Medicine of Paris, known to be bitterly opposed to the procedure. Ten years later, an edict of Parliament prohibited transfusion experiments on humans. Soon thereafter, the Royal Society in England disapproved transfusion practices, as did the magistrates in Rome. This eclipse of overt interest in transfusion therapy lasted 150 years.[125]

In the meantime, an international debate had been initiated as to who and which country should be credited with the first transfusion. Throughout 1667 and 1668, many around Europe contributed to the debate in the form of letters and published pamphlets. Most fell neatly into pro-Denis or anti-Denis camps, although a few were prepared to express an open mind. The controversy is reviewed in detail by Moore.[127]

England's claim was based on Lower's thoroughly documented dog-to-dog transfusions in 1665. The French claimed that the idea had been proposed 10 years earlier and that human transfusions were first done by Denis. National prestige seemed to be at stake even though the treatment was admittedly less than uniformly successful. A considerable exchange of letters between Denis and Henry Oldenburg,[133] the secretary of the Royal Society, took place in late 1667 and 1668 with publication in the *Proceedings of the Society*. Denis had sent a letter to the *Philosophical Transactions*, in London, the official publication of the Royal Society, describing his first transfusion and this was actually printed dated July 22, 1667. However, its publication did not take place until September because the editor, Oldenberg, was incarcerated in the Tower of London on suspicion of treason. Fortunately, he was declared innocent. (Few editors can claim so valid an excuse for delays in publication.[125])

Nevertheless, considering that Lower did not perform his first human transfusion until November of that year, there seems little question that Denis was the first to perform transfusion of a human being.[124] The best that Oldenburg could contend was that the "English might well have been first if they had not been so tender in hazarding the life of man, "a post hoc solicitude with no foundation in fact.[125] The controversy regarding priority long remained in doubt and was not really resolved satisfactorily. It finally seemed to be accepted that Lower, of England, deserved the credit for doing and fully describing the first animal transfusions, whereas Denis, of France, was credited with the first successful transfusions in humans.[125] Denis should also be credited with the first accurate and detailed description of a hemolytic transfusion reaction!

It was not until the late 19th century that successful transfusions were reported, again by an English obstetrician, William Blundell. Transfusion did not become commonly used until almost a decade following Landsteiner's discovery of the ABO blood groups.[124–126]

REFERENCES

1. Pirofsky B: The hemolytic anemias—historical review and classification. In Pirofsky B (ed): Autoimmunization and the Autoimmune Hemolytic Anemias. Baltimore, MD: Williams & Wilkins, 1969:3–20.
2. Dacie JV: Auto-immune haemolytic anaemia AIHA: Warm-antibody syndromes. I: "idiopathic" types: History and clinical features. In The Haemolytic Anaemias, 3rd ed., vol. 3, The Auto-Immune Haemolytic Anaemias. New York: Churchill Livingstone, 1992:6–53.
3. Dacie JV: The life span of the red blood cell and circumstances of its premature death. In Wintrobe MM (ed): Blood, Pure and Eloquent. New York: McGraw-Hill, 1980:211–255.
4. MacK P, Freedman J: Autoimmune hemolytic anemia: A history. Transfus Med Rev 2000;14:223–233.
5. Dacie SJ: The immune haemolytic anaemias: A century of exciting progress in understanding. Br J Haematol 2001; 114:770–785.
6. Nydegger UE, Kazatchkine MD, Miescher PA: Immunopathologic and clinical features of hemolytic anemia due to cold agglutinins. Semin Hematol 1991;28:66–77.
7. Packman CH: The spherocytic haemolytic anaemias. Br J Haematol 2001;112:888–899.
8. Silverstein AM: The Donath-Landsteiner autoantibody: The incommensurable languages of early immunologic dispute. Cell Immunol 1986;97:173–188.
9. Wintrobe MM: Blood, Pure and Eloquent. New York: McGraw-Hill, 1980.
10. Wintrobe MM: The lessons of history. In Wintrobe MM (ed): Blood, Pure and Eloquent. New York: McGraw-Hill, 1980:719–726.
11. Galen C: Volume VIII. In Kuhn DCG (ed): Opera Omnia. Lipsiae 1824:356.
12. Wintrobe MM: Milestones on the path of progress. In Wintrobe MM (ed): Blood, Pure and Eloquent. New York: McGraw-Hill, 1980:1–31.
13. Andral G: Essai d'Hematologie Pathologique. Paris, France: Fortin et Masson, 1943.
14. Vogel J: Upon the colour of the urine. Med Tmes Gazette 1853;7:378.
15. Hughes-Jones NC, Gardner B: Red cell agglutination: The first description by Creite (1869) and further observations made by Landois (1875) and Landsteiner (1901). Br J Haematol 2002;119:889–893.
16. Creite A: Versuche uber die Wirkung des Serumeiweisses nach Injection in das Blut. Zeitschrift für Rationelle Medicin 1869;36:90–108.
17. Landois L: Die Transfusion des Blutes. Leipzig, 1875.

17a. Gottlieb AM, Karl Landsteiner: The melancholy genius: His time and his colleagues, 1868–1943. Transfus Med Rev 1998;12:18–27.

17b. Schwarz HP, Dorner F: Karl Landsteiner and his major contributions to haematology. Br J Haematol 2003;121:556–565.

18. Landsteiner K: Zur Kenntness der antifermentiven lytischen und agglutinierenden Wirkungen des Blutserums und der Lymph. Centralblatt für Bacteriologie 1900;27:357–366.
19. Landsteiner K: Uber Agglutinationserscheinungen normal menschlichen Blutes. Wiener Kinische Wochenschrift 1901;14:1132–1134.
20. Diamond LK: The story of our blood groups. In Wintrobe MM (ed): Blood, Pure and Eloquent. New York: McGraw-Hill, 1980:691–717.
21. Tagarelli A, Piro A, Lagonia P, Tagarelli G: Karl Landsteiner: A hundred years later. Transplantation 2001;72:3–7.
22. Garratty G: Immunohematology is 100 years old. J Lab Clin Med 2000;135:110–111.
23. Vanlair CF, Masius JR: De la microcythemie. Bull Acad R Med Belg 3e Ser 1871;5:515–613.
24. Hayem G: Sur une variete particuliere d'ictere chronique. Ictere infectieux chronique splenomegalique. Presse Med 1898;6:121–125.
25. Minkowski O: Ueber eine hereditare, unter dem bilde eines chronischen icterus mit urobilinurie, splenomegalie und nierensiderosis verlaufende affection. Verhandl Krong f Inn Med 1900;18:316–321.
26. Crosby WH: The pathogenesis of spherocytes and leptocytes (target cells). Blood 1952;7:261–274.
27. Chauffard A: Pathogenie de l'ictere congenital de l'adulte. Semaine Med 1907;27:25–29.
28. Haden RL: The mechanism of the increased fragility of the erythrocytes in congenital hemolytic jaundice. Am J Med Sci 1934;188:441–449.
29. Chauffard A, Fiessinger N: Ictere congenital hemolytique avec lesions globulaires. Soc Med Hosp Paris 1907;24:1169–1178.
30. Chauffard A: Les icteres hemolytique. Semaine Medicale 1908;28:49–52.
31. Lajtha LG: The common ancestral cell. In Wintrobe MM (ed): Blood, Pure and Eloquent. New York: McGraw-Hill, 1980:81–95.
32. Vaughan VC: On the appearance of certain granules in the erythrocytes of man. J Med Res 1903;10:342–366.
33. Ehrlich P, Morgenroth J: Six landmark communications on hemolysis. Berl Klin Wochenschr 1899;36:6 and 481; 1900; 37:453 and 681; 1901;38:251 and 569. (These also appear in The Collected Papers of Paul Ehrlich, vol 2. New York: Pergamon, 1957, in both German and English translation, and in English alone in Collected Studies on Immunity, C. Bolduan, translator, New York: Wiley, 1906.)
34. Bordet J: Ann Inst Pasteur, Paris 1898;12:688.
35. Ehrlich P: The Collected Papers of Paul Ehrlich, vol. 2, pp. 298–315. New York: Pergamon, 1957.

35a. Silverstein AM: Autoimmunity versus horror autotoxicus: The struggle for recognition. Nat Immunol. 2001;2:279–281.

36. Ehrlich P: The Collected Papers of Paul Ehrlich, vol. 1, p. 253. New York: Pergamon, 1957.
37. Dacie JV: Auto-immune haemolytic anaemia AIHA: Cold-antibody syndromes. V: paroxysmal cold haemoglobinuria (PCH). In The Haemolytic Anaemias, 3rd ed., vol. 3, The Auto-Immune Haemolytic Anaemias. New York: Churchill Livingstone, 1992:329–362.
38. Heddle NM: Acute paroxysmal cold hemoglobinuria. Transfus Med Rev 1989;3:219–229.
39. Rosenbach O: Zur Leher von der periodischen Hamoglobinurie. Dtsch Med Wschr 1879;5:613.
40. Rosenbach O: Beitrag zur Lehre von der periodischen Hamoglobinurie. Berl Klin Wschr 1880;17:132, 151–153.
41. Dressler: A case of intermittent albuminuria and chromaturia. In Major RH (ed): Classic Descriptions of Disease. Springfield, IL: Charles C Thomas, 1939:590–592.

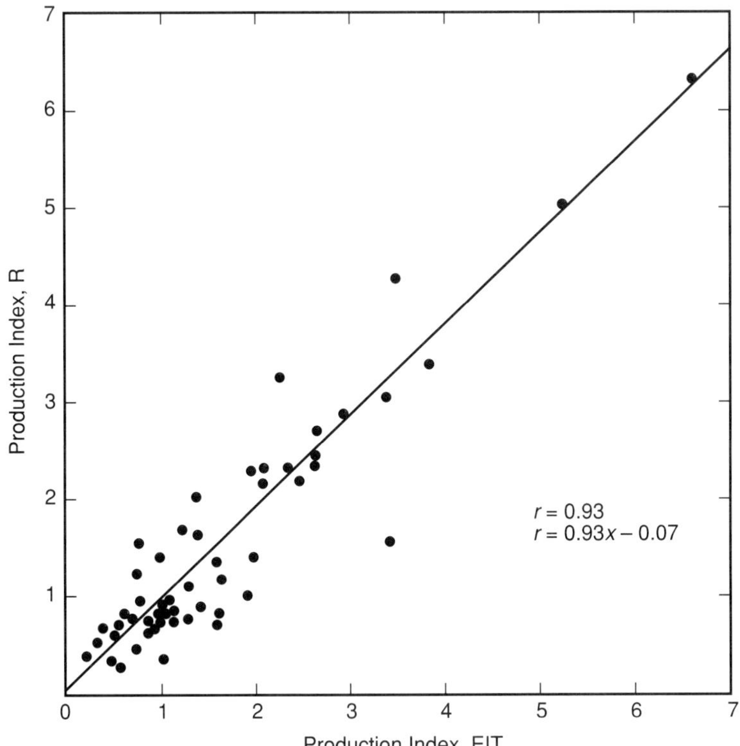

FIGURE 2-8. Comparison between effective RBC production as evaluated by ferrokinetic measurements (EIT) and reticulocyte counts (R). The EIT found in patients was divided by 0.49 to obtain the production index EIT, where 0.49 corresponds to mg iron utilized for RBC production per day in normal individuals. Reticulocyte counts were corrected for hematocrit and for marrow transit time. (From Rhyner K, Ganzoni A: Erythrokinetics: Evaluation of red cell production by ferrokinetics and reticulocyte counts. Eur J Clin Invest 1972;2:96–101.)

TABLE 2-1. COMPARISON OF CALCULATED AND MEASURED ERYTHROCYTE PRODUCTION INDICES

Subject	Age (yr)	Sex	Diagnosis	Hematocrit (%)	Reticulocyte Count (%)	Marrow Transit Time (days)	Production Index (Retic)*	Production Index (EIT)†
1	45	M	Normal	50.0	0.9	3.5	1.00	1.08
2	69	M	Normal	40.0	1.4	3.5	1.12	1.30
3	39	M	Normal	40.0	0.9	3.5	0.76	0.79
4	39	M	Normal	45.0	0.8	3.5	0.80	0.85
5	34	M	Normal	50.0	1.3	3.5	1.78	1.21
6	22	M	Normal	42.0	1.0	3.4	0.90	0.76
Mean				45.0	1.0	3.5	1.06	1.00
SD				4.6	0.2	0.04	0.38	0.23
24	55	M	Hemolytic anemia	31.0	7.8	1.8	2.76	2.65
25	60	F	Hemolytic anemia	30.0	4.7	2.7	2.32	1.94
26	70	F	Hemolytic anemia	36.0	9.6	2.0	4.38	3.47
27	64	F	Hemolytic anemia	33.0	5.7	2.9	3.47	3.81
28	31	M	Hemolytic anemia	38.0	3.9	3.3	3.11	3.38
29	75	F	Hemolytic anemia	16.5	29.0	2.1	6.36	6.57
30	60	F	Hemolytic anemia	18.0	32.0	1.4	5.10	5.22
31	25	F	Hemolytic anemia	20.0	8.3	2.3	2.42	2.57
32	38	M	Hemolytic anemia	35.0	3.9	2.6	2.25	2.45
33	53	M	Hemolytic anemia	33.5	3.7	3.0	2.36	2.04
34	63	F	Hemolytic anemia	28.0	5.8	2.2	2.26	2.06

EIT, erythrocyte iron turnover.
* Production index calculated using corrected reticulocyte counts.
† Production index measured by erythrocyte iron turnover.
Data from Rhyner K, Ganzoni A: Erythrokinetics: Evaluation of red cell production by ferrokinetics and reticulocyte counts. Eur J Clin Invest 1972;2:96–101.

the uncorrected reticulocyte count is greater than 5%. The probability of hemolytic anemia rapidly increases with increasing degrees of reticulocytosis and, if the uncorrected reticulocyte count is greater than 10%, the diagnosis is very likely.

An elevated reticulocyte production index is a more informative indication of the degree of increased erythropoiesis. Within a few days of the development of moderate anemia, RBC production in the marrow may increase to a level three to five times normal.

Under conditions of prolonged stimulation, patients with hemolytic anemia may have rates of 6 to 10 times normal.[11] For patients in the steady state, a reasonable estimate of RBC survival can be made from the reticulocyte count and hematocrit level, as described earlier.

Although an elevated reticulocyte count accurately indicates the presence or absence of hemolytic anemia in a surprisingly high percentage of patients, exceptions do, of course, occur. A reticulocytosis can occur for other reasons, such as blood loss or recent treatment of megaloblastic anemia. However, blood loss causes a problem in differential diagnosis rather infrequently because sustained bleeding that is of sufficient volume and duration to result in a reticulocyte count high enough to cause a strong suspicion of hemolysis can result only from clinically evident blood loss. Similarly, confusing treated megaloblastic anemia with hemolytic anemia is an infrequent clinical problem. In contrast to megaloblastic anemia, treatment of iron deficiency anemia generally produces only a modest reticulocyte response.[8]

In cases in which there is doubt, repeat blood counts will be of value as a persistently elevated absolute reticulocyte count and reticulocyte production index without an increase in hemoglobin and in the absence of blood loss is diagnostic of hemolysis.

RETICULOCYTOPENIA IN PATIENTS WITH HEMOLYTIC ANEMIA

Reticulocytopenia in the presence of hemolytic anemia presents a difficult problem. It is discussed in more depth in Chapter 3.

If the hemolysis is of abrupt onset, at least several days must elapse before the development of a reticulocytosis. Patients with hemolytic anemia that is less acute in onset may also have reticulocytopenia because of bone marrow suppression for various reasons, including autoantibody reactivity against erythroid precursors. Although the initial reticulocyte count may misleadingly suggest that hemolytic anemia is not present, the diagnosis of hemolysis can nevertheless be made simply on the basis of the blood count if serial determinations are made over a period of several days or more. This is true because the combination of hemolysis and reticulocytopenia results in a rapidly falling hemoglobin and hematocrit level, which can result only from hemolysis, provided significant blood loss is excluded.

RBC Morphology

The RBC morphology in the peripheral blood film not only frequently substantiates the impression of hemolysis, but often suggests a specific diagnosis or a limited number of diagnostic possibilities. Morphologic findings are discussed in more detail later (see page 53).

Bilirubin

Bilirubin is formed mainly in the RES system by enzymatic degradation of hemoglobin from senescent RBCs.[25] About 15%, the so-called early labeled pigment or shunt bilirubin, is produced in the liver from nonhemoglobin heme, such as the cytochromes, or in the bone marrow from RBC precursors, as in intramedullary hemolysis or ineffective erythropoiesis. Unconjugated bilirubin in the serum is bound to albumin and is transported to the liver, where it is taken up by hepatic acceptor protein. The hepatic microsomal enzyme, glucuronyl transferase, transforms unconjugated bilirubin to water-soluble conjugated bilirubin, primarily bilirubin diglucuronide, which is then excreted in the bile.[10] In general, the conjugated bilirubin is measured by the direct reacting fraction and the unconjugated bilirubin by the indirect reacting fraction. Hyperbilirubinemias of unconjugated bilirubin are referred to as acholuric jaundice because unconjugated bilirubin cannot be excreted in the urine. In conjugated hyperbilirubinemias a small fraction of serum conjugated bilirubin is excreted in the urine.[26]

Hyperbilirubinemia is usual in hemolytic anemia, but it is not a constant finding, so its absence does not exclude the diagnosis. The indirect reacting fraction is the predominant fraction elevated in the presence of hemolysis. The direct reacting fraction is characteristically elevated in conditions in which true plasma conjugated hyperbilirubinemia results from a reflux of conjugated bilirubin from the liver or biliary tract to the blood. Conjugated hyperbilirubinemia indicates either a physiologic or mechanical obstruction to the flow of bile, which may be located at any point from within the hepatocyte itself to the duodenum. Hepatocellular injury of any type substantially reduces the capacity of the hepatocyte to transport bilirubin into bile. Hence, hemolysis ocurring in the setting of liver disease frequently results in a combination of conjugated as well as unconjugated hyperbilirubinemia.[27]

The plasma concentration of indirect reacting (unconjugated) bilirubin is 0.2 to 0.9 mg/dL for 95% of a normal population, and 99% of such a population will have a value less than 1.0 mg/dL.[27] The upper limit of normal for direct reacting (conjugated) bilirubin in the presence of a normal total plasma bilirubin concentration (<1.2 mg/dL) is 0.2 mg/dL.

Plasma bilirubin turnover studies have indicated that, in patients with chronic hemolysis who are in the steady state, unconjugated bilirubin concentrations in excess of 4 mg/dL do not result from hemolysis per se, but imply a concomitant reduction in hepatic function. This calculation is based on an assumed maximum increase in RBC production by the bone marrow to a rate of eight times the normal rate. This observation does not apply to acute hemolytic episodes, which are non–steady-state situations, in which case the rate of RBC destruction and bilirubin production may be greater.

Many patients with low-grade hemolytic anemia will be found to have unconjugated bilirubin concentrations of less than 1 mg/dL, which are conventionally interpreted as normal. However, Berlin and Berk[27] point out that unconjugated bilirubin levels must be corrected for anemia in a manner analogous to correcting reticulocyte percentages for anemia. They suggest correcting the upper limit of normal for the serum unconjugated bilirubin as follows:

$$\text{Upper limit of normal} = 1.0\ \text{mg/dL} \times \frac{\text{patient's hematocrit}}{45}$$

CLINICAL INTERPRETATION OF UNCONJUGATED HYPERBILIRUBINEMIA

Chronic unconjugated hyperbilirubinemia can be attributable to increased plasma bilirubin turnover, to reduced hepatic bilirubin clearance, or to some combination of the two. Hemolysis is the only source of increased bilirubin turnover in humans. Reduced hepatic bilirubin clearance associated with structural liver disease is almost inevitably accompanied by other biochemical evidence of hepatic dysfunction, including elevated levels of direct bilirubin. An exception to this generalization is Gilbert's syndrome,[27-29] which is an inherited form of mild unconjugated hyperbilirubinemia characterized by decreased bilirubin UDP-glucuronyl transferase activity (UGTA1).[30] Homozygosity for the variant promoter for the *UGTA1* gene, which is associated with Gilbert's syndrome, is frequently encountered in European and African populations with a prevalence of 11% and 19%, respectively.[31]

The greatest importance of the serum bilirubin level in regard to the diagnosis of hemolytic anemia lies in the fact that, if a patient has a significantly elevated serum bilirubin level (characteristically, but not invariably, between 1 and 4 mg/dL), which is almost exclusively of the unconjugated or indirect reacting type, the presence of hemolysis (or Gilbert's syndrome) is almost assured. In other disorders with unconjugated hyperbilirubinemia, such as thalassemia,[32] some cases of sideroblastic anemia,[33] dyserythropoietic jaundice,[34] megaloblastic anemia, and ineffective erythropoiesis,[27] the hyperbilirubinemia is due, at least in part, to hemolysis, including destruction of erythroid precursors in the bone marrow.

Changes in plasma unconjugated bilirubin concentration over time can be an extremely useful indicator of altered physiology. A decline in the plasma unconjugated bilirubin concentration provides early evidence of a decrease in the rate of hemolysis in a patient with hemolytic anemia.[27]

BILIRUBIN VALUES IN PATIENTS WITH HEMOLYTIC ANEMIAS

Tisdale and coworkers[35] performed 77 bilirubin determinations in 46 patients with hemolytic anemia and found that the direct-reacting fraction constituted less than 15% of the total in most patients, especially if the total bilirubin was 4.0 mg/dL or greater. The direct-reacting fraction exceeded 1.2 mg/dL in only five instances unless there was definite evidence of concomitant hepatic disease.

Pirofsky[36] reported that an elevation in serum bilirubin value was one of the most consistent abnormalities noted in patients with AIHA. Total serum bilirubin was determined in 120 patients. An elevated value was found in 66 cases, or 55% of the tested patients. In 57 patients, the indirect bilirubin was increased above normal. In 20 patients, the increased bilirubin value was exclusively of an indirect variety.

Allgood and Chaplin[37] found that the indirect-reacting bilirubin value was less than 1.0 mg/dL in only 13% of 47 patients with AIHA. It varied from less than 0.8 to 8.6 mg/dL, and in 9 of the 47 patients, it was greater than 4 mg/dL. The direct-reacting fraction was significantly elevated in only five patients, and the highest value was 3.6 mg/dL. In two of these patients, there was definite evidence of underlying liver disease; in the other three, it was suspected.

Although indirect-reacting hyperbilirubinemia is characteristic of hemolytic anemia, some authors have reported that an increase in conjugated (direct-reacting) bilirubin does occur in a minority of patients, even in the absence of liver dysfunction.[26,35,36,38] Even less well recognized is the fact that bilirubinuria is seen occasionally in patients with uncomplicated hemolytic jaundice.[35,38]

OTHER ASPECTS OF BILIRUBIN METABOLISM

Within the gastrointestinal tract, bilirubin is further degraded by bacterial action to a series of urobilinogens and a number of other products. Although the conversion of heme to bilirubin and carbon monoxide is quantitative, the further degradation of bilirubin to urobilinogens is not. Hence, measurements of fecal urobilinogen excretion may appreciably underestimate total heme degradation.[27] Although raised values are considered to be valid indications of hemolysis, the tests are difficult to perform accurately and are usually not necessary.

Serum Haptoglobin

Haptoglobin is a dimeric glycoprotein comprising two α chains and two β chains that bind to hemoglobin α dimers. The normal range of serum haptoglobin is about 50 to 150 mg/dL. When RBCs are destroyed in the vascular compartment, the hemoglobin escaping into the plasma is bound to haptoglobin. The haptoglobin-hemoglobin complex is cleared from the plasma with a half-life ($T_{1/2}$) of 10 to 30 minutes.[39] In contrast, free haptoglobin has a half-life of 5 days, so that when large amounts of the rapidly turned over haptoglobin-hemoglobin complex are formed, the haptoglobin content of the plasma is depleted. Haptoglobin is diminished not only in the plasma of patients undergoing frank intravascular hemolysis, but also in the plasma of patients who have accelerated red cell destruction that occurs primarily within macrophages. Presumably, there is either enough intravascular hemolysis in such hemolytic disorders to lower the plasma haptoglobin level or enough leakage from the phagocytic cells into the plasma to bind to haptoglobin. Thus the measurement of haptoglobin in plasma or serum has some usefulness in diagnosing the presence of hemolysis.[39]

SENSITIVITY IN DEMONSTRATION OF HEMOLYSIS

When hemoglobin destruction exceeds two or three times the normal rate, the serum haptoglobin level will usually be low,[7] and even less hemolysis is necessary to result in low serum haptoglobin levels if the hemolysis is primarily intravascular. Indeed, a very small degree of intravascular hemolysis, insufficient to increase the daily turnover of hemoglobin appreciably above normal, can deplete the serum completely of haptoglobin.[7] Thus, the level of serum haptoglobin can be considered a reasonably sensitive indicator of hemolysis, although it must be kept in mind that even greater rates of hemoglobin breakdown may be necessary to depress the level in situations in which there is apparently an increased rate of synthesis, such as in acute or chronic inflammatory disease, neoplasia (including lymphomas), or steroid administration. Also, in severe hepatocellular disease, the serum haptoglobin level may be low, probably as a result of decreased production. Congenital haptoglobin deficiency also occurs, but reports of this disorder are rare.[40]

CLINICAL EXPERIENCES

Marchand and coworkers[41] performed haptoglobin assays on 100 patients with a variety of hematologic and nonhematologic conditions to determine the usefulness of serum haptoglobin in the diagnosis of hemolysis. They found that values of less than 25 mg/dL, as an indication of hemolysis, provided sensitivity and specificity of 83% and 96%, respectively, and that the predictive value for hemolytic disease was 87% (Table 2-2; Fig. 2-9). However, their study population included only 10 cases of AIHA, 6 cases of mechanical hemolysis, 6 cases of megaloblastic anemia, and 2 cases of hypersplenism. (Two patients with megaloblastic anemia and the two patients with hypersplenism had normal values of serum haptoglobin, and these were considered false-negative results.)

Shinton and coworkers[42] found the range of serum haptoglobin in 110 normal subjects to be 33 to 213 mg/dL; 80% of patients with hemolytic disease or megaloblastic anemia had subnormal levels. Subnormal levels were also found in some patients with hemorrhage into the tissues and occasionally in association with other diseases. They concluded that, when taken in conjunction with other clinical and laboratory features, serum haptoglobin measurements can be of diagnostic value.

The serum haptoglobin value after infusion of hemoglobin returns to about half the initial value within 36 hours. Subsequent increments return the concentration nearly to preinfusion levels after 6 to 10 days. This rapid recovery of circulating haptoglobin is of clinical importance, as within 2 days of a transient hemolytic episode, plasma haptoglobin levels may no longer be sufficiently low to be indicative of accelerated red cell destruction.[43]

PATIENTS WITH PROSTHETIC HEART VALVES

Cullhed[44] measured serum haptoglobin in 26 patients with nonoperated aortic valve disease, in 15 patients with a Starr-Edwards aortic prosthesis, in 10 patients with a similar mitral prosthesis, and in 1 patient with a double aortic and mitral prosthesis. In most operated cases, the haptoglobin level was determined 1 year after the operation. Normal values were found in all but two of the nonoperated aortic cases, whereas a low value was the rule in cases with aortic or mitral ball-valve prostheses. The hemoglobin and hematocrit values were normal in all operated patients, and a modest reticulocytosis (2%–4%) was present in only four of the patients with aortic prostheses. Slightly increased serum bilirubin concentrations (1.4 and 1.6 mg/dL, respectively) were found in two aortic cases. The findings of these authors are consistent with the data of Brus and Lewis[7] indicating that small amounts of primarily intravascular hemolysis can deplete the serum of haptoglobin.

HAPTOGLOBIN LEVELS FOLLOWING BLOOD TRANSFUSION

Two groups of investigators studied the effects of blood transfusion on serum haptoglobin levels. Langley and coworkers[45] studied changes in serum haptoglobin values in 21 patients following 29 transfusions of RBC stored for an average of 7.1 days. They found that transfusion produced little effect on the serum haptoglobin. In only three instances was a decrease of more than 25 mg/dL observed. Fink and coworkers[46] measured serum haptoglobin following transfusion of 356 units of RBCs in 120 patients, and also measured serum haptoglobin in 65 patients who were diagnosed as having had a febrile and/or allergic nonhemolytic transfusion reac-

TABLE 2-2. SCREENING FOR HEMOLYSIS WITH A HAPTOGLOBIN CUTOFF OF 25 MG/DL*

	No. of Patients with Haptoglobin ≤25 mg/dL	No. of Patients with Haptoglobin >25 mg/dL	Total
Hemolysis	20	4	24
No hemolysis	3	73	76
Total	23	77	100

* Sensitivity, 83%; specificity, 96%; efficiency, 93%; predictive value of positive result, 87%; and predictive value of negative result, 95%.
From Marchand A, Galen RS, Van Lente F: The predictive value of serum haptoglobin in hemolytic disease. JAMA 1980;243:1909–1911.

tion. In the entire series of 185 patients, there were only four cases in which the pretransfusion level was within normal limits and the post-transfusion level was less than 30 mg/dL. In all four cases, clinical information adequately explained the drop in serum haptoglobin, that is, absorption of hemoglobin into the plasma from a large hematoma. Because low levels of serum haptoglobin have been documented following hemolytic transfusion reactions,[45,46] serum haptoglobin measurement may be considered a diagnostic aid when evaluating a patient for a possible hemolytic transfusion reaction.

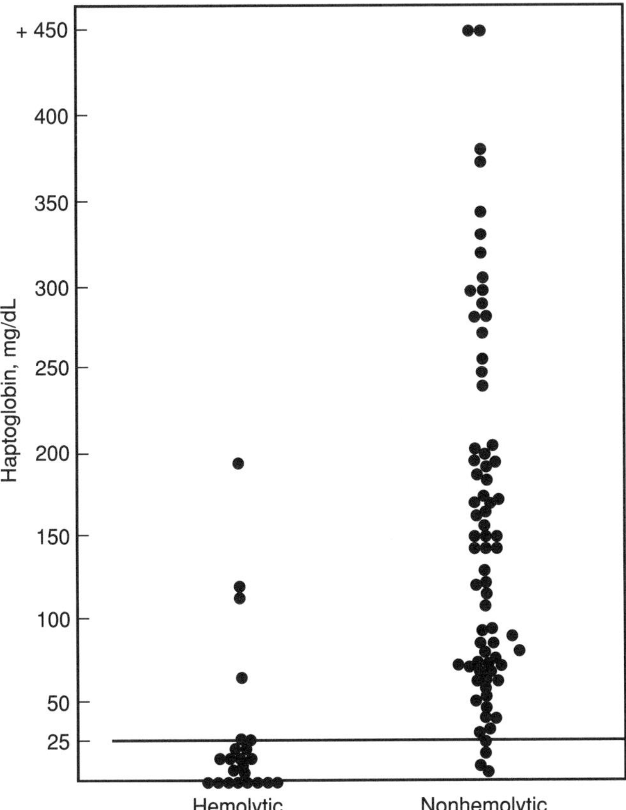

FIGURE 2-9. Serum haptoglobin levels in hemolytic and nonhemolytic disorders. (From Marchand A, Galen RS, Van Lente F: The predictive value of serum haptoglobin in hemolytic disease. JAMA 1980;243:1909–1911.)

Serum Lactic Dehydrogenase

Serum lactic dehydrogenase (LDH) has also been utilized in the diagnosis of hemolytic anemia because RBCs have a high content of the enzyme. Stein[47] studied LDH activity in patients with hemolytic anemia, including patients with primarily intravascular hemolysis (e.g., those with prosthetic heart valves PNH) or primarily extravascular hemolysis (e.g., those with hereditary spherocytosis) (Table 2-3). The degree of elevation in hereditary spherocytosis was modest even with severe hemolysis, although intravascular hemolysis always produced a marked elevation.

Myhre and coworkers[48] performed RBC survival studies with ^{51}Cr-labeled RBCs in patients with various LDH levels several months after insertion of ball-valve aortic and/or mitral prostheses. They found a close correlation between LDH and RBC survival, suggesting that LDH level is a reliable parameter of the degree of intravascular hemolysis (Fig. 2-10). They also used published data from a series of 50 patients with ball-valve prostheses[49] and found that 48 of the 50 observations fell within the 95% confidence interval of their regression line (Fig. 2-11). From these data, the authors suggested that it is possible to approximate the erythrocyte destruction rate from LDH levels for patients with intravascular hemolysis, as indicated in Table 2-4. Similar correlations have not been made in hemolytic disorders with primarily extravascular hemolysis.

An analysis of the sensitivity, specificity, predictive value, and efficiency of LDH and haptoglobin alone or in combination in the diagnosis of hemolysis[41] indicates that haptoglobin and LDH each had a sensitivity of 83%. Requiring either test to be positive yielded a sensitivity of 92%, but for LDH alone, the specificity was only 61% and the predictive value only 40%.

Because LDH is an inexpensive and commonly performed test and has a high degree of sensitivity, it is a good screening test for the evaluation of hemolysis, provided other common causes of an increase are excluded. Isoenzyme fractionation of the elevated LDH in hemolysis may demonstrate increased LD_1 levels that are out of proportion to the LD_2 fraction.[50] Serial determinations of LDH can be performed to

TABLE 2-3. SERUM LACTIC DEHYDROGENASE IN HEMOLYTIC ANEMIA

Patient	Diagnosis	PCV (%)	Reticulocyte Count (%)	Serum LDH (n = 250–800 U/mL)
1	Three artificial heart valves	27	7.4	5,040
2	Two artificial heart valves	27	10.4	4,200
3	One artificial heart valve	25	10.0	8,250
4	Paroxysmal nocturnal hemoglobinuria	24	9.0	9,720
5	Paroxysmal nocturnal hemoglobinuria	12	22.4	22,800
6	Paroxysmal nocturnal hemoglobinuria	27	8.2	8,520
7	Acid ingestion	40	2.1	4,960
8	Chemical abortion	19	3.7	4,400
9	Burns	31	3.0	9,390
10	Vasculitis	27	7.4	7,020
11	Hereditary spherocytosis	28	6.8	700
12	Hereditary spherocytosis	29	10.0	450
13	Hereditary spherocytosis	21	28.4	1,340
14	β-Thalassemia	22	10.5	1,500
15	Sickle cell anemia	18	10.7	2,550

From Stein ID: Serum lactate dehydrogenase isoenzymes: Stability, clearance, and diagnostic application in hemolytic anemia. J Lab Clin Med 1970;76:76–84.

provide an indication of the course of a patient's hemolytic anemia.

Transfusion Requirement

An important method for determining the presence of hemolysis that is frequently ignored and/or misunderstood is an evaluation of a patient's transfusion requirement. This is particularly significant in patients with underlying diseases that affect other indicators of hemolysis. For example, liver disease may affect LDH, bilirubin, and haptoglobin values, and may also diminish the marrow's ability to respond to anemia with a reticulocytosis. Although hemolysis superimposed on liver disease may cause a distinct increase in LDH and bilirubin values, these findings may be difficult to interpret with certainty. In such situations, knowledge of normal transfusion requirements is important, and a significant increase in the absence of bleeding is diagnostic of hemolysis.

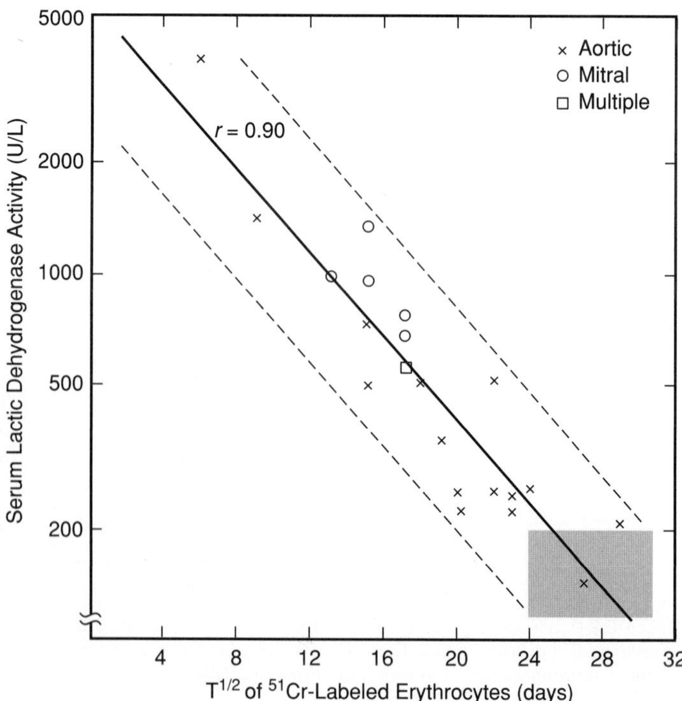

FIGURE 2-10. The correlation between serum lactic dehydrogenase activity (logarithmic scale) and the $T_{1/2}$ of ^{51}Cr-labeled erythrocytes in 21 patients with ball-valve prostheses. The unbroken line indicates the regression line; the broken lines show the 95% confidence interval; and the shaded area shows the normal values. (From Myhre E, Rasmussen K, Anderson A: Serum lactic dehyrogenase activity in patients with prosthetic heart valves: A parameter of intravascular hemolysis. Am Heart J 1997;80:463–468.)

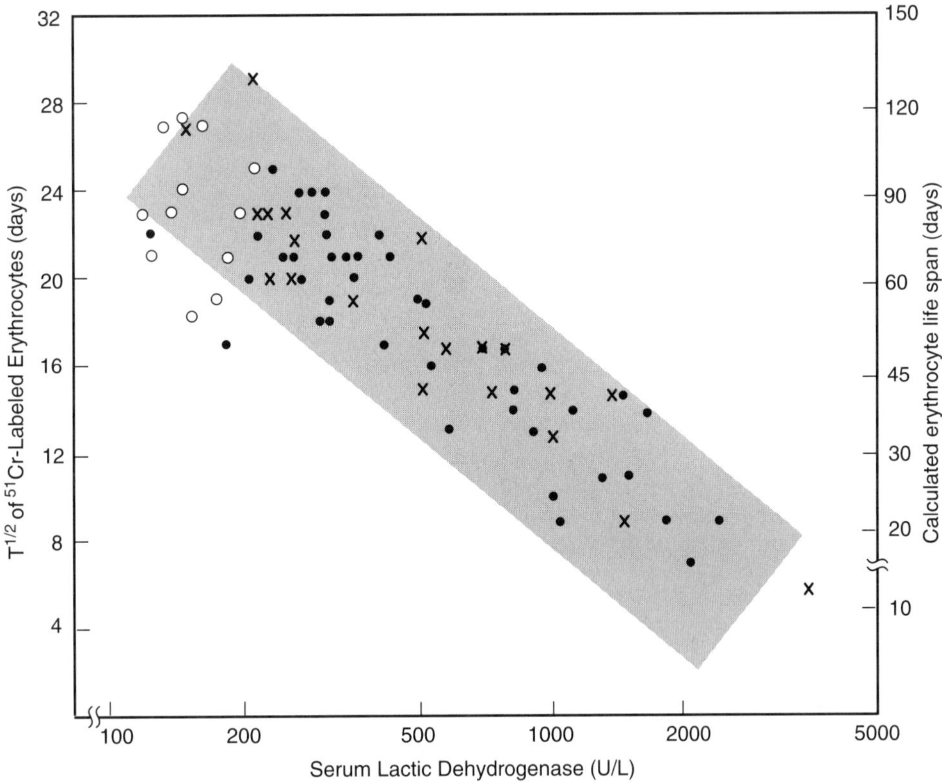

FIGURE 2-11. The relationship between serum lactic dehydrogenase, $T_{1/2}$ of Cr-labeled RBCs and calculated RBC survival in 21 patients with ball-valve prostheses (x); 12 unoperated patients with aortic valvular disease (◦); and recalculated data from 50 patients with ball-valve prostheses (•). The shaded area indicates the 95% confidence interval of our regression line. (From Myhre E, Rasmussen K, Andersen A: Serum lactic dehydrogenase activity in patients with prosthetic heart valves: A parameter of intravascular hemolysis. Am Heart J 1997;80:463–468.)

NORMAL TRANSFUSION REQUIREMENT (Table 2-5)

A 70-kg man has a RBC volume of about 2100 mL (30 mL/kg). If, for convenience, a figure of 100 days is used as the normal RBC life span, he must produce 21 mL of RBCs per day. To maintain a hemoglobin of 10 g/dL (about two thirds of normal) requires an RBC production of 14 mL/day. Freshly obtained RBCs, taken from the circulation of a blood donor, vary in age from 1 to 100 days, and therefore, have an average life expectancy that is one half of normal.[51] Accordingly, the daily requirement of *transfused* RBCs needed to maintain a hemoglobin level of 10 g/dL in a 70-kg male *who is making no RBCs* is 14 × 2, or 28 mL/day, or a requirement of 196 mL/week. One unit of RBCs contains about 180 mL of RBCs, so an average of 1 unit per week will need to be transfused in order to maintain a hemoglobin of 10 g/dL.[51] Because transfusion of RBCs suppresses erythropoiesis,[51] production of RBCs following transfusion may be significantly reduced. In this case, it should be expected that a patient's hemoglobin will return to pretransfusion levels within weeks of a transfusion of 2 or 3 units of RBC; it is incorrect to interpret this as an indication of poor survival of transfused RBCs.

TABLE 2-4. APPROXIMATE RBC DESTRUCTION RATE AS PREDICTED FROM THE SERUM LACTIC DEHYDROGENASE LEVELS

LDH (U/L)	Approximate RBC Destruction Rate (× normal)
<200	1 (range, 0.5–1.5)
200–500	2 (range, 1.5–2.5)
500–1000	3 (range, 2.0–4.0)
>1000	≥4

Modified from Myhre E, Rasmussen K, Andersen A: Serum lactic dehydrogenase activity in patients with prosthetic heart valves: A parameter of intravascular hemolysis. Am Heart J 1997;80:463–468.

INCREASED TRANSFUSION REQUIREMENT AS AN INDICATION OF HEMOLYSIS

The knowledge that transfusion of an average of 1 unit of RBCs per week should be able to maintain a reasonable level of hemoglobin in an adult, even if the patient's marrow is producing no RBCs, indicates that a significantly higher transfusion requirement is proof of shortened survival of transfused RBCs, provided bleeding can be excluded as a cause. In immune hemolytic

TABLE 2-5. TRANSFUSION REQUIREMENTS AS AN INDICATION OF HEMOLYSIS

Calculation of normal transfusion requirements for a 70-kg male whose marrow is producing no RBCs
Normal RBC volume = 30 mL/kg = 2100 mL
If the patient's hemoglobin is 10 g/dL (two thirds of normal), the RBC volume is 1400 mL.
If RBC survival is 100 days, 14 mL of RBCs must be replaced daily to maintain a hemoglobin of 10 g/dL.
Because RBCs obtained from a blood donor are of all ages, average survival of transfused RBCs will be about 50 days.[51]
Therefore, to maintain a hemoglobin of 10 g/dL, 28 mL would have to be transfused daily, or 196 mL/wk.
Each unit of RBCs contains about 180 mL of RBCs.
Thus, about 1 unit of RBCs per week is a normal transfusion requirement for an adult producing no RBCs.
In the absence of bleeding, a significantly increased transfusion requirement indicates hemolysis, i.e., a short RBC survival time of transfused RBCs.

anemias and other hemolytic anemias in which hemolysis is due to an extrinsic mechanism, rather than to an intrinsic red cell defect, transfused normal RBCs will undergo accelerated destruction. An increased transfusion requirement, therefore, can be an important and definitive indicator of a hemolytic anemia.

Further, a rough estimate of RBC survival can be made. For example, if a patient requires 4 units of RBCs per week to maintain a stable hemoglobin, survival of transfused RBCs must be about one fourth of normal. If a patient is also producing RBCs, as indicated by a reticulocytosis, survival of transfused RBCs must be even shorter.

Intravascular Hemolysis

Laboratory findings that indicate that hemolysis is primarily intravascular in nature are helpful in that they suggest that the specific diagnosis is likely to be one of a limited number of disorders, particularly those listed in Table 2-6.

The most remarkable degrees of massive, acute intravascular hemolysis in clinical medicine occur as a result of *Clostridium perfringens* infection.[54-57] The hematocrit may drop very rapidly to levels less than 5%.[56] Indeed, a patient reported by Terebelo and coworkers[57] maintained normal blood pressure, tissue oxygenation, and mentation and survived longer than 4 hours after having been found to have a hematocrit of 0 ("total intravascular hemolysis").[56] The peripheral smear disclosed few intact RBCs. After transfusion of 7 units of RBCs, the hematocrit was 7.2%. Plasma free hemoglobin was responsible for the preservation of tissue oxygenation, intravascular oncotic pressure, and pH.

Constitutional symptoms (fever, backache, etc.) often accompany acute severe intravascular hemolysis. Symptoms may begin shortly after the onset of hemolysis and may be present before the appearance of hemoglobinuria.

A distinctive laboratory finding in intravascular hemolysis is an elevated mean corpuscular hemoglobin concentration (MCHC). This occurs when using an automatic cell counter that calculates the MCHC by dividing the hemoglobin by the product of the mean corpuscular volume (MCV) and RBCs. The presence of plasma free hemoglobin causes the falsely elevated MCHC. Buys and Craven[58] reported two such occurrences in patients with *C. perfringens* infection and commented that other cases have been reported in patients infected with *Leptospira, Toxoplasma,* and *Plasmodium* organisms, as well as in a patient with AIHA.

HEMOGLOBINEMIA AND HEMOGLOBINURIA

The cardinal features of intravascular hemolysis are hemoglobinemia and hemoglobinuria. In normal subjects, hemoglobin breakdown occurs mainly in the cells of the reticuloendothelial system; therefore, the level of free hemoglobin in the plasma is low, ranging from 2 to 5 mg/dL. When hemolysis occurs in the blood, the hemoglobin from the broken down RBCs is liberated into the plasma, causing an increase in plasma hemoglobin values to 100 to 200 mg/dL or even more.

TABLE 2-6. CAUSES OF HEMOGLOBINURIA

Acute Hemoglobinuria
Incompatible blood transfusion
Transfusion of damaged blood (overheating or freezing, bacterial contamination, pump-oxygenation)
Drugs and chemical agents (immune or nonimmune mechanisms)
Paroxysmal cold hemoglobinuria
Acute severe warm antibody AIHA
Passenger lymphocyte syndrome
Clostridium perfringens infection
Malaria ("blackwater fever")
Bartonellosis, babesiosis, leptospirosis, toxoplasmosis
Peritoneal hemorrhage[52]
Severe hypophosphatemia[53]
Snake and spider bites
Cold agglutinin syndrome*
March hemoglobinuria
Microangiopathic hemolytic anemia
Hypotonic bladder irrigation during prostatic surgery
Mistaken intravenous administration of water
Chronic Hemoglobinuria
Paroxysmal nocturnal hemoglobinuria†
Prosthetic cardiovascular materials

*Chronic low-grade intravascular hemolysis is common, with acute hemoglobinuria resulting from exposure to cold.
†Characteristically associated with intermittent episodes of grossly evident hemoglobinuria.

When the plasma hemoglobin level is markedly raised, the plasma has a pink or red color, depending on the concentration of the hemoglobin. When the rise is moderate (e.g., from 10 to 40 mg/dL), this color may be lacking, not only because of the relatively low concentration but also because other pigments, such as bilirubin, which gives a yellow color, and methemalbumin, which gives a brownish color, may mask the pink tint. Also, plasma hemoglobin disappears in 2 to 5 hours after the cessation of hemolysis, whereas methemalbumin has a half-life of 20 hours.[59]

When the level of plasma hemoglobin exceeds the renal threshold, hemoglobin appears in the urine, a condition termed *hemoglobinuria*. The urine may be pink, red, brown, or almost black.[60] It contains two pigments—oxyhemoglobin and methemoglobin—that are produced by auto-oxidation of the hemoglobin in the urinary tract when the urine is acidic. Oxyhemoglobin is bright red, whereas methemoglobin is dark brown; the color of the urine, therefore, depends on the concentration (which is related to the degree of hemolysis) and the relative proportions of the two pigments. Oxyhemoglobin predominates in alkaline urine, whereas methemoglobin is predominant in acidic urine. Hemoglobinuria usually clears within 6 hours of an acute hemolytic episode. It is usually accompanied by albuminuria, which disappears when hemoglobinuria ceases.

The term "blackwater" has been used clinically to describe the dark color of the urine that occurs in some patients with marked hemoglobinuria. The term has most commonly been applied to patients with malaria, in whom hemolysis in association with an acute febrile episode has been called "blackwater fever."

DETECTION OF HEMOGLOBINURIA

Hemoglobin in the urine can be identified by spectroscopic examination and by a positive reaction with benzidine and quaiac. Benzidine-positive pigment in the urine can represent hemoglobin or myoglobin. Usually, the clinical setting strongly suggests one or the other. Myoglobinuria most commonly occurs after crush or other traumatic injury to skeletal muscle, in intoxicated patients subjected to prolonged muscle compression as they lay motionless, and in patients with seizure disorders, although numerous other unusual causes have also been reported.[61,62] Although myoglobinuria can mimic hemoglobinuria, the plasma is less likely to be pink because the small myoglobin molecule is rapidly cleared into the urine with a half-life of approximately 1 to 3 hours.[61,63]

DISTINGUISHING HEMOGLOBINURIA FROM HEMATURIA

Hemoglobinuria is often confused with hematuria (RBCs in the urine), especially when the urine is bright red. The urine in hemoglobinuria is clear, but in hematuria, it is smoky. The microscopic examination of a freshly voided centrifuged specimen will identify hematuria, as the sediment is seen to contain numerous RBCs and the supernatant fluid is clear. Occasionally, however, the specific gravity of the urine is so low (<1.007) that the red cells rupture in the urine and cause the supernatant to turn red. In such cases, the inspection of a carefully collected, centrifuged specimen of blood, with precautions taken to prevent hemolysis, will distinguish the two conditions. In hematuria, the plasma is, of course, of normal color. Accordingly, red plasma plus red (or dark) urine suggests hemoglobin in plasma and urine; clear plasma plus red urine suggests hematuria.

CONSEQUENCES OF HEMOGLOBINURIA

In some patients with acute intravascular hemolysis, the kidneys are damaged, giving rise to acute renal failure secondary to acute tubular necrosis. This condition is characterized clinically by oliguria, which may progress to anuria, uremia, and sometimes, death. Acute tubular necrosis is classically seen following intravascular hemolysis, especially when hemolysis is severe. Urinary output should be monitored in all cases of acute hemoglobinuria in order to allow early detection of the onset of oliguria.

Hemopexin and Methemalbumin

Free heme that is released into the circulation is bound in a 1:1 ratio to the plasma glycoprotein hemopexin, which is cleared from the plasma with a half-life of 7 to 8 hours.[64] A decrease in the hemopexin level signifies intravascular red cell destruction.

Large quantities of hemoglobin that cannot be bound by available haptoglobin or hemopexin are oxidized to methemoglobin.[59] The heme in this form loses its close affinity for the globin part of the molecule and is bound by circulating albumin to form methemalbumin. It is not rapidly removed from the circulation ($T_{1/2}$ = 20 hours), and its presence is considered to be a sign of significant intravascular hemolysis.[59] Methemalbumin may be suspected simply by visual inspection because it gives the plasma a golden to brown color, depending on its concentration. More definitive identification may be accomplished by biochemical tests.

Hemosiderinuria

Hemoglobinuria results in the deposition in the renal tubules of iron-containing granules that are derived from the breakdown of absorbed hemoglobin and that are known as hemosiderin. Hemosiderin appears in the urine, probably as a result of the desquamation of tubular cells, and can be demonstrated by staining a centrifuged urine sediment for iron. Hemosiderinuria is most likely to be seen in patients with chronic intravascular hemolysis, such as occurs in mechanical hemolytic anemias, and it is especially typical of paroxysmal nocturnal hemoglobinuria (PNH), in which hemosiderinuria persists even when hemoglobinuria is absent. Indeed, an early term for PNH was "hemolytic anemia with perpetual hemosiderinuria."[65]

Transient hemosiderinuria also occurs in acute hemoglobinuria, but it is not found at the onset of a hemolytic attack, as the pigment has to be absorbed by the tubular cells of the kidney and reexcreted, a process that takes at least 48 hours.[64] The interval during which hemosiderinuria may be found following completion of a transient hemolytic episode has not been determined, although it has been demonstrated that more than 50% of the ^{59}Fe initially present in the kidneys still remained 2 weeks after an intravenous injection of ^{59}Fe-labeled hemoglobin.[66]

Other Tests

Fehr and Knob[67] have evaluated the use of RBC creatine as an indicator of the severity of hemolytic disease. In patients with steady-state hemolysis, there was a better correlation between RBC survival and red cell creatine than there was between RBC survival and the reticulocyte count. Only 3 of 21 patients with hemolytic disease had nomal creatine levels, and these 3 patients had the least reduced ^{51}Cr half-life values (18.1 to 20 days). The authors suggest that this simple chemical assay may be used to obtain a useful estimation of RBC survival.

For further evidence of hemolysis, one might assess the patient for erythroid hyperplasia of the bone marrow or perform RBC survival studies with ^{51}Cr or ^{32}P-diisopropyl fluorophosphate (DFP)-labeled RBCs.[51] Also, measurement of the rate of endogenous production of carbon monoxide (CO) may be used to calculate the RBC life span,[68-70] and Vreman and coworkers[71] suggest that advances in techniques used for measurement of CO may stimulate the study of hemolysis. However, at present these tests are not generally applied in clinical medicine to establish the presence or absence of hemolysis.

Burns and coworkers[72] have suggested that measurement of RBC adenylate kinase (EAK) is a highly sensitive and specific test for the diagnosis of hemolytic anemia. They studied 25 patients with sickle cell disease, hemolytic transfusion reactions, or thrombotic thrombocytopenic purpura, and compared EAK levels in those patients with levels found in normal subjects. The normal range was 0 to 3.5 units (mean, 0.5); in patients with hemolysis, the mean level was 62.4 units (range of 0 to 298). The diagnostic sensitivity was 96%, with a specificity and accuracy of 97%.

Zeiler and coworkers[73] used flow cytometry to determine the survival of transfused and autologous RBCs in a patient with severe warm antibody AIHA. The patient was group A, Rh+, and the authors transfused group A, Rh– RBCs in order to enable the distinction between autologus and transfused RBCs. The life span of autologous RBCs, measured on two consecutive days, was 69 and 64 hours, whereas the life span of transfused RBCs decreased from 186 hours to 25 hours. They demonstrated that the life span of transfused RBCs almost normalized following splenectomy: a life span of 43 days at postsplenectomy day 3 and a life span of 87 days at postsplenectomy day 69.

Summary and Comments Concerning the Value of Laboratory Tests to Determine the Presence of Hemolysis

Hemolytic anemias are relatively uncommon, and hemolysis is unlikely to be suspected on clinical grounds when a patient presents with a previously undiagnosed anemia. An elevated reticulocyte count should strongly suggest hemolysis, but reticulocyte counts may not be part of the initial complete blood count. The presence of hemolysis may unexpectedly become evident on the basis of laboratory tests ordered for reasons other than for the evaluation of anemia, such as bilirubin, LDH, or compatibility tests, when a blood transfusion is considered to be indicated. In patients with autoimmune or drug-induced immune hemolytic anemias, the laboratory indicators of hemolysis are usually quite evident and, once considered, the presence of hemolysis is usually easily confirmed by simple tests. These tests include reticulocyte count, review of the peripheral blood film, serum bilirubin (direct and indirect) determinations, LDH measurement, and haptoglobin measurement. A more extensive battery of tests is generally not necessary, and one should proceed to determining the cause of the hemolysis, as indicated in the following section.

Hemoglobinemia and hemoglobinuria are definitive indicators of hemolysis, and their presence should precipitate an urgent evaluation of the patient. However, one should be aware that hemolyzed plasma may also be caused by in vitro lysis during or following venipuncture. Thus, the first step in evaluation should be to obtain a repeat blood sample and, in addition, to inspect the urine visually. Hemoglobinemia is generally accompanied by hemoglobinuria, so that if a urine sample has a normal color, in vitro lysis of the blood sample is to be suspected.

Hemoglobinuria is a much less common clinical finding than hematuria, so when the urine is red, the color is often assumed to be the result of the latter. Centrifugation of the urine specimen will usually allow a distinction to be made as to whether the red color is due to RBCs or hemoglobin. In hematuria, the supernatant is clear (although in unusual cases and in the presence of a low specific gravity of the urine, there may be lysis of RBCs in the urine, causing the supernatant to be red). Visual inspection of plasma (or serum) is helpful because hemoglobinemia and/or methemalbuminemia will accompany hemoglobinuria, whereas the plasma will be of normal color in patients with hematuria.

Of the easily performed and very valuable tests for determining the presence of hemolysis, the most underutilized may be inspection of the peripheral blood film. RBC morphology often strongly suggests hemolysis and may suggest a specific diagnosis or a limited number of diagnostic possibilities (see page 53).

In some complex clinical settings, the usual tests indicating hemolysis may yield misleading or uninterpretable results. For example, treatment with chemotherapy may supppress the reticulocyte count, and liver disease may cause hyperbilirubinemia, elevated serum LDH levels, and low serum haptoglobin levels. In such settings, tests that can be used to determine the presence of hemolysis are serial hemoglobin and hematocrit determinations (and, when the marrow is not suppressed, reticulocyte counts). One must keep in mind that there are only two ways to lose RBCs: bleeding and hemolysis. Accordingly, a marked drop in hemoglobin in a patient who has no evidence of significant blood loss strongly suggests hemolysis. Because blood loss is much more common than hemolysis, there is a tendency to misinterpret minor amounts of blood loss, such as that indicated by a weakly positive stool guaiac test, as being an adequate explanation for a severe anemia or a marked drop in hemoglobin in patients in whom hemolysis is not anticipated.

A definitive indicator of hemolysis that is often misunderstood or ignored is the transfusion requirement. In the absence of bleeding, a significantly increased transfusion requirement is diagnostic of hemolysis (see Table 2-5). Another indicator of hemolysis is the presence of a persistent elevation of the reticulocyte count without an increase in the hemoglobin and hematocrit levels, unless chronic bleeding is present.

ESTABLISHING A TENTATIVE DIAGNOSIS OF THE CAUSE OF THE HEMOLYTIC ANEMIA

When it has been established that the patient has a hemolytic anemia, the cause of the hemolysis should be sought next. One should consider the differential diagnosis of hemolytic anemias and develop a preliminary diagnosis. Hemolytic anemias have been classified in a number of ways. Traditionally, they are divided into intracorpuscular and extracorpuscular defects or into hereditary and acquired disorders. Efforts have been made to extend these classifications by incorporating knowledge of the site of the basic defect in reference to the RBC membrane.[74,75] Thus, hemolytic disorders may be caused by intracellular abnormalities, defects of the RBC membrane, or extracellular abnormalities. Taking into account all the information stated earlier, the authors have developed a classification system, presented in Table 2-7, which considers not only the site of the basic defect, but also the hereditary or acquired nature of many of the recognized causes of hemolytic anemia.

Although such a classification is comprehensive, it is rather cumbersome, and many of the disorders listed are extremely rare. Thus, when determining the cause of a patient's hemolytic anemia, it is more practical to emphasize consideration of a limited number of relatively common disorders. The comparatively simple classification presented in Table 2-8 is useful for this purpose.

As the number of causes of hemolytic anemia is large, even when considering the simplified classification, it is evident that it is useful to have a more restricted list of possibilities in mind before performing specific diagnostic tests. A tentative or working diagnosis should be formulated after careful consideration of four important points:

1. A review of the clinical history and physical examination, especially as they relate to various possible causes of hemolysis
2. A review of the peripheral blood film
3. Findings of intravascular hemolysis
4. The results of a direct antiglobulin test (DAT)

History and Physical Examination

Because hemolytic anemia is often not suspected on the basis of the initial history and physical examination, it is important to review them with emphasis on specific points after a diagnosis of hemolysis has been made.

A history of anemia or of splenectomy in members of the family suggests a hereditary hemolytic anemia. If present in successive generations, an autosomal disorder (such as hereditary spherocytosis) or a condition that is manifested in the heterozygous state (such as the unstable hemoglobins) should be considered. The most common hereditary RBC enzyme defects—glucose-6-phosphate dehydrogenase deficiency and pyruvate kinase deficiency—are clinically manifested in the sex-linked hemizygous or rare homozygous state, respectively. In these instances, the examination of other family members is of obvious importance. A history of jaundice at birth and long-standing or recurring anemia and/or jaundice may also be obtained in cases of hereditary hemolytic states.

In contrast, the presence of acquired hemolysis may be indicated by the knowledge of a previously normal blood count or by a history of acute onset of constitutional symptoms, such as fever, malaise, or pain in the back, legs, or abdomen.

A history of red or dark colored urine suggests the presence of hemoglobinuria. The relationship, if any, of hemoglobinuria to sleep (PNH), cold (cold agglutinin syndrome or PCH), and exertion (march hemoglobinuria) should also be noted.

Details relating to drug intake or exposure to chemicals must be obtained, as hemolysis can result from a direct toxic effect on red cells, oxidative injury (especially when an enzyme defect or unstable hemoglobin is present), or immunologic damage. However, an accurate history of ingestion of drugs may not always be easy to obtain. Several types of hemolytic anemia have been described in alcoholism, particularly when there is associated liver disease.[76-80]

TABLE 2-7. CLASSIFICATION OF HEMOLYTIC ANEMIAS

Intracellular Abnormalities	Membrane Abnormalities	Extracellular Abnormalities
Hereditary		
Enzyme defects Glucose-6-phosphate dehydrogenase, pyruvate kinase deficiency, triosephosphate isomerase deficiency, glucose phosphate isomerase deficiency, 2,3-diphosphoglycerate mutase deficiency, etc. Globin disorders Defects in globin structure (sickle cell anemia, hemoglobin S-C disease, hemoglobin S-D disease, hemoglobin C disease, etc.; unstable hemoglobins such as hemoglobin Hammersmith, Bristol, Santa Ana, Madrid) Defects in globin synthesis (thalassemias) Heme disorders (porphyrias) Hepatoerythropoietic porphyria Congenital erythropoietic porphyria	Hereditary spherocytosis Hereditary stomatocytosis Rh_{null} syndrome Hereditary elliptocytosis Abnormal cation permeability Hydrocytosis and dessiccytosis High phosphatidyl choline hemolytic anemia Calcium leak with extreme microcytosis Muscular dystrophies Congenital dyserythropoietic anemias	Lipid abnormalities Abetalipoproteinemia (acanthocytosis) Lecithin:cholesterol acyltransferase (LCAT) deficiency
Acquired		
Environmental factors influencing metabolism Hypophosphatemia Wilson's disease (high serum copper) Uremia Severe iron deficiency anemia	Paroxysmal nocturnal hemoglobinuria Membrane lipid abnormalities Liver disease Clostridial infection Anorexia nervosa Vitamin E deficiency Lead poisoning	Immune hemolytic anemias Autoimmune Alloimmune Drug-induced Drugs (nonimmune) Chemicals, venoms Mechanical hemolytic anemia Prosthetic cardiovascular materials March hemoglobinuria Microangiopathic hemolytic anemia Thrombotic thrombocytopenic purpura Hemolytic uremic syndrome Malignant hypertension Carcinomatosis Hemangioma Heat (severe burns) Infectious agents Malaria, babesiosis, bartonellosis, Bacteria: *Clostridium perfringins* (welchii), *Mycoplasma pneumoniae* Viral: HIV, CMV, EBV, measles, mumps, varicella, Hypersplenism
Hereditary Factor	**Hereditary and Acquired**	**Acquired Factor**
Metabolic defects (Enzymopathies especially glucose 6-phosphate dehydrogenase deficiency)	In conjunction with	Oxidant drugs, favism, infections (e.g., viral hepatitis), diabetic ketoacidosis
Unstable hemoglobins (Zürich, H, Torino, Köln, Shepherds Bush, etc.)	In conjunction with	Oxidant drugs, infections

CMV, cytomegalovirus; EBV, Epstein-Barr virus; HIV, human immunodeficiency virus.

Symptoms and signs suggestive of systemic lupus erythematosus, lymphomas, chronic lymphocytic leukemia, or infections are important because of the association of AIHAs with these diseases. Raynaud's phenomenon and, less frequently, cold urticaria may be present in autoimmune AIHAs caused by cold antibodies. Occasionally, infections are associated with a hemolytic state (see Chapter 3), or they may provoke acute hemolysis in subjects with an intrinsic red cell defect.

Microangiopathic hemolytic anemia is suggested by the presence of certain underlying disorders, as indicated in Table 2-9.

TABLE 2-8. A SIMPLIFIED CLASSIFICATION OF HEMOLYTIC ANEMIAS

Hereditary hemolytic anemias
- Hereditary spherocytosis
- Hereditary elliptocytosis
- Thalassemias
- Hemoglobinopathies
- Enzyme deficiency hemolytic anemias

Acquired hemolytic anemias
- Immune hemolytic anemias
  - Autoimmune hemolytic anemias (AIHAs)
    - Warm antibody AIHA
    - Cold agglutinin syndrome
    - Paroxysmal cold hemoglobinuria
    - Direct antiglobulin test negative AIHA
    - Combined warm and cold AIHA
  - Alloimmune hemolytic anemias
    - Hemolytic disease of the fetus and newborn
    - Hemolytic transfusion reactions
  - Drug-induced immune hemolytic anemia
- Drug-induced hemolytic anemias (nonimmunologic mechanisms)
  - Direct toxic effect
  - Idiosyncrasy mechanism
- Hemolysis associated with transplantation
- Hemolytic anemias associated with numerous irregularly contracted erythrocytes in the blood film
  - Mechanical hemolytic anemia
  - Microangiopathic hemolytic anemias
- Paroxysmal nocturnal hemoglobinuria
- Miscellaneous
  - Infectious agents (uncommon)
    - Protozoal parasites: malaria
    - Bacteria: *Clostridium perfringens* (*welchii*)

The classic physical findings of hemolytic anemia are pallor, jaundice, and splenomegaly. However, in milder degrees of hemolysis, these findings are often absent. Leg ulcers or their residual pigmentation, typically over the malleoli, may be present in chronic hemolytic anemias. Thickening of the skull as a result of bone marrow expansion may occur in severe hereditary hemolytic states, and a radiologic examination will show thinning of cortical bone with expansion and trabeculation of the medulla, sometimes with the typical hair-on-end appearance.

Although splenomegaly occurs in many hemolytic anemias, massive splenomegaly suggests thalassemia major, lymphoma, myelofibrosis, or chronic leukemias. Purpura may be seen in hemolytic anemias associated with systemic lupus erythematosus, thrombotic thrombocytopenic purpura, or Evans's syndrome.

The Peripheral Blood Film

The peripheral blood film is often very helpful in suggesting a specific diagnosis or a limited number of diagnostic possibilities. Spherocytes may be a prominent feature in several hemolytic anemias, as indicated in Table 2-9 and in Figures 2-12 and 2-13. Basophilic stippling, due to clumping of ribosomes, is encountered in many anemias but is prominent in β-thalassemias, and coarse stippling is seen in lead poisoning. Hypochromic RBCs associated with a hemolytic state suggest thalassemic disorders, hemoglobinopathies, lead poisoning, and chronic intravascular hemolysis with urinary loss of iron. Target cells (Fig. 2-14) are present in patients with thalassemia or some of the hemoglobinopathies, especially hemoglobins C and E. They may also be found in patients with obstructive jaundice or hepatitis. Target cell formation is more pronounced after splenectomy. Sickle cells (Fig. 2-15) are seen in patients with sickle cell anemia.

Fragmented RBCs (Fig. 2-16) are typically seen in microangiopathic, mechanical, and some drug-induced hemolytic anemias; irregularly contracted red cells of less characteristic appearance are also present in other hemolytic anemias (see Table 2-9). In hereditary elliptocytosis (or ovalocytosis) (Fig. 2-17), 50% to 90% of the RBCs are oval. In normal subjects, less than 15% of RBCs are oval, and such cells are also present in a wide variety of anemias, including iron deficiency, thalassemia, megaloblastic anemia, and myelofibrosis. However, the degree of elliptocytosis is most marked in the hereditary form.

Cold agglutinin syndrome is suggested by the finding of gross agglutination in blood films made at room temperature, especially if agglutination is not present when the same sample of blood is warmed to

TABLE 2-9. DIFFERENTIAL DIAGNOSIS IN HEMOLYTIC ANEMIAS ASSOCIATED WITH SPHEROCYTOSIS OR NUMEROUS IRREGULARLY CONTRACTED ERYTHROCYTES

Spherocytes
- Hereditary spherocytosis
- Immune hemolytic anemias
  - Alloimmune hemolytic anemia, especially ABO hemolytic disease of the newborn and hemolytic transfusion reactions
  - Autoimmune hemolytic anemia, especially warm antibody AIHA
  - Drug-induced hemolysis (some cases)
- Severe burns
- *Clostridium perfringens* (*welchii*) septicemia
- Hypophosphatemia

Fragmented erythrocytes (schistocytes, helmet cells, burr cells)
- Chemical or drug-induced hemolytic anemia (some cases)
- Mechanical hemolytic anemia (prosthetic cardiovascular materials)
- Traumatic hemolytic anemia (March hemoglobinuria)
- Microangropathic hemolytic anemia
  - Hemolytic uremic syndrome
  - Thrombotic thrombocytopenic purpura
  - Disseminated intravascular coagulation
  - Malignant hypertension
  - Disseminated malignancy

Less characteristic irregularly contracted erythrocytes
- Severe megaloblastic anemia
- Severe iron deficiency
- Thalassemia major

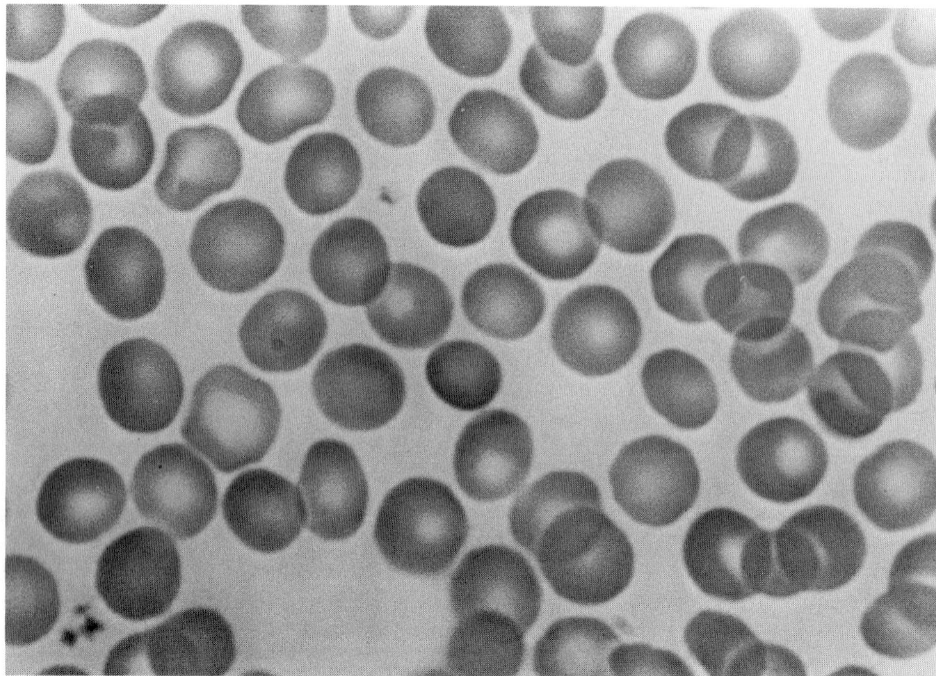

FIGURE 2-12. Hereditary spherocytosis. Numerous densely staining microspherocytes are present.

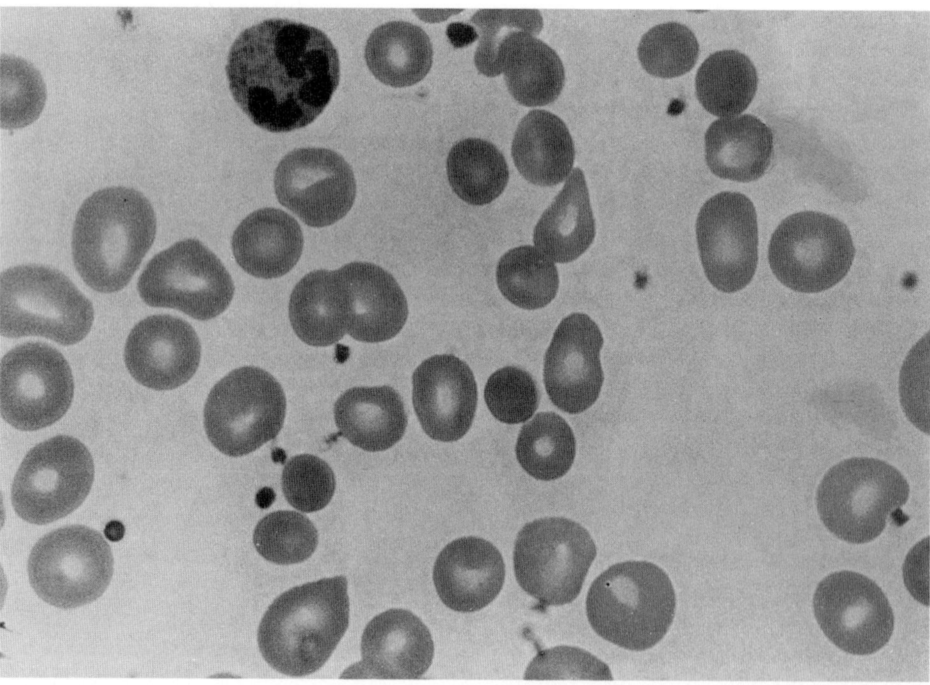

FIGURE 2-13. Warm antibody autoimmune hemolytic anemia. Spherocytes are evident, and the degree of poikilocytosis is generally more marked than in hereditary spherocytosis as a result of the interaction of antibody and/or complement-sensitized RBCs with macrophages.

37°C prior to making the blood film (Figs. 2-18 and 2-19). Erythroblasts are not infrequently present in the peripheral blood of patients with hemolytic anemia, particularly in infants and children. Stomatocytes are present in small numbers in many blood smears, but they occur in larger numbers in a rare hemolytic anemia associated with increased red cell sodium permeability[81] and in alcoholic liver disease.[82] Acanthocytes are characteristically seen in hereditary abetalipoproteinemia, chronic liver disease, and

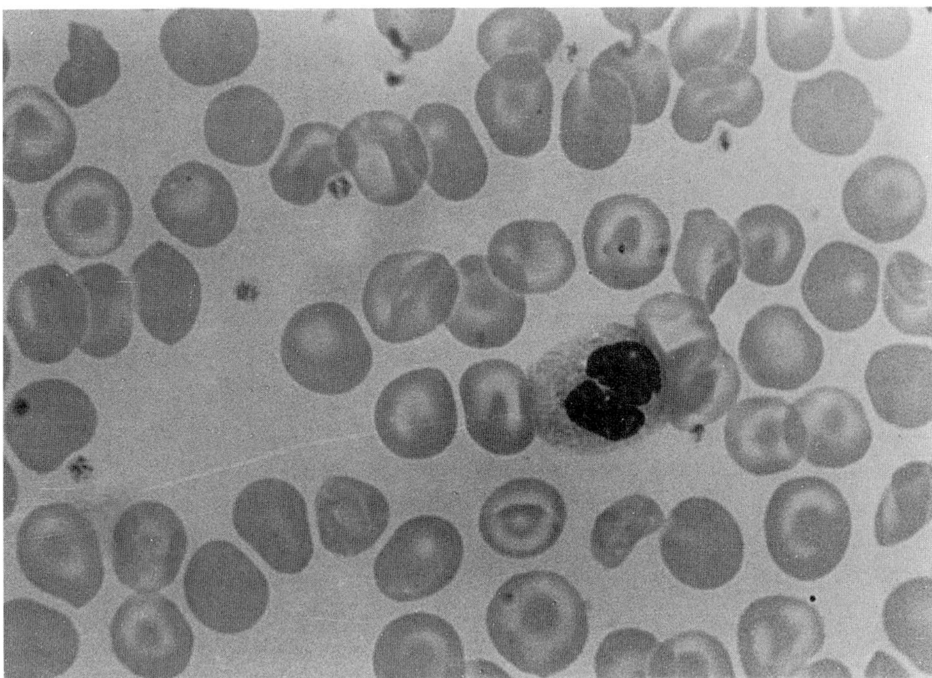

FIGURE 2-14. Hemoglobin C. Numerous target cells are present. Hemoglobin electrophoresis indicated that the patient was heterozygous for hemoglobin C.

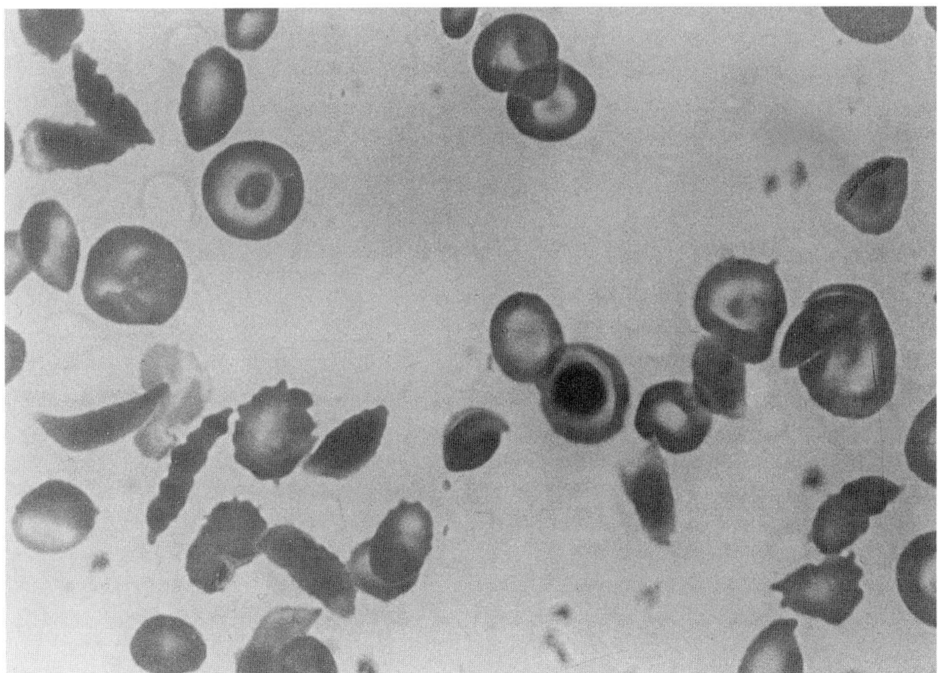

FIGURE 2-15. Hemoglobin S. Anisocytosis, poikilocytosis, and several sickle cells are illustrated.

certain inherited neurologic disorders, and in association with the inheritance of certain RBC antigen polymorphisms.[83]

It is also true that findings in the peripheral blood film other than RBC morphology may suggest the cause of a patient's hemolytic anemia. For example, examination of the film may indicate the presence of chronic lymphatic leukemia or infectious mononucleosis. Also, a marked decrease in platelets in a patient with hemolytic anemia who has numerous fragmented RBCs in the peripheral blood film suggests a diagnosis of thrombotic thrombocytopenic

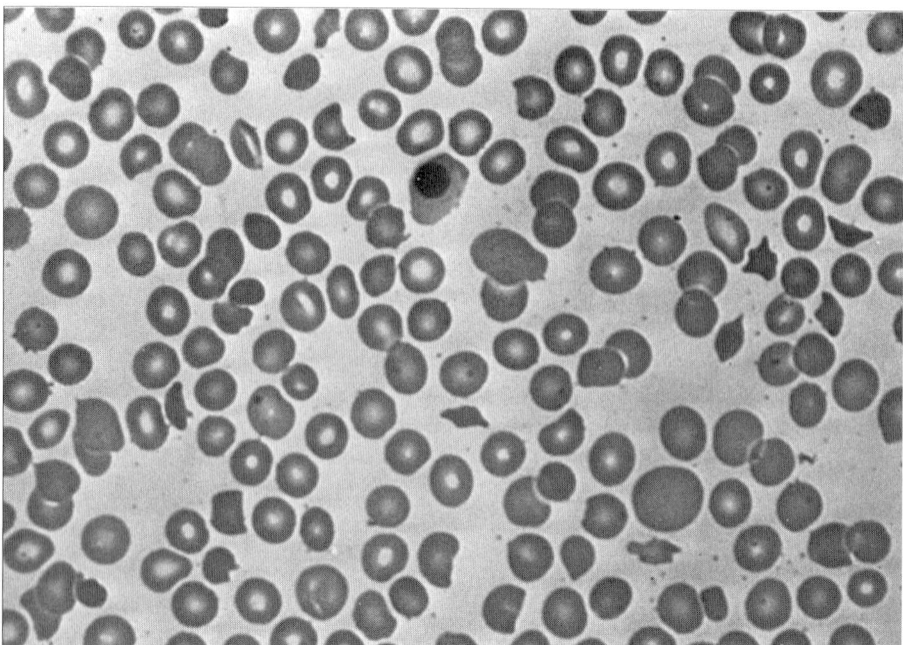

FIGURE 2-16. Thrombotic thrombocytopenic purpura. Numerous fragmented RBCs and a marked decrease in the number of platelets are characteristic features of the disorder. A nucleated RBC is also present.

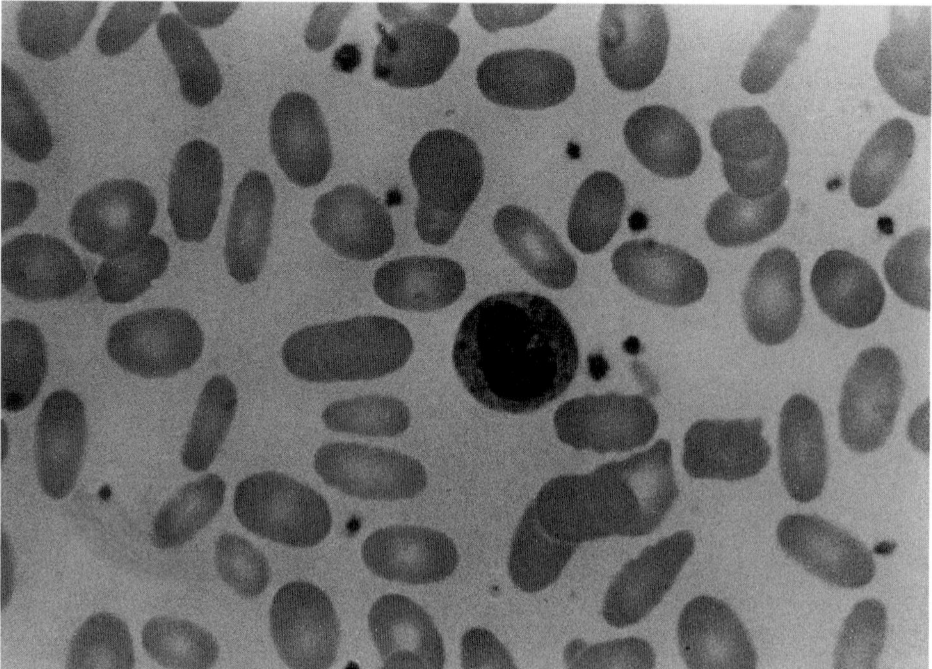

FIGURE 2-17. Hereditary elliptocytosis. Occasionally, elliptocytes may be seen in a variety of anemias, but herediatry elliptocytosis is characterized by the marked degree of elliptocytosus illustrated here. About 15% of patients with hereditary elliptocytosis have hemolytic anemia.

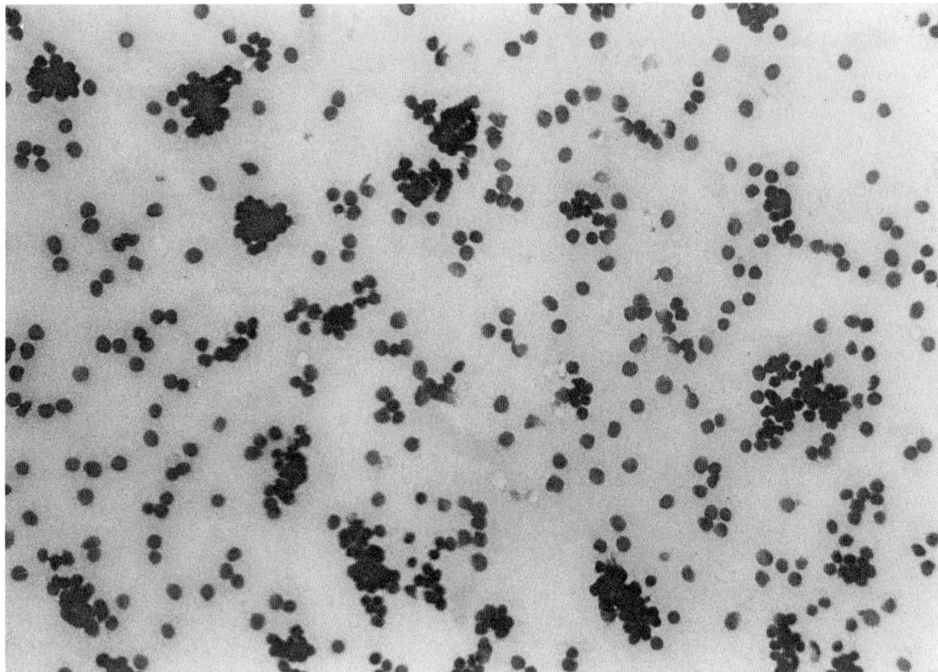

FIGURE 2-18. Cold agglutinin syndrome. The blood film was made at room temperature, and gross autoagglutination is evident.

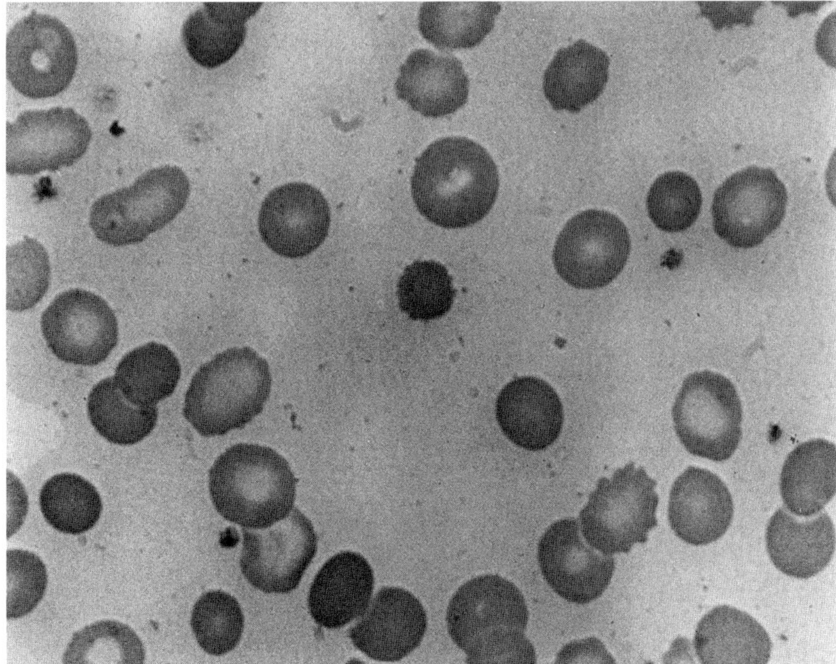

FIGURE 2-19. Cold agglutinin syndrome. Same patient as in Figure 2-18, but the blood film was made strictly at 37°C. Autoagglutination is not present. There is an occasional microspherocyte, moderate poikilocytosis, and anisocytosis with some macrocytes that are probably reticulocytes.

purpura or the hemolytic uremic syndrome, and thrombocytopenia in the presence of spherocytes suggests Evans's syndrome.

Intravascular Hemolysis

The presence of hemoglobinemia and hemoglobinuria, that is, intravascular hemolysis, is an important clinical finding. Such a finding indicates the likelihood that severe hemolysis is taking place and that certain disorders should be considered as the most probable diagnostic possibilities (see page 48 and Table 2-6).

The Direct Antiglobulin Test

The direct antiglobulin test (DAT) should be performed in every patient in whom the presence of hemolysis has been established. Although some exceptions to this rule might be considered, as when the diagnosis of a congenital hemolytic anemia is evident, the DAT is a simple, quick, inexpensive test that yields useful information.

A positive result on a DAT in a patient with hemolytic anemia does, of course, indicate that the most likely diagnosis is one of the immune hemolytic anemias.[84] It should be emphasized that determination of the presence or absence of hemolysis, as described earlier in this chapter, should logically precede the performance of the DAT. The purpose of the latter test is to indicate the presence or absence of an immune etiology in patients known to have hemolytic anemia (Table 2-10). Indeed, the predictive value of a positive DAT for determining whether or not a patient has immune hemolytic anemia is 83% in a patient with hemolytic anemia but only 1.4% in a patient without hemolytic anemia.[84]

Although the result of the DAT in a patient with hemolytic anemia generally indicates whether or not the hemolytic anemia is immunologically mediated, a positive DAT may occur as a coincidental finding in patients with hemolytic anemia caused by nonimmune mechanisms, and some patients with immune hemolytic anemias have a negative DAT.[85]

Moreover, although a positive DAT is quite unusual in perfectly healthy persons, positive reactions are obtained in a significant number of hospitalized patients who do not have hemolytic anemia.[85] These findings emphasize that careful evaluation is required before a precise diagnosis can be made in patients who have a hemolytic anemia and a positive DAT test. The details of such an evaluation are discussed in Chapters 5 and 6.

TABLE 2-10. SCREENING PATIENTS WITH HEMOLYTIC ANEMIA FOR ACQUIRED IMMUNE HEMOLYTIC ANEMIA (AIHA)

	Positive DAT	Negative DAT	Total
AIHA	24	1	25
No AIHA	5	70	75
Total	29	71	100

Positive value of a positive result = (24/29) × 100 = 83%.
Positive value of a negative result = (70/71) × 100 = 99%.
Modified from Kaplan HS, Garratty G: Predictive value of direct antiglobulin test results. Diagn Med 1985;8:29–33.

SPECIFIC CONFIRMATORY TESTS

On the basis of the evaluation indicated thus far, a provisional diagnosis or a limited number of diagnostic possibilities can usually be established with reasonable certainty. It is beyond the scope of this text to describe the details of the use of specific confirmatory tests for a wide variety of nonimmune hemolytic anemias. However, a few examples are cited to illustrate the use of the principles advocated in this chapter.

If, in a patient with hemolytic anemia, the history suggests a hereditary hemolytic anemia, the physical examination reveals splenomegaly, the peripheral blood film reveals spherocytes, features of intravascular hemolysis are absent, and the DAT is negative, a tentative diagnosis of hereditary spherocytosis is warranted. A family history may reveal a similar diagnosis in other family members. Osmotic fragility and autohemolysis tests will yield characteristic abnormalities, although similar results may be obtained in patients who have spherocytosis as a result of acquired disease. Further specialized testing is rarely needed to confirm the diagnosis, although tests may be performed to identify characteristic membrane abnormalities.[86,87]

If an adult patient with hemolytic anemia manifesting for the first time has a history of repeated episodes of dark urine and abdominal pain, a blood film that reveals no characteristic abnormalities, laboratory tests indicating features of intravascular hemolysis, and a negative DAT, the tentative diagnosis of PNH may be made. In past years, the diagnosis was based on the results of Ham's acidified serum test, with the sucrose hemolysis test serving as a screening test. More recently, flow cytometry using antibodies to the glycosylphosphatidylinositol-anchored proteins CD55 and CD59 has been proposed as the standard diagnostic test.[88-90] Further relevant tests include the documentation of hemoglobinuria and hemosiderinuria.

Another example is that of a patient who has an acquired hemolytic anemia; does not have a history of recent blood transfusion or drug ingestion; has an acute onset of systemic symptoms, such as fever, malaise, and aching in the back and legs; a physical examination that reveals splenomegaly; a blood film revealing spherocytosis; no evidence of hemoglobinuria; and a strongly positive DAT. An AIHA is the most likely diagnosis, and details of further diagnostic tests that should be performed are described in later chapters.

REFERENCES

1. Petz LD. The diagnosis of hemolytic anemia. In: Bell CA (ed): A Seminar on Laboratory Management of Hemolysis. Washington, DC: American Association of Blood Banks, 1979:1–27.
2. Erslev AJ: Compensated hemolytic anemia. Blood 1995;86:3612–3613.
3. Finch C: Regulators of iron balance in humans. Blood 1994;84:1697–1702.
4. Erslev AJ, Silver RK: Compensated hemolytic anemia. Blood Cells 1975;1:509.
5. Petz LD, Garratty G: Acquired Immune Hemolytic Anemias, 1st ed. New York: Churchill Livingstone, 1980.
6. Andersen MN, Gabrieli E, Zizzi JA: Chronic hemolysis in patients with ball-valve prostheses. J Thorac Cardiovasc Surg 1965;50:501–510.
7. Brus I, Lewis SM: The haptoglobin content of serum in haemolytic anaemia. Br J Haematol 1959;5:348.
8. Wallerstein RO: Laboratory evaluation of anemia. West J Med 1987;146:443–451.
9. Todd D: Diagnosis of haemolytic states. Clin Haematol 1975;4:63–81.
10. Hillman RS, Finch CA: The detection of anemia. In Red Cell Manual. Philadelphia: FA Davis, 1969:39–65.
11. Hillman RS, Finch CA: Erythropoiesis: Normal and abnormal. Semin Hematol 1967;4:327–336.
12. Hillman RS: Characteristics of marrow production and reticulocyte maturation in normal man in response to anemia. J Clin Invest 1969;48:443–453.
13. Hillman RS, Finch CA: The misused reticulocyte. Br J Haematol 1969;17:313–315.
14. Chen Y-H, Wang SC: A simple model for estimating the hemolytic rate in patients with sickle cell anemia. J Lab Clin Med 1985;105:201–208.
15. McCurdy PR, Sherman AS: Irreversibly sickled cells and red cell survival in sickle cell anemia: A study with both DF32P and 51CR. Am J Med 1978;64:253–258.
16. Milner PF, Charache S: Life span of carbamylated red cells in sickle cell anemia. J Clin Invest 1973;52:3161–3171.
17. Rhyner K, Ganzoni A: Erythrokinetics: Evaluation of red cell production by ferrokinetics and reticulocyte counts. Eur J Clin Invest 1972;2:96–101.
18. Peebles DA, Hochberg A, Clarke TD: Analysis of manual reticulocyte counting. Am J Clin Pathol 1981;76:713–717.
19. Greenberg ER, Beck R: The effects of sample size on reticulocyte counting and stool examination. Arch Pathol Lab Med 1984;108:396–398.
20. Brecher G, Schneiderman M: A time-saving device for the counting of reticulocytes. Am J Clin Pathol 1950;20:1079–1083.
21. Davis BH, Bigelow NC: Automated reticulocyte analysis: Clinical practice and associated new parameters. Diagn Hematol 1994;8:617–630.
22. Davis BH, Bigelow NC: Flow cytometric reticulocyte analysis and the reticulocyte maturity index. Ann N Y Acad Sci 1993;677:281–292.
23. Davis H, Ornvold K, Bigelow N: Flow cytometric reticulocyte maturity index: A useful laboratory parameter of erythropoietic activity in anemia. Cytometry 1995;22:35–39.
24. Chang C, Kass L: Clinical significance of immature reticulocyte fraction determined by automated reticulocyte counting. Am J Clin Pathol 1997;108:69–73.
25. Moseley RH. Approach to the patient with jaundice. In Humes HD (ed): Kelly's Textbook of Internal Medicine, 45th ed. Philadelphia: Lippincott Williams & Wilkins, 2000:782–791.
26. Maldonado JE, Kyle RA, Schoenfield LJ: Increased serum conjugated bilirubin in hemolytic anemia. Postgrad Med 1974;55:183–190.
27. Berlin NI, Berk PD: Quantitative aspects of bilirubin metabolism for hematologists. Blood 1981;57:983–999.
28. Bosma PJ, Chowdhury JR, Bakker C, et al: The genetic basis of the reduced expression of bilirubin udp-glucuronosyltransferase 1 in Gilbert's syndrome. N Engl J Med 1995;333: 1171–1175.
29. Kaplan M, Hammerman C, Rubaltelli FF, et al: Hemolysis and bilirubin conjugation in association with UDP-glucuronosyltransferase 1A1 promoter polymorphism. Hepatology 2002;35:905–911.
30. Iolascon A, Perrotta S, Coppola B, Carbone R, Miraglia DG: Frequency of Gilbert's syndrome associated with UGTA1 (TA)(7) polymorphism in Southern Italy. Haematologica 2000;85:335–336.
31. del Giudice EM, Perrotta S, Nobili B, Specchia C, d'Urzo G, Iolascon A: Coinheritance of Gilbert syndrome increases the risk for developing gallstones in patients with hereditary spherocytosis. Blood 1999;94:2259–2262.
32. White P, Coburn RF, Williams WJ, Goldwein MI, Rother ML, Shafer BC: Carbon monoxide production associated with ineffective erythropoiesis. J Clin Invest 1967;46:1986–1998.
33. Horne MK, Rosse WF, Flickinger EG, Saltzman HA: "Early-peak" carbon monoxide production in certain erythropoietic disorders. Blood 1975;45:365–375.
34. Berendsohn S, Lowman J, Sundberg D, Watson CJ: Idiopathic dyserythropoietic jaundice. Blood 1964;24:1.
35. Tisdale WA, Klatskin G, Kinsella ED: The significance of the direct-reacting fraction of serum bilirubin in hemolytic jaundice. Am J Med 1959;26:214.
36. Pirofsky B: General Laboratory Observations. Autoimmunization and the Autoimmune Hemolytic Anemias. Baltimore: Williams & Wilkins Company, 1969:65.
37. Allgood JW, Chaplin H, Jr: Idiopathic acquired autoimmune hemolytic anemia. A review of forty-seven cases treated from 1955 through 1965. Am J Med 1967;43:254–273.
38. Schalm L, Weber AP: Jaundice with conjugated bilirubin in hyperhaemolysis. Acta Med Scand 1964;176:549.
39. Beutler E: Production and destruction of erythrocytes. In Beutler E, Lichtman MA, Coller BS, Kipps TJ, Seligsohn U (eds): Williams Hematology, 6th ed. New York: McGraw-Hill, 2001:355–368.
40. Manoharan A: Congenital haptoglobin deficiency. Blood 1997;90:1709a–1709.
41. Marchand A, Galen RS, Van Lente F: The predictive value of serum haptoglobin in hemolytic disease. JAMA 1980; 243:1909–1911.
42. Shinton NK, Richardson RW, Williams JDF: Diagnostic value of serum haptoglobin. J Clin Pathol 1965;18:114–118.
43. Noyes WD, Garby L: Rate of haptoglobin synthesis in normal man: Determinations by the return to normal levels following hemoglobin infusion. Scand J Clin Lab Invest 1967;20:33–38.
44. Cullhed I: Serum haptoglobin in cases with Starr-Edwards ball-valve prosthesis. Acta Med Scand 1967;181:321–325.
45. Langley GR, Owen JA, P Adanyi R: The effect of blood transfusions on serum haptoglobin. Br J Haematol 1962;8:392–399.
46. Fink DJ, Petz LD, Black MB: Serum haptoglobin: A valuable diagnostic aid in suspected hemolytic transfusion reaction. JAMA 1997;199:615–618.
47. Stein ID: Serum lactate dehydrogenase isoenzymes: Stability, clearance, and diagnostic application in hemolytic anemia. J Lab Clin Med 1970;76:76–84.
48. Myhre E, Rasmussen K, Andersen A: Serum lactic dehydrogenase activity in patients with prosthetic heart valves: A parameter of intravascular hemolysis. Am Heart J 1997;80:463–468.
49. Walsh JR, Starr A, Ritzmann LW: Intravascular hemolysis in patients with prosthetic valves and valvular heart disease. Circulation 1969;39(Suppl. 1):135–140.
50. Domen RE: An overview of immune hemolytic anemias. Cleve Clin J Med 1998;65:89–99.
51. The transfusion of red cells. In Mollison PL, Engelfriet CP, Contreras M (eds): Blood Transfusion in Clinical Medicine, 10th ed. Oxford: Blackwell Science, 1997:278–314.
52. Martin-Nunez G, Fernandez-Galan MA, Lopez-Lopez R, Gonzalez-Hurtado JA: Peritoneal haemorrhage mimicking intravascular haemolysis. Br J Haematol 2001;115:238.
53. Melvin JD, Watts RG: Severe hypophosphatemia: A rare cause of intravascular hemolysis. Am J Hematol 2002;69:223–224.
54. Jimenez M, Sanz C, Alvarez A, Pereira A: Massive intravascular haemolysis in a patient with Clostridium perfringens sepsis. Vox Sang 2002;82:214.

55. Garcia-Suarez J, de Miguel D, Krsnik I, Barr-Ali M, Hernanz N, Burgaleta C: Spontaneous gas gangrene in malignant lymphoma: An underreported complication? Am J Hematol 2002;70:145–148.
56. Chaplin H: Abdominal pain, total intravascular hemolysis, and death in a 53-year-old woman. Am J Med 1990;88:667–674.
57. Terebelo HR, McCue RL, Lenneville MS: Implication of plasma free hemoglobin in massive clostridial hemolysis. JAMA 1982;248:2028–2029.
58. Buys S, Craven C: MCHC in intravascular hemolysis. Am J Hematol 1990;33:282–283.
59. Kimber RJ: An approach to the diagnosis of haemolytic anaemia. Med J Aust 1974;2:532–535.
60. Berman LB: When the urine is red. JAMA 1977;237:2753–2754.
61. Slater MS, Mullins RJ: Rhabdomyolysis and myoglobinuric renal failure in trauma and surgical patients: A review. J Am Coll Surg 1998;186:693–716.
62. Hroncich ME, Rudinger AN: Rhabdomyolysis with pneumococcal pneumonia: A report of two cases. Am J Med 1989;86:467–468.
63. Hillman RS, Finch CA: Differential Diagnosis of Anemia. In Red Cell Manual. Philadelphia: FA Davis, 1969:112.
64. Sears DA: Disposal of plasma heme in normal man and patients with intravascular hemolysis. J Clin Invest 1970;49:5–14.
65. Marchiafava E: Anemia emolitica con emosiderinuria perpetua. Policlinico, Sez med 1928;35:109–120.
66. Pimstone NR: Renal degradation of hemoglobin. Semin Hematol 1972;9:31–42.
67. Fehr J, Knob M: Comparison of red cell creatine level and reticulocyte count in appraising the severity of hemolytic processes. Blood 1979;53:966–976.
68. Coburn RF, Williams WJ, Kahn SB: Endogenous carbon monoxide production in patients with hemolytic anemia. J Clin Invest 1966;45:460–468.
69. Engel RR, Rodkey FL, Krill CE: Carboxyhemoglobin levels as an index of hemolysis. Pediatrics 1971;47:723–730.
70. Landaw SA, Winchell HS: Endogenous production of 14CO: A method for calculation of RBC lifespan in vivo. Blood 1970;36:642–656.
71. Vreman HJ, Mahoney JJ, Stevenson DK: Carbon monoxide and carboxyhemoglobin. Adv Pediatr, 1995;42:303–334.
72. Burns ER, Kale A, Murthy VV: Diagnosis of the hemolytic state using serum levels of erythrocyte adenylate kinase. Am J Hematol 2000;64:180–183.
73. Zeiler T, Muller JT, Hasse C, Kullmer J, Kretschmer V: Flow cytometric determination of RBC survival in autoimmune hemolytic anemia. Transfusion 2001;41:493–498.
74. Ballas SK: Disorders of the red cell membrane: A reclassification of hemolytic anemias. Am J Med Sci 1978;276:4–22.
75. Catlett JP, Petz LD: Hemolytic anemias. In Humes HD (ed): Kelly's Textbook of Medicine, 4th ed. Philadelphia: Lippincott Williams & Wilkins, 2000:1769–1788.
76. Eichner ER: The hematologic disorders of alcoholism. Am J Med 1973;54:621–630.
77. Straus DJ: Hematologic aspects of alcoholism. Semin Hematol 1973;10:183–194.
78. Petz LD: Hematologic aspects of liver disease. Curr Opin Gastroenterol 1989;5:372–377.
79. Morse EE: Mechanisms of hemolysis in liver disease. Ann Clin Lab Sci 1990;20:169–174.
80. Kristensson AA, Wallersted S, Alling C, Cederblad G, Magnusson B: Haematological findings in chronic alcoholics after heavy drinking with special reference to haemolysis. Eur J Clin Invest 1986;16:178–183.
81. Zarkowsky HS, Oski FA, Sha'afi R, Shohet SB, Nathan DG: Congenital hemolytic anemia with high sodium, low potassium red cells. I. Studies of membrane permeability. N Engl J Med 1968;278:573–581.
82. Douglass CC, Twomey JJ: Transient stomatocytosis with hemolysis: A previously unrecognized complication of alcoholism. Ann Intern Med 1970;72:159–164.
83. Gallagher PG: Acanthocytosis, stomatocytosis, and related disorders. In Beutler E, Lichtman MA, Coller BS, Kipps TJ, Seligsohn U (eds): Williams Hematology, 6th ed. New York: McGraw-Hill, 2001:519–526.
84. Kaplan HS, Garratty G: Predictive value of direct antiglobulin test results. Diagn Med 1985;8:29–33.
85. Garratty G: The significance of IgG on the red cell surface. Transfus Med Reviews 1987;1:47–57.
86. Gallagher PG, Forget BG: Hereditary spherocytosis, elliptocytosis, and related disorders. In Beutler E, Lichtman MA, Coller BS, Kipps TJ, Seligsohn U (eds): Williams Hematology. New York: McGraw-Hill, 2001:503–518.
87. Dacie J: The Haemolytic Anaemias, 3rd ed. vol. 1, The Hereditary Haemolytic Anaemias. New York: Churchill Livingstone, 1985.
88. Hall SE, Rosse WF: The use of monoclonal antibodies and flow cytometry in the diagnosis of paroxysmal nocturnal hemoglobinuria. Blood 1996;87:5332–5340.
89. van der Schoot CE, Huizinga TW, van 't Veer-Korthof ET, Wijmans R, Pinkster J, von dem Borne AE: Deficiency of glycosyl-phosphatidylinositol-linked membrane glycoproteins of leukocytes in paroxysmal nocturnal hemoglobinuria, description of a new diagnostic cytofluorometric assay. Blood 1990;76:1853–1859.
90. Beutler E: Paroxysmal nocturnal hemoglobinuria. In Beutler E, Lichtman MA, Coller BS, Kipps TJ, Seligsohn U (eds): Williams Hematology, 6th ed. New York: McGraw-Hill, 2001:419–424.

CHAPTER 3

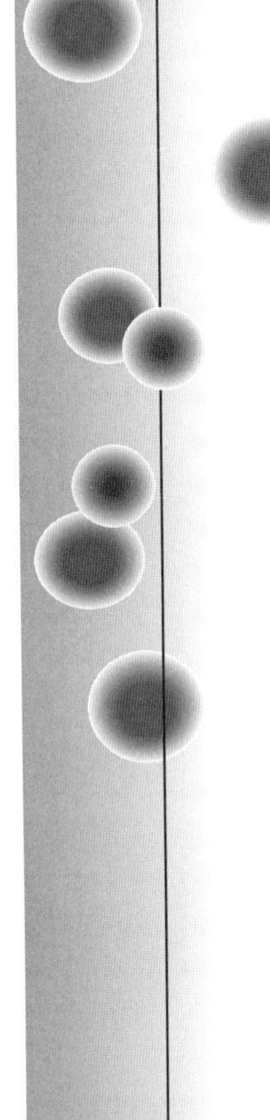

Classification and Clinical Characteristics of Autoimmune Hemolytic Anemias

CLASSIFICATION

In this chapter we present a classification of immune hemolytic anemias and review the clinical manifestations of each of the autoimmune hemolytic anemias (AIHAs).

Numerous classifications of immune hemolytic anemias have been proposed.[1] The purpose of a classification of any group of diseases should be to divide that group into clinically distinctive categories. The rather simple classification listed in Table 3-1 serves this purpose well because the clinical manifestations, prognosis, and therapy differ among the diagnostic groups listed. Table 3-2 outlines some of these distinctions.

The following are some comments about the classification listed in Table 3-1. The majority of cases of AIHA are mediated by *warm-reactive autoantibodies*, that is, antibodies that display optimal reactivity with human red blood cells (RBCs) at 37°C and that are usually of the immunoglobulin G (IgG) class. In contrast, *cold agglutinin syndrome* (CAS) is generally caused by IgM autoantibodies that exhibit maximal reactivity at 4°C. The distinction between cold and warm AIHAs (WAIHAs) is important, because the prognosis and management differ significantly.

We refer to AIHA as *idiopathic* if it is unassociated with any demonstrable underlying disease. If the AIHA is associated with an additional disorder and there is reason to suspect that the association is not merely fortuitous, we refer to the AIHA as *secondary*. AIHA associated with infections is generally transient and remits after resolution of the infectious disease. In patients with an associated lymphoproliferative disorder, the course of the AIHA is less predictable. A significant distinction between idiopathic and secondary cases of CAS is that the IgM cold agglutinin in patients with secondary disease associated with infections is a polyclonal protein, in contrast to the monoclonal antibody that is characteristically found in patients with idiopathic disease or with an underlying lymphoproliferative disorder.

Some patients have both warm and cold autoantibodies in their sera, and the serologic characteristics of these antibodies may satisfy the criteria for both warm antibody AIHA and CAS. We refer to these cases as instances of "combined cold and warm AIHA," or "mixed AIHA."

Paroxysmal cold hemoglobinuria (PCH) is distinct from cold agglutinin disease. The causative antibody is an IgG immunoglobulin with specificity that differs from that found in cold agglutinin disease. The antibody is best detected in vitro by its ability to cause hemolysis of normal RBCs in a two-step procedure, which requires incubation in the cold

TABLE 3-1. CLASSIFICATION OF IMMUNE HEMOLYTIC ANEMIAS

Autoimmune hemolytic anemias (AIHAs)
- Warm antibody AIHA
  - Idiopathic
  - Secondary (e.g., chronic lymphocytic leukemia, lymphomas, systemic lupus erythematosus)
- Cold agglutinin syndrome
  - Idiopathic
  - Secondary
    - Nonmalignant disorders (e.g., mycoplasma pneumoniae infection, infectious mononucleosis, other virus infections)
    - Malignant disorders (e.g., lymphoproliferative disorders)
- Paroxysmal cold hemoglobinuria
  - Idiopathic
  - Secondary
    - Viral syndromes
    - Syphilis
  - Combined cold and warm AIHA ("mixed AIHA")
  - Atypical AIHA
    - AIHA with a negative direct antiglobulin test
    - Warm antibody AIHA caused by IgM or IgA autoantibodies
  - Drug-induced immune hemolytic anemia
    - Drug-related antibody identifiable
    - Drug-induced AIHA
  - Alloantibody-induced immune hemolytic anemia
    - Hemolytic transfusion reactions
    - Hemolytic disease of the fetus and newborn

TABLE 3-2. SOME CHARACTERISTIC FEATURES OF AUTOIMMUNE AND DRUG-INDUCED IMMUNE HEMOLYTIC ANEMIAS

Warm Antibody Autoimmune Hemolytic Anemia

Clinical manifestations: Variable, usually symptoms of anemia, occasionally acute hemolytic syndrome
Prognosis: Fair, with significant mortality
Most effective therapies: Steroids, splenectomy, immunosuppressive drugs

Cold Agglutinin Syndrome

Clinical manifestations: Moderate chronic hemolytic anemia in middle-aged or elderly person, often with signs and symptoms exacerbated by cold
Prognosis: Good, usually a chronic and quite stable anemia
Most effective therapies: Avoidance of cold exposure, immunosuppressive drugs

Paroxysmal Cold Hemoglobinuria

Clinical manifestations: Acute hemolytic anemia, often with hemoglobinuria, particularly in a child with history of recent viral or viral-like illness
Prognosis: Excellent after initial stormy course
Therapy: Not well defined; steroids empirically and transfusions if required

Drug-Induced Immune Hemolytic Anemia

Clinical manifestations: Variable, most commonly subacute in onset, but occasionally acute hemolytic syndrome
Prognosis: Excellent
Therapy: Stop drug; occasionally a short course of steroids empirically

followed by incubation at 37°C in the presence of complement.

The ingestion of some drugs causes hemolytic anemia, in which the causative antibody can be shown to have specificity for the drug or its metabolites. We do not consider these cases of drug-induced immune hemolytic anemia to be autoimmune disorders because the antibody does not have specificity for autoantigens. In other quite remarkable cases, the ingestion of a drug causes the development of RBC autoantibodies, that is, the antibody in the patient's serum and in an eluate from the patient's red cells reacts with red cells similarly to autoantibodies in idiopathic warm antibody AIHA, and no relationship between the drug and the antibody can be demonstrated in vitro. Such cases are appropriately termed *drug-induced AIHA*.

The alloantibody-induced hemolytic anemias are reviewed in Chapters 13 and 14.

CLINICAL CHARACTERISTICS OF AUTOIMMUNE HEMOLYTIC ANEMIAS

Warm Antibody AIHA

INCIDENCE

In Portland, Oregon, Pirofsky[2] reported findings in patients who were referred from a population of 2.3 million in the Pacific Northwest of the United States over an 8-year period. He concluded that the minimum annual incidence of AIHA is 1:80,000 population. Similarly, data obtained from a hospital in Odense, Denmark, that received all medical cases from a population of 230,000 indicated an annual incidence of about 1:75,000 population.[2] A study during a 5-year period in one of Sweden's health care regions indicated an incidence of 2.6:100,000 persons per year.[3] Also, Sokol and coworkers[4] reported a series of 1694 patients with RBC autoantibodies and stated that the incidence of AIHA was about 1:41,000. These authors included patients who had hemolysis in the absence of anemia and commented that the relatively high incidence they observed was probably due to the inclusion of patients with mild and compensated hemolysis.

WAIHA is by far the most common type of AIHA and represented 70.3% of the 347 patients in our series[1] (Table 3-3). Dacie and Worlledge[5] reported 284 patients with AIHA, and 70% of the cases were WAIHA. Engelfriet and coworkers[6] reported that 83% of their 2390 cases of AIHA were caused by warm autoantibodies and, in another 0.4%, both warm and cold autoantibodies were present. Sokol and coworkers[4] classified 60% of their patients as having warm autoantibodies (excluding drug-induced immune hemolytic anemia) and another 7.5% as having both warm and cold autoantibodies.

TABLE 3-3. INCIDENCE OF VARIOUS KINDS OF ACQUIRED IMMUNE HEMOLYTIC ANEMIAS IN OUR SERIES OF 347 PATIENTS

	No. of Patients	Percent of Total
Warm AIHA	244*	70.3
Cold agglutinin syndrome	54	15.6
Paroxysmal cold hemoglobinuria	6	1.7
Drug-induced IHA	43	12.4

IHA, immune hemolytic anemia; AIHA, autoimmune hemolytic anemia; WAIHA, warm AIHA.
* Includes 30 patients with WAIHA induced by α-methyldopa.

AGE DISTRIBUTION

Subjects of all ages are affected, from infants in the first few months of life to elderly people.[7] Pirofsky[8] reported ages of onset of 1 month to 87 years. Of these patients, 73% were over 40 years of age, and the peak incidence appeared between the ages of 60 and 70.

Sokol and coworkers[4] reported that, except for a childhood peak of paroxysmal cold hemoglobinuna (PCH), there is a general increase in incidence throughout life, with a dramatic rise occurring after the age of 50 (Fig. 3-1). Böttiger and Westerholm[3] also found a marked increase in incidence after the age of 50.

As might be anticipated, the underlying disease process has a marked effect on the age distribution. In Allgood and Chaplin's[9] report of idiopathic cases, the peak incidence was in the fourth to seventh decades, with the mean age of onset of 48.6 years. However, patients with secondary warm antibody AIHA associated with chronic lymphatic leukemia (CLL) or systemic lupus erythematosus (SLE) have the age distribution of the underlying disease. This finding emphasizes that clinical features of AIHA occurring in association with other diseases are frequently dominated by underlying pathologic states.

AIHA in the young is not a rarity, and a large body of literature is available that describes such patients. Although clinical and laboratory findings in children are quite similar to those in adults, there are some distinctive features, which are emphasized in Chapter 9.

SEX DISTRIBUTION

Most observers have reported a somewhat higher incidence in females than in males. In idiopathic cases of WAIHA, Allgood and Chaplin[9] reported that 60% of 47 patients were female; Dausset and Colombani[10] reported that 61% of 93 patients were female; Pirofsky[2] indicates that 64% of 44 patients were female; Dacie[7] reported 58% of 108 patients were female; Dacie and Worlledge[5] reported that 59% of 111 patients were female; and, in the series reported by Böttiger and Westerholm,[3] women predominated in all age groups with the exception of the youngest (0 to 14 years), in which the sex distribution was even.

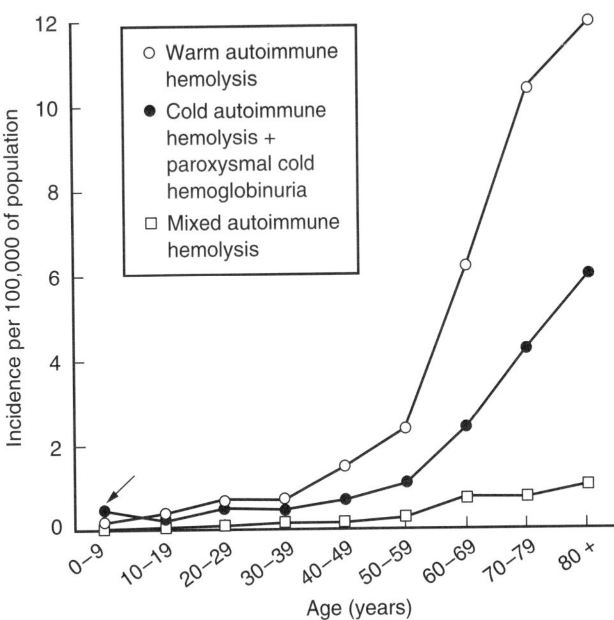

FIGURE 3-1. Incidence of acquired immune hemolytic anemia per 100,000 of population at risk, related to age at presentation. The early childhood peak of cold autoimmune hemolysis (arrow) is largely due to patients with paroxysmal cold hemoglobinuria. (From Sokol RJ, Booker DJ, Stamps R: The pathology of autoimmune haemolytic anaemia. J Clin Pathol 1992;45:1047–1052.)

In secondary WAIHA, the percentages are more varied, perhaps depending on the incidence of underlying diseases seen in referral centers. For example, Pirofsky[2] reported that 80% of cases associated with SLE occurred in females, whereas a male predominance was found when patients with lymphoproliferative disorders were analyzed.

CLINICAL MANIFESTATIONS (Table 3-4)

WAIHA is an extremely variable disorder, and almost every grade of severity may be encountered. In some patients, the onset is slow and insidious over a period of months, with the ultimate emergence of symptomatic anemia. In other patients, the onset is sudden, with fever, abdominal or back pain, malaise, and manifestations of rapidly increasing anemia. In severe anemia, neurologic manifestations may occur that progress from obtundation to coma and death. In children, the disease frequently appears as an acute and sometimes fulminating disorder.[11,12] Although such acute manifestations are serious and present difficult problems in management, they may be of short duration, with complete recovery within a few weeks.[11-13]

Symptoms that relate directly to the presence of anemia and that resolve on improvement in the level of hemoglobin include dizziness, palpitations, and dyspnea on exertion. In more severely affected patients, the intensity of the anemia often leads to serious dyspnea and incapacity.[7] Angina, edema, and frank congestive heart failure occur in a small percentage of patients. At the other end of the scale, the

TABLE 3-4. WARM ANTIBODY AUTOIMMUNE HEMOLYTIC ANEMIA—CHARACTERISTIC CLINICAL MANIFESTATIONS

Symptoms

Symptoms of anemia
- Fatigue
- Weakness
- Dyspnea on exertion

Fever
Abdominal or back pain
Malaise
Dark urine

Physical Signs

Jaundice
Splenomegaly
Hepatomegaly
Lymphadenopathy
Venous thromboembolism

Laboratory Findings

Anemia
Abnormal red blood cell morphology
- Spherocytosis, anisocytosis, poikilocytosis, polychromatophilia, autoagglutination

Reticulocytosis (reticulocytopenia in some patients)
Thrombocytopenia ("Evans's syndrome")
Leukocytosis (leukopenia in some patients)
Urine may contain bile pigments (and/or hemoglobin in patients with brisk hemolysis)
Erythroid hyperplasia in the bone marrow

patient may be free from symptoms and not be significantly anemic, despite definitive evidence of hemolysis.

A history of dark urine may be elicited; this condition may result from the presence of bile pigments or hemoglobinuria (see Chapter 2). Hemolytic jaundice is classically regarded as acholuric but, in seriously ill patients, significant amounts of conjugated bilirubin may circulate in the plasma, and bile pigment may appear in the urine.[7] Furthermore, urobilinogen frequently darkens the color of the urine, especially on standing. Hemoglobinuria may cause the urine to be pink, red, brown, or almost black, depending on the concentration and relative proportions of oxyhemoglobin, which is bright red, and methemoglobin, which is dark brown. The final color of the urine is determined by the concentration of hemoglobin, the pH of the urine, and duration of contact between hemoglobin and urine.[14] Hemoglobinuria is quite unusual in adults, but it is a prominent finding in the most seriously ill patients. It is much more common in children.

In patients with secondary AIHA, the associated pathologic state may cause the most prominent of the patient's symptoms and obscure the symptoms of the hemolytic anemia. Considering the diversity of underlying diseases associated with AIHA, a complete list of presenting symptoms would be encyclopedic and of little or no value. However, considering only those symptoms that may relate specifically to the hemolytic state, weakness is the most common complaint; it occurred in 87% of Pirofsky's series.[2] Other common symptoms are fever and jaundice, although neither of these symptoms occurs in a majority of patients.

PHYSICAL SIGNS

The diagnosis of anemia on the basis of physical signs is remarkably difficult, and the classic observation of pallor is quite unreliable. Jaundice is more commonly observed; it occurred as a presenting sign in 39% of the patients in Pirofsky's series.[2]

Splenomegaly was present in 57% of patients with idiopathic WAIHA reported by Allgood and Chaplin,[9] and in just over 50% of the patients with either idiopathic or secondary AIHA reported by Pirofsky.[2] Dameshek and Schwartz[15] reviewed the data in 40 recorded cases of AIHA and reported that the spleen could be palpated in 28 (70%). The organ is generally firm, nontender, and only slightly to moderately enlarged. It is unusual for an enlarged spleen to reach the umbilicus and, on the whole, the degree of splenomegaly is less than that found in hereditary spherocytosis.

Hepatomegaly has been reported in about one third[8] to two thirds[16] of the patients with idiopathic AIHA, and the organ is usually firm and nontender. Liver enlargement is generally moderate, and massive hepatomegaly is rare. However, liver function may be seriously affected in very seriously ill patients and, in fatal cases, has usually been described as enlarged.[17] Shirey and coworkers,[18] for instance, described a female patient aged 22 who had recurrent episodes of intravacular hemolysis. Her liver progressively enlarged and its function deteriorated. Eventually, she died in hepatic coma. The liver failure was attributed to autoagglutination within the liver sinuses. The antibody responsible was a warm-reacting IgM (see Chapter 5).

The incidence of lymphadenopathy varies in reported series, depending, at least in part, on the relative proportion of idiopathic and secondary cases. In idiopathic AIHA, the lymph nodes are usually not enlarged.[7] However, Pirofsky[2] reported that lymphadenopathy was present in 23% of the patients with idiopathic WAIHA and 37% of the patients with secondary AIHA, a majority of whom had lymphoproliferative disorders. Indeed, enlargement of the various reticuloendothelial structures was the most consistent abnormality on physical examination, and only 26% of all patients manifested no enlargement of the spleen, liver, or lymph nodes.

Thromboembolism. Venous thromboembolism (VTE) has long been recognized as a cause of morbidity and mortality in AIHA, and an illustrative case reported by Swisher[19] is illustrated in Figure 3-2. VTE have been reported to be responsible for or contributed to the death of 3% to 10% of patients with AIHA.[9,10,20]

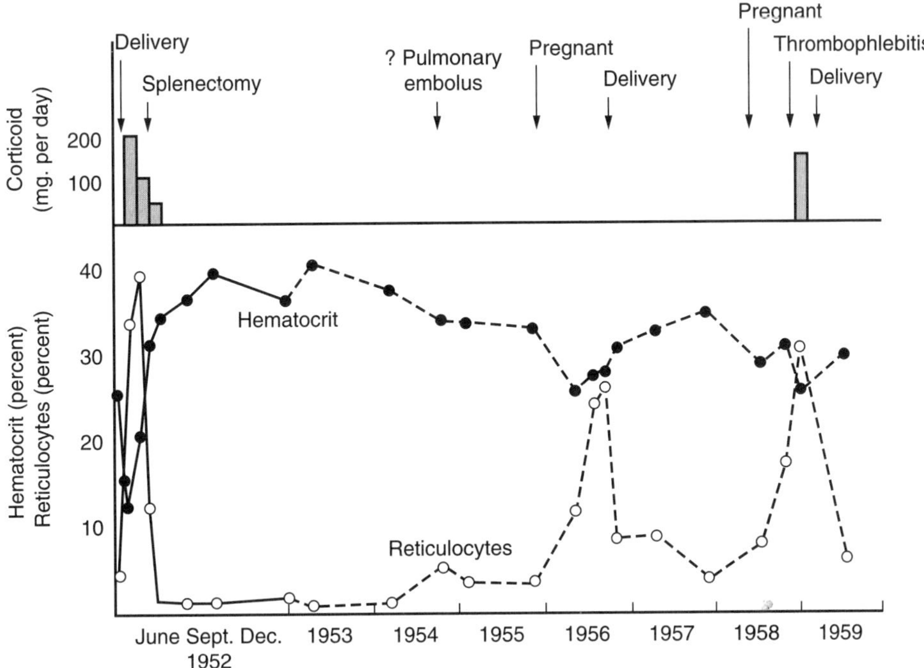

FIGURE 3-2. Clinical course of idiopathic acquired immune hemolytic anemia in a 25-year-old woman through repeated pregnancies. (From Swisher SN: Acquired hemolytic disease. Postgrad Med 1966;40:378–386.)

Pullarkat and coworkers[21] prospectively studied 30 patients with AIHA and found that 8 (27%) had a documented VTE, all of which were confirmed by objective imaging studies. In four patients the VTE occurred with the initial hemolytic crisis, and in three patients thrombotic events occurred with relapse of their AIHA. One patient developed a deep vein thrombosis and pulmonary embolus 3 weeks after laparoscopic splenectomy. The authors determined that 19 of the 30 patients (63%) with AIHA had antiphospholipid (Apl) antibodies, 9 (31%) were positive for the lupus anticoagulant (LAC), and 17 (57%) had anticardiolipin (aCL) antibodies. Seven patients had both LAC and aCL. In the patients with aCL, five were positive for IgG and 12 had IgM. None had detectable IgA aCL.

Venous thromboembolic events were observed in five of the nine patients (63%) positive for LAC. This was statistically significant with a calculated relative risk of 7.5 (95% confidence interval [CI], 1.25 to 45.2, $P = 0.03$) compared with the patients with VTE and no detectable LAC. No significant association was found between the presence of aCL and the development of VTE. Further data have been provided by Kokori and coworkers,[22] who found that the patients with SLE who had AIHA were more likely to have thrombotic episodes than were SLE patients without AIHA. Galli and coworkers[22a] reviewed the medical literature from 1988 to 2000 to formally establish the risk of lupus anticoagulants and anticardiolipin antibodies for arterial and venous thrombosis. They calculated the odds ratio with 95% confidence interval of lupus anticoagulants and/or anticardiolipin antibodies for thrombosis in 4184 patients and 3151 controls. They concluded that lupus anticoagulants have an odds ratio for thrombosis 5 to 16 times higher than controls and that they are strong risk factors for thrombosis regardless of the site and type of thrombosis. Their detection in patients with SLE and/or previous thrombosis is therefore justified. Analysis of anticardiolipin antibodies was more complex because of the effects of isotypes and titer, but it appeared that medium or high titer IgG anticardiolipin antibodies helps identify patients at risk for thrombosis. However, these researchers pointed out that there is an urgent need to harmonize investigational methods.

Thrombosis in hemolytic anemia has largely been attributed to disruption and loss of the RBC membrane, resulting in surface exposure of the negatively charged phosphatidylserine (PS). Exposed RBC PS is thought to promote thrombosis by providing a surface for formation of the tenase and prothrombinase complexes.[21] In addition to AIHA, VTE complications have also been reported in patients with inherited hemolytic anemias, including hereditary spherocytosis and thalassemia major.[23,24] However, the incidence of thrombosis appears to be much lower in inherited hemolytic anemia.

Additional reports of thrombotic events in patients with AIHA have been reported including upper extremity arterial thrombosis[25,26]; superior sagittal sinus thrombosis associated with Evans's syndrome[27]; mesenteric and portal vein thrombosis[28]; in patients with cold and WAIHA,[29,30] of whom one had multiple pulmonary emboli and extensive deep venous thrombosis of the iliofemoral vessels leading to frank gangrene requiring an above-knee amputation[30]; in a patient with cold agglutinin disease[31]; in association with human immunodeficiency virus (HIV) infection[32]; and after blood transfusion in patients with HIV infection.[32,33]

Although prophylactic anticoagulation is not indicated for patients with LAC in the absence of prior thrombosis,[34] Pullarkat and coworkers[21] suggest prophylactic anticoagulation for all patients with AIHA who are positive for LAC, at least during episodes of hemolysis.

THE BLOOD PICTURE

Anemia. The degree of anemia is variable, but it is not infrequently severe. Allgood and Chaplin[9] reported that the initial hemoglobin concentration in 21 of 47 patients was less than 7 g/dL. Although only a moderate anemia may be present on admission, a meticulous follow-up is required, particularly when the patient is first observed. Progression of the severity of the anemia frequently occurs before therapy becomes effective, and the fall in hemoglobin and hematocrit may be rapid, justifying the terms "acute hemolytic anemia" or "hemolytic crisis." Indeed, Pirofsky[8] emphasizes that among 213 patients, the lowest hematocrit ranged from 7.5% to 41.5%, but with a medium value of only 19%. A hematocrit of 15% or less was observed in 49 patients! Similarly, Crosby and Rappaport[35] reported hemoglobin values of 5 g/dL or less in 15 of 34 patients. Characteristically, the anemia is macrocytic rather than normocytic, with the macrocytosis being associated with a raised reticulocyte count.

Blood Films. Anisocytosis is usually a marked feature; this is brought about by the presence of microspherocytes with reduced RBC diameter and macrocytes, which are the reticulocytes. Poikilocytes are generally not conspicuous in AIHA. However, in some patients small numbers of pear-shaped RBCs may be present. Polychromasia is often obvious, reflecting the height of the reticulocyte count.[36]

Spherocytosis is often easily recognized in the blood film of patients with WAIHA. However, they are not always present, at any rate to a marked degree, even if the patient is actively hemolyzing.[36]

Autoagglutination in vitro is a phenomenon occasionally observed, particularly in more severely affected patients.[37] The agglutination typically consists of rather fine clumps of RBCs that may be visible to the naked eye on close observation and, in contrast to those caused by cold agglutinins, they do not change after incubation at 37°C (see Chapter 5).

The presence in the peripheral blood of monocytes (or rarely neutrophils) that have phagocytosed RBCs is a pointer to an autoimmune hemolytic anemia. Erythrophagocytosis is most easily seen in films made from the buffy coat of peripheral blood. Sometimes, however, so many erythrophages are present that they can be found without too much difficulty in films of whole uncentrifuged blood. Numerous case reports in the older medical literature emphasized the presence of erythrophagocytosis.[7,38-43] One wonders if inspection of the blood film has become a less common skill among physicians in modern times (see page 76).

Erythroblasts, mainly polychromatic normoblasts, are often present in the peripheral blood of patients with WAIHA. They are present in large numbers when hemolysis is severe and if the reticulocyte count is markedly raised. The largest numbers are seen in patients in whom increased hemolysis and anemia have persisted after splenectomy. Then the erythroblast count may even exceed the total leukocyte count.[36]

Leukocytes. The white blood cell (WBC) count is normal in more than half of the patients with idiopathic AIHA[2,9] but, of course, it varies greatly among patients with secondary AIHA, depending on the underlying disease. Even in patients with idiopathic disease, a range of values extending from 1400 to 37,000/μL was obtained in Pirofsky's series.[2] Leukocyte counts of less than 2000/μL were observed in 6 of 38 patients. The latter results occurred in a pattern of peripheral pancytopenia with hypoplastic or normal bone marrows and may be a manifestation of an immune pancytopenia.

In acute hemolytic episodes, however, leukocytosis is frequent, with counts usually ranging from 15,000 to 25,000/μL. This finding is chiefly the result of an increase in neutrophils with occasional metamyelocytes and myelocytes as part of a leukemoid reaction.

Counts considerably in excess of the preceding figures have been reported, especially in children. The highest WBC count in Pirofsky's series[2] was in a 2½-year-old infant in whom the count was 37,000/μL, chiefly lymphocytes. Twenty-two of 46 patients reported by Habibi and coworkers[13] had leukocytosis with total WBC counts as high as 40,000/μL and with promyclocytes and myelocytes accounting for up to 20% of the total.

Liesveld and coworkers[44] reviewed the initial leukocyte counts of 108 patients with various types of autoimmune hemolysis. The counts ranged from 1.5 to 137 × 10^9/L; the mean was 10.6 × 10^9/L, and the median was 9.0 × 10^9/L. Forty percent of the patients had initial counts exceeding 11 × 10^9/L. (Three patients with chronic lymphocytic leukemia were excluded from the analysis.)

A reaction to "stress" plus stimulation by products of intravascular hemolysis are probably important factors in producing the leukocytosis, and similar rises have been reported in instances of hemolysis that are not caused by an immune mechanism.[36]

Platelets. Platelet counts are usually normal in idiopathic WAIHA. A minority of patients have thrombocytosis that, on occasion, reaches impressive heights. Allgood and Chaplin[9] reported that 24% of their patients had thrombocytosis at the time of presentation, with the highest value recorded being 1,900,000/μL. Pirofsky[8] reported that 17% of his patients with AIHA in the absence of malignant lymphoid disease had thrombocytosis, with the highest value being greater than 1,000,000/μL. In the series of Liesveld and coworkers,[44] 16 of 85 patients had thrombocytosis (platelet count >400,000/μL). Thirteen of these patients had warm autoantibodies, two had secondary cold-antibody AIHA, and one patient had both warm and cold autoantibodies. Heisel and Ortega[45] recorded a mean platelet count at diagnosis of 421,000/μL (range, 191,000 to 583,000/μL) in 9 children who had acute AIHA and a mean count of 195,000/μL (range, 13,000 to 795,000/μL) in 16 children who had chronic AIHA (10 had counts <150,000/μL at diagnosis). In contrast, Habibi and coworkers[13] did not mention the occurrence of thrombocytosis in their review of 80 children with AIHA, and Crosby and Rappaport,[35] who tabulated the platelet counts of 29 patients, recorded only two counts above 400,000/μL.

Evans's Syndrome. Thrombocytopenia occurs in some patients in all large series of WAIHA. In 1949, Evans and Duane[46] called attention to this association, and the simultaneous occurrence of thrombocytopenia and AIHA is now well recognized and is frequently referred to as "Evans's syndrome." Dausset and Colombani,[10] in a review of 83 patients with idiopathic WAIHA, encountered thrombocytopenic purpura in 11 (13.2%). Allgood and Chaplin[9] reported thrombocytopenia in 3 of 47 patients at the time of diagnosis of the hemolytic anemia; 3 others either had a history of thrombocytopenia, or thrombocytopenia developed at some time after the diagnosis of AIHA was made. Subsequently, many other reports of patients having both AIHA and severe thrombocytopenia have been described,[47-52] and it is now realized that low platelet counts are found quite commonly in AIHA and that clinically obvious purpura is not infrequent.[7]

Evans and coworkers[53] suggested that there exists a spectrum-like relationship between acquired hemolytic anemia and thrombocytopenic purpura; on the one hand, acquired hemolytic anemia with sensitization of the RBCs is often accompanied with thrombocytopenia, whereas, on the other hand, primary thrombocytopenic purpura is frequently accompanied with RBC sensitization with or without hemolytic anemia. Indeed, in addition to these clinical observations, Zucker-Franklin and Karpatkin[54] presented data indicating that autoimmune mechanisms may be directed against RBCs as well as platelets in most patients with severe idiopathic autoimmune thrombocytopenia. They noted that routine blood smears of patients with chronic autoimmune idiopathic thrombocytopenic purpura (ITP) commonly showed platelets larger than normal with many giant forms, but Coulter-counter volume measurements of platelets also revealed a distinct peak in the area in which particles with volumes much below those of normal platelets would be located. By electron microscopy, RBCs as well as platelet fragments were found in the 27,000 × *g* plasma sediment of 15 patients with severe disease. These fragments were not observed in the plasma sediment of 12 normal subjects, 2 healthy asplenic subjects, 3 patients with thrombocytopenia of nonimmunologic origin, and 2 with ITP in remission. They concluded that, in addition to destroying platelets, their patients had subclinical hemolysis.

AIHA and thrombocytopenia do not necessarily appear at the same time.[2] A number of cases have been reported in which AIHA supervened in patients who had undergone splenectomy several years earlier for thrombocytopenic purpura.[7] Waugh[55] described a patient who died of fulminating hemolytic anemia and who had undergone splenectomy for chronic thrombocytopenic purpura 4 years previously. Allgood and Chaplin[9] mentioned one patient who developed AIHA 25 years after splenectomy for thrombocytopenic purpura, and they emphasized that the two disorders may be entirely unrelated in respect to time of onset and response to steroid therapy and/or splenectomy.

Pui and coworkers[56] concluded that the combination of ITP and AIHA is rare in childhood. Among 164 instances of ITP and 15 instances of AIHA, 11 patients were found to have this combination. Three were found to have SLE, one had aplastic anemia, and seven had Evans's syndrome. Neutropenia, at times associated with bacterial infections, occurred in four of the latter patients. Unlike most cases of ITP or AIHA in childhood, the clinical course of Evans's syndrome was usually chronic and relapsing. Treatment including corticosteroids, splenectomy, and immunosuppressive agents was generally unsatisfactory. In view of the frequent presence of antibodies directed at RBCs, platelets, neutrophils, and lymphocytes, the authors suggested that *immunopancytopenia* may be a better term for this condition (see later).

Mathew and coworkers[51] conducted a retrospective survey to assess the demography, presentation, clinical course, and treatment response of children with Evans's syndrome. Information was analyzed from a detailed questionnaire completed by pediatric hematologists mainly in the United States and Canada. The questionnaire sought information regarding demographics, findings at presentation, approach to diagnosis, treatments used (with specific reference to splenectomy, corticosteroids, and intravenous immunoglobulin [IVIG]), course of the disease with emphasis on recurrences, and status at last follow-up. Forty-two patients (22 males and 20 females) were included in the study. The median age was 7.7 years (range, 0.2 to 26.6 years). At presentation, thrombocytopenia (32 patients) and anemia (28) were common; neutropenia occurred in 10 and pancytopenia in 6. Patients received a median of 5 (range, 0 to 12) modalities of treatment. Courses of IVIG and corticosteroids were given to almost all patients; responses were varied, but the effects lasted as long as 2 years. Splenectomy was performed for 15 patients, but the median duration of response was only 1 month. Other treatments included cyclosporine, vincristine, danazol, azathioprine, cyclophosphamide, and plasmapheresis. The course of the disease was characterized by recurrent thrombocytopenia, hemolytic anemia, and neutropenia. After a median follow-up of 3 years, 3 patients had died, 20 had active disease on treatment, 5 had persistent disease (not on treatment), and 14 had no evidence of disease. The authors concluded that Evans's syndrome is a chronic and recurrent condition that is often refractory to IVIG, corticosteroids, and splenectomy. Responses to other agents have been anecdotal and inconclusive. They suggested that a prospective study involving these agents is needed to determine optimal therapeutic combinations.

Savasan and coworkers[52] reported 11 patients (10 boys and 1 girl) with Evans's syndrome with a median follow-up time of 8 years who were evaluated retrospectively. Six patients had either persistent hepatosplenomegaly or generalized lymphadenopathy, or both. In five patients, an increase in lymph node and/or spleen size was observed during the exacerbations of cytopenias. Seven patients had quantitative serum immunoglobulin abnormalities at the time of presentation. There were associated systemic manifestations in nine patients. Various forms of treatment were used with mixed results. Four patients died from sepsis and haemorrhage; four had complete recovery—two after splenectomy. The authors concluded that Evans's syndrome is a heterogeneous disorder with significant morbidity and mortality. There was a high incidence of quantitative serum immunoglobulin abnormalities, lymphoid hyperplasia, and associated systemic manifestations, suggesting that Evans's syndrome may represent a stage of a more broad spectrum, generalized immune dysregulation.

Crosby[57] and Crosby and Rappaport[35] have pointed out that the prognosis appears worse when thrombocytopenia is present in AIHA. Of the patients they reviewed, 12 of 17 patients with thrombocytopenia died, compared with 5 of 16 patients who did not have thrombocytopenia. Chertkow and Dacie[58] derived a similar conclusion from their data, but Allgood and Chaplin[9] found no relationship between initial platelet count and mortality. The high death rates referred to in the earlier reports of Crosby and coworkers and Chertkow and Dacie were derived from data regarding patients for most of whom the only available treatment was blood transfusion or splenectomy.[7] Whether thrombocytopenia affects prognosis using modern therapy is uncertain.

IMMUNOPANCYTOPENIA

Some patients with AIHA have developed immune leukopenia and thrombocytopenia as well. Although the publication by Evans and Duane[46] is generally cited as a description of Evans's syndrome, which is defined as AIHA and thrombocytopenia, two of the five such patients reported by these authors also had leukopenia. Indeed, the authors suggested that the leukopenia and thrombocytopenia were probably due to "an immune body" with a broader range of activity than the RBCs or to a separate immune substance or substances more specific for platelets and WBCs.

Fagiolo[59] studied platelet and leukocyte counts and leukocytotoxic and platelet antibodies in 32 patients with AIHA. Leukopenia was present in 59.4%, thrombocytopenia in 59.4%, and leukothrombocytopenia in 40.5% of the cases. Specific antibodies for granulocytes were found in 81.3%, and platelet antibodies in 90.6%. The AIHA, leukopenia, and thrombocytopenia generally presented a dissociated evolution and a different response to immunosuppressive treatment. The leukopenia of two and the thrombocytopenia of six patients appeared at varied time intervals after the AIHA or the detection of leukocyte and platelet antibodies. Thrombocytopenic purpura was present in six patients, in two of these since infancy. The authors suggested that AIHA may be a complex autoimmune syndrome that may involve leukocytes and platelets as well as RBCs, with synthesis of autoantibodies specific for different blood cells.

Pegels and coworkers[60] used an immunofluorescence test for autoantibodies to study 24 patients with Evans's syndrome and an additional 29 patients with both ITP and idiopathic neutropenia (INP) but without AIHA. The direct immunofluorescence test on platelets and/or on granulocytes was positive in all patients with a cytopenia, but the sera of only 17 patients with Evans's syndrome and 15 of the other patients contained platelet- or granulocyte-specific autoantibodies. From absorption and elution experiments, the authors concluded that the autoantibodies were directed against antigens specific for the various peripheral blood cells, that is, RBCs, platelets, and granulocytes, and that they were not cross-reacting.

Miller and Schultz Beardsley[61] described three children with, concurrently or successively, neutropenia, thrombocytopenia, and AIHA. One of them developed reticulocytopenia. The DAT was positive and antiplatelet and antileukocyte antibodies were present. In two of the children it was possible to show that the anti-RBC and antiplatelet antibodies were separate entities that did not cross-react.

Chapman and coworkers[62] described the development of autoimmune thrombocytopenia followed by AIHA in a woman with measles. An IgM platelet autoantibody was detected using a fluorescent-labeled antiglobulin technique. The thrombocytopenia resolved spontaneously, although the platelet autoantibody persisted and platelet survival remained shortened, suggesting a compensated thrombocytolytic state. An IgG granulocyte autoantibody was present transiently, although the patient was never neutropenic. The AIHA was due to an IgM cold autoantibody (anti-I), which was active up to 30°C, and an IgG warm autoantibody, which was detectable only when she was severely anemic. After an initial blood transfusion, the anemia resolved and the RBC autoantibodies disappeared. The platelet, granulocyte, and red cell autoantibodies were cell specific and not a single cross-reacting antibody.

Wiesneth and coworkers[63] investigated four patients with combined immunocytopenia of unknown origin. Two patients with pancytopenia had alloantibodies and autoantibodies against RBCs, granulocytes, and thrombocytes. Two other patients with granulocytopenia and thrombocytopenia showed alloantibodies and autoantibodies against granulocytes and thrombocytes. All patients went into a transient or persistent remission under immunosuppressive therapy. The normalization of peripheral blood counts correlated with the disappearance of antibodies, suggesting that the cytopenias

TABLE 3-5. CLINICAL FEATURES OF FIVE PATIENTS WITH AIHA AND RETICULOCYTOPENIA

Patient	Age (yr)/ Sex	Hematocrit on Admission (%)	Duration of Reticulocytopenia (days)	Transfusion (U)	Outcome
1	52/F	10	10	19	Recovery
2	78/F	9	4	2	Recovery
3	53/F	10	90	53	Compensated status
4	39/M	9	8	5	Compensated status
5	49/F	8	160	84	Compensated status

From Conley CL, Lippman SM, Ness PM, Petz LD, Branch DR, Gallagher MT: Autoimmune hemolytic anemia with reticulocytopenia and erythroid marrow. N Engl J Med 1982;306:281–286.

were caused by an antibody-mediated autoimmune mechanism.

BONE MARROW FINDINGS

As in other hemolytic anemias, the bone marrow normally undergoes hypertrophy that is roughly proportional to the intensity of the hemolysis.[36] The hypertrophy is primarily due to hyperplasia of erythropoietic cells, with the result that the erythroid/myeloid ratio may even exceed unity. The erythropoiesis is typically normoblastic in type and is usually present even in the presence of reticulocytopenia[36,44] (see later). With severe hemolysis, erythropoiesis tends to become abnormal: In some cases there is a tendency for the nuclei of mature normoblasts to break up into two or more lobes of varying size and for Howell-Jolly bodies to be present in the cytoplasm of some of the normoblasts. Overt megaloblastic erythropoiesis certainly occurs,[9] as in other types of hemolytic anemia, but it has not been reported often.

RETICULOCYTES

As in other types of hemolytic anemias, a persistently raised reticulocyte count is a typical and characteristic finding in patients with WAIHA (see Chapter 2). However, reticulocytosis is not uniformly present and, indeed, reticulocytopenia is recognized as an important, although uncommon, manifestation of AIHA. Diagnosis is more difficult because AIHA does not seem to be a logical consideration in the presence of reticulocytopenia.

Reticulocytopenia. Liesveld and coworkers[44] reviewed data on 109 consecutive patients with various types of autoimmune hemolysis, of whom 51 had WAIHA. The reticulocyte counts ranged from 0.4% to 92% (Fig. 3-3). Twenty percent of the patients had an initial count of less than 4%, and 37% had an initial reticulocyte production index of less than 2 times basal. Eighty-eight cases had serial reticulocyte measurements, and in only 15% of patients did the reticulocyte production index remain less than 2 times basal. Thus, in most cases, the initially low reticulocyte production index probably represented a lag in marrow responsiveness to hemolytic stress. However, in some cases, the reticulocytopenia may be prolonged.[36,64-71]

AIHA with reticulocytopenia should be considered a medical emergency. Conley and coworkers[64,72] described five patients with AIHA in whom reticulocytopenia was associated with life-threatening anemia. Each of the patients had a hematocrit of 10% or less on admission (Table 3-5). The patients survived

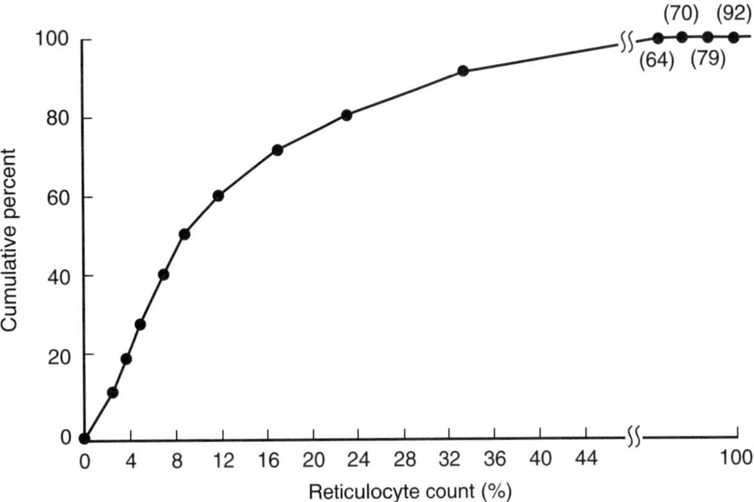

FIGURE 3-3. Cumulative percentage of first uncorrected reticulocyte percentage count obtained at diagnosis in 108 cases. Approximately 20% of patients had an initial reticuloycyte count of less than 4%. (From Liesveld JL, Rowe JM, Lichtman MA: Variability of the erythropoietic response in autoimmune hemolytic anemia: Analysis of 109 cases. Blood 1987;69: 820–826.)

patients followed up who had chronic hemolysis, five showed persistence of both IgG warm autoantibodies and high-thermal amplitude cold autohemagglutinins, whereas two lost their cold autohemagglutinins and showed serologic findings indistinguishable from those of warm antibody AIHA.

Nusbaum and Khosla[218] reported a patient with AIHA and a positive DAT for IgG. They believed that the patient had combined cold and warm antibody AIHA. However, no information was provided about the DAT results using anticomplement reagents or the thermal amplitude of the patient's cold agglutinin. Without this information, it is impossible to ascertain whether their patient had combined cold and warm AIHA or warm antibody AIHA.

Freedman and coworkers[30] reported a patient with AIHA who had three concomitant red cell autoantibodies: a low-titer, high-thermal amplitude IgM anti-I cold agglutinin; an IgG warm panagglutinating autoantibody; and an IgM warm hemolysin. The cold agglutinin reacted at 4°C to a titer of 64 in saline and 256 in albumin, and reacted up to 37°C. In addition, a strong IgG complement-binding platelet antibody was demonstrated. The patient also had thrombophlebitis and developed gangrene of his right foot and lower leg, requiring an above-knee amputation. After the administration of prednisone, the patient's hemolysis resolved and there was no recurrence of hemolysis.

Kajii and coworkers[219] reported that 3 of 46 patients (6.5%) with AIHA satisfied the diagnostic criteria for mixed-type AIHA. All of the cold autoantibodies were IgM-κ and showed high titer and high thermal amplitude.

SECONDARY COLD AND WARM AIHA

De Angelis and coworkers[220] described a young HIV-infected patient who presented with a severe AIHA with both warm and cold autoantibodies. Serologic findings indicated the presence of a low-titer, high thermal amplitude anti-I cold-reacting antibody and a pan-reactive warm autoantibody.

Similarly, Koduri and coworkers[221] described three acutely ill men with acquired immune deficiency syndrome (AIDS) who presented with fever, splenomegaly, and severe AIHA with both warm and cold autoantibodies. However, no information was provided by the authors regarding the thermal amplitude of the cold agglutinins, so it is uncertain that these were clinically important cold antibodies.

Chen and coworkers[222] reported a 49-year-old woman with primary biliary cirrhosis, sicca syndrome, and mixed-type AIHA. She presented with life-threatening anemia and was successfully treated with blood transfusions and pulse methylprednisolone therapy.

Gologan and coworkers[223] reported a patient with Waldenström's macroglobulinemia who also had WAIHA. During a period of compensated hemolysis after treatment, there appeared a severe hemolytic attack induced by transitory cold agglutinins with high thermal amplitude.

Vick and coworkers[224] described a patient with chronic lymphocytic leukemia/small cell lymphoma who developed mixed type AIHA 3 weeks after her fifth cycle of fludarabine. Prompt treatment with corticosteroids and minimal blood transfusions led to marked improvement.

CAUTIONS CONCERNING THE DIAGNOSIS OF COLD AND WARM AIHA

The diagnosis of mixed cold and warm antibody AIHA is sometimes made on the basis of inadequate serologic studies.[218,221] As emphasized in Chapters 5 and 6, appropriate characterization of the serum antibodies must be made before determining the specific type of AIHA present. An important source of potential error is suggested by our data,[1] which indicate that 35% of patients with WAIHA have cold agglutinins reactive at 20°C. However, a large majority of these cold agglutinins are clinically insignificant, and we found that only 5% reacted at 37°C. Unless one can document a cold autoantibody with a high thermal amplitude (>30°C) in association with a warm autoantibody, a diagnosis of cold and warm ("mixed") AIHA is not warranted.

Some reports of cold and WAIHA do, indeed, describe patients with serologic findings of warm AIHA in association with *classic* serologic findings of CAS, that is, a high titer cold autoantibody with a high thermal amplitude.[1,30,214,215,219] However, other reports describe WAIHA plus cold autoantibodies with normal cold agglutinin titers, but of high (30°C to 37°C) thermal amplitude[217,225] (and we have personally observed numerous such cases). Finally, some authors report "mixed" AIHA but do not characterize the cold autoantibody other than stating that it was reactive in the cold and at warm temperatures.[216,226]

In Chapter 6, we review our experience with the diagnosis of "cold and warm" AIHA and discuss the appropriate extent of serologic testing.

CLINICAL COURSE

Some authors suggest that patients with cold and warm AIHA have a more severe onset and more chronic course than patients with other categories of AIHA. However, a comprehensive comparison with the clinical course of patients with warm or cold AIHAs has not been made.

MANAGEMENT

Initial therapy of mixed cold and warm AIHA is corticosteroids with additional measures as may become necessary depending on the patient's course (see Chapter 11). Morselli and coworkers[227] described the successful use of rituximab in a patient with mixed AIHA associated with an overt malignant lymphoproliferative disease who relapsed after a course of corticosteroids.

AIHA Associated with a Negative DAT

This topic is reviewed in Chapter 9.

Secondary Autoimmune Hemolytic Anemias

AIHAs are classified as secondary for any of several reasons. One reason is the association of AIHA with an underlying disease with a frequency greater than can be explained by chance alone. For example, all authors agree that the incidence of WAIHA is higher in patients with CLL and SLE than in the general population.

Another criterion for categorizing a given case of AIHA as secondary is the reversal of the hemolytic anemia simultaneously with the correction of the associated disease. Ovarian tumors are a good example; well-documented cases of cure of the AIHA after surgical removal of the tumor have been reported.[228-231]

Still another reason for suspecting a relationship between the occurrence of AIHA and an associated disease consists of evidence of immunologic aberration as part of the underlying disorder, especially if the associated disease is thought to have an autoimmune pathogenesis. However, when the coexistence of two immunologic disorders in a single patient is infrequent, the pathogenetic significance is conjectural and interpretations vary. For example, rheumatoid arthritis is an extremely common disorder and reports of an associated AIHA are infrequent, so the combination may well be coincidental.[232] Allgood and Chaplin[9] noted the presence of ulcerative colitis and rheumatoid arthritis in some of their patients but still considered the AIHA idiopathic, whereas Pirofsky[2] included these and numerous other disorders among patients classified as having secondary AIHA. In ulcerative colitis, reports of resolution of the hemolytic anemia after colectomy,[233-235] the association of ulcerative colitis with other immunologically mediated abnormalities, and the frequent sequential development of immunologic abnormalities in a single patient lend weight to the suggestion that ulcerative colitis and AIHA should be considered as only two parts of a complex, immunologically mediated multisystem disease state.[2] In general, the evidence for a relationship between immunologic disorders, including immune deficiency states, and AIHA is strong,[2,236-242] although the pathogenetic basis for such a relationship has not been clarified.

The significance of the relationship between other associated diseases and AIHA is far less clear in many reported cases of "secondary" AIHA. Occasionally reported associated diseases include leukemias other than CLL, thyroid disease, myeloproliferative disorders, pernicious anemia, cirrhosis of the liver, and many bacterial infections. Hemolysis in many cases of secondary hemolytic anemia is not caused by an immune mechanism. Dacie[243] has reviewed both immune and nonimmune secondary hemolytic anemias and provides many case reports, including those in the older medical literature.

RELATIVE INCIDENCE OF IDIOPATHIC AND SECONDARY TYPES OF WARM ANTIBODY AIHA

Many reports of the relative incidence of idiopathic and secondary forms of AIHA are available. The reported incidence varies significantly, possibly depending on the nature of the center to which cases were referred and also in regard to an interpretation of what constitutes a related underlying disorder. Reports suggesting that idiopathic cases are more frequent include those of Dacie and Worlledge,[5] Dausset and Colombani,[10] and Sokol and coworkers.[4] An approximately equal incidence is suggested by the reviews of Dameshek and Komninos,[244] Evans and Weiser,[245] Bell and coworkers,[189] and Engelfriet and coworkers.[6] Reports suggesting that secondary cases are more common are those of Chaplin and Avioli[246] and Pirofsky.[2,8] Pirofsky's data are heavily influenced by the fact that his patient population was characterized by many patients with leukemia and lymphoma who were undergoing constant medical follow-up. Table 3-10 summarizes data available in these cited series.

TABLE 3-10. COMPARATIVE INCIDENCE OF IDIOPATHIC AND SECONDARY WARM ANTIBODY AUTOIMMUNE HEMOLYTIC ANEMIA

Reference	No. of Cases	Idiopathic		Secondary	
		No.	%	No.	%
Dameshek and Komninos[244]	43	21	50	22	50
Dacie and Worlledge[5]	199	111	56	88	44
Dausset and Colombani[10]	106	83	78	23	22
Evans and Weiser[245]	37	15	41	22	59
Bell et al.[189]	37	18	49	19	51
Pirofsky[2,8]	234	44	19	190	81
Engelfriet et al.[6]	539	245	45	294	55
Sokol et al.[4] (excluding drug induced)	1694	1034	61	660	39
Total	2889	1571	54	1318	46

TABLE 3-11. CLASSIFICATION OF 1834 PATIENTS WITH AUTOIMMUNE HEMOLYTIC ANEMIA (AIHA), BASED ON SEROLOGIC FINDINGS AND DISEASE ASSOCIATION

Condition	WAIHA	CAS	PCH	Mixed AIHA
Idiopathic AIHA	617	344	11	82
Drug-Related AIHA	140	0	0	0
Neoplasia				
Lymphoid neoplasms				
Chronic lymphocytic leukemia	63	13	0	0
Acute lymphoblastic leukemia	1	4	0	0
Non-Hodgkin's lymphoma	32	22	0	8
Angioimmunoblastic lymphadenopathy	1	1	0	0
Myeloma	4	1	0	0
Macroglobulinemia	2	3	0	0
Thyinoma	1	0	0	0
Hodgkin's disease	10	4	0	4
Ovarian tumours	4	0	0	0
Carcinoma (nonovarian)	67	23	0	6
Acute nonlymphoid leukemias	5	4	0	0
Chronic myeloid leukemia	5	1	0	1
Myelofibrosis	12	0	0	3
Myelodysplastic syndromes	23	4	0	3
Other neoplasms	3	2	0	0
Infection				
Pneumonia—*Mycoplasma*	0	29	0	1
Pneumonia—"viral" and unspecified	2	13	0	1
Infectious mononucleosis	0	6	0	0
Infectious hepatitis	1	1	0	0
Tuberculosis	0	1	0	0
Syphilis	0	0	1	0
Infection—unspecified	13	11	7	3
Collagen Diseases				
Systemic lupus erythematosus	17	8	0	3
Rheumaroid arthritis	34	9	0	3
Polyarteritis nodosa	1	0	0	0
Other Immune-Based and Miscellaneous Disorders				
Ulcerative colitis	19	1	0	1
Thyrotoxicosis	3	1	0	1
Myxedema	1	0	0	0
Chronic active hepaticis	2	0	0	0
Pernicious anemia	7	1	0	0
Diabetes mellitus	8	3	0	0
Sarcoidosis	1	0	0	0
Myasthenia gravis	1	0	0	0
AIHA Associated with Pregnancy	22	15	0	1
AIHA Associated with Chronic Renal Failure	29	12	0	6

Modified from Sokol RJ, Booker DJ, Stamps R: The pathology of autoimmune haemolytic anaemia. J Clin Pathol 1992; 45:1047–1052.

The data of Sokol and coworkers,[4] which indicate the classification of 1834 patients with autoimmune hemolysis, are indicated in Table 3-11. The authors stressed that their series included patients who had hemolysis but who were not anemic. Most of the patients had warm autoantibodies (Table 3-12).

The following sections provide information about secondary AIHA found in association with specific disorders. Further details about management of secondary AIHAs are found in Chapter 11.

OVARIAN TUMORS

Hemolytic anemia associated with ovarian tumors has been recognized since the report of West-Watson and Young in 1938.[247] Their patient had hemolytic anemia and failed to improve after splenectomy. In an attempt to find a hypothetical accessory spleen, the patient underwent further abdominal surgery, at which time an ovarian dermoid cyst was discovered and excised. Excision of the cyst was promptly followed by

TABLE 3-12. SEROLOGIC DISTRIBUTION OF 1834 PATIENTS WITH AUTOIMMUNE HEMOLYTIC ANEMIA

Autoantibody Type	No. (%)
Warm	1151 (62.8)
Cold	
Cold agglutinin disease	537 (29.3)
Paroxysmal cold hemoglobinuria	19 (1.0)
Mixed (warm plus cold)	127 (6.9)

Modified from Sokol RJ, Booker DJ, Stamps R: The pathology of autoimmune haemolytic anaemia. J Clin Pathol 1992;45:1047–1052.

remission of the anemia. Particular notice was taken of this result, and in subsequent years numerous case reports[230,248,249-251] and reviews[228,229,231,252] of AIHA in association with ovarian tumors have been published.

Carreras Vescio and coworkers[252] reviewed 29 published cases in 1983 and added one case of their own[228-231,247,248,252-274] (Table 3-13). Although most of the patients studied were adults (average age, 40 years), the case reported by Allibone and Collins[257] was of a girl only 4 years old. Twenty of the 30 ovarian tumors were teratomas, including 17 dermoid cysts. In three cases, the tumors were reported as cysts, not further described; in one patient, a probable theca-cell tumor was diagnosed, and the remaining patients had malignant neoplasms. In addition, the authors mentioned that two cases of dermoid tumors in organs other than the ovary have been associated with AIHA: one was localized in the hilus of the spleen[275] and the other one in the mesentery.[276] A further case of AIHA and dermoid cyst of the mesentery was reported by Buonanno and coworkers.[277]

An important feature of AIHA in association with ovarian tumors is the striking resistance of the AIHA to any therapeutic approach other than the surgical removal of the tumor. In 16 of the cases in the report of Carreras Vescio and coworkers,[252] the hemolytic anemia was first treated with steroids, which produced only a slight and transient improvement in six instances. In seven patients, splenectomy was performed before excision of the ovarian tumor, but only three patients derived some benefit. In three instances, excision of the ovarian tumor was carried out together with splenectomy; in all three cases surgery was followed by complete recovery. In all of the cases, the ovarian tumor was eventually excised, and this was followed by a generally total and rapid remission of the AIHA, except that only partial benefit occurred in three patients who had malignant tumors with metastatic disease. In one patient who had a malignant tumor with metastatic disease, complete remission of the anemia did occur after removal of the tumor and chemotherapy.

The DAT was positive in 22 cases, negative in only 3; data were not reported in the remaining 5 patients. Most patients had IgG autoantibodies, some exhibiting specificity including anti-e, anti-c anti-E, and anti-dl. In three patients an autoantibody of anti-I specificity was reported.

At least three hypotheses have been put forward to explain the association of AIHA and ovarian tumors: (1) the presence in the tumor of substances foreign to the host that stimulate development of cross-reacting antibodies, (2) the binding of substances secreted by the tumor to the RBCs with production of antibodies reactive with the coated RBCs, and (3) the tumor itself could produce red cell antibody. The latter hypothesis is supported by De Bruyere and coworkers,[230] who found that ovarian cyst fluid from a patient with AIHA contained IgG antibodies of the same specificity as in the patient's serum. Similar findings have been reported by other authors.[231,274]

In conclusion, the association of AIHA with ovarian tumors is rare but its recognition is obviously important. The possibility should be considered in all women who develop AIHA of unknown origin, particularly if the AIHA is not responsive to standard therapeutic measures.

ULCERATIVE COLITIS

The association of AIHA with ulcerative colitis was first reported in 1955 by Lorber and coworkers.[278] Although the association of the two disorders is quite uncommon, there is undoubtedly a pathogenetic relationship because the AIHA has almost invariably gone into remission after colectomy, even when hemolysis is refractory to other therapeutic approaches.[233,235,279]

The incidence of AIHA in patients with ulcerative colitis in various reports has varied between 0.6% and 1.7%.[234,280-282] A positive DAT without hemolysis is found in an additional 2% of patients.[282] Also, one must be aware that patients taking sulfasalazine as therapy for ulcerative colitis have developed hemolytic anemia,[283] although such cases do not have an immune basis.[284,285]

Dacie[243] provided a detailed summary of cases of AIHA in patients with ulcerative colitis that were published up to 1979 (Table 3-14), and, in 1994, Ramakrishna and Manoharan[235] reported two patients, and summarized data on 38 cases previously described in the English literature (Table 3-15). The treatment and outcome and DAT status after therapy are summarized in Table 3-16. The therapeutic approaches that did not include colectomy resulted in a remission of AIHA in about 50% of patients. In contrast, all 16 patients who had splenectomy combined with colectomy or colectomy alone went into remission of their AIHA. Patients who have developed AIHA many years after undergoing total colectomy for severe ulcerative colitis refractory to medical management have been successfully treated with corticosteroids and/or immunomodulators.[281,286]

There is general agreement that the initial therapy for AIHA in association with ulcerative colitis should be steroid therapy, as it has been successful in about

TABLE 3-13. REPORTED CASES OF HEMOLYTIC ANEMIA ASSOCIATED WITH OVARIAN TUMORS

Patient	Age (yr)	Duration of Illness	Splenomegaly	Palpable Tumor	Hemoglobin (g/100 mL)	Reticulocytes (%)	Coombs Test	Corticosteroids	Splenectomy	Tumor Excision	Histologic Diagnosis
1	44	2 mo	+	+	3.6	45	+	—	No response	Remission	Teratoma
2	19	2 yr	+	+	5.0	15	+	—	At time of tumor excision	Remission	"Cyst"
3	47	5 mo	+	+	5.1	46	?	—	Transient response	Remission	Dermoid
4	35	1 mo	?	+	5.0	10	+	—	—	Slow response	Pseudomucinous cystadeno-carcinoma
5	40	?	+	+	4.3	16	+	—	No response	Died at operation	Dermoid
6	4	3 mo	?	+	7.0	39	0	—	—	Remission	Dermoid
7	61	9 mo	0	0	5.2	20	?	—	—	Died of transfusion	Dermoid
8	53	?	0	?	6.5	78	+	No response	—	Remission	Dermoid
9	54	?	0	+	PCV: 23%	58	+	No response	—	Remission	Dermoid
10	40	?	+	?	4.3	74	+	Transient response	Transient response	Remission	Dermoid
11	26	1 yr	+	+	3.6	26	+	—	—	Remission	Teratoma
12	44	9 mo	+	+	4.0	50	+	No response	No response	Remission	Dermoid
13	61	2 yr	+	+	PCV: 37%	39	+	No response	—	Remission	Teratoma
14	23	1 yr	0	+	6.8	11	+	—	—	Remission	"Cyst"
15	39	4 mo	?	?	?	?	+	—	—	Remission	Cystic degeneration
16	49	?	?	?	?	?	?	No response	No response	Remission	Dermoid
17	45	?	?	+	?	?	+	—	—	Remission	Dermoid
18	30	4 mo	+	+	3.5	74	+	Partial response	—	Remission	Dermoid
19	28	?	+	+	6.7	5.7	?	Partial response	—	Partial response	Papillary adenocarcinoma
20	48	3 mo	+	+	4.2	9.7	0	No response	—	Remission	Dermoid
21	36	1 yr	+	+	PCV: 14%	8.6	+	Partial response	—	Incomplete	Anaplastic carcinoma
22	52	9 mo	0	0	6.8	11	+	No response	At time of tumor excision	Remission	Dermoid
23	54	?	?	?	?	?	?	?	?	Partial response	Adenocarcinoma
24	64	1 yr	0	+	4.75	10.2	+	No response	—	Transient response	"Epithelio-sarcomatoid" tumor
25	41	1 yr	+	0	3.8	4.2	0	—	At time of tumor excision	Remission	Theca-granulosa
26	32	8 mo	+	+	3.5	50	+	No response	Transient response	Remission	Dermoid
27	35	1 mo	+	+	5.5	6.5	+	—	—	Remission	Dermoid
28	47	4 mo	0	+	4.8	60	+	Partial response	—	Remission	Dermoid
29	34	1 mo	0	+	10.3	1.9	+	Partial response	—	Remission	Dermoid
30	29	3 mo	0	+	7.3	5.2	+	No response	—	Remission	Anaplastic carcinoma

Modified from Carreras Vescio LA, Toblli JE, Rey JA, Assaf ME, Deinaria HE, Marletta J: Autoimmune hemolytic anemia associated with an ovarian neoplasm. Mediciria (B Aires) 1983;43:415–424.

TABLE 3-14. CASE REPORTS IN CHRONOLOGIC ORDER OF AUTOIMMUNE HEMOLYTIC ANEMIA (AIHA) ASSOCIATED WITH ULCERATIVE COLITIS (UC)

Patient	Age (yr)/Sex of Patient	Time of Onset of AIHA after Onset of UC	Minimum Hb (g/dL)	Maximum Reticulocyte Count (%)	Serologic Findings: DAT; Specificity of Autoantibody	Treatment and Response to Treatment; Other Findings
1	28/F	5 mo	8.2	10.4	DAT 3+. Anti-e; also allo–anti-D and allo–anti-E and a panantibody	Partial response to cortisone and ACTH; further improvement followed subtotal colectomy. Blood loss had contributed to her anemia
2	44/F	19 mo	9.0	2	DAT 1+. Panantibody active against enzyme-treated cells	ACTH controlled intestinal bleeding. Probably no significant hemolysis
3	44/F	21 yr	6.0	72	DAT 4+. Panantibody; also allo–anti-E	Splenectomy led to a good but incomplete remission. DAT 1+ 5 yr later
4	17/F	6 mo	10.8	0.8	DAT weak (±) pos. Panantibody; also allo–anti-E and allo–anti-K	No treatment needed for mild anemia, except transfusion before colectomy
5	31/F				DAT pos. Anti-e + f eluted	Patient had had rheumatic heart disease. DAT neg 6 weeks after colectomy
6	35/F	6 yr	9.0	6.0	DAT 4+. Antibody 7S γG; no specificity demonstrated	^{51}Cr T_{50} 9 days. A high incidence of gastrointestinal disorders and allergies in patient's family, including pernicious anemia
7	23/M	6 mo	4.0	—	DAT and IAT pos	Splenectomy; after postoperative complications, a normal blood picture
8	21/M	1 yr	Hematocrit 18%	—	DAT pos	Rheumatoid arthritis 1 year before UC. Splenectomy (spleen weighed 1850 g); good response
9			10.3	1.8	DAT 3+	RBC survival normal
10	57/M	11 yr after severe UC treated succesfully by colectomy and protectomy	10.2	9.7	DAT strong pos	Remission after prednisone therapy, although DAT remained pos

TABLE 3-14. CASE REPORTS IN CHRONOLOGIC ORDER OF AUTOIMMUNE HEMOLYTIC ANEMIA (AIHA) ASSOCIATED WITH ULCERATIVE COLITIS (UC)—CONT'D

Patient	Age (yr)/Sex of Patient	Time of Onset of AIHA after Onset of UC	Minimum Hb (g/dL)	Maximum Reticulocyte Count (%)	Serologic Findings: DAT; Specificity of Autoantibody	Treatment and Response to Treatment; Other Findings
11	23/F	2 yr	4.4	52	DAT pos. IgG; antibody predominantly anti-e	Remission after prednisone therapy
12	18–58/3M, 2F	3–225 mo	Hematocrit 16.1%	6.3	DAT pos	Four patients died 2–7 mo after onset of pos DAT.
13	42/F	1 yr	5.0	18	DAT strong pos	Hemolysis failed to respond to medical treatment. Rapid emission followed total colectomy
14	32/M	3 yr after colectomy for UC	2.58 × 10^{12}/L RBCs	22.5	DAT pos. IgG; anti-e	Complete recovery from hemolysis after proctectomy
15	23/F	Known case of UC	9.8	7	DAT pos. IgG; anti-e	Hemolysis responded to prednisone therapy
16	30/F	1 yr after onset of mild UC	7.8	80	DAT pos. Anti-Rh	Hemolysis responded to splenectomy
17	36/F	Shortly after onset	8.0	11.5	DAT pos. IgG; anti-e or anti-C	Large doses of corticosteroids and 6MP needed to control hemolysis; remitted after 5 yr; UC also quiescent
18	35/F	10 yr	11.0	2	DAT and IAT strong pos	DAT became neg 4 days after total colectomy
19	34/F	7 yr	Hematocrit 21%	44	DAT 4+. IgG; anti-Rh (neg with Rh_{null} cells)	Incomplete response of hemolysis to prednisone; remission followed splenectomy
20	12/M	1 mo	Hematocrit 26%	7.8	DAT 4+. Nonspecific	Incomplete response of hemolysis to prednisone; remission followed splenectomy. Total colectomy when aged 23; 1 yr later hematocrit 51%
21	24/F	Simultaneous onset of UC and AIHA	Hematocrit 25.5%	5	DAT 4+. IgG; anti-Rh (neg with Rh_{null} cells)	Incomplete response of hemolysis to prednisone and cyclophosphamide. Splenectomy ineffective. Hematocrit stabilized at at 35% after coloproctectomy

TABLE 3-14. CASE REPORTS IN CHRONOLOGIC ORDER OF AUTOIMMUNE HEMOLYTIC ANEMIA (AIHA) ASSOCIATED WITH ULCERATIVE COLITIS (UC)—CONT'D

Patient	Age (yr)/Sex of Patient	Time of Onset of AIHA after Onset of UC	Minimum Hb (g/dL)	Maximum Reticulocyte Count (%)	Serologic Findings: DAT; Specificity of Autoantibody	Treatment and Response to Treatment; Other Findings
22	29/F	5 yr	7.2	24	DAT pos	Incomplete response of hemolysis to prednisone; improved after splenectomy and azathioprine
23	30/F	4.5 yr	9.3	20	DAT pos	Total proctocolectomy and splenectomy. 2.5 yr later no evidence of hemolysis
24	23/M	1.5 yr	Hematocrit 15.6%	52	DAT 4 +	Incomplete response to prednisone. Splenectomy; 4 mo later no evidence of hemolysis

Modified from Dacie JV: The Haemolytic Anaemias, 3rd ed. vol. 4, Secondary or Symptomatic Haemolytic Anemias. New York: Churchill Livingstone, 1995.

half of the cases.[234,287] Several authors suggest that patients unresponsive to steroids should undergo total proctocolectomy directly, even in the absence of active colonic disease.[283,288] Other authors recommend splenectomy before total colectomy.[234,281] Proctocolectomy has the added advantage of removing the risk of primary colonic cancer in longstanding ulcerative colitis[289] and avoids the risks of splenectomy (see Chapter 11).

Mechanism of AIHA. The mechanism of the AIHA in patients with ulcerative colitis remains obscure. Proposed theories include the following[287]: (1) alteration of RBC antigen in the gastrointestinal tract resulting in the production of antibodies against the altered antigens, which may react with the patient's native RBCs; (2) absorption of non-RBC antigens through the diseased colon with the development of antibodies that cross-react with the patient's RBCs; (3) interaction of anticolon antibodies with RBC antigens; and (4) nonspecific stimulation of the immune system with the appearance of a clone of immunocompetent cells producing anti-RBC antibodies.[233,290,291]

TABLE 3-15. PATIENTS WITH AUTOIMMUNE HEMOLYTIC ANEMIA (AIHA) AND ULCERATIVE COLITIS (UC)

Clinical Features		Patients, n
Sex	Male	16
	Female	24
Age range (yr)	12–40	28
	41–60	12
Activity of colitis at the time of AIHA episode	Active	36
	Inactive	4
	AIHA followed colectomy	2
	UC diagnosed after AIHA	2
DAT	Positive	40
	IgG only	15
	IgG and complement	3
	Complement only	1
	Not specified	21
Specificity	Known	8
	Anti-e	6
	Anti-E	1
	Anti-C	1
	Unknown	32

Modified from Ramakrishna R, Manoharan A: Auto-immune haemolytic anaemia in ulcerative colitis. Acta Haematol 1994;91:99–102.

Yates and coworkers[292] studied the ability of mononuclear cells extracted from the colon, draining lymph nodes, peripheral blood, and spleen of a patient with severe AIHA to produce RBC autoantibodies. They demonstrated that in vitro cultures of mononuclear cells of the colon produced immunoglobulin spontaneously, showing the presence of activated B cells and plasma cells, but anti–red cell activity could not be demonstrated. However, mononuclear cells transferred to SCID mice did produce IgG with anti–red cell activity. The authors concluded that the colon is the source of RBC autoantibodies in such patients.

LYMPHOPROLIFERATIVE DISORDERS

The records of 637 patients with lymphoproliferative disorders and 346 patients with myeloproliferative disorders were retrospectively analyzed for the presence of coexistent autoimmune derangements.[293] The frequency of autoimmune perturbations in lymphoproliferative diseases (51 cases; 8.0%) was significantly higher than in myeloproliferative diseases (6 cases; 1.7%; $P < 0.0001$). Rheumatic disorders, autoallergic hematologic manifestations, and other organ-specific autoimmune derangements were responsible for about one third each of the observed disturbances. These data are similar to those of Miller,[294]

TABLE 3-16. PATIENTS WITH AUTOIMMUNE HEMOLYTIC ANEMIA AND ULCERATIVE COLITIS

Treatment	Total No. of Patients	Outcome: Grade of Response I	II	III
Steroids	18	5	2	11
Steroids + immunosuppressives	16	7	3	6
Steroids + danazol	1	—	1	—
Splenectomy	8	1	3	4
Splenectomy + colectomy	6	6	—	—
Colectomy	10	10	—	—

Grade I, hemolysis and colitis in remission, and DAT either negative (n = 12) or weakly positive (n = 8) or unknown (n = 9); grade II, hemolysis in remission, colitis activity unknown or not responsive, DAT status unchanged: grade III, unresponsive or unknown hemolytic and colitis status.

Modified from Ramakrishna R, Manoharan A: Auto-immune haemolytic anaemia in ulcerative colitis. Acta Haematol 1994;91:99–102.

who observed diffuse connective tissue diseases and autoimmune hemolytic anemias in 6.8% of his lymphoma patients.

Autoimmune diseases that preceded the onset of malignancy occurred in lymphoproliferative and myeloproliferative disorders with a comparable frequency without significant differences between individual subgroups of lymphoproliferative diseases. In contrast, autoimmune complications developing in the course of the neoplastic disease were significantly more frequent in lymphoproliferative (4.9%) than in myeloproliferative disorders (0.3%; $P < 0.0005$). Here marked differences were observed between individual lymphoma entities, the rate of concomitant autoimmune derangements ranging from zero to over 15%.

Chronic Lymphocytic Leukemia. CLL is not only a malignant disease but also a complex immunologic disorder. The immune dysregulation that is a hallmark of CLL manifests itself, on the one hand, in an immunodeficiency state and, on the other hand, in an excess of autoimmune phenomena.[295]

AIHA is the most common autoimmune disease associated with CLL, and CLL is the most common of the known causes of AIHA.[6,295] Various reports indicate that AIHA occurs in 5% to 37% of CLL patients.[295-301] The figures are highly dependent on the duration and extent of disease.[295] Table 3-17 summarizes six of the largest series evaluating the relationship of AIHA and malignancy.[295,302] CLL is the diagnosis in 15% of all warm antibody AIHA patients and half of the malignant cases, and is exceeded only by idiopathic cases. In contrast, these data indicate that CAS is only rarely associated with CLL. However, later reports regarding the incidence of AIHA in patients with CLL indicated that hemolysis mediated by IgM cold antibodies was found in 7 of 52 cases (13%) by Mauro and coworkers[296] and in 13 of 76 patients (17%) by Sokol and coworkers.[4]

When CLL is associated with AIHA, the CLL is rarely occult. In collected series of more than 500 patients, the AIHA antedated the diagnosis of CLL in a single patient.[295] A higher lymphocyte count, older age, and male gender are significantly linked with an increased rate of AIHA at CLL diagnosis.[296] Also, therapeutic approaches, such as radiation and alkylating agents, particularly purine analogues, have been considered as risk factors for the occurrence of AIHA. It is generally thought that fludarabine may predisopose to AIHA by inducing a marked lymphocytopenia, particularly of $CD4^+$ lymphocytes, with a T-cell subset imbalance that may favor the emergence of autoreactive T cells (see Chapter 8).

The mean time from diagnosis of CLL to AIHA is 4.1 years; lymphadenopathy is present in 88%; splenomegaly is present in 94%, and it is massive

TABLE 3-17. AUTOIMMUNE HEMOLYTIC ANEMIA (AIHA) AND MALIGNANCY

	n	Idiopathic (%)	Total Associated with Malignancy (%)	CLL (%)	NHL (%)	HD (%)	WM/MM (%)	ALL/AML (%)	Other (%)	Infection (%)
Warm AIHA	1463	47	31	15	4	3	2	3	5	0
Cold AIHA	392	48	21	1	6	3	2	2	10	24

CLL, chronic lymphocytic leukemia; NHL, non-Hodgkin's lymphoma; HD, Hodgkin's disease; MM, multiple myeloma; WM, Waldenstrom's macroglobulinemia; ALL, acute lymphocytic leukemia; AML, acute myeloid leukemia; AIHA, autoimmune hemolytic anemia.

From Diehl LF, Ketchum LH: Autoimmune disease and chronic lymphocytic leukemia: Autoimmune hemolytic anemia, pure red cell aplasia, and autoimmune thrombocytopenia. Semin Oncol 1998;25:80–97.

in 20%. The peripheral blood smear demonstrates microspherocytes, polychromasia, and anisocytosis. Normoblasts are present in about one third of patients, and there is even an occasional early myeloid cell—all changes typical of stimulated erythropoiesis. The peripheral blood film virtually always contains the findings consistent with CLL.[295,303]

Serologic Findings. In the great majority of cases of CLL complicated by AIHA, the responsible autoantibodies have been of the warm type and similar in class, specificity, and behavior in vitro to those associated with idiopathic AIHA. Engelfriet and coworkers[304] reported that of 130 patients with AIHA who had an underlying malignant disease, 79 had CLL and that all had formed warm antibodies. The serologic findings in 11 cases with warm AIHA and CLL reported by Dacie[243] are listed in Table 3-18. However, there have been some reports of cold antibody AIHA in association with CLL.[243,305,306] Ruzickova and coworkers[307] reported a patient with a 7-year history of idiopathic CAS in whom B-CLL subsequently developed. They determined that the B-CLL had developed from the patient's cold agglutinin–producing B-cell population.

Prognosis. Several studies have shown that CLL patients with AIHA represent a poor prognosis category,[297,301,308] whereas a more recent study by Mauro and coworkers[296] found in a multivariate analysis that AIHA has no independent effect on survival probability. However, two independent factors were significantly related to better survival probability of CLL patients with AIHA: the IgG class of the autoantibody and the occurrence of AIHA at the time of CLL diagnosis. Patients with IgM autoantibody identified a small group with very poor survival. In these cases, the IgM autoantibody was a warm agglutinin, optimally reactive at 37°C (Fig. 3-6).

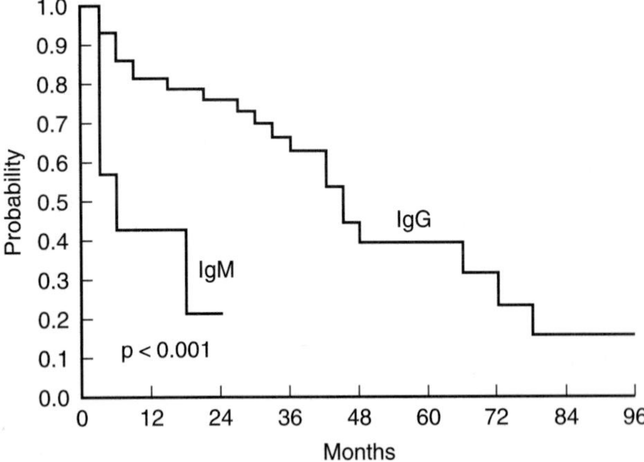

FIGURE 3-6. Actuarial survival probability of chronic lymphatic leukemia patients from autoimmune hemolysis diagnosis according to the Ig class of the autoantibody. Percent surviving at 2 years: IgG (45 patients), 76% (SE, ±6.6); (7 patients), 21% (SE, ±17) ($P < 0.001$). (From Mauro FR, Foa R, Cerretti R, Giannarelli D, Coluzzi S, Mandelli F, et al.: Autoimmune hemolytic anemia in chronic lymphocytic leukemia: Clinical, therapeutic, and prognostic features. Blood 2000;95: 2786–2792.)

Pathophysiology. Although pathogenic RBC autoantibodies in CLL patients with AIHA occasionally may be made by the clone of malignant B cells,[309-312] they are generally produced by remnant normal B cells.[295,296,309,313] The autoantibodies are generally polyclonal, and the Ig isotypes of autoantibodies found in RBC eluates usually differ from that of the Ig expressed by the malignant B-cell clone.

The development of antierythrocyte autoantibodies in CLL patients may reflect a generalized defect in the homeostatic mechanisms that prevent generation of antiself humoral immunity.[295,309] According to this hypothesis, autoantibodies arise not from polyclonal B-cell activation, but rather from a pathologic immune response to self-antigen.[309]

Barcellini and coworkers[314] studied 69 B-CLL patients and 53 controls using a recently developed mitogen-stimulated DAT (MS-DAT), which is able to disclose latent anti-RBC autoimmunity in AIHA. They investigated the prevalence of anti-RBC autoimmunity by MS-DAT and the pattern of cytokine production by PHA-stimulated whole blood cultures. In B-CLL the prevalence of anti-RBC autoimmunity was 28.9% by MS-DAT, compared with 4.3% by the standard DAT. Production of numerous cytokines was significantly increased in all B-CLL patients compared with controls. They concluded that their data were consistent with the hypothesis that autoimmune phenomena in B-CLL are associated with an imbalance toward a Th-2–like profile. The elevated prevalence of anti-RBC autoimmunity found by MS-DAT suggests that an underestimated latent autoimmunity exists in B-CLL.

Hodgkin's Disease. AIHA is an uncommon occurrence in patients with Hodgkin's disease. In 1967, Eisner and coworkers[315] reported 10 patients with Hodgkin's disease who had a positive DAT. Overt hemolytic anemia was present in eight of the patients, and the incidence of AIHA in a series of 219 patients was 2.7%. With one exception, all of the patients had advanced disease at the time of detection of the positive DAT.

Levine and coworkers[316] reviewed 71 cases of Hodgkin's disease and found three who had AIHA (4.2%). A positive DAT without hemolysis was found in an additional 4 patients. These authors emphasized that all of their patients had active disease at the time a positive DAT was first noted, although there have been reports of AIHA in patients with limited stage disease.[317-319] In some patients the AIHA was diagnosed 3 or more years before the diagnosis of Hodgkin's disease,[320-324] whereas in other patients AIHA has supervened after a long interval after the diagnosis of Hodgkin's disease.[325-329]

Xiros and coworkers[330] found only 1 patient with AIHA among 492 patients with Hodgkin's disease (0.2%). Additional case reports of patients with AIHA in Hodgkin's disease have appeared in the medical literature,[243,331-334] including cases in children.[317,335-338] Most reports indicated that the presence of AIHA does not signal a bad prognosis.[316,339]

TABLE 3-18. SEROLOGIC FINDINGS IN AUTOIMMUNE HEMOLYTIC ANEMIA ASSOCIATED WITH CHRONIC LYMPHOCYTIC LEUKEMIA

		DAT		IAT	Agglutination			Lysis					
					Normal RBCs (titer)		Papainized Normal RBCs (titer)	PNH RBCs	Papainized PNH RBCs	Papainized Normal RBCs			
Patient	Age (yr)/ Sex	Anti-γ G	Anti-non-γ	37°C	2–4°C	20°C	37°C	37°C	37°C	Stored 37°C	Fresh 37°C	Type of Autoantibody	Specificity of Autoantibody
1	71/M	+++	—	+	. . .	<1	+	—	—	—	—	Warm	Anti-e + NS
2	57/M	++	—	+	<1	<1	64	—	—	—	—	Warm	NS
3	73/F	++++	—	+	16	<1	1024	—	++	+	—	Warm	NS
4	77/M	++	—	—	<1	<1	<1	—	—	—	—	Warm	NS
5	51/F	+++	++	—	<1	<1	16	. . .	. . .	. . .	. . .	Warm	? NS
6	58/M	++	+	+	<1	<1	16	. . .	. . .	. . .	. . .	Warm	NS
7	65/M	+++	+	++	<1	<1	16	—	—	—	—	Warm	NS
8	68/F	+++	—	—	. . .	. . .	1	—	—	—	—	Warm	NS
9	72/M	+++	—	—	. . .	<1	<1	—	—	—	—	Warm	NS
10	53/M	++	—	—	<1	<1	<1	—	—	—	—	Warm	. . .
11	65/M	—	+±	—	. . .	<1	1	. . .	. . .	±	—	Warm	NS

++++ denotes strong naked-eye agglutination or haemolysis; +++, ++, +±, +, and ± denote lesser degrees of agglutination of hemolysis; . . . denotes no observation; NS denotes no specificity demonstrated.
Modified from Dacie JV: The Haemolytic Anaemias, 3rd ed. vol. 4, Secondary or Symptomatic Haemolytic Anaemias. New York: Churchill Livingstone, 1995.

Autoantibody Specificity. In almost all patients with AIHA associated with Hodgkin's disease, the autoantibody has been found to be warm in type and not distinctly separable in respect of antibody class and specificity from the warm antibodies responsible for idiopathic AIHA.[243] An exceptional case was reported by Brain and coworkers,[323] who described a patient who had had a cold-antibody AIHA for approximately 4 years before recurrence of severe anemia and enlarging lymph nodes led to the diagnosis of an anaplastic type of Hodgkin's disease. The autoantibody was a high thermal amplitude anti-I.

In 1972, Garratty and coworkers[340] described the presence of an autoantibody with anti-I^T specificity in an American patient with Hodgkin's disease. The antibody in this patient was of the IgG class, was transient in nature, and was not associated with overt hemolysis. In a later report, Garratty and coworkers[328] reported three patients with Hodgkin's disease who had AIHA associated with an IgG auto-anti-I^T. Antibody of this specificity was not found in 50 patients with Hodgkin's disease who had a negative DAT, nor was it found in a group of 70 patients with AIHA associated with a variety of underlying diseases, including non-Hodgkin's lymphoma.

However, not all patients with auto-anti-I^T have Hodgkin's disease. Freedman and coworkers[341] reported a patient who did not have Hodgkin's disease but who had AIHA due to an autoagglutinin of anti-I^T specificity. The antibody was of the IgM class, bound complement, and reacted optimally at 37°C. Haffleigh and coworkers[342] described the presence of anti-I^T occurring in three patients who did not have Hodgkin's disease, although two had non-Hodgkin's lymphoma. None of these patients had evidence of shortened red cell survival. Levine and coworkers[316] also found one patient with anti-I^T in whom overt hemolytic anemia was not present, but reported two additional cases with anti-I^T in patients who did have active hemolysis.

AIHA caused by cold agglutinins of anti-I^T specificity have also been reported by Postoway and coworkers[343] and by Ramos and coworkers.[344] In both cases the cold agglutinin reacted with cord (i) > adult (I) > adult (i). The patient reported by Postoway and coworkers[343] was a 73-year-old woman with non-Hodgkin's lymphoma who developed hemolytic anemia with a positive DAT caused by C3. A cold agglutinin was present that reacted to a titer of 256 against cord RBCs and was reactive up to 37°C. The patient reported by Ramos and coworkers[344] was a 54-year-old man who had progressively severe cold AIHA for 9 months. The DAT was weakly positive for IgM and C3d, and the serum gave a bi-thermic ("Donath-Landsteiner–like") reaction and contained a cold agglutinin with wide thermal amplitude and anti-I^TP specificity, reacting to a titer of 640 against cord cells. The patient was treated aggressively but died of sepsis during an unsuccessful trial of chlorambucil. Autopsy revealed disseminated non-Hodgkin's lymphoma.

TABLE 3-19. SUMMARY OF THE CHARACTERISTICS OF 16 PATIENTS WITH NON-HODGKIN'S LYMPHOMA AND AUTOIMMUNE HEMOLYTIC ANEMIA

	n (%)
Age (yr)	
Median	68
Range	33–82
Sex	
Male	4 (25)
Female	12 (75)
Stage of NHL	
II	4 (25)
III	2 (12.5)
IV	10 (62.5)
AIHA	
Warm	13 (81)
Cold	3 (19)
Serum Ig	
IgG	5 (31)
IgM	4 (25)
Median time of response for NHL (days)	65
Median time of response for AIHA (days)	9
Follow-up (mos)	
Median	14.5
Range	3–38

From Sallah S, Sigoumas G, Vos P, Wan JY, Nguyen NP: Autoimmune hemolytic anemia in patients with non-Hodgkin's lymphoma: Characteristics and significance. Ann Oncol 2000;11:1571–1577.

Non-Hodgkin's Lymphomas. The association between AIHA and non-Hodgkin's lymphoma (NHL) has been described in both B- and T-cell disorders. Sallah and coworkers[345] found AIHA in 16 of 501 patients (3%) with NHL. (Patients with small lymphocytic lymphoma and angioimmunoblastic lymphadenopathy with dysproteinemia were excluded from their analysis.) A similar prevalence was reported by Gronbaek and coworkers.[346] The occurrence of AIHA was not statistically significant among the four stages of NHL ($P = 0.722$).[345] In comparison with the cohort of 501 patients with NHL evaluated during the study period, patients with NHL and AIHA were more likely to have T-cell NHL (33% versus 14%; $P = 0.047$), as has also been reported by other investigators.[347,348]

Sallah and coworkers described the clinical, laboratory, and pathologic features of their 16 patients with NHL and AIHA (Table 3-19). They found that the diagnosis of AIHA preceded that of NHL in nine patients, while in seven patients AIHA occurred either at the time of diagnosis of NHL or during the course of the disease. Resolution of the AIHA was achieved in 14 patients at a median time of only 9 days. However, AIHA subsequently recurred in six patients. In five of these patients, the recurrence of AIHA coincided with that of NHL, while in one patient, it reappeared shortly after splenectomy and during hospitalization for sepsis. Both NHL and AIHA were refractory to chemotherapy in two of the three patients with cold agglutinin disease. The patients with NHL who did not develop AIHA had better overall survival and median survival compared with the NHL/AIHA group ($P = 0.006$ and $P = 0.0001$, respectively) (Fig. 3-7)

CAS in Non-Hodgkin's Lymphoma. Although patients with CAS constitute the minority of cases of secondary AIHA in NHL, a number of reports have emphasized this association.[349-355] Isbister and coworkers[356] described four patients with lymphoproliferative disorders who developed severe CAS. In three of the patients, the cold antibody was in low titer (8 to 64) at 4°C, but had a wide thermal range (30°C to 37°C); the fourth patient's cold antibody was present to a titer of 2084 at 4°C. In two patients, the antibody was a panagglutinin, and in the other two, including the patient with a high titer antibody, the specificity was anti-I. Despite a fulminant hemolytic presentation in all four cases, resolution of hemolysis occurred after splenectomy or corticosteroid therapy.

Economopoulos and coworkers[351] reviewed 370 patients with NHL and found that 23 (6.2%) had AIHA, 4 of whom (1.1%) had cold-reacting antibodies. These cases were all associated with IgM-κ serum paraproteins, and the specificity of the autoantibody was anti-I in three of the four cases. All of the patients had low-grade lymphomas with splenomegaly and bone marrow involvement, and all had profound hemolytic anemia. Three of the four patients responded to glucocorticoids and alkylating agents, whereas the fourth patient responded poorly and died with generalized lymphoma and active AIHA. Pascali[352] observed CAS in 3 of 62 (4.8%) patients with NHL. Monoclonal IgM-λ proteins were present in two patients and IgM-κ in the other.

Also, see Waldenström's Macroglobulinemia (page 113).

Development of Lymphoproliferative Disorders as a Complication of AIHA. Sallah and coworkers[357] evaluated 107 patients with idiopathic or secondary AIHA and found that 19 (18%) eventually developed malignant lymphoproliferative disorders. The median time to develop malignancy was 26.5 months (range, 9 to 76 months). Using multivariate analysis, advanced age ($P = 0.005$), underlying autoimmune diseases ($P = 0.002$), and the presence of serum gammopathy ($P = 0.45$) were risk factors for future development of lymphoproliferative disorders in these patients. Also, serum monoclonal IgM protein was a significant predictor ($P = 0.0001$). More than one third of the patients in this study had underlying autoimmune diseases, and immunosuppression had been used on an intermittent or continuous basis to manage immune phenomena in these patients. Thus, it is possible that immunosuppressants potentiate the risk of lymphoproliferative disorders in a subset of patients with AIHA and autoimmune disorders.

A further case was reported by Jasty and coworkers,[358] who described a 9-month-old boy who had Evans's syndrome and was treated with IVIG and corticosteroids. The infant eventually had recurrent fevers, hepatosplenomegaly, pulmonary nodules, and parenchymal central nervous system lesions. Results of a lung biopsy revealed a polyclonal lymphoproliferative disease, and polymerase chain reaction analysis showed the presence of the EBV genome in the lung nodules. The infant died from progressive lung disease 6 months after the initial symptoms of Evans's syndrome.

Chaplin[359] described two patients who had had CAS for 10 and 7½ years, respectively, before developing malignant lymphomas. Both patients had

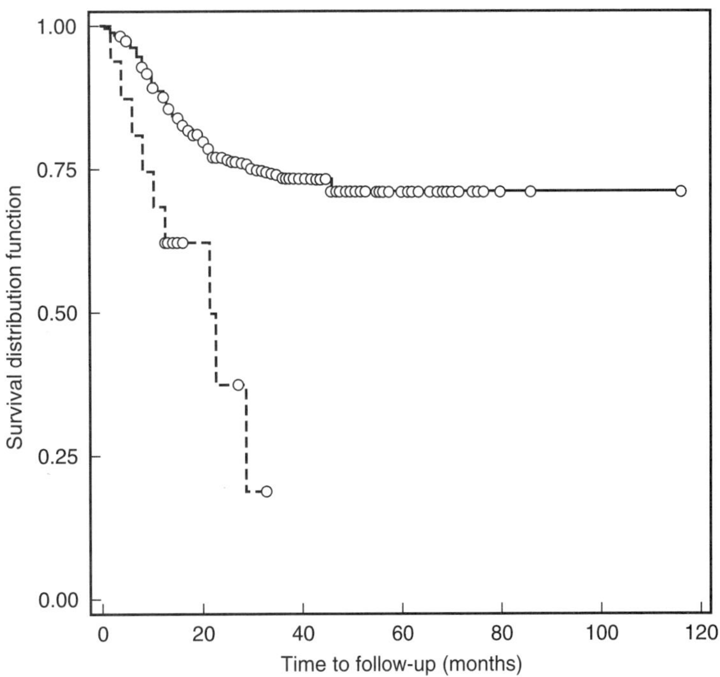

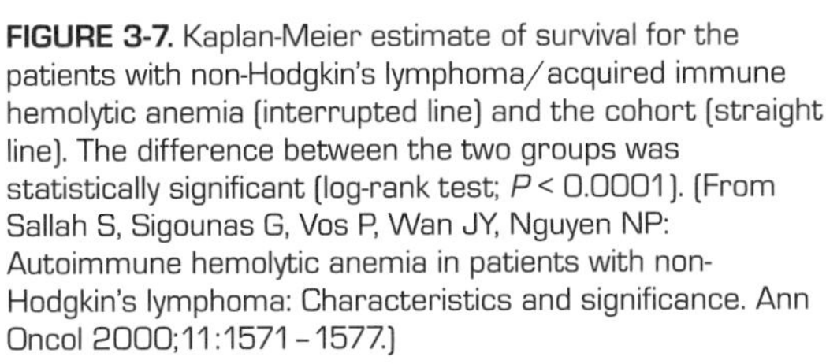
FIGURE 3-7. Kaplan-Meier estimate of survival for the patients with non-Hodgkin's lymphoma/acquired immune hemolytic anemia (interrupted line) and the cohort (straight line). The difference between the two groups was statistically significant (log-rank test; $P < 0.0001$). (From Sallah S, Sigounas G, Vos P, Wan JY, Nguyen NP: Autoimmune hemolytic anemia in patients with non-Hodgkin's lymphoma: Characteristics and significance. Ann Oncol 2000;11:1571–1577.)

received chlorambucil as treatment for their hemolytic anemia, with the cumulative doses being 14.0 and 6.6 g. Otto and coworkers[360] described the development, in a 66-year-old man who had had CAS of IgM-κ type for about 11 years, of increasing numbers of malignant cells in his bone marrow. The findings were interpreted as indicating a slow but progressive change toward malignancy. Kamiyama and coworkers[361] described two patients who developed NHL 7½ and 8 years, respectively, after having initially presented with AIHA.

SYSTEMIC LUPUS ERYTHEMATOSUS

Approximately 8% of patients with WAIHA have SLE.[22] Conversely, about 10% of patients with SLE have AIHA.[22,362-369] Budman and Steinberg[370] reported that the DAT was positive in 18% to 65% of patients in various published series of patients with SLE, but only about 10% of these patients had clinically significant hemolysis. When the DAT was positive in a patient whose SLE was quiescent, it was positive with anti-C sera but negative with anti-IgG sera; in patients with overt hemolysis, the DAT was more commonly positive with both anti-C and anti-IgG sera. Rarely, the DAT was positive only with anti-IgG serum. Mongan and coworkers[371] reported similar findings.

AIHA may be the sole presenting sign of SLE and predate the appearance of other disease manifestations by several years.[370,372-374] Videbaek,[374] for instance, cited patients in whom AIHA was present for 2, 3, and 6 years, respectively, before SLE was diagnosed. More commonly, although hemolytic anemia is the dominant feature from the onset, symptoms suggestive of SLE are also present from the start of the patient's illness. In other cases, at least some of the signs and symptoms of SLE are established before the onset of clear-cut hemolytic anemia.[243] Pirofsky[2] reported a simultaneous onset of SLE and AIHA in five of his patients, preexisting SLE in six, and AIHA antedating the onset of SLE in four patients, with the mean interval being 34 months. In some cases anemia may be minimal and the symptoms of SLE dominate the clinical picture; in other cases the reverse is true.[243]

Kokori and coworkers[22] reported 50 episodes of AIHA in 41 patients with SLE. They found that AIHA occurred as the initial disease manifestation in 27 of the patients (66%). A second hemolytic episode occurred in seven patients (of whom six had presented with AIHA), and a third episode occurred in two patients (of whom one had presented with AIHA). The time to recurrence was not affected significantly by any of the measured immunologic or clinical characteristics of SLE.

Typically, the RBC autoantibodies have been reported to be warm ones. The warm antibodies appear to differ significantly in their serologic reactions from those found in most cases of AIHA of idiopathic origin in that they characteristically fix complement and there has been no evident specificity.[243] Although most cases of AIHA in SLE are associated with warm autoantibodies, Nair and coworkers[375] reported a woman with CAS that developed during the course of SLE. The cold antibody titer was 4096 and the autoantibody had anti-I specificity.

A low level of serum complement is commonly found in SLE. As shown in Table 3-20, the level was low or very low in six out of seven cases tested among a series of patients reported by Dacie.[243]

It is not certain whether AIHA portends a more benign or more severe prognosis for patients with SLE. Two studies found that AIHA was associated with increased mortality,[367,376] but AIHA was not an independent predictor of mortality once other manifestations (e.g., thrombocytopenia and renal disease) were taken into account. Other studies either found no association of AIHA with adverse outcomes or suggested that it may be associated with a more benign course.[22,364,366]

Antiphospholipid Syndrome. AIHA can also be part of the antiphospholipid syndrome (APS), which is characterized by arterial and venous thrombosis, recurrent pregnancy loss, and thrombocytopenia in the presence of antiphospholipid antibodies (aPL).[377,378] These antibodies are identified as lupus anticoagulant (LAC), which prolongs phospholipid-dependent coagulation tests, or as aCL detected by immunoassays. This entity, first described by Hughes in 1983 in patients with SLE,[379] may also appear in patients with no underlying disease, and such patients are diagnosed as having primary APS.

There are well-documented associations between aPL and abnormalities of specific cellular components of the blood, such as thrombocytopenia, hemolytic anemia, and leukopenia.[378] Win and coworkers[380] tested 474,545 normal blood donors and identified 42 with a positive DAT and observed 3 with positive DATs and false-positive VDRL tests, all of whom expressed raised levels of aPL. Moreover, some studies have demonstrated a significant correlation between aCL or LAC and DAT-positive hemolytic anemia in patients with SLE.[381-386] The hemolytic anemia of SLE was found to be associated with IgM aCL, IgG aCL, or aCL of both isotypes.[381,383,384] However, the role of the aCL in the pathogenesis of AIHA is not precisely understood.[381,387]

Kokori et al.[22] found that patients with AIHA, compared with SLE patients with other causes of anemia, were more likely to have elevated titers of IgG aCL (odds ratio [OR] = 5.8; 95% CI, 1.4 to 24) and thrombosis (OR = 4.6; 95% CI, 1.0 to 21). AIHA at the onset of SLE was independently associated with renal involvement (OR = 5.4; 95% CI, 1.0 to 28), thrombocytopenia (OR = 7.3; 95% CI, 1.1 to 48), and possibly thrombotic episodes during follow-up (OR = 11; 95% CI, 0.8 to 160) compared with controls who had other types of anemia at the onset of SLE.

Fong and coworkers[388] determined aCL levels in 17 Asian female SLE patients with AIHA and 29 Asian female SLE patients without AIHA. Both IgG and IgM isotypes were measured by ELISA. Elevated IgM

TABLE 3-20. SEROLOGIC DATA IN 15 CASES OF AUTOIMMUNE HEMOLYTIC ANEMIA ASSOCIATED WITH SYSTEMIC LUPUS ERYTHEMATOSUS

		Antiglobulin Test			Agglutination				Lysis			
		Direct			Normal RBCs (titer)		Papainized Normal RBCs (titer)	Papainized PNH RBCs	Papainized PNH RBCs	Papainized Normal RBCs		
Patient	Age (yr)/ Sex	Anti-γ G	Anti-non-γ†	Indirect 37°C	2–4°C	20°C	37°C	37°C	37°C	Stored 37°C	Fresh 37°C	Remarks
1	29/F	++	†	–	16	4	4	–	–	–	–	Complement* 21 units
2	17/F	+++	†	++	16	4	16	–	++	+	+	Complement 15 units; anticoagulant present
3	10/F	++	†	+	128	4	4	–	+	–	–	Complement 7 units
4	24/F	++	†	–	16	1	4	+++			–	
5	23/F	++	†	–	16	<1	4	–	+	+	+	Complement 104 units
6	26/F	+++	+	+	8	1	64	++		–	–	Complement 16 units
7	13/M	++	+	–	1	<1	1	–	+++	+	±	Complement 57 units
8	14/F	+++	++	–	1	<1	4					Anticoagulant present
9	15/F	++++	++++	++	16	1	4	+	+++	+++	+	Complement 45 units
10	52/M	–	±	–	<4	<1	1	–	+±	+±	–	
11	25/F	+++	+++	++	8	<1	8	++	+++	++	±	
12	40/F	++	+±	–	. . .	<1	4	–	±	–	–	
13	19/F	+++	+++	++	256	4	64			++		
14	24/F	+++	+++	–	16	<1	8			++±		
15	22/F	++±	++±	++++	4	1	16			++		

* Normal range of serum complement activity = 70–150 units.
† Specific anti–non-γ serum was not used, but the reaction was only partially inhibited by the addition of human γ-globulin to the antiglobulin serum.
Modified from Dacie JV: The Haemolytic Anaemias, 3rd ed. vol. 3, Secondary or Symptomatic Haemolytic Anaemias. New York: Churchill Livingstone, 1995.

titers were seen in 11 (64.7%) AIHA patients and 6 (20.7%) control patients ($P < 0.01$). There was no significant difference in IgG aCL titers between the two groups.

Arvieux and coworkers[389] studied sera from patients with SLE to determine the relationship of their antiphospholipid activity to their anti-RBC and complement activation properties. Forty-nine percent of the sera had aPL as demonstrated by ELISA. A cellular radioimmunoassay was used for the detection of immunoglobulin and C3 binding to erythrocytes. The authors found that the levels of IgG aPL correlated with hypocomplementemia and with immunoglobulin binding, and they concluded that some aPL subsets may bind to RBCs, thus accounting for the observed association of these antibodies with positive DATs.

Hazeltine and coworkers[382] detected aCL in 14 of 65 patients (22%) with SLE using an ELISA method. Both aCL and LAC activity were associated with positive DATs and low serum C4 levels. Analysis of RBC eluates and absorption studies suggested that some aCL may act as anti-RBC antibodies, likely directed at membrane phospholipid epitopes.

Davidyuk and coworkers[390] analyzed the plasma from patients with APS for their effect on the growth of allogeneic hematopoietic precursor cells using a microtiter colony assay. They found that the IgG fractions from four patients' plasma demonstrated enhanced BFU-E growth inhibitory activity and concluded that IgG autoantibodies reacting with immature RBC elements may be present in patients with APS but that further study was necessary to determine their role, if any, in the anemia frequently seen in this disorder.

Antiphospholipid Antibodies in Idiopathic AIHA. In addition to patients who have AIHA in association with SLE, isolated cases have been reported of apparently idiopathic AIHA associated with aPL. Cabral and coworkers[385] reported the presence of IgM aPL antibodies in serum and on the RBCs of a patient with idiopathic AIHA during the time of hemolysis but not when hemolysis abated. They demonstrated that purified IgM antibody could bind to bromelain-treated RBCs and induce complement-mediated lysis, suggesting a pathogenic role for the antibody. Subsequently, similar cases have been reported by other investigators.[389,391-393]

Guzman and coworkers[394] studied by ELISA the presence of aPL in sera from 18 patients with idiopathic AIHA and 14 patients with nonautoimmune hemolysis. They found IgM anticardiolipin antibodies in four AIHA patients and none of the patients with nonautoimmune hemolysis. Also, IgG aCL were detected in six patients with AIHA and in one patient with nonautoimmune hemolysis. The authors suggested that the aPL do not represent a secondary phenomenon caused by the release of membrane components but rather that they may play a role in the autoimmune hemolytic process.

Lang and coworkers[392] studied aCL (IgG and IgM) by ELISA in 74 SLE patients without AIHA, 22 SLE patients with AIHA, 50 patients with idiopathic WAIHA, 52 patients with cold antibody AIHA, and 50 healthy controls. They found that the mean IgG and IgM aCL titers in SLE patients without AIHA were significantly elevated compared with the values in healthy controls, and the mean aCL levels in SLE patients with AIHA were higher than in SLE patients without AIHA. Interestingly, the mean aCL levels of patients with both warm and cold idiopathic AIHA were also significantly elevated compared with healthy controls. On the basis of these data, the authors speculated that aCL are involved in the pathogenesis of autoantibody-induced RBC destruction per se irrespective on an underlying SLE.

Latagliata and coworkers[393] reported a case of APS that presented with the clinical and laboratory signs of AIHA in the absence of manifestations typically related to APS. The diagnosis of APS was made only after the occurrence of a sudden severe heart failure due to an intraventricular thrombus requiring a surgical approach. The authors suggested that an accurate thrombophilic screening is warranted in patients with apparently idiopathic AIHA.

On the basis of these studies, one may suggest that aPL antibodies may identify a subgroup of AIHA patients different from those characterized by antibodies directed against Rh-related polypeptides, band-3 glycoprotein, and other membrane proteins.[395-397]

The therapy of AIHA associated with aPL antibodies is similar to that of idiopathic AIHA. Font and coworkers[378] emphasized the usefulness of splenectomy in the treatment of refractory cytopenias (AIHA and/or thrombocytopenia) associated with aPL, with a high rate of response after follow-up and no postoperative complications in reported cases.[378,398]

COLLAGEN DISORDERS OTHER THAN SLE

A number of cases describing the association of AIHA and rheumatoid arthritis have been reported.[232,399-404] However, Estrata and coworkers[232] reported that the incidence of AIHA in patients with rheumatoid arthritis has not been shown to exceed that in the general population. Also, the prevalence of rheumatoid arthritis in patients with AIHA approximates that in the general population. On the basis of these data, it is difficult to establish a relationship between AIHA and rheumatoid arthritis.[232] Similarly, there are occasional case reports of AIHA in association with scleroderma.[404-414]

THYMOMA

Thymoma, occasionally in association with pure red cell aplasia, has been reported to occur in patients with AIHA, and thymectomy has been reported to be beneficial in some such patients (see Chapter 11).

AIHA AND CARCINOMA

Although there are a number of reports of both AIHA and carcinoma in the same subject,[415-429] the association is uncommon, and the question arises as to whether it is a chance event. Sokol and coworkers[213] analyzed the incidence of RBC autoantibodies (with or without active hemolysis) and carcinoma in a region with a general population of 4,662,500, and concluded that the association was highly significant ($P < 0.0005$). Patients with RBC autoantibodies and confirmed carcinoma were found together 12 to 13 times more often than expected from their relative frequencies. Autoantibodies occurred with a wide variety of carcinomas, with the relative incidence largely reflecting tumor incidence (Table 3-21). Further evidence for an association derives from reports of remission of the AIHA with removal of the tumor,[2,252,419,423-425,427,428,430-432] and its relapse with the appearance of metastases[425,431,433]; on specific absorption of autoantibody by tumor cells[430]; on a close temporal relation of onset of both diseases[434]; and on unusual age at presentation.[434]

Sokol and coworkers[213] reviewed findings in 160 patients with carcinoma and autoantibodies, 86 of whom had hemolysis (Table 3-22). All serologic types of autoantibody were found, and the ratio of warm:cold/mixed types (7:3:1) was similar to that generally found in large series of patients with AIHA. They found that 37 (43%) had metastatic disease and 28 died within a few months of presentation. These findings suggest that RBC autoantibodies occur when there is a large tumor mass and metastatic disease, and therefore portend a poor prognosis.

AIHA AFTER VACCINATION

Active immunization stimulates the immune system to produce antigen-specific humoral and cellular immunity.[435] Because autoimmune diseases also involve the stimulation of the immune system against certain antigens in the individual, it is not surprising that some concerns have arisen as to whether immunizations may lead to the development of autoimmune diseases. A temporal association between an influenza vaccine program in the United States in 1976 and an epidemic of Guillain-Barré syndrome caused interest to be focused on the vaccine-autoimmunity cause-effect relationship. The incidence of Guillain-Barré syndrome in the vaccinated population was 5 to 6 times higher than in the nonvaccinated population.[436] More recent examples of such concerns range from whether hepatitis B immunization causes multiple sclerosis to whether early infant immunization may cause type 1 diabetes mellitus.[435] Evidence for immunizations leading to autoimmune diseases come from several sources including animal studies, single and multiple case reports, and epidemiologic studies. On the other hand, Offit and Hackett[436a] have indicated that well-controlled epidemiologic studies do not support the hypothesis that vaccines cause chronic autoimmune disease.

The only hematologic disease for which there are substantial data suggesting that immunization may be causative in some cases is immune thrombocytopenia.[435,436] Nevertheless, the medical literature is filled with many case reports of a wide range of autoimmune illnesses temporally associated with vaccinations,[435] including cases of vaccination-associated immune hemolytic anemia.

TABLE 3-21. DETAILS OF PATIENTS WITH ERYTHROCYTE AUTOANTIBODIES AND CARCINOMA

Site of Primary Tumor	No. of Patients	M/F	Age Range (yr)	Median
Breast	20	0/20	44–85	67
Lung	18	15/3	43–83	68
Pharynx	1	1/0	45	
Esophagus	8	4/4	50–73	62
Stomach	12	9/3	66–89	72
Cecum	2	0/2	72–83	
Colon	15	6/9	64–92	76
Rectum	15	9/6	60–85	73
Liver	1	0/1	68	
Pancreas	7	2/5	61–81	64
Adrenal	1	1/0	44	
Kidney	3	2/1	37–79	69
Ureter	1	1/0	70	
Bladder	8	6/2	51–81	68
Prostate	14	14/0	56–83	71
Ovary	10	0/10	55–77	65
Uterus	3	0/3	59–67	65
Cervix	8	0/8	25–89	49
Skin and mucous membranes (squamous cell carcinoma)	5	2/3	62–73	69
Breast and colon (different histology)	1	0/1	51	
Unknown	7	4/3	40–71	64

Modified from Sokol RJ, Booker DJ, Stamps R: Erythrocyte autoantibodies, autoimmune haemolysis, and carcinoma. J Clin Pathol 1994;47:340–343.

TABLE 3-22. SEROLOGIC PATTERN OF ERYTHROCYTE AUTOANTIBODIES IN PATIENTS WITH CARCINOMA AND NUMBERS WITH EVIDENCE OF HEMOLYSIS

	Type of Erythrocyte Autoantibodies and No. of Patients (No. with Definite or Strong Evidence of Autoimmune Hemolysis)		
Size of Primary Tumor	**Warm**	**Cold**	**Mixed**
Breast	12 (11)	6 (4)	2 (2)
Lung	7 (6)	7 (3)	4 (4)
Pharynx	1 (0)	0 (0)	0 (0)
Esophagus	7 (1)	1 (0)	0 (0)
Stomach	9 (4)	2 (2*)	1 (1)
Cecum	1 (0)	0 (0)	1 (1)
Colon	9 (3)	5 (2)	1 (1)
Rectum	8 (7)	5 (5)	2 (2)
Liver	1 (0)	0 (0)	0 (0)
Pancreas	4 (1)	2 (2)	1 (1)
Adrenal	0 (0)	1 (1)	0 (0)
Kidney	2 (0)	0 (0)	1 (1)
Ureter	0 (0)	1 (0)	0 (0)
Bladder	6 (4)	2 (0)	0 (0)
Prostate	10 (5)	3 (1)	1 (1)
Ovary	8 (4)	2 (0)	0 (0)
Uterus	2 (0)	1 (0)	0 (0)
Cervix	5 (0)	3 (0)	0 (0)
Skin and mucous membranes (squamous cell carcinoma)	3 (1)	1 (0)	1 (1)
Breast and colon	1 (0)	0 (0)	0 (0)
Unknown	3 (2)	4 (2)	0 (0)
Total	99 (49)	46 (22)	15 (15)

* In one patient, the autoantibody was of Donath-Landsteiner type and showed evidence of specificity within the P blood group system.
Modified from Sokol RJ, Booker DJ, Stamps R: Erythrocyte autoantibodies, autoimmune haemolysis, and carcinoma. J Clin Pathol 1994;47:340–343.

Warm Antibody AIHA after Vaccination. A number of cases of warm antibody AIHA in association with vaccination have been reported.[2,13,67,104,437-444] Among the earliest reported cases are those of Kobl,[437] who reported a case of AIHA after smallpox vaccination; the case reported by Dameshek and Schwartz,[438] which followed poliomyelitis vaccination; and that of Pirofsky,[2] which occurred after vaccination with a live measles preparation.

More recently, Downes and coworkers[443] reported a patient who developed fatal AIHA after DPT vaccination and summarized the reports of seven previously reported cases. Including the authors' patient, these cases included 3 girls and 5 boys ranging in age from 6 weeks to 7 years. Hemolytic anemia occurred in two patients after the first vaccine, in four patients after the second vaccine, and in one patient after the third vaccine. Onset of hemolysis after vaccination ranged from 5 days to 6 weeks. Admission hemoglobin levels ranged from 2.3 to 9.4 g/dL (median, 4.90 g/dL). Time to recovery ranged from 3 weeks to 4 months. The authors' patient was admitted to the hospital in extremis with a hemoglobin of 2.3 g/dL and disseminated intravascular coagulation and was the only patient who had a fatal outcome.

Olcay and coworkers[67] reported a 4-month-old girl who had received BCG vaccination when 2 months old, and DPT and oral polio vaccines at 2 and again at 3 months of age. AIHA developed 1 month later, at which time the patient was admitted to the hospital with a hemoglobin of 2.7 g/dL, a hematocrit of 8.5%, and a reticulocyte count of 0.2%. She received multiple transfusions and did not respond to methylprednisolone therapy of 7 days' duration but was successfully treated with a combination of immunosuppressive therapy consisting of cyclophosphamide, 6-mercaptopruine, intravenous immunoglobulin, and prednisolone. The authors did not find an increase in the patient's reticulocyte count (maximum, 0.8%) during multiple determinations during the subsequent 19 weeks even though the hemoglobin improved to between 12 and 13.4 g/dL.

Seltsam and coworkers[444] reported a 20-month-old girl who developed hemolytic anemia 2 weeks after her third inoculation with oral polio vaccine. She recovered within 2 weeks, and 4 months later received DPT vaccine without incident. However, at age 27 months she developed exanthema and fever shortly after a combined vaccination against mumps, rubella, and measles. Two weeks later, she was admitted to the hospital because of jaundice, hemoglobinuria, and signs of hemolysis with a hemoglobin of 5.7 g/dL. The DAT was strongly positive for C3d at the time of the hemolytic episodes but not between the two episodes. However, no RBC antibodies were detected at any time. She was treated with antibiotics, prednisolone, and blood transfusions and recovered within 2 weeks.

A second patient reported by Seltsam and coworkers[444] was a 21-month-old boy with an uneventful medical history who was inoculated with a combination of six vaccines, including the fourth doses of DPT and *Hemophilus influenzae* vaccines, and the third against polio and hepatitis B. Four days later, he became pale and jaundiced and was admitted to the hospital with a hemoglobin of 3.7 g/dL. He was treated with prednisolone and recovered. The DAT was strongly positive using anti-IgG, and weakly positive using anti-C3d. The authors give few serologic details stating only that the IAT was positive with RBCs tested (11 panel cells) and at a follow-up 4 months later RBC antibodies were not detected in the serum or eluate.

Other Types of AIHA after Vaccination. Martinez and Domingo[445] reported a case of Evans's syndrome apparently triggered by recombinant hepatitis B vaccine. Two days after receiving his second dose of hepatitis B vaccine, a 33-year-old man, who was a chronic HbsAg carrier, presented with acute abdominal pain, polyarthralgia affecting his hands and feet, chills, and fever. He had had no reaction to the first dose of vaccine. His hemoglobin was 5.0 g/dL, the reticulocyte count was 20%, and the platelet count was 11,000/μL. The DAT was positive using anti-IgG and anti-C3 sera. The authors did not report the presence or absence of red cell antibodies but did find circulating immune complexes and IgG platelet-bound antibodies suggesting an immune mechanism for the thrombocytopenia. The patient was treated with corticosteroids and recovered over a period of 2 months.

Bunch and coworkers[169] described a 19-month-old girl who, 6 weeks before her admission, was immunized with live attenuated measles vaccine. Three weeks later she developed a mild illness with a morbilliform rash, conjunctivitis, and rhinorrhea, and during the next week she also developed hemoglobinuria. On admission the hemoglobin was 3.3 g/dL, reticulocytes 5%, and platelets 498,000/μL. The DAT was strongly positive. A diagnosis of paroxysmal cold hemoglobinuria was made because the serum contained a typical Donath-Landsteiner antibody characterized as a biphasic, complement-fixing IgG antibody with anti-P specificity. The antibody sensitized RBCs up to 25°C. Syphilis was excluded by negative Wassermann reactions and VDRL screening tests in the patient and both of her parents. The measles complement-fixing antibody titer was high at a level of 128. The patient was kept warm and transfused with RBCs warmed to approximately 37°C. The DAT and Donath-Landsteiner tests became negative within 1 week and she recovered promptly and completely.

Comments. Immune hemolysis after vaccination is very rare, and serologic evidence suggesting a relationship of the AIHA to the vaccine has been reported only once. Haneberg and coworkers[441] reported antibodies to tetanus and diphtheria toxoids and pertussis in heat eluates from one infant suggesting that these antibodies were bound to the RBCs. However, available data are certainly insufficient to indicate either the presence or absence of a causal relationship between vaccination and hemolytic anemia.[446]

Although the reported cases could all be coincidental because vaccination is such a common event, a cause-and-effect relationship cannot be ruled out.

AIHA AND INFECTIOUS AGENTS

Although AIHA in association with upper respiratory infections and unspecified "viral" syndromes or "flu-like illness" is common, the incidence of AIHA after well-documented specific infections is relatively uncommon. In the series of 1223 patients reported by Sokol and Hewitt,[208] infectious mononucleosis and mycoplasma pneumonia were the only two infectious diseases that were documented in more than three patients. Nevertheless, there are well-documented instances in which viral, bacterial, parasitic, and other infectious agents have been associated with immune hemolytic anemia. (Infections associated with PCH were reviewed earlier.)

There are a number of mechanisms by which infections may result in hemolysis on an immune basis.[447,448] Among these are that the infection may result in the production of either cold- or warm-reacting RBC autoantibodies; antibody-antigen complexes specifically related to the infectious agent may coat the RBCs, which then act as an "innocent bystander"; the infectious agent may result in exposure of RBC antigens, which are normally hidden, to naturally occurring antibodies (polyagglutination).

Seitz and coworkers,[448] using an immunofluorescence test, studied 96 children with hemolytic anemia and found that the RBC membrane was altered in vivo in a majority of patients by nonspecific adsorption of foreign material released from infectious microorganisms. In addition, additive binding of complement was detectable by the antiglobulin test. Accordingly, they suggested the adsorption of microbial antigens to the RBC surface as one of the causes for RBC destruction during infection-associated hemolytic anemia.

Additional details regarding the mechanisms by which autoantibodies are produced in response to viral infection have been reviewed by Morrow and coworkers[449] and by Meite and coworkers.[450] Experimental data have suggested that viruses trigger an autoimmune humoral response by a number of distinct mechanisms, including polyclonal B-lymphocyte activation, antigenic mimicry, modification of self-antigen, production of anti-idiotypic antibodies, or enhancement of major histocompatibility complex molecule expression on potential antigen-presenting cells. They also presented data indicating that viruses can trigger the onset of AIHA by enhancing the pathogenicity of autoantibodies. This observation may indicate how different viruses can trigger similar clinical autoimmune diseases.[450]

Specificity of Autoantibodies in AIHA Secondary to Infectious Agents. In postinfection cold antibody AIHAs, there is a striking relation between the specificity of the cold antibody and the underlying infectious agent.[451] Cold antibodies of anti-I specificity are found in infections with *M. pneumoniae,* whereas cold antibodies of anti-i specificity frequently occur in infections with EBV. AIHA associated with varicella or rubella infections have commonly been reported to have anti-Pr specificity. However, exceptions to these findings have also been reported, as indicated later.

***Mycoplasma pneumoniae* Infections.** A rise in the cold agglutinin titer occurs frequently after *M. pneumoniae* infection. From 33% to 76% of patients with *M. pneumoniae* infection have a cold agglutinin titer greater than 64 or have a fourfold or greater increase in titer during convalescence.[452,453] An acute cold agglutinin response is sometimes seen in viral infections such as influenza A and infectious mononucleosis, but very high titers are seen almost exclusively in mycoplasma infections. Usually the magnitude of the cold agglutinin response is related to the clinical severity of the pneumonia,[452-454] although severe anemia has been reported in association with clinically mild pneumonia.[455]

Although overt hemolytic anemia is uncommon in patients with *M. pneumoniae* infection, subclinical hemolysis may be rather common as indicated by the fact that a significant fall in hemoglobin concentration (>2 g/dL) has been observed in 12.8% of patients in one series,[456] and elevated reticulocyte counts (>2%) were found in 64% of infections.[457] A small minority of patients respond to the infection in an exaggerated way, that is, they produce cold antibodies of unusually high titer and which react at an unusually high temperature.[458] When hemolytic anemia occurs in association with *M. pneumoniae* infection, it does so usually in the second or third week of the patient's illness. The patient may already be recovered from his respiratory infection, but becomes ill once more with increasing pallor and jaundice.[459] A rapid onset of hemolysis is frequently observed, and abnormal IgM cold agglutinins (which characteristically have anti-I specificity) are present. Exposure to cold may precipitate hemolysis.[109] The hemolysis may be severe,[460] and even life threatening.[455] Splenomegaly is generally present; acrocyanosis and hemoglobinuria are unusual,[2] although massive hemoglobinuria with acute intravascular hemolysis has been reported.[461] Gangrene of the extremities is rare but has been well described in the older medical literature.[462-465] Other unusual manifestations of the disease are renal failure,[466-468] nephrotic syndrome,[469] mucocutaneous lesions including erythema multiforme and Stevens-Johnson syndrome,[470] disseminated intravascular coagulation, myocarditis, pericarditis, myositis, polyarthritis, meningoencephalitis, cranial and peripheral neuropathy, hepatitis, and pancreatitis.[471]

In recent years postmycoplasma hemolytic anemia seems to have been reported less frequently.[459] In part this may be due to the fact that the disorder is no longer the novelty it was in earlier years, but also, effective antibiotic treatment of the infection has perhaps diminished the incidence of hemolysis. Nevertheless, case reports continue to appear in the medical literature.[455,470,472-474]

Hemolysis is self-limiting and usually resolves in 2 to 3 weeks. However, the hemolytic anemia may proceed at an alarming rate and, indeed, fatalities have been reported.[475,476]

Although AIHA associated with *M. pneumoniae* infection is almost always caused by cold agglultinins, Louie and coworkers[477] reported a patient with severe hemolysis who had both a high titer, high thermal amplitude cold agglutinin, and an IgG warm agglutinin. The DAT was strongly positive with anti-IgG and anti-C3, and the patient's hemolysis persisted despite declining thermal amplitude and titer of the cold agglutinin. The DAT remained positive with anti-IgG, and there was an excellent response to prednisone, leading the authors to conclude that the warm IgG antibody was responsible for the patient's AIHA.

Mechanism of Development of Anti-I in* Mycoplasma pneumoniae *Infection. The cold agglutinin produced in response to human infection with *M. pneumoniae,* as well as the antibody found in idiopathic CAS, usually have specificity for the blood group I antigen contained in red cell glycoproteins. The mechanism by which cold agglutinins are elicited by *M. pneumoniae* has been studied by several groups of investigators. One proposed mechanism is that the organism itself possesses an I-like antigen that stimulates the formation of cross-reacting anti-I antibodies. An alternative hypothesis is that the organism acts on and modifies the I antigen on the RBC membrane so that it becomes unusually autoantigenic. Evidence has been presented to support both hypotheses.

Schmidt and coworkers[478] found that 18 of 25 strains of mycoplasma blocked or destroyed the I antigen receptors on normal RBCs as judged by subsequent agglutinability of the cells by an anti-I present in the serum of an I-negative individual. These investigators also inoculated 27 volunteers with *M. pneumoniae* vaccine and found that the thermal amplitude of anti-I in their serum was increased in 12 and the titer of the anti-I was increased in 4.[479] Feizi and coworkers[480] found that 9 of 28 (32%) rabbits inoculated with OI cells and *M. pneumoniae* developed fourfold or greater rises in cold-agglutinin titers. Loomes and coworkers[481] suggested that anti-I antibodies might arise in *M. pneumoniae* infection in response to a modification of the "self"-antigen-I as a result of its interaction with the organism. They reported that the interaction of *M. pneumoniae* with human erythrocytes is mediated by long chain oligosaccharides of sialic acid joined by alpha 2-3 linkage to the terminal galactose residues of poly-*N*-acetyllactosamine sequences of Ii antigen type.

In contrast, several groups of investigators presented evidence that *M. pneumoniae* does bear an I-like antigen. Costea and coworkers[353,482] injected suspensions of *M. pneumoniae* into rabbits and found that they stimulated the formation of cold agglutinins. They also reported that the cold agglutinins thus formed reacted with the micro-organism as well as with the animals' RBCs. This group of investigators also found that, although intact *M. pneumoniae* organisms were unable to absorb cold agglutinins from the sera of patients who had mycoplasma pneumonia, a mycoplasma lipopolysaccharide was able to reduce titers sixfold or more. They concluded that the antigens in *M. pneumoniae* with which cold agglutinins react are hidden in the organism's limiting membrane and that the development of cold agglutinins in man is due to immunization by cross-reacting antigens.[483] These conclusions were supported by the later work of Lind[484] and Janney and coworkers.[485]

Management. Management includes keeping the patient warm. This is particularly important since chilling is likely to cause an increase in hemolysis.[108,109,459] In patients with severe anemia, the hospital room should be warmed to as high a temperature as is tolerable, and mittens and warm slippers worn as well. One group even resorted to the use of a NASA space suit to provide constant warmth in a rare patient with profound disease.[486,486a] If blood transfusion becomes necessary, the principles and techniques reviewed for CAS in Chapter 10 should be followed. Corticosteroid therapy is usually not indicated because such therapy is generally ineffective in CAS and the hemolysis frequently is not severe and can be expected to subside spontaneously. Nevertheless, several patients with severe hemolytic anemia due to mycoplasma-induced cold agglutinin disease have responded to high-dose corticosteroids.[471,472,487,488]

Tetracycline, erythromycin, and other antibiotics are effective against *M. pneumoniae*,[489] but at the time hemolysis begins, the pneumonia may be resolved. Nevertheless, in some patients who delay seeking medical attention for their respiratory symptoms, antibiotic therapy has seemed to promptly resolve both the pneumonia and the hemolytic anemia (see Chapter 11).

Infectious Mononucleosis (Epstein-Barr Virus). Infectious mononucleosis is a common disorder, and AIHA developing during its course is a well-recognized entity. However, AIHA does not occur commonly, and Dacie and Worlledge[5] concluded that fewer than 1:1000 patients with infectious mononucleosis develop overt hemolysis. Einzig and Neerhout[490] pointed out that acute hemolytic anemia was not noted in five large series comprising 1113 patients. Other studies indicate an incidence of 2% to 3%.[491,492]

Clinical Findings. Acute pharyngitis often brings the patient to the physician. The classic features of the disorder are fever lasting up to 3 weeks or more, lymphadenopathy, splenomegaly, and florid, atypical lymphocytosis along with malaise that may be slow to resolve. Coupled with a positive heterophil antibody reaction or "Monospot test," these features are enough for diagnosis in most cases. The diagnosis is verified by the presence of EBV antibodies.[493]

Some of the clinical features of hemolytic anemia occurring in association with infectious mononucleosis are listed in Table 3-23. The signs of hemolysis usually develop 1 to 2 weeks after the onset of the illness, although in some cases features of infectious mononucleosis and hemolytic anemia develop simultaneously. Most of the patients who develop AIHA are at first acutely ill, with high fever, and then become weak, anemic, and jaundiced, and may have hemoglobinuria.[494,495] About 74% of patients have a palpable spleen and an enlarged liver.[496]

Anemia is usually mild and self-limiting,[497] although severe, life-threatening hemolysis has been reported.[495,497,498] The peripheral blood film may contain spherocytes and, in unusual instances, autoagglutination and erythrophagocytosis.[499] The WBC count is generally above normal and a varying, but often large, proportion of the cells are abnormal lymphocytes typical of infectious mononucleosis.

Palanduz and coworkers[500] reported a 7-year-old girl who developed AIHA and fulminant hepatic failure associated with EBV infection; the patient recovered after corticosteroids and supportive therapy.

Several patients have been described who developed signs of overt hemolysis during an attack of infectious mononucleosis and were subsequently found to have previously inapparent hereditary spherocytosis.[501-506] Except in the patient reported by DeNardo and Ray,[503] evidence of an autoimmune cause of the hemolysis was lacking. Instead, the hemolysis was attributed to the fact that infections, perhaps of any type, are a well-known cause of exacerbation of hemolysis in hereditary spherocytosis.

TABLE 3-23. CLINICAL FINDINGS IN HEMOLYTIC ANEMIA ASSOCIATED WITH INFECTIOUS MONONUCLEOSIS

Onset of hemolysis in relation to the onset of infectious mononucleosis	1 wk (28%)
	7–13 days (44%)
	14–21 days (15%)
	21 days (13%)
Duration of hemolysis	<1 mo (71%)
	1–2 mo (25%)
	>2 mo (4%)
Enlargement of spleen	Palpable (74%)
	Non palpable (26%)
Enlargement of liver	Palpable (74%)
	Non palpable (26%)

Serologic Findings. The DAT is generally positive, although some cases with a negative DAT have been described.[497,498] The sera often contain a cold antibody that agglutinates cord-blood RBCs more strongly than adult RBCs, that is, anti-i. In 1965, Jenkins and coworkers[507] and Calvo and coworkers[508] reported the first cases of hemolytic anemia in infectious mononucleosis apparently mediated by the temporary production of a high thermal amplitude cold agglutinin of anti-i specificity. The latter authors also described the presence of anti-i cold agglutinins in 23 of 38 uncomplicated cases of infectious mononucleosis. Other reports confirmed and extended these findings.[496,509-513]

However, the finding of anti-i of high thermal amplitude is not a uniform finding in patients with AIHA associated with infectious mononucleosis. Wilkinson and coworkers[514] reported three patients and emphasized how variable the antibody pattern might be. The serologic findings in the first patient were considered to be characteristic: his serum agglutinated cord i RBCs to a titer of 512 at 4°C and to titers of 64 at 22°C and 4 at 31°C; it also agglutinated adult I RBCs to a titer of 64 at 4°C and 2 at 22°C. The two other patients had formed anti-i antibodies, but they were of low titer at 4°C and did not cause agglutination at 22°C. The fact that the antibodies were not reactive at physiologic temperatures made it unlikely that they were the cause of the patients' AIHA. In none of the patients were warm autoantibodies detected.

Woodruff and McPherson[495] described a patient who had developed severe intravascular hemolysis. His serum agglutinated both i cord and I adult cells to titers at 4°C of 128 and 64, respectively; at room temperature, the titers were 16 and 32, and at 37°C, 0 and 4.

Lee and coworkers[515] suggested that the Lewis status of the patient is important in the development of hemolysis in infectious mononucleosis. They made this suggestion because of finding two patients with infectious mononucleosis and AIHA who were Le(a–b–), and two other patients with a history of infectious mononucleosis and AIHA who were Le(a–b–) and Le(a+b–), respectively. Of the four patients, three were nonsecretors and the fourth likely to be so. The authors pointed out that the Lewis status of these four patients varies significantly from that of other patients with uncomplicated infectious mononucleosis and from the known distribution of the Lewis type in the white population.

Bowman and coworkers[499] reported the presence of a potent cold-reacting auto-anti-N with increased thermal amplitude in the serum of a patient with severe immunohemolytic anemia after infectious mononucleosis.

Patients in whom the Donath-Landsteiner reaction has been positive have been reported by several groups of investigators.[176,177,516] Wishart and Davey[176] reported a 17-year-old male whose serum contained a high-thermal-amplitude cold antibody which agglutinated RBCs to a titer of 256 in the cold. The Donath-Landsteiner reaction was positive, and it remained so for at least 7 weeks. The antibody did not have any identifiable specificity. Burkhart and Hsu[177] described a 23-year-old man in whom the Donath-Landsteiner reaction was positive. The antibody in his serum was identified as anti-i and was an IgM globulin. The titer at 4°C with i (cord) RBCs was 16,384 and with I RBCs was 512. At 22°C the titer with the i RBCs was 64; at 32°C it was zero. The cold-warm (4°C to 37°C) procedure using i cells was positive to a titer of 64.

Management. Management of patients with AIHA associated with infectious mononucleosis is reviewed in Chapter 11. Of note here is the variable response to blood transfusion that has been reported. The patients of Silber and coworkers[497] and Tonkin and coworkers[498] had severe hemolysis, but no problems were encountered with blood transfusion. In contrast, Perkin and coworkers[517] reported that their patient received five units of compatible blood and had symptoms of a hemolytic transfusion reaction, including back pain, dyspnea, and fever. Furthermore, his hemoglobin concentration increased by only 3.4 g/dL.

Cytomegalovirus Infection. Zuelzer and associates[518,519] were among the first to emphasize the relationship between cytomegalovirus (CMV) infection and hemolytic anemia. They studied 22 children with CMV, 18 of whom had positive DATs, and concluded that the presence of CMV in immunohemolytic anemia was not fortuitous. They described an association between episodes of lymphadenitis due to CMV and periods of hemolysis. However, not all patients developed autoantibodies, and they suggested that RBC antibody production was a secondary phenomenon without clinical significance.

Subsequent reports of CMV infection with associated hemolytic anemia have also been variable regarding the presence or absence of RBC autoantibodies. Kantor and coworkers[520] recorded the clinical and immunologic findings in 10 patients who had developed postperfusion CMV infection; three of them developed transient hemolytic anemia. The DAT was positive in two of seven patients tested, and the cold agglutinin titer was raised to 512 and 2048 in two patients. Harris and coworkers[521] and van Spronsen and Breed[522] described patients with CMV-associated hemolytic anemia and thrombocytopenia, but DATs were negative and there were no RBC antibodies in the patients' sera.

Although hemolytic anemia with a positive DAT in association with spontaneous CMV infection is rare in adults, Salloum and Lundberg[523] reported two such patients and reviewed the findings in six patients reported by others.[524-527] Although the DAT was positive in all patients, serum antibodies were found in only two of the eight cases.[524,527] The authors suggested that the true incidence of immunohemolytic anemia associated with CMV infection may be underestimated because CMV serology is not routinely obtained as a part of hemolysis work-up. Subsequently, Gavazzi and coworkers[528] reported an unusual case of primary CMV infection manifested by severe hemolysis in an immunocompetent adult. The responsible mechanism for the hemolysis was unclear because no RBC antibodies were demonstrated and the DAT was positive "with a low titer" due to complement and IgG. The authors emphasized that severe, multiorgan CMV infection may occur even in immunocompetent adults,[529] but hemolysis seems to be rare even in these patients.

Horwitz and coworkers[527] reported two patients with hemolysis in previously healthy adults with CMV infections. In one patient, the DAT was positive using anti-IgG serum, but the only serum antibody was a weakly reactive low-molecular-weight cold agglutinin. In the other patient, the DAT was negative and no RBC autoantibodies were found. The authors reviewed data from 20 additional patients with CMV infection who had been studied in their laboratory during an 11-year period. They concluded that there had been evidence for subclinical hemolysis in at least 50% of patients. DATs had been carried out on 10 patients and were positive in only 3. Ten patients had cold-agglutinin titers of less than 56, but in no case was the thermal amplitude reported. The authors concluded that the mechanism responsible for hemolysis was obscure.

Dietz[530] reported a 21-year-old man who developed fever, fatigue, precordial chest pain, marked shortness of breath, and dyspnea on minimal exertion. He had enlarged lymph nodes in the inguinal and axillary areas, an enlarged liver, and a palpable spleen. CMV titers (determined by complement fixation) showed an increase from 8 to 512, and the titer of CMV-IgM antibodies was 128. Cultures of a buccal smear and of urine on human fibrobast monolayer medium grew CMV. He developed hemolytic anemia with a drop in hematocrit from 48.5% to 35% with a reticulocyte count of 8.5%. During the episode of hemolysis, the DAT was positive, but no results of tests for serum antibodies are described. Similarly, Berlin and coworkers[531] reported an adult woman who developed CMV and hemolytic anemia with the hemoglobin falling from 12.3 to 8.3 g/dL. However, serologic results are incompletely documented; the DAT was negative, and the IAT was negative against adult RBCs but "weakly reactive" against human cord RBCs. On this basis the authors assumed that the "anti-i" initiated the hemolytic process.

Reller[532] reported a patient with hemolytic anemia that developed during a CMV infection in a previously healthy 30-year-old woman. There was an abrupt fall in hematocrit followed by an increased reticulocyte count and erythroid hyperplasia in the bone marrow. The patient's cold agglutinin titer increased from 16 to "at least" 512 during the illness and demonstrated anti-I specificity. Results of antiglobulin tests were not provided.

Aguado and coworkers[533] reported a patient with multiple myeloma and monoclonal cryoglobulinemia who developed severe hemolytic anemia after CMV infection. The DAT was positive using anti-IgM, anti-C, and anti-IgA, but negative using anti-IgG. The serum contained anti-i to a titer of 128 at 4°C, 32 at 22°C, and 1 at 37°C. The anti-i disappeared when the complement-fixation antibody titers against CMV decreased. Berlin and coworkers[531] reported a patient with spontaneous CMV infection who developed hemolysis and whose serum reacted with cord erythrocytes to a titer of 128 and reacted more weakly against adult RBCs. However, the DAT was negative and no thermal amplitude studies were performed so that the significance of the serum antibody is obscure.

CMV is also only rarely found in children with AIHA. CMV infection was not found among the 42 children with AIHA reported by Sokol and coworkers,[11] and Habibi and coworkers[13] found CMV infection in only 1 of 80 children. The patient reported by McCarthy and coworkers[534] was complicated by CMV infection, although how significant the infection was in causation hemolysis is unclear. Murray and coworkers[535] described two infants with severe CMV-associated WAIHA. The authors demonstrated anti-CMV IgG antibody in one case and suggested a possible causal relationship between AIHA and CMV infection. Both patients were ultimately treated with intravenous CMV immune globulin, with subsequent improvement. Hausler and coworkers[536] reported a 9-month-old infant with congenital HIV-1 infection who presented with severe AIHA and a high CMV viral plasma load. After successful therapy of hemolysis, CMV was not detected in the plasma, which suggested a causal relationship between the hemolysis and CMV infection.

Human Immunodeficiency Virus. Anemia occurs frequently among patients seropositive for HIV, but its multifactorial origin complicates its differential diagnosis.[537-539] The most frequent form of anemia in AIDS has the characteristics of anemia of chronic disease.[538,540] Other causes include opportunistic infections, B19 parvovirus infection, myelosuppressive drugs, thrombotic thrombocytopenic purpura, hypersplenism, marrow infiltration with tumor, iron deficiency, and blood loss anemia.[538,540,541] Also, endogenous erythropoietin concentrations are frequently low and reticulocytopenia is a common finding.[538] In addition, many autoimmune aberrations have been described in individuals with AIDS.[449] Although some of these abnormalities, such as hypergammaglobulinemia and the presence of circulating immune complexes, are only generalized indicators of faulty immunoregulation or even a direct consequence of infection, more specific clinical and pathologic evidence of autoimmunity, including the development of AIHA, has been associated with HIV infection.

Prevalence of Positive Direct Antiglobulin Tests. Most reports indicate that patients with AIDS commonly have a positive DAT.[542-546] The positive DATs may be due to hyperglobulinemia,[542] circulating immune complexes,[544,547] or anti-RBC autoantibodies.[537,543,548] Toy and coworkers[542] reported that the prevalence of a positive DAT was 18% (10 of 55) in AIDS patients compared with 0.6% in general hospital patients during a 2-year period. In the series of Zon and coworkers,[544] the prevalence of a positive DAT in patients with HIV antibodies was 21%, and McGinnis and coworkers[543] found positive results in 12 of 28 (43%) patients with AIDS.

Bordin and coworkers[545] tested blood samples on 239 patients with HIV infection and found a positive DAT in 16.7%. They further studied 67 patients using an enzyme-linked antiglobulin test to measure more accurately the number of IgG molecules per RBC. They found that 30 of the 67 individuals had increased numbers (mean, 155) compared with normal controls and with patients with hypergammaglobulinemia due to multiple myeloma or chronic liver disease. The authors suggested that some AIDS patients may have specific binding of IgG on the surface of their RBCs, rather than nonspecific uptake.

In contrast, Lepennec and coworkers[549] found positive DATs in only 14 of 185 (7.5%) individuals with asymptomatic HIV infection, and van der Lelie and coworkers[550] detected no RBC-bound immunoglobulins in any of their 16 patients, although platelet-bound immunoglobulins were demonstrated by immunofluorescence in all of the patients, and granulocyte-bound immunoglobulins were found in 12.

Immune Hemolytic Anemia. Despite the frequent occurrence of a positive DAT, AIHA is uncommon in patients with HIV infection.[220,548,549,551,552] Nevertheless, a number of case reports have been published.[32,33,536,537,548,553-564] Most patients have had WAIHA, although some reports included patients who had cold antibodies[537,555,557,560-562] or both cold and warm antibodies.[220]

Immune hemolysis may be clinically and serologically indistinguishable from idiopathic WAIHA,[548] although some special features deserve comment. Reticulocytosis, which is characteristic of non-AIDS–related AIHA, is often lacking in HIV-infected patients[537,538,540,556,560,564] despite bone marrow erythroid hyperplasia.[537,564] The levels of erythropoietin may be low and therapy with erythropoietin may be of significant benefit.[538,540]

Koduri and coworkers[221] reported four men with advanced HIV infection (AIDS) and AIHA (Table 3-24). All patients presented with an acute onset of severe AIHA, fever, and splenomegaly. The DAT was positive in all four patients using anti-IgG, and was positive in three patients with anti-C3. The IAT was positive in all, and the serum and red cell eluate showed a panagglutinin in each patient. Three of the patients were reported to have had mixed warm and cold autoantibody hemolytic anemia, based on the fact that there was strong agglutination of reagent RBCs at 22°C, although no thermal amplitude studies were performed. Shortly after admission, two patients died of severe anemia. Two patients responded to prednisone therapy and were in remission from AIHA for 15 and 30 months, respectively, at the time of the report.

Some reported cases of immune hemolysis in association with HIV infection have been caused by drug administration. Fatal acute immune hemolysis has been caused by ceftriaxone[565] and has also been reported in a patient receiving indinavir, a protease inhibitor.[566] In the latter case, the causation of immune hemolysis by the drug is not clear because hemolysis did not appear until 10 months after therapy was begun, and no serum red cell antibodies were described. The drug was implicated nonetheless because of a positive DAT caused by complement, and because of relapse of hemolysis within 24 hours after reintroduction of the drug. The authors suggested caution in the use of protease inhibitors in such patients (see Chapter 8).

Diagnosis and Management. The diagnosis of AIHA may be missed in patients with AIDS because anemia of other causes is very common, whereas AIHA is uncommon.[539] Also, reticulocytopenia may tend to obscure the diagnosis. A high transfusion requirement may be an important indication of the development of AIHA (see Chapter 2), and RBC autoantibodies may first be discovered by the transfusion service.

Treatment of AIHA in HIV-infected patients has generally been successful.[537] Patients may respond well to corticosteroid therapy,[220,537,548,555,557] splenectomy,[537] zidovudine,[559] and blood transfusion.[556,557]

Reports of an increased incidence of thromboembolic events in HIV-positive persons[567-571] suggest that there may be an additional hazard of transfusion therapy in these individuals. Hemolysis results in generation of thromboplastic substances from the erythrocyte stroma and may lead to intravascular coagulation.[572] (Also see pages 64–66 for a discussion of thrombotic events in AIHA.) The increased volume of circulating RBCs after transfusion of a patient with AIHA will result in an increased amount of RBC destruction even though the rate of cell destruction is unchanged. In patients with a hypercoagulable state, this may lead to thrombotic events. Indeed, Saif and coworkers[32] reported a patient with HIV-associated AIHA who developed a pulmonary embolism after transfusion of one unit of RBCs. Although the pulmonary embolism may well have been a coincidental finding, the authors cited two other reports of thromboembolism in patients with HIV-associated AIHA.[26,573] They also cited the case of Bilgrami and coworkers,[33] although the latter report described DIC rather than thromboembolism.

Varicella (Chickenpox). AIHA is a very rare complication of chickenpox, although a number of such cases have been reported.[574-581]

In most instances of varicella-associated AIHA, the hemolysis develops after the onset of chickenpox.[575-579] Northoff and coworkers[579] described the occurrence of a transient attack of acute hemolysis affecting a 43-year-old woman during the acute phase of disease. Her hemoglobin fell from 14.4 to 11.1 g/dL, and her serum contained a monotypic IgG-κ cold antibody which had anti-Pr_{1h} specificity. The DAT was positive

TABLE 3-24. CLINICAL AND LABORATORY DATA IN FOUR PATIENTS WITH AIDS AND AUTOIMMUNE HEMOLYTIC ANEMIA

Patient	Medications*	Temp (°C)	CD4 (×10⁶/L)	DAT		CA (titer)	Hb (g/dL)	MCV (fL)	Reticulocytes (%)	White Blood Cells (×10⁹/L)	Platelets (×10⁹/L)	TB/DB (mg/dL)	LDH (IU/L)
				IgG	C3								
1	None	39.0	10	4+	+	160	2.0	119	11	16.8	130	3.0/0.5	642
2	ZDV, 3TC	38.9	120	4+	Neg†	4+	3.4	97	18	7.3	149	2.4/0.4	916
3	D4T, 3TC, RIT, SAQ	38.3	55	4+	+	Neg	4.7	117	32	15.3	174	6.4/0.9	916
4	ZDV, 3TC, RIT, SAQ	38.9	13	3+	3+	4+	4.1	124	23	17.2	324	7.5/3.7	722

Temp, body temperature on admission; CD4, CD4+ T-lymphocyte count; IgG, direct antiglobulin test using IgG antiserum; C3, direct antiglobulin test using C3b–C3d antiserum; CA, cold agglutinins; MCV, mean cell volume; TB, total serum bilirubin; DB, direct serum bilirubin; LDH, serum lactate dehydrogenase; Neg, negative.

* Antiretroviral medications at the time of admission: ZDV, zidovudine; 3TC, lamivudine; D4T, stavudine; RIT, ritonavir; SAQ, saquinavir.

† C3d Coombs negative.

Modified from Koduri PR, Singa P, Nikolinakos P: Autoimmune hemolytic anemia in patients infected with human immunodeficiency virus. Am J Hematol 2002;70:174–176.

with anti-C but negative with anti-IgG, -IgA, and -IgM. The patient's serum agglutinated all RBCs tested at 22°C, but not at 37°C; the antibody titer at 0°C was 256.

In contrast, the patient reported by Friedman and Dracker[576] developed AIHA in the convalescent phase of his illness, and the patient reported by Terada and coworkers[574] developed AIHA during the incubation period. The latter patient was a 2-year-old boy who was admitted to the hospital with a hemoglobin level of 7.3 g/dL, a reticulocyte count of 8.2%, and other laboratory evidences of hemolysis. On the second day after admission, chickenpox vesicles were found mainly on his trunk, and the patient was treated with acyclovir. The course of both the chickenpox and the hemolytic anemia were mild. The case is unusual in that the specificity of the cold antibody was anti-I. The patient reported by Johnson[578] also had a benign course and recovered after a short course of corticosteroids.

The only fatal case was reported by Herron and coworkers,[577] although the significance of the AIHA in regard to her demise is uncertain. Their patient was a 39-year-old woman who had an extensive exanthematous rash and varicella pneumonia with widespread pulmonary infiltrates in the chest radiograph. On admission. there was no evidence of hemolysis, her hemoglobin was normal, and no RBC antibodies were found. Three days later her hemoglobin dropped to 9.1 g/dL and cold agglutinins of anti-Pr specificity were found with a titer of 128 at 0°C. She ultimately developed multiorgan failure and died 3 weeks after admission.

In the case reported by Parashar and coworkers,[580] the association of AIHA with chickenpox seems less certain. These authors reported an Indian boy who developed persistent fever with progressive jaundice 1 month after having chickenpox. After 1 month of these symptoms, he was admitted with severe DAT-positive AIHA.

Terada and coworkers[574] reviewed reports of chickenpox and hemolytic anemia and found four patients who had anti-Pr cold agglutinins.[576-579] Other specificities that have been reported include "complete antibody,"[575] "warm and cold antibody,"[580] biphasic anti-P (Donath-Landsteiner antibody),[581] anti-DC,[582] and anti-I.[574]

The patient reported by Kaiser and Bradford[581] is unique in that the patient developed paroxysmal cold hemoglobinuria during the prodromal stage of chickenpox.

Ziebold and coworkers[583] conducted a survey of severe complications in immunologically normal children with varicella throughout Germany during a 1-year period. They estimated that the incidence of severe chickenpox complications was 8.5:100,000 children but found only 6 of 119 reported severe complications consisted of hematologic abnormalities. Of these, 5 children had thrombocytopenia and one child developed anemia and neutropenia that lasted for at least 3 months. However, the anemia was not further characterized.

Rubella. Konig and coworkers[451] reported a 5-year-old boy who developed severe hemolytic anemia after serologically ascertained rubella infection. The hemoglobin dropped to 4.2 g/dL, and he required RBC transfusion. Although the DAT was negative throughout the disease, the authors attributed the hemolysis to the presence of an IgG-λ-monotypic cold antibody with anti-Pr specificity.

Kadota and coworkers[584] described a 24-year-old man who presented with dark urine and general malaise. On the fourth day of illness general exanthema and retroauricular lymph nodes were recognized. Although the exanthema disappeared, signs of hemolysis requiring hospitalization became apparent. Rubella was confirmed by the presence of high titer rubella antibodies, and cold agglutinins were present to a titer of 2048. However, as in the case of Konig and coworkers, the DAT was negative.

A series of 13 patients with hemolytic anemia after rubella were described by Ueda and coworkers,[585] but there is little documentation of an immune cause of the hemolysis. The indirect antiglobulin test was positive in only two of the 13 cases, and the DAT was positive in only 3 of the 11 cases in which it was performed.

Miyazaki and coworkers[586] reported a 7-month-old patient with congenital rubella who had a hemoglobin of 6.8 g/dL and a positive DAT which revealed IgM and C3 on the RBCs. The IAT was also said to be positive although no details are provided. Also, the LDH was 7760 units (normal range, 100 to 200 units). However, the reticulocytes were 0.1%, and the bone marrow revealed a marked paucity of erythroid cells so that the evidence for hemolysis as a significant cause of the patient's anemia is inconclusive. The patient was treated with corticosteroids and transfusions and died at 9 months of age.

Cold antibodies of anti-Pr specificity have commonly been associated with infections with rubella infection.[451,587,588] Konig and coworkers[451] reviewed the reports of seven patients with rubella and cold antibodies and found that anti-Pr specificity was present in six[451,587-592] (Table 3-25). An additional case was reported by Kadota and coworkers.[584]

Parvovirus B19. AIHA is among the least common of the numerous clinical associations with human parvovirus B19 infection.[593] Indeed, AIHA is not even mentioned in some extensive reviews of the clinical manifestations of infection with this virus.[90,594] Nevertheless, there have been a few case reports suggesting that infection with parvovirus B19 may have resulted in AIHA.[29,82,174,595,596]

Bertrand and coworkers[82] described a 12-year-old boy who was admitted to the hospital with pancytopenia and an erythroblastopenic marrow with normal granulocytic maturation and rare megakaryocytes. He also had a positive DAT. The patient was transfused and the thrombocytopenia and neutropenia spontaneously resolved within 3 days. However, the positive DAT persisted and he developed a high reticulocyte count and bilirubinemia. The authors

platelets in chronic lymphocytic leukemia (CLL). Nouv Rev Fr Hematol 1988;30:403–406.
302. Diehl LF, Bolan CD, Weiss RB: Hemolytic anemia and cancer. Cancer Treat Rev 1996;22:33–73.
303. Kyle RA, Kiely JM, Stickney JM: Acquired hemolytic anemia in chronic lymphocytic leukemia and the lymphomas. Survival and response to therapy in twenty-seven cases. Arch Intern Med 1959;104:929–936.
304. Engelfriet CP, Ouwehand WH, van 't Veer MB, Beckers DO, Maas N, von dem Borne AE. Auto-immune haemolytic anaemias. Bailliere's Clin Immunol Allergy 1987;1:251–267.
305. Greally JF, Whelan CA, O'Connell L, O'Gorman D: Cold agglutinins in a case of chronic lymphatic leukaemia. A study of the lymphocyte surface. Acta Haematol 1977;57:206–210.
306. Schwartz TB, Jager BV: Cryoglobulinemia and Raynaud's syndrome in a case of chronic lymphocytic leukemia. Cancer 1949;2:319–328.
307. Ruzickova S, Pruss A, Odendahl M, et al: Chronic lymphocytic leukemia preceded by cold agglutinin disease: Intraclonal immunoglobulin light-chain diversity in V(H)4–34 expressing single leukemic B cells. Blood 2002;100(9):3419–3422.
308. Foon KA, Rai KR, Gale RP: Chronic lymphocytic leukemia: New insights into biology and therapy. Ann Intern Med 1990;113:525–539.
309. Kipps TJ, Carson DA: Autoantibodies in chronic lymphocytic leukemia and related systemic autoimmune diseases. Blood 1993;81:2475–2487.
310. Centola M, Lin K, Sutton C, et al: Production of anti-erythrocyte antibodies by leukemic and nonleukemic B cells in chronic lymphocytic leukemia patients. Leuk Lymphoma 1996;20:465–469.
311. Sthoeger ZM, Sthoeger D, Shtalrid M, Sigler E, Geltner D, Berrebi A: Mechanism of autoimmune hemolytic anemia in chronic lymphocytic leukemia. Am J Hematol 1993;43:259–264.
312. Silberstein LE, Litwin S, Carmack CE: Relationship of variable region genes expressed by a human B cell lymphoma secreting pathologic anti-Pr2 erythrocyte autoantibodies. J Exp Med 1989;169:1631–1643.
313. Efremov DG, Ivanovski M, Burrone OR: The pathologic significance of the immunoglobulins expressed by chronic lymphocytic leukemia B-cells in the development of autoimmune hemolytic anemia. Leuk Lymphoma 1998;28:285–293.
314. Barcellini W, Montesano R, Clerici G, et al: In vitro production of anti-RBC antibodies and cytokines in chronic lymphocytic leukemia. Am J Hematol 2002;71:177–183.
315. Eisner E, Ley AB, Mayer K: Coombs'-positive hemolytic anemia in Hodgkin's disease. Ann Intern Med 1967;66:258–273.
316. Levine AM, Thornton P, Forman SJ, et al: Positive Coombs test in Hodgkin's disease: Significance and implications. Blood 1980;55:607–611.
317. May RB, Bryan JH: Autoimmune hemolytic anemia and Hodgkin disease. J Pediatr 1976;89:428–429.
318. Case Records of the Massachusetts General Hospital. New Engl J Med 1978;298:1407–1412.
319. Majumdar G: Unremitting severe autoimmune haemolytic anaemia as a presenting feature of Hodgkin's disease with minimum tumour load. Leuk Lymphoma 1995;20:169–172.
320. Bowdler AJ, Glick IW: Autoimmune hemolytic anemia as the herald state of Hodgkin's disease. Ann Intern Med 1966;65:761–767.
321. Cazenave JP, Gagnon JA, Girouard E, Bastarache A: Autoimmune hemolytic anemia terminating seven years later in Hodgkin's disease. Can Med Assoc J 1973;109:748–749.
322. Bjorkholm M, Holm G, Merk K: Cyclic autoimmune hemolytic anemia as a presenting manifestation of splenic Hodgkin's disease. Cancer 1982;49:1702–1704.
323. Brain MC, et al: A case of malignant lymphoma with cold agglutinins. Br Med J 1969;iii:33–37.
324. Fernandez O, Morales E, Toledo J: Autoimmune processes terminating 24 years later in Hodgkin's disease. Br J Haematol 1992;81:308–309.
325. Guerra L, Najman A, Homberg JC, Duhamel G, Andre R: Multiple autoantibodies in the course of Hodgkin's disease: Interpretation of erythroblastopenia. Nouv Rev Fr Hematol 1969;9:601–610.
326. Decker BL, Rukes JM, et al: Hodgkin's disease with hemolytic anemia;complications of sternal puncture;treatment with ACTH and cortisone. Amer Pract 1951;2:885–890.
327. Blajchman MA, Gordon H: Successful pregnancy in a patient with Hodgkin's disease complicated by warm autoimmune hemolytic anemia and anti-e alloimmunization. Transfusion 1972;12:276–279.
328. Garratty G, Petz LD, Wallerstein RO, Fudenberg HH: Autoimmune hemolytic anemia in Hodgkin's disease associated with anti-I^T. Transfusion 1974;14:226–231.
329. Lawe JE: Successful exchange transfusion of an infant for AIHA developing late in mother's pregnancy. Transfusion 1982;22:66–68.
330. Xiros N, Binder T, Anger B, Bohlke J, Heimpel H: Idiopathic thrombocytopenic purpura and autoimmune hemolytic anemia in Hodgkin's disease. Eur J Haematol 1988;40:437–441.
331. Brady-West DC, Thame J, West W: Autoimmune haemolytic anaemia, immune thrombocytopenia, and leucopenia. An unusual presentation of Hodgkin's disease. West Indian Med J 1997;46:95–96.
332. Kedar A, Khan AB, Mattern JQ, Fisher J, Thomas PR, Freeman AI: Autoimmune disorders complicating adolescent Hodgkin's disease. Cancer 1979;44:112–116.
333. McKenna W, Lampert I, Oakley C, Goldman J: Pel-Ebstein fever coinciding with cyclical haemolytic anaemia and splenomegaly in a patient with Hodgkin's disease. Scand J Haematol 1979;23:378–380.
334. Weitberg AB, Harmon DC: Autoimmune neutropenia, hemolytic anemia, and reticulocytopenia in Hodgkin's disease. Ann Intern Med 1984;100:702–703.
335. Chu J-Y: Autoimmmune hemolytic anemia in childnood Hodgkin's disease. American Journal of Pediatric Hematology/Oncology 1982;4:125–128.
336. Ertem M, Uysal Z, Yavuz G, Gozdasoglu S: Immune thrombocytopenia and hemolytic anemia as a presenting manifestation of Hodgkin disease. Pediatr Hematol Oncol 2000;17:181–185.
337. Shah SJ, Warrier RP, Ode DL, Lele HE, Yu LC: Immune thrombocytopenia and hemolytic anemia associated with Hodgkin disease. J Pediatr Hematol Oncol 1996;18:227–229.
338. Carpentieri U, Daeschner CW, III, Haggard ME: Immunohemolytic anemia and Hodgkin disease. Pediatrics 1982;70:320–321.
339. Kalmanti M, Polychronopoulou S: Autoimmune hemolytic anemia as an initial symptom in childhood Hodgkin's disease. Pediatr Hematol Oncol 1992;9:393–395.
340. Garratty G, Haffleigh B, Dalziel J, Petz LD: An IgG anti-I^T detected in a Caucasiaon American. Transfusion 1972;12:325–329.
341. Freedman J, Newlands M, Johnson CA: Warm IgM anti-I^T causing autoimmune haemolytic anaemia. Vox Sang 1977; 32:135–142.
342. Hafleigh EB, Wells RF, Grumet FC: Nonhemolytic IgG anti-I^T. Transfusion 1978;18:592–597.
343. Postoway N, Capon S, Smith L, Rosenbaum D, Garratty G: Cold agglutinin syndrome caused by anti-I^T: Joint Congress of the International Society of Blood Transfusion and the American Association of Blood Banks Book of Abstracts. S337. 1990. (Abstract)
344. Ramos RR, Curtis BR, Eby CS, Ratkin GA, Chaplin H: Fatal outcome in a patient with autoimmune hemolytic anemia associated with an IgM bithermic anti-I^TP. Transfusion 1994;34:427–431.
345. Sallah S, Sigounas G, Vos P, Wan JY, Nguyen NP: Autoimmune hemolytic anemia in patients with non-Hodgkin's lymphoma: Characteristics and significance. Ann Oncol 2000;11:1571–1577.
346. Gronbaek K, D'Amore F, Schmidt K: Autoimmune phenomena in non-Hodgkin's lymphoma. Leuk Lymphoma 1995;18:311–316.
347. Coiffier B, Berger F, Bryon PA, Magaud JP: T-cell lymphomas: Immunologic, histologic, clinical, and therapeutic analysis of 63 cases. J Clin Oncol 1988;6:1584–1589.

348. Horning SJ, Weiss LM, Crabtree GS, Warnke RA: Clinical and phenotypic diversity of T cell lymphomas. Blood 1986; 67:1578–1582.
349. Bassan R, Pronesti M, Buzzetti M, et al: Autoimmunity and B-cell dysfunction in chronic proliferative disorders of large granular lymphocytes/natural killer cells. Cancer 1989;63:90–95.
350. Liaw YS, Yang PC, Su IJ, Kuo SH, Wang CH, Luh KT: Mucosa-associated lymphoid tissue lymphoma of the lung with cold-reacting autoantibody-mediated hemolytic anemia. CHEST 1994;105:288–290.
351. Economopoulos T, Stathakis N, Constantinidou M, Papageorgiou E, Anastassiou C, Raptis S: Cold agglutinin disease in non-Hodgkin's lymphoma. Eur J Haematol 1995;55:69–71.
352. Pascali E: Monoclonal gammopathy and cold agglutinin disease in non-Hodgkin's lymphoma. Eur J Haematol 1996;56:114–115.
353. Costea N, Yakulis VJ, Heller P: The mechanisms of induction of cold agglutinins by M: Pneumoniae. Blood 34, 829 (Abstract 15), 1968. (Abstract)
354. Mainwaring CJ, Walewska R, Snowden J, et al: Fatal cold anti-i autoimmune haemolytic anaemia complicating hairy cell leukaemia. Br J Haematol 2000;109:641–643.
355. Bar BM, Reijnders FJ, Keuning JJ, Bal H, van Beek M: Primary malignant lymphoma of the uterine cervix associated with cold-reacting autoantibody-mediated hemolytic anemia. Acta Haematol 1986;75:232–235.
356. Isbister JP, Cooper DA, Blake HM, Biggs JC, Dixon RA, Penny R: Lymphoproliferative disease with IgM lambda monoclonal protein and autoimmune hemolytic anemia: A report of four cases and a review of the literature. Am J Med 1978;64: 434–440.
357. Sallah S, Wan JY, Hanrahan LR: Future development of lymphoproliferative disorders in patients with autoimmune hemolytic anemia. Clin Cancer Res 2001;7:791–794.
358. Jasty R, Strouse PJ, Castle VP: Fatal lymphoproliferative disease as a complication of Evans syndrome. J Pediatr Hematol Oncol 2000;22:460–463.
359. Chaplin H, Jr. Lymphoma in primary chronic cold hemagglutinin disease treated with chlorambucil. Arch Intern Med 1982;142:2119–2123.
360. Otto S, Borzonyi M, Eckhardt S, Mohay A, Gergely J, Kellner R: Immunochemical and ultrastructural investigations in a patient with cold-agglutinine-active monoclonal IgMK-gammopathy. Blut 1977;34:299–304.
361. Kamiyama R, Saitoh K, Hirosawa S, Yamaguchi H, Tsukada T: Two patients with autoimmune disease developing into non-Hodgkin's lymphoma. Nippon Ketsueki Gakkai Zasshi 1986;49:915–921.
362. Voulgarelis M, Kokori SI, Ioannidis JP, Tzioufas AG, Kyriaki D, Moutsopoulos HM: Anaemia in systemic lupus erythematosus: Aetiological profile and the role of erythropoietin. Ann Rheum Dis 2000;59:217–222.
363. Harvey AM, Shulman LE, Tumulty PA, et al: Systemic lupus erythematosus. Review of the literature and clinical analysis of 138 cases. Medicine 1854;33:291–437.
364. Nossent JC, Swaak AJ: Prevalence and significance of haematological abnormalities in patients with systemic lupus erythematosus. Q J Med 1991;80:605–612.
365. Worlledge S: Immune haemolytic anaemias. In Hardisty RM, Weatherall DJ (eds): Blood and Its Disorders. Oxford: Blackwell Scientific, 1982:479–513.
366. Alger M, Alarcon-Segovia D, Rivero SJ: Hemolytic anemia and thrombocytopenic purpura: Two related subsets of systemic lupus erythematosus. J Rheumatol 1977;4:351–357.
367. Ward MM, Pyun E, Studenski S: Mortality risks associated with specific clinical manifestations of systemic lupus erythematosus. Arch Intern Med 1996;156:1337–1344.
368. Alarcon-Segovia D, Deleze M, Oria CV, et al: Antiphospholipid antibodies and the antiphospholipid syndrome in systemic lupus erythematosus: A prospective analysis of 500 consecutive patients. Medicine (Baltimore) 1989;68:353–365.
369. Deleze M, Alarcon-Segovia D, Oria CV, et al: Hemocytopenia in systemic lupus erythematosus: Relationship to antiphospholipid antibodies. J Rheumatol 1989;16:926–930.
370. Budman DR, Steinberg AD: Hematologic aspects of systemic lupus erythematosus: Current concepts. Ann Intern Med 1977;86:220–229.
371. Mongan ES, Leddy JP, Atwater EC, Barnett EV: Direct antiglobulin (Coombs) reactions in patients with connective tissue diseases. Arthritis Rheum 1967;10:502–508.
372. Michael SR, Vural IL, Bassen FA, Schaefer L: The hematologic aspects of disseminated (systemc) lupus erythematosus. Blood 1951;6:1059–1072.
373. Wasserman LR, Stats D, Schwartz L, Fudenberg H: Symptomatic and hemopathic hemolytic anemia. Am J Med 1955;18:961–989.
374. Videbaek A: Auto-immune haemolytic anaemia in systemic lupus erythematosus. Acta Med Scand 1962;171:187–194.
375. Nair K, Pavithran K, Philip J, Thomas M, Geetha V: Cold haemagglutinin disease in systemic lupus erythematosus. Yonsei Med J 1997;38:233–235.
376. Drenkard C, Villa AR, Alarcon-Segovia D, Perez-Vazquez ME: Influence of the antiphospholipid syndrome in the survival of patients with systemic lupus erythematosus. J Rheumatol 1994;21:1067–1072.
377. Asherson RA, Cervera R, Piette JC, et al: Catastrophic antiphospholipid syndrome: Clues to the pathogenesis from a series of 80 patients. Medicine (Baltimore) 2001;80:355–377.
378. Font J, Jimenez S, Cervera R, et al: Splenectomy for refractory Evans' syndrome associated with antiphospholipid antibodies: Report of two cases. Ann Rheum Dis 2000;59:920–923.
379. Hughes GR: Thrombosis, abortion, cerebral disease, and the lupus anticoagulant. Br Med J (Clin Res Ed) 1983;287: 1088–1089.
380. Win N, Islam SI, Peterkin MA, Walker ID: Positive direct antiglobulin test due to antiphospholipid antibodies in normal healthy blood donors. Vox Sang 1997;72:182–184.
381. Sthoeger Z, Sthoeger D, Green L, Geltner D: The role of anticardiolipin autoantibodies in the pathogenesis of autoimmune hemolytic anemia in systemic lupus erythematosus. J Rheumatol 1993;20:2058–2061.
382. Hazeltine M, Rauch J, Danoff D, Esdaile JM, Tannenbaum H: Antiphospholipid antibodies in systemic lupus erythematosus: Evidence of an association with positive Coombs' and hypocomplementemia. J Rheumatol 1988;15:80–86.
383. Deleze M, Oria CV, Alarcon-Segovia D: Occurrence of both hemolytic anemia and thrombocytopenic purpura (Evans' syndrome) in systemic lupus erythematosus. Relationship to antiphospholipid antibodies. J Rheumatol 1988;15:611–615.
384. Hammond A, Rudge AC, Loizou S, Bowcock SJ, Walport MJ: Reduced numbers of complement receptor type 1 on erythrocytes are associated with increased levels of anticardiolipin antibodies. Findings in patients with systemic lupus erythematosus and the antiphospholipid syndrome. Arthritis Rheum 1989;32:259–264.
385. Cabral AR, Cabiedes J, Alarcon-Segovia D: Hemolytic anemia related to an IgM autoantibody to phosphatidylcholine that binds in vitro to stored and to bromelain-treated human erythrocytes. J Autoimmun 1990;3:773–787.
386. Cervera R, Font J, Lopez-Soto A, et al: Isotype distribution of anticardiolipin antibodies in systemic lupus erythematosus: Prospective analysis of a series of 100 patients. Ann Rheum Dis 1990;49:109–113.
387. Alarcon-Segovia D: Pathogenetic potential of antiphospholipid antibodies. J Rheumatol 1988;15:890–893.
388. Fong KY, Loizou S, Boey ML, Walport MJ: Anticardiolipin antibodies, haemolytic anaemia and thrombocytopenia in systemic lupus erythematosus. Br J Rheumatol 1992;31: 453–455.
389. Arvieux J, Schweizer B, Roussel B, Colomb MG: Autoimmune haemolytic anaemia due to anti-phospholipid antibodies. Vox Sang 1991;61:190–195.
390. Davidyuk G, Goldsby RA, Dearden MT, Stec TC, Andrzejewski C: Autoantibodies to immature erythrocytes in

patients with the anti-phospholipid antibody syndrome. Transfusion 42, 103S: 2002. (Abstract)
391. Del Papa N, Meroni PL, Barcellini W, et al: Antiphospholipid antibodies cross-reacting with erythrocyte membranes: A case report. Clin Exp Rheumatol 1992;10:395–399.
392. Lang B, Straub RH, Weber S, Rother E, Fleck M, Peter HH: Elevated anticardiolipin antibodies in autoimmune haemolytic anaemia irrespective of underlying systemic lupus erythematosus. Lupus 1997;6:652–655.
393. Latagliata R, Celesti F, Bongarzoni V, et al: Intracardiac thrombus in a patient with autoimmune hemolytic anemia leading to a diagnosis of antiphospholipid syndrome. Acta Haematol 2002;107:170–172.
394. Guzman J, Cabral AR, Cabiedes J, Pita-Ramirez L, Alarcon-Segovia D: Antiphospholipid antibodies in patients with idiopathic autoimmune haemolytic anemia. Autoimmunity 1994;18:51–56.
395. Barker RN, Casswell KM, Reid ME, Sokol RJ, Elson CJ: Identification of autoantigens in autoimmune haemolytic anaemia by a non-radioisotope immunoprecipitation method. Br J Haematol 1992;82:126–132.
396. Victoria EJ, Pierce SW, Branks MJ, Masouredis SP: IgG red blood cell autoantibodies in autoimmune hemolytic anemia bind to epitopes on red blood cell membrane band 3 glycoprotein. J Lab Clin Med 1990;115:74–88.
397. Leddy JP, Falany JL, Kissel GE, Passador ST, Rosenfeld SI: Erythrocyte membrane proteins reactive with human (warm-reacting) anti-red cell autoantibodies. J Clin Invest 1993;91:1672–1680.
398. Galindo M, Khamashta MA, Hughes GR: Splenectomy for refractory thrombocytopenia in the antiphospholipid syndrome. Rheumatology (Oxford) 1999;38:848–853.
399. Vaughan JH, Barnett EV, Leddy JP: Autosensitivity diseases Immunologic and pathogenetic concepts in lupus erythematosus, rheumatoid arthritis and hemolytic anemia. N Engl J Med 1966;275:1426–1432.
400. Pollock JG, Fenton E, Barrett KE: Familial autoimmune haemolytic anaemia associated with rheumatoid arthritis and pernicious anaemia. Br J Haematol 1970;18:171–182.
401. Durance RA, Hamilton EB: Myasthenia gravis, rheumatoid arthritis, vitiligo, and autoimmune haemolytic anaemia. Proc R Soc Med 1971;64:61–62.
402. Chapman AH: Concurrent development of acute autoimmune haemolytic anaemia with rheumatoid arthritis. Proc R Soc Med 1972;65:1013–1015.
403. Suda T, Oike S, Omine M, Naruse T, Tsuchiya J: Haemolytic anaemia due to warm type autohaemagglutin in a patient with rheumatoid arthritis. Nippon Ketsueki Gakkai Zasshi 1977;40:466–471.
404. Maharaj D: Autoimmune haemolytic anaemia associated with rheumatoid arthritis and paroxysmal nocturnal haemoglobinuria. Acta Haematol 1986;75:241.
405. Chaves FC, Rodrigo FG, Franco ML, Esteves J: Systemic sclerosis associated with auto-immune haemolytic anaemia. Br J Dermatol 1970;82:298–302.
406. Rosenthal DS, Sack B: Autoimmune hemolytic anemia in scleroderma. JAMA 1971;216:2011–2012.
407. Ivey KJ, Hwang YF, Sheets RF: Scleroderma associated with thrombocytopenia and Coombs-positive hemolytic anemia. Am J Med 1971;51:815–817.
408. Loft B, Olsen F: Autoimmune haemolytic anaemia with positive Ham and Crosby's test and scleroderma. A case report. Scand J Haematol 1973;11:131–134.
409. Sumithran E: Progressive systemic sclerosis and autoimmune haemolytic anaemia. Postgrad Med J 1976;52:173–176.
410. Jones E, Jones JV, Woodbury JF, Carr RI, Skanes V: Scleroderma and hemolytic anemia in a patient with deficiency of IgA and C4: A hitherto undescribed association. J Rheumatol 1987;14:609–612.
411. Pettersson T, von Bonsdorff M: Auto-immune haemolytic anaemia and thrombocytopenia in scleroderma. Acta Haematol 1988;80:179–180.
412. Lugassy G, Reitblatt T, Ducach A, Oren S: Severe autoimmune hemolytic anemia with cold agglutinin and sclerodermic features—favorable response to danazol. Ann Hematol 1993;67:143–144.
413. Wanchu A, Sud A, Bambery P: Linear scleroderma and autoimmune hemolytic anaemia. J Assoc Physicians India 2002;50:441–442.
414. Andrews J, Hall MA: Dermatomyositis-scleroderma overlap syndrome presenting as autoimmune haemolytic anaemia. Rheumatology (Oxford) 2002;41:956–958.
415. Ellis LD, Westerman MP: Autoimmune hemolytic anemia and cancer. JAMA 1965;193:962–964.
416. Holland PV, Menken M, Berlin NI: Autoimmune hemolytic anemia, acute leukemia, and carcinoma of the lung. Sodium phosphate P 32 treatment of polycythemia vera. Arch Intern Med 1967;120:341–344.
417. Miura AB, Shibata A, Akihama T, Endo Y, Sugawara M: Autoimmune hemolytic anemia associated with colon cancer. Cancer 1974;33:111–114.
418. Najafi JA, Guzman LG: Tumor induced autoimmune hemolytic anemia in bronchogenic carcinoma: Case reports. Mil Med 1979;144:754–756.
419. Spira MA, Lynch EC: Autoimmune hemolytic anemia and carcinoma: an unusual association. Am J Med 1979;67: 753–758.
420. Inoue Y, Kaku K, Kaneko T, Matsumoto N: Autoimmune hemolytic anemia and gastric cancer: Case report and review of the literature. Nippon Ketsueki Gakkai Zasshi 1983; 46:836–841.
421. Venzano C, De Micheli A, Cavallero GB: Autoimmune hemolytic anemia associated with hypernephroma. Haematologica 1985;70:59–61.
422. Honan W, Balazs J, Jariwalla AG: Autoimmune haemolytic anaemia (AHA) and lung carcinoma. Br J Clin Pract 1986;40:35–36.
423. Girelli G, Adorno G, Perrone MP, et al: Kidney carcinoma revealed by autoimmune hemolytic anemia. Haematologica 1988;73:309–311.
424. Adorno G, Girelli G, Perrone MP, et al: A metastatic breast carcinoma presenting as autoimmune hemolytic anemia. Tumori 1991;77:447–448.
425. Hibino S, Stoller RG, Jacobs SA: Autoimmune haemolytic anaemia associated with transitional cell carcinoma. Lancet 1992;340:373.
426. Nakao A, Iwagaki H, Notohara K, et al: Successful resection of rectal carcinoma in an Evans' syndrome patient followed by predonisolone and high-dose immunoglobulin: Report of a case. Acta Med Okayama 2001;55:253–257.
427. Lands R, Foust J: Renal cell carcinoma and autoimmune hemolytic anemia. South Med J 1996;89:444–445.
428. Kamra D, Boselli J, Sloane BB, Gladstone DE: Renal cell carcinoma induced Coombs negative autoimmune hemolytic anemia and severe thrombocytopenia responsive to nephrectomy. J Urol 2002;167:1395.
429. Cao L, Kaiser P, Gustin D, Hoffman R, Feldman L: Cold agglutinin disease in a patient with uterine sarcoma. Am J Med Sci 2000;320:352–354.
430. Gordon PA, Baylis PH, Bird GW: Tumour-induced autoimmune haemolytic anaemia. Br Med J 1976;1:1569–1570.
431. Bradley GW, Harvey M: Haemolytic anaemia with hypernephroma. Postgrad Med J 1981;57:46–47.
432. Kornberg A, Naparstek E, Hershko C: Cryopathic haemolytic anaemia associated wtih uterus myomatosus. Acta Haematol 1980;63:235.
433. Johnson P, Gualtieri RJ, Mohler DN, Carpenter JT: Autoimmune hemolytic anemia associated with a hypernephroma. South Med J 1985;78:1129–1131.
434. Wortman J, Rosse W, Logue G: Cold agglutinin autoimmune hemolytic anemia in nonhematologic malignancies. Am J Hematol 1979;6:275–283.
435. Chen RT, Pless R, Destefano F: Epidemiology of autoimmune reactions induced by vaccination. J Autoimmun 2001;16:309–318.

436. Cohen AD, Shoenfeld Y: Vaccine-induced autoimmunity. J Autoimmun 1996;9:699–703.
436a. Offit PA, Hackett CJ: Addressing parents' concerns: Do vaccines cause allergic or autoimmune diseases? Pediatrics 2003;111:653–659.
437. Kolbl H: Klinik und Therapie der akuten erworbenen hamolytischen Anamien im Kindesalter. Ostdeutsch Z Kinderheilk 1955;11:27.
438. Dameshek W, Schwartz R: Hemolytic mechanisms. Ann NY Acad Sci 1959;77:589.
439. Gedikoglu AG, Cantez T: Haemolytic-anaemia relapses after immunisation and pertussis. Lancet 1967;2:894–895.
440. Bossi E, Wagner HP: Autoimmune hemolytic anemia and cytomegalovirus infection in a six- months-old child, treated with azathioprine. Helv Paediatr Acta 1972;27:155–162.
441. Haneberg B, Matre R, Winsnes R, Dalen A, Vogt H, Finne PH: Acute hemolytic anemia related to diphtheria-pertussis-tetanus vaccination. Acta Paediatr Scand 1978;67:345–350.
442. Johnson ST, McFarland JG, Casper JT, et al: An unusual case of autoimmune hemolytic anemia following DPT vaccination. Transfusion 1989;29:50S.
443. Downes KA, Domen RE, McCarron KF, Bringelsen KA: Acute autoimmune hemolytic anemia following DTP vaccination: Report of a fatal case and review of the literature. Clinical Pediatrics 2001;40:355–358.
444. Seltsam A, Shukry-Schulz S, Salama A: Vaccination-associated immune hemolytic anemia in two children. Transfusion 2000;40:907–909.
445. Martinez E, Domingo P: Evans's syndrome triggered by recombinant hepatitis B vaccine. Clin Infect Dis 1992;15:1051.
446. Howson CP, Fineberg HV: Adverse events following pertussis and rubella vaccines. Summary of a report of the Institute of Medicine. JAMA 1992;267:392–396.
447. Berkowitz FE: Hemolysis and infection: Categories and mechanisms of their interrelationship. Rev Infect Dis 1991;13:1151–1162.
448. Seitz RC, Buschermohle G, Dubberke G, Herbrand R, Maiwald M, Hellwege HH: The acute infection-associated hemolytic anemia of childhood: Immunofluorescent detection of microbial antigens altering the erythrocyte membrane. Ann Hematol 1993;67:191–196.
449. Morrow WJ, Isenberg DA, Sobol RE, Stricker RB, Kieber-Emmons T: AIDS virus infection and autoimmunity: A perspective of the clinical, immunological, and molecular origins of the autoallergic pathologies associated with HIV disease. Clin Immunol Immunopathol 1991;58:163–180.
450. Meite M, Leonard S, Idrissi ME, Izui S, Masson PL, Coutelier JP: Exacerbation of autoantibody-mediated hemolytic anemia by viral infection. J Virol 2000;74:6045–6049.
451. Konig AL, Schabel A, Sugg U, Brand U, Roelcke D: Autoimmune hemolytic anemia caused by IgG lambda-monotypic cold agglutinins of anti-Pr specificity after rubella infection. Transfusion 2001;41:488–492.
452. Murray HW, Masur H, Senterfit LB, Roberts RB: The protean manifestations of Mycoplasma pneumoniae infection in adults. Am J Med 1975;58:229–242.
453. Chanock RM: Mycoplasma infections of man. N Engl J Med 1965;273:1257–1264.
454. Denny FW, Clyde WA, Jr, Glezen WP: Mycoplasma pneumoniae disease: Clinical spectrum, pathophysiology, epidemiology, and control. J Infect Dis 1971;123:74–92.
455. Daxbock F, Zedtwitz-Liebenstein K, Burgmann H, Graninger W: Severe hemolytic anemia and excessive leukocytosis masking mycoplasma pneumonia. Ann Hematol 2001;80:180–182.
456. Ali NJ, Sillis M, Andrews BE, Jenkins PF, Harrison BD: The clinical spectrum and diagnosis of Mycoplasma pneumoniae infection. Q J Med 1986;58:241–251.
457. Feizi T: Cold agglutinins, the direct coombs' test and serum immunoglobulins in Mycoplasma pneumoniae infection. Ann N Y Acad Sci 1967;143:801–812.
458. Jacobson LB, Longstreth GF, Edgington TS: Clinical and immunologic features of transient cold agglutinin-hemolytic anemia. Am J Med 1973;54:514–521.
459. Dacie JV: Auto-immune haemolytic anaemia (AIHA): Cold-antibody syndromes III: Haemolytic anaemia following mycoplasma pneumonia. In The Haemolytic Anaemias, 3rd ed. vol. 3, The Auto-Immune Haemolytic Anaemias. New York: Churchill Livingstone, 1992: 296–312.
460. Linz DH, Tolle SW, Elliot DL: Mycoplasma pneumoniae pneumonia. Experience at a referral center. West J Med 1984; 140:895–900.
461. Smith GN, Weir WR: Cold agglutinins accompanying Mycoplasma pneumoniae infection. Br Med J 1980;281: 1391–1392.
462. Platt WR, Ward DS: Cold isohemagglutinins. Their association with hemolytic anemia and multiple thromboses in primary atypical pneumonia: A brief review of the clinical and laboratory problems involved. Am J Clin Path 1945;15:202–209.
463. Carey RM, Wilson JL, Tamerin JA: Gangrene of feet and hemolytic anemia associated with cold hemagglutinins in atypical pneumonia. Harlem Hosp Bull 1948;1:25–32.
464. Stats D, Wasserman LR, Rosenthal N: Hemolytic anemia with hemoglobinuria. Amer J Clin Path 1948;18:757–777.
465. Kumar S, Singh MM, Bhatia BB: Symmetrical peripheral gangrene in acquired hemolytic anemia. Acta haemat (Basel) 1958;19:369–377.
466. Schulman P, Piemonte TC, Singh B: Acute renal failure, hemolytic anemia, and Mycoplasma pneumoniae. JAMA 1980;244:1823–1824.
467. Lawson DH, Lindsay RM, Sawers JD, et al: Acute renal failure in the cold-agglutination syndrome. Lancet 1968;2:704–705.
468. Shibasaki T, Gomi H, Ohno I, Ishimoto F, Sakai O: A case of chronic renal failure followed by cold agglutinin due to Mycoplasma pneumoniae infection. Nephron 1991;57:249–250.
469. Poth JL, Sharp GS, Schrier SL: Cold agglutinin disease and the nephrotic syndrome. JAMA 1970;211:1989–1992.
470. Cherry JD: Anemia and mucocutaneous lesions due to Mycoplasma pneumoniae infections. Clin Infect Dis 1993;17 (Suppl. 1):S47–S51.
471. Chu CS, Braun SR, Yarbro JW, Hayden MR: Corticosteroid treatment of hemolytic anemia associated with Mycoplasma pneumoniae pneumonia. South Med J 1990;83:1106–1108.
472. Tsuruta R, Kawamura Y, Inoue T, Kasaoka S, Sadamitsu D, Maekawa T: Corticosteroid therapy for hemolytic anemia and respiratory failure due to Mycoplasma pneumoniae pneumonia. Intern Med 2002;41:229–232.
473. Chan LY, Chan JC: Mycoplasma pneumoniae infection presenting as haemolytic anaemia. Br J Hosp Med 1997;58:170.
474. Fink FM, Dengg K, Kilga-Nogler S, Schonitzer D, Berger H: Cold haemagglutinin disease complicating Mycoplasma pneumoniae infection in a child under cytotoxic cancer treatment. Eur J Pediatr 1992;151:435–437.
475. Tanowitz HB, Robbins N, Leidich N: Hemolytic anemia. Associated with severe Mycoplasma pneumoniae pneumonia. N Y State J Med 1978;78:2231–2232.
476. Maisel JC, Babbitt LH, John TJ: Fatal Mycoplasma pneumoniae infection with isolation of organisms from lung. JAMA 1967;202:287–290.
477. Louie EK, Ault KA, Smith BR, Hardman EL, Quesenberry PJ: IgG-mediated haemolysis masquerading as cold agglutinin-induced anaemia complicating severe infection with mycoplasma pneumoniae. Scand J Haematol 1985;35:264–269.
478. Schmidt PJ, Barile MF, McGinniss MH: Mycoplasma (Pleuropneumonia-like organismns) and blood group I: Associations with neoplastic disease. Nature (Lond) 1965;205: 371–372.
479. Smith CB, McGinniss MH, Schmidt PJ: Changes in erythrocyte I agglutinogen and anti-I-agglutinins during Mycoplasma pneumoniae infection in man. J Immunol 1967;99:333–339.
480. Feizi T, Taylor-Robinson D, Shields MD, Carter RA: Production of cold agglutinins in rabbits immunized with human erythrocytes treated with Mycoplasma pneumoniae. Nature 1969;222:1253–1256.
481. Loomes LM, Uemura K, Childs RA, et al: Erythrocyte receptors for Mycoplasma pneumoniae are sialylated oligosaccharides of Ii antigen type. Nature 1984;307:560–563.

482. Costea N, Yakulis V, Heller P: Experimental production of cold agglutinins in rabbits. Blood 1965;26:323–339.
483. Costea N, Yakulis VJ, Heller P: Inhibition of cold agglutinins (anti-I) by M: pneumoniae antigens. Proc Soc Exp Biol Med 1972;139:476–479.
484. Lind K: Production of cold agglutinins in rabbits induced by Mycoplasma pneumoniae, Listeria monocytogenes or Streptococcus MG. Acta Pathol Microbiol Scand [B] Microbiol Immunol 1973;81:487–496.
485. Janney FA, Lee LT, Howe C: Cold hemagglutinin cross-reactivity with Mycoplasma pneumoniae. Infect Immun 1978;22: 29–33.
486. Bartholomew JR, Bell WR, Shirey RS: Cold agglutinin hemolytic anemia: Management with an environmental suit. Ann Intern Med 1987;106:243–244.
486a. Ness PM, Bell WR, Shirey RS: Transfusion medicine illustrated. Novel management of cold agglutinin disease. Transfusion 2003;43:839.
487. Turtzo DF, Ghatak PK: Acute hemolytic anemia with Mycoplasma pneumoniae pneumonia. JAMA 1976;236:1140–1141.
488. Lindstrom FD, Stahl-Furenhed B: Autoimmune haemolytic anaemia complicating Mycoplasma pneumoniae infection. Scand J Infect Dis 1981;13:233–235.
489. Helms CM: Infections caused by Mycoplasma pneumoniae and the genital mycoplasmas. In: Humes HD, et al (eds): Kelly's Textbook of Internal Medicine. New York: Lippincott Williams & Wilkins, 2000:2110–2113.
490. Einzig MJ, Neerhout RC: Hemolytic anemia in infectious mononucleosis. Clin Pediatr (Phila) 1969;8:171–173.
491. Hoagland RJ: Infectious Mononucleosis. New York: Grune & Stratton, 1967.
492. Boughton CR: Glandular fever. A study of a hospital series in Sydney. Med J Aust 1970;2:529–535.
493. Pagano JS: Epstein-Barr virus and the infectious mononucleosis syndrome. In: Humes HD (ed): Kelly's Textbook of Internal Medicine. Philadelphia: Lippincott Williams & Wilkins, 2000:2179–2185.
494. Dacie JV: Auto-immune haemolytic anaemia (AIHA): Cold-antibody syndromes IV: Haemolytic anaemia following infectious mononucleosis and other viral infections. In The Haemolytic Anaemias, 3rd ed. vol. 3, The Auto-Immune Haemolytic Anaemias. New York: Churchill Livingstone, 1992:313–328.
495. Woodruff RK, McPherson AJ: Severe haemolytic anaemia complicating infectious mononucleosis. Aust N Z J Med 1976;6:569–570.
496. Worlledge SM, Dacie JV: Haemolytic and other anaemias in infectious mononucleosis. In: Carter RL, Penman HG (eds): Infectious Mononucleosis: Oxford: Blackwell Scientific, 1969:82–98.
497. Silber M, Richards JD, Jacobs P: Life-threatening haemolytic anaemia and infectious mononucleosis: A case report. S Afr Med J 1985;67:183–185.
498. Tonkin AM, Mond HG, Alford FP, Hurley TH: Severe acute haemolytic anaemia complicating infectious mononucleosis. Med J Aust 1973;2:1048–1050.
499. Bowman HS, Marsh WL, Schumacher HR, Oyen R, Reihart J: Auto anti-N immunohemolytic anemia in infectious mononucleosis. Am J Clin Pathol 1974;61:465–472.
500. Palanduz A, Yildirmak Y, Telhan L, et al: Fulminant hepatic failure and autoimmune hemolytic anemia associated with Epstein-Barr virus infection. J Infect 2002;45:96–98.
501. Young LE, Izzo MJ, Platzer RF: Hereditary spherocytosis. I: Clinical hematologic and genetic features in 28 cases, with particular reference to the osmotic and mechanical fragility of incubated erythrocytes. Blood 1951;6:1073–1098.
502. Bean RHD: Haemolytic anaemia complicating infectious mononucleosis, with report of a case. Med J Aust 1957;1: 386–389.
503. DeNardo GL, Ray JP: Hereditary spherocytosis and infectious mononucleosis, with acquired hemolytic anemia: Report of a case and review of the literature. Amer J Clin Path 1963; 39:284–288.
504. Godal HC, Skaga E: Aggravation of congenital spherocytosis during infectious mononucleosis. Scand J Haematol 1969;6: 33–35.
505. Gehlbach SH, Cooper BA: Haemolytic anaemia in infectious mononucleosis due to inapparent congenital spherocytosis. Scand J Haematol 1970;7:141–144.
506. Taylor JJ: Haemolysis in infectious mononucleosis: Inapparent congenital spherocytosis. Br Med J 1973;4:525–526.
507. Jenkins WJ, Koster HG, Marsh WL, Carters RL: Infectious mononucleosis: An unsuspected source of anti-i. Brit J Haemat 1965;11:480–483.
508. Calvo RS, Stein W, Kochwa S, Rosenfield RE: Acute hemolytic anemia due to anti-i: Frequent cold agglutinins in infectious mononucleosis. Journal of Clinical Investigation 44, 1033. 1965. (Abstract)
509. Rosenfield RE, Schmidt PJ, Calvo RC, McGinniss MH: Anti-i, a frequent cold agglutinin in infectious mononucleosis. Vox Sang 1965;10:631–634.
510. Wollheim FA, Williams RC, Jr: Studies on the macroglobulins of human serum. I: Polyclonal immunoglobulin class M (IgM) increase in infectious mononucleosis. N Engl J Med 1966;274:61–67.
511. Troxel DB, Innella F, Cohen RJ: Infectious mononucleosis complicated by hemolytic anemia due to anti-i. Am J Clin Pathol 1966;46:625–631.
512. Burkart PT, Hsu TC: IgM cold-warm hemolysins in infectious mononucleosis. Transfusion 1979;19:535–538.
513. Gronemeyer P, Chaplin H, Ghazarian V, Tuscany F, Wilner GD: Hemolytic anemia complicating infectious mononucleosis due to the interaction of an IgG cold anti-i and an IgM cold rheumatoid factor. Transfusion 1981;21:715–718.
514. Wilkinson LS, Petz LD, Garratty G: Reappraisal of the role of anti-i in haemolytic anaemia in infectious mononucleosis. Br J Haematol 1973;25:715–722.
515. Lee CH, Hagen MA, Chong BH, Grace CS, Rozenberg MC: The Lewis system and secretor status in autoimmune hemolytic anemia complicating infectious mononucleosis. Transfusion 1980;20:585–588.
516. Ellis LB, Wollenman OJ, Stetson RP: Autohemagglutinins and hemolysins with hemoglobinuria and acute hemolytic anaemia, in an illness resembling infectious mononucleosis. Blood 3, 419–429. 1948. (Abstract)
517. Perkin RL, Fox AD, Richards WL, King MH: Acute hemolytic anemia secondary to infectious mononucleosis. Can Med Assoc J 1979;121:1095–1097.
518. Zuelzer WW, Stulberg CS, Page RH, Teruya J, Brough AJ: Etiology and pathogenesis of acquired hemolytic anemia. Transfusion 1966;6:438–461.
519. Zuelzer WW, Mastrangelo R, Stulberg CS, Poulik MD, Page RH, Thompson RI: Autoimmune hemolytic anemia: Natural history and viral-immunologic interactions in childhood. Am J Med 1970;49:80–93.
520. Kantor GL, Goldberg LS, Johnson BL, Jr, Derechin MM, Barnett EV: Immunologic abnormalities induced by postperfusion cytomegalovirus infection. Ann Intern Med 1970;73:553–558.
521. Harris AI, Meyer RJ, Brody EA: Cytomegalovirus-induced thrombocytopenia and hemolysis in an adult. Ann Intern Med 1975;83:670–671.
522. van Spronsen DJ, Breed WP: Cytomegalovirus-induced thrombocytopenia and haemolysis in an immunocompetent adult. Br J Haematol 1996;92:218–220.
523. Salloum E, Lundberg WB: Hemolytic anemia with positive direct antiglobulin test secondary to spontaneous cytomegalovirus infection in healthy adults. Acta Haematol 1994;92:39–41.
524. Coombs RR: Cytomegalic inclusion-body disease associated with acquired autoimmune haemolytic anaemia. Br Med J 1968;2:743–744.
525. Houston MC, Porter LL, III, Jenkins DE, Jr, Flexner JM: Acute immune hemolytic anemia in adults after cytomegalovirus infection. South Med J 1980;73:1270–1274.
526. Horwitz CA, Henle W, Henle G, et al: Clinical and laboratory evaluation of cytomegalovirus-induced mononucleosis in pre-

viously healthy individuals: Report of 82 cases. Medicine (Baltimore) 1986;65:124–134.
527. Horwitz CA, Skradski K, Reece E, et al: Haemolytic anaemia in previously healthy adult patients with CMV infections: Report of two cases and an evaluation of subclinical haemolysis in CMV mononucleosis. Scand J Haematol 1984;33:35–42.
528. Gavazzi G, Leclercq P, Bouchard O, Bosseray A, Morand P, Micoud M: Association between primary cytomegalovirus infection and severe hemolytic anemia in an immunocompetent adult. Eur J Clin Microbiol Infect Dis 1999;18:299–301.
529. Eddleston M, Peacock S, Juniper M, Warrell DA: Severe cytomegalovirus infection in immunocompetent patients. Clin Infect Dis 1997;24:52–56.
530. Dietz AJ, Jr: Cytomegalovirus infection with carditis, hepatitis, and anemia. Postgrad Med 1981;70:203–208.
531. Berlin BS, Chandler R, Green D: Anti-"i" antibody and hemolytic anemia associated with spontaneous cytomegalovirus mononucleosis. Am J Clin Pathol 1977;67:459–461.
532. Reller LB: Granulomatous hepatitis associated with acute cytomegalovirus infection. Lancet 1973;7793.:20–22.
533. Aguado JM, Castrillo JM, Sanz J, Serrano J: Severe haemolytic anaemia due to cold anti-"i" antibodies associated with cytomegalovirus infection. Postgrad Med J 1990;66:392–394.
534. McCarthy LJ, Danielson CF, Fernandez C, et al: Intensive plasma exchange for severe autoimmune hemolytic anemia in a four-month-old infant. J Clin Apheresis 1999;14:190–192.
535. Murray JC, Bernini JC, Bijou HL, Rossmann SN, Mahoney DH, Jr, Morad AB: Infantile cytomegalovirus-associated autoimmune hemolytic anemia. J Pediatr Hematol Oncol 2001;23:318–320.
536. Hausler M, Schaade L, Hutschenreuter G, Hannig U, Kusenbach G: Severe cytomegalovirus-triggered autoimmune hemolytic anemia complicating vertically acquired HIV infection. Eur J Clin Microbiol Infect Dis 2000;19:57–60.
537. Telen MJ, Roberts KB, Bartlett JA: HIV-associated autoimmune hemolytic anemia: Report of a case and review of the literature. J Acquir Immune Defic Syndr 1990;3:933–937.
538. Kreuzer KA, Rockstroh JK: Pathogenesis and pathophysiology of anemia in HIV infection. Ann Hematol 1997;75:179–187.
539. Claster S: Biology of anemia, differential diagnosis, and treatment options in human immunodeficiency virus infection. J Infect Dis 2002;185 (Suppl. 2):S105–S109.
540. Coyle TE: Hematologic complications of human immunodeficiency virus infection and the acquired immunodeficiency syndrome. Med Clin North Am 1997;81:449–470.
541. Hambleton J: Hematologic complications of HIV infection. Oncology (Huntingt) 1996;10:671–680.
542. Toy PT, Reid ME, Burns M: Positive direct antiglobulin test associated with hyperglobulinemia in acquired immunodeficiency syndrome (AIDS). Am J Hematol 1985;19:145–150.
543. McGinniss MH, Macher AM, Rook AH, Alter HJ: Red cell autoantibodies in patients with acquired immune deficiency syndrome. Transfusion 1986;26:405–409.
544. Zon LI, Arkin C, Groopman JE: Haematologic manifestations of the human immune deficiency virus (HIV). Br J Haematol 1987;66:251–256.
545. Bordin JO, Kerbauy J, Souza-Pinto JC, et al: Quantitation of red cell-bound IgG by an enzyme-linked antiglobulin test in human immunodeficiency virus-infected persons. Transfusion 1992;32:426–429.
546. De Angelis V, Biasinutto C, Pradella P, Vaccher E, Spina M, Tirelli U: Clinical significance of positive direct antiglobulin test in patients with HIV infection. Infection 1994;22:92–95.
547. Inada Y, Lange M, McKinley GF, et al: Hematologic correlates and the role of erythrocyte CR1 (C3b receptor) in the development of AIDS. AIDS Res 1986;2:235–247.
548. Simpson MB, Delong N: Autoimmune hemolytic anemia in a patient with acquired immune deficiency syndrome. Blood 70, 127A: 1987. (Abstract)
549. Lepennec PY, Lefrere JJ, Rouzaud AM, Rouger P: Red cell autoantibodies in asymptomatic HIV-infected subjects. Transfusion 1989;29:465–466.
550. van der Lelie J, Lange JM, Vos JJ, van Dalen CM, Danner SA, dem Borne AE: Autoimmunity against blood cells in human immunodeficiency-virus (HIV) infection. Br J Haematol 1987;67:109–114.
551. Scadden DT, Zon LI, Groopman JE: Pathophysiology and management of HIV-associated hematologic disorders. Blood 1989;74:1455–1463.
552. Saif MW: HIV-associated autoimmune hemolytic anemia: An update. AIDS Patient Care STDS 2001;15:217–224.
553. Schreiber ZA, Loh SH, Charles N, Abeebe LS: Autoimmune hemolytic anemia in patients with the acquired immunodeficiency syndrome (AIDS). Blood 62, 117A: 1983. (Abstract)
554. Miller KD, Gralnik HR, Rick ME: Hematologic problems in patients with AIDS and ARC: The NIH experience. Blood 70, 124A: 1987. (Abstract)
555. Puppo F, Torresin A, Lotti G, Balleari E, Orlando G, Indiveri F: Autoimmune hemolytic anemia and human immunodeficiency virus (HIV) infection. Ann Int Med 1988;109:249–250.
556. Rapoport AP, Rowe JM, McMican A: Life-threatening autoimmune hemolytic anemia in a patient with the acquired immune deficiency syndrome. Transfusion 1988;28:190–191.
557. Gaffuri L, Repetto L, Rossi E, Oliva C, Rosso R, Rizzo F: Haemolytic anaemia with positive cryoglobulin test in a HIV positive man. Eur J Cancer 1991;27:304.
558. Taneja-Uppal N, Rappaport S, Berger BJ, Davidson E, Rahal JJ: Human immunodeficiency virus (HIV) infection and hemolytic anemia. Ann Intern Med 1989;111:340–341.
559. Tongol JM, Gounder MP, Butala A, Rabinowitz M: HIV-related autoimmune hemolytic anemia: Good response to zidovudine. J Acquir Immune Defic Syndr 1991;4:1163–1164.
560. Pan A, Pirola F, Bergonzi C, Petrini C, Carnevale G: Reticulocytopenic immune hemolytic anemia in an AIDS patient. Int Conf AIDS 1992;8:120.
561. Romo M, Martin VC, Guerra JL, Marinas C, de Diego T: IgM cryoagglutinin with biphasic hemolysin activity in a patient with AIDS: Sangre (Barc) 1991;36:165–166.
562. Lopez Dupla JM, Rodriguez PA, Martinez MP, de Castro CJ, Lavilla UP, Gil AA: Hemolytic anemia due to cold-reacting antibodies: association with human immunodeficiency virus infection and non-Hodgkin's lymphoma. Med Clin (Barc) 1992;98:502–504.
563. Dollus C, Dalle JH, Reviron M, Leverger G, Lasfargues G, Courpotin C: Pediatric case of HIV associated autoimmune hemolytic anemia. Int Conf AIDS 1993;9:450.
564. Sukthankar AD, Bowman CA, Carey M, Radcliffe KW: HIV infection with haemolytic anaemia. Genitourin Med 1997;73:66–69.
565. Borgna-Pignatti C, Bezzi TM, Reverberi R: Fatal ceftriaxone-induced hemolysis in a child with acquired immunodeficiency syndrome. Pediatr Infect Dis J 1995;14:1116–1117.
566. Prazuck T, Semaille C, Roques S: Fatal acute haemolysis in an AIDS patient treated with indinavir. AIDS 1998;12:531–533.
567. Capron L, Kim YU, Laurian C, Bruneval P, Fiessinger JN: Atheroembolism in HIV-positive individuals. Lancet 1992;340:1039–1040.
568. Pinilla J, Hill AR: Thromboembolism associated with acquired immunodeficiency syndrome. CHEST 1992;102:1634.
569. Pulik M, Lionnet F, Couderc LJ, Matheron S, Saimot AG: Thromboembolic disease and human immunodeficiency virus infection. Blood 1993;82:2931.
570. Cohen JR, Lackner R, Wenig P, Pillari G: Deep venous thrombosis in patients with AIDS: N Y State J Med 1990;90:159–161.
571. Saif MW, Bona R, Greenberg B: AIDS and thrombosis: Retrospective study of 131 HIV-infected patients. AIDS Patient Care STDS 2001;15:311–320.
572. Haemolytic transfusion reactions. In: Mollison PL, Engelfriet CP, Contreras M (eds): Blood Transfusion in Clinical Medicine, 10th ed. Oxford: Blackwell Science Ltd, 1997:358–389.
573. Ries M, Simon S, Hummer HP, Leipold G: Acute mesenteric vein thrombosis. A rare complication after splenectomy due to autoimmune hemolytic anemia in childhood. Monatssch Kinderheilkd 1993;141:779–781.
574. Terada K, Tanaka H, Mori R, Kataoka N, Uchikawa M: Hemolytic anemia associated with cold agglutinin during

chickenpox and a review of the literature. J Pediatr Hematol Oncol 1998;20:149–151.
575. Borbolla L, Chediak B: Anemia hemolitica de etiologia viral revision de la literature. Rev Cubana Pediatr 1953;25: 557–564.
576. Friedman HD, Dracker RA: Cold agglutinin disease after chicken pox. An uncommon complication of a common disease. Am J Clin Pathol 1992;97:92–96.
577. Herron B, Roelcke D, Orson G, Myint H, Boulton FE: Cold autoagglutinins with anti-Pr specificity associated with fresh varicella infection. Vox Sang 1993;65:239–242.
578. Johnson AM: Cold agglutinin disease after chickenpox. Am J Clin Pathol 1992;98:271–272.
579. Northoff H, Martin A, Roelcke D: An IgG kappa-monotypic anti-Pr 1h associated with fresh varicella infection. Eur J Haematol 1987;38:85–88.
580. Parashar S, Bhandary S, Menezes S, et al: Auto immune haemolytic anaemia. J Assoc Physicians India 1981;29:679–682.
581. Kaiser AD, Bradford WL: Severe hemoglobinuria in a child occurring in the prodromal stage of chickenpox. Arch Pediatr 1929;46:571–577.
582. Sanchis CJ, Carbonell UF: Autoimmune hemolytic anemia with anti-DC specificity following a primary infection by Varicella virus. Haematologica 1997;824:508–509.
583. Ziebold C, von Kries R, Lang R, Weigl J, Schmitt HJ: Severe complications of varicella in previously healthy children in Germany: A 1-year survey. Pediatrics 2001;108:E79.
584. Kadota Y, Fujinami S, Tagawa Y, et al: Haemolytic anaemia caused by anti-Pra following rubella infection. Transfusion Med 1993;3:207–209.
585. Ueda K, Shingaki Y, Sato T, Tokugawa K, Sasaki H: Hemolytic anemia following postnatally acquired rubella during the 1975–1977 rubella epidemic in Japan. Clin Pediatr (Phila) 1985;24:155–157.
586. Miyazaki S, Ohtsuka M, Ueda K, Shibata R, Goya N: Coombs positive hemolytic anemia in congenital rubella. J Pediatr 1979;94:759–760.
587. Konig AL, Keller HE, Braun RW, Roelcke D: Cold agglutinins of anti-Pr specificity in rubella embryopathy. Ann Hematol 1992;64:277–280.
588. Geisen HP, Roelcke D, Rehn K, Konrad G: High titer cold agglutinins with anti-pr specificity after rubella infection. Klin Wochenschr 1975;53:767–772.
589. Roelcke D, Ebert W, Geisen HP: Anti-Pr3: serological and immunochemical identification of a new anti-Pr subspecificity. Vox Sang 1976;30:122–133.
590. Habibi B, Cregut R, Brossard Y, Veron P, Salmon C: Auto-anti-Pra: A "second" example in a newborn. Br J Haematol 1975;30:499–505.
591. Roelcke D, Kreft H: Characterization of various anti-Pr cold agglutinins. Transfusion 1984;24:210–213.
592. Brody M, Kreysel HW: Cold agglutinin syndrome after rubella infection. Kinderarztl Prax 1992;60:134–136.
593. Torok TJ: Unusual clinical manifestations reported in patients with parvovirus B19 infection. In: Anderson LJ, Young NS (eds): Human Parvovirus B19. Basel: Karger, 1997:61–92.
594. Brown KE: Human parvovirus B19 epidemiology and clinical manifestations. In: Anderson LJ, Young NS (eds): Human Parvovirus B19. Basel: Karger, 1997:42–60.
595. Kunimi M, Ishikawa K, Tsutsumi H, Hirai M, Kumakawa T, Mori M: Parvovirus infection and hemolytic anemia. Am J Hematol 1994;46:159–160.
596. Smith MA, Shah NS, Lobel JS: Parvovirus B19 infection associated with reticulocytopenia and chronic autoimmune hemolytic anemia. Am J Pediatr Hematol Oncol 1989;11:167–169.
596a. de la Rubia J, Moscardo F, Arriaga F, Monteagudo E, Carreras C, Marty ML: Acute parvovirus B19 infection as a cause of autoimmune hemolytic anemia. Haematologica 2000;85:995–997.
597. Petz LD: Hematologic aspects of liver disease. Curr Op Gastroenterol 1989;5:372–377.
597a. Ramos-Casals M, Garcia-Carrasco M, Lopez-Medrano F, et al: Severe autoimmune cytopenias in treatment-naive hepatitis C virus infection: Clinical description of 35 cases. Medicine (Baltimore) 2003;82:87–96.
598. Chao TC, Chen CY, Yang YH, Chen PM, Chang FY, Lee SD: Chronic hepatitis C virus infection associated with primary warm-type autoimmune hemolytic anemia. J Clin Gastroenterol 2001;33:232–233.
599. Srinivasan R: Autoimmune hemolytic anemia in treatment-naive chronic hepatitis C infection. J Clin Gastroenterol 2001;32:245–247.
600. Fellermann K, Stange EF: Chronic hepatitis C, common variable immunodeficiency and autoimmune hemolytic anemia. Coincidence by chance or common etiology? Hepatogastroenterology 2000;47:1422–1424.
601. Landau A, Castera L, Buffet C, Tertian G, Tchernia G: Acute autoimmune hemolytic anemia during interferon-alpha therapy for chronic hepatitis C. Dig Dis Sci 1999;44:1366–1367.
602. Kazuta Y, Watanabe N, Sagawa K, et al: A case of autoimmune hemolytic anemia induced by IFN-beta therapy for type-C chronic hepatitis. Fukushima J Med Sci 1995;41:43–49.
603. Hizawa N, Kojima J, Kojima T, et al: A patient with chronic hepatitis C who simultaneously developed interstitial pneumonia, hemolytic anemia and cholestatic liver dysfunction after alpha-interferon administration. Intern Med 1994;33:337–341.
604. Hirashima N, Mizokami M, Orito E, et al: Chronic hepatitis C complicated by Coombs-negative hemolytic anemia during interferon treatment. Intern Med 1994;33:300–302.
605. Moccia F, Tognoni E, Boccaccio P: Autoimmune hemolytic anemia in chronic hepatitis C virus infection: An unusual extrahepatic autoimmune manifestation. Ann Ital Med Int 2001;16:256–259.
606. Longo F, Hastier P, Buckley MJ, Chichmanian RM, Delmont JP: Acute hepatitis, autoimmune hemolytic anemia, and erythroblastocytopenia induced by ceftriaxone. Am J Gastroenterol 1998;93:836–837.
607. Kondo H, Kajii E, Oyamada T, Kasahara Y: Direct antiglobulin test negative autoimmune hemolytic anemia associated with autoimmune hepatitis. Int J Hematol 1998;68:439–443.
608. Ibe M, Rude B, Gerken G, Meyer zum Buschenfelde KH, Lohse AW: Coombs-negative severe hemolysis associated with hepatitis A. Z Gastroenterol 1997;35:567–569.
609. Melendez HV, Rela M, Baker AJ, et al: Liver transplant for giant cell hepatitis with autoimmune haemolytic anaemia. Arch Dis Child 1997;77:249–251.
610. Perez-Atayde AR, Sirlin SM, Jonas M: Coombs-positive autoimmune hemolytic anemia and postinfantile giant cell hepatitis in children. Pediatr Pathol 1994;14:69–77.
611. Weinstein T, Valderrama E, Pettei M, Levine J: Early steroid therapy for the treatment of giant cell hepatitis with autoimmune hemolytic anemia. J Pediatr Gastroenterol Nutr 1993;17:313–316.
612. Brichard B, Sokal E, Gosseye S, Buts JP, Gadisseux JF, Cornu G: Coombs-positive giant cell hepatitis of infancy: Effect of steroids and azathioprine therapy. Eur J Pediatr 1991;150:314–317.
613. Bernard O, Hadchouel M, Scotto J, Odievre M, Alagille D: Severe giant cell hepatitis with autoimmune hemolytic anemia in early childhood. J Pediatr 1981;99:704–711.
614. Hartman C, Berkowitz D, Brik R, Arad A, Elhasid R, Shamir R: Giant cell hepatitis with autoimmune hemolytic anemia and hemophagocytosis. J Pediatr Gastroenterol Nutr 2001;32: 330–334.
615. Hadzic N, Portmann B, Lewis I, Mieli-Vergani G: Coombs positive giant cell hepatitis—a new feature of Evans' syndrome. Arch Dis Child 1998;78:397–398.
616. Gurudu SR, Mittal SK, Shaber M, Gamboa E, Michael S, Sigal LH: Autoimmune hepatitis associated with autoimmune hemolytic anemia and anticardiolipin antibody syndrome. Dig Dis Sci 2000;45:1878–1880.
617. Hume R, Williamson JM, Whitelaw JW: Red cell survival in biliary cirrhosis. J Clin Pathol 1970;23:397–401.
618. Shichiri M, Koyama W, Tozuka S, Sakamoto S, Kanayama M: Primary biliary cirrhosis. A patient with adverse reactions to tiopronin and autoimmune hemolytic anemia with reticulocytopenia. Arch Intern Med 1984;144:89–91.

619. Orlin JB, Berkman EM, Matloff DS, Kaplan MM: Primary biliary cirrhosis and cold autoimmune hemolytic anemia: Effect of partial plasma exchange. Gastroenterology 1980;78:576–578.
620. Buonanno G, Castaldo C, Izzo GN: Cold agglutinin disease and cryoglobulinemia: Report of two cases. Haematologica 1985;70:174–177.
621. Lachaux A, Bertrand Y, Bouvier R, Dumont C, Pinzaru M, Hermier M: Intravenous immunoglobulin therapy in an infant with autoimmune hemolytic anemia associated with necrotic hepatitis and peliosis. J Pediatr Gastroenterol Nutr 1996;22: 99–102.
622. Perseghin P, Balduini CL, Piccolo G, et al: Guillain-Barré syndrome with autoimmune hemolytic anemia following acute viral hepatitis. Ital J Neurol Sci 1985;6:447–450.
623. Yoshioka K, Miyata H: Autoimmune haemolytic anaemia in an asymptomatic carrier of hepatitis B virus. Arch Dis Child 1980;55:233–234.
624. Tibble JA, Ireland A, Duncan JR: Acute auto immune haemolytic anaemia secondary to hepatitis A infection. Clin Lab Haematol 1997;19:73–75.
625. Williams AJ, Marsh J, Stableforth DE: Cryptogenic fibrosing alveolitis, chronic active hepatitis and autoimmune haemolytic anaemia in the same patient. Br J Dis Chest 1985;79:200–203.
626. Pounder RE: Pancreatic exocrine deficiency, chronic active hepatitis and familial autoallergic haemolytic anaemia. Proc R Soc Med 1974;67:323–324.
627. Panush RS, Wilkinson LS, Fagin RR: Chronic active hepatitis associated with eosinophilia and Coombs'-positive hemolytic anemia. Gastroenterology 1973;64:1015–1019.
628. Lightwood AM, Scott GL: Autoimmune haemolytic anaemia due to red cell antibodies of different specificities in a patient with chronic hepatitis. Vox Sang 1973;24:331–336.
629. Pengelly CD, Jennings RC: Active chronic hepatitis and haemolytic anaemia associated with Rh-specific antibodies. Postgrad Med J 1971;47:683–686.
630. Cuesta B, Fernandez J, Pardo J, Paramo JA, Gomez C, Rocha E: Evan's syndrome, chronic active hepatitis and focal glomerulonephritis in IgA deficiency. Acta Haematol 1986;75:1–5.
631. Christophers SR, Bentley C: Phagocytosis of red cells in blackwater fever. JAMA 1908;50:1383.
632. Zuckerman A: Autoimmunization and other types of indirect damage to host cells as factors in certain protozoan diseases. Experimental Parasitology 1964;15:138–183.
633. Daniel-Ribeiro CT, Zanini G: Autoimmunity and malaria: What are they doing together? Acta Trop 2000;76:205–221.
634. Woodruff AW, Ansdell VE, Pettitt LE: Cause of anaemia in malaria. Lancet 1979;1:1055–1057.
635. Facer CA, Bray RS, Brown J: Direct Coombs antiglobulin reactions in Gambian children with Plasmodium falciparum malaria. I: Incidence and class specificity. Clin Exp Immunol 1979;35:119–127.
636. Facer CA: Direct Coombs antiglobulin reactions in Gambian children with Plasmodium falciparum malaria. II: Specificity of erythrocyte-bound IgG. Clin Exp Immunol 1980;39:279–288.
637. Facer CA: Direct antiglobulin reactions in Gambian children with P: Falciparum malaria. III: Expression of IgG subclass determinants and genetic markers and association with anaemia. Clin Exp Immunol 1980;41:81–90.
638. Abdalla S, Weatherall DJ, Wickramasinghe SN, Hughes M: The anaemia of P: Falciparum malaria. Br J Haematol 1980;46: 171–183.
639. Drouin J, Rock G, Jolly EE: Plasmodium falciparum malaria mimicking autoimmune hemolytic anemia during pregnancy. Can Med Assoc J 1985;132:265–267.
640. Brown KN, Berzins K, Jarra W, Schetters T: Immune responses to erythrocytic malaria. Clinics in Immunology and Allergy 1986;6:227.
641. Lee SH, Looareesuwan S, Wattanagoon Y, et al: Antibody-dependent red cell removal during P: Falciparum malaria: The clearance of red cells sensitized with an IgG anti-D. Br J Haematol 1989;73:396–402.
642. Neva FA, Sheagren JN, Shulman NR, Canfield CJ: Malaria: Host-defense mechanisms and complications. Ann Intern Med 1970;73:295–306.
643. Looareesuwan S, Merry AH, Phillips RE, et al: Reduced erythrocyte survival following clearance of malarial parasitaemia in Thai patients. Br J Haematol 1987;67:473–478.
644. Jeje OM, Kelton JG, Blajchman MA: Quantitation of red cell membrane associated immunoglobulin in children with Plasmodium falciparum parasitaemia. Br J Haematol 1983;54:567–572.
645. Berzins K, Wahlgren M, Perlmann P: Studies on the specificity of anti-erythrocyte antibodies in the serum of patients with malaria. Clin Exp Immunol 1983;54:313–318.
646. Wahlgren M, Berzins K, Perlmann P, Bjorkman A: Characterization of the humoral immune response in Plasmodium falciparum malaria. I: Estimation of antibodies to P: Falciparum or human erythrocytes by means of microELISA. Clin Exp Immunol 1983;54:127–134.
647. Lundgren K, Wahlgren M, Troye-Blomberg M, Berzins K, Perlmann H, Perlmann P: Monoclonal anti-parasite and anti-RBC antibodies produced by stable EBV-transformed B cell lines from malaria patients. J Immunol 1983;131:2000–2003.
648. Topley E, Knight R, Woodruff AW: The direct antiglobulin test and immunoconglutinin titres in patients with malaria. Trans R Soc Trop Med Hyg 1973;67:51–54.
649. Rosenberg EB, Strickland GT, Yang SL, Whalen GE: IgM antibodies to red cells and autoimmune anemia in patients with malaria. Am J Trop Med Hyg 1973;22:146–152.
650. Wenisch C, Spitzauer S, Florris-Linau K, et al: Complement activation in severe Plasmodium falciparum malaria. Clin Immunol Immunopathol 1997;85:166–171.
651. Lefrancois G, Bouvet E, Le Bras J, Vroklans M, Simonneau M, Vachon F: Anti-erythrocyte autoimmunisation during chronic falciparum malaria. Lancet 1981;2:661–664.
652. Ritter K, Kuhlencord A, Thomssen R, Bommer W: Prolonged haemolytic anaemia in malaria and autoantibodies against triosephosphate isomerase. Lancet 1993;342:1333–1334.
653. Conrad ME: Pathophysiology of malaria. Hematologic observations in human and animal studies. Ann Intern Med 1969;70:134–141.
654. Merry AH, Looareesuwan S, Phillips RE, et al: Evidence against immune haemolysis in falciparum malaria in Thailand. Br J Haematol 1986;64:187–194.
655. Petz LD: The expanding boundaries of transfusion medicine. In Nance SJ (ed): Clinical and Basic Science Aspects of Immunohematology. Arlington, VA: American Association of Blood Banks, 1991:73–113.
656. Gajewski JL, Petz LD, Calhoun L, et al: Hemolysis of transfused group O red blood cells in minor ABO-incompatible unrelated-donor bone marrow transplants in patients receiving cyclosporine without posttransplant methotrexate. Blood 1992;79:3076–3085.
657. Petz LD, Calhoun L, Shulman IA, Johnson C, Herron RM: The sickle cell hemolytic transfusion reaction syndrome. Transfusion 1997;37:382–392.
658. Kokkini G, Vrionis G, Liosis G, Papaefstathiou J: Cold agglutinin syndrome and hemophagocytosis in systemic leishmaniasis. Scand J Haematol 1984;32:441–445.
659. Pontes De Carvalho LC, Badaro R, Carvalho EM, et al: Nature and incidence of erythrocyte-bound IgG and some aspects of the physiopathogenesis of anaemia in American visceral leishmaniasis. Clin Exp Immunol 1986;64:495–502.
660. Kobayakawa T, Louis J, Izui S, Lambert PH: Autoimmune response to DNA, red blood cells, and thymocyte antigens in association with polyclonal antibody synthesis during experimental African trypanosomiasis. J Immunol 1979;122: 296–301.
661. Wolf CFW, Resnick G, Marsh WL, Benach J, Habicht G: Autoimmunity to red blood cells in babesiosis. Transfusion 1982;22:538–539.
662. Homer MJ, Aguilar-Delfin I, Telford SR, III, Krause PJ, Persing DH: Babesiosis. Clin Microbiol Rev 2000;13:451–469.

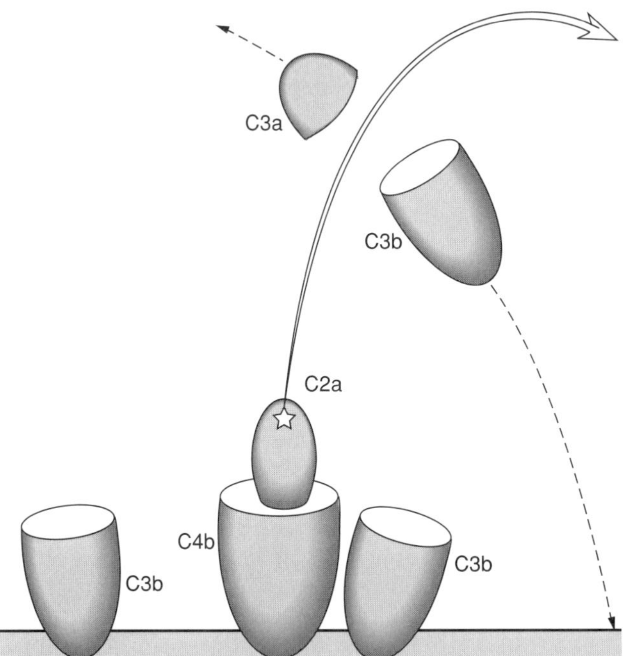

FIGURE 4-4. C3 convertase ($\overline{\text{C4b2a}}$) cleaves C3 into fragments: C3a anaphylotoxin, which circulates in the plasma, and C3b, which can attach to cell membranes. Some C3b molecules will fall close to $\overline{\text{C4b2a}}$ complexes and will form a new enzyme, $\overline{\text{C4b2a3b}}$ or C5 convertase.

The Membrane Attack Complex (MAC). C5b appears to bind C6 and C7 by adsorption (see Fig. 4-5). The resulting trimolecular complex attaches to the cell membrane and binds C8 and C9 (Fig. 4-6). Fully assembled, MAC consists of about 20 protein molecules, including one molecule of C5b, C6, C7, and C8 and multiple molecules of C9. It has a molecular weight of about 1.7 million. The end result of the pathway is lysis of the cell.

Electron microscopy shows that lesions start appearing in the cell membrane at the C8 stage, although the cell does not lyse until C9 is complexed.[12] Mayer[13] proposed the so-called "doughnut" hypothesis; a stable hole is produced by the assembly of a rigid, doughnut-shaped structure in the lipid bilayer of the cell membrane. The hole forms a channel connecting the inside of the cell with the extracellular fluid. The outside of the doughnut could be composed of nonpolar peptides, that is, protein chains that are hydrophobic; the interior would need polar peptides so that it could be hydrophilic. He suggested that C5b, C6, C7, C8, and C9 may be the proteins that form the doughnut or funnel shape, penetrating the lipid bilayer of the membrane.[13] The cell then lyses either by direct egress of the hemoglobin or, more commonly, through colloid osmotic pressure.[13] Water and sodium enter the cell with resultant swelling; the membrane of the swollen cell becomes permeable to macromolecular substances, including intracellular proteins and nucleotides. Once intracellular contents have diffused out, the membrane seals again and effectively becomes an empty sac. The cellular remnant is removed from the circulation by phagocytosis.

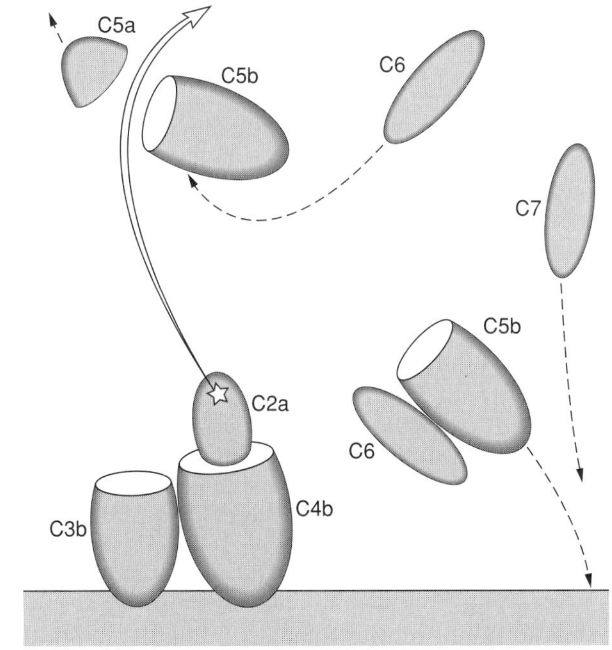

FIGURE 4-5. C5 convertase ($\overline{\text{C4b2a3b}}$) cleaves C5 into two fragments: C5a anaphylotoxin, which circulates in the plasma, and C5b, which is capable of absorbing C6 and C7. The trimolecular complex can attach to cell membranes, initiating the formation of the membrane attack complex (MAC).

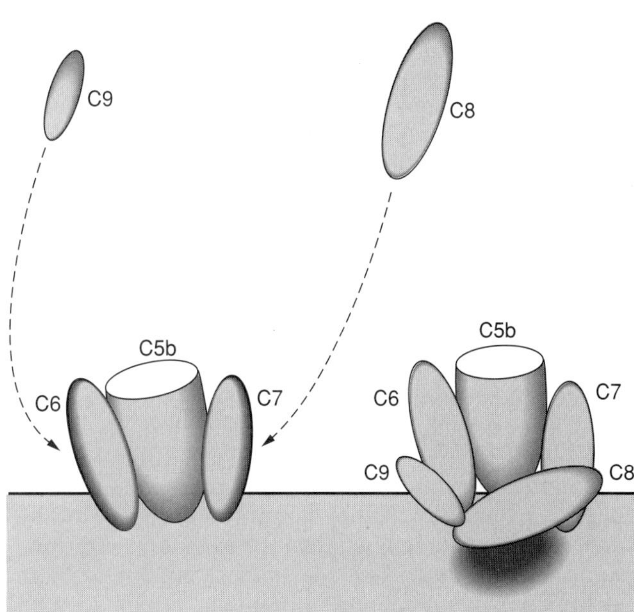

FIGURE 4-6. C5b67 absorbs C8. This complex is inserted into the bilipid layer of the membrane. Finally, C9 is absorbed, forming the final membrane attack complex (MAC), leading to lysis of the cell.

Several regulatory proteins that affect MAC function have been described, including C8-binding protein (C8bp) or homologous destruction factor, membrane inhibitor of reactive lysis (MIRL, CD 59), and S protein in plasma.

THE ALTERNATIVE PATHWAY OF COMPLEMENT ACTIVATION

In 1954, Pillemer and his coworkers[14] showed that properdin, a substance present in normal plasma, would react with a wide variety of naturally occurring polysaccharides and lipopolysaccharides to activate complement, without the presence of antibody. Several other factors present in normal plasma (e.g., C3, factor A, and factor B) were found to be necessary for the reaction. They suggested that this might be an important in vivo defense mechanism in an unimmunized host. Very few scientists accepted Pillemer's theories at that time, particularly when work emerged on the structure of immunoglobulins and the differences between different immunoglobulin (Ig) classes in complement activation were described. Many investigators believed that the in vitro complement activation that Pillemer had described as attributable to zymosan (a yeast extract) was actually the result of a naturally occurring IgM antibody to zymosan, and thus the complement activation was antibody dependent.[15] The theory of an antibody-independent complement activation mechanism lay fallow for about 10 to 15 years and then was gradually resurrected.[16]

In 1968, Gewurz and coworkers[17] showed that endotoxin and immune complexes could consume C3-C9 without affecting C1, C2, or C4 levels. Schur and Becker[18] demonstrated that the $F(ab')_2$ fragments of rabbit antibody (i.e., rabbit IgG antibody that had the Fc fragment digested away but had both of its antigen-combining sites intact) could fix complement. Sandberg and colleagues[19] showed that guinea pig immune complexes made with IgG1 or IgG2 antibodies would fix complement; this was of great interest because guinea pig IgG1 antibodies are known not to activate C1 (i.e., the antibody does not have a binding site for C1 on its Fc fragment). In addition, the IgG1 antigen-antibody complexes led to the preferential fixation of C3-C9 with very little fixation of C1, C4, and C2. Ellman and coworkers[20] discovered a strain of guinea pigs that were genetically deficient in C4. This strain added to the evidence accumulating in support of Pillemer's original hypothesis, suggesting an alternative complement-activation pathway. The $F(ab')_2$ and endotoxin experiments could be duplicated by the addition of the appropriate antigen-antibody complexes or endotoxins to serum of animals totally deficient in C4. Bacterial endotoxins and immune complexes depleted the C4-deficient guinea pig sera of the later complement components, which seemed to prove without doubt that an alternative pathway must be operative.[21]

About this time, Muller-Eberhard's group was studying the interaction of cobra venom and complement. In 1903, Flexner and Noguchi demonstrated that cobra venom abolished the hemolytic activity of serum.[22] It was shown later that this factor could be isolated from cobra venom, and that it not only inactivated C3 but potentially activated the complement system at the C3 reaction step, leading to the formation of C5b-9. Studies on cobra venom led to the description of the C3 activator system, with its various factors, many of which could be equated with factors described originally by Pillemer. The C3 activator system was integrated with the properdin system, providing a basis for an alternative pathway of complement activation.[22]

The alternative pathway leads to the formation of C5 convertase and thus the self-assembling C5b-9 complex, with eventual cell damage, just as in the classical pathway.

Reaction Mechanism of the Alternative Complement Pathway. Table 4-2 lists some activators of the alternative pathway. All investigators agree that the alternative pathway can be activated in vitro without immunoglobulin (e.g., by endotoxin, inulin, zymosan), but the ability of nonaggregated immunoglobulin to activate the alternative pathway was controversial for years. It now seems clear that antibody can play a role in activation of the alternative pathway. Most workers agree that aggregated IgA can activate the pathway,[23] but there are differing reports in the literature on the ability of aggregated IgG to activate the pathway.[24] One has to be cautious of interpreting some of the data, as preparations of immunoglobulins can be contaminated with endotoxin, which alone can activate the pathway. Evidence for the role of antibody independent from its classical pathway function has accrued from experiments with purified proteins of the alternative pathway, sera genetically deficient in C2 and C4, and chelating agents specific for calcium so as to prevent activation of C1.

Five major proteins (factors P, $\overline{P}$, B, $\overline{B}$, $\overline{D}$) are involved solely in alternative pathway activity[25] (Table 4-3). Only five of these proteins are essential for initiation and amplification because these events occur in the absence of properdin. Of these five proteins, three (C3, factor B, and factor D) are required for the generation of the initial enzyme and the amplifying enzyme of the pathway. The other two proteins (factor H and factor I) are regulators of C3 convertase; they suppress C3 convertase formation in the fluid phase and confine enzyme formation to the surface of activators. Activation of the pathway consists of initiation and amplification. Initiation is nonspecific, inasmuch as it

TABLE 4-2. ACTIVATORS OF THE ALTERNATIVE COMPLEMENT PATHWAY

Immunoglobulins	IgA (aggregated) IgG and IgE (see text)
Polysaccharides	Inulin, agar, endotoxin, yeast, cell walls
Miscellaneous	Cobra venom factor, trypsin

TABLE 4-3. PROTEINS PARTICIPATING IN THE ALTERNATIVE PATHWAY

Component	Symbol	Molecular Weight	Electrophoretic Mobility	Synonyms
Properdin	P	184,000	γ	–
Activated P	$\overline{P}$	184,000	γ	–
Proactivator	B	93,000	β	PA, GBG
Activated B	$\overline{B}$	63,000	γ	C3A,GGG,211,Bb
Proactivator Convertase	$\overline{D}$	24,000	α	PAse, GBGase
C3	C3	180,000	β	Factor A, HSF
C3b	C3b	171,000	α2	HSFa
C3b Inactivator	C3b INA	88,000	β	
β1H	β1H	180,000	β	

does not require immunoglobulin or an antibody-like recognition factor. Initiation appears to be a two-step process involving (1) random binding of C3b through its labile binding site to an activator, and (2) discriminatory interaction of the bound C3b with surrounding surface structures. The random event is the result of the action of the initial C3 convertase, which is a fluid-phase enzyme.

No one has yet described an initiator of the alternative pathway that fulfills the role of antibody in the classical pathway. Lachman and coworkers[25,26] suggested that C3b is formed continuously at a low level in a "tick-over" mechanism involving an enzyme. It has also been suggested that the first molecule of metastable C3b may be formed in a nonenzymatic fashion, and that may then be followed by an enzymatic step. Native C3 undergoes spontaneous alteration in neutral buffer at 37°C. Following this alteration, a free sulfhydryl group appears that is not present in native C3. The product, $C3(H_2O)$, is a form of uncleaved C3 in which the thioester has been hydrolyzed. $C3(H_2O)$ exhibits all the functional properties of C3b, including the ability (unlike native C3) to bind to C3b receptors. $C3(H_2O)$ is structurally distinct from C3b in that it contains an intact α-chain, rather than the α′-chain of C3b that lacks the C3a domain. Unlike native C3, the α-chain of $C3(H_2O)$ is susceptible to cleavage by factor I. Factor I cleaves the α-chain of $C3(H_2O)$ into fragments of 76,000 and 40,000 d. The larger fragment contains the 67,000-d piece of the α-chain of iC3b plus the covalently linked 9000-d C3a domain of the α-chain.

In the presence of magnesium, $C3b(H_2O)$ and factor B form a reversible complex which, if activated by the serine protease factor D, becomes the initial C3 convertase C3,Bb. This transient C3 convertase can cleave C3 in the fluid phase into C3a and C3b. Following C3a removal, C3b expresses a highly reactive site. Metastable C3b can bind covalently to a variety of sugars and attach to cell surfaces.

The spontaneous formation of $C3(H_2O)$ and thus the initial C3 convertase provide a mechanism for the continuous low-level supply of metastable C3b. It has been suggested that a random initiation mechanism operates in the alternative pathway as compared to the nonrandom initiation of the classical pathway. A unique feature of the alternative pathway is a C3b-dependent positive feedback mechanism of amplication. Each newly formed C3b molecule has the potential to form more C3 convertase ($C\overline{3bBb}$) and thus more C3b.

A discriminatory interaction occurs after binding of C3b to particles (e.g., cells). When bound to a nonactivator of the alternative pathway, C3b is able to bind factor H and becomes inactivated through the combined effects of factors H and I. When bound to an activator, control is restricted because C3b is relatively resistant to inactivation by factors H and I. In contrast, binding of factor B to C3b and the formation of C3 convertase are unaffected by the nature of the surface. As a consequence of the discriminatory phase of initiation, C3 convertase formation on the activator occurs, and amplification through the solid phase C3 convertase commences. Through the additional enzymatic cleavage of C3, more C3b attaches to the membrane; receptor function is thought to reside in at least two critically oriented and closely spaced C3b molecules. The role of the second C3b molecule is to bind C5 and to modify it for cleavage by Bb. Binding of activated factor B to the C3b-doublet receptor results in generation of the labile C5 convertase, $\overline{C3b,Bb}$ (which also acts on C3). The C5 convertase can activate properdin (P) nonenzymatically. Properdin is not an essential component for activation of the pathway, but confers an increased degree of stability on $\overline{C3b,Bb}$, and its presence results in more rapid amplification of bound C3b.

Once C3 is activated in the alternative pathway, the molecular consequences seem to be identical to those of the classical pathway. The alternative pathway has not yet been incriminated in many immunohematologic problems; this may relate to the fact that it is very inefficient in the lysis of human RBCs as compared to the classical pathway.[27] It is of interest to note that the RBCs of patients with PNH can be shown to hemolyze through the alternative pathway as well as the classical pathway.[28] It is also of interest to note that activation of the alternative pathway by autologous RBC stroma has been described.[29] Complement activation is controlled by

TABLE 4-4. PHYSICAL AND FUNCTIONAL PROPERTIES OF THE COMPLEMENT REGULATORY PROTEINS

State	Protein	Subunits	MW (kD)	Serum (μg/mL)	Biological Activity
Soluble	C1-INH	1	110	200	
	C4bp	8	500	250	Accelerates decay of $C\overline{4b2a}$
	Factor H	1	150	450	Accelerates decay of $C\overline{4b2a}$
	Factor I	2 (αβ)	80	35	Cleavage of C3b
	S protein	1	83	500	Binds fluid phase C5b-7
	Sp-40,40	2	70	50	Binds fluid phase C5b-7
Membrane	CR1	1	160–250		Accelerates decay of C3/C5
	CD55	1	70		Accelerates decay of C3/C5
	MCP	1	45–70		Accelerates decay of C3/C5
	HRF/MIP	1	65		Control of MAC formation
	CD59	1	20		Control of MAC formation

a number of regulatory proteins; these are shown in Table 4-4.

THE MANNOSE-BINDING LECTIN PATHWAY OF COMPLEMENT ACTIVATION

A mannose-binding lectin (MBL), a pattern-recognition molecule of the innate immune system, binds to arrays of terminal mannose groups on a variety of bacteria. This reaction can initiate complement activation.[30,31] MBL interacts with two serine proteases: MSPI, which cleaves C3 directly, and MASP2, which cleaves and activates C3 and C4. This pathway is relevant to bacteria, but not RBCs.

IN VIVO EFFECTS OF RED CELL–BOUND COMPLEMENT

If the complement cascade goes to completion (i.e., MAC formation), then the RBC is hemolyzed. When hemoglobin is released into the plasma, it rapidly combines with haptoglobin to form a complex that is cleared within a few hours by the reticuloendothelial system. When the haptoglobin system is saturated, free hemoglobin circulates in the plasma. Some of it is oxidized and bound to albumin as methemalbumin. Methemalbumin appears about 3 to 6 hours following a hemolytic episode and remains in the plasma for about 24 hours. This dark brown pigment may mix with free hemoglobin, leading to brownish-colored plasma. When plasma contains about 20 mg of hemoglobin per 100 mL, it will appear slightly pink or light brown, if examined in a thickness of about 1 cm. If present on the order of 1 mg per mL, the plasma will appear red.[7] Both the hemoglobin-haptoglobin complex and the methemoglobin are broken down in the reticuloendothelial system to form bilirubin, which will then appear in the plasma (maximum concentrations are usually not attained for 3 to 6 hours after a hemolytic episode). When the plasma hemoglobin level exceeds 1 mg per 100 mL, hemoglobin may be excreted in the urine, producing hemoglobinuria. During this process, some hemoglobin may be absorbed by the renal tubules, splitting off iron, which may eventually (i.e., several days later) appear in the urine as hemosiderin (also see Chapter 2).

Although most blood group antibodies to RBC antigens are IgG1 and/or IgG3, and are thus theoretically capable of activating C1, most do not activate complement efficiently enough to cause RBC lysis and/or complement coating of the RBC. Table 4-5 shows the usual complement-activating efficiency of some RBC alloantibodies. The relative efficiencies probably relate to the number and location of antigen sites on the RBC membrane. For instance, there are at least a million A or B sites on the membrane of A and B RBCs, and the A and B antigens extend from the membrane, providing optimal conditions for IgG doublet formation and complement activation. In contrast, there are only about 30,000 Rh(D) sites, and these are at the membrane surface.

If the RBC is not hemolyzed, it can circulate as a C3b-coated cell. C3b can interact with the macrophage CR1 receptor, leading to phagocytosis. Most complement-coated RBCs are destroyed in the liver by the Kupffer cells; they are also destroyed in the spleen, but the liver has more macrophages than the spleen. This is in contrast to the dominant role of the spleen in the destruction of IgG-coated RBCs. The spleen is more efficient than the liver in the destruction of IgG-coated RBCs because of the reduction of monomeric plasma IgG (which competes for macrophage Fc receptors) due to hemoconcentration. As there is no C3b or iC3b in normal plasma, there is no competition for the macrophage complement (CR1 and CR3) receptors in the liver; thus the splenic macrophages have no more efficiency that the Kupffer cells in the destruction of C3-coated RBCs. C3b does not remain on the red cell very long. If the C3b-coated red cell does not interact, or if the interaction with a C3b receptor on a macrophage is inefficient, the cell-bound C3b is denatured. Naturally occurring complement control enzymes factors H and I cleave C3b molecules,

TABLE 4-5. COMPLEMENT-ACTIVATING EFFICIENCY OF RBC ANTIBODIES

	Does Antibody Cause:		
Specificity	In Vitro or In Vivo RBC Complement Sensitization?	In Vitro Hemolysis?	In Vivo Complement-Mediated Intravascular Hemolysis?
Anti-A, -B	Usually	Often	Usually
Anti-Rh	No	No	No
Anti-I, -i	(Yes)*	Rarely†	Rarely†
Anti-Le^a	Usually	Sometimes	Rarely
Anti-M, -N	No	No	No
Anti-P_1	Sometimes	Rarely	No
Anti-K	Sometimes (19%)	No	No
Anti-Fy^a	Sometimes (13%)	No	No
Anti-Jk^a	Sometimes (46%)	Rarely	Rarely
Anti-S	Sometimes (33%)	No	No
Anti-Vel	Often	Sometimes	Sometimes
Anti-PP_1P^k	Often	Sometimes	Sometimes

*In vitro sensitization occurs commonly when conditions are optimal (e.g., low temperature, low ionic strength, or with enzyme-treated RBCs). In vivo sensitization is rare, occurring only when antibody is of high thermal amplitude (30°C–37°C).
†Only when antibody is of high titer and thermal range.

first forming iC3b, then a second cleavage breaks away C3c, leaving only C3dg on the RBC membrane. C3dg can be further cleaved in vitro, using trypsin, to C3d (Fig. 4-7). It should be noted that many earlier reports relating to the end in vivo cleavage product use the term C3d when it is now known to be C3dg. C3d is only formed when C3dg is cleaved in vitro with enzymes, such as trypsin.

Macrophages have receptors for iC3b (CR1 and CR3/CD 11b/CD 18) in addition to C3b (CR1/CD35), but do not seem to have receptors (or have inefficient receptors) for C3dg or C3d; thus C3b- or iC3b-coated RBCs can be destroyed by macrophages within the reticuloendothelial system. In vivo relationships of complement activation to AIHA are discussed later in this chapter.

EXTRAVASCULAR IMMUNE RED CELL DESTRUCTION

If RBCs become sensitized with IgG, or if RBCs are sensitized with complement but do not proceed through the cascade completely to lysis, then they may be destroyed or damaged within the RES; this system is capable of removing up to about 400 mL of RBCs per day.[7] It is believed that sensitized RBCs are destroyed, within the RES, predominantly by macrophages. Macrophages arise primarily from bone marrow precursors, probably the promonocyte. After a short period of maturation in the bone marrow, monocytes are released into the blood stream. After spending a few days in the peripheral circulation, they migrate to the tissues and there mature functionally and morphologically to become typical histiocytic or exudative macrophages[32] (Fig. 4-8). They are particularly prominent in the liver (Kupffer cells), lung (alveolar macrophages), spleen, and bone marrow. The survival time of mature tissue macrophages is thought to be several weeks, or even months.[32] Immune red cell destruction occurs predominantly in the spleen and the liver.[7]

Macrophage Receptors

Macrophages have receptors on their membranes that specifically recognize certain classes of immunoglobulins (either monomeric [i.e., not complexed with antigen] or in an immune complex), and certain complement components. The receptors are for IgG,[33-38] IgA,[39-43] C3,[44-46] and C4.[45-47]

IgG Fc Receptors (FcγR). FcγRs are members of the immunoglobulin superfamily. There are three classes of Fc receptors: FcγRI, FcγRII, and FcγRIII. Macrophages possess all three classes[36-38] (Fig. 4-9). The three classes are encoded by eight genes localized on chromosome 1 at q21-23. There are at least 12 FcγR isoforms and various genetic polymorphisms.[36-38]

FcγRI (CD64). FcγRI is a 70-kD integral membrane glycoprotein expressed predominantly on macrophages and monocytes. It binds IgG1 and IgG3 with high affinity, binds IgG4 with a lower affinity, but has little or no affinity for IgG2. It has a high affinity (kD = 10^{-8} to 10^{-9} M) for monomeric IgG. This receptor is important in the cytoxic lysis of IgG-sensitized RBCs. Interferon regulates FcγRI expression and thus increases antibody-dependent, cell-mediated cytotoxicity (ADCC) efficiency. As it is continually reacting with monomeric IgG in vivo, FcγRI does not appear to participate in the initial stages of adherence of IgG-sensitized RBCs to the

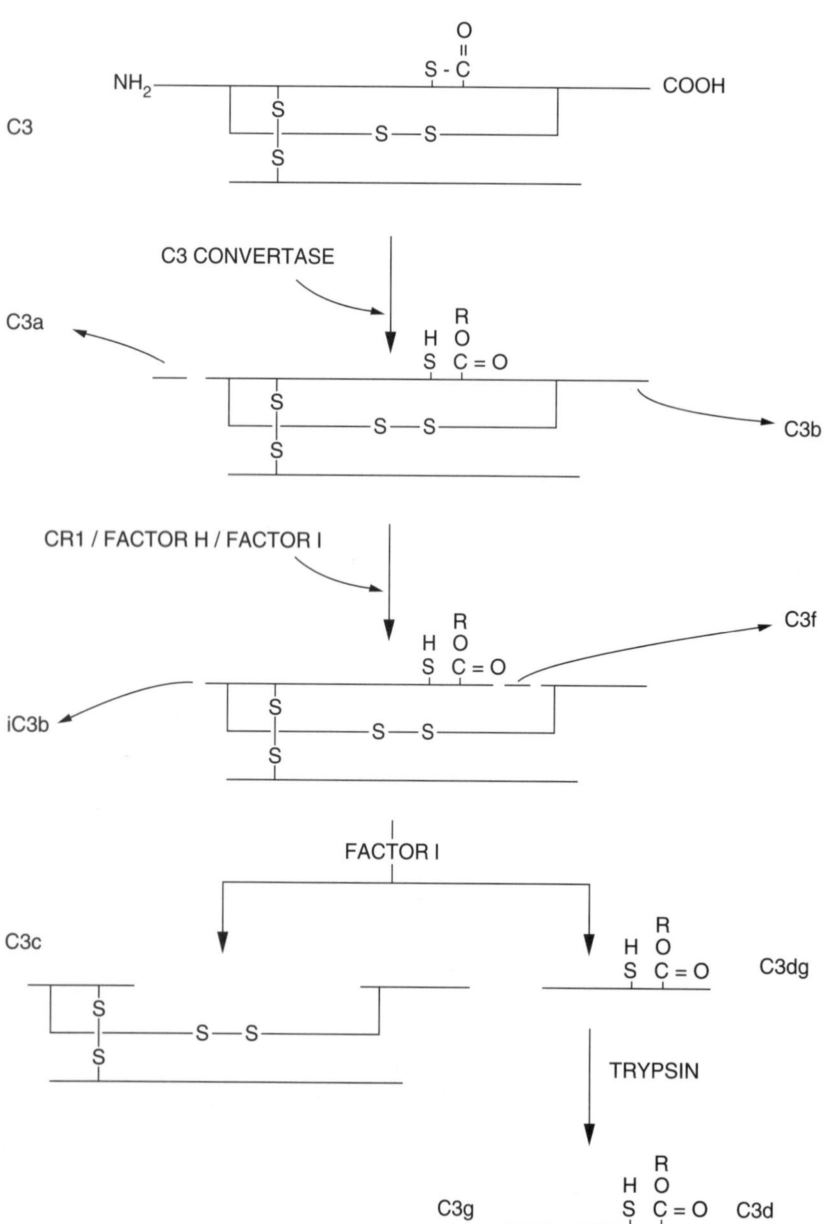

FIGURE 4-7. The enzymatic cleavage pathways of C3. (Reprinted from Freedman J, Semple JW: Complement in transfusion medicine. In Garratty G (ed): Immunobiology of Transfusion Medicine. New York: Dekker, 1994, by courtesy of Marcel Dekker Inc.)

macrophage. It has been suggested that adherence begins with FcγRII and RIII, leading to stripping of the monomeric IgG from FcγRI and subsequent activation of FcγRI to participate in the phagocytic event.

FcγRII (CD32). FcγRII is a 40-kD integral membrane glycoprotein that is found on most circulating blood cells, except RBCs, in the human circulation. It binds all four subclasses, but IgG1 and IgG3 usually bind far more efficiently than IgG2 or IgG4. It has a low affinity for monomeric IgG. There is a genetically determined polymorphism of the FcγRII receptor demonstrable by its interaction with mouse monoclonal IgG1. Three allotypes have been described: IIa^{HR}, IIa^{LR}, and IIb1 (HR = high reactivity with mouse IgG1; LR = low reactivity with mouse IgG1). All three allotypes have a high affinity for IgG3. Allotypes IIa^{HR} and IIb1 have a very low affinity for IgG2, but IIa^{LR} has a similar affinity for IgG2 as for IgG1 (less than for IgG3, but far greater than for IgG4). The IIa^{LR} allotype is found in only 30% of whites, but is present in almost 85% of Japanese.[33] This polymorphism explains why some individuals' macrophages interact efficiently enough with RBCs coated with human IgG2 antibodies to cause AIHA; one would expect to find IgG2-associated AIHA more commonly in the Japanese. FcγRII has a low affinity for its ligands, but is important in phagocytosis, antibody dependent cell mediated cytotoxicity (ADCC) superoxide, and lysosomal enzyme production. FcγRII-mediated ADCC is enhanced by IFN-γ. There are three isoforms (RIIA, RIIB, and RIIC) of FcγRII. RIIA induces phagocytosis; RIIB and RIIC only induce adherence of EA to

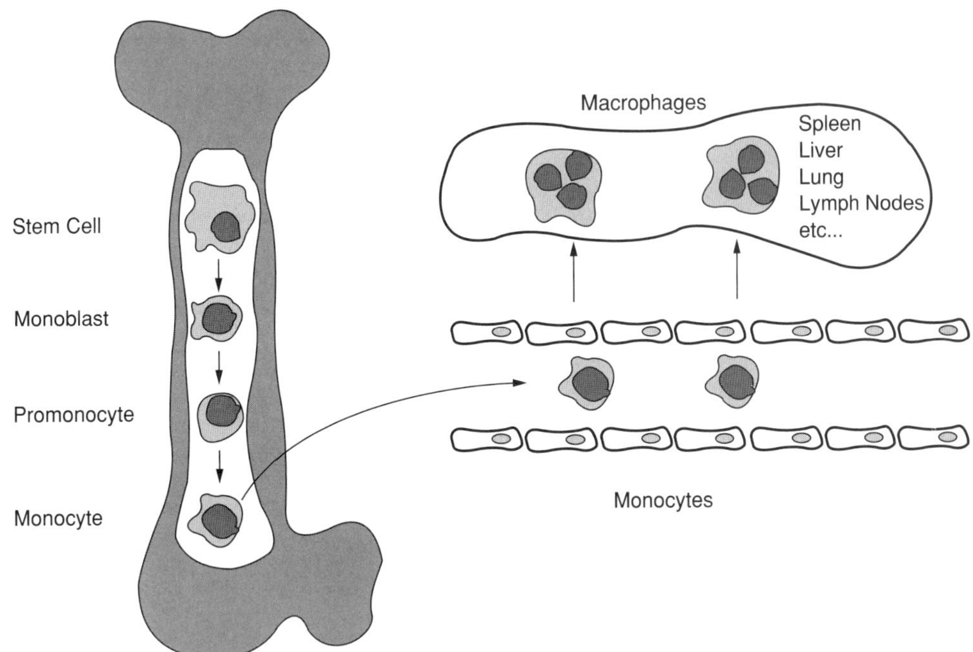

FIGURE 4-8. Mononuclear phagocyte cell lineage. Hematopoietic stem cells in the bone marrow give rise to monoblasts that divide and produce promonocytes. The promonocytes differentiate into monocytes that leave the bone marrow and circulate in the blood. The monocytes migrate into tissues where they differentiate into macrophages. (Reprinted from Horsewood P, Kelton JG: Macrophage-mediated cell destruction. In Garratty G (ed): Immunobiology of Transfusion Medicine. New York: Dekker, 1994:435–464, by courtesy of Marcel Dekker Inc.)

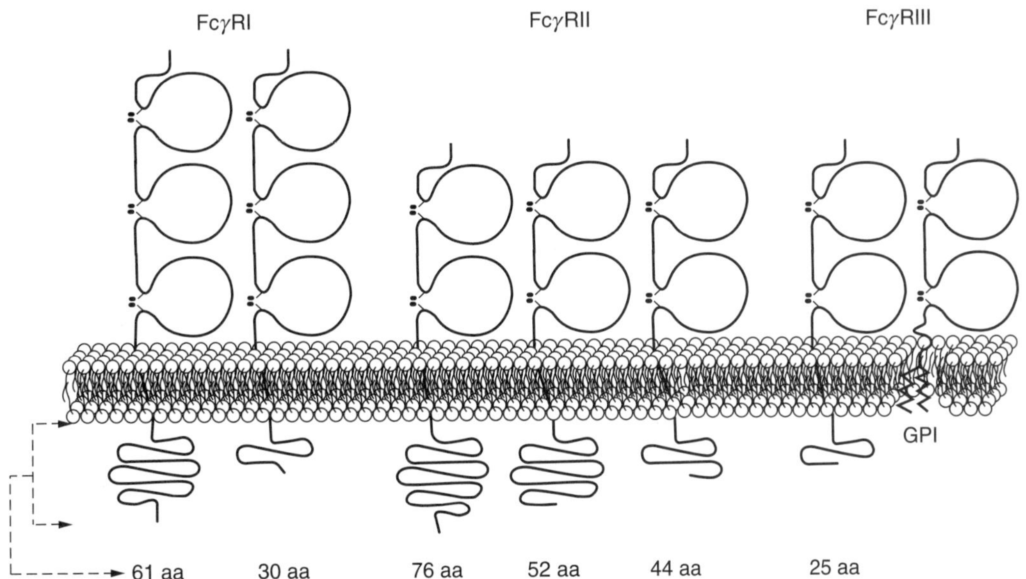

FIGURE 4-9. Schematic diagram of the three classes of membrane Fcγ receptors. The FcγRI integral membrane receptors comprise three immunoglobulin C2 domains and a crytoplasmic tail of either 61 or 30 amino acids (aa). The FcγRII integral membrane receptors have two extracellular immunoglobulin domains and a cytoplasmic tail of 76, 52, or 44 amino acids. The integral membrane FcγRIII that is present on macrophages and NK cells has two immunoglobulin domains and a 25-amino acid cytoplasmic tail. The FcγRIII present on neutrophils is a glycosylphosphatidylinositol (GPI)–linked molecule lacking a cytoplasmic tail, and it has two extracellular immunoglobulin domains. (Reprinted from Horsewood P, Kelton JG: Macrophage-mediated cell destruction. In Garratty G (ed): Immunobiology of Transfusion Medicine. New York: Dekker, 1994:435–464, by courtesy of Marcel Dekker Inc.)

macrophages.[38] Indik and coworkers[38] found that FcγRIIA consistently mediated higher levels of phagoctyosis than FcγRI or RIII.

FcγRIII (CD16). FcγRIII is a 45- to 65-kD membrane glycoprotein present on a subpopulation of monocytes, macrophages, neutrophils, eosinophils, and natural killer (NK) cells. It binds IgG1 and IgG3, but not IgG2 or IgG4. It has a low affinity for monomeric IgG (kd $<10^{-7}$ M). Two FcγRIII genes have been identified. The FcRIIIA gene codes for a transmembrane glycoprotein expressed on macrophages and NK cells. The FcRIIIB gene codes for a glycosylphosphatidylinositol (GPI)-

linked protein expressed on neutrophils only; this protein carries the NA1/NA2 neutrophil-specific antigen. The macrophage FcγRIII can mediate phagocytosis of IgG-coated RBCs.

IgA Fc Receptors. Although early work suggested that macrophages did not have an IgA receptor, such a receptor (FcαR) has now been described by several groups.[39-43] One IgA receptor (Fcα/μR) has recently been shown to crossreact with IgM.[47a] Its clinical significance in RBC destruction is unknown.

Complement Receptors

There are three complement receptors on macrophages: CR1, CR3, and CR4[45,46] (Fig. 4-10).

Complement Receptor Type 1 (CR1 [CD35]). CR1 is found on most circulating cells, including RBCs. It is a large (190 to 280 kD) molecule projecting above the glycocalyx of the membrane. The extracellular part of the molecule is composed of four long homologous repeats, each of which is composed of seven short consensus repeats. Each of the long repeats constitutes a separate receptor site, except for the one nearest the membrane. The repeat furthest from the membrane is the C4b3b receptor. The two more centrally located repeats are receptors for C3b. CR1, on macrophages, can participate in phagocytosis of sensitized RBCs, but a second signal (e.g., IgG and Fc receptor) is usually required. CR1 acts as a receptor for C3b, iC3b, C4b, and C1q. C3b interactions are the most efficient. C4b and C1q are very inefficient.

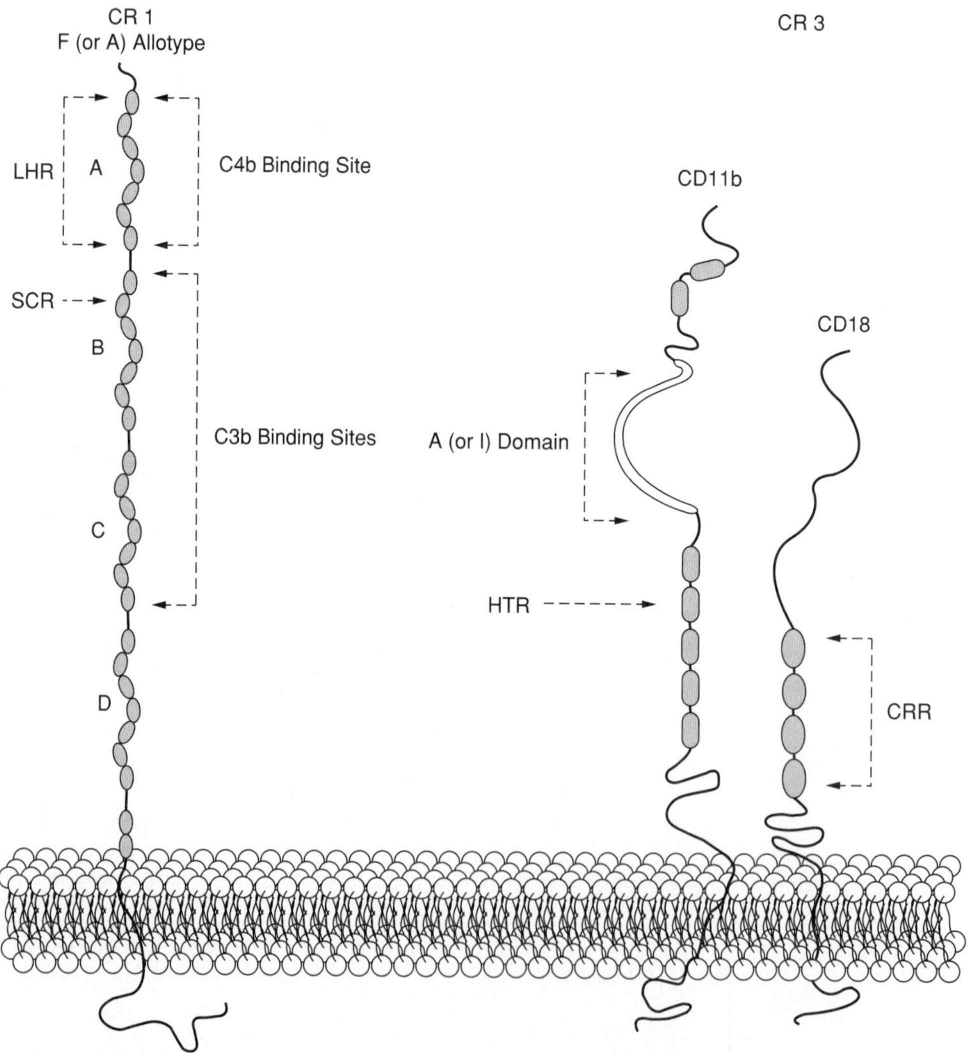

FIGURE 4-10. Schematic diagram of the structure of the CR1 and CR3 complement receptors. The CR1 F (also known as A) allotype is shown. It is a single-chain glycoprotein organized into four (A–D) long homologous repeats (LHRs), each composed of seven short consensus repeats (SCRs). The terminal LHR binds C4b and the two central LHRs bind C3b. CR3 is a noncovalently linked heterodimer composed of an α chain (CD11b) and a β chain (CD18). The α chain (CD11b) contains seven homologous tandem repeats (HTR), the second and third of which are split by an additional A (also called interactive, I) domain that may contain the C3 ligand-binding site. The β chain (CD18) has a cysteine-rich region (CRR) consisting of four tandem repeats. (Reprinted from Horsewood P, Kelton JG: Macrophage-mediated cell destruction. In Garratty G (ed): Immunobiology of Transfusion Medicine. New York: Dekker, 1994:435–464, by courtesy of Marcel Dekker Inc.)

Red cells have relatively few CR1 receptors (500–700/red cell), but as there are so many RBCs in the body, they become the major CR1-carrying cell population. This suggests a major role for RBCs in clearing complement (C3b, iC3b)-carrying immune complexes from the circulation. These complexes are stripped from the RBCs by high-affinity CR3 receptors on macrophages in the RES, particularly Kupffer cells in the liver. The RBCs appear not to be harmed by this process and return to the circulation (see later section).

The Knops system blood group antigens are found on the CR1 molecule.[48]

Complement Receptor Type 3 (CR3 [CDIIb/CD18]). CR3 is the receptor for iC3b. It is widely distributed (e.g., in macrophages, monocytes, follicular dendritic cells, neutrophils, and eosinophils). CR3 is a member of the integrin superfamily of adhesion molecules. It can mediate phagocytosis and lysis of iC3b-coated RBCs; like CR1, a second signal is probably required for phagocytosis. CR3 is also involved in killing of cells by NK cells.

Complement Receptor Type 4 (CR4). CR4 is closely related to CR3 and also recognizes iC3b. Like CR1 and CR3, to participate in phagocytosis, CR4 needs an additional signal.

Macrophage Interactions with RBCs Coated with Immunoglobulin and/or Complement

The attachment of appropriately sensitized RBCs to macrophages can be easily visualized in vitro. Sometimes, there is a so-called rosette formation whereby the macrophage becomes ringed by sensitized RBCs, like petals on a flower (Fig. 4-11).[49] Upon attachment to the macrophage, the RBCs usually undergo considerable distortion and deformity in the region of the attachments.[49] The sensitized RBC may become completely engulfed by the macrophage and may be destroyed internally (Fig. 4-12), or a portion of the RBC may become internalized (Figs. 4-13 and 4-14),

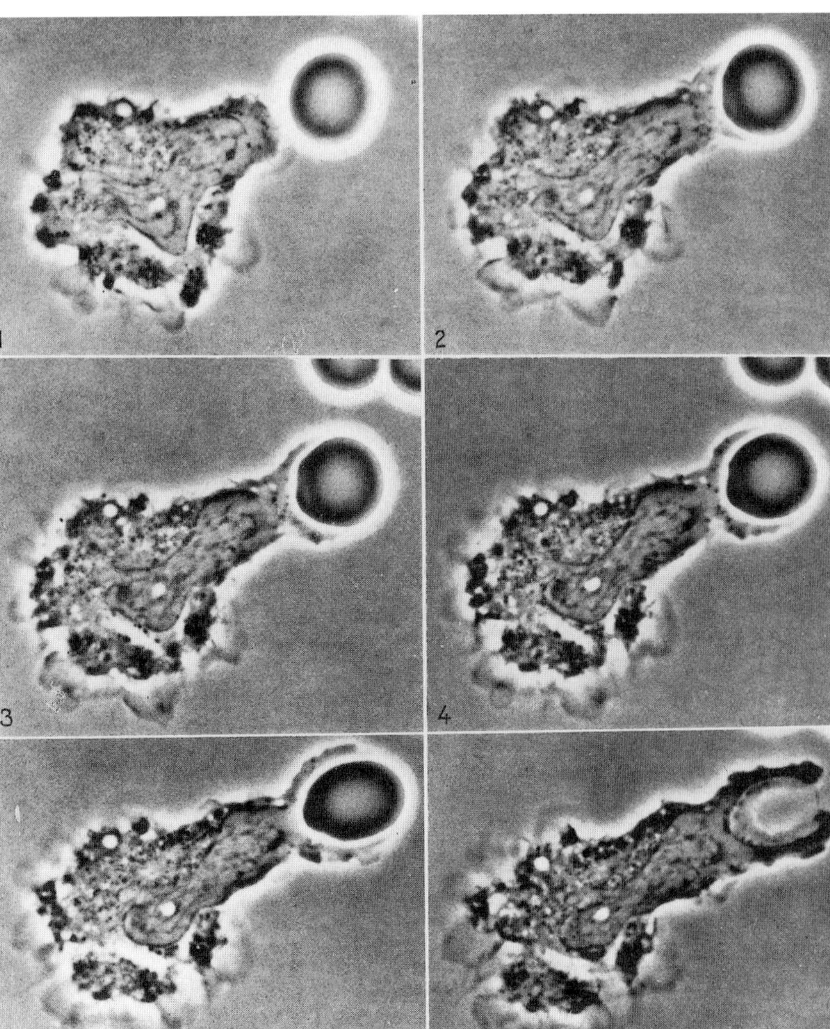

FIGURE 4-11. Scanning electron micrograph illustrating the interaction of antibody-coated red cells and phagocytic white cell. The white cell is surrounded by sensitized red cells forming a rosette (courtesy of Dr. W. Rosse).

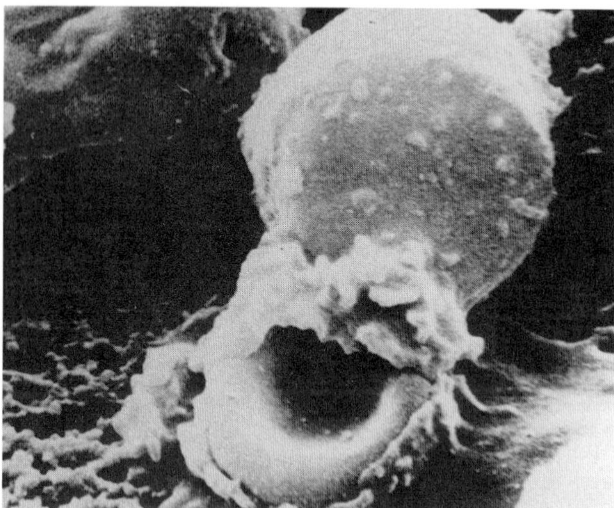

FIGURE 4-12. Scanning electron micrograph illustrating the reaction of a phagocytic white cell with an antibody-coated red cell. Only a small exposed area remains of a nearly ingested red cell. (Reproduced from Rosse WF, de Boisfleury A, and Bessis M: The interaction of phagotic cells and red cells modified by immune reactions: Comparison of antibody and complement coated red cells. Blood Cells 1975;1:345, by permission of Springer-Verlag.)

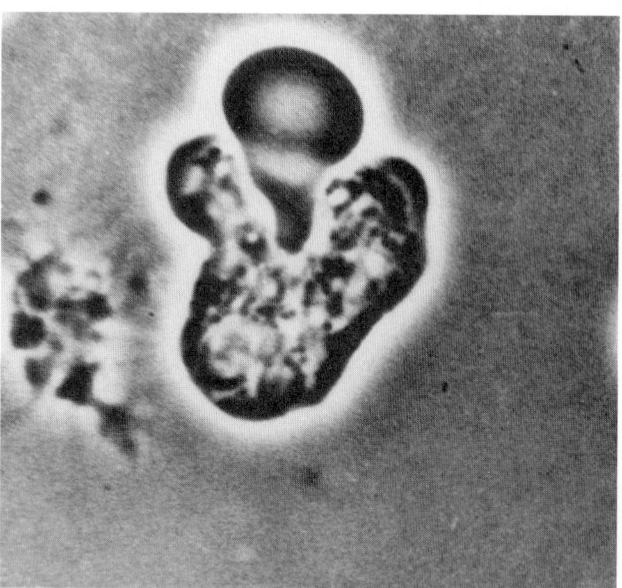

FIGURE 4-13. Phase-contrast photomicrograph illustrating the interaction of an antibody-coated red cell and a phagocytic white cell. The red cell, having been taken by the metapod, is deformed as the metapod flows along its sides. (Reproduced from Rosse WF, de Boisfleury A, and Bessis M: The interaction of phagotic cells and red cells modified by immune reactions: Comparison of antibody and complement coated red cells. Blood Cells 1975;1:345, by permission of Springer-Verlag.)

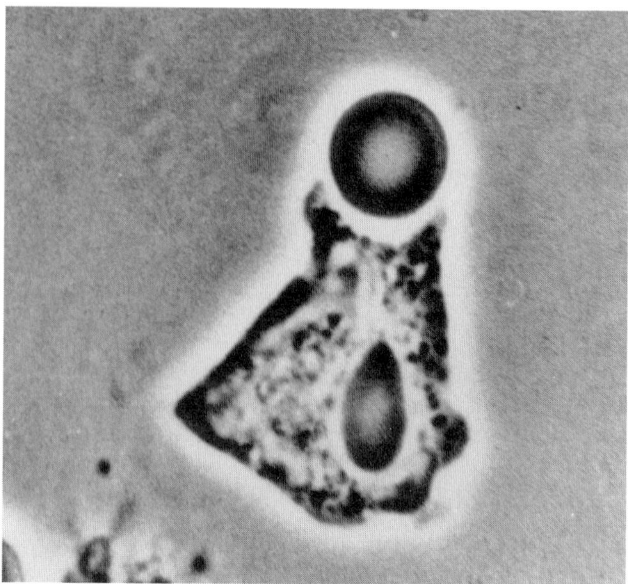

FIGURE 4-14. Further interaction between the phagocytic white cell and the antibody-coated red cell results in internalization of a portion of red cell. (Reproduced from Rosse WF, de Boisfleury A, and Bessis M: The interaction of phagotic cells and red cells modified by immune reactions: Comparison of antibody and complement coated red cells. Blood Cells 1975;1:345, by permission of Springer-Verlag.)

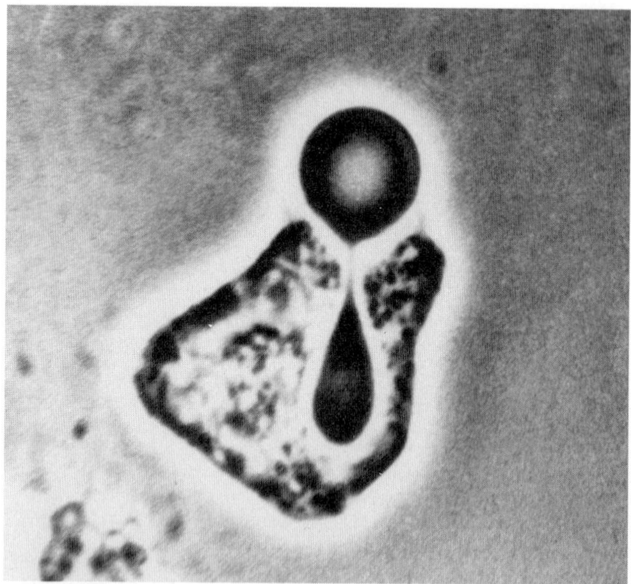

FIGURE 4-15. The separation of the internal and external portions of the red cell is complete; the portion of the red cell outside the macrophage may escape and circulate as a spherocyte. (Reproduced from Rosse WF, de Boisfleury A, and Bessis M: The interaction of phagotic cells and red cells modified by immune reactions: Comparison of antibody and complement coated red cells. Blood Cells 1975;1:345, by permission of Springer-Verlag.)

resulting in loss of membrane protein and lipids. The portion of the RBC outside the macrophage may escape and circulate as a spherocyte[50] (Fig. 4-15). The membrane of this spherocytic RBC is rigid owing to the loss of protein and lipids; thus the RBC is unable to change its shape readily to traverse the fine channels of the spleen and so is susceptible to early destruction.[51-53] Once attached to the macrophage, a sensitized RBC may also be destroyed or damaged by enzymes released by the macrophage (ADCC). Figure 4-16 summarizes the possible interactions of a sensitized RBC with macrophages.

MACROPHAGE/MONOCYTE CYTOTOXICITY

Since the incrimination of macrophages as the major effector cell in immune RBC destruction, the emphasis

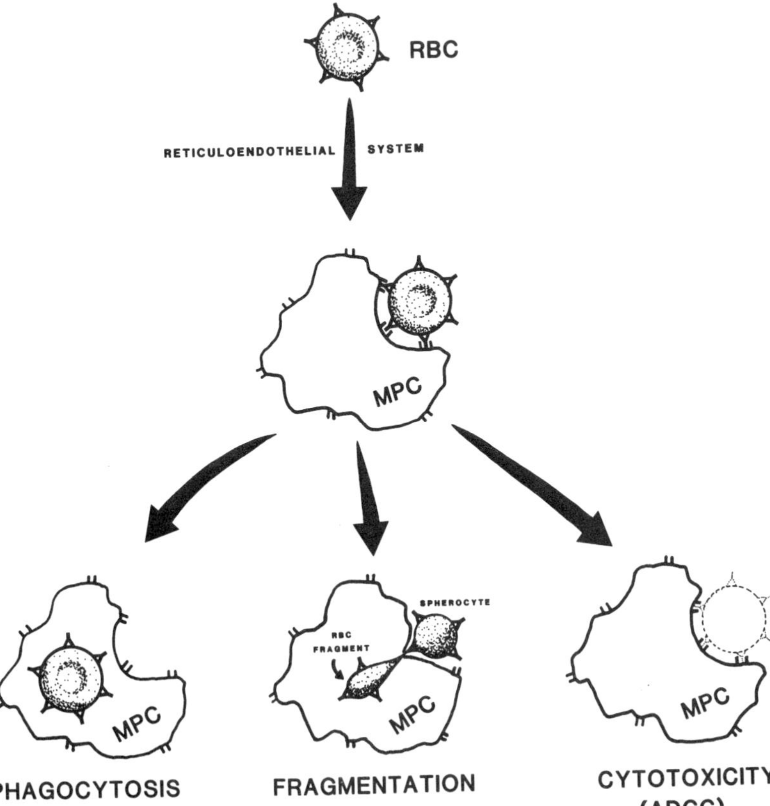

FIGURE 4-16. Immune RBC destruction by cellular mechanisms.

has been on phagocytosis. However, recent studies have suggested that an extracellular mechanism is also operative and that the cytotoxic properties of the macrophage may be more important than first thought.[54] Most of the interactions are similar to those described previously for ADCC by lymphocytes: (1) specific recognition and cell adherence; (2) intimate contact stimulating membrane phagocytosis and triggering release of specific macrophage cytotoxin; (3) specific macrophage cytotoxin acting directly on the target cell membrane.

There are many publications showing that monocytes/macrophages can cause lysis (ADCC) of RBCs sensitized with anti-A, anti-B, or anti-D.[55-70] For instance, Kurlander and colleagues[56] were able to demonstrate in vitro monocyte-mediated lysis of human RBCs sensitized with IgG anti-Rh (D) and anti-A or -B. Cells sensitized with only human complement components (even up to 80,000 molecules per RBC) were not lysed, but complement (C3b or C3d) sensitization augmented IgG-mediated lysis and reduced the amount of IgG necessary to produce lysis. Without complement, 1000 to 1500 molecules of anti-D per RBC were necessary for lysis; less than 1000 molecules were necessary when complement was present in addition to IgG on the RBC. IgG anti-A or anti-B was 5- to 10-fold less efficient in promoting phagocytosis or lysis per molecule of IgG bound; however, because of the greater antigen density of A and B, more than 100,000 molecules of IgG per RBC could be bound, producing equivalent lysis of anti-D sensitized cells. Even after degradation of C3b to C3d, complement augmentation persisted.

Engelfriet's group[54,67-70] has suggested that cytotoxicity may play a more important role than phagocytosis in immune RBC destruction. Using ^{51}Cr-labeled human RBCs sensitized with anti-D, they were able to demonstrate cytotoxicity by monocytes, independent of phagocytosis. An interesting finding was that the cytotoxicity, but not the phagocytosis, was inhibited by hydrocortisone.[70] The release of lysosomal enzymes by the monocytes was also inhibited by hydrocortisone; a significant correlation was found between lysosomal enzyme release and lysis.[70] The authors concluded that lysosomal enzymes released by monocytes, when incubated with Rh-sensitized RBCs, were responsible for lysis of these RBCs. The lysis occurred only over a short range, probably at the site of attachment of the red cell, because only RBCs bound to the monocyte were lysed. Thus, in vivo IgG-sensitized RBCs may attach to macrophages in the spleen and be lysed external to the macrophage, without phagocytosis occurring. This direct lysis (ADCC) would not require complement.

Unlike other investigators,[71-85] Fleer and coworkers[67,68] were not able to demonstrate lysis of Rh-sensitized cells by lymphocytes. Another important effect noted by Fleer and coworkers[59] was the development of an increased osmotic fragility of a considerable part of the nonlysed Rh-sensitized red cells; osmotically more fragile RBCs considerably outnumbered, lysed, and ingested RBCs. A correlation with increased osmotic fragility and severity of autoimmune hemolytic anemia had been described previously.[86] The presence of spherocytes has, for years, been said to be a hallmark of AIHA; the spherocytes are now thought to be formed through fragmentation of the sensitized RBCs by macrophages[49] (see Figs. 4-13 to 4-15). It has also been assumed that the increased osmotic fragility is due to the presence of spherocytes; it may well be that the damage to the RBC membrane caused by cytotoxicity, without fragmentation and spherocyte formation, may also contribute to the increased fragility.

Extravascular red cell destruction leads to the appearance, in the plasma and urine, of breakdown products of hemoglobin, such as bilirubin and urobilinogen.[7] Occasionally, laboratory tests may show some results that are associated with intravascular lysis (e.g., hemoglobinemia and hemoglobinuria), even though no complement-mediated lysis has occurred. For instance, hemoglobinemia and hemoglobinuria are relatively common following destruction of large volumes of Rh-incompatible blood (see Chapter 14). The Rh antibodies in these cases have never been shown to fix complement. As macrophages (and possibly, lymphocytes) are known to destroy sensitized RBCs by extracellular cytotoxicity (ADCC) in addition to phagocytosis, this may explain the noncomplement-mediated hemoglobinemia and hemoglobinuria associated with extravascular lysis. In addition, or perhaps alternatively, hemoglobin may be released into the blood stream following fragmentation of the RBCs during phagocytosis, particularly when large amounts of blood are rapidly destroyed (e.g., several units).[5] Most alloantibodies (e.g., Rh, Kell, Duffy) other than ABO and the few rare antibodies mentioned previously destroy RBCs extrasvascularly. Most of the RBC destruction associated with AIHA is extravascular (e.g., warm antibody AIHA, which comprises almost 70% of all AIHA). In addition, many of the drug-induced hemolytic anemias (e.g., those caused by methyldopa or penicillin) are primarily associated with extravascular red cell destruction.

Many factors may affect immune red cell destruction.[6] The more important factors are listed in Table 4-6. Some of these factors are discussed relative to: (1) RBCs sensitized with Ig alone, and (2) RBCs sensitized with complement, with or without Ig present.

TABLE 4-6. FACTORS THAT INFLUENCE THE PATHOGENICITY OF RBC ANTIBODIES

Characteristics of antibody
Class
Subclass
Specificity
Thermal range
Complement-activating efficiency
Affinity
As yet unknown qualitative characteristics
Quantity of RBC-bound IgG and/or complement
Characteristics of target antigen
Quantity of antigen on membrane
Distribution of antigen on membrane
Presence of antigen in tissues and/or body fluids
Type of complement present on circulating RBCs
Activity of reticuloendothelial system

DESTRUCTION OF RED CELLS SENSITIZED WITH IgG ALONE

RBCs sensitized by IgG only are destroyed predominantly in the spleen. Although the liver is a much larger organ, it has been shown that the spleen is nearly 100 times more efficient at removing Rh (IgG)–sensitized RBCs.[7] About 20 to 30 µg of anti-Rh per milliliter of RBCs will lead to complete clearance in a single passage through the spleen (T_{50} of 20 minutes), but in the absence of the spleen, the cells are removed by the liver with a T_{50} of about 5 hours.[7] Lo Buglio and coworkers[49] showed that the reaction between the Fc receptor on human monocytes and macrophages with IgG-sensitized RBCs could specifically be inhibited with IgG, or its Fc fragment, in solution. They suggested that the free IgG in plasma competes with RBC–bound IgG for receptors on the monocyte/macrophage surface. At hematocrit levels in excess of 75%, comparable to those encountered in the splenic red pulp, plasma had little inhibitory effect. It was suggested that plasma skimming enhanced entrapment of antibody-coated RBCs in vivo; the fact that the spleen is notable for both erythroconcentration and for efficient trapping of IgG-coated RBCs supported this interpretation. Other investigators[54,87-89] have confirmed the inhibitory effect of even small amounts of normal plasma or serum.

Fleer and coworkers[87] published data supporting the hypothesis of Lo Buglio and coworkers,[49] that is, that the efficiency of splenic destruction was related to the hemoconcentration (loss of plasma) that occurs in the spleen. They were able to show that the in vitro interaction between monocytes and IgG Rh–sensitized RBCs was completely inhibited by low concentrations of IgG (e.g., 30 to 100 µg/mL); however, the interaction with IgG anti-A–sensitized RBCs was not inhibited by IgG. They suggested that this difference was probably quantitative. The higher the number of IgG antibody molecules per sensitized RBC, the less the interaction between the sensitized RBC and monocyte was inhibited by IgG. Kelton and coworkers[88] showed that there was a significant relationship between the concentration of IgG in the serum and the rate of clearance of antibody-sensitized RBCs ($r = 0.51$, $p < 0.1$). Using ^{51}Cr-labeled IgG (Rh)–sensitized RBCs, they showed that patients with hypergammaglobulinemia had the slowest Fc-dependent clearance, whereas those with hypogammaglobulinemia had the most rapid clearance. The unusually rapid clearance in a patient with hypogammaglobulinemia could be returned to normal by raising the concentration of IgG in the serum. This would seem to support the observations by Lo Buglio and coworkers[49] and Fleer and coworkers,[87] but does not agree with the findings reported by Scornik and coworkers.[90] The latter showed that IgG-sensitized RBCs were rapidly cleared from the circulation of patients with myeloma, despite serum IgG concentrations that were several times higher than normal. They concluded that the current explanations derived from in vitro experiments were insufficient to explain the IgG-dependent clearance of RBCs in the presence of free IgG.

Fleer and coworkers[87] reported that the number of sensitized RBCs per monocyte also had a strong influence on the inhibitory effect of IgG. When the number of sensitized RBCs per monocyte was increased from 1 to 32, the percentage of inhibition by a fixed amount of IgG (50 μg/mL) decreased significantly. This in vitro effect was only evident when relatively weakly sensitized RBCs were used and when the in vivo destruction of these weakly sensitized RBCs was confined to the spleen. As a considerable hemoconcentration occurs in this organ, it is conceivable that a highly sensitized RBC to macrophage ratio is accomplished. A high ratio may allow interaction between weakly sensitized RBCs and splenic macrophages, despite the presence in vivo of a high concentration of IgG. Kurlander and Rosse[89] also reported that the amount of phagocytosis was greatly influenced by the proportion of sensitized RBCs, when in the presence of plasma IgG.

Quantitative Factors. Generally speaking, there appears to be a direct relationship between the amount of IgG on RBCs and the amount of in vivo RBC destruction. This is generally true for alloantibodies, but there are many exceptions to this when autoantibodies are studied. Mollison[7] has clearly shown that if different quantities of a single example of an allo anti-Rh are used to sensitize RBCs in vitro, there is a good correlation between the amount of IgG sensitizing the red cell and the rate of in vivo clearance (Fig. 4-17). Constantoulakis and colleagues[91] also showed this, but in studying autoantibody sensitization, they were not able to establish a close correlation between the amount of antibody on the RBC and the rate of destruction determined by ^{51}Cr. In contrast to this, Rosse[92] found that the amount of RBC–bound IgG was generally proportional to the rate of RBC destruction, although many exceptions could be found. In a given patient, the rate of destruction was closely related to the concentration of IgG antibody detected on the membrane; this is of some value in follow-up evaluation of an individual patient during response to therapy (see Chapter 11). It has been known for some time that RBCs sensitized with the same amounts of IgG autoantibody can have markedly different cell survival times. For example, Constantoulakis and coworkers[91] reported two different RBC samples with approximately 0.9 μg of IgG antibody nitrogen on each having a T_{50} of 45 minutes

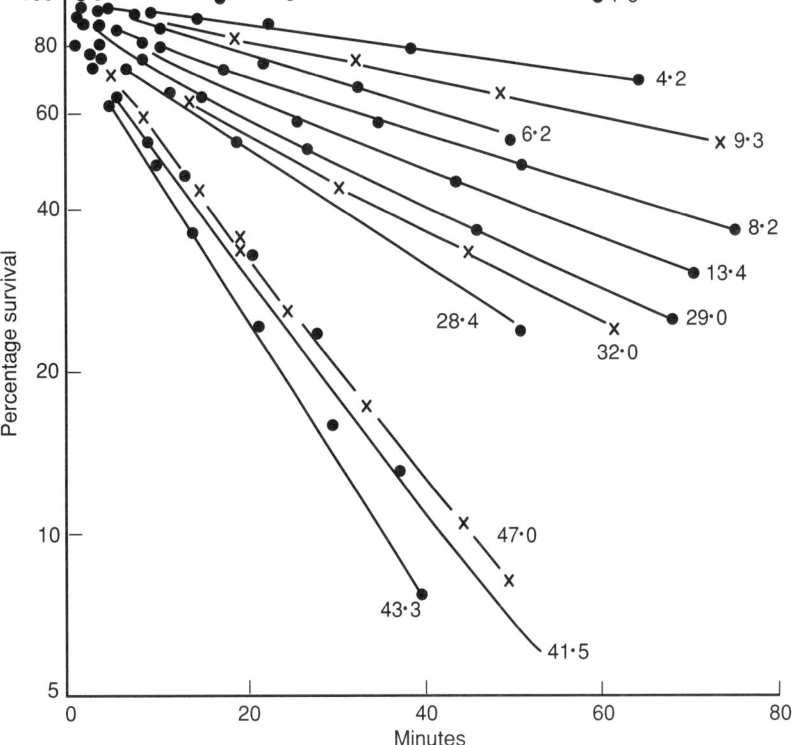

FIGURE 4-17. Survival of Rh-positive RBCs sensitized in vitro with varying amounts of a particular anti-Rh (Avg). Purified IgG, prepared from Avg serum, was used to sensitize the RBCs. The figures against each slope are the estimates of the amount of antibody on the RBCs at the time of injection (expressed as grams of antibody per milliliter red cells). In three cases (x) the estimates were made by using labeled anti-Rh. (From Mollison PL, Crome P, Hughes-Jones NC, Rochna E: Rate of removal from the circulation of red cells sensitized with different amounts of antibody. Brit J Haematol 1965;11:401.)

be detectable in the plasma. This may well explain the RBC survival collapse curve noted when small volumes (<10 mL) of ^{51}Cr-labeled RBCs are injected into previously nonimmunized individuals,[7] but it is more difficult to extend this as an explanation for DAT-negative AIHA and hemolytic transfusion reactions with no detectable antibody. In these conditions, one would think that antibody would eventually appear in the plasma, but perhaps antibody could be continually adsorbed by macrophages.[210]

IN VIVO AGGLUTINATION OF RED CELLS

Before the role of the macrophage was fully appreciated, aggregation or agglutination of RBCs in vivo was believed to play a major role in immune RBC destruction. It was commonly believed that RBCs sensitized with nonagglutinating antibodies (e.g., IgG Rh) could be aggregated in the spleen where the protein concentration was high, and that these aggregates or agglutinates would be held up in the spleen and thus be more susceptible to destruction by macrophages. There is very little evidence to support this theory as a major cause of immune RBC destruction, but it may play a role in some circumstances. Romano and Mollison[211] showed that RBCs coated with as little as 110 to 190 IgG anti-A molecules/RBC would agglutinate if mixed with plasma and rocked on a tile. By contrast, the minimum amount of IgG anti-Rh required for agglutination under these conditions was about 19,000 IgG molecules/RBC. Complement-binding by RBCs coated with IgG anti-A could be demonstrated only when the amount of antibody on the cells was at least 5134 IgG molecules/RBC. Since, in ABO hemolytic disease, the amount of antibody on the cells is frequently less than 0.6 µg/mL (approximately 200 IgG molecules per red cell), it seems that RBC destruction in this syndrome is not caused by the activation of complement, but may be due to the sequestration of agglutinated cells. Mollison and coworkers[7] have also suggested that some noncomplement-binding IgM alloantibodies, active at 37°C (e.g., examples of anti-c and anti-M), may destroy RBCs in vivo because agglutinates may become trapped in small blood vessels and eventually suffer metabolic damage. Such suggestions may also be relevant to questions that are often asked about the potential of cold antibodies to cause clinical problems in patients undergoing cardiac surgery using hypothermia (see Chapter 9).

REFERENCES

1. Fairley NH: The fate of extracorpuscular circulating haemoglobin. Br Med J 1940;2:213.
2. Dacie JV: The Haemolytic Anaemias, 2nd ed. Part II, The Auto-Immune Haemolytic Anemias. New York: Grune & Stratton, 1962.
3. Aschoff L: Ergebn inn. Med Kinderheilk 1924;26:1.
4. van Furth R, Cohn ZA, Hirsch JG, et al: The mononuclear phagocyte system: A new classification of macrophages, monocytes, and their precursor cells. Bull WHO 1972;46:845.
5. Garratty G: The significance of complement in immunohematology. CRC Crit Rev Clin Lab Sci 1984;20:25.
6. Garratty G: Factors affecting the pathogenicity of red cell auto- and alloantibodies. In Nance SJ (ed): Immune Destruction of Red Blood Cells. Arlington, Va: American Association of Blood Banks, 1989:109.
7. Mollison PL, Engelfriet CP, Contreras M: Blood Transfusion in Clinical Medicine, 10th ed. Boston, Mass: Blackwell Scientific, 1997.
8. Müller-Eberhard HJ: Complement. Ann Rev Biochem 1975;44:697–724.
9. Walport MJ: Complement. N Engl J Med 2001;344:1058–1067.
10. Borsos T, Rapp HR: Hemolysin titration based on fixation of the activated first component of complement: Evidence that one molecule of hemolysin suffices to sensitize an erythrocyte. J Immunol 1965;95:559.
11. Humphrey JH, Dourmashkin RR: Electron microscope studies of immune cell lysis. In Wolstenholme GEW, Knight J (eds): Complement. Boston: Little, Brown, 1965:175.
12. Humphrey JH, Dourmashkin RR: The lesions in cell membranes caused by complement. Adv Immunol 1969;11:75–115.
13. Mayer MM: Mechanism of cytolysis by complement. Proc Natl Acad Sci USA 1972;69:2954–2958.
14. Pillemer L, Blum L, Lepow IH, et al: The properdin system and immunity. I. Demonstration and isolation of a new serum protein, properdin, and its role in immune phenomena. Science 1954;120:279.
15. Nelson RA: An alternative mechanism for the properdin system. J Exp Med 1958;108:515.
16. Lepow IH: Louis Pillemer, properdin, and scientific controversy. J Immunol 1980;125:471–475.
17. Gewurz H, Shin HS, Mergenhagen SE: Interactions of the complement system with endotoxin lipopolysaccharides: Consumption of each of the six terminal complement components. J Exp Med 1968;128:1049–1057.
18. Schur PH, Becker EL: Pepsin digestion of rabbit and sheep antibodies: The effect of complement fixation. J Exp Med 1963;118:891.
19. Sandberg AL, Oliveira B, Osler AG: Two complement interaction sites in guinea pig immunoglobulins. J Immunol 1971; 106:282–285.
20. Ellman L, Green I, Frank MM: Genetically controlled total deficiency of the fourth component of complement in the guinea pig. Science 1970;170:74–75.
21. Frank MM, May JE, Gaither T, Ellman L: In vitro studies of complement function in sera of C4 deficient guinea pigs. J Exp Med 1971;134:176–187.
22. Flexner S, Noguchi H: Snake venom in relation to hemolysis, bacteriolysis, and toxicity. J Exp Med 1903;6:277.
23. Götze O, Müller-Eberhard HJ: The alternative pathway of complement activation. Adv Immunol 1976;24:1–35.
24. Schreiber RD, Pangburn MK, Lesavre PH, Müller-Eberhard HJ: Initiation of the alternative pathway of complement: Recognition of activators by bound C3b and assembly of the entire pathway from six isolated proteins. Proc Natl Acad Sci USA 1978;75:3948–3952.
25. Lachman PJ, Oldroyd RG, Milstein C, Wright BW: Three rat monoclonal antibodies to human C3. Immunology 1980;41:503.
26. Lachman PJ, Pangburn MK, Oldroyd RG: Breakdown of C3 after complement activation. J Exp Med 1982;156:205–216.
27. May JE, Green I, Frank MM: The alternate complement pathway in cell damage: Antibody-mediated cytolysis of erythrocytes and nucleated cells. J Immunol 1972;109:595–601.
28. Götze O, Müller-Eberhard HJ: Paroxysmal nocturnal hemoglobinuria: Hemolysis initiated by the C3 activator system. N Engl J Med 1972;286:180.
29. Poskitt TR, Fortwengler HP, Lunskis BJ: Activation of the alternative complement pathway by autologous red cell stroma. J Exp Med 1973;138:715–722.

30. Turner MW: Mannose-binding lectin: The pluripotent molecule of the innate immune system. Immunology Today 1996; 17:532–540.
31. Stahl PD, Ezckowitz RA: The mannose receptor is a pattern recognition receptor involved in host defense. Curr Opin Immunol 1998;10:50–55.
32. van Furth R: Origin and kinetics of monocytes and macrophages. Semin Hematol 1970;7:125.
33. Huber H, Fudenberg HH: Receptor sites of human monocytes for IgG. Int Arch Allergy 1968;34:18.
34. Huber H, Douglas SD, Nusbacher J, Kochwa S, Rosenfield RF: IgG subclass specificity of human monocyte receptor sites. Nature 1970;229:419.
35. Abramson N, Gelfand EW, Jandl JH, Rosen FS: The interaction between human monocytes and RBCs. Specificity for IgG subclasses and IgG fragments. J Exp Med 1970;132:1207–1215.
36. van de Winkel JGJ, Capel PJA: Human IgG Fc receptor heterogeneity: Molecular aspects and clinical implications. Immunol Today 1993;14:215–221.
37. Ravetch JV, Bolland S: IgG Fc receptors. Ann Rev Immunol 2001;19:275–290.
38. Indik ZK, Park JG, Hunter S, Schreiber AD: The molecular dissection of Fcγ receptor mediated phagocytosis. Blood 1995;86:4389–4399.
39. Fanger MW, Shen L, Pugh J, Bernier GM: Subpopulations of human peripheral granulocytes and monocytes express receptors for IgA. Proc Natl Acad Sci USA 1980;77:3640–3644.
40. Gauldie J, Richards C, Lamontagne L: Fc receptors for IgA and other immunoglobulins on resident and activated alveolar macrophages. Mol Immunol 1983;20:1029.
41. Maliszewski CR, March CJ, Schoenborn MA, Gimpel S, Shen L: Expression cloning of a human Fc receptor for IgA. J Exp Med 1990;172:1665–1672.
42. Shen L: Receptors for IgA on phagocytic cells. Immunol Res 1992;11:273–282.
43. Morton HC, van Egmond K, van de Winkel JGJ: Structure and function of human IgA Fc receptors (FcαR). Crit Rev Immunol 1996;16:423–440.
44. Huber H, Polley M, Linscott W, Fudenberg HH, Muller-Eberhard H: Human monocytes: Distinct receptor sites for the third component of complement and for immunoglobulin. G Science 1968;162:1281–1283.
45. Wright SD: Receptors for complement and the biology of phagocytosis. In Gallin JI, Goldstein IM, Snyderman R (eds): Inflammation: Basic Principles and Clinical Correlates, 2nd ed. New York: Raven Press, 1992:477.
46. Sim RB, Walport MJ: C3 receptors. In Whaley K (ed): Complement in Health and Disease. Boston: MTP Press Ltd, 1987:125.
47. Cooper NR: Immune adherence by the fourth component of complement. Science 1969;165:396–398.
47a. Shibuya A, Sakamoto N, Shimizu Y, et al: Fc α/μ receptor mediates endocytosis of IgM-coated microbes. Nat Immunol 2000;1:441–446.
48. Moulds JM: Association of blood group antigens with immunologically important proteins. In Garratty G (ed): Immunobiology of Transfusion Medicine. New York: Marcel Dekker Inc., 1994:273.
49. Lo Buglio AF, Cotran R, Jandl JH: Red cells coated with immunoglobulin G: Binding and sphering by mononuclear cells in man. Science 1967;158:1582–1585.
50. Brown DL, Nelson DA: Surface microfragmentation of RBCs as a mechanism for complement-mediated immune spherocytosis. Br J Haematol 1973;24:301.
51. Weed RI: The importance of erythrocyte deformability. Am J Med 1970;49:147–150.
52. Cooper RA: Loss of membrane components in the pathogenesis of antibody-induced spherocytosis. J Clin Invest 1972;51: 16–21.
53. Mohandas N, de Boisfleury A: Antibody-induced spherocytic anemia. I. Changes in red cell deformity. Blood Cells 1977;3:187.
54. Engelfriet CP, von dem Borne AEG Kr, Beckers D, et al: Immune destruction of RBCs. In Bell CA (ed): A Seminar on Immune-mediated Cell Destruction. Washington, DC: American Association of Blood Banks, 1981:93.
55. Holm G, Hammarstrom S: Haemolytic activity of human blood monocytes: Lysis of human erythrocytes treated with anti-A serum. Clin Exp Immunol 1973;13:29.
56. Kurlander RJ, Rosse WF, Logue WL: Quantitative influence of antibody and complement coating of RBCs on monocyte-mediated cell lysis. J Clin Invest 1978;61:1309–1319.
57. Milgrom H, Shore SL: Lysis of antibody-coated human RBCs by peripheral blood mononuclear cells. Cell Immunol 1978;30:178–187.
58. Fleer A, Roos D, von dem Borne AEG Kr, Engelfriet CP: Cytotoxic activity of human monocytes towards sensitized RBCs is not dependent on the generation of reactive oxygen species. Blood 1979;54:407–411.
59. Randazzo B, Hirschberg T, Hirschberg H: Cytotoxic effects of activated human monocytes and lymphocytes to anti-D-treated human erythrocytes in vitro. Scand J Immunol 1979;9:351–358.
60. Yust I, Goldsher N, Greenfeld R, Rabinovitz M: Hemolysis due to human antibody-dependent cell-mediated cytotoxicity. Israel J Med Sci 1980;16:174–180.
61. Koller CA, LoBuglio AF: Monocyte-mediated antibody-dependent cell-mediated cytotoxicity: the role of the metabolic burst. Blood 1981;58:293–299.
62. Sagone AL Jr, Klassen DK, Decker MA, Clark L, Metz EN: Characteristics of the metabolic response of human monocytes to RBCs sensitized with anti-D alloantibodies. J Lab Clin Med 1981;98:382–395.
63. Todd RF III, Torchia RA, Peterson KE, Leeman EL: Binding and lysis of antibody-coated human erythrocytes by activated human monocytes. Clin Immunol Immunopathol 1984;30: 413–429.
64. Yust I, Frisch B, Goldsher N: Antibody-dependent cell-mediated cytotoxicity (ADCC) of penicillin-treated human red blood cells. Br J Haematol 1981;47:443–452.
65. Yust I, Frisch B, Goldsher N: Antibody-dependent cell-mediated cytotoxicity and phagocytosis of autologous red blood cells in alphamethyldopa-induced haemolysis. Scand J Haematol 1986;36:211–216.
66. Samdal HH, Michaelsen TE, Heier HE, Nordhagen R: Antibody dependent cell mediated cytotoxicity against anti-D sensitized human erythrocytes. APMIS 1988;96:250–256.
67. Fleer A, van der Hart M, von dem Borne AEG Kr, Engelfriet CP: Monocyte-mediated lysis of human erythrocytes. In Eijsvoogel VP, Roos D, Zeimaker WP, eds:. Leucocyte Membrane Determinants Regulating Immune Reactivity. New York: Academic Press, 1976:675.
68. Fleer A, van der Hart M, von dem Borne AEG Kr, Engelfriet CP: Mechanism of antibody-dependent cytotoxicity by human blood monocytes towards IgG-sensitized erythrocytes. Eur J Clin Invest 1976;6:333.
69. Fleer A, Koopman MJ, von dem Borne AEG Kr, Engelfriet CP: Monocyte-induced increase in osmotic fragility of human RBCs sensitized with anti-D alloantibodies. Br J Haematol 1978;40:439–446.
70. Fleer A, van Schaik MLJ, von dem Borne AEG Kr, Engelfriet CP: Destruction of sensitized erythrocytes by human monocytes in vitro. Effects of cytochalasin B, hydrocortisone and colchicine. Scand J Immunol 1978;8:515–524.
71. Hinz CF Jr, Chickosky JF: Lymphocyte cytotoxicity for human erythrocytes. In Schwarz MR (ed): 6th Leucocyte Culture Conference, University of Washington, 1971. New York: Academic Press, 1972:699.
72. Kurnick JT, Grey HM: Relationship between immunoglobulin-bearing lymphocytes and cells reactive with sensitized human erythrocytes. J Immunol 1975;115:305–307.
73. Shaw GM, Levy PC, LoBuglio AF: Human lymphocyte antibody-dependent cell-mediated cytotoxicity (ADCC) toward human red blood cells. Blood 1978;52:696–705.
74. Kurlander RL, Rosse WF, Ferreira E: Quantitative evaluation of antibody-dependent lymphocyte-mediated lysis of human RBCs. Am J Hematol 1979;6:295–311.

75. Lajos J, Benczur M, Nemák P: Characteristics of different Rhesus alloantibodies in lymphocyte dependent (K cell) cytotoxicity to human erythrocytes. Vox Sang 1979;36:240–243.
76. Kurlander RL, Rosse WF: Lymphocyte-mediated lysis of antibody coated human RBCs in the presence of human serum. Blood 1979;53:1197–1202.
77. Shaw GM, Aminoff D, Balcerzak SP, LoBuglio AF: Clustered IgG on human red blood cell membranes may promote human lymphocyte antibody-dependent cell-mediated cytotoxicity. J Immunol 1980;125:501–507.
78. Bakás T, Kimber I, Ringwald G, Moore M: K cell mediated haemolysis: Influence of large numbers of unsensitized cells on the antibody-dependent lysis of anti-D-sensitized erythrocytes by human lymphocytes. Br J Haematol 1984;57:447–455.
79. Sándor J, Lajos J, Braun J: Lymphocyte killer activity in individuals sensitized against anti-D assessed by direct ADCC lysis of O, Rh-positive erythrocytes. Vox Sang 1986;51:310–313.
80. Kumpel BM, Leader KA, Merry AH, et al: Heterogeneity in the ability of IgG1 monoclonal anti-D to promote lymphocyte-mediated red cell lysis. Eur J Immunol 1989;19:2283–2288.
81. Holm G: Lysis of antibody-treated human erythrocytes by human leukocytes and macrophages in tissue culture. Int Arch Allergy 1972;43:671.
82. Milgrom H, Shore SL: Lysis of antibody coated human RBCs by peripheral blood mononuclear cells. Altered effector cell profile after treatment of target cells with enzymes. Cell Immunol 1978;30:178.
83. Urbaniak SJ: Lymphoid cell dependent (K-cell) lysis of human erythrocytes sensitized with rhesus alloantibodies. Br J Haematol 1976;33:409–413.
84. Northoff H, Kluge A, Resch K: Antibody dependent cellular cytotoxicity (ADCC) against human erythrocytes, mediated by blood group alloantibodies: A model for the role of antigen density in target cell lysis. Z Immun Forsch 1978;154:15.
85. Handwerger BS, Kay NW, Douglas SD: Lymphocyte-mediated antibody-dependent cytolysis: Role in immune hemolysis. Vox Sang 1978;34:276–280.
86. von dem Borne AEG Kr, Engelfriet CP, Beckers D, van Loghem JJ: Autoimmune haemolytic anaemia with incomplete warm autoantibodies. Clin Exp Immunol 1971;8:377–388.
87. Fleer A, van der Meulen FW, Linthout E, von dem Borne AEG Kr: Destruction of IgG-sensitized erythrocytes by human blood monocytes: Modulation of inhibition by IgG. Br J Haematol 1978;39:425.
88. Kelton JG, Singer J, Rodger C, et al: The concentration of IgG in the serum is a major determinant of Fc-dependent reticuloendothelial function. Blood 1985;66:490–495.
89. Kurlander RJ, Rosse WF: Monocyte-mediated destruction in the presence of serum of RBCs coated with antibody. Blood 1979;54:1131–1139.
90. Scornik JC, Salinas MC, Drewinko B: IgG dependent clearance of red blood cells in IgG myeloma patients. J Immunol 1975; 115:901–903.
91. Constanoulakis M, Costea N, Schwartz RS, Dameshek W: Quantitative studies of the effect of red blood cell sensitization on in vitro hemolysis. J Clin Invest 1963;42:1790.
92. Rosse WF: Correlation of in vivo and in vitro measurements of hemolysis in hemolytic anemia due to immune reactions. Prog Hematol 1973;8:51–75.
93. Garratty G: The clinical significance (and insignificance) of red-cell-bound IgG and complement. In Wallace ME, Levitt JS (eds): Current applications and interpretation of the direct antiglobulin test. Arlington, Va: American Association of Blood Banks, 1988:1.
94. Garratty G: The significance of IgG on the red cell surface. Trans Med Rev 1987;1:47.
95. Garratty G: Effect of cell-bound proteins on the in vivo survival of circulating blood cells. Gerontology 1991;37:68–94.
96. Horsewood P, Kelton JG: Macrophage-mediated cell destruction. In Garratty G (ed): Immunobiology of Transfusion Medicine. New York: Marcel Dekker Inc., 1994:435–464.
97. Hughes-Jones NC, Polley MJ, Telford R, Gardner B, Kleinschmidt G: Optimal conditions for detecting blood group antibodies by the antiglobulin test. Vox Sang 1964;9:385.
98. van der Meulen FW, de Bruin HG, Goosen PCM et al: Quantitative aspects of the destruction of RBCs sensitized with IgG1 autoantibodies: an application of flow cytofluorometry. Br J Haemat 1980;46:47.
99. Garratty G, Nance SJ: Correlation between in vivo hemolysis and the amount of red cell-bound IgG measured by flow cytometry. Transfusion 1990;30:617-21.
100. Merry AH, Thomson EE, Rawlinson VI, Stratton F: A quantitative antiglobulin test for IgG for use in blood transfusion serology. Clin Lab Haemat 1982;4:393.
101. Merry AH, Thomson EE, Rawlinson VI, Stratton F: Quantitation of IgG on erythrocytes: correlation of number of IgG molecules per cell with the strength of the direct and indirect antiglobulin tests. Vox Sang 1984;47:73-81.
102. Dubarry M, Charron C, Habibi B, Bretagne Y, Lambin P: Quantitation of immunoglobulin classes and subclasses of autoantibodies bound to RBCs in patients with and without hemolysis. Transfusion 1993;33:466-71.
103. Lynen R, Neuhaus R, Schwarz DWM, et al: Flow cytometric analyses of the subclasses of red cell IgG antibodies. Vox Sang 1995;69:126-30.
104. Sokol RJ, Hewitt S, Booker DJ, Bailey A: Red cell autoantibodies, multiple immunoglobulin classes, and autoimmune hemolysis. Transfusion 1990;30:714-17.
105. Sokol RJ, Hudson G: Quantiation of red cell-bound immunoprotein. Transfusion 1998;38:782-95.
106. Sokol RJ, Hewitt S, Booker DJ, Bailey A: Erythrocyte autoantibodies, subclasses of IgG and autoimmune haemolysis. Autoimmunity 1990;6:99-104.
107. Engelfriet CP, von dem Borne AEG Kr, Beckers D, van Loghem JJ: Autoimmune haemolytic anaemia. Serological and immunochemical characteristics of the autoantibodies: Mechanisms of cell destruction. Ser Haematol 1974;8: 328–347.
108. Fabijanska-Mitek, Lopienska H, Zupanska B: Gel test application for IgG subclass detection in auto-immune haemolytic anaemia. Vox Sang 1997;72:233–237.
109. Engelfriet CP, Overbeeke MAM, von dem Borne AEG Kr: Autoimmune hemolytic anemia. Semin Hematol 1992;29:3.
110. Nance S, Bourdo S, Garratty G: IgG2 red cell sensitization associated with autoimmune hemolytic anemia. Transfusion (abstract) 1983;23:413.
111. Roush GR, Rosenthal NS, Gerson SL, et al: An unusual case of autoimmune hemolytic anemia with reticulocytopenia, erythroid dysplasia, and an IgG2 autoanti-U. Transfusion 1996;36:575–580.
112. von dem Borne AEG Kr, Beckers D, Van der Meulen W, Engelfriet CP: IgG4 autoantibodies against erythrocytes, without increased haemolysis: A case report. Br J Haematol 1977;37:137.
113. Zupanska B, Thomson EE, Merry AH: Fc receptors for IgG_1 and IgG_3 on human mononuclear cells—An evaluation with known levels of erythrocyte-bound IgG. Vox Sang 1986;50:97–103.
114. Schreiber AD, Frank MM: Role of antibody and complement in the immune clearance and destruction of erythrocytes. I. In vivo effects of IgG and IgM complement fixing sites. J Clin Invest 1972;51:575–582.
115. Schreiber AD, Frank MM: Role of antibody and complement in the immune clearance and destruction of erythrocytes. II. Molecular nature of IgG and IgM complement fixing sites and effects of their interaction with serum. J Clin Invest 1972;51: 583–589.
116. Cutbush M, Mollison PL: Relation between characteristics of blood-group antibodies in vitro and associated patterns of red cell destruction in vivo. Br J Haematol 1958;4:115.
117. Burton MS, Mollison PL: Effect of IgM and IgG iso-antibody on red cell clearance. Immunology 1968;14:861.
118. Engelfriet CP, von dem Borne AEG Kr, Giessen M, et al: Autoimmune haemolytic anaemias. I. Serological studies with pure anti-immunoglobulin reagents. Clin Exp Immunol 1968;3:605–614.

119. Wager O, Haltia K, Rasauen JA, Vuopio P: Five cases of positive antiglobulin test involving IgA warm type autoantibody. Ann Clin Res 1971;3:76–85.
120. Stratton F, Rawlinson VI, Chapman SA, et al: Acquired hemolytic anemia associated with IgA anti-e. Transfusion 1972;12:157–161.
121. Worlledge SM, Blajchman MA: The autoimmune haemolytic anaemias. Br J Haematol 1972;23(S):61.
122. Sturgeon P, Smith LE, Chun HMT, et al: Autoimmune hemolytic anemia associated exclusively with IgA of Rh specificity. Transfusion 1979;19:324–328.
123. Suzuki S, AmanoT, Mitsunaga M, et al: Autoimmune hemolytic anemia associated with IgA autoantibody. Clin Immunol Immunopathol 1981;21:247–256.
124. Wolf CFW, Wolf DJ, Peterson P, et al: Autoimmune hemolytic anemia with predominance of IgA autoantibody. Transfusion 1982;22:238–240.
125. Clark DA, Dessypris EN, Jenkins DE Jr, Krantz SB: Acquired immune hemolytic anemia associated with IgA erythrocyte coating: Investigation of hemolytic mechanisms. Blood 1984;64:1000–1005.
126. Kowal-Vern A, Jacobson P, Okuno T, Blank J: Negative direct antiglobulin test in autoimmune hemolytic anemia. Am J Pediatr Hematol Oncol 1986;8:349–351.
127. Reusser P, Osterwalder B, Burri H, Speck B: Autoimmune hemolytic anemia associated with IgA—Diagnostic and therapeutic aspects in a case with long-term follow-up. Acta Haematol 1987;77:53–56.
128. Girelli G, Perrone MP, Adorno G, et al: A second example of hemolysis due to IgA autoantibody with anti-e specificity. Haematologica 1990;75:182–183.
129. Göttsche B, Salama A, Mueller-Eckhardt C: Autoimmune hemolytic anemia associated with an IgA autoanti-Gerbich. Vox Sang 1990;58:211–214.
130. Sokol RJ, Booker DJ, Stamps R, et al: Autoimmune hemolytic anemia due to IgA class autoantibodies. Immunohematology 1996;12:14–19.
131. Sokol RJ, Booker DJ, Stamps R, Booth JR, Hook V: IgA red cell autoantibodies and autoimmune hemolysis. Transfusion 1997;37:175–181.
132. Petz LD, Garratty G: Acquired Immune Hemolytic Anemias, 1st ed. New York: Churchill Livingstone, 1980.
133. Gilliland BC, Leddy JP, Vaughan JH: The detection of cell-bound antibody on complement-coated human RBCs. J Clin Invest 1970;49:898–906.
134. Leddy JP, Bakemeier RF, Vaughan JH: Fixation of complement components to autoantibody eluted from human RBC. J Clin Invest 1965;44:1066.
135. Mantovani B, Rabinovitch M, Nussenzweig V: Phagocytosis of immune complexes by macrophages: Different roles of the macrophage receptor sites for complement (C3) and for immunoglobulin (IgG). J Exp Med 1972;135:780–792.
136. Griffin FM, Jr, Bianco C, Silverstein SC: Characterization of the macrophage receptor for complement and demonstration of its functional independence from the receptor for the Fc portion of immunoglobulin G. J Exp Med 1975;141:1269–1277.
137. Bianco C, Griffin FM Jr, Silverstein SC: Studies of the macrophage complement receptor. J Exp Med 1975;141: 1278–1290.
138. Scornik JC, Drewinko B: Receptors for IgG and complement in human spleen lymphoid cells: Preferential binding of particulate immune complexes through complement receptors. J Immunol 1975;115:1223–1226.
139. Ehlenberger AG, Nussenzweig V: Immunologically-mediated phagocytosis: Role of C3 and Fc receptors. In Litwin SD, Christian CL, Siskind GW (eds): Clinical Evaluation of Immune Function in Man. New York: Grune & Stratton, 1976:47.
140. Munn LR, Chaplin H JY, Jr: Rosette formation by sensitized human RBCs—Effects of source of peripheral leukocyte monolayers. Vox Sang 1977;33:129–142.
141. Jaffe CJ, Atkinson JP, Frank MM: The role of complement in the clearance of cold agglutinin-sensitized erythrocytes in man. J Clin Invest 1976;58:942–949.
142. Griffin FM, Silverstein SC: Segmental response of the macrophage plasma membrane to a phagocytic stimulus. J Exp Med 1974;139:323–336.
143. Nicholson GC, Masouredis SP, Singer SJ: Quantitative two dimensional ultrastructural distribution of Rho (D) antigenic sites on human erythrocyte membranes. Proc Natl Acad Sci 1971;68:1416–1420.
144. Masouredis SP, Sudora EJ, Mahan L, Victoria EJ: Antigen site densities and ultrastructural distribution patterns of red cell Rh antigens. Transfusion 1976;16:94–106.
145. Victoria EJ, Muchmore EA, Sudora EJ, Masouredis SP: The role of antigen mobility in anti-Rh (D) induced agglutination. J Clin Invest 1975;56:292–301.
146. Brown DL, Lachmann PJ, Dacie JV: The in vivo behavior of complement-coated RBCs: Studies in C6-deficient, C3-depleted and normal rabbits. Clin Exp Immunol 1970; 7:401–421.
147. Brown DL: The behavior of phagocytic cell receptors in relation to allergic red cell destruction. Ser Haematol 1974;7:3.
148. Logue G, Rosse W: Immunologic mechanisms in autoimmune hemolytic disease. Semin Hematol 1976;113:277.
149. Fischer J, Petz LD, Garratty G, Cooper N: Correlations between quantitative assay of red cell bound C3, serologic reactions, and hemolytic anemias. Blood 1974;44:359–373.
150. Lewis SM, Dacie JV, Szur L: Mechanisms of haemolysis in the cold-haemagglutinin syndrome. Br J Haematol 1960;6:164.
151. Mollison PL: The role of complement in haemolytic processes in vivo. In Wolstenholme GEW, Knight J (eds): Complement. London: Churchill, 1965:323.
152. Wellek B, Hahn HH, Opferkuch W: Evidence for macrophage C3d-receptor active in phagocytosis. J Immunol 1975;114: 1643–1645.
153. Reynolds HY, Atkinson JP, Newball HH, Frank MM: Receptors for immunoglobulin and complement on human alveolar macrophages. J Immunol 1975;114:1813–1819.
154. Ehlenberger AG, Nussenzweig V: Synergy between receptors for Fc and C3 in the induction of phagocytosis by human monocytes and neutrophils. Fed Proc Fed Am Soc Exp Biol 1975;34:854.
155. Atkinson JP, Frank MM: Studies on the in vivo effects of antibody interaction of IgM antibody and complement in the immune clearance and destruction of erythrocytes in man. J Clin Invest 1974;54:339–348.
156. Müller-Eberhard HJ: Complement and phagocytosis. In Bellanti JA, Delbert HD (eds): The Phagocytic Cell in Host Resistance. New York: Raven Press, 1975:87.
157. Bianco C: Plasma membrane receptors for complement. In Good RA, Day SB (eds): Comprehensive Immunology. New York: Plenum Press, 1975:69.
158. Griffin FM Jr, Griffin JA, Leider JE, Silverstein SC: Studies on the mechanism of phagocytosis. I. Requirements for circumferential attachment of particle-bound ligands to specific receptors on the macrophage plasma membrane. J Exp Med 1975;142:1263–1282.
159. Rosse WF, De Boisfleury A, Bessis M: The interaction of phagocytic cells and RBCs modified by immune reactions. Comparison of antibody and complement coated RBCs. Blood Cells 1975;1:345.
160. Atkinson JP, Frank MM: Role of complement in the pathophysiology of hematologic diseases. Prog Hematol 1977;10: 211–245.
161. Boyer JT: Complement and cold agglutinins. II. Interactions of the components of complement and antibody within the haemolytic complex. Clin Exp Immunol 1967;2:241–252.
162. Engelfriet CP, von dem Borne AEG Kr, Beckers D, Reynierse E, van Loghem JJ: Autoimmune haemolytic anaemias. V. Studies on the resistance against complement haemolysis of the RBCs of patients with chronic cold agglutinin disease. Clin Exp Immunol 1972;11:255–264.
163. Evans RS, Turner E, Bingham M: Chronic hemolytic anemia due to cold agglutinins: The mechanism of resistance of RBCs to C′ hemolysis by cold agglutinins. J Clin Invest 1967; 46: 1461–1474.
164. Evans RS, Turner E, Bingham M: Studies with radio iodinated cold agglutinins of ten patients. Am J Med 1965;38:378.

165. MacKenzie MR: Monocytic sensitization in autoimmune hemolytic anemia. Clin Res (abstract) 1975;23:132.
166. Kay NE, Douglas SD: Monocyte-erythrocyte interaction in vitro in immune hemolytic anemias. Blood 1977;59:889–897.
167. Douglas SD, Schmidt ME, Siltzbach HE: Monocyte receptor activity in normal individuals and patients with sarcoidosis. Immunol Commun 1972;1:25–38.
168. Gallagher MT, Branch DR, Mison A, Petz LD: Evaluation of reticuloendothelial function in autoimmune hemolytic anemia using an in vitro assay of monocyte-macrophage interaction with erythrocytes. Exp Hematol 1983;11:82–89.
169. Kelton JG: Impaired reticuloendothelial function in patients treated with methyldopa. N Engl J Med 1985;313:596.
170. Branch DR, Gallagher MT, Shulman IA, et al: Reticuloendothelial cell function in α-methyldopa-induced hemolytic anemia. Vox Sang 1983;45:278–287.
171. Frank MM, Hamburger MI, Lawley TJ, Kimberly RP, Plotz PH: Defective reticuloendothelial system Fc-receptor function in systemic lupus erythematosus. N Engl J Med 1979;300:518.
172. Atkinson JP, Frank MM: The effect of bacillus calmette-guerin-induced macrophage inactivation on the in vivo clearance of sensitized erythrocytes. J Clin Invest 1974;53:1742–1749.
173. Rhodes J: Altered expression of human monocyte Fc receptors in malignant disease. Nature 1977;265:253–255.
174. Arend WP, Mannik M: Quantitative studies on IgG receptors on monocytes. In van Furth R (ed): Mononuclear Phagocytes in Immunity, Infection, and Pathology. Oxford: Blackwell Scientific, 1975:303.
175. Kölbl H: Klinik und therapie der akuten erworbenen hämolytischen anämien im kindesalter. Ostdeutsch Z Kinderheilk 1955;11:27.
176. Dameshek W, Schwartz R: Hemolytic Mechanisms. Ann NY Acad Sci 1959;77:589.
177. Gedikoglu AG, Cantez T: Haemolytic anaemia relapses after immunisation and pertussis. Lancet 1967;2:894–895.
178. Pirofsky B: Infectious disease and autoimmune hemolytic anemia. In Pirofsky B (ed): Autoimmunization and the Autoimmune Hemolytic Anemias. Baltimore: Williams & Wilkins, 1969:153.
179. Bossi E, Wagner HP: Autoimmune hemolytic anemia and cytomegalovirus infection in a six month old child, treated with azathioprine. Helv Paediat Acta 1972;27:155-62.
180. Rosse WF: Correlation of in vivo and in vitro measurements of hemolysis in hemolytic anemia due to immune reactions. Prog Hematol 1973;8:51–75.
181. Bunch CF, Schwartz CM, Bird GWG: Paroxysmal cold haemoglobinuria following measles immunization. Arch Dis Child 1975;47:299.
182. Zupanska B, Lawkowicz W, Górska B, et al: Autoimmune hemolytic anemia in children. Br J Haematol 1976;34: 511–520.
183. Haneberg B, Matre R, Winsnes R, et al: Acute hemolytic anemia related to diptheria-pertussis-tetanus vaccination. Acta Paediatr Scand 1978;67:345–350.
184. Johnson ST, McFarland JG, Casper JT, Oshima S, Gottschall JL: An unusual case of autoimmune hemolytic anemia following DPT vaccination (abstract). Transfusion 1989;29:50S.
185. Garratty G: Basic mechanisms of in vivo cell destruction. In Bell CA (ed): A Seminar on Immune-mediated Cell Destruction. Washington, DC: American Association of Blood Banks, 1981:1.
186. Garratty G, Vengelen-Tyler V, Postoway N, et al: Hemolytic transfusion reactions (HTR) associated with antibodies not detectable by routine procedures (abstract). Transfusion 1982;22:429.
187. Gilsanz F, de la Serna FJ, Moltó L, Alvarez-Mon M: Hemolytic anemia in chronic large granular lymphocytic leukemia of natural killer cells: Cytotoxicity of natural killer cells against autologous RBCs is associated with hemolysis. Transfusion 1996;36:463–466.
188. Zipursky A, Brown EJ: The ingestion of IgG-sensitized erythrocytes by abnormal neutrophils. Blood 1974;43:737–742.
189. Gelfand EW, Abramson N, Segel GB, Nathan DG: Buffy-coat observations and red-cell antibodies in acquired hemolytic anemia. N Engl J Med 1971;284:1250–1252.
190. Spiva DA, George JN, Sears DA: Acute autoimmune hemolytic anemia due to a low molecular weight IgM cold hemolytic associated with episodic lymphoid granulomatous vasculitis. Am J Med 1974;56:417–428.
191. Djaldetti M, Elion D, Bessler H, Fishman P: Paroxysmal cold hemoglobinuria. Am J Clin Pathol 1975;63:804–810.
192. Wolach B, Heddle N, Barr RD, et al: Transient Donath-Landsteiner haemolytic anaemia. Br J Haematol 1981;48:425–434.
193. Lau P, Sererat S, Moore V, McLeish K, Alousi M: Paroxysmal cold hemoglobinuria in a patient with Klebsiella pneumonia. Vox Sang 1983;44:167–172.
194. Hernandez JA, Steane SM: Erythrophagocytosis by segmented neutrophils in paroxysmal cold hemoglobinuria. Am J Clin Pathol 1984;81:787–789.
195. Uzokwe CO, Gwynn AM, Gorst DW, Adamson AR: Infectious mononucleosis complicated by haemolytic anaemia due to the Donath Landsteiner antibody and by severe neutropenia. Clin Lab Haematol 1993;15:137.
196. Friedman HD, Dracker RA: Intravascular erythrophagocytosis. JAMA 1991;265:1082.
197. Dameshek W: Autoimmunity: Theoretical aspects. Ann NY Acad Sci 1965;124:6–28.
198. Götze O, Muller-Eberhard HJ: Lysis of erythrocytes by complement in the absence of antibody. J Exp Med 1970;132:898–915.
199. Salama A, Mueller-Eckhardt C: Delayed hemolytic transfusion reactions. Transfusion 1984;24:188–193.
200. Salama A, Mueller-Eckhardt C: Binding of fluid phase C3b to nonsensitized bystander human RBCs: A model for in vivo effects of complement activation on blood cells. Transfusion 1985;25:528–534.
201. Petz LD: The expanding boundaries of transfusion medicine. In Nance SJ (ed): Clinical and Basic Science Aspects of Immunohematology. Arlington, Va: American Association of Blood Banks, 1991:73.
202. Thompson RA, Rowe DS: Reactive haemolysis—A distinctive form of red cell lysis. Immunology 1968;14:745.
203. Lachmann PJ, Thompson RA: Reactive lysis: The complement-mediated lysis of unsensitized cells. II. The characteristics of activated reactor as C56 and the participation of C8 and C9. J Exp Med 1970;131:643–657.
204. Yachnin S, Ruthenberg JM: The initiation and enhancement of human red cell lysis by activators of the first component of complement and by first component esterase; studies using normal RBCs and RBCs from patients with paroxysmal nocturnal hemoglobinuria. J Clin Invest 1965;44:518.
205. Sirchia G, Ferrone S, Mercuriali F: Leukocyte antigen-antibody reaction and lysis of paroxysmal nocturnal hemoglobinuria erythrocytes. Blood 1970;36:334–336.
206. Boyden SV, Sorkin E: The adsorption of antigen by spleen cells previously treated with antiserum in vitro. Immunology 1960;3:272.
207. Sunada M, Suzuki S, Ota Z: Reticuloendothelial cell function in autoimmune hemolytic anemia (AIHA): Studies on the mechanism of peripheral monocyte activation. Acta Med Okayama 1985;5:375–384.
208. Hymes KB, Schuck MP, Karpatkin S: Regulation of autoimmune anti-platelet antibody-mediated adhesion of monocytes to platelet GPIIb/BPIIIa: effect of armed monocytes and the Mac-1 receptor. Blood 1990;75:1813–1819.
209. Griffiths HL, Kumpel BM, Elson CJ, Hadley AG: The functional activity of human monocytes passively sensitized with monoclonal anti-D suggests a novel role for FcγRI in the immune destruction of blood cells. Immunology 1994;83:370.
210. Garratty G: Novel mechanisms for immune destruction of circulating autologous cells. In Silberstein CE (ed): Autoimmune disorders of blood. Bethesda, Md: American Association of Blood Banks, 1996:79–114.
211. Romano EL, Mollison PL: Red cell destruction in vivo by low concentrations of IgG anti-A. Br J Haematol 1975;29:121–127.

CHAPTER 5

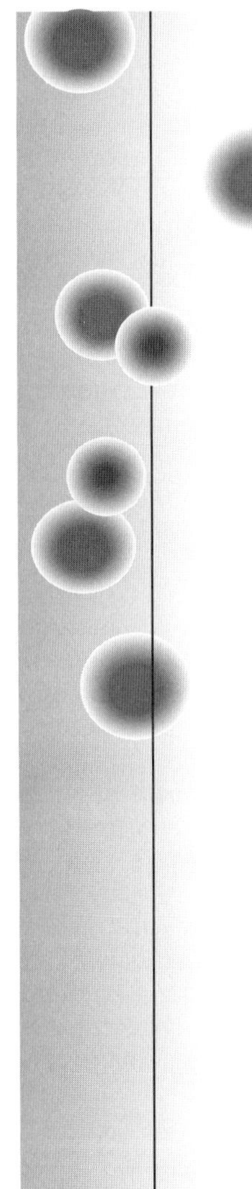

Differential Diagnosis of Immune Hemolytic Anemias

As indicated in Chapter 2, the laboratory evaluation of a patient who has an acquired hemolytic anemia should include a direct antiglobulin test (DAT), which, if positive, allows a presumptive diagnosis of an immune hemolytic anemia (IHA). The physician must then differentiate among the various causes of IHA, which are listed in Table 3-1.

We begin the discussion of the differential diagnosis by emphasizing distinctive clinical and laboratory findings. The approach to the laboratory diagnosis of each kind of autoimmune hemolytic anemia (AIHA) includes a narrative overview that omits technical details but explains the significance of the results of the tests described in Chapter 6. We discuss results of screening tests, more definitive tests, and characteristic findings in patients with IHAs of various types (i.e., warm antibody AIHA (WAIHA), cold agglutinin syndrome (CAS), paroxysmal cold hemoglobinuria (PCH), and combined cold and warm AIHA). This includes a review of some atypical serologic findings such as AIHA caused by IgM warm autoantibodies or IgG cold autoantibodies. (AIHA associated with a negative DAT is discussed in Chapter 9.) Although the differential diagnosis of IHAs is based on clinical and serologic findings, we also review some basic science aspects of the autoantibodies, including their immunoglobulin class and subclass and the immunochemistry of cold autoantibodies.

DISTINCTIVE CLINICAL AND ROUTINE LABORATORY FEATURES

Some of the clinical and routine laboratory findings in patients with IHAs are sufficiently distinctive as to strongly suggest the type of IHA that is present. The following observations merit particular emphasis because they are most helpful.

Association with Exposure to Cold

A history of acrocyanosis and/or hemoglobinuria on exposure to cold in an elderly patient with an acquired hemolytic anemia strongly suggests a diagnosis of CAS. However, although reports in the early medical literature on CAS stressed these disease manifestations, we find that they are absent in a majority of patients. Their absence in most patients with CAS who have been diagnosed in recent years perhaps is attributable to the fact that CAS was the last type of AIHA to be well characterized, and, initially, only those patients with the most severe disease were so diagnosed. A review of earlier serologic studies supports this impression. In Dacie's[1] series of

26 patients published in 1962, all but 2 had cold agglutinin titers of 4000 or greater, whereas in our series, 43% of patients had a cold agglutinin titer less than 1000 (see later).

Although one might assume that PCH is commonly precipitated by exposure to cold, this is only occasionally true. Indeed Wolach and coworkers[2] pointed out that the most common form of PCH is the transient type, secondary to infection (e.g., in childhood), and this is rarely paroxysmal, is only occasionally clearly precipitated by cold, and is not invariably expressed as hemoglobinuria (although the latter finding is very common).[3]

Autoagglutination

Autoagglutination is a finding that may be noted by technologists in all sections of the laboratory, not just those in the blood transfusion or immunohematology laboratories. Indeed, cold autoagglutinins that react strongly at room temperature cause such striking findings that they are difficult to ignore. Autoaggutination visible to the naked eye occurring at room temperature is characteristic of CAS, but may also be noted in about one third of patients with WAIHA.[4] Although the autoagglutination caused by such cold agglutinins is often 2+ to 4+, it almost always completely disperses after a few minutes of incubation at 37°C (Fig. 5-1), whereas that caused by warm autoantibodies is usually much weaker and will not disperse at 37°C. If the blood sample has been obtained from a patient known to have hemolytic anemia, such simple observations offer an important clue to the correct diagnosis.

However, a common error is the overinterpretation of cold agglutination. Many cold antibodies are reactive at room temperature but are clinically benign, albeit somewhat of a nuisance in the laboratory. The criteria for distinguishing clinically benign cold agglutinins from those pathologic cold agglutinins capable of causing CAS are discussed later.

Drug Ingestion

A temporal history of drug ingestion may suggest the etiology of the patient's IHA. A critical aspect of evaluation of a patient with IHA is the elicitation of a history of drug ingestion, which, in some instances, may have occurred a week or more before the onset of hemolysis, or be a single dose given for surgery (e.g., cefotetan). Knowledge of the drugs that have been implicated as a cause of drug-induced IHA is essential (see Chapter 8).

Many drug-induced IHAs can be distinguished from AIHA by laboratory findings, that is, the demonstration of a drug-dependent red blood cell (RBC) antibody. However, the administration of some drugs causes hemolytic anemia that is serologically indistinguishable from cases of idiopathic WAIHA. We refer to the latter cases as drug-induced AIHA, and cases wherein a drug-dependent antibody can be identified we refer to as drug-induced IHA. The most common drug at present to cause AIHA is fludarabine (see Chapter 8).

Alloantibody-Induced Immune Hemolytic Anemia

Alloantibody-induced hemolytic anemias include hemolytic disease of the newborn and hemolytic transfusion reactions. The clinical setting usually strongly suggests these diagnoses. Although autoantibody-induced hemolytic disease of the newborn can occur as a result of transplacental passage of a mother's IgG warm autoantibody, this is very unlikely unless the mother has obvious and quite severe WAIHA (see Chapter 9).

Also, when hemolysis occurs in the immediate aftermath of an RBC transfusion, the diagnosis of an acute hemolytic transfusion reaction is quite evident. However, distinguishing a delayed hemolytic transfusion from AIHA is difficult on occasion.[4-7] This differential diagnosis is discussed in Chapter 9.

Hemoglobinemia and Hemoglobinuria

Hemoglobinuria (hemoglobin in the urine) is far less common than hematuria (RBCs in the urine), and a very common clinical error is the assumption that a patient's red urine is caused by hematuria. It should be remembered that hemoglobinuria, associated with hemolytic anemia, cannot occur without hemoglobinemia. If red urine is present without hemoglobinemia, it should be suspected that the cause is hematuria

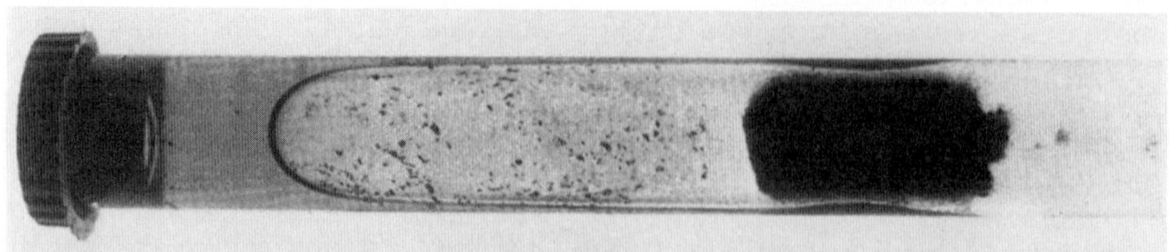

FIGURE 5-1. An anticoagulated blood sample from a patient with cold agglutinin syndrome. The cold agglutinin reacted to a titer of 2048 at 4°C and 512 at 20°C in saline. The figure shows a huge mass of agglutinated red cells in an anticoagulated blood sample that had been placed at 4°C. Such agglutination is often mistaken for a clot. However, agglutination completely disperses after incubation at 37°C for 5 to 10 minutes.

and not hemolysis. The presence of hemoglobinemia and hemoglobinuria should alert the clinician to a specific group of diagnoses and, when considered in association with the clinical setting, often makes the specific diagnosis evident (see Table 2-6 of Chapter 2). The most common associated diagnoses are probably a hemolytic transfusion reaction and severe acute WAIHA, although hemoglobinuria may occur in patients with CAS, especially after exposure to cold. Also, drug-induced HA caused by cefotetan and ceftriaxone are commonly associated with hemoglobinemia and hemoglobinuria (see Chapter 8).

Hemoglobinuria and hemoglobinemia are much more common in children (see Chapter 9). In children, both warm and cold AIHA can be the cause. In a child, PCH should be suspected and a Donath-Landsteiner (DL) test performed whenever an acute severe hemolytic anemia occurs with hemoglobinemia and hemoglobinuria. Indeed, hemoglobinuria is a common presenting manifestation of PCH[3] so that this becomes an important diagnostic clue.

Red Blood Cell Morphology and Erythrophagocytosis

One of the easily performed and very valuable tests for determining the specific diagnosis in a patient with hemolytic anemia is examination of the peripheral blood film. RBC morphology often strongly suggests a specific diagnosis or a limited number of diagnostic possibilities (see Chapter 2, page 53).

Red cell adherence and erythrophagocytosis by neutrophils are prominent findings in PCH but are seen rarely in other forms of immune-mediated hemolytic anemia. Erythrophagocytosis is rarely observed in the peripheral blood film of the more common WAIHA. When it is observed, monocytes, not neutrophils, are more often involved (see Chapter 3, page 76).

Association with *Mycoplasma pneumoniae*

If a patient with *Mycoplasma pneumoniae* infection develops AIHA, the diagnosis of CAS must be strongly suspected because AIHA in this setting is almost always caused by cold agglutinins (see Chapter 3, page 100).

LABORATORY DIAGNOSIS OF IMMUNE HEMOLYTIC ANEMIAS

Even in the presence of valuable clinical clues that may suggest a specific diagnosis, the confirmation of the precise diagnosis of the type of IHA present depends on the laboratory. The serologic tests to be performed determine whether the patient's RBCs are coated with immunoglobulin G (IgG), complement components, or both. The performance of the DAT supplies such information. Further tests must be performed to determine the characteristics of the antibodies in the patient's serum and in a RBC eluate. In addition to the DAT, we usually perform an "AIHA screen," which is an elaboration of the routine antibody screen performed for pretransfusion testing. The full technical details of this are given in Chapter 6. In summary, the patient's serum is tested against a pool of untreated and enzyme (e.g., ficin)-treated allogeneic group O RBCs and autologous RBCs at 20°C (room temperature can be used) and 37°C (all stages strictly at 37°C). A duplicate set of tubes is used with added fresh complement (pooled normal sera) at optimal pH (6.5 to 6.8) for lysis. After incubation, the tubes are inspected for hemolysis, agglutination, and sensitization (antiglobulin test using polyspecific antiglobulin serum).

The results of this screen usually indicate whether we are dealing with a cold autoagglutinin, a "warm" autoantibody, or possibly a combination of both. Other points of interest are whether there is a hemolysin present and whether it is a "cold" or "warm" hemolysin. If agglutination occurs at 20°C, a cold agglutinin titer and thermal amplitude are performed.

With the results of the DAT, AIHA screen, and possibly a cold agglutinin titer/thermal amplitude, we usually have a very good idea of whether we are dealing with WAIHA or CAS. Sometimes the patient's history and results of the DAT/AIHA screen will lead to further tests such as the DL test for PCH, or detection of drug-dependent antibodies.

The full battery of tests described above and in Chapter 6 are perhaps best done by specialists (e.g., a reference laboratory), but for most cases, the DAT, antibody screen as performed routinely in pretransfusion testing, together with a cold agglutinin titer, can yield enough information to support a diagnosis of WAIHA or CAS. For instance, the addition of complement (at pH 6.5 to 6.8) is useful only in a small percentage of cases (see Tables 5-1 and 5-2).

Significance of the DAT in the Differential Diagnosis of Immune Hemolytic Anemias

The DAT using polyspecific and monospecific antiglobulin reagents provides useful information in the evaluation of a patient with IHA. However, the results must always be interpreted in conjunction with clinical and other laboratory data to avoid erroneous conclusions. As indicated in Chapter 6, a positive DAT occurs in situations other than IHAs. A positive DAT does not necessarily indicate the presence of autoantibody; furthermore, even if autoantibody is present, the patient may or may not have a hemolytic anemia. Thus, an independent assessment must be made to determine the presence or absence of hemolytic anemia, and the role of the DAT

TABLE 5-1. RESULTS OF SERUM SCREENING IN 244 PATIENTS WITH WARM ANTIBODY AIHA

	Serum (% Positive Reactions)	Acidified Serum and Acidified Complement (% Positive Reactions)
20°C, Untreated RBCs		
Lysis	0.4	0.8
Agglutination	34.8	34.8
20°C, Enzyme Treated		
Lysis	1.6	2.5
Agglutination	78.6	78.6
37°C, Untreated RBCs		
Lysis	0.4	0.4
Agglutination	4.9	4.9
Indirect antiglobulin test	57.4	57.4
37°C, Enzyme Treated		
Lysis	8.6	12.7
Agglutination	88.9	88.9

is to aid in the evaluation of the etiology of hemolysis when present.

Kaplan and Garratty[8] used a predictive value (PV) model (Table 5-3) to evaluate the value of the DAT in predicting whether a patient has AIHA. The reported incidence of positive DATs in random hospital patients has ranged from approximately 1% up to 15% but is usually 7% to 8%, when the antiglobulin reagent contains optimal anti-C3d activity.[9] The prevalence of AIHA in this group has not been determined, but if we arbitrarily assign a figure of 1:1000—an almost 100-fold increase over that of the general population—we can calculate the PV of a positive DAT.

TABLE 5-2. RESULTS OF SERUM SCREENING IN 57 PATIENTS WITH COLD AGGLUTININ SYNDROME

	Serum (% Positive Reactions)	Acidified Serum and Acidified Complement (% Positive Reactions)
20°C, Untreated RBCs		
Lysis	2.0	14.3
Agglutination	98	98
20°C, Enzyme Treated		
Lysis	24.5	93.8
Agglutination	100	100
37°C, Untreated RBCs		
Lysis	0	0
Agglutination	10.7	10.7
Indirect antiglobulin test	5.4	5.4
37°C, Enzyme Treated		
Lysis	12.2	22.5
Agglutination	28.6	28.6

Sensitivity of the test is 96% to 98% because only 2% to 4% of patients with AIHA have a negative DAT (see Chapter 9), but specificity is about 92% to 93% (100% minus the 7% to 8% incidence). Of 10,000 patients, there would be 10 true positives (TPs) and no false negatives (FNs). A total of 690 would be FPs (7% of 9990), leaving 9300 TNs. Thus, the PV of a positive DAT is 1.4%. Clearly, even in a hospital population, the DAT should not be used to screen for AIHA; it would be wasteful to let positive results trigger other serologic and biochemical tests. Performing a DAT as part of a differential diagnosis of hemolytic anemia is another picture entirely (see Table 5-3). If a patient with hemolytic anemia has a positive DAT, sensitivity remains at 98% and specificity at 93%, but disease prevalence changes markedly. We have assumed that one fourth, or 25 of 100, cases of hemolytic anemia may be autoimmune. If 4% of AIHAs are DAT-negative, then there would be 1 FN and 24 TP. Five (7% of 75) would be FP and 71 would be TN. Thus, the PV of a positive DAT is 83%, which is clearly useful. The 99% PV of a negative result is also quite important in this setting.

Numerous complexities may be considered regarding the DAT, and highly detailed classifications of AIHA have been based on DAT results.[10-12] However, we believe that excessively detailed testing adds little to a clinically significant classification of IHAs. Prognosis and appropriate therapy cannot be correlated with classifications based on the results of the DAT even when it is performed with a large battery of antisera to immunoglobulins and complement components.

Results Using Polyspecific and Monospecific Antiglobulin Reagents in Patients with AIHAs

It is convenient to first perform the DAT with a polyspecific antiglobulin serum, which is defined as one that must contain anti-IgG and anti-C3d and may contain antibodies to other complement components (e.g., C3b, C3c, and C4) and to other immunoglobulins (e.g., IgA and IgM). A positive result in a patient with acquired hemolytic anemia generally indicates that the patient's RBCs are coated with IgG, C3dg, or both.

Using monospecific anti-IgG and anti-C3, it is then a simple matter to determine which of these two proteins are coating the patient's RBCs. The significance of such results is outlined in Tables 5-4 and 5-5.

THE ANTI-COMPLEMENT COMPONENT OF POLYSPECIFIC ANTIGLOBULIN SERUM

One point that is evident that must be emphasized is that the performance of the DAT with an antiglobulin serum that does not contain anti-C3d will frequently result in misleadingly negative results in patients with IHAs. This is true in all patients with CAS, 13% of patients with WAIHA, essentially all patients with

TABLE 5-3. USING A PREDICTIVE VALUE MODEL TO EVALUATE THE VALUE OF THE DAT IN DIAGNOSING AIHA

	Patients with Positive Test Result	Patients with Negative Test Result	Totals
Patients with disease	True positives (TP)	False negatives (FN)	TP + FN
Patients without disease	False positives (FP)	True negatives (TN)	FP + TN
Totals	TP + FP	FN + TN	TP + FP + TN + FN

Sensitivity: Percent positivity in disease:

$$\frac{TP}{TP + FN} \times 100$$

Predictive value of a positive result:

$$\frac{TP}{TP + FP} \times 100$$

Specificity: Percent negativity in absence of disease:

$$\frac{TN}{FP + FN} \times 100$$

Predictive value of a negative result:

$$\frac{TN}{TN + FN} \times 100$$

Screening Random Hospital Patients and Patients with Hemolytic Anemia (HA) for a Diagnosis of AIHA

	Positive DAT		Negative DAT		Total	
	Random	HA	Random	HA	Random	HA
AIHA	10	24	0	1	10	25
No AIHA	690	5	9300	70	9990	75
Total	700	29	9300	71	10,000	100

PV of a positive result for random patients = (10/700) × 100 = 1.4%
PV of a positive result for patients with HA = (24/29) × 100 = 83%
[PV of a negative test = (70/71) × 100 = 99%]

PCH, and many instances of drug-induced IHAs. Altogether 26% of the patients in our series had a positive DAT caused only by complement sensitization of the RBCs[4] (see Table 5-5). Other reported series of patients with AIHA yielded comparable information. For instance, Dacie and Worlledge[13] reported that 33% of 29 patients with AIHA had RBCs sensitized only with complement components.

In regard to antibodies against other complement components in antiglobulin serum, we have occasionally found patients whose RBCs are sensitized with C4d but not C3d. However, none of these patients has had hemolytic anemia.[14,15] Patients with IHA frequently have C4d on their RBCs in addition to C3d, but in testing hundreds of patients with AIHA, we have not observed a single patient with hemolysis whose RBCs had C4d but not C3d. We know of no experience contrary to this in the medical literature.

TABLE 5-4. TYPICAL DIRECT ANTIGLOBULIN TEST RESULTS IN PATIENTS WITH IMMUNE HEMOLYTIC ANEMIAS

Type of Immune Hemolytic Anemia	Anti-IgG	Anti-C3
Autoimmune Hemolytic Anemias		
Warm antibody AIHA		
67%	+	+
20%	+	0
13%	0	+
Warm antibody AIHA associated with systemic lupus erythematosus	+	+
Cold agglutinin syndrome (100%)*	0	+
Paroxysmal cold hemoglobinuria (100%)	0	+
Drug-induced Immune Hemolytic Anemias		
Drug-dependent antibodies		
Penicillin and first-generation cephalosporins	+	(+)
Second- and third-generation cephalosporins	+	+
Associated with "immune complex mechanism"	(+)	+
Drug-independent antibodies	+	(+)
Drug-induced nonimmunologic adsorption of proteins	+	(+)
Hemolytic Disease of Fetus/Newborn	+	0
Hemolytic Transfusion Reactions	+	(+)

(+) = Sometimes positive
* We detected IgG +C3 on the RBCs of one patient with CAS because the patient was on methyldopa therapy and made IgG autoantibodies.

TABLE 5-5. RESULTS OF DIRECT ANTIGLOBULIN TEST WITH ANTI-IgG AND ANTI-C3 IN 347 PATIENTS WITH AIHA AND DRUG-INDUCED IMMUNE HEMOLYTIC ANEMIA

	Percentage*	
IgG (no C3)	23	73% have IgG on RBC (IgG (no C3) + IgG + C3)
IgG + C3	50	
C3 (no IgG)	26.4	76.4% have C3 on RBC (IgG + C3 + C3 (no IgG))

* Two patients (0.6%) had only IgA present on their RBCs.

Therefore, anti-C4 appears to be superfluous in antiglobulin serum used for detection and differential diagnosis of IHA. Similarly, although with less extensive data available, antibodies to other complement components in antiglobulin serum (C5, C6, C8) have proven to be of little significant clinical value.[14,16,17] One exception was a single report suggesting that C5, without the presence of C3d, may sometimes be on the RBCs of rare patients with AIHA.[18]

SIGNIFICANCE OF ANTI-IgM AND ANTI-IgA IN ANTIGLOBULIN SERUM

Even with potent antisera, RBC-bound IgM is difficult to detect with the antiglobulin test.[4,19,20] Fortunately, IgM antibodies that cause IHA characteristically fix complement that is much more readily detected. AIHA associated with warm IgM autoantibodies without the presence of IgG occurs on rare occasions and is discussed later in this chapter and in Chapter 9.

Anti-IgA and anti-IgM that are standardized for the DAT are not readily available in the United States. Nevertheless, one can standardize immunologic reagents for use in the DAT to detect for detection of IgA and IgM (see Chapter 6, page 210). These reagents are of significance in evaluating exceptional patients with AIHA, particularly those whose AIHA is associated only with IgA autoantibodies or warm IgM autoantibodies. IgM sensitization of RBCs is more readily detected using flow cytometry than by the DAT[21-24]; flow cytometry is also useful for detecting RBC-bound IgA.[25]

IgA antibodies only infrequently play a role in RBC sensitization, and in such cases, other immune globulins and/or complement components are almost always, although not invariably, found on the cell surface as well. Occasionally patients with WAIHA have a DAT that is positive only with anti-IgA. The clinical and hematologic features of WAIHA associated only with IgA autoantibodies are very similar to AIHA associated with warm IgG autoantibodies. Because WAIHA associated with IgA autoantibodies usually presents as AIHA with a negative DAT, such cases are discussed in Chapter 9.

Antiglobulin Test Titrations and Scores

The amount of protein sensitizing RBCs can be judged in a semiquantitative way by simply testing the RBCs with dilutions of antiglobulin serum. The strength of agglutination at each dilution of the antiglobulin serum can then be used to develop an antiglobulin test titration score. For example, 4+ agglutination may be assigned a value of 10; 3+ agglutination, a value of 8; 2+, a value of 6; 1+, a value of 4; and ½+, a value of 2. More accurate ways of measuring the amount of RBC-bound proteins using radiolabeled antiglobulin serum, ELISA, and flow cytometry[26-32] have largely replaced the use of antiglobulin test titrations and scores. Nevertheless, some useful information has been gained using this technique in the past.

For example, clinical remission of AIHA is frequently associated with a significant decrease in the strength of the DAT, although this may not be evident if one uses only a single dilution of the antiglobulin serum. It should be noted that these dilutions were performed using raw antiglobulin sera, not commercial products, which are already diluted optimally for routine use. The 1:128 dilution in Table 5-6 is probably close to undiluted commercial anti-IgG. Table 5-6 illustrates the results of testing a patient's RBCs with dilutions of anti-IgG during relapse and during clinical remission. The decrease in strength of sensitization of the RBCs is not obvious with the 1:128 dilution (or undiluted commercial anti-IgG) but is obvious after using a series of dilutions of the anti-IgG. Chaplin[33,34] has reported similar observations. The fact that the DAT is often markedly reduced in strength during remission is frequently missed because DAT titrations are now rarely performed.

There have been published studies on the relationship between antiglobulin test titration scores and quantitative measurements of RBC sensitization. We used an immunochemical method to quantitate the number of C3 molecules bound to human RBCs in vitro or in vivo, and then compared these results with the antiglobulin test and the antiglobulin test titration scores.[35] As illustrated in Figures 5-2 and 5-3, a wide range of cell-bound C3 molecules may result in a 2+ to 4+ DAT using a single dilution of antiglobulin serum. In contrast are the data illustrated in Figures 5-4 and 5-5, which indicate that antiglobulin test scores correlated quite well with the immunochemical assessment of the number of molecules per RBC. There is also a good correlation between the antiglobulin test titration scores and quantitative measurements of RBC bound IgG with RBCs sensitized with fewer than 1000 molecules of IgG per RBC as is illustrated in Figure 5-6.

Fischer and colleagues[35] further studied 25 patients who had positive DATs that were caused at least in

TABLE 5-6. ANTIGLOBULIN TEST TITRATIONS IN A PATIENT WITH WAIHA IN RELAPSE AFTER REMISSION INDUCED BY CORTICOSTEROID THERAPY

Reciprocals of Dilutions of Our Anti-IgG*	128	256	512	1024	2048	4096	Score
Relapse	4+	4+	4+	3+	2+	1+	48
Remission	4+	2+	1+	0	0	0	18

Agglutination reactions are graded as ½+ to 4+.
* Raw (undiluted) "homemade" anti-IgG (see text above).

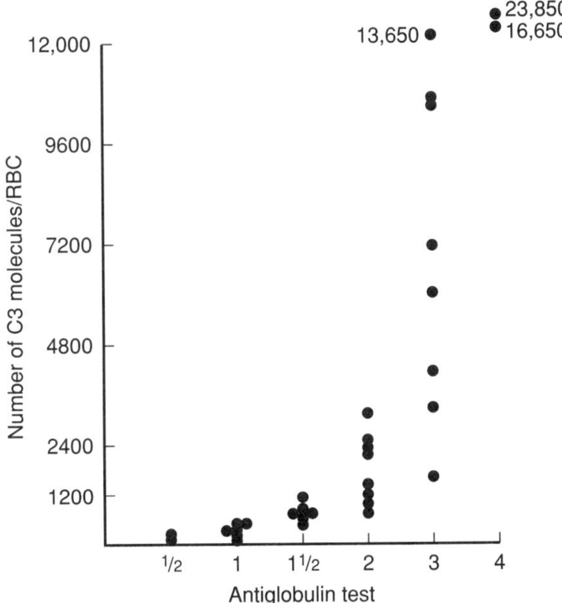

FIGURE 5-2. The relationship between the number of C3 molecules per red cell and the antiglobulin test using a single dilution of anti-C3 antiserum. C3-sensitized RBCs were prepared in vitro using Le[a] antibody in varying dilutions. (From Fischer JT, Petz LD, Garratty G, Cooper NR: Correlations between quantitative assay of red-cell bound C3, serologic reactions, and hemolytic anemia. Blood 1974;44:359.)

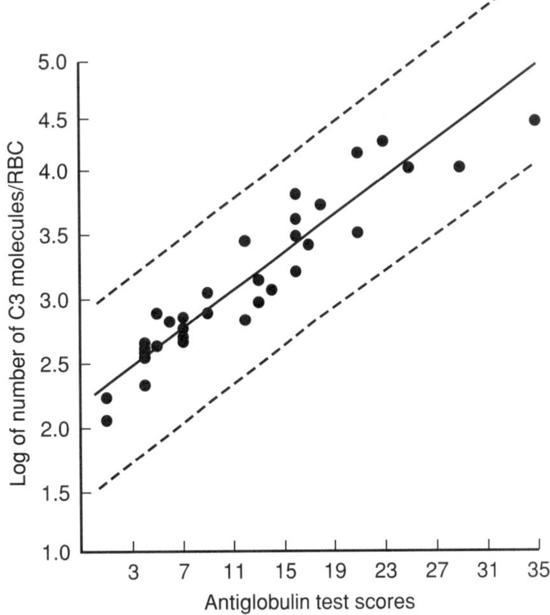

FIGURE 5-4. Correlation between antiglobulin titration scores and the quantitative assay of cell-bound C3 (in vitro sensitized RBCs). The linear regression coefficient with 95 percent confidence limits is 0.071 ± 0.005. The coefficient of correlation by linear regression (r) = 0.83, significant at the 1 percent level. (From Fischer JT, Petz LD, Garratty G, Cooper NR: Correlations between quantitative assay of red-cell bound C3, serologic reactions, and hemolytic anemia. Blood 1974;44:359.)

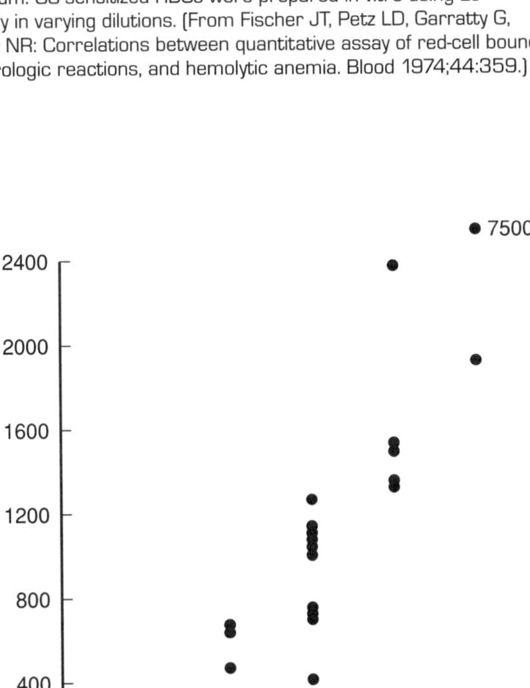

FIGURE 5-3. The relationship between the number of C3 molecules per RBC and the antiglobulin test using a single dilution of anti-C3. C3-sensitized RBCs were obtained from patients having a positive DAT caused at least in part by RBC sensitization by C3. (From Fischer JT, Petz LD, Garratty G, Cooper NR: Correlations between quantitative assay of red-cell bound C3, serologic reactions, and hemolytic anemia. Blood 1974;44:359.)

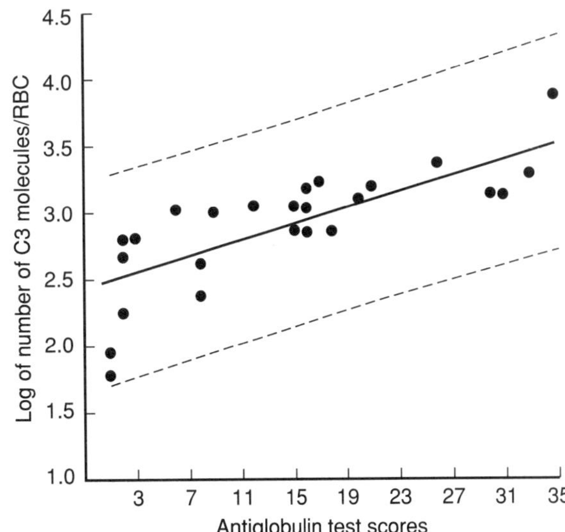

FIGURE 5-5. Correlation between DAT titration scores and the quantitative assay of cell bound C3 (RBCs sensitized in vivo). The linear regression coefficient with 95 percent confidence limits is 0.031 ± 0.012. The coefficient of correlation by linear regression (r) = 0.66, significant at the 1 percent level. (From Fischer JT, Petz LD, Garratty G, Cooper NR: Correlations between quantitative assay of red-cell bound C3, serologic reactions, and hemolytic anemia. Blood 1974;44:359.)

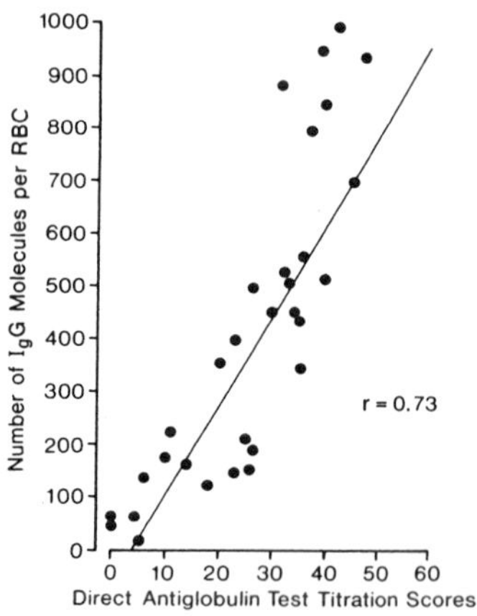

FIGURE 5-6. Correlation between antiglobulin test titration scores and a quantitative immunochemical assay of red cell bound IgG.

part by RBC-bound C3. Only 2 of 14 patients with less than 1100 molecules of C3 per RBC had hemolytic anemia, whereas 8 of 11 patients with at least 1100 molecules of C3 per RBC did have overt hemolysis. The presence or absence of hemolysis was not explained by variations in the amount of IgG on these patients' RBCs as assessed by the antiglobulin test using monospecific anti-IgG (Table 5-6).

Garratty and Nance[29] showed that flow cytometry was more efficient at differentiating the degree of RBC sensitization with IgG than test titration scores, when RBCs were strongly sensitized (e.g., 4+ antiglobulin tests). Table 5-8 shows the results.

The significance of semiquantitative or quantitative measurements of the amount of IgG or C3 on the RBC membrane must not be exaggerated. Rosse[36,37] and Garratty and Nance[29] demonstrated that the amount of antibody detected on the RBC membrane was generally proportional to the rate of RBC destruction, but exceptions to this correlation were frequent. Indeed, in an individual patient, it is impossible to predict the presence or absence of a shortened RBC life span on the basis of measures of RBC bound immunoglobulins. The in vivo significance of a given degree of RBC sensitization by autoantibodies varies greatly, even among antibodies of the same immunoglobulin class.[29]

Warm Antibody AIHA

In WAIHA, there is no diagnostic pattern of DAT reactivity. Most commonly, positive reactions are obtained both with anti-IgG and anti-C3, but in a minority of cases, only IgG or C3 is found on the patient's RBCs. Using these antisera to test the RBCs of 244 patients with WAIHA, we found 67% had RBC-bound IgG and C3; 20% had RBC-bound IgG but no C3; and 13% had RBC-bound C3 but no IgG[10] (see Table 5-4). Worlledge and Blajchman[38] found that 48% had RBC-bound IgG+ C3; 39% had IgG but no C3; 11% had C3 but no IgG; and 2% had only IgA. Sokol and coworkers[39] found only 24% of their AIHA patients to have RBC-bound IgG+ C3 and 61% had IgG alone. These differences might be due to the amount of anti-C3dg in the anti-C3 used for the DAT. Other patterns may also be found if additional antiglobulin sera are used (e.g., anti-IgA and -IgM)[4] (Table 5-9).

Hsu and coworkers[19] studied 34 patients with positive DATs using an AutoAnalyzer, which was more sensitive than the routine DAT. None of the 16 patients without hemolytic anemia had RBC-bound C3 or IgM; 88% had RBC-bound IgG; and 25% had RBC-bound IgA (2 patients had only IgA detected on the RBCs). RBC-bound IgG was detected on the RBCs of 11 of 13 patients (85%) with AIHA; 61% had RBC-bound C3; 69% had RBC-bound IgA; and 61% had RBC-bound IgM. The authors emphasized that hemolytic anemia appeared to be associated commonly with RBC-bound C3, IgA, and IgM in addition to IgG, in contrast to the patients without hemolytic anemia. They noted that RBC-bound IgM was not detected when the hemolytic anemia was in partial or complete remission. It should be emphasized that the AutoAnalyzer may detect RBC-bound proteins not detectable by the routine DAT, even when anti-IgM is used. It is interesting to note that Lalezari and coworkers[40] found that the RBCs from patients with hemolytic anemia due to methyldopa therapy had RBC-bound IgM (and C1q) in addition to IgG. When the hemolysis stopped, no RBC-bound IgG was detectable. Patients with positive DATs but no hemolytic anemia did not have RBC-bound IgM. The RBC-bound IgM was only detectable using an AutoAnalyzer. It was suggested that the RBC-bound IgM was monomeric. No one has confirmed this interesting finding.

Ben-Izhak and coworkers[41] suggested that the presence of more than one class of immunoglobulin on RBCs, detectable by the standard DAT, was associated with severe hemolytic anemia. They found that 36% of 25 patients with AIHA had IgM or IgA in addition to IgG on their RBCs. These patients appeared to respond less well to steroid therapy. Using an enzyme-linked antiglobulin test (ELAT), Sokol and coworkers[42] showed that multiple immunoglobulins could be detected on 35% of 153 patients who were suspected of having AIHA. Only 7.2% showed the same results when the standard DAT (anti-IgG+ anti-C3) was used. Using ELAT, the following immunoglobulins were detected: 23% of the RBCs were sensitized with IgG and IgM; 5.8% were sensitized with IgG plus IgA; and 8% were sensitized with IgG, IgM, and IgA. RBC-bound IgG was present in larger amounts than IgM or IgA in 63% of the samples. Compared with IgG sensitization alone, multiple immunoglobulins were significantly associated with larger quantities (>800 molecules/RBC) of IgG, multiple IgG subclasses, IgG+C3d bound to RBCs, and with serum haptoglobin levels of less than 0.1 g/L. The latter association was still significant when higher levels of RBC-bound IgG and IgG subclass pattern were taken into account. In RBC samples

TABLE 5-7. RESULTS OF ASSAYS OF RBC-BOUND C3 IN 25 PATIENTS AND CORRELATION WITH CLINICAL AND SEROLOGICAL DATA

	Disease	DAT (Anti-C3)	No. of C3 Molecules per RBC	DAT (Anti-C3) Titration Score	Hemolytic Anemia	Hct	Hgb	Reticulocytes (%)	DAT (Anti-IgG)
1.	SLE	½+	60	1	No	41.7	14.8	—	1+
2.	Iron deficiency anemia	½+	90	1	No	21.1	7.0	3	0
3.	Normal	1+	180	2	No	39.8	14.0	—	0
4.	SLE	1+	235	8	Yes	30.2	10.4	4.8	1+
5.	Hypertension	2+	410	7	No	44.4	15.8	—	3+
6.	DIIHA[a] (Aldomet)	1+	465	2	Yes	37.5	12.6	3.1	4+
7.	Normal	1+	625	2	No	42.0	—	—	0
8.	SLE	1+	630	3	No	41.5	13.4	—	0
9.	Vasculitis	2+	700	16	No	40.0	14.1	2	0
10.	SLE	2+	720	18	No	44.0	14.7	—	2+
11.	SLE	2+	735	15	No	42.2	14.3	—	2+
12.	SLE	2+	1010	8	No	41.7	14.8	—	0
13.	WAIHA (post-splenectomy)	2+	1050	6	No	42.0	13.2	—	2+
14.	Chronic active hepatitis	2+	1075	15	No	40.1	13.3	—	2+
15.	DIIHA[a] (penicillin)	2+	1100	16	Yes	11.0	3.6	26	2+
16.	Acute lymphocytic leukemia	2+	1125	11	Yes	17.0	4.5	0.3[b]	3+
17.	PCH	3+	1260	21	Yes	35.0	11.2	6.3	0
18.	SLE	3+	1335	30	No	26.7	8.5	2.1	1+
19.	WAIHA	3+	1340	31	Yes	31.0	9.3	10.2	0
20.	Rheumatoid arthritis	3+	1510	15	No[c]	34.0	10.0	2.0	3+
21.	SLE	3+	1560	21	No	38.0	12.9	0.8	4+
22.	WAIHA	2+	1710	16	Yes	33.0	10.7	1.5	1+
23.	CAS	4+	1910	33	Yes	24.0	7.8	9.2	0
24.	CAS	3+	2375	19	Yes	20.5	7.1	4.4	0
25.	CAS	4+	7500	35	Yes	22.4	7.8	11.6	0

[a] DIIHA, drug-induced immune hemolytic anemia.
[b] Hemolysis was present as indicated by an excessive transfusion requirement without evidence of blood loss. The patient's low reticulocyte response was presumably related to his acute leukemia.
[c] Later this patient developed overt hemolytic anemia, with the hematocrit level falling to as low as 10 percent and the reticulocytes increasing to a maximum of 30%.
Data from Fischer JT, Petz LD, Garratty G, Cooper NR: Correlations between quantitative assay of red cell-bound C3, serologic reactions, and hemolytic anemia. Blood 1974;44:359–373.

TABLE 5-8. ANTIGLOBULIN TEST TITRATION SCORES AND FLOW CYTOMETRIC ANALYSIS OF RBCs SENSITIZED IN VITRO WITH DILUTIONS OF ANTI-D

Anti-D Dilution	Indirect Antiglobulin Test	Titration Score	Fluorescence per RBC	Percentage of Fluorescence
1:5	4+	68	212.0	100
1:10	4+	68	183.2	100
1:20	4+	62	130.1	100
1:40	4+	65	84.7	99.4

Data from Garratty G, Nance SJ: Correlation between in vivo hemolysis and the amount of red cell-bound IgG measured by flow cytometry. Transfusion 1990;30:617–621.

with multiple immunoglobulin sensitization, there was no significant relationship ($p > 0.05$) between haptoglobins of less than 0.1 g/L and RBC-bound C3d or multiple IgG subclasses. The authors concluded that RBC sensitization with multiple immunoglobulin classes, even when undetected by the DAT, may be an important factor in determining the severity of AIHA.

Sokol and coworkers[43] extended the above in 404 patients with warm-reactive RBC autoantibodies on 590 occasions. Multiple immunoglobulins were detected by enzyme-linked DATs in 218 samples (37%), but in only 87 (15%) by DAT (i.e., by agglutination). RBC-bound C3d was detected on the RBCs of 64% of the patients. Compared with IgG coating alone, multiple immunoglobulins were significantly associated with larger quantities (>800 molecules/RBC) of IgG, multiple IgG subclasses, IgG3 and C3d bound to the cells, and with serum haptoglobin levels of less than 0.1 g/L. The latter association was still significant when higher levels of RBC-bound IgG and subclass pattern were taken into account. It was concluded that multiple immunoglobulin coating, even when undetected by agglutination methods, is a major cause of hemolysis; it is part of a more generalized autoimmune response and acts with other factors such as the quantity of bound IgG, the IgG subclass pattern, and complement; it also has an important hemolytic effect in its own right.

TABLE 5-9. DAT RESULTS IN 104 PATIENTS WITH WAIHA USING SEVERAL MONOSPECIFIC ANTIGLOBULIN SERA

	Percentage
IgG only	18.3
C3 only	10.6
IgA only	1.9
IgM only	0*
IgG and C3	46.2
IgG and C3 and IgA	12.5
IgG and C3 and IgA and IgM	1.9
IgG and IgA	2.9
IgG and IgM	0*
IgG and IgM and C3	3.9
IgG and IgA and IgM	0*
C3 and IgA	1.9
C3 and IgM	1.9
IgG present alone or together with other proteins	85.6
C3 present alone or together with other proteins	78.9
IgA present alone or together with other proteins	21.2
IgM present alone or together with other proteins	7.7

* Since studying these 104 patients, we have encountered rare patients who have IgM but no C3 on their RBCs.

Cold Agglutinin Syndrome

In contrast to the variable findings in WAIHA, the DAT in CAS is invariably positive with anti-C3. Equally important is the fact that reactions are almost always negative with anti-IgG; that is, a positive DAT with anti-IgG essentially excludes CAS as the sole diagnosis (see Table 5-4).

Paroxysmal Cold Hemoglobinuria

PCH is caused by an IgG complement fixing antibody but, nevertheless, the DAT is usually positive only with anti-C3 (see Table 5-4). If RBCs are washed at 37°C, no RBC-bound IgG is detected. Negative reactions with anti-IgG are probably caused by the fact that the DL antibody readily elutes from the RBC membrane during in vitro washing, whereas complement components remain fixed to the cell membrane. Dacie and Worlledge[13] reported that if the patient's RBCs are washed in saline at 10°C or below, the DAT may be positive using anti-IgG antiserum as well as anti-C3. Gottsche and coworkers[44] reported that the DAT was positive using anti-IgG in 6 of 22 patients (27%) if the RBCs were washed at 20°C but invariably negative if RBCs were washed at 37°C. The DAT will be positive at the time of a paroxysm of hemoglobinuria and for a variable duration of time thereafter.[13,44]

Drug-Induced Immune Hemolytic Anemia

DAT results in patients with drug-induced IHAs varies and generally correlates with the mechanism of development of the drug-induced antibodies (see Chapter 8). Typically, when penicillin or first-generation cephalosporins cause IHA by the "drug-adsorption mechanism," the DAT is positive with anti-IgG; a minority of patients may have RBC-bound complement detected as well. The DATs associated with IHA due to second- and third-generation cephalosporins are usually strongly positive due to IgG plus C3 or, less commonly, C3 with no IgG sensitization.[45] Drugs causing IHA via the "immune complex mechanism" characteristically result in the DAT being positive with anti-C3, but in a minority of instances RBC-bound IgG and/or IgM may also be present. Patients with drug-induced AIHA usually have positive DATs associated with IgG sensitization; a few patients may also have weak C3 sensitization. Drug-induced nonimmunologic adsorption of proteins may cause the DAT to be positive as a result of a multitude of proteins on the RBC surface (e.g., IgG, IgM, IgA, C3, and albumin).

Systemic Lupus Erythematosus

Systemic lupus erythematosus (SLE) deserves particular consideration, because many patients with this disorder have C3 on their RBCs even when no evidence of hemolysis exists. Budman and Steinberg[46] reported that the DAT was positive in 18% to 65% of patients in various published series of patients with SLE but only about 10% of these patients had clinically significant hemolysis. When the DAT was positive in a patient whose SLE was quiescent, it was positive with anti-C3 but negative with anti-IgG; in patients with overt hemolysis, the DAT was more commonly positive with both anti-C3 and anti-IgG as indicated in Table 5-4. Rarely, the DAT was positive only with anti-IgG. Mongan and coworkers[47] reported similar findings.

An Approach to the Characterization of Antibodies in the Serum and Eluates from RBCs of Patients with AIHA

Although the DAT provides useful information, the definitive diagnosis rests on the characterization of the antibodies present in the patient's serum and in an eluate from the patient's RBCs. It is wise to initiate such studies with screening tests to develop a preliminary diagnosis and then to perform additional tests as are necessary for confirmation of the diagnosis and for the exclusion of alternative possibilities.

Although the differential diagnosis of IHAs appears complex (see Table 3-1), the initial evaluation can often be simplified in concept by keeping the following points in mind.

The differentiation between idiopathic and secondary AIHA is *not* based on serologic tests but instead concerns the usual tests pertinent to the diagnosis of SLE, chronic lymphocytic leukemia, lymphomas, etc.

Drug-induced IHA may in some cases be excluded on the basis of the patient's history. However, histories of drug administration are notoriously inaccurate (see Chapter 8). For example, if the drug was given during surgery, the patient may not be aware of having received it and its administration may be indicated only in obscure locations (e.g., anesthesiologists notes) in the medical record. Also, with some drugs (e.g., second- and third-generation cephalosporins), the hemolytic anemia may not develop for a week or more following drug administration. If drug-induced IHA is a plausible diagnosis, additional studies are often necessary to demonstrate the drug-related red cell antibody. These tests are discussed separately in Chapter 8.

If a patient has an acquired hemolytic anemia with a positive DAT but no RBC antibodies are demonstrable in either the serum or RBC eluate, such findings lend weight to a diagnosis of a drug-induced hemolytic anernia. This is true because drug-dependent antibodies will give negative results in serologic studies unless the offending drug is in the in vitro test system. However, one must also keep in mind that drug-induced IHAs are very uncommon, whereas positive DATs that yield nonreactive eluates are quite common. Indeed, up to 80% of all positive DATs yield nonreactive eluates as occurs when the DAT is due to nonimmunologic uptake of IgG onto the patient's RBCs.

Alloantibody-induced IHAs (hemolytic disease of the newborn and acute hemolytic transfusion reactions) are usually made evident by the clinical setting. However, a delayed hemolytic transfusion reaction may not be obvious because the hemolysis may develop at least several days following the transfusion (see Chapter 9).

Thus, depite the lengthy list of diagnostic possibilities, it is usually optimal to perform the initial serologic tests with only three diagnostic considerations in mind: WAIHA, CAS, and PCH.

If findings are not characteristic of any of these diagnoses, the patient may have a drug-induced IHA (Chapter 8), or an atypical hemolytic anemia, such as AIHA with a negative DAT (Chapter 9), AIHA caused by IgM warm autoantibodies (see later, page 180), AIHA associated with IgA autantibodies (Chapter 9), or AIHA caused by IgG cold autoantibodies (see later, page 190). Collectively, such cases constitute only a small percentage of cases of IHAs, but nevertheless are an important group of patients.

Using the "AIHA Screen" as an Aid in the Differential Diagnosis of AIHA. Although a routine blood bank antibody screen, together with a cold agglutinin titer, can sometimes provide enough information to help in the differential diagnosis of AIHA, we find more extended testing is necessary to be certain of the diagnosis. We have found the "AIHA screen," described in detail in Chapter 6 and in summary on page 169 of this chapter, to be immensely helpful in classifying difficult cases.

Tables 5-1 and 5-2 show the results we obtained in the sera from 244 patients with WAIHA and 54 patients with CAS, respectively. Sera from patients with PCH often show negative test results at all phases of the AIHA screen (see later). Thus, although there are obvious differences in the AIHA screen results, there is also overlap between WAIHA and CAS, indicating that other data (e.g., DAT and cold agglutinin titer/thermal amplitude) are necessary to finalize the diagnosis. The AIHA screen has been very useful in helping classify unusual cases. For instance, the finding of a hemolysin at 37°C, but not 20°C, may help classify a patient as WAIHA when other results are suggestive of CAS (e.g., complement but no IgG on patient's RBCs, and a 4+ cold autoagglutinin at room temperature). On the other hand, a hemolysin at

20°C, in the presence of a similar DAT and agglutination patterns, may be more suggestive of CAS, which would be confirmed by a high thermal amplitude (≥30°C) agglutinin.

Characteristic Serology of WAIHA

Autoantibodies causing WAIHA are usually IgG but can be IgM or IgA. As discussed on pages 180–182, these proteins can be present together; it is rare for only IgM or IgA to be the cause of AIHA (see Table 5-9). Table 5-1 shows the characteristics of the antibodies associated with 244 cases of WAIHA. Because the patient's RBCs are adsorbing warm autoantibodies continuously, autoantibodies are usually only found in the serum when all autoantigens are saturated. Only about 60% of patients' sera will react with saline-suspended RBCs, but a higher percentage will react in the presence of potentiators (e.g., polyethylene glycol) or enzyme-treated RBCs (Table 5-1).

Some sera contain warm hemolysins, which react optimally at 37°C but may react at 20°C. The hemolysis is enhanced by adding fresh complement at pH 6.5 to 6.8 to the patients' sera. Von dem Borne and coworkers[48] showed that such hemolysins were usually IgM autoantibodies; they were maximally reactive at a pH of 6.5, and 7 of 11 (64%) reacted optimally at 30°C; 4 of 11 reacted optimally at 37°C.[48] We found that about one third of sera from patients with WAIHA contain IgM cold autoagglutinins that can react quite strongly at 20°C (or room temperature) but have a normal cold agglutinin titer at 4°C and do not react at 30°C. We do not think that these are pathogenic but may be naturally occurring cold antibodies that become boosted (e.g., raised thermal amplitude) during the pathogenic autoimmune response.

A diagnosis can usually be reached on the basis of the serologic tests described thus far. Despite the seemingly complicated nature of the foregoing, the usual or "typical" essential diagnostic tests that lead to a reasonably confident diagnosis of WAIHA may be very simply summarized as follows: (a) the presence of an acquired hemolytic anemia, (b) a positive DAT, and (c) an unexpected antibody in the serum and eluate that reacts optimally at 37°C. The antibody usually reacts with all normal RBCs but, in some cases, it can readily be shown to react preferentially with antigens on the patient's own RBCs.

Examples of typical serologic findings in a patient with WAIHA are listed in Table 5-10.

When performing tests for lysis in vitro, one must keep in mind that the patient's serum is frequently deficient in complement, so it is advisable to add fresh complement. This is conveniently done by adding an equal volume of ABO compatible normal serum, which has been shown to contain no unexpected antibodies, to the patient's serum. Figure 5-7 shows the effects of different storage conditions on serum complement levels.

It is logical and convenient to perform tests for specificity of the autoantibody using the screening test that gave the strongest reactions. Usually this test is the IAT or agglutination of enzyme-treated RBCs.

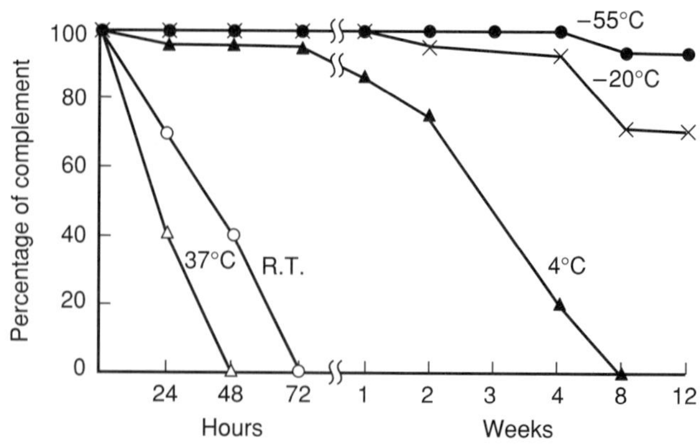

FIGURE 5-7. Average complement activity of 12 normal sera as measured by antiglobulin test assay after storage at various temperatures. (From Garratty G: The effects of storage and heparin on the activity of serum complement, with particular reference to the detection of blood group antibodies. Amer Clin Pathol 1970;54:531.)

IgG SUBCLASS OF RBC-BOUND IgG

Nance and Garratty[49] and Garratty[50] reported the IgG subclass of the autoantibody on RBCs of 167 individuals with positive IATs (46 patients with AIHA, and 32 patients and 89 blood donors with a positive DAT but no hemolytic anemia). Table 5-11 shows the results. In all three groups the RBCs were sensitized with predominantly IgG1 autoantibodies (89%, 85%, and 87%, respectively); usually IgG1 was the only subclass present. IgG2 was present alone, or together with other subclasses, on the RBCs of 5.8% of donors, and 15.6% and 26.2%, respectively, of the RBCs from patients, without and with AIHA. IgG2 was not found often as the only subclass on the RBCs, but it is interesting to note that one patient with hemolytic anemia had only IgG2 detected on the RBCs. IgG3 was detected on the RBCs of 7% of donors, and 13% and 29%, respectively, of the RBCs of patients without and with AIHA; similar to IgG2, it was unusual to find IgG3 alone on the RBCs. IgG4 was detected on the RBCs of 12% of donors, and 13% and 24% of patients without and with AIHA, respectively, of the RBCs; it was detected as the sole sensitizing subclass in only five cases, and all were blood donors. Dacie[51] found a similar distribution of IgG subclasses on the RBCs of 57 patients with AIHA. Most of our results were similar to those reported by Engelfriet and coworkers[52] except for our one unusual case of IgG2-associated AIHA, and the cases with IgG3 sensitization associated with no obvious hemolytic anemia. Engelfriet and coworkers[52] found that IgG3 sensitization was always associated with overt hemolysis. As can be seen in Table 5-11, although IgG3 sensitization was far more common (29%) in patients with hemolytic anemia than in donors or patients without AIHA, we found six (7%) DAT-positive blood donors and four (13%) patients with IgG3 RBC sensitization, but no obvious signs of hemolytic anemia. Engelfriet and coworkers[53] reported on the subclass of RBC-bound IgG of 746 patients with a positive DAT. The patients were not categorized into those with and

TABLE 5-10. SEROLOGIC FINDINGS IN A TYPICAL PATIENT WITH WARM ANTIBODY AUTOIMMUNE HEMOLYTIC ANEMIA

Screening Tests for Serum Antibody

			Controls	
	Serum	**AS + AC**	**AC Alone**	**Auto***
20°C, Untreated Cells				
Lysis	0	0	0	0
Agglutination	0	0	0	0
20°C, Papainized Cells				
Lysis	0	0	0	0
Agglutination	2+	2+	0	2+

	Serum			Controls	
	Saline	**Alb**	**AS + AC**	**AC Alone**	**Auto* with Alb**
37°C, Untreated Cells					
Lysis	0	0	0	0	0
Agglutination	0	1+	0	0	1+
IAT	1+	3+	1+	0	3+
37°C, Papainized Cells					
Lysis	0	NT	0	0	0
Agglutination	3+	NT	2+	0	3+

Specificity of Antibody in Serum and Eluate

Serum: no obvious specificity (all routine panel RBCs reacting 1+ to 2+)
Eluate: no obvious specificity (all routine panel RBCs reacting 3+)
Cold agglutinin titer: not performed (no agglutination in screening tests at 20°C)
Other data:all serum autoantibody removed by warm autoadsorptions (see Chapter 10)
Summary: findings typical of WAIHA
Follow-up: rapid improvement of anemia over two week period of prednisone therapy

AS, acidified serum; AC, acidified complement; Alb, albumin; NT, not tested
* Auto, patient's own RBCs.

those without hemolytic anemia. Ninety-six percent had IgG1 on their RBCs, 12% had IgG2, 13% had IgG3, and 3% had IgG4 on their RBCs. Although 74% had only IgG1 on their RBCs, IgG2, IgG3, and IgG4 were usually present with other subclasses (0.7% had only IgG2, 2% had only IgG3, and 0.9% had only IgG4 on their RBCs).[53]

TABLE 5-11. IgG SUBCLASS OF AUTOANTIBODIES ON DAT+ RBCs OF BLOOD DONORS AND PATIENTS WITH AND WITHOUT AIHA

IgG Subclass	Blood Donors (%) (n = 46)	Patients (%) No AIHA (n = 89)	Patients (%) AIHA (n = 32)
IgG1 alone	81	72	50
IgG2 alone	1.3	6.3	2.2
IgG3 alone	2.6	6.3	6.6
IgG4 alone	6.5	0	0
IgG1 with other subclasses	7.9	12.5	37
IgG2 with other subclasses	4.5	9.4	24
IgG3 with other subclasses	4.5	6.3	22
IgG4 with other subclasses	5.6	12.6	24

Data from Garratty G: Autoimmune hemolytic anemia. In Garratty G (ed): Immunobiology of transfusion medicine. New York: Dekker, 1994:493–521; and Nance S, Garratty G: Subclass of IgG on red cells of donors and patients with positive direct antiglobulin tests (abstr). Transfusion 1983;23:413.

Nance and Garratty[49] reported that eluates made from DAT+ RBCs often contained extra subclasses not detected by the DAT using anti-IgG1, -IgG2, -IgG3, and -IgG4. They also found that generally, the stronger the DAT, the greater was the incidence of multiple IgG subclasses and the degree of hemolytic anemia; 39% of patients with AIHA had multiple subclasses detected on their RBCs compared with only 13 of patients/donors without hemolytic anemia. All these findings were confirmed by Sokol and coworkers.[54] Sokol and coworkers[54] used an ELAT to subclass the IgG eluted from the RBCs of 304 patients on 426 occasions. IgG1 was most common, being found in 98% of cases and as the sole subclass in 64%; multiple subclasses occurred in 34.5%. The IgG subclass pattern possibly changed with time ($p < 0.02, > 0.01$), populations being compared at 6 and 12 months. There was a highly significant and important correlation between multiple IgG subclasses and multiple immunoglobulin coating; in our further studies, this necessitated the use of samples where only cell-bound IgG was increased. Multiple IgG subclasses strongly correlated with larger amounts of cell-bound IgG, groups with more than 2 and less than 1 OD unit by the ELAT being compared (approximately more than 800 and less than 400 molecules IgG per red cell, respectively). Multiple subclasses ($p < 0.05, > 0.01$), but not IgG3, were possibly associated with low haptoglobin levels; significance was reached, however, if the multiple immunoglobulin effect was ignored. They concluded that IgG subclass interrelationships are clearly complex and require strictly defined populations for their study.

Dubarry and coworkers[55] used a solid-phase ELAT to quantitate immunoglobulin classes and IgG subclasses of IgG eluted from RBCs of DAT-positive patients. Three groups were analyzed: Group 1 included 23 patients with AIHA associated with warm autoantibodies of IgG class; group 2 included 11 patients without anemia but with a positive DAT; and group 3 included 10 healthy DAT-negative subjects. The mean number of IgM and IgA molecules per RBC was low in the three groups. IgG1 predominated in all groups except in two patients with AIHA, in whom IgG3 made up at least 50% of total IgG. The mean number of IgG1, IgG2, and IgG4 molecules per RBC in group 1 was about three times that in group 2, whereas the mean number of IgG3 molecules per RBC was 10 times as high ($p < 0.001$). It follows that IgG3 was more common in patients of group 1, but it was also detected in patients of group 2.

Lynen and coworkers[56] studied quantitation and determination of IgG subclass of RBC-bound IgG of 65 patients using a newly developed gel centrifugation test (GCT) and flow cytometry (FC). The GCT involved using dilutions of the antiglobulin sera, including subclass antisera. The dilutions were selected by comparison of the GCT, flow cytometry, and clinical findings. The amount of IgG on the RBCs as determined by GCT dilution cards correlated with FC ($r = 0.70$, $p < 0.0001$). IgG subclass results as determined by GCT IgG subclass cards were confirmed by FC in 14 cases with an anti–IgG-γ chain titer ≥300, whereas IgG subclass cards were not suitable in cases with anti-IgG-γ chain titers less than 300. In 44 patients with 2+ or 3+ DAT in the GCT and anti–IgG-γ chain titer ≤30, no hemolysis was observed, whereas hemolysis occurred in 13 of 14 patients with an anti–IgG-γ chain titer ≥300. GCT data obtained by IATs with anti-D sera were concordant with FC results. They concluded that there is a correlation between the amount of RBC-bound IgG and immune hemolysis. The GCT cards that detect the anti–IgG-γ chain may be useful to predict hemolysis in patients with a 2+ or 3+ DAT in the GCT. The diagnostic value of GCT cards for IgG subclass testing needs to be investigated further.

WAIHA Associated with IgM Autoantibodies

An unusual but important catergory of WAIHA consists of cases associated with IgM warm autoantibodies[48,57-76] (also see Chapter 9, page 331). IgM warm autoantibodies may agglutinate untreated and/or enzyme-treated RBCs, hemolyze untreated and/or enzyme-treated RBCs, and sensitize RBCs so that IgM and/or complement is detectable by the antiglobulin test. Patients may be divided into four groups.

Patients with Warm IgM Autoantibodies Associated with RBC-Bound Complement. Routinely, RBCs are only tested with anti-IgG and anti-C3 (C3d). From 6% to 13% of RBCs from patients with WAIHA have been reported to react with anti-C3 (C3d) but not with anti-IgG.[1,4,33] In most cases it is not known how the C3 came to be on the RBCs. If anti-IgM is used for the DAT, sometimes RBC-bound IgM can be detected, and it is assumed that the IgM autoantibody may have activated complement causing RBC-bound C3 (C3dg). We found that 2% of patients with WAIHA associated with RBC-bound C3 also had RBC-bound IgM.[4] Sokol and coworkers[58] only found 1 of 355 patients with WAIHA to have IgM+ C3 on their RBCs. Several cases of WAIHA due to IgM warm autoantibodies associated with a positive routine DAT due to RBC-bound C3 (C3d) have been reported[58-67]; sometimes the IgM was only detectable by tests more sensitive than the DAT.[22-24] As the amount of anti-C3d in commercial AGS is variable, these patients could present as DAT-negative AIHA. IgM autoantibodies were detectable in the serum of most patients and sometimes in eluates made from the patients' RBCs. Some investigators commented on the difficulty of obtaining reactive eluates. Dorner and coworkers[68] could only demonstrate the RBC-bound IgM autoantibody if it was eluted into albumin or serum. Ellis and coworkers[69] studied the most suitable elution method for IgM in 42 patients with AIHA associated with RBC-bound IgM; heat (56°C) elution was found superior to acid stromal, organic solvent, or freeze-thaw methods. Although all of the patients' sera contained pentameric forms of IgM, and 64% contained oligomeric forms of IgM, only pentameric IgM was eluted from the RBCs. Thus, it was concluded that low molecular weight IgM was not the cause of in vivo hemolysis in these 42 patients.

Patients with Easily Detectable IgG Autoantibodies, and IgM Autoantibodies that May Not Be Detected by Routine Tests. If routine procedures are used to test the RBCs and serum of this group, the results associated with this group would be those most commonly found in idiopathic WAIHA (e.g., IgG or IgG+C3 detected on the RBCs; agglutination and perhaps lysis of enzyme-treated RBCs; a positive IAT with untreated and enzyme-treated RBCs). These results are obtained because anti-IgM is not used routinely for the DAT and IAT, and the immunoglobulin class of the serum antibody(ies) is (are) not usually determined. When anti-IgM was used, we found that RBC-bound IgM was detected on 8% of the RBCs of patients with WAIHA.[4] None of the 104 patients had only IgM on the RBCs; 2% had IgG+IgA+C3+IgM; 4% had IgG+IgM+C3; and 2% had IgM+C3. If more sensitive tests are applied, then RBC-bound IgM is detected more often. Vos and coworkers[77] showed that 42% of eluates prepared from the RBCs of 55 patients with WAIHA contained IgM and/or IgA in addition to the IgG detected by the DAT. Using the AutoAnalyzer,

Hsu and coworkers[19] found that 8 of 11 (73%) patients with WAIHA, associated with IgG-positive DATs, had RBC-bound IgM present in addition. None of 16 DAT-positive patients without AIHA had RBC-bound IgM. Using ELAT, Sokol and coworkers[78,79] detected IgM on the RBCs of 39 of 102 (38%) patients with WAIHA, associated with IgG-positive DATs.

We found that 5% of sera from patients with WAIHA would agglutinate, and 0.4% would hemolyze, untreated RBCs at 37°C. Ninety percent of the sera agglutinated enzyme-treated RBCs, and 9% to 13% would hemolyze enzyme-treated RBCs, at 37°C.[4] We did not prove that these results were due to IgM autoantibodies, but the characteristics are what might be expected of IgM rather than IgG antibodies. von dem Borne and colleagues[48,71] showed that autoantibodies that hemolyze enzyme-treated RBCs at 37°C are IgM, and that such antibodies, by themselves, cause only slight to moderate in vivo RBC destruction. Wolf and Roelcke[61] studied eight sera containing warm hemolysins against enzyme-treated RBCs; none of these agglutinated or hemolyzed untreated RBCs at 37°C. Seven of the eight antibodies were shown to be IgM (one had an IgG component and one an IgA component in addition); one appeared to be IgG, without IgM or IgA. In three sera the IgM were shown to be monoclonal proteins (κ light chains only). Only one of these eight patients had RBC-bound IgG detectable by the DAT; five had a positive DAT due to RBC-bound complement, and two had negative DATs. Wolf and Roelcke[72] also presented evidence to suggest that the targets for IgM warm hemolysins belong to a newer group of phospholipase susceptible RBC antigens and that this specificity emphasizes that they are a separate category of warm autoantibodies.

The relative pathogenic role of IgG versus IgM autoantibodies in patients with AIHA associated with the above findings is not clear, but there are some publications[73-75] where the IgM warm autoantibody shows the characteristics associated with WAIHA associated with IgM warm autoantibodies without IgG being associated (as described in the section above), suggesting that the IgM autoantibody was pathogenic.

Patients with Warm IgM Autoantibodies and a Negative DAT. Some authors have demonstrated IgM on the RBCs of patients who have AIHA but have a negative routine DAT.[18,21,70] Such cases are quite unusual and are reviewed in Chapter 9 in the segment on AIHA with a negative DAT.

Severe (Sometimes Fatal) Hemolytic Anemia Associated with Warm IgM Autoantibodies Directed Against Determinants on Glycophorins. We know of seven cases of severe WAIHA associated with IgM antibodies directed against determinants on glycophorins [En^a,[23] Pr,[23] N,[64] Ge,[66] and Wr^b[23,74]]. Table 5-12 shows some data from these patients.

TABLE 5-12. RESULTS OF TESTING RBCs AND SERA FROM PATIENTS WITH WARM IgM AUTOANTIBODIES DIRECTED AGAINST DETERMINANTS ON GLYCOPHORINS

Case No. (Ref.)	DAT	Eluate	Spontaneous Agglutination of Patients' RBCs	Serum	Clinical Course
1 (70)	Negative		No	IgM agglutinin 4+ at 37°C; (IAT at 37°C was negative); anti-En^a	? Pure red cell aplasia. Remission of AIHA.
2 (23)	2+ (C3), no IgG	IgM, 37°C, (3+) agglutinin	Yes	IgM agglutinin 3+ at 37°C; anti-En^{a}FS. Only reactive at low pH (e.g., pH 6.5) or in the presence of albumin.	Intravascular lysis → hematocrit <2%; died.
3 (23)	3+ (C3), no IgG, IgM, or IgA	Nonreactive	No	IgM agglutinin 2+ at 37°C; 37°C lysin; anti-En^{a}FR. Better reactions at low pH or in the presence of albumin.	Lymphoma. Died following transfusion of 5 U.
4 (23)	1/2+ C3. No IgG, IgM, or IgA by DAT but IgM by flow cytometry.	IgM, 37°C, (4+) agglutinin	Yes	IgM agglutinin 3+ at 37°C; no lysin; anti-Pr	Intravascular lysis. Plasma exchange. IVIG. Remission.
5 (74)	1+ (IgG + C3)	Anti-Wr^b reacting by IAT	Not recorded	IgM agglutinin 4+ at 37°C (LISS); and 4+ IAT 37°C lysis (LISS only); anti-Wr^b	Hemoglobin dropped from 7 g to 4 g % in 24 hr. Patient died.
6 (64)	4+ (C3 + IgA) (IgM by flow cytometry)	IgM, 37°C, anti-N	Yes	IgM agglutinin 3+ at RT (1 + at 37°C). Only reactive if pH <7.0. Anti-N	Hb 3.9 g/dL; hct 13%. Transfused 7 units. Died on day 5.
7 (66)	3+ (C3 no IgG) (IgM by flow cytometry)	IgM agglutininating; anti-Ge	Yes	No detectable antibody	Hb 4.4 g/dL. Transfused 4 units. Treated with steroids. Hb ↑ 13 g/dL. Discharged on day 6.

It should be noted that the patients' RBCs spontaneously agglutinated when centrifuged in two of the cases, which led to difficulties in performing DATs and RBC typing. Treatment of the RBCs with dithiothreitol (DTT) overcame the spontaneous agglutination but because of the effect of DTT on RBC-bound IgM, the DATs using anti-IgM were unreliable. It is interesting to note that following DTT treatment, with subsequent diminished spontaneous agglutination, IgM could sometimes still be detected (especially by flow cytometry).[23] This would suggest that RBC-bound IgM monomers are still present following DTT treatment.[23] Further work using anti-IgM by flow cytometry, which does not involve centrifugation of the RBCs, showed that RBC-bound IgM could be detected by this approach.[23,24,66,80]

Several points are worth emphasizing concerning the serology. Although these antibodies were very effective in vivo, they had unusual in vitro characteristics. Two of the DATs were only weakly positive, and one was negative. Although the serum antibodies agglutinated RBCs strongly, they sometimes did not react by the IAT, thus they appear to be low affinity antibodies susceptible to the washing process. We have also encountered this phenomenon with an IgM alloanti-En^a that caused a fatal hemolytic transfusion reaction.[81] Two of the autoanti-En^a, that caused fatal hemolysis, reacted only at low pH (e.g., 6.5) or in the presence of 30% albumin.[23] Although one example of auto anti-Wr^b caused fatal hemolysis, it was detected poorly in systems using normal ionic strength saline.[74]

Brain and coworkers[76] published an interesting hypothesis as to why autoantibodies directed at epitopes on glycophorin A were associated with such severe hemolytic anemia. The inexplicable severity of a WAIHA associated with anti-Pr led them to test the hypothesis that the hemolysis was primarily due to a change in the function of glycophorin A, on which the Pr antigen is located. The lectins *Maclura pomifera* and wheat germ agglutinin that bind to glycophorin A induced hemolysis of normal RBCs in vitro. Lectin binding led to an increase in RBC membrane permeability to sodium and potassium, the former resulting in an influx of water and subsequent hemolysis. The response was glycophorin A specific as concanavalin A, which binds to band 3, did not cause hemolysis and peanut agglutinin only did so after removal of RBC sialic acid. The lectin-induced cation leak was not mediated by activation of cation channels as the inhibitors, tetrodotoxin, amiloride, and 4,4'-diisothiocyanate stilbene 2,2'-disulfonate, had no effect, suggesting that the hemolysis was due to exacerbation of the inherent cation permeability of the RBC membrane. A human IgAγ anti-Pr autoantibody and a mouse anti-human glycophorin A antibody increased RBC permability to sodium. The role of glycophorin A in stabilizing and, upon aggregation, destabilizing the phospholipids bilayer was discussed.[76]

Typical Serology of WAIHA Associated with IgM Autoantibodies. Garratty and coworkers[24] reported on the serology of 41 patients with AIHA associated with IgM warm autoantibodies. Problems were often encountered when the patient's RBCs were used for ABO/Rh typing and/or DAT, as 61% of the RBCs spontaneously agglutinated when centrifuged. This spontaneous agglutination could be overcome by treating the patient's RBCs with DTT.[82]

Most of the patients had a positive DAT but some presented as a DAT-negative AIHA.[24] Most (90%) of the patients had detectable RBC-bound C3 on their RBCs; 60% had only C3 detectable on their RBCs; 17% had IgG+ C3. Only 28% reacted with an anti-IgM standardized for use by the routine DAT (see Chapter 6), but 82% of the RBCs that were nonreactive with anti-IgM had RBC-bound IgM detected by a flow cytometric method.[23,24]

Most (91%) of the sera contained IgM, 37°C-reactive autoagglutins. Untreated and enzyme-treated RBCs were lysed by 13% and 58% of the sera, respectively. One interesting finding was that the autoantibodies were sometimes difficult to detect even though the patient had severe (sometimes fatal) hemolytic anemia. Sometimes the autoantibodies would only react or were enhanced considerably at a low pH and/or in the presence of albumin (e.g., 30% bovine albumin). The antibodies often reacted optimally at 30°C (rather than the expected 37°C). More (39%) autoantibodies had clearly defined specificities than are usually seen with WAIHA (see Chapter 7). Eight of the autoantibodies had clear-cut Rh specificity (e.g., an anti-c agglutinin), two had senescent cell antigen specificity, and there was one each showing anti-En^a, -Wr^b, -Pr, -N, -Ge, and -I^T specificity.[24]

Characterization of Antibodies in the Cold Agglutinin Syndrome

Cold agglutinins that satisfy, the "classic" characteristics described for antibodies in CAS, often produce striking in vitro findings and make their presence known in several sections of the clinical laboratory. These cold agglutinins have a titer of 1000 to 16,000 or higher in saline at 4°C (normal is <64), and cause *in vitro* agglutination of anticoagulated blood at room temperature that is grossly evident to the naked eye. Indeed, all the RBCs may be bound in one huge agglutinate, which may be mistaken by the uninitiated as a clot (see Fig. 5-1). Preparation of adequate blood smears at room temperature becomes impossible because of gross agglutination of RBCs, and blood counts in automated blood cell counters produce nonsense numbers.[83-86] Also, if a sample is sent to the blood transfusion service for compatibility testing, the cold agglutinins are immediately apparent and special knowledge will be required to circumvent the problems that they produce. For anyone who has observed just one similar case previously, the diagnosis of CAS comes immediately to mind.

However, other patients with an elevated cold agglutinin titer have no evidence of hemolysis. Even though these antibodies are clinically benign, they may react at room temperature, causing some of the in vitro problems previously described. The converse is also true; that is, we frequently encounter patients who do not have striking increases in their cold agglutinin titer yet appear to have CAS since they have an acquired hemolytic anemia, a DAT that is positive only with anticomplement sera, a moderate elevation of cold agglutinin titer and thermal amplitude, and no other definable cause of hemolysis after extensive evaluation and long-term follow-up. Further complicating the situation is the fact that about 30% of the patients with WAIHA also have a modest to moderate elevation of cold agglutinin titer and/or thermal amplitude and, especially if characteristic or "typical" serologic findings of WAIHA are not present, the patient may be erroneously diagnosed as having CAS.

Therefore, the mere observance of cold autoagglutination is not diagnostic of CAS, and when they are encountered, the task is to determine whether the patient has clinically insignificant albeit abnormal cold agglutinins, has WAIHA with an associated but probably insignificant elevation of cold agglutinin titer or thermal amplitude, or has CAS. A rather common diagnostic error is overdiagnosis of CAS in patients who have benign cold antibodies and pathogenic warm autoantibodies. Also, in rare patients, characteristic findings of both WAIHA and CAS occur simultaneously (see Chapter 3, "Combined Cold and Warm AIHA" and later in this chapter, page 191).

Table 5-2 shows the AIHA screen results associated with CAS.

Additional Comments Regarding Serologic Tests. Cold agglutinins that are reactive at room temperature are frequently encountered and are noticed because they cause difficulty in compatibility testing and cause agglutination visible to the naked eye in an anticoagulated blood sample, as well as other of the in vitro phenomena previously described. Commonly it is assumed that such cold agglutinins must be potent enough to cause in vivo shortening of RBC survival and, if the patient has a hemolytic anemia, a diagnosis of CAS is made without further characterization of the antibody. However, such patients may have WAIHA accompanied by a clinically insignificant cold agglutinin. Thermal amplitude studies and other serologic tests are necessary to determine the correct diagnosis.

If a patient has a positive DAT due to only complement sensitization, and very high titer cold agglutinin (>1000 at 4°C), CAS is very likely to be the correct diagnosis and, in these cases, thermal amplitude studies are not as critical. However, many cold agglutinins in patients with CAS have a titer that is 1000 or less at 4°C in saline (see Tables 5-13 and 5-14), and it is in these patients that determination of thermal amplitude is extremely important. Characterization of the patient's cold agglutinin is crucial in order to avoid diagnostic errors.

The specificity of the antibody in 54 patients with CAS in our series is indicated in Table 5-13. Although such specificity results are of interest, they are not essential either for diagnosis or for the selection of blood for transfusion. Other specificities are discussed in Chapter 7.

Development of Criteria to Distinguish Benign Cold Agglutinins from Those Associated with In Vivo Hemolysis. To develop guidelines that may be of value in the diagnosis of CAS, we studied various characteristics of cold agglutinins in patients with CAS and in patients without hemolytic anemia. As with most RBC antibodies, it is difficult to predict the in vivo significance from in vitro tests, and it is obvious that the titer of an antibody when tested at 4°C is not a direct measurement of its clinical importance.

Our study characterized cold agglutinins by various techniques, but it emphasized the reactivity of the antibody at various temperatures against red cells suspended in saline or in 30% albumin medium.[87] The use

TABLE 5-13. COLD AGGLUTININ TITERS AND SPECIFICITIES OF 135 ANTIBODIES FROM PATIENTS WITH CAS

	No. of Patients (%)			
Titers	**San Francisco**	**Los Angeles**	**United Kingdom**	**Total**
<1000 (range = 8–512)	23 (43)	29 (45)	0	52 (39)
1000–8000	27 (50)	30 (46)	7 (44)	64 (47)
16,000–64,000	3 (5)	6 (9)	7 (44)	16 (12)
125,000–512,000	1 (2)	0	2 (12)	3 (2)
Total	54	65	16	135
Specificities				
Anti-I	49 (91)			
Anti-i	4 (7)			
Unidentified	1 (2)			

San Francisco: data extracted from ref. 4
United Kingdom: data extracted from ref. 1
Los Angeles: From Garratty G, unpublished data of samples submitted, 1981–2002.

TABLE 5-14. TITERS AND THERMAL AMPLITUDE (WITH OR WITHOUT ALBUMIN) IN 32 PATIENTS—RELATIONSHIP TO HEMOLYTIC ANEMIA

Patient	Hemolytic Anemia	4°C		30°C		37°C	
		Saline	Albumin	Saline	Albumin	Saline	Albumin
1	Yes	2560	5120	1	640	0	320
2	Yes	5120	10240	1	640	0	160
3	Yes	2560	5120	4	320	0	80
4	Yes	2560	5120	20	320	0	20
5	Yes	1280	1280	10	160	1	1
6	Yes	10240	10240	1	40	0	1
7	Yes	640	1280	1	20	0	1
8	Yes	640	5120	10	160	0	10
9	Yes	640	2560	1	40	0	1
10	Yes	2560	5120	1	10	0	1
11	Yes	1280	1280	1	10	0	1
12	Yes	8192	4096	128	128	8	16
13	Yes	1024	256	0	1	0	0
14	Yes	1024	2048	0	2	0	1
15	Yes	640	2560	0	10	0	1
16	Yes	640	1280	0	40	0	1
17	Yes	1280	5120	0	20	0	1
18	Yes	1024	256	0	4	0	2
19	Yes	640	640	0	1	0	0
20	Yes	640	640	0	1	0	0
21	Yes	2048	1024	0	8	0	1
22	Yes	320	320	0	10	0	0
23	Yes	320	320	0	1	0	0
24	Yes	256	1024	1	4	0	1
25	Yes	256	512	1	2	0	0
26	Yes	256	512	0	4	0	0
27	Yes	128	1024	1	1	0	0
28	Yes	8	128	0	1	0	1
29	No	320	320	0	0	0	0
30	No	320	640	0	0	0	0
31	No	1280	2560	0	0	0	0
32	No	320	20	0	0	0	0

Data from Garratty G, Petz LD, Hoops JK: The correlation of cold agglutinin titrations in saline and albumin with haemolytic anaemia. Br J Haemat 1977;35:587–595.

of 30% albumin medium was based on the report of Haynes and Chaplin,[88] who described an enhancing effect of albumin on cold agglutinins that was particularly striking in one patient. This patient had a hemolytic anemia associated with only a modestly elevated cold agglutinin titer of 128 at 4°C using saline-suspended RBCs, but a titer of 131,000 in the presence of bovine albumin. We studied 32 patients who had elevated cold agglutinin titers and positive DATs due to complement sensitization of their RBCs. Twenty-eight of these patients had an associated hemolytic anemia.

We found that testing for cold hemolysins in vitro did not differentiate clinically important antibodies from benign cold agglutinins. Although sera from all patients with CAS caused lysis of enzyme-treated RBCs at 20°C, sera from 3 of the 4 patients without hemolytic anemia also caused in vitro lysis.

The cold agglutinin titer at 4°C, when performed in saline or albumin, did not correlate with the presence or absence of hemolysis, but determination of the thermal range did prove helpful.[87] Table 5-14 shows the comparative titrations using saline and albumin at 4°C, 30°C, and 37°C in the 32 patients who were divided into 4 groups. Patients 1 to 12 all had hemolytic anemia associated with high titer cold agglutinins at 4°C, and all sera reacted at 30°C with saline-suspended RBCs. The sera of two patients (5 and 12) reacted at 37°C with saline-suspended red cells, and all 12 reacted at 37°C in the presence of albumin.

Patients 13 to 21 all had hemolytic anemia associated with cold agglutinins of high titer at 4°C, but none of the sera from these 9 patients reacted at 30°C unless albumin was present in the incubation mixture. In the presence of albumin all nine reacted at 30°C, and five of the nine reacted also at 37°C.

Patients 22 to 28 all had hemolytic anemia but normal to moderately increased cold agglutinin titers at 4°C (i.e., not more than about two tubes above our upper limit of normal). Three of the 7 sera reacted at 30°C with saline-suspended RBCs, and all 7 reacted in the presence of albumin. Two of the 7 (14 and 28) reacted at 37°C in the presence of albumin.

Patient 28 is of considerable interest because he had severe hemolytic anemia associated with a cold agglutinin titer of only 8 at 4°C when saline-suspended RBCs were tested (normal cold agglutinin titers at 4°C range up to 64 in our laboratory). In the presence of albumin the cold autoantibody reacted to a titer of 128 at 4°C and up to 37°C. These tests were reproducible even with very strict control of temperature. This patient had a strongly positive DAT due to complement sensitization. In addition to the cold agglutinin, the serum contained a cold hemolysin, reacting optimally at 20°C against enzyme-treated RBCs. The DL test was negative. The reactions at 30°C and 37°C in the presence of albumin showed anti-I specificity, and the reactions were inhibited by 2-mercaptoethanol. No other antibody activity at 37°C could be demonstrated in the serum or in an eluate prepared from the patient's red cells. Thus, it appeared that all reactions were due to the IgM cold autoantibody with a high thermal maximum and that no warm autoantibodies optimally reactive at 37°C were present. No other cause of hemolysis was found in this patient.

Patients 29 to 32 all had increased cold agglutinin titers at 4°C but no associated hemolytic anemia. None of these sera reacted at 30°C or 37°C, even in the presence of albumin. Thus, all patients with hemolytic anemia had cold agglutinins that reacted at 30°C in albumin in contrast to negative reactions in patients without hemolytic anemia. Based on the empiric findings in this report, it appears that reactivity of a cold agglutinin at 30°C in albumin may be the optimal means for distinguishing clinically insignificant cold agglutinins from those associated with in vivo hemolysis.

An additional point of significance in this study was that we excluded IgG antibody activity in 22 of the 28 sera that reacted at 30°C in the presence of albumin by treating them with 2-mercaptoethanol. It was concluded that IgG antibodies were not causing the original agglutination reactions observed at 30°C or 37°C.

Isbister and coworkers[89] reported three interesting patients who had lymphoproliferative disease with immunoglobulin M lambda (IgMλ) monoclonal proteins and severe AIHA. These three patients had cold autoagglutinins of low titer (8, 8, and 64) at 4°C; all three autoagglultinins reacted strongly at 30°C and weakly at 37°C. All patients had only complement detectable on their RBCs. In two patients, splenectomy led to a remission; the third patient responded to steroids.

It should be noted that we proposed this means of distinguishing benign cold agglutinins from those causing CAS more than 25 years ago. We had every expectation that exceptions to the "rule of thumb" that we suggested would be found, and that more precise criteria would subsequently be reported. In contrast, our suggested criteria have served as remarkably good guidelines for diagnosis.

However, two exceptional patients have been reported who had high titer, high thermal amplitude cold agglutinins but not hemolytic anemia. Sniecinski and coworkers[90] reported a patient who had a cold antibody that had both a high titer (greater than 4096 at 4°C) and a wide thermal range (4°C to 37°C). The patient was closely followed over a 3-year period and no evidence of hemolysis was ever documented, despite a persistence of a positive DAT and the cold autoagglutinin. Similarly, Arndt and coworkers[91] reported a patient who did not have evidence of hemolysis although he had an auto-anti-B reacting to a titer of 8192 at 4°C and 16 at 30°C. The anti-B caused weak hemolysis of group B enzyme-treated but not untreated RBCs in vitro.

Sokol and coworkers[92] studied 221 patients who had cold autoagglutinins that reacted to ≥30°C, in the presence of albumin. They found they could divide them into three groups. Group 1 contained 116 (52%) individuals in whom hemolysins were never detected, and the 74 (34%) patients in group 2 had monophasic hemolysins alone, whereas both monophasic and biphasic hemolysins were detected in the 31 (14%) group 3 patients. There was a significantly higher proportion of patients in groups 2 and 3 with haptoglobin levels less than 0.1 g/L compared with groups 1 and 2, respectively. DAT results showed that the autoimmune response became more complex and IgM predominant through groups 1 to 3, resulting in an increasing ability to activate complement, which was reflected in increasing hemolysin activity and number of patients with active hemolysis. The 31 patients in group 3 were mostly elderly (median age, 71 years at presentation) and the majority had chronic CAS, several in association with lymphoid neoplasms or carcinomas; only four had acute CAS. It would appear that these results are in conflict with our results and conclusions,[87] but it should be pointed out that the two studies were very different. We studied the titers and thermal amplitude of cold autoagglutinins in patients who were suspected of having CAS. Sokol and coworkers[92] studied random cold antibodies from patients referred to their blood center for antibody investigations, from 1984 to 1996. The predictive value of our findings was high in our patients; we would not expect the predictive value to be high in Sokol's patient population. For instance, many warm autoantibodies (i.e., optimally reactive at 37°C), or alloantibodies will react at 30°C in the presence of albumin. Nevertheless, the findings of Sokol and coworkers[92] are of interest as they showed that the demonstration of hemolysins correlated better with the presence of hemolytic anemia (based on lowered haptoglobin levels) than thermal amplitude and cold agglutinin titers. As Table 5-2 shows, we found that only 2% or 24.5% of sera from CAS patients hemolyzed untreated or enzyme-treated RBCs, respectively, at 20°C without added complement. When complement was added (at optimal pH), then 14% and 94% of the sera hemolyzed untreated or enzyme-treated RBCs, respectively. So, it appears that a hemolysin test at 20°C, when performed optimally (i.e., added complement, optimal pH, enzyme-treated RBCs), has a very good predictive value but this is not as easy for a nonspecialist laboratory to perform as it is to test for agglutination at 30°C in the presence of albumin.

Essential Diagnostic Tests for CAS. On the basis of the preceding findings we offer the following approach to the diagnosis of CAS. The diagnosis must be considered in all patients with acquired hemolytic anemia who have a positive DAT using anti-C3 and a negative DAT using anti-IgG. A practical initial serum screening procedure is to test the ability of the patient's serum to agglutinate saline-suspended normal red cells at 20°C (or room temperature) after incubation for 30 to 60 minutes (Chapter 6). This recommendation is based on data illustrated in Table 5-2 namely, that the sera of essentially all patients in our series who had CAS caused agglutination of saline-suspended red cells at 20°C. If this screening test is negative, CAS is extremely unlikely; if positive, further studies are necessary to determine the thermal amplitude of the antibody.

When CAS appears to be a possible diagnosis on the basis of the preceding evaluation, studies of the thermal range of reactivity of the antibody in saline and albumin are indicated. It is also convenient to determine possible Ii blood group specificity of the antibody simultaneously (see Chapter 6). The titer of the cold agglutinin in CAS is invariably highest at 4°C and progressively decreases at higher temperatures. Of particular note are the reactions at 30°C and 37°C. If the former is positive in saline or albumin, the antibody may well be of pathogenetic significance, that is, it may be causing short red blood cell survival in vivo. If the reaction at 37°C is also positive in the presence of albumin (as was true in 19 of the 28 [68%] patients in Table 5-14) or when albumin is not present (2 of 28 patients [7.1%]), the antibody will cause problems in the compatibility testing (see Chapter 10).

Using clinical information, the results of the DAT, and the preceding screening tests, a reasonably confident assessment of the presence or absence of CAS may be made. CAS may be diagnosed if the following are present: (1) clinical evidence of acquired hemolytic anemia, (2) a positive DAT caused by sensitization with C3, (3) a negative DAT using anti-IgG, (4) the presence of a cold autoagglutinin with reactivity up to at least 30°C in saline or albumin. Although a cold agglutinin will be present to a titer of ≥256 at 4°C, except in very unusual cases, we would emphasize that the cold agglutinin titer is not the critical aspect of diagnosis. Indeed, a screening test can be performed in which one observes for agglutination at 30°C using a single tube with the patient's undiluted serum and normal RBCs.

An alternative diagnosis must be sought for patients who do not satisfy all these criteria.

An example of typical findings in a patient with CAS are given in the following case report with serologic findings listed in Tables 5-15A and B.

PATIENT 1: A 52-year-old woman sought medical attention because she noted that her fingers turned blue on exposure to cold. This sign was associated with mild discomfort under her fingernails and a sensation of tingling. The findings resolved quickly upon warming. She had no other complaints and, in particular, had no symptoms of fatigue. Approximately 1 year previously her hematocrit was 35%. There was no history of blood loss. Site appeared neither acutely nor chronically ill, and a physical examination revealed no abnormal findings.

Laboratory data revealed a hemoglobin level of 9.6 mg/dL, hematocrit 25%, white cells 7700/µL with a normal differential, platelets 392,000/µL, and reticulocytes 15.6%. Total bilirubin was 1.2 mg/dL; direct reacting bilirubin was 0.21 mg/dL, serum iron was 107, and total iron binding capacity was 199 µg/dL. Urinalysis revealed specific gravity of 1.009, and there was no proteinuria or glycosuria; a test for Bence Jones protein was negative. Tests for occult blood in the stool were negative. Antinuclear antibody was negative. Total protein was 7.6 g/dL; serum electrophoresis indicated that there was no M component.

TABLE 5-15A. SEROLOGIC FINDINGS IN A TYPICAL PATIENT WITH COLD AGGLUTININ SYNDROME

DAT: Polyspecific antiglobulin serum: 4+ Anti-IgG: negative Anti-C3: 3+

	Screening Tests for Serum Antibody		
	Serum	**AS + AC***	**Control AC**
20°C, Untreated Cells			
Lysis	0	2+	0
Agglutination	4+	4+	0
20°C, Papainized Cells			
Lysis	0	4+	0
Agglutination	4+	4+	0
37°C, Untreated Cells			
Lysis	0	0	0
Agglutination	0	0	0
37°C, Papainized Cells			
IAT	0	0	0
Agglutination	0	0	0

* AS, acidified serum; AC, acidified complement

TABLE 5-15B. TITER, THERMAL RANGE, AND SPECIFICITY OF COLD AGGLUTININ USING SALINE-SUSPENDED RBCs

Dilution Patient Serum	1	2	4	8	16	32	64	128	256	512	1024	2048	4096	Titer
4°C														
adult OI	4+	4+	4+	4+	4+	4+	4+	4+	$2\frac{1}{2}$+	1+	1+	1+	0	2048
cord Oi	4+	4+	4+	4+	4+	4+	$3\frac{1}{2}$+	2+	2+	1+	1+	0	0	1024
adult Oi	4+	4+	4+	4+	$3\frac{1}{2}$+	$3\frac{1}{2}$+	$2\frac{1}{2}$+	2+	1+	0	0	0	0	512
25°C														
adult OI	4+	4+	3+	$2\frac{1}{2}$+	2+	$1\frac{1}{2}$+	1+	(1)+	0	0	0	0	0	128
cord Oi	3+	1+	0	0	0	0	0	0	0	0	0	0	0	2
adult Oi	2+	0	0	0	0	0	0	0	0	0	0	0	0	1
30°C														
adult OI	1+	0	0	0	0	0	0	0	0	0	0	0	0	1
cord Oi	0	0	0	0	0	0	0	0	0	0	0	0	0	0
adult Oi	0	0	0	0	0	0	0	0	0	0	0	0	0	0
37°C														
adult OI	0	0	0	0	0	0	0	0	0	0	0	0	0	0
cord Oi	0	0	0	0	0	0	0	0	0	0	0	0	0	0
adult Oi	0	0	0	0	0	0	0	0	0	0	0	0	0	0

Specificity:
Serum: anti-I
Eluate: not tested
Cold agglutinin titer: 2048 vs. adult OI RBCs at 4°C
Cold agglutinin thermal amplitude: up to 30°C
Summary: Findings characteristic of cold agglutinin syndrome
Follow-up: Chronic moderately severe anemia with no change in serologic reactions in seven years

The laboratory technologists noted that 4+ agglutination occurred at room temperature (23°C) and that there was no agglutination at 37°C. Hemolysis was present in serum samples collected at room temperature. The DAT was positive. Smears of aspirated bone marrow revealed gross clumping and were inadequate for interpretation. Sections revealed normoblastic erythropoiesis and no evidence of an infiltrative process, although an occasional focus of mature lymphocytes was seen.

Her serologic findings are indicated in Tables 5-15A and B. Although the antibody was only minimally reactive at 30°C without albumin, it caused 4+ agglutination at that temperature in the presence of 30% albumin and reacted against adult OI RBCs even at 37°C. The clinical and serologic findings were considered diagnostic of CAS.

Her course initially was quite stable, although she had exacerbations in cold weather, particularly when she also had an upper respiratory infection. Six years later she developed a sore throat, malaise, chilly sensations, and a fever of 101°F. Her hematocrit dropped to 16% and reticulocytes dropped to 3.5%. Site was admitted to the hospital and placed in a warmed room, and she wore gloves and warm stockings continuously. A bone marrow aspiration revealed striking erythroid hyperplasia with normal megakaryocytes and granulocytic precursors. Occasional plasma cells were present, but there was no lymphocytic infiltration. Her hematocrit reached a low of 14%, but then gradually improved. She was discharged from the hospital when the hematocrit reached 20%, and a progressive increase to 31% was noted as she was followed as an outpatient.

In subsequent years her usual hematocrit level became somewhat lower, usually in the range of about 24%. Therapy with chlorambucil was initiated at a time when her hematocrit had dropped to 18%. A bone marrow biopsy at this time revealed multiple nodules of mature lymphocytes; the biopsy was interpreted as indicating the presence of it lymphoma. However, no abnormal physical findings were present and, in particular, there was no hepatosplenomegaly or lymphadenopathy. Her hematocrit improved to 24% during therapy with 8 mg chlorambucil daily, during which time she was also more meticulous about avoiding cold. Chlorambucil was gradually increased to 10 mg per day and she subsequently developed pancytopenia and reticulocytopenia. Her hematocrit reached a nadir of 12.5%; white cells 2500/µL; platelets 88,000/µL; and reticulocytes 2.0%. She was treated with transfusions of 2 units of RBCs on three occasions in order to keep her hematocrit at about 20%, after which her marrow function spontaneously improved. Her pancytopenia resolved and her hematocrit remained stable at about 24%. A repeat bone marrow examination revealed marked improvement, and nodules of lymphocytes were no longer apparent, although the total number of lymphocytes was increased above normal.

Nine years after she first presented, her disease was stable and she had received no further transfusions. Her hematocrit level remained about 24% to 26%, she received no specific therapy, and she continued to work daily. She still noticed acrocyanosis on exposure to mild cold. There were no new physical findings.

Serologic evaluations performed in intervals throughout her course revealed a minimal diminution in the strength of the DAT using anti-C3 but the cold agglutinin titer and thermal amplitude were essentially unchanged.

As we have already indicated, the ability of cold antibodies to cause lysis at 20°C (of enzyme-treated RBCs with added complement at optimal pH) was a characteristic of essentially all antibodies from patients with CAS, but it was also a characteristic of antibodies from some patients with no evidence of in vivo hemolysis. Thus, positive tests for lysis at 20°C are not diagnostic of CAS. What is more important is that cold antibodies will cause a decreasing amount of lysis at progressively higher temperatures. If results for lysis are more strongly positive at 37°C than at 20°C or 30°C, a warm hemolysin that may be a separate antibody must be suspected.

Immunochemistry and Molecular Analysis of Cold Autoagglutinins Associated with CAS

With rare exceptions, pathogenic cold agglutinins are IgM. They exhibit a reversible, thermal-dependent equilibrium reaction with RBCs, with association being favored at lower temperatures. The thermal amplitude depends on the concentration and equilibrium constant of the antibody. The cold agglutinins associated with chronic idiopathic CAS found in older individuals are almost always monoclonal IgM proteins. Antibodies of the most common specificity (anti-I) almost always have only κ light chains; rare examples of anti-i often have only λ light chains.[93-98] The demonstration of the exclusive, or virtually exclusive, occurrence of κ chains in anti-I cold agglutinins was the first example of a relationship between antibody specificity and light chain type. Amino acid sequence studies, and the studies of the N-terminal amino acid, of light chains isolated from cold agglutinin light chains identified glutamic acid as the N-terminal amino acid, indicating that they belong to the subgroup VκII.[99,100] A restriction within the heavy μ-chains has also been demonstrated by peptide mapping heavy chains of 14 isolated cold agglutinins.[98] Thirteen of the 14 belonged to one μ subgroup, as shown by the lack of a particular peptide in 40% of monoclonal M-globulins without known antibody activity.[98]

Further immunochemical studies of the heavy chains of IgM cold agglutinins indicated that the μ chains of different cold agglutinins share antigenic determinants not found on IgM molecules lacking cold agglutinin activity. These specific antigenic determinants appeared to be present on the heavy chains of monoclonal proteins of both anti-I and anti-i specificities,[101] and there is one report of similar structural characteristics of a restricted polyclonal protein from a patient with *Mycoplasma pneumoniae* infection.[102] Furthermore, antisera specific for the heavy chains of IgM cold agglutinins cross-react with heavy chains of IgA cold agglutinins, which suggests that there is a common idiopathic specificity.[101]

Gergely and coworkers[103] studied the variable regions of four anti-I and two anti-Pr cold autoagglutinins. Results showed that the heavy chains of four IgM anti-I cold agglutinins were exclusively V_HI subgroups and their light chains were exclusively VκII subgroups. In contrast, the light chains of two cold agglutinins with anti-Pr specificity were not VκII, whereas their heavy chains were not restricted to a single subgroup. The amino acid sequences at the first hypervariable region of light chains (positions 25 to 35) were similar in two of the four anti-I cold agglutinins. These sequences were different from that of the light chain of another cold agglutinin with anti-Pr specificity. These results supported the concept that only antibodies with the same specificity can share similar primary structure at their antigen-combining sites.

IgG V_H genes are classified into families according to sequence homology. At first it was thought that most of them could be assigned to three major groups: V_HI, V_HII, and V_HIII. DNA analysis has revealed the presence of three additional V_H families: V_HIV, V_HV, and V_HVI. Pascual and coworkers[104] and Silverman and Carson[105] showed that anti-I cold autoagglutinins exclusively use heavy chains that derive from the V_HIV family. Pascual and coworkers[104] and Silberstein and coworkers[106] confirmed that pathologenic anti-I cold autoagglutinins are encoded by the V_H4.21 heavy chain gene. Pascual and coworkers[104] showed that a nucleotide change in H chain CDR1 results in the substitution of an aspartic acid residue for glycine at position 31, suggesting that this amino acid might be critical to the recognition of I antigen on the RBC. Silberstein and coworkers[106] studied anti-I and anti-i cold agglutinins from B-cell clones and from the peripheral circulation of patients with lymphoproliferative syndromes. Sequence analyses of expressed variable region genes indicated that both anti-i and anti-I specificities from B-cell clones from two patients were encoded by the V_H4.21 or a very closely related V_H4 heavy chain gene, whereas the expressed light chain genes differed. The anti-i–secreting B cells expressed unmutated germline-encoded V_H4.21 and VκI gene sequences. The V_H region gene encoding anti-I has the closest homology (97%) to the V_H4.21 germline gene and differs at the protein level by only three amino acids. In contrast, although V_L region gene encoding anti-I is most homologous (96%) to the VκIII, kv328 germline gene, there are seven amino acid differences due to nonrandom replacement mutations, which suggests a role for antigen-mediated selection in the anti-I response of this individual. These studies were extended by a structural survey of 20 additional cold agglutinins using antipeptide antibodies specific for determinants V_H and V_L regions. All anti-I and anti-i cold agglutinins were shown to express V_H4 heavy chains, and 14 of 17 cold agglutinins expressed a previously described V_H4 second hypervariable region determinant, termed *VH-4-HV2a*. It was also found that 13 of 14 anti-I cold agglutinins used VκIII light chains, whereas the anti-i cold agglutinins used light chains from at least three V_L families. Taken together, the data show that anti-i and anti-I cold agglutinins probably both derive from the V_H4.21 gene (or a closely related gene). Furthermore, the restricted V_H and different V_L gene use in anti-i and anti-I may reflect the close structural relationship of the i and I antigens. Silverman and coworkers[105] demonstrated that many anti-I have κIII L chains that express primary sequence-dependent Id determinants linked to the germline gene *Humkv325* or a nearly identical gene.

The study of the structures of cold agglutinating autoantibodies has centered around determining gene segment usage encoding the variable regions by sequence analysis, and detecting the presence of variable region idiotopes (Id) using anti-idiotopic antibodies (anti-Id).[107,108] It has been determined that there are both naturally occurring, nonpathogenic anti-I/i cold agglutinins, and pathogenic anti-I/i cold agglutinins derived from B cell clonal expansions. Despite attempts to correlate antibody subclass, complement-fixing ability, or antibody titer with the presence or absence of hemolysis,[29,50,109,110] it remains unclear what structural properties distinguish "benign" autoantibodies from hemolytic ones.[107]

Initial studies of the structure of these antibodies focused on the constant regions of the immunoglobulin molecules. Later studies focused on studying the structural diversity of the variable regions of these autoantibodies through the use of anti-idiotypic reagents and by direct nucleotide sequencing of the rearranged immunoglubulin variable region genes.[107]

Naturally occurring IgM cold agglutinins are commonly found in low titers and have no pathological significance. These nonpathogenic autoantibodies are thought to be the product of either random rearrangement of the immunoglobulin gene segments in the bone marrow and/or produced as a result of molecular mimicry with structures on the surface of infectious agents.[108] These autoantibodies have been shown to be polyreactive and encoded by the V_H3 gene segments V3-15 and V3-48[111] and V_H4 family gene segments including V4-49, V4-29, and V4-34.[111,112] Some anti-i antibodies from the normal B cell repertoire were V4-34 encoded, and selected antibodies had similar avidities to pathogenic V4-34 encoded autoantibodies. Therefore, while autoantibodies with anti-I/i specificity are encoded by some members of the V_H4 and V_H3 families, they are not associated with disease.[108]

In contrast, cold agglutinins produced in chronic lymphoproliferative conditions are exclusively encoded by the V4-34 gene segment in association with different D and J_H gene segments.[105,113-116] The V4-34 encoded regions of pathogenic cold agglutinins have been found in both germline configuration and somatically mutated. This use of a single gene segment in antibodies directed against an autoantigen is very rare in immunology, and suggests that the V4-34 gene segment is required to encode the anti-I/i specificity.[110,115] Also, a monoclonal anti-idiotypic antibody termed "9G4" has been described, which recognizes an idiotypic determinant present on the heavy chain of both anti-I and anti-i cold agglutinins as well as on neoplastic B cells secreting cold agglutinins. The 9G4 idioptype was present on all 48 pathogenic anti-I/i cold agglutinins studied.[113,116] However, natural/benign cold agglutinins do not express the 9G4 idiotope.[107]

Thus, available data suggest a diverse B-cell origin of natural cold agglutinins, which infers that B-cell clones secreting natural cold agglutinins do not necessarily represent precursors of the monoclonal B-cell expansions secreting pathogenic cold agglutinins. The differences between benign and pathogenic cold agglutinins have not been completely characterized, and further study should provide insights into our understanding of what makes an autoantibody pathogenic.[108]

Occasionally, cold agglutinins are cryoprecipitable.[117-125] Cryoprecipitable anti-I has been observed, and at least one third of anti-i cold agglutinins are cryoprecipitable.[124] In 50 patients with CAS, the total concentration of IgM varied from 0.7 to 24.5 mg/mL.[125] In most of the patients, the cold agglutinin accounts for the entire elevation of serum IgM above normal levels. In two patients studied by Harboe,[125] a homogeneous protein remained in the serum after adsorption with RBC stroma in the cold. This finding was shown to be due to the presence of an additional monoclonal protein without cold agglutinin activity, thus indicating that these were instances of biclonal gammopathy.

Many investigators have noted similarities of laboratory findings in patients with CAS and patients who have monoclonal IgM proteins without cold agglutinin activity. In both instances, bone marrow findings may consist of increased numbers of abnormal lymphoid and plasma cells,[126] although Dacie[1] and Firkin and coworkers[127] reported no excess of plasma cells in patients with CAS. Schubothe[128] analyzed 14 patients with CAS and found 9 had bone marrow lymphocyte counts exceeding 25%; it exceeded 40% in six patients. In one patient, there was an impressive progression of lymphocytic infiltration of the marrow 4 years after the onset of the disease. On the basis of these similarities, some investigators think that a typical case of CAS is probably a variant of Waldenström's macroglobulinemia in which the IgM M-component has cold agglutinin activity. However, there are many differences between CAS and patients with macroglobulinemia without cold agglutinin activity (see Chapter 3).

In 1982, Crisp and Pruzanski[129] reported on patients with cold autoagglutinins. Among 78 patients with persistent cold agglutinins, 31 had lymphoma, 13 had Waldenström's macroglobulinemia, 6 had chronic lymphocytic leukemia, and 28 had chronic CAS. The average age was over 60 years. Patients with chronic CAS had more hemolytic crises, bleeding, and Raynaud's phenomena and less frequently lymphadenopathy or hepatosplenomegaly. The frequency of anemia, positive DAT test results, cryoglobulinemia, and Bence Jones proteinuria was similar in the various groups. Survival time from diagnosis was on average 2 years in lymphoma, 2.5 years in Waldenström's macroglobulinemia, more than 6 years in chronic lymphocytic leukemia, and more than 5 years in chronic CAS. Anti-I was common in chronic CAS (74%) and uncommon in other groups (32% to 33%). Anti-i and other cold agglutinins were rare in chronic CAS and common in lymphoma and Waldenström's macroglobulinemia. In chronic cold agglutinin disease and in Waldenström's macroglobulinemia, cold agglutinins usually had κ light chains, 92% and 71%, respectively, whereas in lymphoma, 71% of cold agglutinins had λ light chains. The type of light chains related to the specificity of cold agglutinins: 58% of IgM/κ were anti-I and 75% of IgM/λ had other specificities. Cold agglutinins were cytotoxic to autologous and allogeneic lymphocytes. Occasionally, more autologous than allogeneic cells were killed, implying that the former may be precoated in vivo with the antibodies. Crisp and Pruzanski[129] concluded that conditions with persistent cold agglutinins are a spectrum that varies from "benign" chronic cold agglutinin disease to malignant lymphoma. Marked differences in the light chain type of cold agglutinins, specificity toward membranous antigens, and severity of clinical manifestations were noted in benign and malignant varities.

IgG and IgA Cold Autoagglutinins. Although CAS is almost always caused by an IgM autoantibody, there are a number of reports of cases in which the cold autoagglutinin was of the IgG immunoglobulin class.[130-141] Included among such cases are those with biclonal antibodies, for example, a combination of IgG and IgM autoantibodies. Occasionally, IgA autoagglutinins are found as well.

Roelcke and coworkers[133] described two children with transient CAS who had IgG cold agglutinins. Mygind and Ahrons[134] reported two patients with first trimester abortion and idiopathic CAS. Using sucrose gradient ultracentrifugation and 2 mercaptoethanol treatment, the authors demonstrated the presence of IgM as well as IgG cold agglutinins. Moore and Chaplin[135] described a patient with severe AIHA whose RBCs were strongly coated with IgG and C3d. In addition to a typical IgM anti-I cold agglutinin of modest titer, the serum contained a lambda IgG antibody that bound more strongly to RBCs at 4°C (titer 64) than at 37°C (titer 4). The patient improved following splenectomy, but the authors were not successful in demonstrating IgG or IgM antibodies in a concentrated splenic extract.

Ratkin and coworkers[130] estimated by radial immunodiffusion the IgG, IgA, and IgM concentration in eluates that had been prepared in a carefully standardized and controlled way from normal RBCs that had been sensitized at 0°C by exposure to 19 different high-titer cold antibodies, 14 of which had been derived from patients with CAS. As expected, the IgM concentrations were 32 to 4800 times the concentrations of residual Ig predicted to be present in the fluid in which the RBCs were suspended after the last washing. Seventeen of the 19 eluates contained 9 to 660 times the predicted concentration of IgG and 6 of the 19 eluates contained 12 to 226 times the expected concentrations of IgA. These findings certainly suggest that IgG cold antibodies are not infrequently present in sera containing high-titer cold antibodies alongside the characteristic and usually dominant IgM antibodies. Less commonly, IgA cold antibodies are present as well.

Freedman and Newlands[136] investigated two women, aged 23 and 30, respectively. The first gave a 10-year history of chronic AIHA and the second gave a 1-year history of AIHA; in both instances the onset of hemolysis had been acute. Both cases had IgM autoantibodies that were cold agglutinins with anti-I specificity and were complement binding. Both cases also had IgG nonagglutinating autoantibodies that were of wide thermal range and also had anti-I specificity, but were not complement binding. The RBCs of both patients were coated with C4/C3d and IgG

Dellagi and coworkers[131] performed immunologic studies in a case of chronic AIHA associated with a cold agglutinin that had a titer of only 16. Despite the low titer cold agglutinin, there was prominent autoagglutination of RBCs soon after blood collection. The authors demonstrated that the cold agglutinin was directed against the Pr RBC antigen and was not reduced by mercaptoethanol treatment of the serum; the antibody reacted up to 37°C. They concluded that the chronic AIHA was related to low titer monoclonal IgG cold agglutinins with anti-Pr activity.

Silberstein and coworkers[137] reported a patient with IgG κ and IgM κ immunoglobulins, both possessing cold agglutinin activity. In view of the predominance of the IgG cold agglutinin, splenectomy was recommended for treatment and in the subsequent 30 months no additional therapy was necessary.

Szymanski and coworkers[138] described a 65-year-old man with severe hemolytic anemia of 2 months' duration who had IgG and IgM lambda agglutinins in his serum. Their thermal optimum was unusual, the titers with adult group O cells being 16 at 4°C, 128 at 22°C, and 1 at 37°C. They did not bind complement in vitro, consistent with the finding that the patient had negative DAT using anti-C3d. Their specificity could not be determined. The patient responded to corticosteroid therapy and remained well without treatment 14 months after the hemolytic episode. The authors suggested that the presence of IgG cold agglutinins may be predictive of a favorable response to corticosteroid therapy.

Silberstein and coworkers[132] reported six patients whose serum cold agglutinin was not inactivated or was incompletely inactivated with the IgM-reducing agent dithiothreitol. In five of these patients, isolation of the antibodies revealed that two patients had predominantly IgG cold-reactive antibody, which was associated with smaller amounts of IgM in one patient and with IgA in the other; two patients had predominantly IgM cold agglutinin with lesser amounts of cold-reactive IgG; and one patient had an IgG cold agglutinin only.

Curtis and coworkers[139] reported a 21-year-old man with fulminant CAS who was hospitalized with hemoglobinemia, hemoglobinuria, a hemoglobin concentration of 3.3 gm/dL, a negative DAT with polyspecific and anti-C3d reagents, a negative DL test, and a cold agglutinin titer of 80. He failed to respond to corticosteroids, multiple plasma exchanges, and cyclophosphamide; he required 54 transfusions in 10 days to maintain a hemoglobin concentration of 6.0 to 10.0 g/dL. He improved dramatically after a splenectomy was performed. The wide thermal amplitude cold agglutinin proved to be an IgG1 κ antibody with Pr^a specificity. The patient's serum exhibited normal complement activation. When the DAT was carried out at 0°C to 4°C, the result was strongly positive for IgG; the IAT at 0°C to 4°C was positive with the patient's serum diluted 1 in 640. Within 6 months, he was in complete remission and receiving no therapy. The patient is remarkable for his requirement for many transfusions and for DATs that were consistently negative for C3d.

Angevine and coworkers[142] described a patient with reticulum sarcoma who had acrocyanosis associated with cold exposure. He had a negative DAT and no hemolytic anemia. He had a cold agglutinin with titers of 1024 to 4096. The antibody was found to be IgA (kappa light chains only). We described a similar case.[143] Our patient first developed symptoms of acrocyanosis associated with the cold, 21 years before being diagnosed as having multiple myeloma associated with a monoclonal IgA paraprotein. He had a negative DAT and no hemolytic anemia, but had a cold autoagglutinin with a titer of 16,000; the specificity was anti-Pr. An IgA anti-Pr autoagglutinin in a patient with myeloma was previously described by Roelcke and Dorow in 1968.[144] The IgA cold agglutinins described by Angevine and coworkers[142] and Garratty and coworkers[143] were studied further by Roelcke[144,145]; both were confirmed as having anti-Pr_1 specificity. Further examples of IgA anti-Pr have been described by Roelcke and coworkers.[146,147]

Tschirhart and coworkers[148] reported a patient with CAS whose serum contained a biclonal IgA and IgM gammopathy, with identical findings demonstrable in the patient's RBCs eluate. The authors commented that serum electrophoresis suggested that their patient had a monoclonal gammopathy, and only immunofixation electrophoresis demonstrated the presence of biclonal immunoglobulins.

Patients Who Have Warm and Cold Autoantibodies

As mentioned previously, approximately one third of WAIHA patients have cold agglutinins that can react quite strongly at room temperature but have normal titer (at 4°C) and do not react at 30°C and 37°C. We do not think such antibodies are pathogenic, but sometimes patients with WAIHA have cold antibodies that react up to 30°C or above; such antibodies may be pathogenic. We reviewed the clinical and hematological findings of such patients in Chapter 3 (pages 79–81). Serologically, the patients fall into three groups. The first group have IgG and C3 on their RBCs, and their sera may contain IgG 37°C-reactive antibodies together with high-titer high thermal amplitude cold autoagglutinins (i.e., the combined serology of classic WAIHA and CAS).[4,39,149-155] The second group usually have IgG and/or C3 on their RBCs, and their sera contain IgG 37°C-reactive antibodies together with cold autoagglutinins of normal titer, but in contrast to the one third of WAIHA mentioned above, the cold autoagglutinins react at 37°C and/or 30°C. There are only three published reports that relate to this group and the report by Sokol and coworkers[155] does not give any cold agglutinin titers, so some of the patients may belong in group 1. Shulman and coworkers[154] believe that up to 8% of WAIHA may belong to this group. Table 5-16 shows the serological results of 39 patients we believe fit in this group. In these patients we believe the cold autoagglutinin, although of normal titer, could have played a role in the hemolytic process. It is of interest to note that Isbister and coworkers[89] described four patients with lymphoproliferative disease, with IgM λ monoclonal proteins and severe AIHA, who had low-titer high thermal amplitude cold autoagglutinins but no IgG autoantibodies. These findings support the findings we have that such antibodies can play a pathogenic role and that this role may be significant.

Laboratory Diagnosis of Paroxysmal Cold Hemoglobinuria

ESSENTIAL DIAGNOSTIC TESTS

The diagnosis of PCH or the exclusion of that diagnosis in the laboratory is usually considerably easier than that of either WAIHA or CAS. The essential laboratory test is the Donath-Landsteiner (DL) test, which is described in detail in Chapter 6, page 223). A positive test is illustrated in Figure 3-4. A negative test excludes the diagnosis of PCH and a positive test is, with rare exceptions (described below), diagnostic of the disorder.

The autoantibody associated with PCH is termed a *biphasic hemolysin*, that is to say, it sensitizes RBCs in the cold but only hemolyzes them when the RBCs reach 37°C. The diagnostic test is the DL test where RBCs are incubated with the patient's serum at 0°C (e.g., melting ice) and then moved to 37°C for a further incubation. No lysis occurs following the incubation at 0°C, and no lysis occurs if the incubation is carried out only at 37°C. The thermal amplitude of this antibody is usually less than 20°C, that is to say, the antibody will give a positive DL test only when the initial incubation is <20°C; stronger results will occur as the temperature of the initial incubation is lowered. Rare patients have been described when the DL test is positive when the first incubation phase is as high as 32°C, or their DL antibody would sensitize RBCs up to 37°C, as detected by the IAT (see below).[156-158]

The autoantibody may sometimes agglutinate RBCs in addition to giving a positive DL test.[1] The agglutination is usually of low titer (<64) at 4°C, and of low thermal amplitude (<20°C). The antibody is IgG but is usually only detectable by the IAT if, following incubation of the patient's serum and

TABLE 5-16. SEROLOGY OF 39 PATIENTS WITH WARM AND COLD AUTOANTIBODIES

Patients	DAT	IAT (Polyspecific AGS)	Autoagglutinin		Titers			Lysins		Notes
			20°C	37°C	4°C	30°C	37°C	20°C (UT/ET)	37° (UT/ET)	
1	IgG/C3	2+	3½+	3+	64	2	1	0/2+	0/3+	
2	IgG/C3	Micro+	3+	0	2	[2+]	0	0/0	0/0	Anti-En[a] or –Pr
3	IgG/C3	1+	4+	1	32	[2+]	[1½+]	0/1+	0/2+	
4	IgG/C3/IgM	3½+	3½+	1½	16	8	4	0/0	0/0	
5	IgG/C3	Micro+	2½+	0	16	1	1	0/0	0/0	
6	IgG/C3/IgM	Micro+	3+	0	32	1	0	0/2+	0/3+	
7	IgG/C3	0	3½+	0	64	1	0	0/½+	0/0	
8	IgG/C3	3+	0/4+ (I/i)	0	2/64 (I/i)	0/16 (I/i)	0	NT	NT	Anti-i
9	IgG/C3	1+	3+	1	4	1	0	0/0	0/2+	
10	IgG/C3	0	3+	1½	128	4	1	0/0	0/1+	
11	IgG/C3	Micro+	4+	0	32	1	0	0/0	0/Trace	
12	IgG/C3/IgM/IgA	2+	4+	2	32	4	2	0/1+	0/2+	
13	IgG/C3	3+	4+	1	16,000	[3+]	[1+]	NT	NT	
14	IgG/C3	0+	2½+	0	8	1	1	0/0	0/2	
15	IgG/C3	1+	3½+	0	128/1024 (I/i)	0/1 (I/i)	0	0/3+	0/0	Anti-i
16	IgG/C3	Micro+			32	2	1	0/0	0/0	Probable anti-I[T]
17	IgG/C3	1+	3½+	2½	64	1	1	0/0	0/0	
18	IgG/C3	Micro+	4+	0	64	4	0	0/0	0/0	IgG cold agglutinin
19	IgG/C3	0	3+	0	16	0	0	NT	NT	Reactive at 30°C in presence of albumin
20	IgG/C3	1+	3½+	1	128	1	1	0/2	0/3+	
21	C3	1+	3½+	3½	64	16	2	0/0	0/4+	
22	C3	Micro+	3½+	2	64	[2+]	[2+]	0/4	0/4+	20°C lysin titer = 1; 37°C lysin titer = 16
23	C3	Micro+	4+	1	128	2	2	0/0	0/2+	IgM warm + cold antibodies
24	C3	½+	3½+	1	8	1	1	0/½+	0/3+	
25	IgG/C3/IgM	½+	1+	0	128	1	1	0/0	0/0	
26	IgG/C3/IgM/IgA	1–2+	3+	2+	4	2	1	0/2+	0/4+	
27	IgG/C3/IgM	½+	2+	0	16	1	1	0/2+	0/3+	
28	IgG/C3	2½+	1½+	1+	16–32	1	1	0/1+	0/0	
29	IgG/C3/IgM	1½+	1+	0	32	1	0	0/0	0/0	
30	IgG/C3/IgM/IgA	2+	4+	0	128	1	1	tr/2+	0/1+	
31	IgG/C3/IgM	1+	3+	1+	32	1	1	0/0	0/0	
32	IgG	3+	1+	0	1	[2½+]	[1½]	0/0	0/0	Low affinity IgG anti-Pr (reactions at 30°C only in presence of albumin at low pH)
33	C3	0	3+	1½+	16	4	2	0/1+	0/4+	
34	IgG/C3/IgM	0	2–3½+	1+	16	1	1	0/0	0/trace	
35	IgA	1–2+ (anti-IgA)	3+	2½+	8	4	2	0/0	0/0	
36	IgG	0	4+	0	2	0	0	0/0	0/0	Low affinity RBC-bound IgG antibody. Agglutination at 30°C in presence of albumin.
37	IgG/C3/IgM	1+	2½+	1½+	32	1	1	0/1+	0/3½+	
38	IgG/C3/IgM/IgA	1+	2½+	0	32	2	NT	0/0	0/0	
39	IgG/C3	0	2½+	½+	8	2	?	0/0	0/0	

From Garratty G, Arndt P, Leger R: Previously unpublished data.
UT = untreated RBCs; ET = enzyme-treated RBCs; [ ] = reaction with undiluted serum; titer not available.

RBCs at 0°C, the RBCs are washed with ice-cold saline and ice-cold antiglobulin serum is used. Indeed, Dacie[1] has found that the IAT was a more sensitive way of demonstrating antibody activity than looking for lysis. Such agglutination tests must be carefully controlled because many sera give positive results under these circumstances if a polyspecific antiglobulin serum is used, due to the presence in human sera of the normal incomplete cold antibody. It is important, therefore, to be sure that monospecific anti-IgG antiglobulin serum is used.

Since PCH is quite rare, one may justifiably question the advisability of performing a DL test routinely in patients with acquired hemolytic anemia. Our own attitude is to be liberal with the indications for performance of the test since it is simple to perform and its inclusion avoids diagnostic errors. We certainly feel that the performance of the test is indicated in any child, any patient with hemoglobinuria, patients with a history of hemolysis exacerbated by cold, and in all cases with "atypical" serologic findings. If positive results are obtained in the DL test, determination of the specificity of the autoantibody is indicated. All cases of PCH we have encountered in the last 30 years were associated with anti-P specificity. Sokol and coworkers[159] found anti-P specificity in 27 of 30 (90%) patients with PCH; specificity was not clearly defined in the other three cases. Nevertheless, rare reports of other specificities said to be associated with PCH have been reported (see below and Chapter 7, page 254). RBCs necessary for determining anti-P specificity are rare but, with the assistance of reference laboratories, specificity testing can be carried out. It should be noted that the DL test must be used to determine specificity.

Typical findings in a patient with PCH are presented in the following case report and in Table 5-17.

PATIENT 2: A 4½-year-old boy was in good health until 10 days prior to admission to the hospital, at which time he developed a cough and sore throat. Three days prior to admission, he developed a fever of 102°F, headache, myalgia, abdominal pain, vomiting, and diarrhea. He was treated with oral penicillin. Two days prior to admission he began passing dark urine, and the next day he was noted to be jaundiced. His parents noted that his urine output was scanty.

On admission to the hospital he was not in acute distress. Temperature was 37°C, pulse 120, respirations 30, and blood pressure 110/50 mg Hg. Physical examination was unremarkable. His hematocrit was 31.9%, bilirubin 2.4 mg/dL total and 0.2 mg/dL direct reacting, and the lactic dehydrogenase (LDH) 2868 units. The urine was brown, specific gravity 1.017, pH 5.5, hemoglobin test 3+, protein 3+, bilirubin negative, and only 2 RBCs were present per high-power field. The creatinine was 2.6 mg/dL, the sodium was 132 mEQ, potassium 5.9 mEQ, chloride 102 mEQ, and the carbon dioxide 8 mEQ/L.

During the next 24 hours he was anuric. At this point his hemoglobin was 7.0 g/dL; the hematocrit 19.6%; reticulocytes 1.1%; and the white count was 17,400 with 59% neutronphils, 2% bands, 29% lymphocytes, 8% monocytes, and 2% eosinophils. The platelet count was 214,000/μl. The peripheral blood film showed moderate numbers of spherocytes and poikilocytes. The blood urea nitrogen was 192 mg, and the creatinine 6.0 mg/dL. Total bilirubin was 2.3 mg/dL, and haptoglobin 20 mg/dL. The DAT was 3+. Cultures of blood, urine, throat, stool, and cerebral spinal fluid failed to reveal pathogenic bacteria.

Serologic findings are summarized in Table 5-17 and were diagnostic of PCH.

The hospital course was marked by 10 days of oliguria necessitating peritoneal dialysis twice. Thereafter, the urine output was normal (>60 mL/kg/day), and his creatinine decreased from a high of 12.9 to 1.9 mg/dL at the time of discharge. Therapy with prednisone was begun on the fourth hospital day at a dose of 2 mg/kg/day for 1 week, after which it was gradually decreased and then discontinued. The patient's hemoglobin level dropped to 4.3 g/dL on the day after admission, and he was transfused with 95 mL of P+ RBCs without clinical symptoms of a reaction and with transient benefit. Two days later his hemoglobin had again dropped to 4.8 g/dL, and he received 160 mL of RBCs, which raised his hemoglobin to 8.6 g/dL. The following day his reticulocyte count was 5.1%, and thereafter his hemoglobin level remained stable and he required no further transfusions.

Follow-up examination 2 months later revealed a hemoglobin level of 13.3 g/dL, hematocrit 38.6%, reticulocytes 38.6%, creatinine 0.4 mg/dL, urinalysis normal, and a 24-hour protein excretion of 50 mg.

Cautions Regarding the Interpretation of the DL Test. The DL test is essentially diagnostic for PCH, but one must be cautious when using sera from patients with CAS. This is true because about 15% of sera from patients with CAS contain monophasic cold hemolysins that will hemolyze untreated RBCs at around 20°C. Up to 95% of such sera will cause direct lysis of enzyme-treated red cells at 20°C.[4] During the performance of the DL test, there is a brief period of time when cells and serum are at room temperature after being moved from the ice bath to a 37°C water bath. Dacie[1] has reported slight hemolysis in the DL test using 2 sera containing high-titer cold agglutinins (titers of 4000 and 64,000, respectively).

We retrospectively tested 20 sera from patients with CAS who had monophasic cold hemolysins, against untreated red cells, and found three (15%) of them to give false weakly positive DL tests. In all other aspects these patients had symptoms and serology that was typical of CAS, rather than PCH. It should be emphasized that many other patients with CAS did not have positive DL tests, even when powerful monophasic cold lysins were present in their sera. It should also be noted that the monophasic lysins were detected in the presence of fresh complement at pH 6.5 whereas the DL

TABLE 5-17. SEROLOGIC FINDINGS IN A PATIENT WITH PCH

Direct Antigloublin Test: Polyspecific Antiglobulin Serum: 2+
Anti-IgG: negative   Anti-C3: 2+

Screening Tests for Serum Antibody	Serum	AS + AC*	Control AC Alone
20°C, Untreated Cells			
Lysis	0	0	0
Agglutination	0	0	0
20°C, Papainized Cells			
Lysis	0	1+	0
Agglutination	1+	1+	0
37°C, Untreated Cells			
Lysis	0	0	0
Agglutination	0	0	0
37°C, Papainized Cells			
IAT	0	0	0
Agglutination	0	0	0

*AS, acidified serum; AC, acidified complement
Specificity of serum and eluate:
Serum: anti-P
Eluate: not done
Cold agglutinin titer: normal
Donath-Landsteiner test: positive
Summary: Findings diagnostic of paroxysmal cold hemoglobinuria
Follow-up: Rapid improvement in anemia and in renal function after initial episode of intravascular hemolysis and renal failure. Two months later the DAT was weakly positive with anti-C3 (titer 16, score 7) and the Donath-Landsteiner test was negative.

test was performed without acidification of the serum. If enzyme-treated RBCs are used for the DL test, as suggested by some investigators,[3] the false-positive rate might be higher. We caution that if enzyme-treated red cells are used for the DL test, a control for monophasic lysis set up in parallel should be mandatory.

Performing the DL Test in Patients with Hemoglobinemia. It may be impossible to determine if in vitro hemolysis has occurred in the DL test if the patient's serum is red because of marked hemoglobinemia. In this case, a simple procedure is to perform the cold phase of the DL test using the patient's serum, but after incubation at 4°C, carefully replace the patient's serum with fresh normal acidified serum before moving to the 37°C phase of the test. As a control, a similar tube can be kept at 4°C after replacing the patient's serum with normal serum, or one may replace the patient's serum with inactivated serum before the 37°C phase. Also, if it is known that the specificity of the antibody is anti-P and P-negative RBCs are available, they may be used in the DL test as a control. Another simple technical aid is to compare the size of the RBC buttons following centrifugation. If these approaches fail, then a "cold IAT" can be performed.

Comparison of PCH and CAS. CAS and PCH are generally quite distinct disorders, and typical findings in each syndrome are compared in Table 5-18. A few similar features may result in the blurring of the distinction between the two disorders, especially in some unusual cases. Clinically, similarities result from the fact that acrocyanosis and hemoglobinuria may develop in either disorder after exposure to cold. In addition, both syndromes have been reported to occur after *Mycoplasma pneumoniae* infection, although PCH following infection with this organism is rare.

In the laboratory, some exceptions to the typical findings listed in Table 5-15 occur. For example, patients with the CAS may have a cold agglutinin titer less than 500 (see Table 5-14). The thermal range of the autoantibody has been reported as high as 32°C to 37°C in three exceptional cases,[156-158] and there are several reports of DL antibodies reactive at temperatures of 18°C to 25°C.[159-161] These antibodies do not require incubation at 0°C as in the DL test and may cause "monophasic" lysis at room temperature. There are rare reports of the specificity of the DL antibody being reported as anti-I or anti-HI, similar to that frequently found in CAS; we suspect that these patients may have had false-positive DL tests due to monophasic lysins.

Although the preceding findings may seem to add an air of uncertainty to the differentiation between the two disorders, it is rare that the distinction is actually difficult, either on clinical grounds or in the laboratory. Clinically, PCH is an acute hemolytic anemia associated with marked constitutional symptoms; modern case reports describe the disorder almost exclusively in children or young adults, and it is almost always transient. In contrast, CAS generally occurs in middle-aged or elderly persons, the patient's symptoms are frequently just those of anemia, and the disorder is chronic except in the minority of patients who have transient CAS following *Mycoplasma pneumoniae* infection or other infectious diseases.

In the laboratory, a positive DL test should be considered diagnostic of PCH unless a cold agglutinin that is of high thermal amplitude and is a potent hemolysin is present. When such antibodies cause weakly positive reactions in the DL test, the reactions should be interpreted as a "false-positive" DL test in a patient with CAS.

Opposite findings occur in patients with PCH. That is, even if the thermal range of a DL antibody is high

TABLE 5-18. COMPARISON OF TYPICAL CHARACTERISTICS OF THE ANTIBODY IN COLD AGGLUTININ SYNDROME WITH THE DONATH-LANDSTEINER ANTIBODY OF PAROXYSMAL COLD HEMOGLOBINURIA

	Cold Agglutinin Syndrome	Donath-Landsteiner Antibody
Titer (4°C)	High (>500)	Moderate (<64)
Thermal range	High (>30°C)	Moderate (<20°C)
Bithermic lysis (Donath-Landsteiner test)	Negative	Positive
Immunoglobulin class	IgM	IgG
Specificity	Anti-I or i	Anti-P

enough to result in monophasic lysis, maximal lysis will occur if an incubation at 0°C precedes incubation at 37°C. Also, specificity tests are usually of value in separating the two disorders, and the antibody in PCH is of the IgG immunoglobulin class, in contrast to the antibody in CAS, which is almost always IgM. A further means of distinguishing these disorders is that in PCH the peripheral blood film frequently reveals striking RBC adherence and erythrophagocytosis by neutrophils, whereas this we have not found this to be true in CAS. Further tests in the laboratory will reveal that RBCs from patients with PCH will be phagocytosed by monocytes in an in vitro monocyte monolayer assay (see Chapter 3, page 76).

Autoantibodies with Unusual Characteristics in Patients Who Have Been Diagnosed as Having PCH

The characteristic DL antibody causes hemolysis in the classic biphasic hemolysin test, is of the IgG immunoglobulin class and has anti-P specificity. These laboratory findings in association with the typical clinical findings described above allow for a confident diagnosis of PCH. However, some antibodies in patients in whom a diagnosis of PCH has been made do not have anti-P specificity, and/or are IgM, or have other unusual characteristics.

DL Antibodies with Specificity Other Than Anti-P

Bird and coworkers[160] suggested that the definition of PCH be restricted to cases in which the autoantibody demonstrated specificity within the P blood group system, usually anti-P. Dacie stated[1] that, in his view, anti-P specificity is an essential criterion for labeling an autoantibody as a DL antibody. However, biphasic antibodies showing other blood group specificities have been described including anti-I,[162-164] anti-p[165] (which may be anti-Gd), anti-"Pr-like,"[166] anti-i,[167] and anti-HI.[168] The IgG nature of the anti-p,[165] one anti-I,[162] the anti-i,[167] and anti-"Pr-like"[166] were confirmed, thus lending support to their being classified as DL antibodies.

DL Antibodies with Unusual Activity

Although, as mentioned above, DL antibodies commonly cause sensitization to agglutination by antiglobulin serum when tested at 4°C with anti-IgG,[1] some DL antibodies have unusual properties. Lindgren and coworkers[157] described a patient whose serum gave a strongly positive DL test when the initial incubation phase was 0°C or 20°C, but was negative at 30°C and 37°C. The serum also reacted strongly by IAT at 37°C with anti-IgG. The 37°C tests were repeated several times with strict control of the temperature at all phases of testing. The serum reacted with all RBCs tested except those that were PP_1P^k negative and P^k positive; thus, the specificity was anti-P. After treatment of the patient's serum with 2-mercaptoethanol, it still gave a positive DL test and reacted at 37°C with anti-IgG by the IAT, indicating that the autoantibody was IgG. Nordhagen[158] described two similar cases in which the serum gave a positive DL test with anti-P specificity. In both patients, the antibodies also reacted by the IAT at 37°C when the tests were read with anti-IgG. Sabio and coworkers[169] also reported a patient whose serum contained a biphasic hemolysin with anti-P specificity, and which also reacted by IAT at 37°C. The patients described by the above authors all had clinical findings typical of PCH.

Lau and coworkers[170] reported a patient in whom erythrophagocytosis was noted on a routine blood smear. The hematocrit subsequently decreased from 30% to 23% in 24 hours and hemoglobinemia and hemoglobinuria became evident. The DL test was strongly positive with both the patient's serum and the RBC eluate, and was inhibited by globoside but not by other glycosphingolipids. The highest temperature of the initial erythrocyte sensitization was 10°C. The autoantibody agglutinated P-positive reagent RBCs incubated in LISS medium at 22°C and in the antiglobulin phase. Further testing confirmed anti-P specificity of the antibody. Both heat and ether eluates agglutinated P-positive but not P-negative RBCs at 4°C and 22°C, but failed to react at 37°C and in the antiglobulin phase.

IgM Antibodies Giving a Positive DL Test

Rarely, patients with IgM agglutinating antibodies with biphasic hemolytic properties have been diagnosed as having PCH. Nakamura and coworkers[163] reported a patient with a biphasic hemolysin of the IgM immunoglobulin class with anti-I specificity, Ramos and coworkers[171] reported a patient with a positive DL test whose serum contained a single IgM cold autoantibody with I^T and P specificities (anti-I^TP), and Zamora and coworkers[172] reported a patient with an IgM agglutinating antibody with biphasic hemolytic properties having anti-P specificity. Lippman and coworkers[173] also reported a patient with a biphasic anti-IgM autohemolysin. It is difficult to determine whether or not these cases represent instances in which an IgM cold agglutinin with hemolytic properties caused a false-positive DL test, as described above.

Antibodies with Unique Characteristics

Even more atypical are the following. Bastrup-Madsen and Petersen[174] reported a case of benign idiopathic monoclonal gammopathy with cold sensitivity due to the presence of an IgG monoclonal protein that gave a positive DL test. The patient had episodes of hemoglobinuria and developed urticarial wheals in cold weather. On one occasion Bence Jones proteinuria was demonstrated. That the gammopathy was of the benign type was supported by the fact that no rise was seen in the M-protein level or plasma cell count at a follow-up examination 6½ years after the onset of the cold sensitivity.

von dem Borne and coworkers[175] reported a case of AIHA associated with IgM monoclonal cold autoagglutinins and monophasic hemolysins with anti-P specificity.

Judd and coworkers have described an example of a pH-dependent autoanti-P[176] and two examples of autoanti-P that were reactive only at low ionic strength.[177]

Mensinger and coworkers[178] reported a patient who developed a fatal case of hemolytic anemia. Her serum contained an IgM anti-P agglutinin in combination with an IgG anti-P monophasic lysin that reacted up to 32°C. However, the presence of a biphasic lysin could not be confirmed. Thus, this is a unique case in which an antibody of anti-P specificity caused lysis in vitro, but did not give a positive DL test.

Comments on the definition of PCH. By far the most common case of PCH has characteristic clinical and laboratory findings. However, uncertainty arises when findings are atypical, as in the cases cited above. For example, some authors[1,160] indicate that a diagnosis of PCH is not warranted unless an antibody of anti-P specificity can be demonstrated, whereas other investigators have reported cases as examples of PCH even though the biphasic hemolysin had specificity other than anti-P.

When an IgM antibody gives a positive DL test, the possibility that the hemolysis in vitro was actually a false-positive test caused by a monophasic hemolysin must be carefully excluded. Even if false-positive tests are excluded, should patients with IgM antibodies be diagnosed as having PCH, especially if the antibodies demonstrate specificity other than anti-P and the clinical findings are not typical?

Still other investigators report DL antibodies that are monoclonal, antibodies that react only under very special in vitro testing conditions, or antibodies with anti-P specificity that do not cause biphasic hemolysis.

Thus, there seems to be no strong consensus as to what it is that defines PCH. Among the cases with atypical features described above, we feel most comfortable in accepting a diagnosis of PCH when the antibody gives a characteristic biphasic hemolysis test and is of the IgG immunoglobulin class, even if the specificity is not the characteristic anti-P. If the antibody also causes agglutination, and/or reacts by IAT at 20°C to 37°C, this would not negate a diagnosis of PCH. However, it is probably best to not definitively diagnose PCH when the clinical findings are atypical and the antibody is IgM or has unique characteristics.

REFERENCES

1. Dacie JV: The Haemolytic Anaemias. Part II. Auto-Immune Haemolytic Anaemias, 2nd ed. London: J & A Churchill Ltd., 1962.
2. Wolach B, Heddle N, Barr RD, Zipursky A, Pai KR, Blajchman MA: Transient Donath-Landsteiner haemolytic anaemia. Br J Haematol 1981;48:425–434.
3. Heddle NM: Acute paroxysmal cold hemoglobinuria. Transfus Med Rev 1989;3:219–229.
4. Petz LD, Garratty G: Acquired Immune Hemolytic Anemias, 1st ed. New York: Churchill Livingstone, 1980.
5. Croucher BEE, Crookston MC, Crookston JH: Delayed haemolytic transfusion reactions simulating auto-immune haemolytic anaemia. Vox Sang 1967;12:32.
6. Croucher BEE: Differential diagnosis of delayed hemolytic transfusion reaction. In Bell CA (ed): A Seminar on Laboratory Management of Hemolysis. Washington, DC: American Association of Blood Banks, 1979:151–160.
7. Worlledge SM: The interpretation of a positive direct antiglobulin test. Brit J Haemat 1978;39:157–162.
8. Kaplan HS, Garratty G: Predictive value of direct antiglobulin test results. Diagnostic Med 1985;8:29–32.
9. Garratty G: The significance of IgG on the red cell surface. Transfus Med Rev 1987;1:47–57.
10. Jeannet M: Specificity of the antiglobulin test in "auto-immune" hemolytic anemias. Helv Med Acta 1966;33:151–163.
11. Gerbal A, Homberg JC, Rochant H, Perron L, Salmon C: Autoantibodies in acquired hemolytic anemia. I. Analysis of 234 cases. Nouv Rev Fr Hematol 1968;8:155–157.
12. Gerbal A, Homberg JC, Rochant H, Perron L, Salmon C: The auto-antibodies of acquired hemolytic anemias. II. Nature, specificity, clinical interest and mechanism of formation. Nouv Rev Fr Hematol 1968;8:351–368.
13. Dacie JV, Worlledge SM: Auto-immune hemolytic anemias. In Brown EB, Moore CV (eds): Progression in Hematology. New York: Grune & Stratton, 1969:82–120.
14. Garratty G, Petz LD: The significance of red cell bound complement components in development of standards and quality assurance for the anti-complement components of antiglobulin sera. Transfusion 1976;16:297–306.
15. Petz LD, Garratty G: Complement in immunohematology. Prog Clin Immunol 1974;2:175–190.
16. Kerr RO, Dalmasso AP, Kaplan ME: Erythrocyte-bound C5 and C6 in autoimmune hemolytic anemia. J Immunol 1971;107:1209–1210.
17. Salama A, Bhakdi S, Mueller-Eckhardt C, et al: Deposition of the terminal C5b-9 complement complex on erythrocytes by human red cell autoantibodies. Br J Haematol 1983;55:161–169.
18. Salama A, Bhakdi S, Mueller-Eckhardt C: Evidence suggesting the occurrence of C3-independent intravascular immune hemolysis. Transfusion 1987;27:49–53.
19. Hsu TC, Rosenfield RE, Burkart P, Wong KY, Kochwa S: Instrumented PVP-augmented antiglobulin tests. II. Evaluation of acquired hemolytic anemia. Vox Sang 1974;26:305–325.
20. Garratty G, Petz LD: An evaluation of commercial antiglobulin sera with particular reference to their anticomplement properties. Transfusion 1971;11:79–88.
21. Garratty G: Autoimmune hemolytic anemia. In Garratty G (ed): Immunobiology of transfusion medicine. New York: Dekker, 1994:493–521.
22. Arndt P, Garratty G: Use of flow cytometry for detection of IgM on RBCs showing spontaneous agglutination (abstr). Transfusion 1994;34:68S.
23. Garratty G, Arndt P, Domen R, et al: Severe autoimmune hemolytic anemia associated with IgM warm autoantibodies directed against determinants on or associated with glycophorin A. Vox Sang 1997;72:124–130.
24. Garratty G, Arndt P, Leger R: Serological findings in autoimmune hemolytic anemia associated with IgM warm autoantibodies (abstr). Blood 2001;98:61a.
25. Talano J-AM, Johnson ST, Friedman KD, et al: Serologic characteristics of three cases of IgA mediated autoimmune hemolytic anemia (AIHA) confirmed by flow cytometry (abstr). Blood 2002;100:283a.
26. Merry AH, Thomson EE, Rawlinson VI, Stratton F: Quantitation of IgG on Erythrocytes: Correlation of number of IgG

molecules per cell with the strength of the direct and indirect antiglobulin tests. Vox Sang 1984;47:73–81.
27. Hazlehurst DD, Hudson G, Sokol RJ: A quantitative ELISA for measuring red cell-bound immunoglobulins. Acta Haematol 1996;95:112–116.
28. Kumpel BM: A simple nonisotopic method for the quantitation of red cell-bound immunoglobulin. Vox Sang 1990;59:34–38.
29. Garratty G, Nance SJ: Correlation between in vivo hemolysis and the amount of red cell-bound IgG measured by flow cytometry. Transfusion 1990;30:617–621.
30. Dubarry M, Charron C, Habibi B, Bretagne Y, Lambin P: Quantitation of immunoglobulin classes and subclasses of autoantibodies bound to red cells in patients with and without hemolysis. Transfusion 1993;33:466–471.
31. Jeje MO, Blajchman MA, Steeves K, et al: Quantitation of red cell-associated IgG using an immunoradiometric assay. Transfusion 1984;24:473–476.
32. Chaplin H, Nasongkla M, Monroe MC: Quantitation of red blood cell-bound C3d in normal subjects and random hospitalized patients. Br J Haematol 1981;48:69–78.
33. Chaplin H Jr: Clinical usefulness of specific antiglobulin reagents in autoimmune hemolytic anemias. Progr Hematol 1973;8:25–49.
34. Chaplin H, Avioli LV: Grand rounds: Autoimmune hemolytic anemia. Arch Intern Med 1977;137:346–351.
35. Fischer JT, Petz LD, Garratty G, Cooper NR: Correlations between quantitative assay of red cell-bound C3, serologic reactions, and hemolytic anemia. Blood 1974;44:359–373.
36. Rosse WF: Quantitative immunology of immune hemolytic anemia. I. The fixation of C1 by autoimmune antibody and heterologous anti-IgG antibody. J Clin Invest 19791;50:727–733.
37. Rosse WF: Quantitative immunology of immune hemolytic anemia. II. The relationship of cell-bound antibody to hemolysis and the effect of treatment. J Clin Invest 1971;50:734.
38. Worlledge SM, Blajchman MA: The autoimmune haemolytic anaemias. Br J Haematol 1972;23(Suppl.):61.
39. Sokol RJ, Hewitt S, Stamps BK: Autoimmune haemolysis: An 18-year study of 865 cases referred to a regional transfusion centre. Br Med J (Clin Res Ed) 1981;282:2023–2027.
40. Lalezari P, Louie JE, Fadlallah N: Serologic profile of alphamethyldopa-induced hemolytic anemia: Correlation between cell-bound IgM and hemolysis. Blood 1982;59:61–68.
41. Ben Izhak C, Shechter Y, Tatarsky I: Significance of multiple types of antibodies on red blood cells of patients with positive direct antiglobulin test: A study of monospecific antiglobulin reactions in 85 patients. Scand J Haematol 1985;35:102–108.
42. Sokol RJ, Hewitt S, Booker DJ, et al: Enzyme linked direct antiglobulin test in patients with autoimmune haemolysis. J Clin Pathol 1985;38:912–914.
43. Sokol RJ, Hewitt S, Booker DJ, Bailey A: Red cell autoantibodies, multiple immunoglobulin classes, and autoimmune hemolysis. Transfusion 1990;30:714–717.
44. Gottsche B, Salama A, Mueller-Eckhardt C: Donath-Landsteiner autoimmune hemolytic anemia in children: A study of 22 cases. Vox Sang 1990;58:281–286.
45. Arndt PA, Leger RM, Garratty G: Serology of antibodies to second- and third-generation cephalosporins associated with immune hemolytic anemia and/or positive direct antiglobulin tests. Transfusion 1999;39:1239–1246.
46. Budman DR, Steinberg AD: Hematologic aspects of systemic lupus erythematosus: Current concepts. Ann Intern Med 1977;86:220–229.
47. Mongan ES, Leddy JP, Atwater EC, Barnett EV: Direct antiglobulin (Coombs) reactions in patients with connective tissue diseases. Arthritis Rheum 1967;10:502–508.
48. von dem Borne AEG Jr, Engelfriet CP, Beckers D, et al: Autoimmune haemolytic anaemias. II. Warm haemolysins–serological and immunochemical investigations and ^{51}Cr studies. Clin Exp Immunol 1969;4:333–343.
49. Nance S, Garratty G: Subclass of IgG on red cells of donors and patients with positive direct antiglobulin tests (abstr). Transfusion 1983;23:413.
50. Garratty G: Factors affecting the pathogenicity of red cell auto- and alloantibodies. In Nance SJ (ed): Immune Destruction of Red Blood Cells. Arlington, VA: American Association of Blood Banks, 1989:109–169.
51. Dacie JV: Autoimmune hemolytic anemia. Arch Intern Med 1975;135:1293–1300.
52. Engelfriet CP, von dem Borne AEG, Beckers D, et al: Immune destruction of red cells. In Bell CA (ed): A Seminar on Immune-Mediated Cell Destruction. Washington, DC: American Association of Blood Banks, 1981:93–130.
53. Engelfriet CP, Overbeeke MA, dem Borne AE: Autoimmune hemolytic anemia. Semin Hematol 1992;29:3–12.
54. Sokol RJ, Hewitt S, Booker DJ, et al: Erythrocyte autoantibodies, subclasses of IgG and autoimmune haemolysis. Autoimmunity 1990;6:99–104.
55. Dubarry M, Charron C, Habibi B, et al: Quantitation of immunoglobulin classes and subclasses of autoantibodies bound to red cells in patients with and without hemolysis. Transfusion 1993;33:466–471.
56. Lynen R, Krone O, Legler TJ, et al: A newly developed gel centrifugation test for quantification of RBC-bound IgG antibodies and their subclasses IgG1 and IgG3: Comparison with flow cytometry. Transfusion 2002;42:612–618.
57. Salama A, Mueller-Eckhardt C: Autoimmune haemolytic anaemia in childhood associated with noncomplement binding IgM autoantibodies. Br J Haematol 1987;65:67–71.
58. Sokol RJ, Booker DJ, Stamps R: Autoimmune hemolytic anemia caused by warm-reacting IgM-class antibodies. Immunochemistry 1998;14:53–58.
59. Freedman J, Newlands M, Johnson CA: Warm IgM anti-IT causing autoimmune haemolytic anaemia. Vox Sang 1977;32:135–142.
60. Freedman J, Wright J, Lim FC, et al: Hemolytic warm IgM autoagglutinins in autoimmune hemolytic anemia. Transfusion 1987;27:464–467.
61. Wolf MW, Roelcke D: Incomplete warm hemolysins. I. Case reports, serology, and immunoglobulin classes. Clin Immunol Immunopathol 1989;51:55–67.
62. Araguas C, Martin-Vega C, Massague I, de Latorre FJ: "Complete" warm hemolysins producing an autoimmune hemolytic anemia. Vox Sang 1990;59:125–126.
63. Hamilton T, Hoffer J, Reid ME, et al: Transient IgM autoantibody with apparent anti-c specificity (abstr). Transfusion 1993;33:545.
64. Garratty G, Arndt P, Tsuneta R: Fatal hemolytic anemia associated with antoanti-N (abstr). Transfusion 1994;34:205.
65. Friedmann AM, King KE, Shirey RS, et al: Fatal autoimmune hemolytic anemia in a child due to warm-reactive immunoglobulin M antibody. J Pediatr Hematol Oncol 1998;20:502–505.
66. Sererat T, Veidt D, Arndt P, et al: Warm autoimmune hemolytic anemia associated with an IgM autoanti-Ge. Immunochemistry 1998;14:26–29.
67. Nowak-Wegrzyn A, King KE, Shirey RS, Chen AR, McDonough C, Lederman HM: Fatal warm autoimmune hemolytic anemia resulting from IgM autoagglutinins in an infant with severe combined immunodeficiency. J Pediatr Hematol Oncol 2001;23:250–252.
68. Dorner IM, Parker CW, Chaplin H Jr: Autoagglutination developing in a patient with acute renal failure: Characterization of the autoagglutinin and its relation to transfusion therapy. Br J Haematol 1968;14:383–394.
69. Ellis JP, Sokol RJ: Detection of IgM autoantibodies in eluates from red blood cells. Clin Lab Haematol 1990;12:9–15.
70. Brunt D, Greenfield T, Simon K, et al: An auto anti-En^a mimicking an allo anti-En^a associated with pure red cell aplasia (abstr). Transfusion 1983;23:408.
71. von dem Borne AEG Kr, Engelfriet CP, Reynierse E, Beckers D, van Loghem JJ: Autoimmune haemolytic anaemia. VI. 51 Chromium survival studies in patients with different kinds of warm autoantibodies. Clin Exp Immunol 1973;13:561–571.
72. Wolf MW, Roelcke D: Incomplete warm hemolysins. II. Corresponding antigens and pathogenetic mechanisms in

autoimmune hemolytic anemias induced by incomplete warm hemolysins. Clin Immunol Immunopathol 1989;51:68–76.
73. Shirey RS, Kickler TS, Bell W, Little B, Smith B, Ness PM: Fatal immune hemolytic anemia and hepatic failure associated with a warm-reacting IgM autoantibody. Vox Sang 1987;52:219–222.
74. Dankbar DT, Pierce SR, Issitt PD, et al: Fatal intravascular hemolysis associated with autoanti-Wrb (abstr). Transfusion 1987;27:534.
75. McCann EL, Shirey RS, Kickler TS, Ness PM: IgM autoagglutinins in warm autoimmune hemolytic anemia: A poor prognostic feature. Acta Haematol 1992;88:120–125.
76. Brain MC, Prevost JM, Pihl CE, Brown CB: Glycophorin A-mediated haemolysis of normal human erythrocytes: Evidence for antigen aggregation in the pathogenesis of immune haemolysis. Br J Haematol 2002;118:899–908.
77. Vos GH, Petz LD, Fudenberg HH: Specificity and immunoglobulin characteristics of autoantibodies in acquired hemolytic anemia. J Immunol 1971;106:1172–1176.
78. Sokol RJ, Hewitt S, Booker DJ, et al: Small quantities of erythrocyte bound immunoglobulins and autoimmune haemolysis. J Clin Pathol 1987;40:254–257.
79. Sokol RJ, Hewitt S, Booker DJ, et al: Enzyme linked direct antiglobulin tests in patients with autoimmune haemolysis. J Clin Pathol 1985;38:912–914.
80. Garratty G, Postoway N, Nance S, Arndt P: Detection of IgG on red cells of patients with suspected direct antiglobulin test negative autoimmune hemolytic anemia (AIHA). Book of Abstracts of the ISBT/AABB Joint Congress, 87. 1990 (abstr).
81. Postoway N, Anstee DJ, Wortman M, Garratty G: A severe transfusion reaction associated with anti-EnaTS in a patient with an abnormal alpha-like red cell sialoglycoprotein. Transfusion 1988;28:77–80.
82. Reid ME: Autoagglutination dispersal utilizing sulphydryl compounds. Transfusion 1978;18:353–355.
83. Hattersley PG, Gerard PW, Caggiano V, Nash DR: Erroneous values on the Model S Coulter Counter due to high titer cold autoagglutinins. Am J Clin Pathol 1971;55:442–446.
84. Petrucci JV, Dunne PA, Chapman CC: Spurious erythrocyte indices as measured by the model S Coulter counter due to cold agglutinins. Am J Clin Pathol 1971;56:500–502.
85. DeLange JA, Eernisse GJ, Veltkamp JJ: Cold agglutinins and the Coulter Counter Model S. Am J Clin Pathol 1972; 58:599–600.
86. Lawrence C, Zozicky O: Spurious red-cell values with the Coulter Counter. N Engl J Med 1983;309:925–926.
87. Garratty G, Petz LD, Hoops JK: The correlation of cold agglutinin titrations in saline and albumin with haemolytic anaemia. Br J Haemat 1977;35:587–595.
88. Haynes CR, Chaplin H Jr: An enhancing effect of albumin on the determination of cold hemagglutinins. Vox Sang 1971;20: 46–54.
89. Isbister JP, Cooper DA, Blake M, et al: Lymphoproliferative disease with IgM Lambda monoclonal protein and autoimmune hemolytic anemia. Am J Med 1978;64:434–440.
90. Sniecinski I, Margolin K, Shulman I, Oien L, Meyer E, Branch DR: High-titer, high-thermal-amplitude cold autoagglutinin not associated with hemolytic anemia. Vox Sang 1988;55:26–29.
91. Arndt P, Do G, Garratty G, Kuriyan M, Strair R: A high titer, high thermal amplitude auto anti-B associated with acrocyanosis but no obvious hemolytic anemia. Transfusion 2003; 43:1133–1137.
92. Sokol RJ, Booker DJ, Stamps R, et al: Cold haemagglutinin disease: clinical significance of serum hemolysins. Clin Lab Haematol 2000;22:337–344.
93. Harboe M, Lind K: Light chain type of transiently occurring cold haemagglutinins. Scand J Haematol 1966;3:269.
94. Harboe M, Furth R, van Schubothe H, et al: Exclusive occurrence of κ-chains in isolated cold agglutinins. Scand J Haematol 1965;2:259.
95. Cooper AG, Worlledge SM: Light chains in chronic cold hemagglutinin disease. Nature 1967;214:799.
96. Feizi T: Lambda chains in cold agglutinins. Science 1967; 156:1111.
97. Capra JP, Kehoe JM, Williams RC Jr, et al: Light chain sequences of human IgM cold agglutinins. Proc Natl Acad Sci USA 1972;69:40.
98. Cooper AG, Chavin SI, Franklin FC: Predominance of a single mu chain subclass in cold agglutinin heavy chains. Immunochemistry 1970;7:479.
99. Edman P, Cooper AG: Amino acid sequence at the N-terminal end of a cold agglutinin kappa chain. Fed Eur Biochem Soc Lett 1968;2:33.
100. Cohen S, Cooper AG: Chemical differences between individual cold agglutinins. Immunology 1968;15:93.
101. Williams RC Jr: Cold agglutinins: studies of primary structure, serologic activity, and antigenic uniqueness. Ann NY Acad Sci 1971;190:330.
102. Jacobson LB, Longstreth GF: Clinical and immunologic features of transient cold agglutinin hemolytic anemia. Am J Med 1973;54:514.
103. Gergely J, Wang AC, Fudenberg HH: Chemical analyses of variable regions of heavy and light chains of cold agglutinins. Vox Sang 1973;24:432–440.
104. Pascual V, Victor K, Lesz D, et al: Nucleotide sequence analysis of the V regions of two IgM cold agglutinins. J Immunol 1991;146:4386.
105. Silverman GJ, Carson DA: Structural characterization of human monoclonal cold agglutinins: Evidence for a distinct primary sequence-defined VH4 idiotype. Eur J Immunol 1990;20:351.
106. Silberstein LE, Jefferies LC, Goldman J, et al: Variable region gene analysis of pathologic human autoantibodies to the related i and I red blood cell antigens. Blood 1991;78:2372.
107. Silberstein LE: B-Cell Origin of Cold Agglutinins. In Atassi MZ (ed): Immunobiology of Proteins and Peptides VII. New York: Plenum Press, 1994:193–205.
108. Potter KN: Molecular characterization of cold agglutinins. Transfus Sci 2000;22:113–119.
109. Rosse WF, Adams JP: The variability of hemolysis in the cold agglutinin syndrome. Blood 1980;56:409–416.
110. Schreiber AD, Herskovitz BS, Goldwein M: Low-titer cold-hemagglutinin disease: Mechanism of hemolysis and response to corticosteroids. N Engl J Med 1977;296:1490–1494.
111. Jefferies LC, Carchidi CM, Silberstein LE: Naturally occurring anti-i/I cold agglutinins may be encoded by different VH3 genes as well as the VH4.21 gene segment. J Clin Invest 1993;92:2821–2833.
112. Schutte ME, van Es JH, Silberstein LE, Logtenberg T: VH4.21-encoded natural autoantibodies with anti-i specificity mirror those associated with cold hemagglutinin disease. J Immunol 1993;151:6569–6576.
113. Pascual V, Victor K, Randen I, et al: Nucleotide sequence analysis of rheumatoid factors and polyreactive antibodies derived from patients with rheumatoid arthritis reveals diverse use of VH and VL gene segments and extensive variability in CDR-3. Scand J Immunol 1992;36:349–362.
114. Pascual V, Victor K, Spellerberg M, Hamblin TJ, Stevenson FK, Capra JD: VH restriction among human cold agglutinins: The VH4-21 gene segment is required to encode anti-I and anti-i specificities. J Immunol 1992;149:2337–2344.
115. Leoni J, Ghiso J, Goni F, Frangione B: The primary structure of the Fab fragment of protein KAU, a monoclonal immunoglobulin M cold agglutinin. J Biol Chem 1991;266:2836–2842.
116. Grillot-Courvalin C, Brouet JC, Piller F, et al: An anti-B cell autoantibody from Wiskott-Aldrich syndrome which recognizes i blood group specificity on normal human B cells. Eur J Immunol 1992;22:1781–1788.
117. Poldre P, Pruzanski W, Chiu HM, et al: Fulminant gangrene in transient cold agglutinemia associated with *Escherichi coli* infection. Can Med Assoc J 1985;132:261–263.
118. Crisp D, Pruzanski W: B-cell neoplasms with homogeneous cold-reacting antibodies (cold agglutinins). Am J Med 1982;72:915–922.
119. Pruzanski W, Cowan PH, Parr DM: Clinical and immunochemical studies of IgM cold agglutinins with lambda type light chains. Clin Immunol Immunopathol 1974;2:234–245.

120. Ferriman DG, Dacie JV, Keele KD, et al: The association of Raynaud's phenomena, chronic haemolytic anaemia, and the formation of cold antibodies. Quart J Med 1951;20:275.
121. Rorvik K: The syndrome of high-titre cold haemagglutination; a survey and a case report. Acta Med Scand 1954; 148:299.
122. Gaddy CG, Powell LW: Raynaud's syndrome associated with idiopathic cryoglobulinemia and cold agglutinins: Report of a case and discussion of classification of cryoglobulinemia. Arch Intern Med 1958;102:468.
123. Umlas J, Kaufman M, MacQueston C, et al: A cryoglobulin with cold agglutinin and erythroid stem cell suppressant properties. Transfusion 1991;31:361–364.
124. Pruzanski W, Shumak KH: Biologic activity of cold-reacting autoantibodies (first of two parts). N Engl J Med 1977; 297:538–542.
125. Harboe M: Cold auto-agglutinins. Vox Sang 1971;20:289–305.
126. Ritzman SE, Levin WC: Cold agglutinin disease: A type of primary macroglobulinemia: A new concept. Tex Rep Biol Med 1962;20:236.
127. Firkin BG, Blackwell JB, Johnston GA: Essential cryoglobulinaemia and acquired haemolytic anaemia due to cold agglutinins. Aust Ann Med 1959;8:151.
128. Schubothe H: The cold hemagglutinin disease. Semin Hematol 1966;3:27.
129. Crisp D, Pruzanski W: B-cell neoplasms with homogeneous cold-reacting antibodies (cold agglutinins). Am J Med 1982;72:915–922.
130. Ratkin GA, Osterland CK, Chaplin H Jr: IgG, IgA, and IgM cold-reactive immunoglobulins in 19 patients with elevated cold agglutinins. J Lab Clin Med 1973;82:67–78.
131. Dellagi K, Brouet JC, Schenmetzler C, Praloran V: Chronic hemolytic anemia due to a monoclonal IgG cold agglutinin with anti-Pr specificity. Blood 1981;57:189–191.
132. Silberstein LE, Berkman EM, Schreiber AD: Cold hemagglutinin disease associated with IgG cold-reactive antibody. Ann Intern Med 1987;106:238–242.
133. Roelcke D, Anstee DJ, Jungfer H, Nutzenadel W, Webb AJ: IgG-type cold agglutinins in children and corresponding antigens: Detection of a new Pr antigen: Pra. Vox Sang 1971;20: 218–229.
134. Mygind K, Ahrons S: IgG cold agglutinins and first trimester abortion. Vox Sang 1972;23:552–560.
135. Moore JA, Chaplin H Jr: Autoimmune hemolytic anemia associated with an IgG cold incomplete antibody. Vox Sang 1973;24:236–245.
136. Freedman J, Newlands M: Autoimmune haemolytic anaemia with the unusual combination of both IgM and IgG autoantibodies. Vox Sang 1977;32:61–68.
137. Silberstein LE, Shoenfeld Y, Schwartz RS, Berkman EM: A combination of IgG and IgM autoantibodies in chronic cold agglutinin disease: Immunologic studies and response to splenectomy. Vox Sang 1985;48:105–109.
138. Szymanski IO, Teno R, Rybak ME: Hemolytic anemia due to a mixture of low-titer IgG lambda and IgM lambda agglutinins reacting optimally at 22°C. Vox Sang 1986;51: 112–116.
139. Curtis BR, Lamon J, Roelcke D, Chaplin H: Life-threatening, antiglobulin test-negative, acute autoimmune hemolytic anemia due to a noncomplement-activating IgG1 kappa cold antibody with Pra specificity. Transfusion 1990;30:838–843.
140. Goldberg LS, Barnett EV: Mixed gamma G-gamma M cold agglutinin. J Immunol 1967;99:803–809.
141. Ambrus M, Bajtai G: A case of an IgG-type cold agglutinin disease. Haematologia 1969;3:225–235.
142. Angevine CD, Anderson BR, Barnett EV: A cold agglutinin of the IgA class. J Immunol 1966;96:578.
143. Garratty G, Petz LD, Brodsky I, et al: An IgA high-titer cold agglutinin with an unusual blood group specificity within the Pr complex. Vox Sang 1973;25:32–38.
144. Roelcke D, Dorow W: Besonderheiten der Reaktionswerte eines mit Plasmocytom-gA-Paraprotein identischen Kälteagglutinins. Klin Wschr 1968;46:126.
145. Roelcke D: Serological studies on the Pr1/Pra antigens using dog erythrocytes: Differentiation of Pra from Pr1 and detection of a Pr1 heterogeneity: Pr1h/Pr1d. Vox Sang 1973;24:354.
146. Roelcke D: Specificity of IgA cold agglutinins: Anti-Pr1. Eur J Immunol 1973;3:206–212.
147. Roelcke D, Hack H, Kreft H, et al: IgA cold agglutinins recognize Pr and Sa antigens expressed on glycophorins. Transfusion 1993;33:472–475.
148. Tschirhart DL, Kunkel L, Shulman IA: Immune hemolytic anemia associated with biclonal cold autoagglutinins. Vox Sang 1990;59:222–226.
149. Moake JL, Schultz DR: Hemolytic anemia associated with multiple alloantibodies and low serum complement. Am J Med 1975;58:431–437.
150. Crookston JH: Hemolytic anemia with IgG and IgM autoantibodies and alloantibodies. Arch Intern Med 1975;135:1314–1315.
151. Freedman J, Lim FC, Musclow E, et al: Autoimmune haemolytic anaemia with concurrence of warm and cold red cell autoantibodies and a warm hemolysin. Transfusion 1985;25:368–372.
152. Kajii E, Miura Y, Ikemoto S: Characterization of autoantibodies in mixed-typed autoimmune hemolytic anemia. Vox Sang 1991;60:45–52.
153. Patten E, Reuter FP: Evan's syndrome: possible benefit from plasma exchange. Transfusion 1980;20:589–593.
154. Shulman IA, Branch DR, Nelson JM, et al: Autoimmune hemolytic anemia with both cold and warm autoantibodies. JAMA 1985;253:1746–1748.
155. Sokol RJ, Hewitt S, Stamps BK: Autoimmune haemolysis: mixed warm and cold antibody type. Acta Haematol 1983; 69:266–274.
156. Ries CA, Garratty G, Petz LD, et al: Paroxysmal cold hemoglobinuria: Report of a case with an exceptionally high thermal range Donath-Landsteiner antibody. Blood 1971;38:491–499.
157. Lindgren S, Zimmerman S, Gibbs F, Garratty G: An unusual Donath-Landsteiner antibody detectable at 37°C by the antiglobulin test. Transfusion 1985;25:142–144.
158. Nordhagen R: Two cases of paroxysmal cold hemoglobinuria with a Donath-Landsteiner antibody reactive by the indirect antiglobulin test using anti-IgG. Transfusion 1991;31:190–191.
159. Sokol RJ, Booker DJ, Stamps R: Erythropoiesis: paroxysmal cold haemoglobinuria: A clinico-pathological study of patients with a positive Donath-Landsteiner test. Hematology 1999;4:137–164.
160. Bird GW, Wingham J, Martin AJ, et al: Idiopathic nonsyphilitic paroxysmal cold haemoglobinuria in children. J Clin Pathol 1976;29:215–218.
161. Vogel JM, Hellman M, Moloshok RE: Paroxysmal cold hemoglobinuria of nonsyphilitic etiology in two children. J Pediatr 1972;81:974–977.
162. Bell CA, Zwicker H, Rosenbaum DL: Paroxysmal cold hemoglobinuria (P.C.H.) following mycoplasma infection: Anti-I specificity of the biphasic hemolysin. Transfusion 1973;13: 138–141.
163. Nakamura H, Watanabe T, Hayashida T, Ichimaru M: Donath-Landsteiner antibody of the IgM class with anti-I specificity and possible efficacy of azathioprine therapy in paroxysmal cold hemoglobinuria: A case report. Rinsho Ketsueki 1990;31:1548–1552.
164. Green ES, Dvenish A, Bradshaw HH, Davis SG, England JM, Contreras M: Chronic haemolysis caused by an unusual Donath-Landsteiner-like (DL) antibody associated with non-Hodgkin's lymphoma (NHL). Transfusion Med 1990;1 (Suppl. 1):15.
165. Engelfriet CP, Beckers D, von dem Borne AE, et al: Haemolysins probably recognizing the antigen p. Vox Sang 1972;23:176–181.
166. Judd WJ, Wilkinson SL, Issitt PD, et al: Donath-Landsteiner hemolytic anemia due to an anti-Pr-like biphasic hemolysin. Transfusion 1986;26:423–425.
167. Shirey RS, Park K, Ness PM, et al: An anti-i biphasic hemolysin in chronic paroxysmal cold hemoglobinuria. Transfusion 1986;26:62–64.

168. Bell CA, Zwicker H: Donath-Landsteiner hemolysin with anti-HI specificity. Transfusion 1967;7:384.
169. Sabio H, Jones D, McKie VC: Biphasic hemolysin hemolytic anemia: Reappraisal of an acute immune hemolytic anemia of infancy and childhood. Am J Hematol 1992;39:220–222.
170. Lau P, Sererat S, Moore V, et al: Paroxysmal cold hemoglobinuria in a patient with Klebsiella pneumonia. Vox Sang 1983; 44:167–172.
171. Ramos RR, Curtis BR, Eby CS, et al: Fatal autoimmune hemolytic anemia (AHA) associated with IgM bi-thermic anti-P and cold IT. Joint Congress of the International Society of Blood Transfusion and the American Association of Blood Banks Book of Abstracts. S341. 1990.
172. Zamora C, Hernandez-Jorda M, Herrero S, et al: Donath-Landsteiner antibody detectable at 37°C by the antiglobulin test in a HIV+ patient. Transfusion Med 1998;8:278.
173. Lippman SM, Winn L, Grumet FC, et al: Evans' syndrome as a presenting manifestation of atypical paroxysmal cold hemoglobinuria. Am J Med 1987;82:1065–1072.
174. Bastrup-Madsen P, Petersen SH: Monoclonal gammapathy with the M-component behaving like Donath-Landsteiner haemolysin. Scand J Haematol 1971;8:81–85.
175. von dem Borne AE, Mol JJ, Joustra-Maas N, et al: Autoimmune haemolytic anaemia with monoclonal IgM (kappa) anti-P cold autohaemolysins. Br J Haematol 1982;50:345–350.
176. Judd WJ: A pH-dependent auto-agglutinin with anti-P specificity. Transfusion 1975;15:373–376.
177. Judd WJ, Steiner EA, Capps RD: Autoagglutinins with apparent anti-P specificity reactive only by low-ionic-strength salt techniques. Transfusion 1982;22:185–188.
178. Mensinger E, Lerner W, Leger R, et al: Serological profile associated with a fatal case of paroxysmal cold hemoglobinuria (abstr). Transfusion 1995;35:21S.

CHAPTER 6

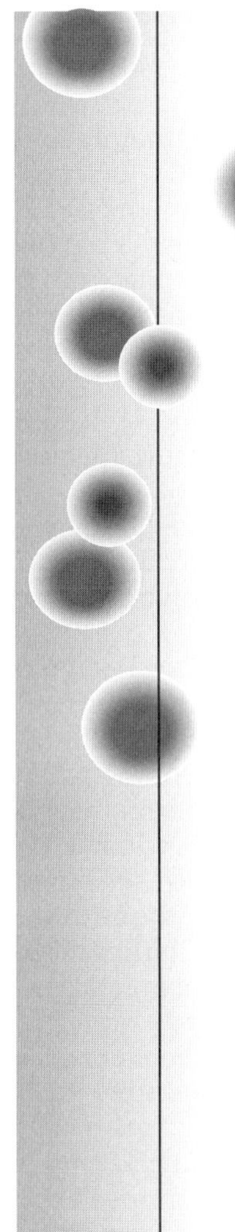

The Serologic Investigation of Autoimmune Hemolytic Anemia

In this chapter, we review the laboratory tests that are of value in the diagnosis of autoimmune hemolytic anemia (AIHA). The rationale for performance of the tests and the interpretation of the results are discussed briefly, and the methods are described in detail. Each of these tests has a place in the diagnostic evaluation of at least some patients with acquired hemolytic anemia, but some of the procedures described in this chapter are indicated only infrequently. Information in this chapter serves as an extension of the discussion in Chapter 5 of the differential diagnosis of the AIHAs. In Chapter 5, no technical details are given, but instead a more detailed narrative description of the step-by-step approach to diagnosis is presented. Additional technical procedures that are relevant to the investigation of drug-induced immune hemolytic anemia and compatibility testing are described in Chapters 8 and 10, respectively.

The AIHAs can be classified into three main groups: (1) those associated with warm autoantibodies (i.e., optimally reactive at 37°C); (2) those associated with cold agglutinins (optimally reactive at 0°C to 4°C, but with a wide thermal range); and (3) those associated with a biphasic cold hemolysin, the Donath-Landsteiner antibody (i.e., paroxysmal cold hemoglobinuria [PCH]). The diagnosis of the specific type of AIHA is made by determining the in vitro characteristics of the autoantibody. Often, the differential diagnosis can be achieved in the laboratory by simple extensions of tests that are used every day in the blood bank. The majority of cases of AIHA can be correctly diagnosed simply by taking into account the clinical findings, the direct antiglobulin test (DAT) using anti-IgG and anti-C3 (containing anti-C3d,g or C3d), a cold agglutinin titer, and a simple antibody screening procedure using careful technique (e.g., strict control of incubation temperatures). However, such abbreviated evaluations lead to a surprising number of misinterpretations and erroneous diagnoses. Therefore, when we encounter a case of hemolytic anemia suspected of having an immune basis, we prefer, as a routine, to perform a panel of screening tests and then to perform more specific tests to develop a more confident diagnosis.

Red cell autoantibodies, like alloantibodies, are usually IgM or IgG; on occasion they may be IgA. In vitro, the IgM antibodies will usually directly agglutinate saline-suspended red blood cells (RBCs) (e.g., the IgM anti-I associated with cold agglutinin syndrome [CAS]); often they will hemolyze RBCs if the conditions are right. For instance, one may have to use enzyme-treated RBCs and/or add fresh complement to demonstrate the lysis. IgG autoantibodies do not often cause direct agglutination of saline-suspended normal RBCs but almost always agglutinate enzyme-treated RBCs or agglutinate untreated RBCs when potentiators (e.g., polyethylene glycol) are present. IgG autoantibodies rarely cause in vitro lysis of RBCs (the IgG auto anti-P biphasic hemolysin, associated with PCH, is an exception) but often sensitize RBCs and can be detected by the antiglobulin test (AGT).

THE ANTIGLOBULIN TEST

In 1945, Coombs and coworkers[1] demonstrated the presence of nonagglutinating Rh alloantibodies (the "incomplete" or "sensitizing" antibodies) in sera, by the antiglobulin reaction.

Principles of the Antiglobulin Test

Red cell autoantibodies and alloantibodies are gamma globulins, usually IgM or IgG. If they are IgM, they usually directly agglutinate saline-suspended RBCs. In contrast, IgG antibodies often do not agglutinate RBCs but react with the corresponding antigens on the RBC membrane, giving a "sensitized" RBC. Thus, chemically speaking, the RBCs are sensitized with gamma globulin.

Coombs and coworkers[1] postulated that if a rabbit was injected with human gamma globulin, the rabbit would form antibodies to the foreign protein, that is, anti-human globulin (AHG). This antiglobulin serum (AGS) after suitable processing (e.g., adsorption of heterophil antibodies) would react specifically with human globulin. More recently, monoclonal AGS that does not contain heterophil antibodies is being used. Thus, if the human globulin, in the form of antibody, is attached to the RBC membrane, the AHG will combine with it, crosslinking the sensitized RBCs and causing agglutination (Fig. 6-1).

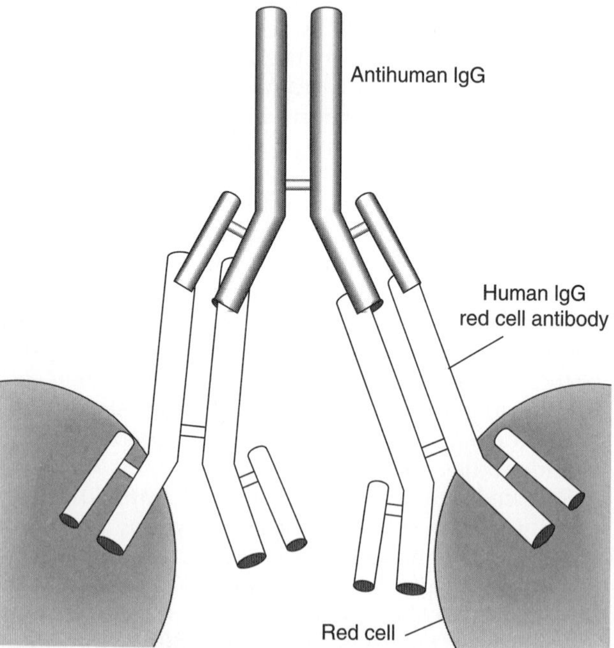

FIGURE 6-1. The antiglobulin test. Antihuman IgG in the antiglobulin serum reacts with red cell bound IgG antibody, which causes the development of a lattice formation and agglutination. Although the reaction is illustrated with IgG-sensitized cells, similar reactions can occur with red cells coated with other proteins (e.g., complement components), provided that appropriate antibodies are present in the antihuman serum.

As shown in Figure 6-1, anti-IgG reacts mainly with the Fc portion (i.e., heavy chains) of human IgG molecules. Antibodies to light chains may be present in polyclonal AGS as well; in a polyspecific AHG, this has no disadvantages and theoretically may be an advantage by forming extra "bridges" across adjacent light chains. In a monospecific anti-IgG, the presence of antibodies to light chains can lead to false-positive results because light chains are shared by IgG, IgM, and IgA; only the heavy chains are specific for each class.

In 1946, Boorman and coworkers[2] and Loutit and Mollison[3] reported that the RBCs from a number of patients with idiopathic acquired hemolytic anemia reacted with AHG. The first application of the test (i.e., detection of Rh antibodies in serum)[1] became known as the indirect antiglobulin test (IAT), and the second application (i.e., detection of in vivo sensitization)[2,3] became known as the DAT. Table 6-1 shows where these two tests can be applied in immunohematology.

In 1947, Coombs and Mourant[4] showed that the component in AGS that reacted with Rh-sensitized RBCs could be inhibited from reacting by the addition of small amounts of human gamma globulin; alpha and beta globulins did not inhibit the reaction. Dacie[5] reported that RBCs from various patients with AIHA reacted differently in the AGT. Some patients reacted better with high dilutions of the AHG (i.e., exhibited a prozone effect), whereas others reacted better with more concentrated AHG. In addition, the addition of purified gamma globulin to the AHG did not inhibit the reaction of the AHG with the RBCs from some patients. The reactions that could be inhibited appeared to be those associated with warm autoantibodies. In contrast, those not inhibited appeared to be associated with high titer cold autoagglutinins; it was

TABLE 6-1. USES OF THE ANTIGLOBULIN TEST

A. Direct antiglobulin test; valuable in diagnosis of
   1. Autoimmune hemolytic anemia
   2. Drug-induced immune hemolytic anemia
   3. Hemolytic transfusion reactions due to alloantibodies
   4. Hemolytic disease of the fetus and newborn
B. Indirect antiglobulin test; useful for
   1. Detection of antibodies in serum
      (a) Antibody detection
      (b) Crossmatching
   2. Detection of antibodies in eluates prepared from sensitized RBCs
   3. Determination of specificity of antibodies
   4. Typing of RBCs
      (a) Testing for weak D phenotypes
      (b) Using antiglobulin reactive typing reagents (e.g., anti-Fy^a, anti-Jk^a, etc.)

suggested that the RBCs from such patients were probably sensitized with antibodies that were non–gamma globulins. Further experiments[6] showed that the non–gamma globulin sensitizing the RBCs was not antibody but complement. The role of complement in immunohematology, and the AGT in particular, has been reviewed previously.[7-10]

Some immune hemolytic anemias are caused by immunoglobulins other than IgG. However, IgM sensitization of RBCs is difficult to detect with the AGT[11,12]; furthermore, IgM antibodies that cause immune hemolytic anemia characteristically, if not invariably, fix complement, which is much more readily detected.[13] IgA antibodies only infrequently play a role in RBC sensitization, and in such cases, other immune globulin and/or complement components are almost always, although not invariably, found on the RBC surface as well.[14-16] Thus, it does not seem reasonable to demand standards for manufacturers that would require the presence of anti-IgM and anti-IgA as a component of polyspecific AGS, although we prefer to have them present. Interested workers, especially those in research and reference laboratories, will continue to be concerned about the unusual instances in which they are of use, but such needs can usually be met by the use of monospecific antisera (carefully standardized for use with RBCs) in selected cases.

To summarize, polyspecific AHG used for the investigation of AIHA must contain anti-IgG and anti-C3d (or anti-C3d,g) and may contain antibodies to other C3 determinants (e.g., C3b, C3c) and C4; antibodies to other immunoglobulins (e.g., IgA or IgM) would be a bonus.

Monospecific Antiglobulin Reagents

Although it is reasonable and perhaps most convenient to perform the initial DAT with a polyspecific AHG, it is advisable to perform further tests with monospecific reagents in all patients who have a positive DAT and who have hemolytic anemia. This is true because such testing provides additional information that is helpful in determining the specific type of immune hemolytic anemia that is present.[17,18] For this purpose, the most important reagents are a monospecific anti-IgG and an anti-C3 containing anti-C3d/C3dg activity (which may contain antibodies against other C3 determinants).[7] Such antisera, licensed in the United States by the Food and Drug Administration (FDA) for use in the DAT, are readily available.

In the unusual instance in which a patient is suspected of having an immune hemolytic anemia but has a negative DAT with AGS containing anti-IgG and anti-C3d, the use of anti-IgM and anti-IgA antibodies may be indicated (see Chapter 9). At the present, antisera of such specificities have not been licensed in the United States for use as AGS (i.e., for use with RBCs), but antisera of these specificities that are manufactured for immunologic use can be used after appropriate standardization (see later).

Significance of a Positive DAT

The results of a DAT should reflect what is happening in vivo, not what has occurred in vitro through the use of inappropriate techniques. For instance, the RBCs from refrigerated clots obtained from normal individuals often have a positive DAT; this sometimes also occurs when testing RBCs from patients' clotted samples left at room temperature. This is commonly due to the presence of a naturally occurring cold nonagglutinating autoantibody ("normal incomplete cold" antibody), which has anti-H specificity and binds complement to the RBCs.[13,19] The commonly found low titer anti-I cold autoagglutinin also plays an additional role in autocomplement sensitization at 4°C. Because of this phenomenon, the results of a positive DAT on RBCs from a cooled clotted sample, when using an anti-complement-containing reagent, should never be accepted without confirming the results on either freshly drawn blood kept at 37°C or in EDTA anticoagulant; the EDTA prevents (by binding calcium needed for C1 activation) any in vitro complement binding but does not interfere with any in vivo bound complement.

A positive DAT, even when due to in vivo sensitization, does not necessarily indicate AIHA, or even that an autoantibody has caused the positive DAT.[20,21] Positive DATs can be obtained (even when warm [37°C] blood or EDTA blood is used) because of many causes; some are listed here.

Causes of Positive DAT

1. *Autoantibodies against intrinsic RBC antigens, leading to sensitization of the RBCs with immunoglobulins and/or complement components.* Hemolytic anemia may or may not be present (see later).
2. *Antibodies against drugs attached to RBC membrane (e.g., penicillin) (see Chapter 8).*
3. *RBC-bound immune complexes, or complement bound to "innocent bystander" RBCs by complement activation remote from RBCs (e.g., anti–drug-drug complex) (see Chapters 8 and 9).*
4. *Nonspecific uptake of protein:* From 1% to 15% of random hospital patients and 0.01% to 0.1% of blood donors have been reported to have positive DATs.[20,21] Many of these positive DATs are thought to be due to nonspecific uptake of IgG from the plasma (cytophilic IgG). Several reports indicate that 65% to 80% of RBCs with positive DATs yield nonreactive eluates, suggesting that no RBC antibodies are present on the cell. Toy and coworkers[22] and Heddle and coworkers[23] showed a relationship between positive DATs yielding nonreactive eluates and elevated plasma gamma globulin levels. Sometimes drugs can modify the RBC membrane, leading to the

adsorption of many proteins, including IgG. An example of this is the positive DAT sometimes associated with cephalosporin administration (see Chapter 8). It is also possible that this is the cause of the positive DAT that have been described associated with some bacterial or viral infections.

5. *Hemolytic transfusion reactions (HTRs):* Delayed HTRs can often be very difficult to differentiate serologically from AIHA (see Chapter 9). Alloantibodies present in the recipient can sensitize the transfused donor RBCs, leading to a positive DAT. If the alloantibody(ies) present in the plasma of the donor react with most RBCs (e.g., antibody to a high frequency antigen or a mixture of antibody specificities), they can appear to be autoantibody.
6. *Passive transfer of alloantibody in transfused products*[24]: Alloantibodies may be present in plasma products (e.g., platelets, IVIg), or even donor RBCs. Such antibodies (including ABO antibodies) can sensitize the recipient's RBCs and sometimes cause an HTR.
7. *Hemolytic disease of the newborn:* Maternal antibodies can cross the placenta and sensitize fetal RBCs (see Chapter 13).
8. *High reticulocyte count:* There have been reports indicating that high reticulocyte counts cause false-positive DATs due to anti-transferrin in the AHG.[25,26] We have not found this to be a problem with modern polyclonal reagents, and this will not occur with monoclonal AGS. Similarly, Chaplin[18] and Worlledge[27] have not found this to be a cause of false-positive results in their series.
9. *Polyagglutinable RBCs:* When the T antigen is exposed on the RBC membrane (e.g., by bacterial infection), a false-positive DAT can occur if sufficient anti-T is present in polyclonal (e.g., rabbit) AHG. We have not observed this in commercially available polyclonal AHG, probably because the rabbit serum is diluted considerably or fractionated in the preparation of the AHG. Monoclonal AGS will not contain anti-T.
10. *Silica, derived from glass, and metallic ions, have been described as a cause of false positive DAT.*[28,29] We have not encountered any examples of this.

Causes of False-Negative DATs

1. Poor technique
   a. Insufficient washing of RBCs will enable residual plasma globulin to inhibit the AHG. To control this, known IgG weakly sensitized RBCs *must* be added to every negative test and recorded as positive (i.e., indicating uninhibited AGS to be present in the tube) before the negative test can be accepted as truly negative.
   b. Use of saline or AGS contaminated with human globulin (1 part in 4000 parts of normal plasma/serum is often sufficient to completely inhibit the anti-IgG in an AHG reagent; this can be controlled as given in a).
   c. Resuspending centrifuged RBCs too vigorously may disperse weak agglutination.
2. AGS does not contain appropriate antibody: As mentioned elsewhere, commercial polyspecific AHG may have insufficient anti-C3d,[7,8,11] anti-IgA,[16,30] or anti-IgM[11,16] to detect these proteins sensitizing a patient's RBCs.
3. Low-affinity antibody sensitizing a patient's RBCs. We occasionally encounter patients with RBCs sensitized with autoantibody that does not seem to "fit" very well; that is, it dissociates very easily, even during routine washing of the RBCs for performance of the DAT. It is important to add the AHG to the washed RBCs immediately after washing and to read the AGTs immediately after centrifugation, as these autoantibodies will elute from the RBCs very rapidly after washing. More of the autoantibody is lost from the RBCs when they are washed at 37°C than at room temperature or below, even though the patient has warm-type AIHA. If we suspect this is occurring, we wash the RBCs in ice-cold low ionic strength or normal ionic strength saline with appropriate controls (e.g., after washing, centrifuge 1 vol of 2% to 5% washed RBCs in 2 vol AHG diluent [if available] or 6% albumin in a separate "control" tube, to ensure that the cells are not agglutinated due to cold autoantibodies).[16] We have encountered several patients with acute AIHA whose DATs were negative when the cells were washed at 37°C, 1+ when washed at room temperature, and 3+ when washed in ice cold saline. It has been suggested that IgG serum alloantibodies and autoantibodies that agglutinate *only* enzyme-treated RBCs are of such low affinity that they wash off untreated RBCs during the washing process of the IAT.[31] Such antibodies may be similar in nature to the autoantibodies discussed earlier that have sensitized the patient's RBCs in vivo.
4. RBC-bound IgG autoantibody may be present in too low a concentration to be detected by the AGT. Before a positive AGT is clearly visible, the RBCs usually must be sensitized with 150 to 500 molecules of IgG per RBC.[32-35] Sometimes, more sensitive techniques will show IgG to be present on the RBC (see Chapter 9 for a full discussion).

IgG and Complement on RBCs of DAT-Negative Healthy Individuals

RBC-BOUND IgG

Gilliland and coworkers[34] and Petz and Garratty,[35] using a complement fixation antiglobulin consumption assay, found 35 or fewer IgG molecules per RBC when testing DAT-negative healthy individuals. Investigators in England and Canada came to very similar conclusions using radiolabeled anti-IgG to measure IgG on the RBCs of healthy individuals. Merry and coworkers[36] found the RBC to have 5 to 90 (mean, 39) IgG molecules per RBC, and Jeje and coworkers[37] found 3.7 to 16 fg of IgG/10^3 RBCs, with a mean of 14 fg/10^3 RBCs, or 31 IgG molecules per RBC. Thus, there seems to be no doubt that normal healthy individuals have IgG on their RBCs, but it is still not clear whether it is present on all or only some RBCs, whether the amount varies a great deal from cell to cell, and whether it serves a physiologic role.

The source of RBC-bound IgG in healthy individuals is not clear. Is the IgG representing IgG RBC autoantibody or nonspecifically bound IgG ("cytophilic IgG"), or are both populations present? If either or both are present, are they present on all RBCs or only on a subpopulation (e.g., older RBCs)?

Kay[38] found that RBCs aged in vitro were phagocytosed when they were incubated in autologous or allogeneic IgG and then incubated with autologous macrophages. In vitro aged RBCs incubated in IgM-, IgA-, and IgG-depleted serum or medium were separated, by density, from freshly drawn human blood. Less than 5% of the young cells were phagocytosed, whereas more than 30% of the old cells were phagocytosed, independent of the incubation medium. In further studies, Kay eluted the immunoglobulin from the older RBCs and showed that it was IgG1 and IgG3. The eluted IgG would reattach only to stored autologous or allogeneic RBCs; after treatment, these cells were phagocytosed by autologous macrophages. No phagocytosis occurred with young RBCs incubated in the eluted IgG. Neuraminidase-treated RBCs incubated in medium were not phagocytosed, but after incubation in eluted IgG, they were phagocytosed. Finally, Kay and coworkers showed that the phenomenon was not due to nonspecific binding of IgG, because adsorption of pooled normal IgG with aged RBCs abolished its phagocytosis-inducing activity; receptor blockade studies showed that the IgG was attaching to the RBCs by its Fab portion. The authors suggested that the cell-bound IgG was a physiologic autoantibody contributing to the maintenance of homeostasis by collaborating with macrophages in the removal of senescent and damaged cells.

Several other publications support the hypothesis of Kay and coworkers. Alderman and coworkers[39] reported that 85% to 95% of older RBCs had membrane-bound IgG, whereas no IgG was detected on the younger RBCs. They confirmed the findings of Kay and coworkers that the IgG eluted from older RBCs would combine in vitro with older RBCs but not young cells. They also demonstrated that the eluted IgG would bind to neuraminidase-treated RBCs, suggesting that the antigenic site revealed during enzyme treatment in vitro is similar to that developing during aging in vivo. Szymanski and coworkers[40] used a sensitive automated AGT to confirm the presence of IgG on normal RBCs. They showed that separated young RBCs had less membrane-bound IgG than older cells. Freedman[41] had similar findings using ^{125}I-labeled anti-IgG. Kay[42] suggested that the senescent cell antigen is derived from band 3, probably via degradation, and that oxidation may be involved. Lutz and coworkers[43] suggested that the antigen is a dimer of band 3. Low and coworkers[44] presented evidence that as hemoglobin begins to denature, it forms hemichromes that crosslink band 3 into clusters, and suggested that it is these clusters that provide the recognition site for antibodies directed against the senescent cell antigen.

RBC-BOUND COMPLEMENT

Complement also has been detected on the RBCs of healthy individuals. Using potent anti-C3d reagents and the standard AGT, Graham and coworkers[45] showed that RBCs from most individuals were coated with C3d; other workers have confirmed this. Using the AutoAnalyzer, Rosenfield and Jagathambal[46] reported 5 to 40 C3 molecules per RBC. Using radiolabeled anti-C3, Freedman and Barefoot[47] reported 207 to 427 C3d molecules per RBC; Chaplin and coworkers[48] reported 50 to 160 C3 molecules per RBC, and Merry and coworkers[49] found 280 to 560 C3d molecules per RBC. The differences among these three reports perhaps reflect the specificity of the anti-C3 used (e.g., the proportion of antibody activity directed against various epitopes, such as C3d or C3dg, on the RBC-bound C3).

Freedman[50] showed that older RBCs, separated from fresh blood, had more C3d on their membrane (as well as IgG, IgM, and IgA) than did younger RBCs; they found no increase in C3b, C4d, C5, or factor B. They also quoted unpublished observations that C3b-coated RBCs have 10% to 15% less free sialic acid than uncoated RBCs and suggested that the accumulation of C3 on older RBCs may relate to their removal from the circulation. They did not believe that the complement was on the RBCs as a result of complement activation by IgG autoantibody (i.e., senescent cell antibody), as RBC-bound C4 was not increased on older cells. This would suggest complement activation by the alternative pathway rather than antibody-mediated classic pathway activation. RBC-bound complement has been shown to accumulate on RBCs stored in vitro. It is of some interest that Szymanski and coworkers[51] found that the 24-hour survival of stored RBCs showed a negative correlation with the length of storage and the amount of RBC-bound C3. They suggested that RBC-bound C3 may contribute significantly to the storage lesion of stored RBCs.

There are many reasons why RBCs may have small amounts of complement on their surface, other than as a result of complement activation by RBC autoantibodies and alloantibodies. One reason may relate to the presence of complement receptor (CR1) on RBCs. This receptor can bind C3b, iC3b, and C4b. Although all of these complement molecules are activation products and might not be expected to be present in healthy individuals, there is increasing evidence that low-level activation may be occurring continually, and small amounts of C3b and its breakdown products, iC3b and C3d,g, may be commonly present in the plasma. It is possible that some of these activation products may bind to the CR1 receptor of RBCs, accounting for a small number of "naturally occurring" RBC-bound complement molecules. It has also been shown that RBCs can be involved as "innocent bystanders" in complement activation remote from the RBC. This might occur in infections or immune complex formation (e.g., in systemic lupus erythematosus). For instance, Salama and Mueller-Eckhardt[52] showed that complement activation by bacteria could lead to complement sensitization of nonsensitized bystander RBCs. It follows that one might expect to find more RBC-bound complement in sick patients than in healthy individuals, and there is good evidence for this (see later). Siegel and coworkers[53] suggested that RBCs were perhaps more important than macrophages in clearing immune complexes from the circulation. They suggested that the main function of the RBC CR1 receptor may be to attract complement-containing immune complexes, leading to macrophage interaction and subsequent clearance. Thus, it is easy to accept that RBCs may be coated with small amounts of complement independent of activation by antibody directed against RBC antigens.

Seemingly Healthy Individuals with Positive DATs Due to IgG and/or C3 Sensitization

It has been known for many years that some apparently normal individuals have positive DATs, but the incidence among normal blood donors varies somewhat in the literature.[54-58] Using an AGS that contained mainly anti-IgG, Weiner[54] reported 18 cases in a British donor population of 60,000 (1:3300). Most of the cases reported by Weiner had strongly positive (>2+) DATs. Habibi and coworkers[55] reported an incidence of 1:13,000 in a large French donor population; 97% of their positive DATs were associated with IgG sensitization. Gorst and coworkers[56] reported 65 donors with positive DATs encountered in a 14-year period (an incidence of approximately 1:14,000 donations, but their figures were not corrected for the incidence in donors, rather than units donated); approximately 50% of these positive DATs were associated with IgG sensitization (23% of these had complement in addition to IgG detectable on the RBCs). Bareford and coworkers[58] reported an incidence of positive DATs in their donor population in Leeds (United Kingdom) over a 20-year period as 1:7500. All of the DAT-positive donors tested had IgG on their RBCs, 12% of these had RBC-bound complement in addition to IgG.

Allen and Garratty[57] found 1:1000 of 1.3 million donors in Los Angeles, tested over a 5-year period, had a positive DAT. Eighty percent of the DAT reactions were 1+ or less (50% were <1+). The difference in reading or recording very weakly positive DATs may account for the higher incidence reported from Los Angeles compared with other areas (Table 6-2 shows agglutination reactions and scores as used by our laboratory at the time most of the data in this book were gathered). This may be particularly true for Europe, where the reported incidences were much lower, because sometimes the results in the reports from the United Kingdom related to DATs performed on tiles and read macroscopically; the DAT results in Los Angeles were from a "spin" tube technique, where all macroscopic negatives were checked microscopically. Approximately 18% of the DAT reactions were graded as 2+, and 3% were graded as 3+ or higher. Sixty-seven percent of the positive DATs were associated with IgG sensitization, 32% had RBC-bound IgG but no complement, 35% had RBC-bound IgG and complement, and 33% had only RBC-bound complement.

Two English studies suggest that it is rare for a positive DAT in blood donors to be associated with hemolytic anemia. Gorst and coworkers[56] recalled 32 donors who had a positive DAT and studied them in detail. Twenty-six (81%) still had a positive DAT 6 months up to 18 years after the initial finding. Seventeen (53%) of the 32 were associated with IgG sensitization; of these, 13 (41%) of the 32 donors still had IgG-sensitized RBCs when retested. They found a strong correlation between increasing age of donors and positive DATs. No clinical abnormalities were detected in any of the 32 donors. All hematologic and biochemical tests, including reticulocyte counts, were normal. One donor, after having a positive DAT for 2 years, suddenly developed WAIHA that required splenectomy for its control. In a similar study, Bareford and coworkers[58] also recalled 26 DAT-positive donors for study. All of the positive DATs were associated with IgG sensitization. Of these donors, 9 (35%) still had a positive DAT 1 to 18 years after the original finding. One of the donors had developed AIHA soon after the initial positive DAT 10 years earlier and required treatment with steroids and splenectomy. One donor had developed ulcerative colitis, one had mild arthritis, and the other five remained in good health. As in the series of Gorst and coworkers,[56] an increasing incidence of positive DATs was noted with increasing age.

Habibi and coworkers[55] followed 63 French DAT-positive donors for 5 years and, in contrast to the UK studies, found 72% of them to have some evidence of increased RBC destruction as evidenced by increased reticulocytes, hyperbilirubinemia, and abnormal $T_{50}Cr$ of labeled RBCs (Cr studies were performed on only 12 of the DAT-positive donors). These 63 were selected from 69 DAT-positive donors detected in 892,000 donors (an incidence of 1:13,000). Almost all (97%) of the positive DATs were associated with IgG sensitization. Seventeen (25%) were due to methyldopa therapy. Only 10% of the donors had a mild anemia (hemoglobin <13 g/dL in men and <12 g/dL in women). Seventeen percent had an increased reticulocyte count, and 12% had hyperbilirubinemia in addition to increased reticulocytes. RBC survival studies were performed on cells of 12 donors, using autologous ^{51}Cr-labeled RBCs, and 61% were found to be abnormal. Twenty-eight percent of the donors had a $T_{50}Cr$ of more than 26 days, and 33% had a $T_{50}Cr$ of less than 24 days (normal $T_{50}Cr$, 30 ± 3 days). These figures suggest that somewhere between 1:18,000 and 1:21,000 (61% to 72% of all DAT-positive donors) of French blood donors

TABLE 6-2. AGGLUTINATION GRADING AND SCORES

Grading	Appearance of Red Cells	Score
++++ or 4+	One large agglutinate; no unagglutinated cells	10
+++ or 3+	Several large agglutinates, few free cells	8
++ or 2+	Large agglutinates in a sea of smaller clumps and some free cells	6
+ or 1+	Many small agglutinates (approximately 20 RBCs per agglutinate)	4
(+) or (1+) or ½+	Scattered small agglutinates in a sea of free cells. Just visible macroscopically	3
± or micro	Small agglutinates visible only microscopically	1
0	No agglutinates seen	0

present with some signs of AIHA. These findings can be contrasted to the findings in England of approximately 1 case of AIHA per 1 million donations (not donors) reported by Gorst and coworkers[56] and 1 case per 5 million donors studied by Bareford and coworkers.[58] Pirofsky[59] reported the incidence of AIHA in the United States as approximately 1:80,000 of the general population, which may be a higher incidence than a typical blood donor population, where most donors are 17 to 70 years old. It should be emphasized that Pirofsky's incidence only relates to patients with clinically obvious hemolytic anemia, in contrast to the French study where individuals with an abnormal laboratory test result (DAT) were carefully studied for any signs of increased RBC destruction (e.g., use of ^{51}Cr-labeled RBCs). Thus, it would seem that increased RBC destruction due to IgG autoantibodies, in blood donors, may be more common than is generally assumed, but many of these have a relatively normal hemoglobin and probably never feel sick enough to go to a physician.

Positive DATs in Hospitalized Patients

Many more patients than donors have positive DATs but may also not have hemolytic anemia. Once again, there is considerable variation in incidence, even in accounts from the United States, where the reported incidence varies from 1% to 15%.[20,21] It is not clear why reports vary so much. Different types of AGS (anti-IgG versus polyspecific) account for some variations, but the major factor may be the types of patients predominating in certain medical centers and the number of patients tested.

Using AGS containing powerful anti-C3d activity, Worlledge and Blajchman,[14] Petz and Garratty,[35] Freedman,[60] and Chaplin and coworkers[48] all reported a 7% to 8% incidence of positive DATs in hospital patients. More than 80% of these were due to complement sensitization, with no IgG detectable. Bohnen and coworkers[61] found an incidence of 1% positive DATs in a 13-year study of hospitalized patients, where 17,110 DATs were performed. Lau and coworkers[62] found a 0.9% incidence of positive DATs when testing 6883 medical and surgical admissions to the hospital. Lau and coworkers[62] used only an anti-IgG reagent, and it is probable that when Bohnen and coworkers[61] performed their study (1950 to 1963), the commercial AGS was predominantly anti-IgG.

The highest incidence was reported by Judd and coworkers,[63] who found 15% of patients undergoing pretransfusion tests to have a positive DAT; 55% of these (8% of a total of 65,000 patients) were associated with IgG sensitization. In a later paper from the same hospital, Judd and coworkers[64] reported a slightly lower incidence (6%) of pretransfusion patients with positive DATs associated with IgG sensitization. Huh and coworkers[65] found 3.5% of pretransfusion samples, or 10% of patients (14,548 pretransfusion blood samples from 6959 patients), had a positive DAT; 68% of these were associated with IgG sensitization (42% IgG only and 26% IgG plus C3), 19% had C3 only on the RBCs, and 14% were said to be equivocal.

Clinical Significance of Positive DATs in Patients

It is difficult to assess the clinical significance of a positive DAT in random patients. If one relates clinical significance only to RBC survival, then a positive DAT associated with IgG is probably more significant than one due to only complement sensitization, but in many patients it may have no significance (e.g., see Toy and coworkers[22] and Heddle and coworkers,[23] discussed later). Bohnen and coworkers[61] found that 60% of their DAT-positive patients had signs of anemia but found it difficult to explain the etiology of the anemia. Reticulocytes were raised above 10% in only 17% of the anemic patients, and above 5% in 31%; these results included defined cases of AIHA. Very little evidence was presented for hemolysis in most of the anemic patients. Of the patients with positive DATs, 39% had received blood transfusions during the previous 2 months, and alloantibodies were detected in 25% of these patients. Eluates were not tested, but it is probable that many of the DATs in this recently transfused population were due to alloantibodies or would have nonreactive eluates (see later).

Toy and coworkers[66] reported that 18% of patients with acquired immune deficiency syndrome (AIDS) had a positive DAT. This contrasted with an incidence of only 0.6% positive DATs in their hospital population. Of the positive DATs in AIDS patients, 80% were associated with IgG sensitization of RBCs. Although all AIDS patients were anemic, no obvious evidence of clinical hemolysis was noted, but no ^{51}Cr-labeld RBC survival studies were performed. Because serum globulin levels were raised in the DAT-positive AIDS patients and eluates from the patients' RBCs were nonreactive, Toy and coworkers[66] suggested that the positive DATs might be due to nonimmune adsorption of IgG onto the patient's RBCs. In a separate study, Toy and coworkers[22] found that elevated serum globulin and blood urea nitrogen levels correlated significantly with positive DATs associated with nonreactive RBC eluates in patients who did not have AIDS. They found 0.7% of their hospital patients to have a positive DAT associated with IgG sensitization, and 79% of these RBCs yielded a nonreactive eluate. Seventy-five percent of these cases had elevated serum globulins, in contrast to 29% of DAT-negative controls. The major causes of elevated serum globulins were liver disease and infection. Heddle and coworkers[23] have also described a correlation with hypergammaglobulinemia and RBC-bound IgG. Fifteen DAT-positive patients with nonreactive eluates had elevated IgG levels (range, 1450 to 7730 mg/dL; mean, 2621 mg/dL). A prospective study of 44 patients with elevated serum IgG levels yielded three positive DATs and these occurred in patients with the highest IgG levels (2381, 3441, and 3520 mg/dL).

These findings are extremely important because they suggest that in a hospital population, most (about 65% to 80%) of the positive DATs due to IgG sensitization are due to nonimmunologic adsorption of plasma IgG and are of no clinical significance. Thus, approximately only 1 in 125 hospital patients have IgG-positive DATs with any potential clinical significance.[20] Positive DATs of potential significance include IgG autoantibodies, drug-induced antibodies, and alloantibodies that may or may not cause increased RBC destruction.

Using radiolabeled anti-C3d, Chaplin and coworkers[67] and Freedman and coworkers[68] showed that random hospitalized patients had more RBC-bound C3 than did healthy individuals. Chaplin and coworkers[67] found that 33% of 313 patients had levels of RBC-bound C3d above the normal range; only 8% of the patients had enough RBC-bound C3 to be detected by the DAT. The great majority of the patients with increased RBC-bound C3d did not have any known autoimmune disease. Freedman and coworkers[68] studied 227 hospitalized patients; 72 (32%) were found to have moderately increased levels of RBC-bound C3d. In contrast to Chaplin and coworkers,[67] Freedman and coworkers[68] found that these increases were more often found in patients with conditions where complement activation might be expected. Twenty-six (13%) of 203 patients had markedly elevated RBC-bound C3d; these patients (>1100 molecules C3d per RBC) almost always had an associated autoimmune disease (e.g., AIHA).

AIHA Associated with a Negative DAT

The most common causes for this are (1) RBC-bound IgG below the threshold of the AGT (i.e., <200 IgG molecules per RBC); (2) RBC-bound IgA and IgM, which are not detectable by most routine reagents used for the DAT; and (3) low-affinity IgG autoantibodies, which are washed off the RBCs during the washing phase of the DAT (see Chapter 9).

DETECTING SMALL AMOUNTS OF RBC-BOUND IgG (AND IgA AND IgM)

Using Flow Cytometry[69]

1. Wash test RBCs and control RBCs four times with 4°C phosphate-buffered saline (PBS). Suspend to 3% to 5% with 4°C PBS. Perform all of the following steps in cold (cold reagents, cold washes, cold incubations in refrigerator or dishpan with ice water) as much as possible.
2. For each RBC sample to be tested, label at least two tubes. Label one tube as a control, and the other(s) with the antisera to be tested (e.g., anti-IgG, anti-IgM, etc.).
3. Place 0.1 mL of 3% to 5% washed RBCs in each tube.
4. Add 0.01 mL of the appropriate dilution of fluorochrome-labeled antisera to the appropriately labeled tubes.
5. Add nothing to the control tubes (background).
6. Vortex all tubes.
7. Incubate 30 minutes (e.g., room temperature for fluorescein isothiocyanate (FITC)-labeled antibodies, 4°C for phycoerythin (PE)-labeled antibodies).
8. Wash RBCs once with 0.2% BSA/PBS for FITC-labeled antibodies or 2% bovine serum albumin (BSA)/PBS for PE-labeled antibodies.
9. Add 0.1 mL PBS to cell button and mix by drawing RBCs up and down, using a small-bore pipette (to break up any small agglutinates that may be present).
10. Add a subsample of each RBC sample to a 12 × 75-mm polystyrene tube containing 1 to 2 mL PBS so that an RBC suspension of approx-imately 0.2% is obtained (flow rate on the flow cytometer should be around 500 to 1000 events per second).
11. Immediately before aspiration into the flow cytometer, mix RBCs by vortexing.
12. Acquire at least 10,000 events for each sample.
13. Analyze data. Place electronic region around the RBC population based on forward versus side scatter cytogram of 1 normal RBC control.
    a. Printout forward versus side scatter cytogram and fluorescence histogram for each sample.
    b. Record median relative fluorescence intensity (RI):

$$RI = \frac{\text{Median fluoresence of RBCs} \pm \text{fluorochrome-labeled antibody}}{\text{Median fluorescence of RBC background control}}$$

    c. Overlay RBC background control fluorescence histogram on top of RBCs + fluorochrome antibody histogram. Use subtract graphs function. Divide number of events after subtraction by number of gated events in RBCs plus fluorochrome antibody. Record this as percent positive result for all samples.

d. Determine mean + 2 SDs for median RI and percent positive for all the control results.

Quality Control

1. RBCs plus nothing (background) control gives an indication of autofluorescence background. The patient's RBC autofluorescence may be increased (compared with the normal donor's RBCs) due to medications, etc. If so, then interpretation of results with fluorochrome-labeled antibodies may be difficult.
2. To control for RBC agglutination (e.g., when testing anti-IgM), test another antiserum expected to be nonreactive (e.g., anti-IgG, anti-IgA) in parallel. If anti-IgG or anti-IgA is reactive, this may indicate the presence of that immunoglobulin on those RBCs. If both anti-IgG and anti-IgA are reactive, that may indicate that RBC agglutination is present. The anti-IgG and anti-IgA results may then be used as background to determine if the anti-IgM results are positive.

Interpretation

1. Patient's RBCs with median RI and percent positive results of greater than mean + 2 SDs of normal controls are positive for the relevant immunoglobulin.
2. Patient's RBCs with only median RI or percent positive results of greater than mean + 2 SDs need to be evaluated individually (e.g., visual inspection of histogram).
3. When testing RBCs with cold or spontaneous agglutination, compare results, for example, of patient's RBCs plus fluorochrome labeled anti-IgM versus patient's RBCs plus fluorochrome labeled antisera expected to be nonreactive.

DIRECT POLYBRENE TEST

Principle

Polybrene (Sigma, St. Louis, MO) is a quarternary ammonium polymer (hexadimethrine bromide) that facilitates detection of RBC antibodies. The RBC sensitization phase occurs in a low ionic medium (LIM). Polybrene is then added to nonspecifically aggregate the RBCs, which permits crosslinking of antibody molecules through close approximation of the RBCs. Hypertonic salt solutions, such as sodium citrate, disperse nonspecific aggregation of the RBCs, but antibody-mediated agglutination of IgG-coated RBCs will persist. The test can then be converted to an AGT if antibody is not detected by the Polybrene effect.

Materials

0.9% NaCl, unbuffered
- 9 g NaCl
- 1 L deionized H_2O
- Store at room temperature

LIM (low ionic medium)
For 100 mL
- 5 g dextrose
- 0.2 g Na_2EDTA
- Bring to 100 mL with deionized H_2O
- Store at 2°C to 8°C

Polybrene (hexadimethrine bromide, a very hygroscopic polymer) has to be stored in a desiccator at (2°C to 8°C)
- 10% Stock solution:
- 1 g hexadimethrine bromide
- Bring to 10 mL with 0.9% unbuffered NaCl
- Store in a plastic container at 2°C to 8°C

Working solution (0.05%, or 1:200 dilution of the 10% stock):
- 0.05 Polybrene stock + 9.95 mL unbuffered NaCl
- Resuspending solution
  - 3.35 g trisodium citrate ($Na_3C_6H_5O_7$)•$2H_2O$
  - 2 g dextrose
  - Bring to 100 mL with deionized H_2O
  - Store at 2°C to 8°C

PBS, pH 7.3
AB plasma
- 5% AB plasma in PBS (v/v)
  - 2 mL AB plasma
  - 38 mL PBS
  - Store at –20°C in 0.5-mL aliquots

12 × 75-mm test tubes
Uniform drop pipettes
D+ RBCs for the controls, 3% to 5% (v/v)
Commercial anti-D diluted in 5% AB plasma so that it does not react by routine tube indirect AGT (e.g., 1:8000). Store frozen at –20°C in 0.5-mL aliquots
Anti-IgG
Antiglobulin control cells

Procedure

1. Label 4 12 × 75-mm tubes for patient's washed RBCs, patient's unwashed RBCs, the positive control, and the negative control.
2. Add 2 drops of 5% AB plasma and 1 drop of the patient's washed 3% to 5% RBCs to the "washed" tube.
3. Add 3 drops of a 1.5% suspension of the patient's unwashed RBCs suspended in autologous plasma to the "unwashed" tube.
4. Add 2 drops of the diluted anti-D and 1 drop of D+ RBCs to the positive control tube.
5. Add 2 drops of 5% AB plasma and 1 drop of D+ RBCs to the negative control tube.
6. To all tubes add 1 mL of LIM. Mix.
7. Incubate 1 minute at room temperature.
8. Add 2 drops of working Polybrene solution to all tubes and mix.

9. After 15 seconds, centrifuge at 1000 × g for 10 seconds.
10. Decant supernatant.
11. Add 2 drops of resuspending solution.
12. Mix gently (shake rack at 45-degree angle) for 10 seconds.
13. Read macroscopically and microscopically within 3 to 5 minutes. Do *not* recentrifuge.
14. Add 1 drop of resuspending solution. Mix.
15. Add 2 drops normal (neat) AB plasma. Mix.
16. Wash 3 times with PBS.
17. Add anti-IgG, centrifuge, and read. Read all macroscopically negative results under the microscope. Record results.
18. Add antiglobulin control cells to all negative tests, centrifuge, read, and record macroscopically positive results.

Interpretation

1. The presence of RBC-bound antibody is recognized by the persistence of agglutination after the Polybrene effect has been neutralized (resuspension phase) and/or by reactivity with anti-IgG.
2. Negative tests indicate the absence of RBC-bound IgG, provided that the positive control was reactive.

Notes

1. Compare tests with the negative control when examining for persistence of agglutination after adding the resuspending solution.
2. The activity of the Polybrene can vary; the reagent is very hygroscopic and reactivity can weaken over time. Reagents should be checked when first put into use after preparation with the anti-D dilution previously used for verification of reactivity. The dilution of the control antibody may need to be adjusted with new lots of Polybrene reagents.
3. Excess citrate can cause dissociation of antibody-dependent RBC agglutinates.
4. Read results shortly after Polybrene is neutralized or negative results will occur.
5. Antibodies in the Kell system sometimes fail to react or are weaker in the Polybrene system (resuspension phase). The antiglobulin phase should enable detection of these antibodies.
6. Antiglobulin reagents containing anti-complement should not be used after Polybrene treatment because complement can be fixed to RBCs in the low ionic phase.

DETECTING RBC-BOUND IgA AND IgM

At present, in the United States, anti-IgA and anti-IgM are not available as licensed reagents for use with RBCs. They are readily available as immunologic reagents and can often be used as long as they are carefully standardized and controlled (e.g., they sometimes contain heterophil antibodies that have to be removed by dilution or adsorption with non-sensitized human RBCs). The quality control must be precise, as agglutination is a far more sensitive technique than some immunologic techniques. Monospecificity by some immunologic techniques (e.g., precipitation or flow cytometry) does not ensure monospecificity by the AGT (e.g., an anti-IgA that does not show any precipitin line against IgG may react 4+ with IgG Rh antibody sensitized RBCs). Thus, anti-IgA must always be shown to be nonreactive *by the AGT* against RBCs strongly sensitized with IgG, IgM, and complement; similarly, anti-IgM must not react with IgG, IgA or complement sensitized RBCs.

Standardization of anti-IgA and anti-IgM. It is difficult to find pure nonagglutinating IgA and IgM blood group antibodies to prepare IgA/IgM-coated RBCs; therefore, we standardize our AHG using a passive agglutination technique. We coat chromic chloride-treated RBCs with purified IgA or IgM proteins and then test these coated RBCs by the regular AGT.

CHROMIC CHLORIDE METHOD FOR COUPLING PROTEINS TO RBCS

Materials

Unbuffered saline (UBS), 0.9% NaCl.
PBS, pH 7.3.
Chromium chloride, 6-hydrate ($CrCl_3•6H_2O$): 1% stock solution prepared in deionized water. Store in dark bottle at 2°C to 8°C.
Antigen or antibody to be coupled to the RBCs (e.g., purified Ig)
Group O RBCs (>24 hours old, <8 days old)
Test tubes, glass (never use plastic)
Appropriate antisera to determine if antigen/antibody is bound to RBCs

Procedure

1. Prepare dilutions of stock $CrCl_3$ in UBS (e.g., 1 in 10, 1 in 20, 1 in 40).
2. Prepare dilutions of antigen or antibody in UBS (e.g., 0.5, 1, 2 mg/mL).
3. Wash and pack RBCs.
4. Label several tubes, one for each of the different combinations of $CrCl_3$ and the antigen or antibody to be used (i.e., a checkerboard titration). Also include a tube (for each $CrCl_3$ dilution) where no antigen/antibody is added, just UBS + RBCs + $CrCl_3$.
5. In the labeled glass test tubes, place 1 vol (e.g., 0.1 mL) antigen or antibody solution and 1 vol packed washed RBCs.
6. Add 1 vol of diluted $CrCl_3$, mixing well during this addition.
7. Mix well for 5 minutes at room temperature.

8. Wash RBCs four times with UBS (do not centrifuge longer than 30 seconds at 1000 × *g*).
9. Resuspend RBCs to 3% to 5% in PBS.
10. Test RBCs against appropriate antibody (e.g., anti-IgA) and 6% albumin.

Quality Control
Reactivity of the antigen or antibody/$CrCl_3$-treated RBCs with specific antibody and not with 6% albumin indicates that the antigen or antibody is coupled to the RBCs. Repeat the $CrCl_3$ treatment with different amounts of antigen/antibody and/or $CrCl_3$ if these results are not obtained.

Interpretation
A checkerboard titration is used to determine the optimal combination of antigen or antibody and $CrCl_3$ concentrations. In general, the higher the Cr ion concentration, the more efficient the coupling, but the more likely it is to also encounter nonspecific aggregation. The amount of $CrCl_3$ that causes aggregation depends on the protein concentration. The optimal amount of $CrCl_3$ is thus a little below that which causes aggregation.

Choose the combination of antigen or antibody/$CrCl_3$ that gives no aggregation of the RBCs tested with 6% albumin and gives the desired strength of reactivity with the appropriate antisera.

Notes
1. The presence of phosphate ions must be avoided during the coupling procedure, because they will result in the precipitation of chromic ions.
2. The source of $CrCl_3 \bullet 6H_2O$ can be important.
3. Aged $CrCl_3$ (3 weeks) is more efficient in coupling than freshly prepared solutions. To ensure even coupling, the $CrCl_3$ should be added dropwise, with constant mixing.
4. The order of addition of reactants is important. The $CrCl_3$ must be added last, as it is rapidly inactivated by protein.

STANDARDIZATION OF ANTICOMPLEMENT AGS

Preparation of RBCs Coated with Various Complement Compounds
The methods below are those we have used successfully in our laboratory. Hoppe[70] described methods recommended to manufacturers of AGS by the FDA.

1. C3b- and C4b-coated RBCs[71]
   a. Using low ionic strength
      i. Prepare 10 mL of 10% sucrose in water. (This can be done simply by adding sucrose to the 1-mL mark of a 10-mL graduated centrifuge tube and then adding water to the 10-mL mark.)
      ii. Add 1 mL of whole blood. This can be fresh blood or ACD or CDP blood that has been stored at 4°C for less than 3 weeks.
      iii. Mix and incubate at 37°C for 15 minutes.
      iv. Wash 4 times.
      v. Resuspend RBCs to 2% to 5%.
   b. Using nonagglutinating Lewis antibodies (e.g., anti-Le^a, anti-Le^b, or anti-Le^a + anti-Le^b) (the amount of complement on the RBCs can be varied by using dilutions of the Lewis antibodies).[71] If the Lewis antibodies have been stored for longer than 48 hours at 4°C or 1 month at –20°C, then the two-stage EDTA AGT described below is optimal but not essential. Freshly collected Lewis antibodies (or Lewis antibodies stored below –50°C) can be used with a routine one-stage indirect AGT (e.g., do not add EDTA and do not perform steps v, vi, and vii).
      i. To 9 vol of Lewis antibody, add 1 vol of neutral EDTA (4.45% K_2 EDTA•$2H_2O$ + 0.3% NaOH).
      ii. Add 1 vol of 50% washed Lewis-positive RBCs.
      iii. Incubate at 37°C for 30 to 60 minutes.
      iv. Wash 4 times.
      v. To button of RBCs, add 5 vol of fresh normal serum as a source of complement.
      vi. Reincubate at 37°C for 15 minutes.
      vii. Wash 4 times.
      viii. Resuspend RBCs to 2% to 5%.
   c. Using anti-I (the amount of complement on the RBCs can be varied by using dilutions of the anti-I).[71]
      i. Titrate an anti-I and select a dilution that agglutinates OI adult RBCs approximately 2+ at 20°C to 25°C. This should yield moderately strongly sensitized RBCs.
      ii. Dilute the anti-I appropriately in a source of complement (i.e., "fresh" inert human serum). For instance, for serum from a patient with a cold agglutinin titer at 4°C of 4000; we dilute this anti-I 1:1000 and 1:100 to prepare weakly and strongly C3b/C4b sensitized RBCs, respectively.
      iii. Add 0.1 vol of 50% washed RBCs.
      iv. Incubate at 20°C to 25°C for 10 to 15 minutes.
      v. Incubate at 37°C for approximately 5 to 10 minutes (to allow agglutination to disperse).
      vi. Wash RBCs 4 times at 37°C.
      vii. Resuspend RBCs to 2% to 5%.

2. C3b (but not C4b)-coated RBCs[72,73]

Diluent Solution A
In a 250-mL flask containing approximately 125 mL distilled water, dissolve:
a. 23.1 g sucrose
b. 173 mg $NaH_2PO_4 \bullet H_2O$

c. 395 mg $Na_2EDTA \cdot 2H_2O$
q.s. to 250 mL with distilled water

Diluent: Solution B
In a 250-mL flask containing approximately 125 mL distilled water, dissolve
23.1 g sucrose
178 mg Na_2HPO_4
395 mg $Na_2EDTA \cdot 2H_2O$
q.s. to 250 mL with distilled water.
Adjust solution A to pH 5.1 by the addition of solution B (e.g., approximately 6.5 mL).

0.4 M $MgCl_2$ Additive
To 10 mL distilled water add 810 mg $MgCl_2 \cdot 6H_2O$.

Coating Procedure
a. Whole ACD or CPD blood may be used equally well. Chill all reactants to ice-water temperature before combining.
b. Place 19 mL diluent in small flask in ice-water bath on magnetic stirrer.
c. With stirrer on, add 1.0 mL ACD or CPD blood dropwise, rapidly.
d. *Immediately* add 0.1 mL $MgCl_2$ additive (i.e., final concentration of added Mg = 0.002 mg).
e. Stir in ice-bath for 1 hour.
f. Wash RBCs 4 times with saline at 0°C.

3. C4b (but not C3b)-coated RBCs[67]
   a. Using low ionic strength method
      i. Add 10 mL of 10% sucrose in water to a 100 X 16-mm tube containing 12 or 15 mg K EDTA.
      ii. Add 1 mL of whole blood as described in 1 (a) (ii) above.
      iii. Incubate at 37°C for 15 minutes.
      iv. Wash 4 times.
      v. Resuspend to 2% to 5%.
4. C3d/C4d, C3d or C4d-coated RBCs[71,74]
   a. RBCs sensitized with C3b/C4b, C3b, or C4b can be prepared by any of the methods described previously.
   b. An equal volume of packed, washed C3b/C4b, C3b, or C4b-coated RBCs is incubated with 0.1% trypsin (pH 7.3) for 30 minutes or inert fresh normal EDTA-treated serum (as a source of factors H and I) for 12 hours at 37°C. Non–complement-sensitized RBCs should also be incubated with the trypsin, or the normal serum, as a negative control.
   c. The RBCs are washed 4 times and resuspended to 2 to 5%.

Once prepared, any of the above complement-sensitized RBCs can be stored frozen in glycerol or liquid nitrogen. If the C3b- or C4b-sensitized RBCs are frozen immediately after preparation, they do not appear to decay to C3d/C4d on storage.

Daily Quality Control of AGS
For daily quality control, polyspecific AHG need only be tested against RBCs weakly sensitized with IgG (e.g., anti-D). Although it could be argued that it would be optimal to test the AHG against complement-sensitized RBCs, it seems unnecessary because *daily* quality control is primarily to ensure that the AGS has not become inactivated by contamination or improper storage. There is no evidence to suggest that the anticomplement activity can be selectively inactivated under the usual conditions of storage in blood banks; in our experience, when any inactivation occurs (e.g., contamination with human serum), the anti-IgG reaction will be a sensitive indicator as long as RBCs *weakly* (approximately 1+) sensitized with IgG-sensitized RBCs are used as indicator cells; many commercially available AGT "check cells" are too strongly sensitized to show minimal to moderate inhibition of the AGS.[75] Some commercial package inserts recommend the use of complement-coated RBCs, in addition to IgG-sensitized RBCs when using polyspecific AGS.

1. Preparation of IgG weakly sensitized RBCs for quality control of AGS
   a. To each of 12 tubes, add 1 mL of saline.
   b. To the first tube, add 1 mL of an IgG anti-D (e.g., a slide and rapid tube anti-D commercial typing reagent), making a 1:2 dilution.
   c. Prepare serial doubling dilutions by mixing saline and antibody, and then transferring 1 mL to the next tube. This is repeated with each tube to the 12th tube, and the final 1 mL is discarded.
   d. To each 1 mL of anti-D, add 10 drops of a 5% suspension of D-positive RBCs to each tube.
   e. Incubate at 37°C for 15 minutes.
   f. Centrifuge, remove, and discard supernatant; wash RBCs 4 times.
   g. Resuspend RBCs to 5%. Add 1 drop of RBCs from each tube to 2 drops of AGS.
   h. Centrifuge tubes and inspect for degree of agglutination, carefully noting the strength of the reaction (see Table 6-2).
   i. Select tubes that show 1+ to 2+ macroscopic agglutination.
   j. As 1+ sensitized RBCs may appear much weaker when added to nonsensitized RBCs in the "check cell" procedure, it is wise to try several of the sensitized cells (1+ or 2+) as a check cell and choose a dilution that yields RBCs that will give about 1+ reactions *following* addition to nonsensitized RBCs.
   k. A large batch of sensitized RBCs can be prepared, washed, and stored in CPD or Alsevers solution at 4°C; these usually last for up to 1 month. Alternatively, prepare a quantity of anti-D at this dilution and freeze it in aliquots suitable for use each day.

DETECTING LOW-AFFINITY AUTOANTIBODIES WITH A COLD LOW IONIC STRENGTH SALINE WASH DAT[16,75,76]

Materials

Test tubes, 10 × 75 mm
Cold anti-IgG
Cold diluent control (e.g., 6% albumin or manufacturer supplied)
Ice-cold low ionic strength saline (LISS) (4°C)
Antiglobulin control cells
Refrigerated centrifuge (e.g., Sorvall RT6000)
Serologic centrifuge

Procedure

1. Label 2 test tubes: one for anti-IgG, one for control.
2. Add 2 drops of cold anti-IgG and cold diluent control to the respective tubes and place the tubes in the refrigerator.
3. Wash the RBCs to be tested 4 times with cold LISS using a refrigerated centrifuge (1000 × *g* for 1 to 2 minutes).
4. Resuspend the RBCs to 3% to 5% in cold LISS.
5. Add 1 drop of RBCs to each of the two tubes from the refrigerator.
6. Mix and centrifuge in a serologic centrifuge for the calibrated time.
7. Inspect macroscopically for agglutination and record results.
8. Inspect macroscopically negative results, microscopically. Record results.
9. To the anti-IgG test, add 1 drop antiglobulin control cells.
10. Centrifuge.
11. Read macroscopically and record positive results with a check mark.

Quality Control

The patient's cold LISS washed RBCs should be nonreactive with the diluent control. A positive test with the control indicates the presence of a cold autoagglutinin and the test is invalid.

Antiglobulin control cells, when added to the anti-IgG test, should be macroscopically reactive. If not, then investigations need to include the quality of the check cells, the efficiency of the washes, and/or the activity of the anti-IgG. Repeat the DAT.

Interpretation

1. A positive result with anti-IgG, in conjunction with a nonreactive diluent control, means that IgG is present on the patient's RBCs.
2. When the routine DAT with anti-IgG is negative or becomes weak/negative on sitting, and the cold LISS wash DAT is positive or stronger, the IgG is low affinity.

Notes

1. A column agglutination technique (e.g., gel) anti-IgG DAT may also enhance reactivity of low-affinity IgG because the patient's RBCs are not washed before performing the test.
2. Washing RBCs at 37°C enhances dissociation of low-affinity autoantibodies, even when they are associated with WAIHA.

STANDARDIZATION OF IgG SUBCLASS ANTISERA FOR USE WITH SENSITIZED RBCs

The only commercial source of IgG subclass antisera standardized for use with RBCs that we know of in the United States are those made by the Netherlands Red Cross. Their recommended methods are a sedimentation or microplate (V wells) AGT methods not generally used in the United States. Some years ago, we tested these antisera for sensitivity and specificity using the routine centrifugation AGT and a capillary tube test and found the methods to be comparable.[77] We found that some methods (e.g., albumin capillary method) that have been used to define the subclass of RBC-bound IgG were inappropriate and led to false-positive results.[77]

Sensitizing RBCs with Antibodies or Purified Proteins of Known Subclass. Rh alloantibodies of known IgG allotype and subclass can be used to coat RBCs, or purified proteins of known subclass can be attached to chromic chloride-treated RBCs.

Preparation of RBCs Coated with Known Subclass

1. Using alloantibodies of known subclass: 0.2 mL of appropriate dilutions of the antibodies are incubated at 37°C for 30 minutes with 0.1 mL of packed RBCs. The cells were then washed four times with saline and resuspended to a 5% suspension.
2. Using purified proteins of known subclass: Protein quantification is performed by diluting the purified proteins in 0.1 M NaOH and measuring absorbance at a wavelength of 280 nm, using a spectrophotometer. Protein concentrations are calculated from a graph of known protein concentrations plotted against optical density at 280 nm. The samples are adjusted to contain 1 mg/mL, and the procedure described on pages 210 to 211 is followed.

Tube AGT Using IgG Subclass AGS

Two drops of the IgG subclass antisera are added to 1 drop of a 5% washed sensitized RBC suspension, mixed, and centrifuged at 1000 × g for 15 seconds. After centrifugation, the button of RBCs is gently resuspended and inspected for agglutination (see Table 6-2).

Sedimentation AGT Using IgG Subclass AGS
One drop of IgG subclass antisera is added to 1 drop of a 5% washed sensitized RBC suspension, mixed, and incubated at 37°C for 1 hour. After incubation, the tubes are gently removed from the water bath and the buttons inspected for a sedimentation pattern. A smooth round button is considered a negative result, and a cell button with a broader irregular border is considered a positive result.

Capillary AGT Using IgG Subclass AGS
Glass capillary tubes measuring 0.4 × 90 mm are used. Equal volumes of IgG subclass antisera and 50% washed sensitized RBCs are drawn into the capillary tube. The tubes are inverted and the end of the capillary containing antisera is inserted in a Sealease holder at a 45° angle. After 15 minutes at room temperature, examine tubes for agglutination (beading, ribbon, or granular appearance). Invert and examine again after 15 minutes. Repeat one more time.

GENERAL SEROLOGIC INVESTIGATIONS

The results obtained in each type of AIHA are discussed in Chapter 5 under the appropriate headings.

Collection of Blood

We collect clotted blood to provide serum, and blood in EDTA to provide RBCs for the DAT, ABO, and Rh phenotyping and for preparation of eluates. If blood has not been kept at 37°C from the time of venipuncture, we incubate blood samples at 37°C for 10 to 15 minutes before we separate the serum (which is separated by centrifugation at 37°C). We perform the DAT and prepare an eluate from the EDTA sample.

Several problems can arise if the blood is not kept at 37°C from the time of bleeding and cold autoantibodies are present:

1. Autoagglutination of the RBCs may occur, leading to difficulties in grouping. This almost always is a reversible phenomenon and can be overcome by incubating the samples at 37°C before processing and testing. However, in rare cases, autoagglutinin may persist at 37°C.
2. Loss of antibody from the serum by in vitro autoadsorption, leading to a false low cold agglutination titer, etc. This is also a reversible phenomenon (see later).
3. Possible direct hemolysis of the RBCs, using antibody and complement, again leading to a false low laboratory value and possible misinterpretation of in vitro hemoglobinemia as being in vivo occurrence. This will occur only in the clotted sample, as EDTA will inhibit any in vitro complement-mediated lysis.
4. If EDTA blood is not used, then in vitro complement autosensitization may occur due to the presence of normal incomplete cold autoantibodies. This may lead to a false-positive result or an increase in the strength of the DAT. EDTA will prevent any in vitro complement sensitization, even if the blood is cooled; thus, any complement detected on the EDTA RBCs represents in vivo sensitization. Nevertheless, we do not routinely bleed our patients into warmed syringes, etc., unless we know we are dealing with a severe case of CAS or PCH. We find that by always warming the samples before separation, we can obtain reliable results in most cases.

Determining the Blood Group of DAT-Positive Patients

The main problem when typing DAT-positive RBCs is that the RBCs may spontaneously agglutinate in the presence of potentiators, including albumin.[78] In the United States, manufacturers are allowed to add up to 8% albumin to any antisera; thus, we use a 10% albumin negative control if a diluent control is not provided by the company and if the protein concentration is not known. If monoclonal reagents are used, the protein concentration is usually lower (e.g., 3%) and the negative control can be adjusted appropriately. There should be no problems in ABO and Rh typing patients with AIHA if certain rules are followed; however, if they are not followed, serious errors can occur. If cold autoantibodies are suspected, the blood samples should be separated at 37°C, and the RBCs should be washed with 37°C warm saline; if the patient has CAS, a 37°C centrifuge will have to be used (see later).

Garratty and coworkers[78] studied how often spontaneous agglutination occurred with various media when the RBCs had a positive DAT. Red cells from 475 individuals (donors and patients) with a positive DAT (66% were ½ to 1+, 19% were 1½+ to 2+, and 15% were 2½+ or greater) were examined for spontaneous agglutination after incubation in various media. Twenty-three percent of the samples showed spontaneous agglutination in commercial Rh control solutions for "slide and rapid tube" reagents, 6% in 30% albumin, 3% in 10% albumin, 2% in 6% albumin, and 1% in saline. Cells suspended in serum were more prone to spontaneous agglutination. The strength of spontaneous agglutination varied; more than 50% of the samples reacted only 1+ or less, approximately 10% reacted greater than 2+. There was not a complete correlation with spontaneous agglutination and the quantity of IgG on the cells, as determined by the AGT. Of the samples showing spontaneous agglutination, 50% were associated with a DAT strength of more than 2+, 27% with a DAT of 1½+ to 2+, and 23% with a DAT of ½+ to 1+. Spontaneous agglutination occurred with the same frequency whether the cells were sensitized with both IgG and C3 or with IgG alone. Surprisingly, 7% of the samples sensitized with C3 but no detectable IgG also demonstrated spontaneous agglutination; this may have been due to RBC-bound IgM. Marked differences in reaction strength were seen with Rh control solutions from different manufacturers, and the degree of spontaneous agglutination was inconsistent with individual products.[78]

Most monoclonal reagents do not usually contain potentiators and usually give reliable results, but problems due to potentiators have been reported.[79] Because of this, and because spontaneous agglutination can occur in low protein solutions (see earlier),[78] we prefer to have a negative control. Ideally, this should be the diluent without the Rh antibody; if this is not available then a negative control containing albumin equivalent to the protein concentration of the antiserum should be used. If this information is not available, then we recommend using 8% to 10% albumin as a control. Rodberg and coworkers[79] reported that one company's monoclonal Rh antisera gave problems with DAT+ patients because a potentiator was present. Monoclonal anti-Rh reagents were used according to manufacturer's directions on untreated and chloroquine-treated DAT+ RBCs. Of 32 DAT+ patients, who appeared to be D+C+c+E+e+ (R_1R_2), 13 still appeared to be R_1R_2 following chloroquine treatment; but 19 appeared to be R_1R_1, R_2R_2, R_0r, or rr following testing of chloroquine-treated RBCs. None of these DAT+ RBCs reacted in the 6% albumin control. RBCs from 2 other DAT+ (3+) patients reacted weaker (1+) than expected with monoclonal anti-e and reacted stronger (3+) after chloroquine treatement (DAT still 2+). These latter results suggest that blocking auto anti-e might have caused the initial weakly positive result with anti-e. Thus, fragile, or weaker than expected, agglutination results obtained when Rh typing DAT+ RBCs with monoclonal anti-Rh reagents must be interpreted with care. Such results might indicate a false positive, or a true weak positive due to a blocking autoantibody. The false-positive results were not indicated by the 6% albumin control recommended by this particular manufacturer.

ABO Group. The washed RBCs are tested in the usual fashion with anti-A, anti-B, and perhaps anti-A,B, but a negative albumin control is also set up. This control should be compared with the tests and if positive indicates either nondispersed autoagglutination or spontaneous agglutination of heavily IgG-sensitized cells in albumin.

The patient's serum is tested against A_1, B, O, and his own cells as usual. If the patient is known to have or appears to have CAS, the serum typing tests should be repeated by a prewarmed technique, strictly at 37°C. At this temperature, all but the weakest ABO agglutinins will usually react well at 37°C but the cold autoantibody will not react. These results may be confirmed (by the normal methods) after the cold autoantibody has been autoadsorbed from the patient's serum. As patients with WAIHA do not often have strong autoagglutinins, problems in ABO typing are rare.

Rh Phenotype. It is useful to Rh phenotype patients with WAIHA, preferably before they are transfused. Monoclonal antisera are preferable to polyclonal reagents as they contain less protein or potentiators, so fewer false-positive results due to spontaneous agglutination occur. Commercial "slide and rapid tube" reagents always contain potentiators (e.g., albumin) and the manufacturers should always make available the diluent containing the potentiator but not the anti-Rh; this must always be tested in parallel as a negative control. If the diluent control is negative then the Rh typing result on the patient is acceptable, even if the DAT is strongly positive. If the control is positive, then the Rh typing will have to be repeated with a "saline tube test" anti-Rh or monoclonal reagents. These reagents are said not to give false-positive reactions with RBCs, even strongly sensitized with IgG. Nevertheless, we believe false-positive reactions may still occasionally occur and we prefer to always use an albumin negative control when using such reagents.

Phenotyping DAT+ RBCs When Spontaneous Agglutination Occurs or When Using Antiglobulin Reactive Antisera

Spontaneous agglutination usually is associated with IgG sensitization but on rare occasions is associated with RBC-bound IgM (see Chapter 9).

Most of the phenotyping approaches are based on methods used to remove IgG from RBCs, but IgM may also be removed. The method should cause minimal or no damage to RBC antigens; careful controls for this are essential. The first method used was gentle heat (e.g., 45°C to 50°C) for 5 to 10 minutes. This is not a very efficient method compared with the later methods but can be used if careful controls are used.

We prefer the EDTA-glycine acid method, which relies on low pH. The method, described by Louie and coworkers,[80] is based on an elution method described by Rekvig and Hannestad[81] and is the basis of a commercial kit called "EGA" (Gamma Biologicals). The method is efficient for typing Rh and most other antigens, but it should be noted that Kell antigens are destroyed or greatly diminished. des Roziers and Squalli[82] found the method of Louie and coworkers[80] to be superior to heat and chloroquine methods. A modification of the Louie method[80] by Byrne[83] uses larger volumes of reagent so that an eluate suitable for testing is also obtained in addition to the treated RBCs.

Chloroquine has been used to inhibit RBC antigen-antibody reactions in vitro and in vivo.[84,85] Mantel and Holtz[85] used chloroquine to elute IgG autoantibodies from RBCs of patients with AIHA. Edwards and coworkers[86] applied this to typing RBCs with a positive DAT. Complete dissociation of IgG antibody occurred in 47 of 56 strongly sensitized RBC samples from patients with positive DAT. They did not observe any apparent loss of ABH, Rh, MNSs, P_1, Lewis, Kell, Duffy, or Kidd antigens. Other workers,[87-89] including ourselves, have observed weakening of some blood group antigens after chloroquine treatment. Fortunately, this is not sufficient to be noticed when using strongly reactive antisera, but if weaker antisera are used, then the reactions may be much weaker than with untreated RBCs. This does not make the technique any less useful as long as weak positive control RBCs (e.g., from heterozygotes) are incubated along with the test cells undergoing the chloroquine treatment.

DISSOCIATION OF IgG AUTOANTIBODY USING A MODIFIED GLYCINE-ACID/EDTA TECHNIQUE[80]

Reagents

10% EDTA [disodium ethylenediamine-tetraacetate (Na_2EDTA)]

0.1 M glycine acid buffer (pH 1.5)
- 0.75 g glycine
- Make up to 100 mL with 0.9% sodium chloride
- Adjust to pH 1.5 using concentrated hydrochloric acid (HCl)

1.0 M Tris-NaCl
- 12.1 g Tris(hydroxymethyl)aminomethane (Tris)
- 5.25 g sodium chloride
- Make up to 100 mL with distilled water

Procedure

1. Wash RBCs 6 times in 0.9% sodium chloride. On the last wash, pack the RBCs well and transfer all supernatant to a tube labeled "last wash."
2. In a test tube, mix together 20 vol of 0.1 M glycine-HCl buffer (pH 1.5) and 5 vol 10% EDTA. *This is the elution reagent.*
3. Place 10 vol of packed RBCs that have been washed 6 times in 0.9% sodium chloride into a 12 × 75-mm glass tube.
4. Add 20 vol of elution reagent to the RBCs, mix well, and incubate at room temperature for 2 minutes. (*Caution:* Overincubation will cause irreversible damage to the RBCs.)
5. After incubation add 1 vol of 1.0 M Tris-NaCl, mix, and immediately centrifuge at 1000 × *g* for 60 seconds.
6. Remove supernatant (now the eluate) into a labeled tube.
7. Using 1.0 M Tris and pH paper, *carefully* adjust the pH of the eluate to between 7.0 and 7.4. (*Caution:* 1.0 M Tris-NaCl is very alkaline, and only a *very small* amount is required to attain the desired pH.)
8. If a precipitate forms in the eluate, centrifuge the eluate and remove the clear supernatant (eluate) into another labeled tube.
9. The eluate may now be used for testing in parallel with the last wash.
10. The acid/EDTA-treated RBCs should be washed at least 3 times in 0.9% sodium chloride before use, and tested by the DAT. If the DAT is negative, the RBCs are ready for use. If the DAT is still positive, repeat treatment (steps 1 to 6) one more time (for a maximum of 2 treatments).

DISSOCIATION OF IgG AUTOANTIBODY USING CHLOROQUINE REAGENT[86]

Materials

PBS, pH 7.3

Chloroquine diphosphate, 200 mg/mL
- 20 g chloroquine diphosphate in 100 mL PBS
- Adjust pH to 5.0 ± 0.1 with 1N or 5N NaOH
- Store at 2°C to 8°C for no more than 1 year

Anti-IgG

Positive and negative control RBCs for the antigen(s) to be tested

Test tubes

Serologic centrifuge

Antiglobulin control cells

Procedure

1. Wash the test and control RBCs in PBS
2. To 1 vol of washed, packed RBCs, add 4 vol of chloroquine.
3. Mix and incubate at room temperature for 30 minutes.
4. Remove a small amount of the chloroquine-treated test RBCs and wash 4 times in PBS.
5. Test with anti-IgG.
   If the anti-IgG is nonreactive, wash the test and control RBCs 4 times in PBS and use for phenotyping.
   If the anti-IgG is reactive, repeat steps 4 and 5 at 30-minute intervals until the anti-IgG is nonreactive or up to 2 hours.
   If the anti-IgG is still reactive after 2 hours of treatment, use a different approach to remove the IgG (e.g., glycine acid/EDTA).
6. Add antiglobulin control cells to all negative tests. Centrifuge and examine for agglutination.

Quality Control

Control RBCs must be treated in the same way as the test RBCs and must give valid typing results. If the antigen activity of the positive control RBCs is diminished, use a different approach to remove IgG from the test RBCs (e.g., glycine acid/EDTA).

If the antiglobulin control cells are not macroscopically positive or react weaker than expected, then repeat the test.

Interpretation
When the procedure is effective, IgG is completely removed from the IgG-coated RBCs and phenotyping is possible.

Notes
1. Incubation of RBCs with chloroquine diphosphate should not exceed 2 hours; hemolysis or loss of antigen activity could occur.
2. IgM is removed, but C3 is not removed from the RBCs by chloroquine.
3. When testing Rh antigens, use high-protein reagents. It has been reported that Rh antigens can be weakened by chloroquine treatment, especially when saline or chemically modified Rh reagents are used.
4. This method is also effective in removing Bg (HLA-related) antigens from RBCs.

PHENOTYPING DAT-POSITIVE RBCS BY ADSORPTION OF ANTISERA

Sometimes the IgG autoantibody will not dissociate after treatment. If this happens, typing can be carried out by measuring the amount of specific antibody left in the typing antiserum after adsorption with the patient's RBCs, and comparing the results with adsorptions using RBCs known to contain the appropriate antigens (RBCs from heterozygotes and homozygotes).

Procedure
1. Add 0.2 mL of the antiserum to 0.2 mL washed, packed RBCs from the patient. To other 0.2-mL aliquots of the antiserum, add 0.2 mL antigen-negative and antigen-positive RBCs, respectively. Mix.
2. Incubate the three adsorption tests at 37°C for 1 hour. Mix occasionally.
3. Centrifuge the three tubes and separate the serum into labeled tubes.
4. Label three sets of 10 × 75-mm tubes. Make twofold dilutions (0.1 mL) of each aliquot of adsorbed antiserum using saline as a diluent.
5. To each dilution of adsorbed antiserum, add 0.1 mL 2% to 5% saline-suspended antigen-positive RBCs.
6. Incubate the 3 sets of titration tubes for 30 minutes at 37°C. Perform AGT on RBCs from all tubes.
7. Compare the results (Table 6-3).

SEROLOGIC INVESTIGATIONS TO HELP IN THE DIFFERENTIAL DIAGNOSIS OF AIHA

In this section, we describe detailed screening tests that may be used in evaluating a patient with possible AIHA. All tests are not necessary in all cases, although care must be taken in the interpretation of abbreviated serologic evaluations. The significance of each step of the diagnostic workup is further discussed in Chapter 5.

To diagnose and classify the patient correctly, several questions have to be answered:

QUESTION 1: *Are the patient's RBCs sensitized with protein?*

To answer this question, the patient's washed RBCs are first tested with a polyspecific AHG. Most commercial AHG will detect IgG sensitization adequately, but approximately 20% to 30% of all AIHA cases have only complement (C3d and C4d) on their RBCs, and rare cases have been described with only IgA or IgM on their cells; as mentioned previously, some commercial polyspecific AGS will not detect IgA and IgM and occasionally will not detect weak C3d sensitization.

Other cases exist (perhaps as many as 5% to 10% of all AIHA cases), where a negative DAT is found in the presence of AIHA (see Chapter 9). Thus, if the DAT is negative and the patient has all the symptoms of AIHA, the diagnosis of AIHA should not be excluded on the results of the DAT.

DAT

1. Wash RBCs (preferably from EDTA blood) 4 times in large volume of saline. (We usually wash 2 or 3 drops of whole blood.)
2. Add 1 drop of 2% to 5% washed RBCs to 2 drops of polyspecific AHG (or add 2 drops of AHG to the dry button from 1 drop of 2% to 5% washed RBCs).
3. Centrifuge tubes at 1000 × *g* RCF for 15 to 20 seconds (time specified by serologic calibration of centrifuge).
4. Inspect tubes for agglutination (we prefer to check all macroscopically negative results for microscopic agglutination).

Controls
We always add 1 drop of the washed patient's RBCs to 2 drops of the AHG diluent (or 5% to 10% albumin if diluent is not available), as a negative control, and centrifuge this along with the test. The DAT is only truly positive if the AHG reacts stronger than the diluent; ideally, of course, the tube containing diluent should be negative. If the negative control is positive, it could be due to cold autoagglutinins or RBC-bound warm IgM autoantibody. To dispense

TABLE 6-3. Jk^{a} TYPING OF PATIENT WITH POSITIVE DIRECT ANTIGLOBULIN TEST USING DIFFERENTIAL ADSORPTION

RBCs Used to Adsorb Anti-Jk^{a} Typing Serum	Dilutions of Adsorbed Anti-Jk^{a} Tested Against Jk (a+b+) RBCs*						
	1	2	4	8	16	32	Score
Jk(a+b+)	2+	1+	1+	½+	0	0	17
Jk(a+b−)	1+	1+	0	0	0	0	8
Jk(a−b+)	3+	3+	2+	2+	1+	0	32
Patient's	2+	1+	0	0	0	0	10

* These results indicate that the patient is probably Jk(a+)

cold autoagglutinins, the EDTA sample should be warmed to 37°C and the RBCs washed with 37°C saline. If the control is still positive, this suggests the presence of an IgM warm autoantibody and the RBCs may have to be treated with 2-mercaptoethanol (2ME)[90] or dithiothreitol (DTT) to prevent spontaneous agglutination.

Red cells presensitized with IgG (e.g., anti-D) should always be added to all negative tests with AHG. After recentrifugation, the tests should now be positive, ensuring that the AGS has not been inhibited (e.g., by inadequate washing). No AGT should ever be called negative without this control.

QUESTION 2: *What proteins are present on the RBCs?*

The RBCs are often sensitized with IgG and complement or IgG alone, and sometimes by complement alone. The presence of these proteins is best detected by performing AGTs using monospecific AGS such as anti-IgG and anticomplement containing anti-C3d. Red cell–bound IgA and IgM are sometimes detected but they are usually present together with IgG and/or complement.

The amount of protein sensitizing the RBCs can be judged in a semiquantitative way. By testing the RBCs of the patient with dilutions of the AHG, one can obtain a relative estimate of the amount of protein sensitizing the RBCs. For instance, the undiluted AHG may show 3+ results on two specimens, but the two may have very different agglutination scores on titration. Agglutination scores correlated very well with results of assays that measured the number of RBC-bound IgG and C3 molecules. Although we have previously emphasized that commercial AGS should never be diluted when used routinely (e.g., for compatibility testing), it is acceptable to dilute these antisera when they are only being used to compare the amount of RBC-bound IgG or C3. We stress once again, they must *never* be diluted when used for antibody detection or crossmatching. More accurate ways of measuring the amount of RBC-bound proteins using radiolabeled AHG, ELISA, and flow cytometry have been described but are rarely useful at a practical clinical level.[91-94]

QUESTION 3: *Does the serum contain antibodies?*

Are they agglutinins or "incomplete"? Do they have hemolytic activity? At what temperature do they react optimally? What is their thermal range? What is their specificity? Are they autoantibodies or alloantibodies?

These questions can be answered by regular serologic techniques (with a few minor additions) used in the blood bank for detection and identification of antibodies.

To aid in the visualization of hemolysis, we use a 10% RBC suspension; to keep the antigen-antibody ratio in a ratio similar to usual, we add 1 vol of the cell suspension to 4 vol of serum. As patients with AIHA may have low serum complement levels, it is advisable to set up a duplicate set of tests to which an equal volume of fresh compatible inert serum has been added as a source of complement. The mixture of patient's serum and complement should be in the pH range 6.5 to 6.8 (i.e., add 0.1 vol of 0.2N HCl to the serum), as this seems to be optimal for the detection of warm and cold hemolysins.

Many warm and cold reacting autoantibodies give enhanced reactions with enzyme-treated RBCs; thus, it is useful to include such cells in the serum screening procedure. Hemolysis of enzyme-treated cells is much more commonly observed than hemolysis of untreated RBCs.

It is extremely important that tests set up at 37°C are kept strictly at 37°C. To do this, the patient's serum, reagent RBCs, and any other reagents (e.g., albumin) are warmed to 37°C separately before mixing. The tests are then centrifuged at 37°C, and the cells are washed in 37°C saline for the AGT. If this is not done carefully (with careful control of the temperature at each stage), then positive results may be misinterpreted, lending to erroneous conclusions regarding the classification of the AIHA and to the clinical significance of the autoantibody.

The approach we give below is optimal; we have been rewarded many times by the extra work involved. On the other hand, a great deal of information can be obtained by routine blood bank techniques (e.g., a DAT using anti-IgG and anti-C3d; antibody screening with one set at RT and one set at 37°C; a cold agglutinin titer at 4°C if RT agglutination is obtained and one tube test of patient's serum plus RBCs plus 30% albumin at 30°C).

The serum may contain:

- No antibodies; they may all have been autoadsorbed onto the patient's RBCs in vivo
- Only autoantibodies
- Autoantibodies plus alloantibodies
- Alloantibodies only

SERUM SCREEN TO DETERMINE SERUM ANTIBODY(IES) CHARACTERISTICS

Purpose

To characterize serum autoantibodies in AIHA as far as the following: Are they agglutinins or sensitizing antibodies? Do they have hemolytic activity? Do they react preferentially at 20°C or at 37°C? Results of this testing, in conjunction with results of the DAT and the titer/thermal amplitude, can aid in the differential diagnosis of WAIHA versus cold AIHA versus warm plus cold AIHA variations.

Principle

The patient's serum is tested with and without acidification and the addition of fresh normal serum (as a source of complement), against untreated and enzyme-treated RBCs (allogeneic and autologous), at 20°C and 37°C (prewarmed).

Specimen Requirements

Patient's serum, about 2 mL

Patient's RBCs, preferably in EDTA; 37°C washed, or DTT/2ME-treated, if appropriate.

Materials

10 × and 12 × 75-mm test tubes

Complement source [pooled normal donor sera, not containing unexpected antibodies, fresh or stored (in aliquots) at –70°C.

RBCs [usually a pool of two commercial antibody detection RBCs (e.g., R_1R_1 + R_2R_2)]. If patient has alloantibodies, then RBCs should lack antigens that would react with alloantibody.

0.1% Ficin, prepared fresh by adding 4.5 mL PBS to 0.5 mL of 1% ficin

37°C water bath

20°C incubator if available

0.2N HCl: 10 mL 1N HCl + 40 mL deionized H_2O

pH meter with pH 7 reference buffer

PBS, pH 7.3

Uniform drop glass pipettes

Serologic centrifuge

37°C serologic centrifuge (if available)

37°C PBS in squeeze bottle

Polyspecific AGS

Antiglobulin control cells

Procedure

1. Turn on 37°C centrifuge to warm up. Place 37°C PBS into a 37°C water bath to warm up. Turn on pH meter.
2. Label two tubes for pooled RBCs, "PC" or "pool," and another 2 tubes for autologous cells, "Auto." Label one of each pair: "UT" (untreated) or "ET" (enzyme-treated).
3. Place 16 drops of 3% to 4% pooled RBCs into each of the two tubes marked "PC" or "pool."
4. Place 16 drops of 3% to 4% washed patient's RBCs into each of the two tubes marked "Auto."
5. Wash RBCs 1 time with PBS.
6. Add 2 vol of 0.1% ficin to 1 vol of the packed RBCs in the "ET" tubes (e.g., 0.2 mL ficin added to 0.1 mL RBCs).
7. Incubate at 37°C for the specified time for that lot (e.g., 15 minutes).
8. Wash 3 times with PBS.
9. Add 6 drops of PBS to each of the packed RBCs in the "UT" tube and the "ET" tube.
10. Place 27 drops of complement into a 12 × 75-mm tube labeled "AC." Add 3 drops 0.2N HCl.
11. Place 9 drops of patient's serum into a 12 × 75-mm tube labeled "ASAC." Add 1 drop 0.2N HCl and 10 drops of AC from step 10.
12. Place approximately 1 mL patient's serum into a 12 × 75-mm tube labeled "S."
13. Determine pH of sera in "S," "ASAC," and "AC" tubes. Record results on the worksheet.
14. If the pH of the sera in the "AC" or "ASAC" tubes is less than 6.5 or greater than 6.8, then adjust accordingly by adding more complement, or complement plus patient's serum (± acidification), respectively. In adjusting the pH of the ASAC, it is important to keep the 1:1 ratio of complement to serum. Record pH and any adjustment made.
15. Label two sets of eight 10 × 75-mm tubes: two tubes are labeled "S" (patient's serum), two tubes are labeled "ASAC" (acidified patient's serum plus AC), two tubes are labeled "AC" (acidified complement), and two tubes are labeled "Auto" (autologous RBCs). One of each pair is labeled "UT" (untreated cells), and the other is labeled "ET" (enzyme-treated cells). One set of eight tubes is labeled "20°C," and the other set of eight tubes is labeled "37°C."
16. Place 4 drops of patient's serum into each of the four tubes labeled "S" and into each of the four tubes labeled "Auto."
17. Place 4 drops of acidified serum plus AC (ASAC) into each of the four tubes labeled "ASAC."
18. Place 4 drops of the AC into each of the four tubes labeled "AC."
19. Place the set of serum tubes labeled "37°C" into the 37°C water bath. Place the set of serum tubes labeled "20°C" and the RBC tubes at 19°C to 21°C.

20. After the 20°C sera tubes and the RBC tubes have reached 19°C to 21°C (e.g., ≥5 minutes' incubation, if necessary), use a uniform drop pipette to add 1 drop of untreated pooled RBCs to each of the S, ASAC, and AC tubes labeled "UT"; 1 drop of the untreated autologous RBCs to the tube labeled "Auto UT"; 1 drop of the enzyme-treated pooled RBCs to each of the S, ASAC, and AC tubes labeled "ET"; and 1 drop of the enzyme-treated autologous RBCs to the tube labeled "Auto ET." Record temperature on worksheet.
21. Move the RBC tubes to 37°C. Make sure a uniform drop pipette is in each tube.
22. After the 37°C sera tubes and the RBC tubes have reached 37°C (≥5 minutes' incubation), add RBCs to sera tubes as in step 20. Record temperature on worksheet.
23. Incubate all tubes for 1 to 2 hours.
24. Gently resuspend the "20°C" set of settled RBCs and record the results (settled reading).
25. Centrifuge the "20°C" set for 15 to 20 seconds (previously calibrated time) at 1000 × *g*.
26. Observe the supernatant carefully for hemolysis, and record results.
27. Gently resuspend the button of cells and observe for agglutination. Record results after centrifugation.
28. Gently resuspend the "37°C" set of settled RBCs and record the results (settled reading). (Read each tube one at a time, returning tubes to 37°C as soon as possible.)
29. Bring the 37°C centrifuge to 37°C ± 2°C by centrifuging (e.g., 1 minute or more).
30. Centrifuge the "37°C" set for 15 to 20 seconds (calibrated time) in the 37°C centrifuge.
31. Maintain the 37°C temperature (i.e., by keeping the tubes in the warm 37°C centrifuge or placing them back into the 37°C incubator).
32. Carefully observe each supernatant for hemolysis. Record results.
33. One tube at a time, gently resuspend the button of cells and observe for agglutination (return tubes to the 37°C incubator or 37°C centrifuge as soon as possible). Record results after centrifugation.
34. Recentrifuge the "37°C" set for 30 to 60 seconds in the 37°C centrifuge.
35. Quickly remove supernatant serum.
36. Wash RBCs 4 times with 37°C saline in the 37°C centrifuge.
37. Add 2 drops PBS to each tube. Draw RBCs up into pipette and dispense 1 drop back into the tube; discard the pipette containing the remainder of the RBCs.
38. Add polyspecific AGS to each of the tubes.
39. Centrifuge for 15 to 20 seconds (calibrated time) at 1000 × *g*. Read for agglutination (macroscopically negative tests should be read microscopically). Record results.
40. Add antiglobulin control cells to all negative tests.
41. Centrifuge.
42. Read for agglutination (macroscopically) and record results.

Quality Control

Antiglobulin control cells are added to check for reactivity/presence of AGS. Reactivity should be macroscopically positive. If the antiglobulin control cells are nonreactive or react weaker than expected, then repeat the test.

The AC tests control for reactivity of the complement source in the test system and are usually nonreactive. If the AC does react, then results of patient's serum plus AC need to be judged taking that background reactivity into account.

Interpretation

Results are interpreted on a case-by-case basis, in conjunction with the results of the titer/thermal amplitude study (if performed) and the DAT. Typical results for warm AIHA and CAS are shown in Tables 6-4, 6-5, and 6-6.

Notes

1. If the patient's serum contains alloantibodies, select RBCs that are antigen negative. If the patient's autoantibody shows a blood group specificity, then select antigen positive test RBCs.
2. If there is no reactivity observed in the 20°C tests, then there is no need to spin or wash the "37°C" tests at 37°C. A cell washer could be used to wash RBCs for the AGT, however, still remove the serum before washing and reduce the RBC volume after washing as in steps 34–37. Performing the IAT on the 10% RBC button can lead to decreased sensitivity.
3. If the 37°C tests are not performed strictly at 37°C, then positive results may be misinterpreted, leading to erroneous conclusions regarding the classification of the AIHA and to the clinical significance of the autoantibody.

COLD AGGLUTININ TITER/THERMAL AMPLITUDE/Ii SPECIFICITY

We usually only perform these tests if agglutination is observed at 20°C in the serum screening. If only the cold agglutinin titer is required, the tests below can be reduced to a single row of dilutions tested against group OI adult RBCs incubated at 4°C. Precautions mentioned below in step k. still apply.

1. Serial dilutions (1 in 1 to 1 in 2048) of the warm (37°C) separated patient's serum are prepared in saline, in 0.5 mL quantitities. The last aliquot to be

TABLE 6-4. TYPICAL RESULTS OF SERUM SCREENING TESTS IN AUTOIMMUNE HEMOLYTIC ANEMIA

			Warm Autoimmune Hemolytic Anemia			
			S	AS + AC	Negative Control AC	Auto
Untreated RBCs	20°C	Lysis	0	0	0	0
		Agglutination	0	0	0	0
	37°C	Lysis	0	0	0	0
		Agglutination	0	0	0	0
		IAT	2+	2+	0	*
Enzyme-treated RBCs	20°C	Lysis	0	0	0	0
		Agglutination	1+	1+	0	1+
	37°C	Lysis	½+	2+	0	½+
		Agglutination	3+	3+	0	3+

S, Patient's serum; AS, patient's serum + 0.1 vol 0.2 N HCl, pH 6.5 to 6.8; AS + AC, Acidified serum + acidified complement (normal inert fresh serum + 0.1 vol 0.2 N HCl, pH 6.5 to 6.8.
*Depends on strength of DAT.

TABLE 6-5. TYPICAL RESULTS OF SERUM SCREENING TESTS IN AUTOIMMUNE HEMOLYTIC ANEMIA

			Cold Agglutinin Syndrome			
			S	AS + AC	Negative Control AC	Auto
Untreated RBCs	20°C	Lysis	1+	3+	0	0
		Agglutination	4+	4+	0	4+
	37°C	Lysis	0	0	0	0
		Agglutination	0	0	0	0
		IAT	0	0	0	*
Enzyme-treated RBCs	20°C	Lysis	2+	4+	0	1+
		Agglutination	4+	X	0	4+
	37°C	Lysis	0	0	0	0
		Agglutination	0	0	0	0

S, Patient's serum; AS, patient's serum + 0.1 vol 0.2 N HCl, pH 6.5 to 6.8; AS + AC, acidified serum + acidified complement (normal inert fresh serum + 0.1 vol 0.2 N HCl, pH 6.5 to 6.8; X, no RBCs left.
*Depends on strength of DAT.

TABLE 6-6. TYPICAL RESULTS OF SERUM SCREENING TESTS IN AUTOIMMUNE HEMOLYTIC ANEMIA

			Paroxysmal Cold Hemoglobinuria			
			S	AS + AC	Negative Control AC	Auto
Untreated RBCs	20°C	Lysis	0	0	0	0
		Agglutination	0	0	0	0
	37°C	Lysis	0	0	0	0
		Agglutination	0	0	0	0
		IAT	0	0	0	‡
Enzyme-treated RBCs	20°C	Lysis	0	2+†	0	0
		Agglutination	1+*	1+*	0	0
	37°C	Lysis	0	0	0	0
		Agglutination	0	0	0	0

S, Patient's serum; AS, patient's serum + 0.1 vol 0.2 N HCl, pH 6.5 to 6.8; AS + AC, acidified serum + acidified complement (normal inert fresh serum + 0.1 vol 0.2 N HCl, pH 6.5 to 6.8).
*Found in 3 of 6 cases we studied.
†Found in 4 of 6 cases we studied.
‡Depends on strength of DAT.

TABLE 6-7. EXAMPLE OF RESULTS OF A COLD AGGLUTININ TITER

	Dilutions of Patient's Serum (×10³)								
	1	2	4	8	16	32	64	128	256
Same pipette or pipette tip	4+	4+	4+	4+	3+	3+	2+	1+	0
Separate pipettes or pipette tip	3½+	3+	2+	1+	½+	0	0	0	0

carried over is kept in case further dilutions are required. It is of prime importance that separate pipettes (or pipette tips) are used to transfer each 0.5 mL aliquot to the next tube when preparing each dilution as "carry over" can give extremely inaccurate high titers if a single pipette or pipette tip is used. (See Table 6-7; patient's correct titer was 8000, not 128,000 as reported to us.)

2. Place three rows of 10 × 75 mm tubes in a rack. The first row is labeled "I." The second row is labeled "i" and the third row is labeled "auto."
3. Starting from the highest dilution (e.g., 2048), dispense 2 drops of diluted serum into three tubes (e.g., 2048I; 2048i and 2048 auto).
4. Prepare three 2% to 5% washed RBC suspensions from group O adult I cells (e.g., pool of two screening cells), group O cord i cells, and the patient's own 37°C washed RBCs. In addition, if the patient is group A or B, it is sometimes useful to test A_1 or B RBCs (this may suggest anti-H, -HI, -A or -B specificity instead of the more common anti-I specificity).
5. Incubate the tubes containing serum dilutions at 37°C until they reach 37°C (5–10 minutes).
6. Incubate aliquots of the washed RBC suspensions at 37°C, along with the serum dilutions, and also allow to reach 37°C.
7. When both RBCs and serum are at 37°C, add 1 drop of cell suspension to each of the appropriate rows. Mix and allow to incubate for up to 2 hours.
8. Either centrifuge strictly at 37°C after 30 minutes to 1 hour or allow the RBCs to sediment at 37°C for 2 hours before reading for agglutination. If the tubes are centrifuged at 37°C, they must be put back in the 37°C water bath immediately after centrifugation and each tube read separately, as quickly as possible, so that no cooling ensues. Similar care must be taken if the cells are allowed to sediment.
9. After reading, move the tubes to a 30°C water bath. Then read the tests following 2 hours sedimentation at 30°C, taking the same care as mentioned above.
10. Next, incubation at room temperature is used; then the tubes can be centrifuged at room temperature after 30 minutes to 1 hour.
11. After reading, incubate the tubes at 4°C. The tubes can either be centrifuged at 4°C (i.e., in a refrigerated centrifuge, validated for serologic methods), after 30 minutes to 1 hour, or left for at least 2 hours (we often leave ours overnight) to sediment at 4°C before reading.

    When reading the 4°C tests, it is important that the rack of tubes is placed in a melting ice bath (following centrifugation or sedimentation) and the tubes read rapidly, one at a time. Table 6-7 shows results from a typical anti-I cold autoagglutinin.

Interpretation

1. Normal cold agglutinin titer is less than 64 in saline at 4°C.
2. Cold agglutinin titers associated with CAS are usually ≥1000 at 4°C.
3. Reactivity of a cold agglutinin at 30°C in albumin distinguishes clinically significant (i.e., associated with in vivo hemolysis) from clinically insignificant cold autoantibodies.[95] If the patient has hemolytic anemia and the agglutinin was nonreactive at 30°C, perform the 30°C test in the presence of albumin (i.e., patient's undiluted serum + 30% albumin + RBCs[95]) to determine the thermal amplitude.
4. Cold agglutinins of normal titer at 4°C (≤64), but of high thermal amplitutde (30°C or 37°C) can be seen in the "mixed type" AIHA (i.e., IgG warm autoantibodies are also present).
5. Some agglutinins in the IgM warm autoimmune category demonstrate optimal reactivity at 20°C to 30°C.
6. A titer difference of more than two tubes and/or a score difference of greater than 10 is considered to indicate a significant difference between results of different RBCs.
7. Stronger reactions with I adult RBCs than with cord RBCs and/or i adult RBCs indicate anti-I specificity.
8. Stronger reactions with cord RBCs than with I adult RBCs indicate anti-i specificity.
9. Anti-I^T reacts strongest with i cord RBCs, less strong with I adult RBCs, and least strong with i adult RBCs.

Notes

1. If only a cold agglutinin titer is required, testing can be limited to a single set of dilutions tested

against a pool of group O adult I RBCs incubated at 4°C for 1–2 hours or overnight.
2. Use separate pipette tips for transferring each aliquot when preparing dilutions as carryover can result in inaccurate titers.
3. It may be desirable to test other RBCs (e.g., i adult RBCs or ABO identical RBCs) in order to determine the autoantibody specificity.
4. Thoroughly mix the patient's serum/plasma before preparing the dilutions. If cryoglobulins are present and precipitated out, the titer result may not be accurate (falsely lower).
5. Settled readings are more accurate after 2 hours of incubation.
6. If the agglutinin reacts at the warmer temperatures (e.g., at 37°C or 30°C) and the titer is not increasing as the temperature is lowered, then the observed titers at the lower temperatures may be due to agglutination carryover. It may be necessary to repeat the titers with separate sets of tubes for each temperature.

Titration of Hemolysins

If hemolysins are detected in the serum screen, it is not usually necessary to quantitate the reaction, but on some occasions (e.g., following effects of therapy), it may be useful information.

1. Make serial dilutions (1 in 2 to 1 in 512) of the patient's serum in "fresh" inert serum as a source of complement (stored serum may be used if correct storage conditions for complement activity are applied.[96] If the serum screen indicates lysis only in AS + AC, then the fresh normal serum should be acidified to pH 6.5 to 6.8. A control tube of the complement alone should also be set up.
2. To 0.2 mL aliquots of each dilution, 1 drop of 10–20% group O RBCs in saline (preferably buffered to pH 7–7.4). If only the enzyme-treated RBCs are hemolyzed in the screening, then these are substituted for the untreated RBCs.
3. The tubes are mixed and incubated for 1 hour. If *cold* hemolysins are being quantitated, then the tubes are incubated at 20°C. If *warm* hemolysins are being quantitated, then the serum dilutions and RBCs are warmed to 37°C separately for approximately 10 minutes, then the cells are added.
4. After incubation, mix the tubes gently (mixing is important) and centrifuge at 1000 RCF for 2 minutes. If warm hemolysins are being measured, then the centrifugation should be at 37°C.
5. Examine the supernatants for lysis and grade the results.

Note

If the patient's serum is already red due to in vivo lysis, then it is a good idea to also take into account the size of the unlysed RBC button (i.e., compare it with the tube containing complement only).

DONATH-LANDSTEINER (DL) TEST

Procedure

1. Place 5 drops of patient's serum into each of 4 tubes, two labeled "test" and two labeled "control."
2. To one of the "test" tubes and one of the "control" tubes, add 2 to 5 drops of fresh normal serum.
3. To a 5th tube (complement control), add 5 drops of fresh normal serum.
4. Add 1 drop of 25% RBCs to each tube.
5. Place the patient's "control" tubes in the 37°C incubator.
6. Place the patient's "test" tubes and the complement control tube in a melting ice bath for 30–60 minutes.
7. After 30–60 minutes, gently mix the tubes in the melting ice and transfer them to the 37°C incubator. Incubate 30 minutes.
8. Gently mix and centrifuge all tubes.
9. Observe for lysis. Record results (hemolysis is graded on a 0 to 4+ scale with 4+ indicating total hemolysis of test RBCs; less than total hemolysis is graded subjectively from weak- to 3+ based on increasing color of supernatant and/or decreasing size of cell button).

Quality Control

The complement control tube is a negative control (no lysis). If the complement alone causes lysis, the test with the added complement is invalid. Repeat the test without complement added (if not already done) or with a new source of complement.

The patient's 37°C only tube is a negative control (no lysis). If the 37°C only tube shows lysis, repeat the test with the 37°C test set up prewarmed; if possible, include a parallel patient's serum control set up precooled at 0°C. Both the 37°C and 0°C controls, set up prewarmed and precooled, respectively, should be negative.

Interpretation

1. Hemolysis in the patient's "test" tube (with or without complement added), without lysis in the control tubes, indicates a positive test. To confirm that the lysis is not a false positive test due to a monophasic lysin, place the patient's 37°C "control" tube(s) at 20°C for 60 minutes.
2. No hemolysis in the patient's "test" tube indicates a negative test.

Notes

1. The test can also be performed by placing samples of the patient's blood into two tubes prewarmed to 37°C. One sample is left to clot at 37°C. The other is placed immediately in melting ice and left undisturbed for 1 hour. It is then moved to 37°C for 30 minutes, centrifuged, and

inspected for hemolysis. This is known as the direct Donath-Landsteiner (DL) Test and is a simple way of performing the test, but rather wasteful of blood, and less sensitive than the indirect test described above.

2. The indication of a positive test is grossly evident in in vitro hemolysis so that presence of marked hemoglobinemia, which is common in the acute stages of PCH, complicates the test. One way to observe for hemolysis when using a test serum that is already pink or red is to note the size of the RBC button after centrifugation. A change in the color of the serum may not be evident, but only a small number of cells may remain indicating that hemolysis has taken place. If a change in the size of the RBC button is not readily apparent when compared to a control tube utilizing the same volume of RBCs, additional variations on the theme should be performed as follows:
3. Since antibody is fixed to the RBCs in the cold phase of incubation and warming is necessary only to allow the complement cascade to proceed, the patient's serum may be replaced by fresh normal ABO compatible serum after the cold incubation. This technique is called a "two-stage" DL test and is useful when the patient's serum is red before performing the test. After incubation for 1 hour at 0°C, the supernatant serum is removed from the settled RBCs (centrifugation is not necessary) and replaced with fresh normal ABO compatible serum. The tube is then incubated at 37°C after gentle mixing and observed for hemolysis as described above. Since a small amount of the patient's serum may remain in the original tube, a control tube utilizing the patient's inactivated (heated to 56°C for 30 minutes) serum followed by replacement with normal inactivated serum will be necessary.
4. Enzyme-treated RBCs can be used for the DL test, but careful controls are necessary. On rare occasions, the DL test is only positive with enzyme-treated RBCs.[97-99]
5. It is also possible to test for the DL antibody by the IAT, although this sometimes presents difficulties because of agglutination at 0°C caused by the DL antibody itself or by a coincidentally occurring IgM cold agglutinin. If direct agglutination after the cold incubation step is absent or weak, the RBCs may then be washed four times in ice-cold saline (to avoid elution of the antibody) and tested with monospecific anti-IgG AGS.[99] Although it is advisable to do the IAT in the cold for maximal reactivity, some antibody may remain fixed to the cells even after incubation at 37°C.[100-102] If pp or P^k RBCs are available, these can serve as controls, since the specificity of DL antibodies is almost always anti-P. Performing the DL test against normal group O, P+ RBCs, and pp or P^k RBCs also defines the specificity of the antibody and further confirms the diagnosis of PCH. This is evidenced by the fact that the AGT is positive on unlysed cells remaining after performing the biphasic hemolysis test.

As a patient recovers from his illness and the antibody gradually weakens in reactivity, the IAT may remain positive indicating that this is a sensitive means of detecting the antibody. The specificity of the antibody as demonstrated by the IAT will be the same as when tested by the classic bithermic hemolysis test.

QUESTION 4: *What is the specificity of the antibody eluted from the patient's RBCs and present in the patient's serum?*

It is essential to prepare an eluate from the RBCs if one wants to characterize (e.g., determine the specificity) of the autoantibody. If RBCs have only complement components demonstrable on them by the DAT, then no antibody is usually detectable in the eluate from the RBCs. If IgG is present on the cells, it can usually be eluted by any of the many elution methods described in the literature. Most of the elution data we published in 1980[35] were based on the ether elution method. In the 1980s, we routinely used a xylene[103] method, and in the 1990s we used an acid elution method (Elu-Kit II, Gamma Biologicals) and later a modification of this method following the findings of some false-positive results using the original method.[104]

If the patient has not been transfused recently, then the eluate should contain autoantibody only; if the specificity is obvious then one can confirm the presence of the matching antigen on the patient's RBCs. If a patient with hemolytic anemia has a positive DAT due to IgG sensitization, and the eluate shows no activity against normal cells, then an association with drugs might be suspected. A good example of this is penicillin-induced hemolytic anemia where the eluate from DAT-positive cells will not react with untreated normal cells, but will react strongly with RBCs treated with penicillin (see Chapter 8). It should be emphasized that, as mentioned previously, up to 80% of eluates prepared from random DAT+ patients are nonreactive and are probably due to uptake of nonantibody proteins.

DETERMINING SPECIFICITY OF AUTOANTIBODIES

Many interesting observations and concepts have been derived from detailed studies of the specificity of autoantibodies in AIHA (see Chapter 7). However, such exhaustive studies are not required for *diagnostic* purposes. Nevertheless, we feel it is useful (if time allows) to perform at least limited specificity studies, especially in patients with suspected WAIHA. This is true because diagnostic error is avoided by confirming that the patient's warm antibody is, indeed, an autoantibody. In some patients, alloantibody(ies) may be detected in addition to autoantibody and it is helpful to have such information available since transfusion may be required. The specificity of the autoantibody may also be of significance with regard to transfusion. Delaying specificity testing until a decision is made that blood is needed for transfusion (at which time the need may be urgent) is not recommended. In still other patients, the initial impression of AIHA may not be substantiated. Antibody found in initial screening tests of the patient's serum may be alloantibody and the DAT may be positive for any of the reasons listed on page 213. If the patient has been transfused recently, a distinction between delayed hemolytic transfusion reactions and AIHA may be difficult, and the specificity of the RBC-bound antibody may be a clue to which is occurring (see Chapter 9). If the patient has received cefotetan recently, the DAT and the apparent autoantibody could be drug induced (see Chapter 8).

DETERMINING SPECIFICITY OF AUTOANTIBODIES ASSOCIATED WITH WARM TYPE AUTOIMMUNE HEMOLYTIC ANEMIA

If the eluate (and/or serum) reacts with all RBCs on a routine panel and no specificity is obvious, the earliest recommended method was to first test dilutions of the eluate (and/or serum) against rr, R_1R_1, and R_2R_2 RBCs.[5] If stronger reactions are obtained with some phenotypes, the results are expressed as a "relative specificity."

Dilution Technique

1. Prepare serial doubling dilutions of eluate (and/or serum) in saline from 1 in 1 to 1 in 512 (e.g., 0.2 aliquots).
2. Starting from highest dilution, transfer 2 drops to three 10 × 75-mm test tubes labeled rr, R_1R_1, R_2R_2.
3. Add 1 drop of 2% to 5% group O rr, R_1R_1, R_2R_2 RBCs to each appropriate row of tubes.
4. Incubate at 37°C for 15 to 60 minutes.
5. Wash 4 times in isotonic saline.
6. Add AGS to button of washed RBCs.
7. Examine for agglutination

Table 6-8 shows results of an eluate that would be interpreted as showing an anti-e of "relative specificity." The major disadvantage of this method is that it assumes that the specificity is within the Rh system, which is not always true (see Chapter 7, and references 105 and 106). In addition, we have often found that when eluates or sera showing results similar to those shown in Table 6-8 (i.e., anti-e of relative specificity) are tested with more RBCs (e.g., more R_2R_2 cells), then the specificity pattern is different. We recommended a modification of this technique[35]; that is, a dilution of the eluate (and/or serum) is selected that gives an approximate 1 to 2+ reaction and that dilution is tested against as many different phenotypes as possible; very rare RBCs lacking high frequency antigens have to be included and possible adsorption/elution studies to define many specificities.[105-109] An additional advantage of this latter approach is that the results may indicate alloantibody (as alloantibody is commonly of higher titer than autoantibody), in addition to autoantibody specificity. Table 6-9 illustrates a case where the undiluted eluate reacted with all cells and the serum appeared to have relative anti-e specificity. A 1 in 64 dilution of the eluate showed relative anti-e specificity and a 1 in 4 dilution of the serum showed an allo anti-K to be present in addition to the anti-"e."

Differential Adsorptions and Elutions

The patient's serum or eluate can be adsorbed with RBCs of known phenotype and the adsorbed serum or eluate tested against a panel. In addition, an eluate prepared from the adsorbing RBCs can be tested against a panel. Such tests are time consuming and need large quantities of RBCs, but have sometimes revealed interesting specificities.[107-109] Descriptions of so-called mimicking autoantibodies have made the interpretations of this method complex. Issitt and coworkers[109] studied 48 autoantibodies with apparent "simple" Rh specificity (anti-e, -E, -D, -C, -Ce, -G) by multiple adsorption tests. The finding that 34

TABLE 6-8. ELUATE SHOWING ANTI-e OF "RELATIVE SPECIFICITY"

	Dilutions of Patient's Eluate							
Phenotype of RBCs	2	4	8	16	32	64	128	256
rr	4+	3+	3+	2+	2+	1+	0	0
R_1R_1	4+	3+	3+	2+	2+	1+	0	0
R_2R_2	3+	2+	1+	0	0	0	0	0

TABLE 6-9. SPECIFICITY TESTING OF ELUATE AND SERUM

IAT on Pooled Screening RBCs	Dilutions 2	4	8	16	32	64	128	256
Eluate	3+	3+	2+	2+	1+	1+	0	0
Serum	2+	1+	0	0	0	0	0	0

	Selected Group O RBCs rr K−	rr K+	r'r K−	R_1R_1 K+	R_1R_1 K−	R_1R_2 K−	R_2R_2 K−	r"r" K−
Eluate neat	3+	3+	3+	3+	3+	3+	3+	3+
Eluate 1in 64	1+	1+	1+	1+	1+	1+	0	0
Serum neat	2+	2+	2+	2+	2+	2+	0	0
Serum 1in 4	0	1+	0	1+	0	0	0	0

(70.8%) of these antibodies could bind to RBCs lacking the antigens that the antibodies appeared to define indicated that the antibodies had different specificities than indicated by initial antibody identification tests. For instance, in contrast to allo-anti-E, autoantibodies that appeared to have anti-E specificity could be adsorbed by E negative RBCs. Those autoantibodies that at first appeared to be directed against the Rh antigens e, E, or c, most often had anti-Hr or anti-Hr_0 specificity (see Chapter 7).

Most autoantibodies in patients with WAIHA have specificity within the Rh system (see Chapter 7). Using rare cells such as -D- and Rh_{null}, Weiner and Vos[107] described specificity against normal cells, partially deleted cells, and deleted cells. Autoantibodies that failed to react with Rh_{null} RBCs and had anti-U specificity have been described. It was suggested that the "Rh-related" autoantibodies that cannot be identified as specific Rh antibodies may be anti-U. We examined eluates from the RBCs of eight patients with AIHA using a panel of extremely rare cells and cross-adsorption and elution techniques.[108] We demonstrated autoantibody specificities not definable without the rare cells, and further defined heterogeneity of the LW antigen. Autoantibodies with U specificity occurred in three eluates only; anti-U was always present with an antibody of another specificity. Six of the eluates contained anti-LW, two anti-nl, five anti-pdl, three anti-dl, and one anti-e. Adsorption and elution studies using the rare Rh-positive LW-negative (Mrs. B) RBCs showed that anti-pdl may in fact represent anti-LW + anti-LW_1 and that Mrs. B may represent a weak variant of LW. Injection of her RBCs into guinea pigs produced an anti-LW that reacted similarly to the antibody produced by injecting Rh-positive LW-positive cells. An analogy to the ABO was suggested: Normal Rh+ RBCs may represent LW_1. Rh-negative LW-positive RBCs may represent LW_2, Mrs. B may represent LW_3, and Rh_{null} cells may represent the only true LW-negative (lw).[105,108]

DETERMINING SPECIFICITY OF AUTOANTIBODIES ASSOCIATED WITH COLD AGGLUTININ SYNDROME

As the specificity associated with CAS is commonly anti-I and less commonly anti-i, the specificity is usually obvious from the results of the cold agglutinin titer/thermal range technique described on page 220. As all adult cells contain some i and all cord cells some I, results are never clear-cut when determining specificity within the Ii "system." Often, at 4°C the i cells will react as strongly as the I cells, and only by performing a titer and thermal range will the specificity become obvious (Table 6-10 shows the results of a typical anti-I). When cord RBCs react stronger than adult RBCs, the specificity may be anti-i but adult i RBCs will have to be tested to confirm that these reactions are due to anti-i rather than anti-I^T (see Chapter 7). The determination of the specificity of the cold agglutinin is often only of academic interest as it is not recommended that the rare i adult blood is obtained for these patients but that they are transfused with normal I adult blood at 37°C (see Chapter 10). If further confirmation of specificity is required (e.g., to determine if antibody is possibly anti-HI, etc.), then the titration/thermal range technique can be extended using more cells, for example, I adult, i cord, and/or i adult RBCs of different ABO types and O_h (Bombay) RBCs. On rare occasions, another specificity, anti-Pr, is observed.[110] This should be suspected if the I adult and i cord (and/or i adult) RBCs react equally at all phases. The Pr antigens are destroyed by proteolytic enzymes. Thus, the cold agglutinin titer can be repeated comparing untreated RBCs with enzyme-treated RBCs (e.g., papain-treated). Both anti-I and anti-i react better with enzyme-treated RBCs, but most anti-Pr will give no reaction, or much weaker reactions. Other antibodies that react with antigens that are destroyed by enzyme-treatment (e.g., M and N) must be excluded by testing a panel of RBCs; anti-Pr

TABLE 6-10. TYPICAL COLD AGGLUTININ TITER/THERMAL RANGE SUGGESTING ANTI-H SPECIFICITY

	4°C		25°C		30°C	
Dilutions of Patients' Sera	Adult RBCs	Cord RBCs	Adult RBCs	Cord RBCs	Adult RBCs	Cord RBCs
2	4+	4+	4+	1+	1+	0
4	4+	4+	4+	1+	1+	0
8	4+	4+	4+	1+	1+	0
16	4+	4+	3+	½+	½+	0
32	4+	4+	2+	0	0	0
64	4+	4+	1+	0	0	0
128	4+	3+	½+	0	0	0
256	3+	3+	0	0	0	0
512	3+	2+	0	0	0	0
1024	2+	1+	0	0	0	0
2048	1+	0	0	0	0	0

TABLE 6-11. SUMMARY OF MOST IMPORTANT SEROLOGIC CHARACTERISTICS ASSOCIATED WITH AIHA

Type	DAT	Eluate	Serologic Characteristics	Antibody Specificity
Warm AIHA	IgG and/or complement (C3dg)	IgG antibody	IAT positive (50% to 90% sera), agglutinating enzyme premodified cells (90%), hemolyzing enzyme premodified cells (13%)	Usually within Rh system; other specificities include LW, U, I^T, K, Kp^b, K13, Ge, Jk^a, En^a, and Wr^b
Cold agglutinin syndrome	Complement (C3dg) alone	Negative	Agglutinating activity up to 30°C in albumin; high titer at 4°C (usually ≥512)	Usually anti-I; other specificities include i, Pr, Gd, and Sd^x
Paroxysmal cold hemoglobinuria	Complement (C3dg) alone	Negative	Biphasic hemolysin (i.e., sensitizing red cells in the cold and then hemolyzing them when moved to 37°C)	Anti-P (i.e., reacts with all normal red cells except p or P^k cells)

will react with all untreated human RBCs on the panel. Further confirmatory tests can be performed using various animal RBCs and neuraminidase-treated RBCs[110] (see Chapter 7).

DETERMINING SPECIFICITY OF AUTOANTIBODIES ASSOCIATED WITH PAROXYSMAL COLD HEMOGLOBINURIA

In our experience and in the experience of Dacie,[5] the specificity of the DL antibody in PCH has always been anti-P. There are isolated reports of other specificities.[105] In contrast to CAS, the specificity may be of clinical importance when transfusing patients with PCH, as this is the only AIHA where the specificity is clear-cut like an alloantibody. Because of this, some workers have suggested that the rare pp RBCs have such better survival that it is worth trying to obtain them for transfusing to PCH patients with severe acute hemolysis.[111,112] However, since obtaining pp RBCs is likely to delay transfusion, which is often needed urgently in PCH patients, we advise using common P positive blood in such instances. Our limited experience has been that common P positive blood, if given at 37°C, gives the expected rise in hematocrit, but if this does not occur then we agree that there is an argument for trying to obtain the blood of the rare pp phenotype. To determine specificity, the patient's serum should be tested against I adult, i cord (and/or i adult), and the rare pp and/or P^k RBCs by the DL test.

REFERENCES

1. Coombs RRA, Mourant AE, Race RR: A new test for the detection of weak and "incomplete" Rh agglutinins. Br J Exp Pathol 1945;26:255.
2. Boorman KE, Dodd BE, Loutit JF, Mollison P: Some results of transfusion of blood to recipients with "cold" agglutinins. Br Med J 1946;i:751.
3. Loutit JF, Mollison PL: Haemolytic icterus (acholuric jaundice) congenital and acquired. J Pathol Bact 1946;58:711.
4. Coombs RRA, Mourant AE, Race RR: In vivo iso-sensitization of RBCs in babies with haemolytic disease. Lancet 1946;i:264.
5. Dacie JV: The Haemolytic Anaemias, 3rd ed. vol. 3, The Auto-immune Haemolytic Anaemias. New York: Churchill Livingstone, 1992.
6. Dacie JV, Crookston JH, Christenson WN: "Incomplete" cold antibodies: Role of complement in sensitization to antiglobulin serum by potentially haemolytic antibodies. Br J Haematol 1957;3:77.
7. Petz LD, Garratty G: Antiglobulin sera—past, present and future. Transfusion 1978;18:257–268.

8. Garratty G: The significance of complement in immunohematology. Crit Rev Clin Lab Sci 1985;20:25.
9. Freedman J: Complement in transfusion medicine. In: Garratty G, ed. Immunobiology of Transfusion Medicine. New York: Dekker, 1994:403–434.
10. Issitt PD, Anstee DJ: Applied Blood Group Serology, 4th ed. Durham, NC: Montgomery Scientific Publications, 1998.
11. Garratty G, Petz LD: An evaluation of commercial antiglobulin sera with particular reference to their anticomplement properties. Transfusion 1971;11:79–88.
12. Burkart P, Rosenfield RE, Hsu TCS, et al.: Instrumented PVP-augmented antiglobulin tests. I. Detection of allogeneic antibodies coating other normal erythrocytes. Vox Sang 1974;26:280.
13. Mollison PL, Engelfriet CP, Contreras M: Blood Transfusion in Clinical Medicine, 10th ed. Oxford: Blackwell Scientific, 1997.
14. Worlledge SM, Blajchman MA: The autoimmune haemolytic anemias. Br J Haematol 1972;23(Suppl.):61.
15. Sokol RJ, Booker DJ, Stamps R: The pathology of autoimmune haemolytic anaemia. J Clin Pathol 1992;45:1047–1052.
16. Garratty G: Autoimmune hemolytic anemias. In: Garratty G, (ed). Immunobiology of Transfusion Medicine. New York: Dekker, 1994:523–551.
17. Petz LD, Garratty G: Laboratory correlations in immune hemolytic anemias. In: Vyas GN, Sites DP, Brecher G, (eds). Laboratory Diagnosis of Immunologic Disorders. New York: Grune & Stratton, 1975.
18. Chaplin H, Jr: Clinical usefulness of specific antiglobulin reagents in autoimmune hemolytic anemias. In: Brown EB, (ed). Progress in Hematology, vol. VIII. New York: Grune & Stratton, 1973.
19. Dacie JV: Occurrences in normal human sera of "incomplete" forms of "cold" autoantibodies. Nature (Lond) 1950;166:36.
20. Garratty G: The clinical significance (and insignificance) of red-cell-bound IgG and complement. In: Wallace ME, Levitt JS, (eds). Current Applications and Interpretation of the Direct Antiglobulin Test. Arlington, VA: American Association of Blood Banks, 1988:1–24.
21. Garratty G: The significance of IgG on the RBC surface. Transfus Med Rev 1987;1:47–57.
22. Toy PTCY, Chin CA, Reid ME, et al: Factors associated with positive direct antiglobulin tests in pretransfusion patients: A case-control study. Vox Sang 1975;49:216-220.
23. Heddle NM, Kelton JG, Turchyn KL, et al: Hypergammaglobulinemia can be associated with a positive direct antiglobulin test, a nonreactive eluate, and no evidence of hemolysis. Transfusion 1988;28:29–33.
24. Garratty G: Problems associated with passively transfused blood group alloantibodies. Am J Clin Pathol 1998;109:769–777.
25. Jandl JH: The agglutination and sequestration of immature RBCs. J Lab Clin Med 1960;55:663.
26. Sutherland DA, Eisentraut AM, McCall MS: The direct Coombs test and reticulocytes. Br J Haematol 1963;9:68–76.
27. Worlledge SM: The interpretation of a positive direct antiglobulin test. Br J Haematol 1978;39:157.
28. Stratton F, Renton PH: Effect of crystalloid solutions prepared in glass bottles on human RBCs. Nature (London) 1955;175:722.
29. Jandl JH, Simmons RL: The agglutination and sensitization of RBCs by metallic cations: Interactions between multivalent metals and the RBC membrane. Br J Haemat 1957;3:19.
30. Sturgeon P, Smith LE, Chun HMT, Hurvitz CH, Garratty G, Goldfinger D: Autoimmune hemolytic anemia associated exclusively with IgA of Rh specificity. Transfusion 1979;19:324–328.
31. Casey FM, Dodd BE, Lincoln PJ: A study of the characteristics of certain Rh antibodies preferentially detectable by enzyme technique. Vox Sang 1972;23:493–507.
32. Hughes-Jones NC, Polley MJ, Telford R, Gardner B, Kleinschmidt G: Optimal conditions for detecting blood group antibodies by the antiglobulin test. Vox Sang 1964;9:385.
33. Dupuy ME, Elliot M, Masouredis SP: Relationship between RBC bound antibody and agglutination in the antiglobulin reaction. Vox Sang 1964;9:40.
34. Gilliland BC: Coombs-negative immune hemolytic anemia. Semin Hematol 1976;13:267–275.
35. Petz LD, Garratty G: Acquired Immune Hemolytic Anemias, 1st ed. New York: Churchill Livingstone, 1980.
36. Merry AH, Thomsen EE, Rawlinson VI, Stratton F: A quantitative antiglobulin test for IgG for use in blood transfusion serology. Clin Lab Haematol 1982;4:393–402.
37. Jeje MO, Blajchman MA, Steeves K, Horsewood P, Kelton JG: Quantification of RBC-associated IgG using an immunoradiometric assay. Transfusion 1984;24:473–476.
38. Kay MMB: Mechanism of removal of senescent cells by human macrophages in situ. Proc Natl Acad Sci USA 1975; 72:3521–3525.
39. Alderman EM, Fudenberg HH, Lovins RE: Binding of immunoglobulin classes to subpopulations of human red blood cells separated by density-gradient centrifugation. Blood 1980;55:817–822.
40. Szymanski IO, Odgren PR, Fortier NL, et al: Red blood cell associated IgG in normal and pathologic states. Blood 1980;55:48–54.
41. Freedman J: Membrane-bound immunoglobulins and complement components on young and old RBCs. Transfusion 1984;24:477–481.
42. Kay MMB: Localization of senescent cell antigen on band 3. Proc Natl Acad Sci USA 1984;81:5753–5757.
43. Lutz HU, Flepp R, Stringaro-Wipf G: Naturally occurring autoantibodies to exoplasmic and cryptic regions of band 3 protein, the major integral membrane protein of human red blood cells. J Immunol 1984;133:2610–2618.
44. Low PS, Waugh SM, Zinke K, et al: The role of hemoglobin denaturation and band 3 clustering in red blood cell aging. Science 1985;227:531–533.
45. Graham HA, Davies DM, Jr, Brower CE: Detection of C3b and C3d on RBC membranes. International Symposium on the Nature and Significance of Complement Activation. Raritan Ortho Research Institute of Medical Sciences, 1976:107–111.
46. Rosenfield RE, Jagathambal K: Antigenic determinants of C3 and C4 complement components on washed erythrocytes from normal persons. Transfusion 1978;18:517–523.
47. Freedman J, Barefoot C: Red blood cell-bound C3d in normal subjects and in random hospital patients. Transfusion 1982;22:511–514.
48. Chaplin H, Nasongkla M, Monroe MC: Quantification of red blood cell-bound C3d in normal subjects and random hospitalized patients. Br J Haematol 1981;48:69–78.
49. Merry AH, Thomsen EE, Rawlinson VI, Stratton F: The quantification of C3 fragments on erythrocytes: Estimation of C3 fragments on normal cells, acquired haemolytic anaemia cases and correlation with agglutination of sensitized cells. Clin Lab Haematol 1983;5:387–397.
50. Freedman J: Membrane-bound imunoglobulins and complement components on young and old RBCs. Transfusion 1984;24:477–481.
51. Szymanski IO, Odgren PR, Valeri CR: Relationship between the third component of human complement (C3) bound to stored preserved erythrocytes and their viability in vivo. Vox Sang 1985;49:34–41.
52. Salama A, Mueller-Eckhardt C: Binding of fluid phase C3b to nonsensitized bystander human RBCs. Transfusion 1985;25:528–534.
53. Siegel I, Liu TL, Gleicher N: The red-cell immune system. Lancet 1981;ii:556–559.
54. Weiner W: "Coombs positive" "normal" people. Proceedings of the Tenth Congress of the International Society of Blood Transfusion, Stockholm, 1964:34–39.
55. Habibi B, Muller A, Lelong F, et al: Auto-immunisation erythrocytaire dans la population "normale." Nouvelle Presse Ed 1980;43:3253–3257.
56. Gorst DW, Rawlinson VI, Merry AH, et al: Positive direct antiglobulin test in normal individuals. Vox Sang 1980;38:99–105.
57. Allan J, Garratty G: Positive direct antiglobulin tests in normal blood donors. Proceedings of the International Society of Blood Transfusion, Montreal, 1980:150 (Abstr).

58. Bareford D, Longster G, Gilks L, et al: Follow-up of normal individuals with a positive antiglobulin test. Scand J Haematol 1985;35:348-53.
59. Pirofsky B: Autoimmunization and the Autoimmune Hemolytic Anemias. Baltimore: Williams & Wilkins, 1969.
60. Freedman J: False-positive antiglobulin tests in healthy subjects and in hospital patients. J Clin Pathol 1979; 32:1014–1018.
61. Bohnen RF, Ultmann JE, Gorman JG, Farhangi M, Scudder J: The direct Coomb's test: Its clinical significance. Ann Intern Med 1968;68:19–32.
62. Lau P, Haesler WE, Wurzel HA: Positive direct antiglobulin reaction in a patient population. Am J Clin Pathol 1975; 65:368–375.
63. Judd WJ, Butch SH, Oberman HA, Steiner EA, Bauer RC: The evaluation of a positive direct antiglobulin test in pretransfusion testing. Transfusion 1980;20:17–23.
64. Judd WJ, Barnes BA, Steiner EA, Oberman HA, Averill DB, Butch SH: The evaluation of a positive direct antiglobulin test (autocontrol) in pretransfusion testing revisited. Transfusion 1986;26:220–224.
65. Huh YO, Lichtiger B: Evaluation of a positive autologous control in pretransfusion testing. Am J Clin Pathol 1985; 84:632–636.
66. Toy PTCY, Reid M, Burns M: Positive direct antiglobulin test associated with hyperglobulinemia in acquired immunodeficiency sydnrome (AIDS). Am J Hematol 1985;19:145–150.
67. Chaplin H, Nasongkla M, Monroe MC: Quantification of red blood cell-bound C3d in normal subjects and random hospitalized patients. Br J Haematol 1981;48:69–78.
68. Freedman J, Ho M, Barefoot C: Red blood cell-bound C3d in selected hospital patients. Transfusion 1982;22:515–520.
69. Garratty G, Arndt PA: Application of flow cytofluorometry to red blood cell immunology. Cytometry 1999;38:259–267.
70. Hoppe PA: Background for current federal requirements for antiglobulin reagents in the United States. In: Chaplin H, Jr (ed). Immune Hemolytic Anemias. New York: Churchill Livingstone, 1984:209.
71. Garratty G, Petz LD: The significance of RBC bound complement components in development of standards and quality assurance for the anti-complement components of antiglobulin sera. Transfusion 1976;16:297–306.
72. Fruitstone MJ: C3b-sensitized erythrocytes (letter). Transfusion 1978;18:125.
73. Chaplin H, Friedman J, Massay A, Monroe MC: Characterization of red blood cells strongly coated in vitro by C3 via the alternative pathway. Transfusion 1980;20:256–262.
74. Moore JA, Chaplin H: Anti-C3d antiglobulin reagents. Transfusion 1974;14:407–415.
75. Garratty G, Arndt PA: Evaluation of IgG sensitized RBCs used for controlling antiglobulin tests. Transfusion 1999;39:104S (abstr).
76. Garratty G: Low affinity autoantibodies: A cause of false negative direct antiglobulin tests. Transfus Today 1991;12:3–4.
77. Postoway N, Garratty G: Standardization of IgG subclass antiserums for use with sensitized RBCs. Transfusion 1983; 23:398–400.
78. Garratty G, Postoway N, Nance S, Brunt D: Spontaneous agglutination of RBCs with a positive direct antiglobulin test in various media. Transfusion 1984;24:214–217.
79. Rodberg K, Tsuneta R, Garratty G: Discrepant Rh phenotyping results when testing IgG-sensitized RBCs with monoclonal Rh reagents. Transfusion 1995;35(Suppl.):67S.
80. Louie JE, Jiang AF, Zaroulis CG: Preparation of intact antibody-free red blood cells in autoimmune hemolytic anemia. Transfusion 1986;26:550 (Abstr).
81. Rekvig OP, Hannestad K: Acid elution of blood group antibodies from intact erythrocytes. Vox Sang 1977;33:280–285.
82. des Roziers NB, Squalli S: Removing IgG antibodies from intact red cells: Comparison of acid and EDTA, heat, and chloroquine elution methods. Transfusion 1997;37:497–501.
83. Byrne PC: Use of a modified acid/EDTA elution technique. Immunohematology 1991;7:46–47.
84. Holtz G, Mantel W, Buck W: The inhibition of antigen-antibody reactions by chloroquine and its mechanism of action. Z Immun Forsch Bd 1973;146:145–157.
85. Mantel W, Holtz G: Characterisation of autoantibodies to erythrocytes in autoimmune haemolytic anaemia by chloroquine. Vox Sang 1976;30:453463.
86. Edwards JM, Moulds JJ, Judd WJ: Chloroquine dissociation of antigen-antibody complexes. Transfusion 1982;22:59–61.
87. Sassetti R, Nichols D: Decreased antigenic reactivity caused by chloroquine. Transfusion 1982;22:537–538.
88. Mallory D, Reid M: Misleading effects of chloroquine (letter). Transfusion 1984;24:412.
89. McShane K, Cronwall S: Chloroquine reduces antigen strength (letter). Transfusion 1985;25:83.
90. Reid ME: Autoagglutination dispersal utilizing sulphydryl compounds. Transfusion 1998;18:353–355.
91. Merry AH, Thomson EE, Rawlinson VI, et al: Quantification of IgG on erythrocytes: correlation of number of IgG molecules per cell with the strength of the direct and indirect antiglobulin tests. Vox Sang 1984;47:73–81.
92. Kumpel BM: A simple non-isotopic method for the quantification of RBC-bound immunoglobulin. Vox Sang 1990; 59:34–38.
93. Dubarry M, Charron C, Habibi B, et al: Quantification of immunoglobulin classes and subclasses of autoantibodies bound to RBCs in patients with and without hemolysis. Transfusion 1993;33:466–471.
94. Garratty G, Nance SJ: Correlation between in vivo hemolysis and the amount of red cell-bound IgG measured by flow cytometry. Transfusion 1990;30:617–621.
95. Garratty G, Petz LD, Hoops JK: The correlation of cold agglutinin titrations in saline and albumin with haemolytic anaemia. Br J Haemat 1977;35:587–595.
96. Garratty G: The effect of storage and heparin on serum complement activity with particular reference to the detection of blood group antibodies. Am J Clin Pathol 1970;54:531–538.
97. Heddle NM: Acute paroxysmal cold hemoglobinuria. Transfus Med Rev 1989;III:219–229.
98. Sokol RJ, Booker DJ, Stamps R: Paroxysmal cold hemoglobinuria and the elusive Donath-Landsteiner antibody. Immunohematology 1998;14:109–112.
99. Worlledge SM, Rousso C: Studies on the serology of paroxysmal cold haemoglobinuria (PCH), with special reference to its relationship with the P blood group system. Vox Sang 1965;10:293–298.
100. Ries CA, Garratty G, Petz LD, et al: Paroxysmal cold hemoglobinuria: report of a case with an exceptionally high thermal range Donath-Lansteiner antibody. Blood 1971;38:491–499.
101. Lindgren S, Zimmerman S, Gibbs F, Garratty G: An unusual Donath-Landsteiner antibody detectable at 37°C by the antiglobulin test. Transfusion 1985;25:142–144.
102. Nordhagen R: Two cases of paroxysmal cold hemoglobinuria with a Donath-Landsteiner antibody reactive by the indirect antiglobulin test using anti-IgG (letter). Transfusion 1991;31:190.
103. Bueno R, Garratty G, Postoway N: Elution of antibody from RBCs using xylene—a superior method. Transfusion 1981; 21:157–162.
104. Leger RM, Arndt PA, Ciesielski DJ, Garratty G: False-positive eluate reactivity due to the low-ionic wash solution used with commercial acid-elution kits. Transfusion 1998;38:565–572.
105. Garratty G: Target antigens for red-cell-bound autoantibodies. In: Nance SJ, (ed). Clinical and Basic Science Aspects of Immunohematology. Arlington, VA: American Association of Blood Banks, 1991:33–72.
106. Garratty G: Specificity of autoantibodies reacting optimally at 37°C. Immunohematology 1999;15:24–40.
107. Weiner W, Vos GH: Serology of acquired hemolytic anemias. Blood 1963;22:606–613.
108. Vos GH, Petz LD, Garratty G, Fudenberg HH: Autoantibodies in acquired hemolytic anemia with special group reference to the LW system. Blood 1973;42:445–453.
109. Issitt PD, Zellner DC, Rolih SD, Duckett JB: Autoantibodies mimicking alloantibodies. Transfusion 1977;17:531–538.

110. Roelcke D: Cold agglutination. Transfus Med Rev 1989; 3:140–166.
111. Rausen AR, LeVine R, Hsu TCS, Rosenfield RE: Compatible transfusion therapy for paroxysmal cold hemoglobinuria. Pediatrics 1975;55:275–278.
112. Rosenfield RE, Jagathambal K: Transfusion therapy for autoimmune hemolytic anemia. Semin Haematol 1976;13:311.

CHAPTER 7

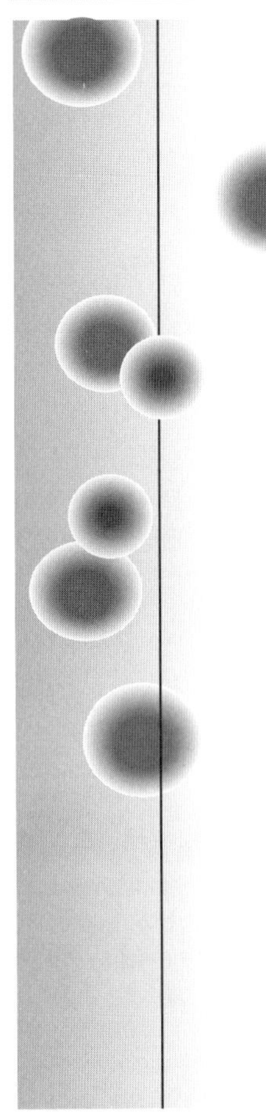

Specificity of Autoantibodies

Up to 1953, autoantibodies were generally considered to be "nonspecific"; that is, they reacted with all human red blood cells (RBCs) tested, although some variation in reaction had been observed.[1,2] The first convincing data suggesting that autoantibody specificity could be defined were presented by Race, Sanger, and Selwyn in 1951.[3]

SPECIFICITIES ASSOCIATED WITH WARM-ANTIBODY TYPE AUTOIMMUNE HEMOLYTIC ANEMIA

Rh and LW Specificity. Using RBCs from the recently discovered rare phenotype –D–, Race and coworkers[3] showed that the "nonspecific" autoantibodies could be subdivided into two groups; one group that reacted with –D– RBCs, and the other that did not; this suggested some Rh specificity. The first example of a clearly specific autoantibody was an autoanti-e in an R_1R_1 patient described by Weiner and coworkers in 1953[4]; others soon followed. Holländer[5] described an autoanti-c in an R_1r patient and showed that an additional "nonspecific" element was also present in the eluate made from the patient's RBCs. In 1953 and 1954, Dacie[6] and Dacie and Cutbush[7] reported specificities on 10 patients with warm-antibody type autoimmune hemolytic anemia (WAIHA): one R_1r patient had autoanti-C+e; the other nine patients had "nonspecific" autoantibodies, but three also had clearly demonstrable autoanti-e and one patient autoanti-e and -D (at different times). Wiener and coworkers[8] suggested that 37°C-reactive ("warm") autoantibodies might be directed against the "nucleus of the Rh-Hr substance." Pirofsky and Pratt, in 1966,[9] compared the reactions of alloanti-Rh and "warm" autoantibodies with RBCs from a large variety of primates and nonprimates and essentially agreed with the findings of Wiener and coworkers[8]; neither Rh alloantibodies nor autoantibodies reacted with nonprimate RBCs or certain primates (e.g., tree shrew, fulvus lemur, and woolly monkey), but both reacted with other primates (ringtail lemur, squirrel monkey, celebes ape, rhesus monkey, baboon, and chimpanzee). The authors concluded that the data strongly suggested that warm autoantibodies have specificity for Rh antigens.[8,9] In the next decade, many other workers reported on autoantibody specificities associated with WAIHA.[10]

With the exception of one anti-B,[11] one anti-Jk^a,[11] and two examples of anti-K,[12,13] all of the specificities reported during this time were associated with Rh. Autoanti-e was the most common reported specificity; it has been pointed out that the reported relative incidence of different specific Rh autoantibodies corresponds well with the incidence of Rh antigens in the population (i.e., e is present on the RBCs of approximately 98% of the population).[10] In 1963 Weiner and Vos[14] expanded the work of Race and coworkers,[3] who used RBCs of the rare phenotype –D– to demonstrate "Rh" specificity. Weiner and Vos[14] studied 60 RBC eluates that were initially thought to be nonspecific; these eluates were tested against RBCs of common phenotypes and rare phenotypes such as –D–, cD–, and the recently discovered Rh_{null}. Adsorptions, elutions (i.e., eluates made from RBCs incubated in vitro with eluates prepared from patients'

TABLE 7-1. AUTOANTIBODIES IN ACQUIRED HEMOLYTIC ANEMIA AND THEIR SEROLOGIC REACTIVITY FOR SELECTED RED BLOOD CELLS (RBCs)

	Anti-nl	Anti-pdl	Anti-dl	"Antigens"
RBCs with common ("normal") phenotypes	+	+	+	nl, pdl, dl
"Partially deleted" cells (–D–/–D– or cD–/cD–)	–	+	+	pdl, dl
"Fully deleted" cells [– – –/– – – (Rh_{null})]	–	–	+	dl

RBCs sensitized in vivo), and titrations were performed, using saline, albumin, enzymes, and indirect antiglobulin tests (IATs). Fifty-three percent of the eluates failed to react with Rh_{null} RBCs, and 18% reacted weaker than with RBCs of common phenotypes. Thus, approximately 70% of the eluates appeared to be reacting with Rh antigens. The patterns of reactivities suggested three different autoantibody types that could be present separately or in combination. They were termed anti-nl (normal), anti-pdl (partially deleted), and anti-dl (deleted) (Table 7-1). The nl determinants were said to be present on RBCs of common phenotypes but not –D–, Dc–, or Rh_{null}; the pdl determinants present on RBCs of common phenotypes, –D–, and Dc–, but not Rh_{null}; and the dl determinants present on RBCs of common phenotypes, –D–, Dc–, and Rh_{null}. Thus, if an autoantibody reacts with all RBCs of common phenotype but not "partially deleted" or "fully deleted" RBCs, the autoantibody would be classified as having anti-nl specificity. If the autoantibody reacts with all RBCs, it may be anti-dl but selective adsorptions may reveal a mixture of anti-dl + pdl, anti-dl + nl, or anti-dl + pdl + nl. In other words, adsorption of a "nonspecific" autoantibody with Rh_{null} RBCs may reveal an antibody only reacting with RBCs of common phenotype (Table 7-2). We confirmed these findings in our own laboratory and collaborated with Vos to extend the original observations.[15-17] It should be pointed out that autoanti-nl, -pdl, and -dl show patterns similar to antibodies of the later-defined specificities shown in Table 7-2, and may be identical specificities.

In a detailed review in 1969, Dacie and Worlledge[18] reviewed results on their series of AIHA patients seen over a 20-year period. Specificity testing of eluates from 98 patients with WAIHA were reported. When tested against a panel of RBCs with common phenotypes, approximately 30% showed obvious Rh specificity (23 anti-e, 4 anti-c, 1 anti-C + D, 1 anti-D + e). When –D– RBCs were added to the panel, an additional 17% could be classified as "Rh" specific (47% of the total) and if Rh_{null} RBCs were added, then an additional 5% could be added, giving a total of 52% showing some "Rh" specificity; results were very similar to those of Weiner and Vos.[14]

Leddy and coworkers[19] studied eluates from RBCs of 46 patients with WAIHA. They used a panel of rare human RBCs including Rh_{null}, –D–, LW negative, and K_o RBCs as well as monkey RBCs (rhesus and stump tailed monkeys). Sixteen of 20 eluates derived from patients whose RBCs were sensitized with both IgG and complement reacted with all RBCs tested. Conversely, 12 of 26 eluates from "IgG only" RBCs did not react with Rh_{null} RBCs, suggesting "Rh" specificity. Leddy and coworkers[19] found four patterns of reactions that suggested a working classification: Group I reacted with RBCs of common phenotype but were negative with Rh_{null} and monkey RBCs, and no complement was fixed in vitro; group II reacted with RBCs of common phenotype and weaker with Rh_{null}, about 25% reacted with monkey RBCs; group III reacted with RBCs of common phenotype and Rh_{null} RBCs equally but did not react with monkey RBCs; group IV reacted equally with RBCs of normal phenotypes, Rh_{null}, and monkey RBCs.

Vos and coworkers[15] studied 24 sera and RBC eluates from WAIHA. They showed that the IAT using untreated RBCs often showed different specificities than tests using ficin. As shown by others, they

TABLE 7-2. ANTI-nl, -pdl, AND -dl AUTOANTIBODIES MAY HAVE A WELL-DEFINED BLOOD GROUP SPECIFICITY IF TESTED AGAINST RED BLOOD CELLS (RBCs) OF RARE PHENOTYPES (E.G., NULL PHENOTYPES OTHER THAN RH_{null})

Anti-nl*	Anti-pdl*	Anti-dl*
-Hr	-Rh29	-En^a
-Hr_0	-LW^a	-Wr^b
-Rh34	-LW^{ab}	-Di^b
	-U	-Ge
		-Kp^b
		-K13
		-Sc1/Sc3
		-Vel
		-AnWj

* Anti-nl, reacts with RBCs of common phenotype, but not –D– or Rh_{null} RBCs; Anti-pdl, reacts with RBCs of common phenotype and –D–, but not Rh_{null} RBCs; Anti-dl, reacts with RBCs of common phenotype, –D–, and Rh_{null} RBCs.

reported that the eluates from RBCs sensitized only with IgG showed clearer specificity than the "IgG+ complement" group; 72% of the "IgG only" group did *not* react with Rh_{null} RBCs, in contrast to 100% of the "IgG+ complement" group reacting with Rh_{null} RBCs in addition to common phenotypes. Additional studies using RBC eluates revealed that no direct correlation could be established between the presence of complement components on the patient's RBCs, as determined by direct antiglobulin testing (DAT), and the intensity of the IAT using anti-IgG serum. On the other hand, the simultaneous presence of anti-nl and anti-dl autoantibodies in eluates was often associated with the presence of complement on the RBCs. They suggested that the presence of complement components in association with anti-nl and anti-dl may be analogous to complement fixation by multiple Rh alloantibodies as described by Rosse.[20]

In a later publication, Vos and coworkers[16] showed that the presence of complement on RBCs, in addition to IgG, seemed to be associated exclusively with autoantibodies of multiple immunoglobulin classes, as well as multiple RBC specificities. Vos postulated that the variability encountered in multiple antibodies may reflect continuous differences in the inciting stimulus resulting from altered configuration of red cell antigenic determinants. Assuming that trapping and processing of antigen are prerequisites for the induction of antibody response, it was postulated that an adequate concentration of anti-nl on the RBCs might block sites inhibiting synthesis of antibody, but not necessarily the enhancement of antibody synthesis for other unblocked antigens on the immunizing RBCs (e.g., anti-pdl and anti-dl). The suggestion that multiple antibody and immunoglobulin formation follows a predetermined sequence of development as a consequence of variability in antigen presentation is not in full agreement with the idea that the disease primarily results from an aberration of the immune mechanism. The authors suggest that WAIHA associated with Rh antibodies may result from a defect in the structural composition of the genome that is rejected by a normal immune mechanism. The subsequent development of additional specificities to other RBC antigens involving multiple immunoglobulin classes does not necessarily indicate the establishment of an aberrant immune apparatus. Sokol and coworkers[21] also reported a correlation of RBC-bound multiple immunoglobulin classes with severity of hemolytic anemia.

In 1975 Dacie[22] reported further data on 121 patients with WAIHA. "Rh" specificity could be demonstrated in 68% of the patients and was as high as 83% if only patients with IgG but no complement on their RBCs were considered; only 37% of patients with IgG and complement on their RBCs showed "Rh" specificity. In an extensive study published in 1976, Issitt and coworkers[23] found "obvious" anti-Rh specificity (specificities seen included anti-D, -C, -E, -c, -e, -f, -Ce, and anti-G) to be present alone in 3 of 87 cases (3.5%), together with autoantibodies of other specificities, such as anti-nl, -pdl, -dl, and anti-Wr^b (see later) in 23 of 87 (26%) cases. Overall, 74% of the autoantibodies reacted as well with –D– and Rh_{null} RBCs as with common phenotypes. This study also confirmed earlier studies[16] in terms of the immunoglobulin class of the autoantibodies and the fact that complement fixation in vivo generally occurs only when autoantibodies with complex specificity, such as anti-pdl or anti-dl, are produced.

In 1967, Celano and Levine[24] demonstrated anti-LW in all six cases of WAIHA that they studied. All six showed "nonspecific" reactions when tested against a panel of RBCs of common phenotype, but when Rh_{null} and Rh+LW– and/or Rh–LW– RBCs were included, one serum showed clear anti-LW specificity. Further adsorption and elution studies on the other five cases revealed the presence of anti-LW, together with a "nonspecific" element. In 1973, we collaborated with Vos to study, in depth, eight eluates made from RBCs of patients with WAIHA.[17] We used a panel of RBCs containing very rare phenotypes (e.g., LW+U–, LW–U+, Rh_{null} LW–U+, Rh_{null} LW–U–) and performed selected adsorption and elution studies. We were able to demonstrate specificities not definable without the use of some of these exotic phenotypes. Three of the eight (38%) eluates were shown to contain anti-U and six of eight (75%) contained anti-LW. The anti-LW and anti-U were always detected together with other antibody specificities. The definition of these antibodies was only possible because we had access to the only known examples of Rh_{null} LW–U+ and Rh+LW–; this also explains why we detected anti-U in 38% of the eluates compared with only 6% reported by Marsh and coworkers.[25] Other rare phenotypes such as the only example of Wr(b-) and K_o RBCs have also revealed new specificities among autoantibodies.

Of particular interest in the Vos and coworkers[17] study was the observation that adsorption and elution studies, including the use of Rh+LW– RBCs, showed that antibodies previously classified as anti-pdl (antibodies reacting with common phenotypes and –D– but not Rh_{null} phenotypes) appeared to be anti-LW + LW_1. We made the analogy to the ABO system, where anti-A can be shown to be anti-A + A_1 by adsorption with A_2 RBCs.[17] We suggested that Rh+LW+ RBCs should be classified as LW_1, Rh–LW+ RBCs as LW_2, and the rare Rh+LW– RBCs as LW_3.[17] In 1981 a new antibody (anti-Ne^a) was found to be part of the LW system.[26] Anti-Ne^a was renamed anti-LW^b and the old anti-LW was renamed anti-LW^a. Sistonen and Tippett[26] suggested that LW_1 (i.e., D+LW+) are of the genotype LW^aLW^a or LW^aLW; LW_2 (D–LW+) are LW^aLW^b; LW_3 are LW^bLW^b or LW^bLW; and LW_4 are *LWLW* (the only true "LW negative"). The antibody LW_4 individuals make is an inseparable anti-LW^{ab}. Thus, the autoanti-LW described previously were probably anti-LW^a or anti-LW^{ab}.[17,27] Transient anti-LW has been described in individuals who produced anti-LW at a time they typed as LW– but were later found to be LW+; these will be described later in the section on "mimicking" antibodies.

It should be noted that many of the above studies used eluates rather than sera from patients with "warm" autoantibodies to define specificity. Autoantibodies present in sera usually show "cleaner" specificity than those eluted from RBCs. Another point to notice is that some study populations were composed of only patients with hemolytic anemia, and others included patients/donors with "warm" autoantibodies but no hemolytic anemia. The clarity of the specificity may vary within these two populations. Unfortunately, some studies did not define the clinical status of their populations. A further difference in clarity of specificity is observed if patients are subdivided into those with only IgG on their RBCs or whether other proteins are present (e.g., complement). For instance, Dacie and Worlledge[18] found that, using a panel of RBCs of common phenotypes, 38% of "IgG alone" DATs were associated with Rh specificity in contrast to only 10% in the "IgG and complement" population. When RBCs of the –D– and Rh_{null} phenotypes were included, 68% of "IgG alone" group showed "Rh" specificity in contrast to 14% of the "IgG and complement" group. Eyster and Jenkins[28] studied eluates from 37 patients. One eluate showed anti-e specificity, another failed to react with some cells but no specificity was obvious; the other 35 reacted with all RBCs tested; of the 35 eluates that reacted with all RBCs, 6 of 12 eluates from RBCs having an "IgG only" positive DAT showed "Rh" specificity, whereas only 6 of 23 "IgG and complement" eluates showed specificity. They also confirmed the experiments of Weiner and Vos[14] by showing that if the "nonspecific" eluates were adsorbed with Rh_{null} RBCs, then the adsorbed serum sometimes demonstrated relative Rh specificity with RBCs of common phenotypes.

SPECIFICITIES ASSOCIATED WITH GLYCOPHORINS

The first undisputed obvious specificity, other than Rh, in patients with WAIHA was described in 1971 when Nugent and coworkers[29] described a patient with an autoantibody with U blood group specificity. Because of the observations of Schmidt and coworkers[30] that Rh_{null} RBCs also have aberrant U antigen, together with some degree of abnormality of the Ss antigens, Marsh and coworkers[25] thought autoantibodies that were being called "Rh" specific because they failed to react with Rh_{null} RBCs should be reexamined. They studied eluates from 50 patients that reacted with all RBCs of common phenotypes; 24 of these eluates reacted significantly weaker with Rh_{null} RBCs and in some of these cases, well-defined specificity for known Rh antigens could be demonstrated (e.g., anti-e). Three of the 24 cases showed autoantibodies that reacted with all RBCs of common phenotype but more weakly with both U– and Rh_{null} RBCs. In two of these cases, adsorption and elution studies resulted in the separation of anti-e and anti-U with an additional "nonspecific" component reacting with Rh_{null} RBCs. Adsorption and elution studies in a third case yielded anti-U and "nonspecific" antibody only. Thus, in 50 eluates, 3 (6%) showed anti-U specificity. Other workers since have also demonstrated autoanti-U specificity associated with WAIHA, and in patients with a positive DATs and no hemolytic anemia.[27] In our study with Vos[17] described previously, we used the only Rh_{null} U+ red cell sample so far described, in addition to an Rh_{null} U– sample, to study eight selected RBC eluates from patients with WAIHA. We were able to demonstrate autoantibodies with U specificity in three of the eight eluates (38%) but they were always present with autoantibodies of other specificity (e.g., anti-LW, -nl, -pdl, -dl, and anti-e). Without the rare Rh_{null} RBCs, it would have been very difficult to demonstrate the presence of the anti-U and this probably accounts for the much higher incidence of autoanti-U detected compared with other series (e.g., Marsh and coworkers[25]).

In 1972, Worlledge[31] reported that approximately 33% of anti-dl autoantibodies failed to react with En(a–) RBCs. She also noted that those anti-dl autoantibodies most likely to fail to react with En(a–) RBCs were the same ones that reacted less strongly with enzyme-treated RBCs than untreated RBCs.[31] A study from the same department in a later report found 44% of 23 "nonspecific" eluates to react weaker, or not at all, with En(a–) RBCs.[22] In 1975, Goldfinger and coworkers[32] reported a case of WAIHA associated with an autoantibody of Wr^b specificity. The antibody was initially noticed to react with all RBCs tested (including many RBCs lacking high-frequency antigens) but gave weaker reactions with heterozygous Wr(a+b+) RBCs than with the common Wr(a–b+) RBCs. The specificity was confirmed by finding a negative reaction against the only known example of Wr(a+b–) RBCs. Issitt and coworkers[23] found that the antibody reacted weakly with En(a–) RBCs. The En(a–) RBCs, when tested with the only known example of anti-Wr^b, were found to type Wr(b–). It was suggested that the anti-En^a specificity reported earlier by Worlledge[31] may perhaps have been anti-Wr^b instead. The only known example of Wr(a+b–) RBCs typed as En(a+), thus anti-Wr^b and anti-En^a do not have the same specificity.

In a detailed study, Issitt and coworkers reported on anti-Wr^b and other autoantibodies responsible for positive DATs in 150 individuals.[23] Of 87 patients with AIHA, 64 eluates (73.6%) had autoantibodies reacting with all RBCs including Rh_{null}. Of these 64 anti-dl autoantibodies, 34 contained autoanti-Wr^b (53.1%). Of 33 patients being treated with methyldopa who had developed positive DATs, 23 had anti-dl autoantibodies (69.7%), 4 (17.4%) of which contained autoanti-Wr^b. Of 30 hematologically normal donors with positive DATs, 23 (76.7%) eluates contained anti-dl autoantibodies and 8 (34.8%) eluates contained autoanti-Wr^b. If autoantibodies not reacting with

Rh_{null} RBCs were included, a total of 46 examples of autoanti-Wr^b were encountered. The incidence of autoanti-Wr^b in each group was 39.1% in AIHA; 12.1% in methyldopa-induced positive DATs, and 26.7% in normal blood donors with positive DATs. These investigators[23] commented that autoanti-Wr^b can cause gross RBC destruction in vivo or can be benign on occasions; it occurs with a higher frequency in AIHA and "normal" donors with positive DATs than in patients with methyldopa-induced positive DATs. We would comment that if the group of AIHA with only IgG on their RBCs (i.e., 38 patients) are analyzed, then the percentage associated with anti-Wr^b is lower, 28.9% compared with 39.1% of the total AIHA. If this group is compared with the methyldopa group (who also have only IgG on their RBCs), then the difference is not as marked (i.e., 28.9% versus 12.1% instead of 39.1% versus 12.1%); this difference is very similar to that seen with the normal donors (70% of whom only had IgG on their RBCs), compared with the methyldopa group (i.e., 26.7% versus 12.1%) (Tables 7-3 and 7-4).

Issitt and coworkers[23] also commented on Worlledge's report[31] concerning autoanti-En^a and the weaker reactions seen with enzyme-treated RBCs. Issitt and coworkers[23] had already shown that the Wr^b antigen was partially denatured by ficin, which would seem to support the concept that the antibodies Worlledge reported might have been anti-Wr^b. However, in tests on the unadsorbed eluates from 110 individuals with autoanti-dl, Issitt and coworkers[23] only found four (3.6%) that failed to react with En(a–) RBCs, a very different incidence than the 33% Worlledge reported.[31] Issitt and coworkers[23] thought that this difference may just reflect a difference in technique as they were able to show that in one case an ether eluate contained anti-Wr^b + anti-dl, whereas a heat eluate from the same RBCs contained only anti-Wr^b. When examples of anti-dl were adsorbed with Wr(a+b–) RBCs, then anti-Wr^b could be demonstrated in 41.8% of eluates, which is much closer to the 33% figure of "anti-En^a" described by Worlledge.[31] Issitt and coworkers[23] believe that technical differences may account for the fact that 73.6% of the 87 AIHA patients had anti-dl, while the incidence in 55 patients studied by Vos and coworkers[17] was 40%. Bell and Zwicker[33] confirmed that autoantibodies may have anti-Wr^b, anti-En^a, or a mixture of both specificities. Several other examples of autoanti-En^a[34-36] and autoanti-Wr^b[37,38] have been described.

Issitt and coworkers[39] tested 119 sera, from patients with autoantibodies, with Di(b–) RBCs. None contained only anti-Di^b but 2 of 74 sera subjected to adsorption were shown to contain an autoanti-Di^b component.

Pr specificity is usually associated with cold autoantibodies (see later) but is on rare occasions associated with WAIHA.[36,40] Anti-En^a, -Pr, and -Wr^b are often

TABLE 7-3. "Rh" SPECIFICITY OF "WARM" AUTOANTIBODIES DEFINED BY USE OF -D-, RH_{null}, U-, AND Wr(b-) RED BLOOD CELLS (RBCs)

Specificity	The Only Autoantibody (% of patients)	Plus Other Autoantibodies (% of patients)
"Simple" (Rh)	4.6	26
anti-nl*	4.6	23
anti-pdl*	3.4	33
anti-dl*	15	56
anti-U	1.2	1.2
anti-Wr^b	2.3	37

* Anti-nl, reacts with RBCs of common phenotype, but not –D– or Rh_{null} RBCs; Anti-pdl, reacts with RBCs of common phenotype and –D–, but not Rh_{null} RBCs; Anti-dl, reacts with RBCs of common phenotype, –D–, and Rh_{null} RBCs.
Modified from Issitt PD, Pavone BG, Goldfinger D, et al: Anti-Wr^b and other autoantibodies responsible for positive direct antiglobulin tests in 150 individuals. Br J Haematol 1976;34:5–18.

TABLE 7-4. THE INCIDENCE OF ANTI-dl, "PURE" AUTOANTI-Wr^b, AND AUTOANTI-Wr^b AS A COMPONENT OF ANTI-dl IN 150 PATIENTS WITH POSITIVE DIRECT ANTIGLOBULIN TESTS (DATs)

	Total No. of Cases Tested	No. of Cases Tested in Which anti-dl Was Present (%)	No. of Cases Tested in Which anti-dl Was Pure anti-Wr^b (%)	No. of Cases Tested in Which the anti-dl Present Contained, anti-Wr^b (%)	Percentage of Cases in Which anti-dl Was Present in Which the anti-dl Was, or Contained, anti-Wr^b
AIHA	87	64 (74)	2 (2)	32 (37)	53
Aldomet-induced positive DATs*	33	23 (70)	0	4 (12)	17
"Normal" donors with positive DATs†	30	23 (77)	2 (7)	6 (20)	35

AIHA, acquired immune hemolytic anemia.
All eluates and sera containing anti-dl were absorbed with Wr(a+b–) RBCs to determine whether autoanti-Wr^b was present. Anti-nl and anti-pdl did not contain autoanti-Wr^b because the D– and Rh_{null} cells used (one or both of which failed to react with these antibodies) were shown to be Wr(b+).
* The majority of these patients showed no evidence of increased rates of RBC destruction in vivo.
† As far as could be determined, none of these donors was undergoing an increased rate of RBC destruction in vivo.
Modified from Issitt PD, Pavone BG, Goldfinger D, et al: Anti-Wr^b and other autoantibodies responsible for positive direct antiglobulin tests in 150 individuals. Br J Haematol 1976;34:5–18.

confused. For instance, when an antibody does not react with enzyme-treated RBCs, anti-En^a, anti-Pr, and anti-Wr^b should be among the list of suspects. If the antibody also fails to react with En(a–) RBCs, which lack glycophorin A, many workers call the antibody anti-En^a. This can be a mistake, as anti-Pr and anti-Wr^b may also not react with En(a–) RBCs. The best way of differentiating anti-En^a and anti-Pr is to test the antibodies against neuraminidase (sialidase)-treated (NT) RBCs. As almost all sera contain anti-T, which will react with NT-RBCs, one has to use an eluate (prepared from RBCs incubated with the serum in vitro) containing the antibody. Anti-En^a will react with NT-RBCs and most anti-Pr will not. Unfortunately, one rare form of anti-Pr (anti-Pr^a) will react with NT-RBCs (see later); thus, the use of NT-RBCs does not always differentiate anti-En^a from anti-Pr. En(a–) RBCs will adsorb anti-Pr^a but not anti-En^a. Thus, to properly differentiate anti-En^a and anti-Pr involves a great deal of work and access to relatively large amounts of the rare En(a–) RBCs. Some anti-En^a do not react with trypsin-, papain-, or ficin-treated RBCs (anti-En^aFS); some react with trypsin-, papain-, and ficin-treated RBCs (anti-En^aFR). As anti-Wr^b does not react with En(a–) RBCs, but does react with trypsin-, papain-, and ficin-treated En(a+) RBCs, it can be confused with anti-En^aFR. The only way of differentiating these two is to use RBCs from the only example of the En(a+) Wr(b–) phenotype; anti-En^aFR will react with these RBCs but anti-Wr^b will not. Because of these difficulties, one has to read the literature very carefully when relying on specificities that are said to be anti-En^a, -Pr, or -Wr^b.

WAIHA associated with M and N autoantibodies is uncommon[41-44]; we described a fatal WAIHA associated with an IgM autoanti-N.[44] A few cases of anti-N associated with renal dialysis, and perhaps stimulated by formalin, were shown to cause shortened in vivo survival of N+ RBCs.[45,46] No cases of AIHA due to autoanti-M have been reported. Four cases of AIHA associated with autoanti-S have been reported.[47-49]

In 1981 Reynolds[50] described the first case of AIHA associated with autoanti-Ge. Several other examples have been reported.[51-55] Three of the four examples presented with negative DATs, and their RBCs, although typing as Ge+ did not react with the patient's own anti-Ge at initial testing[52-54]; they are discussed in the section below on autoantibodies mimicking alloantibodies.

SPECIFICITIES ASSOCIATED WITH THE KELL SYSTEM

As mentioned previously, there were two early reports of anti-K associated with WAIHA.[12,13] In 1972, another case associated with Kell autoantibodies was intensively studied in Warsaw and London.[56] A 17-year-old boy developed severe hemolytic anemia and was treated with steroids and blood transfusion without effect. His DAT was initially negative but during his hospitalization it became weakly positive. During the next several weeks he was treated with steroids, azothioprine, and blood transfusion without much success. During the fourth week of the disease, he had a severe hemolytic transfusion reaction following 500 mL of RBCs. During the fifth week of his disease his RBCs were found to lack K, Kp^a, and Js^a antigens, whereas the antithetical antigens k and Kp^b were only weakly expressed. His serum now contained anti-Kp^b (titer of 256 by albumin technique). Following transfusion of Kp(b–) RBCs, the patient began to improve (^{51}Cr half-life of transfused RBCs was 19 days). Serological tests performed 6 weeks after this first compatible Kp(b–) blood transfusion revealed a very low level of anti-Kp^b in the serum and a weakly positive DAT; anti-Kp^b could be eluted from the cells. The patient's RBCs now reacted strongly with his serum collected 6 weeks previously, although his RBCs were compatible with current serum, unless the RBCs were ficin treated when they reacted weakly. The ^{51}Cr half-life of the patient's RBCs at this time was still short (8.5 days), with most of the RBCs being destroyed in the spleen. During the eighth week of his illness, more Kp(b–) RBCs were transfused; although he had an excellent hematological response, the ^{51}Cr half-life of his own RBCs was only 8.5 days. The patient was discharged in excellent condition after 4 months of hospitalization. By the 16th week, although the DAT was still weakly positive (complement only present on the RBCs), the anti-Kp^b in the serum was undetectable; the Kell phenotype was now normal, K– Kp(a–) Js(a–), with normal expression of k and Kp^b. After 7 months, the ^{51}Cr half-life of his own RBCs was 26 days. The authors suggested that although blocking of the Kp^b antigen could have occurred during the acute phase of the disease, the structure of the antibody molecule must have differed from that which normally has anti-Kp^b specificity because antiglobulin sera reacted with it only weakly (i.e., very weak positive DAT). An alternative and more probable explanation, they thought, was that during the acute stage of the disease, an unknown exogenous factor, such as a virus, disturbed the synthesis of Kell antigens by inhibiting the action of transferases, which are necessary for the full expression of these antigens on RBCs. Another very similar case has been described.[57]

In 1973 we described another association of anti-K with WAIHA.[58] The patient was a 49-year-old white woman who presented in 1971 with intermittent fevers of unknown origin. She was found to have granulomas of the lung and liver and to be anemic. She was treated with tetracycline, isoniazid, and pyridoxine. In December 1972, she was admitted to the hospital with fever and hemolytic anemia. Her DAT was found to be strongly positive. Her hemolytic anemia cleared spontaneously, and by January 1973 she was hematologically normal and has remained so since. When we first studied her serologically at the end of 1972, her DAT was found to be strongly positive due to sensitization with IgG, IgM, and complement. The eluate prepared from her RBCs contained IgG and IgM anti-K. No reactions were obtained against K– RBCs. The patient's serum contained IgG and IgM anti-K, reacting by IAT; enzyme-treated KK RBCs were completely hemolyzed. The serum also contained another IgG antibody reacting by IAT, against 93% of 183 K– samples, including K_o, McLeod, Ch(a–), and Yk(a–) RBCs; positive reactions ranged from 1/2+ to 3+. The serum placed known weak, moderate, and strong Bg(a+) RBCs in order when tested blind and a tail of weak agglutination reactions was observed on titration (i.e., high titer, low avidity). The patient's serum also contained anti-HLA-A2, -B7, and -A28, which have been shown to react with the Bg blood groups on RBCs. The patient's RBCs typed as AB K–k+ Kp(a–b+) Js(a–b+) Ku+ KL+. As Seyfried and coworkers[56] had described an apparent depression of Kell antigens associated with WAIHA, the patient's RBCs were tested by titration against several different anti-K, -k, and -Js^b reagents. No depression of any Kell antigens was noted. Her lymphocytes typed as HLA-A3, 11, 5, and 8. Her lymphocyte autocytotoxicity was negative. When the patient's serum was incubated at 4°C or 37°C with K– RBCs, it was possible to elute anti-K from these RBCs. The reaction was always weaker than the eluate obtained from K+ RBCs. Eluates from these in vitro sensitized RBCs and from the patients own RBCs were also tested for anti-HLA activity with negative results. In 1971, Giblett and coworkers[59] described a possible association between the rare sex-linked chronic granulomatous disease (CGD) and the Kell system, in that there appeared to be a high incidence of the rare K_o phenotype; the association was later found to be with the McLeod phenotype (depressed Kell antigens) rather than K_o.[60]

As our patient presented with granulomas and an unusual serological phenomenon involving Kell, we investigated the family history carefully. We found that the patient had one living healthy son of 26 years of age, but another boy had died at the age of 9. His case history and autopsy findings in retrospect were classic for CGD, although not recognized as such at that time. The patient's leukocytes were tested for their ability to kill *Staphylococci* and *Serratia*. The killing effect was intermediate between leukocytes from a normal individual and a patient with CGD. The leukocytes were also tested by the nitroblue tetrazolium dye reduction test; once again, the results obtained were intermediate between normal and CGD. Both sets of test results are diagnostic for a carrier state of CGD. Marsh and coworkers[60] showed that anti-KL contained an antibody, anti-Kx, that reacted with an antigen present on K_o RBCs. They further described a difference in the Kell antigens on leukocytes from patients with CGD, in that they appear to lack the Kx antigen. Dr. Marsh kindly tested the leukocytes from the patient and showed that they adsorbed anti-Kx from an anti-KL serum much less efficiently than normal leukocytes. The patient's DAT became progressively weaker and, when last tested, was barely positive. The anti-K had also diminished in strength, as had the other antibodies reacting against the K– RBCs. In contrast, the HLA-A2 and 7 titers had not weakened. The ability of the serum to sensitize K– RBCs in vitro with anti-K appeared to diminish in direct relationship to the presence of RBC antibodies in the serum.

To summarize the above case: The patient was a female carrier of CGD who presented with hemolytic anemia associated with RBC sensitization due to anti-K. The patient was K– and we were able to explain why the anti-K sensitized K– RBCs in vivo and in vitro. Although another antibody was present in the serum, we were unable to demonstrate the presence of this antibody together with anti-K in eluates from K– RBCs, so we were unable to classify this as an example of the Matuhasi-Ogata phenomenon,[27] but it is of interest to note that Wilkinson and coworkers[61] described in vitro adsorption of anti-D onto D– RBCs in the presence of anti-Bg and that anti-Bg is highly suspect in our patient's serum. Since reporting this case, Issitt and coworkers[62] reported the phenomenon of autoantibodies with mimicking specificities (see later) and we now believe that the anti-"K" in this case was a "mimicking" antibody. The autoantibody was probably not anti-K but only appeared to be and really had a broader specificity. It appeared to be anti-K because it reacted preferentially with K+ RBCs by the AGT, but adsorption/elution studies showed that it was capable of reacting with K– and K+ cells.

Viggiano and coworkers[63] reported another mimicking anti-K in 1982. Several examples of autoanti-Kp^b have been reported.[56,57,64-66] Several examples were found in patients with weakened Kp^b antigens[56,57,64,65] and are discussed in a later section on autoantibodies mimicking alloantibodies. Other high-incidence antigens in the Kell system have served as targets for RBC autoantibodies.[67-70] Marsh and coworkers[67,68] tested eluates from the RBCs of 950 DAT+ individuals against K_o RBCs, in addition to Rh_{null}, U–, and other RBCs. Four eluates contained autoantibodies to Kell system antigens; two were autoanti-Kp^b, one was autoanti-K13[67], and one was an autoantibody reacting with an undefined high-incidence antigen in the Kell system[68]; the latter patient had no evidence of HA. An example of autoanti-Js^b, enhanced by PEG, has been described[71]; this was not associated with WAIHA.

SPECIFICITIES ASSOCIATED WITH THE KIDD AND DUFFY SYSTEMS

Anti-Jk^a has been reported as an autoantibody on several occasion,[11,72-80] and three examples of autoanti-Jk^b have been reported.[81-83] One of the examples of anti-Jk^a[79] and one of anti-Jk^b[82] were found initially as mimicking antibodies (see later). It is of interest to note that one anti-Jk^a was methyldopa induced,[73] two were associated with Evans's syndrome,[77,79] and one anti-Jk^a and two anti-Jk^b were associated with bacterial infections.[76,80,81] Two examples of autoanti-Jk3 have been described[82,84]; both of these were detected in pregnant women. Issitt and coworkers[85] tested 35 examples of anti-dl with Jk(a–b–) RBCs; none of the eluates contained anti-Jk3.

Four patients with autoanti-Fy^b of the mimicking type have been described[86-88]; the specificity was not always clear as Fy(a+) but not Fy(a–b–) RBCs sometimes reacted.[87]

SPECIFICITIES ASSOCIATED WITH ABO AND Hh SYSTEMS

Although there are many reports in the literature of autoantibodies within the ABO and Hh systems, most of these antibodies were "cold" autoantibodies of no clinical significance. There are several reports of ABO autoantibodies being associated with hemolytic anemia, but most of these involve high thermal amplitude cold autoantibodies reacting optimally at 4°C (see later). There are only a few reports of anti-A or anti-B autoantibodies being associated with WAIHA,[11,89-93] and we find all these reports, except reference 89, lacking in either clinical or serological data to support the suggestion that the ABO autoantibodies caused WAIHA. For instance, there were few data (e.g., indirect bilirubin, reticulocytes, lactic dehydrogenase [LDH], haptoglobins, etc.) to support that a *hemolytic* anemia was occurring in most of these patients. It is also important to always exclude that the patient had not received blood products (e.g., platelets, group O blood) containing ABO antibodies; this was rarely mentioned in any of the publications.

A very unusual case of fatal fulminant intravascular hemolysis associated with an anti-A autoantibody was described by Szymanski and coworkers.[89] A group A_1 patient experienced severe bilateral lumbar pain associated with generalized weakness, jaundice, and lethargy and was admitted the next day semicomatose. The patient was grossly icteric, had splenomegaly, and was severely oliguric. Eighteen hours later acute tachycardia developed, followed by respiratory and cardiac arrest. On admission, the patient was found to have a strongly positive DAT (IgG but no complement). The patient's serum contained antibody(ies) that agglutinated all RBCs tested (A_1, A_2, O adult, and O cord cells) at 22°C and reacted by IAT at 37°C; type O RBCs reacted much weaker. When the patient's serum was diluted 1 in 5, A_1 and A_2 RBCs still reacted (2+ at 4°C) and O RBCs were negative; the reactions with group A RBCs could be inhibited by the addition of porcine A substance. A heat eluate prepared from the patient's IgG sensitized RBCs demonstrated anti-A specificity by IAT at 37°C. It is interesting to note that the patient's medical history was noncontributory until 7 years before the onset of AIHA, when he was hospitalized for myocardial infarction associated with hypotension. Subsequently, clinical gout, obstructive lung disease, glomerulonephritis, and cirrhosis developed. An additional finding of extramedullary hematopoiesis indicated a long-standing hemolytic process. The authors speculated that during this period, anti-A autoantibodies may have combined with A antigen of tissue cells and that such a phenomenon could have contributed to the multisystem disease in a similar way to the humoral antibodies that have been suggested for Goodpasture's syndrome, some cases of glomerulonephritis, fibrosing alveolitis, and chronic active hepatitis.

There are a few reports in the literature that describe anti-A and anti-B in patients who have A and/or B antigens on their RBCs but these antibodies are not true *auto*antibodies (even though the title of the article sometimes uses this term). These are ABO antibodies that developed following transplantation of kidney, liver, or hematopoietic stem cells. The antibodies appear to have been made in the A or B individuals by donor lymphocytes that were infused with the donor organ or donor stem cells. That is to say, "passenger lymphocytes" from a group O donor proliferated in a group A recipient and produced allo-anti-A that would appear to be an autoantibody (see Chapter 12).

Kuipers and coworkers[94] described an IgM monoclonal (kappa) 37°C anti-H associated with malignant lymphoma. The antibody reacted to a titer of 512 at 37°C but no cold agglutinin titers were given; it is possible that this also was a cold autoantibody with a high thermal amplitude.

MISCELLANEOUS TARGETS FOR 37°C REACTIVE AUTOANTIBODIES

In 1972, we described a new target antigen for warm autoantibodies, I^T.[95] Anti-I^T had previously been described as a cold autoagglutinin of no clinical significance.[96] The "T" stood for "transitional" as it was suggested that the putative antigen was a transitional antigen appearing when i developed into I.[96] If only cord (i) and adult (I) RBCs are tested, anti-I^T may appear to be anti-i as cord RBCs react much stronger than adult RBCs, but in contrast to anti-i, adult i RBCs react very weakly (Tables 7-5 and 7-6). We first encountered an example of IgG autoanti-I^T in a boy with Hodgkin's disease but no hemolytic anemia.[95] We later described four cases of WAIHA associated with Hodgkin's disease and IgG autoanti-I^T.[97] We questioned whether I^T was really an antigen transient between i and I, as we could not demonstrate this by testing RBCs from fetuses at different gestation times.[97,98] Hafleigh and coworkers[99] found three examples of IgG autoanti-I^T in patients who did not have Hodgkin's disease or AIHA. Levine and coworkers[100] studied 71 cases of Hodgkin's disease; seven were found to have positive DATs, and four of these were due to IgG autoanti-I^T. Freedman and coworkers[101] described a case of AIHA associated with an IgM anti-I^T, reacting optimally at 37°C.

TABLE 7-5. RELATIVE STRENGTH OF REACTIONS SEEN WITH ANTI-I, ANTI-i, AND ANTI-I^T

	I Adult	i Cord	i Adult
Anti-I	4+	1+	½+
Anti-i	1+	3+	4+
Anti-I^T	1+	4+	½+

Four examples of autoanti-Vel have been described.[102-105] All of the antibodies were IgM. Two of the patients were DAT– and one had no evidence of hemolytic anemia[102]; one patient was DAT– but had severe hemolytic anemia; and two patients were DAT+, one had some evidence for increased RBC destruction[103] and the other had acute hemolytic anemia.[104] Three examples of autoanti-Sc1 and two examples of autoanti-Sc3 have been reported.[106-108] The autoanti-Sc1 were associated with AIHA; the autoanti-Sc3 were associated with positive DATs and anemia, but it was not clear from the data presented whether AIHA was present. One example of autoanti-Xg^a has been reported[109]; the anti-Xg^a was said to be associated with hemolytic anemia; however, although the patient was anemic, no data were presented to support the diagnosis of hemolytic anemia.

Autoantibodies reacting with all RBCs except Lu(a–b–) cells have been reported.[110-112] One example appeared to be benign[110] and the other was associated with hemolytic anemia.[111] Marsh and coworkers[110] showed that RBCs from Lu(a–b–) individuals of the recessive type would react with the antibody but Lu(a–b–) RBCs from individuals of the *In(Lu)* dominant inhibitor type would not react, thus the antibody was not directed against high-incidence Lutheran antigens. The autoantibody was named anti-Wj by Marsh and coworkers,[110] but Wj appears to be the same as the previously described Anton (An) antigen, so the autoantibody is now termed anti-AnWj. An interesting association that is of great interest is that the AnWj antigen has been shown to be a receptor for *Haemophilus influenzae.*[113]

In 1983 Denegri and coworkers[114] described a case of WAIHA due to anti-Rx (initially called anti-Sd^x). This antibody usually occurs as an IgM cold agglutinin, but in the case described by Denegri[114] the antibody had an IgG component in addition to the IgM component. Sullivan and coworkers[115] described a case of WAIHA associated with autoanti-Kx; this is still the only one in the literature.

A "new" autoantibody specificity associated with AIHA was described by Marsh and coworkers[116] in 1985. An IgG autoantibody, from a patient who died of AIHA, reacted with all RBCs of common phenotype, K_o RBCs, and RBCs treated with a dithiothreitol-papain (ZZAP) solution. The antibody did not react with Rh_{null} RBCs or RBCs treated with 2-aminoethylisothiouronium bromide (AET). As ZZAP and AET-treated RBCs exhibit loss of all Kell antigens, behaving like K_o RBCs, the antibody did not appear to be reacting with antigens belonging to the Kell system. The authors suggested that the antibody was reacting with an antigen that is not part of the Kell or Rh system, but an antigen produced by in vitro membrane modification by ZZAP, that is similar to antigens produced by in vivo membrane modifications known to occur on Rh_{null} RBCs.[116]

Table 7-7 lists the specificities that have been described as targets for "warm" autoantibodies.

"MIMICKING ANTIBODIES"

As early as 1956, cases were described where the "wrong" (unexpected) antibody was eluted from the patients' RBCs.[117-119] Fudenberg and coworkers[119] described two cases where antibody eluted from the patients' RBCs had specificity for Rh blood factors not present on the patients' RBCs. Since that time many workers have observed the same phenomenon, particularly anti-E being eluted from E– RBCs. In 1959, Dunsford and Stapleton[120] reported on an anti-D that could be adsorbed and eluted from D– RBCs in vitro at 4°C; the authors suggested that the phenomenon may be associated with the concomitant presence of a cold autoagglutinin.

In a series of reports (1959–1964), Matuhasi[121] and Ogata and Matuhasi[122,123] showed that the "wrong" *allo*antibody can be adsorbed onto RBCs lacking its particular antigen if another *specific* antibody present in the serum is adsorbed onto the cells. They showed that if a mixture of anti-B and anti-D were present in a serum and this serum was incubated with group B, D–

TABLE 7-6. ELUATE FROM RED BLOOD CELLS OF ACQUIRED IMMUNE HEMOLYTIC ANEMIA PATIENT WITH SHOWING ANTI-I^T SPECIFICITY

	Dilutions of Eluate								
Red Blood Cells	2	4	8	16	32	64	128	256	Agglutination Score
I adult	1+	1+	1+	½+	0	0	0	0	18
i adult	2+	1+	½+	0	0	0	0	0	12
i cord	3+	3+	2+	1+	1+	½+	0	0	32

TABLE 7-7. TARGET ANTIGENS FOR "WARM" AUTOANTIBODIES

Rh("Rh", c, C, D, e, E, f, rh_i, G, Hr_0, Rh34, Rh29, Rh39)
LW (LW^a, LW^{ab})
Glycophorin associated (U, M*, N, S, En^a, Pr, Wr^b, Ge2, Ge3, Ge4)
Kell (K, k, Kp^b, K13, Js^b*)
Kidd (Jk^a, Jk^b, Jk3)
Duffy (Fy^b)
Diego (Wr^b, Di^b)
Scianna (Sc1, Sc3)
ABO (A, B)
Hh (H)
Others (Kx, Xg^a*, Co3, Yt^{ab}*, Vel, $AnWj$, I^T, Rx)

"Rh," nonreactive with Rh_{null} red blood cells.
* Not associated, so far, with hemolytic anemia.

RBCs, then an eluate prepared from the group B cells could be shown to contain anti-D as well as anti-B. In 1967, Svardel and coworkers[124] reported the adsorption of anti-e, -f, and -Ce onto the RBCs of a cDE/cDE individual who had autoanti-I present in addition. They suggested this was due to the Matuhasi-Ogata phenomenon. During the next decade, the "Matuhasi-Ogata phenomenon" became a popular term to use when immunohematologists had no other explanation for a particular phenomenon, and in our opinion, it has been greatly overused in the field by workers who usually had very little, if any, evidence to support their hypothesis.

One article appearing in 1969[125] offered data to suggest that the "Matuhasi-Ogata phenomenon" might be responsible for the adsorption of the "wrong" antibody in autoimmune hemolytic anemia. Later studies by Bove and coworkers[126] seemed to exclude this explanation, and indeed, one of the authors (Issitt) of the 1969 publication[125] has also rejected his own earlier hypothesis.[129]

In 1977 Bove and coworkers[126] criticized the suggested basis for the Matuhasi-Ogata phenomenon. These investigators used ^{125}I-labeled IgG antibody and "nonantibody" IgG attached to RBCs and showed that there was no increased adsorption of antibody in the presence of "nonantibody" IgG. They used a hypothetical case: If serum has 1.2 g% IgG and contains 40 µg/mL of IgG anti-D, then 0.33% of the IgG is anti-D. Suppose 1 mL of D– RBCs are added and following incubation the RBCs are well washed and an eluate prepared. Normal RBCs will bind 10 µg IgG/mL of RBCs and eluates are known to contain about 60% of the RBC-bound IgG. Thus, 1 mL eluate should contain about 6 mg IgG; 0.33% (0.02 µg) of this IgG would be anti-D, which is enough to yield a positive antiglobulin test. In summary, Bove and coworkers[126] thought that some IgG is always adsorbed by RBCs during incubation of RBCs with allogeneic serum. This is mainly "nonantibody" IgG but if enough IgG is adsorbed, some of the molecules will be IgG antibody present in the serum and thus may be present in an eluate made from the RBCs. During the elution process, concentration of any antibody present occurs, which will exaggerate the amount of antibody adsorbed. Bove and coworkers[126] did not explain why this phenomenon occurs in only some patients.

In 1977 and 1978, Issitt and coworkers[127,128] suggested that the "wrong" antibodies present in eluates may not have the simple specificity suggested by serological reactions against phenotyped RBCs but perhaps a less obvious, more complex, specificity. Autoantibodies of seemingly "simple" Rh specificity (e.g., anti-D, -C, -c, -E, rh_i [-Ce], and -G), when tested with RBCs having and not having the putative antigens, including –D– and Rh_{null} RBCs, by IAT, were studied by multiple adsorption tests. Seventy-one percent of these antibodies could be adsorbed using RBCs that lacked the specific antigen. Of interest was the finding that if the antibody initially appeared to be autoanti-D, there was a greater than 60% chance that it was a "true" autoanti-D (i.e., not adsorbed by D– RBCs). It was suggested that those autoantibodies that at first appeared to be directed against e, E, or c were only mimicking these specificities and were probably anti-Hr or anti-Hr_0 with a broad specificity. For instance, an autoantibody may only react with E+ RBCs when a panel of RBCs is tested, but the reaction may be due to autoanti-Hr or -Hr_0, mimicking anti-E, because E+ RBCs have more Hr/Hr_0 than E– RBCs. This is comparable in some ways to a weak (e.g., diluted) anti-A reacting with A_1 and not A_2 RBCs; the antibody is not anti-A_1, but only reacting as such, because A_1 RBCs have more antigenic sites than A_2 RBCs, thus reacting better with weak anti-A. Similarly, a weak anti-LW can mimic anti-D because D+ RBCs have more LW sites than D– RBCs. Issitt[129] termed the phenomenon "Matuhasi-Ogata maximus" and the phenomenon reported by Bove and coworkers[126] as "Matuhasi-Ogata minimus."

Issitt and coworkers[127] found that sera of DAT+ patients may contain mimicking autoantibody alone (e.g., autoanti-Hr reacting like anti-E), alloantibody alone (e.g., anti-E) or mimicking autoantibody + alloantibody. They may be differentiated by adsorption; the mimicking antibody will be adsorbed by antigen-negative (e.g., E–) and antigen-positive (e.g., E+) RBCs, whereas the alloantibody will only be adsorbed by antigen-positive (e.g., E+) RBCs. It is important to note that, in contrast to the earlier findings where the "wrong" antibody was eluted from DAT+ RBCs, of the 34 autoantibodies that had "mimicking" specificities (i.e., adsorbed by "antigen-negative" RBCs) studied by Issitt and coworkers,[127] 28 (85%) were found in patients who had the putative antigen present on their RBCs. In 150 patients with a positive DAT and 87 with WAIHA, 4 (2.6%) and 43 (49%), respectively, had autoantibodies with a true "simple" specificity. Since this work with mimicking Rh antibodies, mimicking specificities in many systems have been described[27,34,49-70,128-145] (Table 7-8).

In 1978,[145] we published a report on an unusual patient who not only had the "wrong" antibody eluted from his RBCs but also was classified as a "DAT-negative" AIHA (see Chapter 9). A previously

TABLE 7-8. SPECIFICITIES ASSOCIATED WITH MIMICKING ANTIBODIES

System	Antigens
Rh	D*, C*, E, c, e*, Ce, G, hr^B*
MN	S, En^a*
Lutheran	Lu^b, "high incidence"*
Kell	K, Kp^b*, "high incidence"*
Duffy	Fy^a, Fy^b*
Kidd	Jk^a*, Jk^b, Jk3
Scianna	Sc1*, Sc3*
Colton	Co^a
LW	LW^a*
Gerbich	Ge2, "Ge"*
Miscellaneous	$AnWj$*, Lan

* Associated sometimes with depressed antigens (i.e., autoantibody mimicking alloantibody).

untransfused 20-year-old man presented with a 7-day history of malaise, fatigue, jaundice, dark urine, and splenomegaly. Hemolytic anemia was indicated by a hemoglobin of 8.7 g/dL, reticulocyte count of 8%, bilirubin of 4.3 mg/dL (direct 0.1 mg/dL), and undetectable haptoglobins. Tests for nonimmunological mediated hemolytic anemia were negative. The DAT was repeatedly negative with polyspecific antihuman globulin, anti-IgG, -IgA, -IgM, and anti-C3. The patient's serum contained a weak anti-I, anti-E strongly reactive by IAT, and an antibody reactive against all RBCs tested. The latter antibody reacted weakly by IAT but strongly against enzyme-treated RBCs (titer 160). Eluates from the patient's RBCs only reacted with E+ RBCs. The patient typed E–. The results of serum adsorptions with group O rr, R_1R_1, and R_2R_2 RBCs are illustrated in Table 7-9. Following the first and second adsorptions, the sera reacted only with the R_2R_2 RBCs and following three adsorptions with either rr, R_1R_1, or R_2R_2 RBCs, there was no detectable antibody. These data indicate that the serum antibody could be adsorbed to exhaustion by a variety of Rh phenotypes although the serum reacted only with E+ RBCs.

The results of ether eluates prepared from the group O rr, R_1R_1, and R_2R_2 RBCs used for the adsorptions are presented in Table 7-10. Regardless of the Rh phenotypes used for adsorption, all eluates reacted only with E+ RBCs. This was confirmed by repeated testing with RBCs of varying Rh phenotypes. The possible anti-c previously detected in the patient's serum was apparently too weak to be detected after the adsorption–elution procedures. Similar adsorption and elution procedures were attempted with an eluate prepared from RBCs of the original patient specimen, but the reactions were too weak to interpret with any certainty. The patient was treated with high doses of prednisone. By the twelfth day, his response allowed the medication to be tapered, and 1 month from the onset of treatment, laboratory studies had returned to normal. The DAT remained negative; however, following recovery, anti-E could not be eluted from the RBCs. Anti-E remained in his serum but the titer of

TABLE 7-9. ANTIBODY TITERS (37°C IAT) OF SERUM FROM PATIENT WITH "MIMICKING" ANTI-E

	Red Blood Cells Tested		
Serum	rr	R_1R_1	R_2R_2
Unabsorbed	1	1	64
Absorbed with rr cells			
x1	0	0	8
x2	0	0	2
x3	0	0	0
Absorbed with R_1R_1 cells			
x1	0	0	8
x2	0	0	2
x3	0	0	0
Absorbed with R_2R_2 cells			
x1	0	0	8
x2	0	0	1
x3	0	0	0

From Rand BP, Olson JD, Garratty G, et al: Coombs negative immune hemolytic anemia with anti-E occurring in the red blood cell eluate of an E-negative patient. Transfusion 1978;18:174–180.

the enzyme reactive antibody had decreased to 16. Of particular significance is the decrease in the serum anti–"E-like" antibody titer. In our experience, true alloantibodies usually are not affected during steroid treatment although autoantibodies do decrease in titer. The results suggested that the serum anti–"E-like" antibody in this patient behaved more like an autoantibody than an alloantibody.

Issitt and coworkers[127,128] made some interesting observations on this phenomenon. In 1977[128] they described a patient with similar serology to the patient above, except that their patient had a positive DAT. They suggested that the anti-"E" might represent autoanti-Hr rather than anti-E. They discuss that some Rh alloantibodies are known to show marked preferences for RBCs of certain phenotypes when IATs are performed but that adsorption studies reveal that some weakly, or even nonreactive RBCs carry small amounts of the antigens against which the antibodies are directed. For example, Rosenfield[146] has observed that anti-hr^S reacts better with RBCs from individuals who have *ce* cis genes than with those from individuals who

TABLE 7-10. ANTIBODY TITERS (37°C IAT) OF ELUATES PREPARED FROM THE RED BLOOD CELLS USED FOR ABSORPTION IN TABLE 7-9

	Red Blood Cells Tested		
Eluate from	rr	R_1R_1	R_2R_2
Absorbing rr cells	0	0	4*
Absorbing R_1R_1 cells	0	0	4*
Absorbing R_2R_2 cells	0	0	8*

* Anti E specificity identified by larger panel.
From Rand BP, Olson JD, Garratty G, et al: Coombs negative immune hemolytic anemia with anti-E occurring in the red blood cell eluate of an E-negative patient. Transfusion 1978;18:174–180.

have *Ce cis* genes. In spite of this, almost all CDe/CDe bloods are hr^S+. This means, of course, that in initial studies anti-hr^S might well mimic anti-c or anti-f, but that in adsorption studies CDe/CDe RBCs (which are c–, f–) invariably adsorb anti-hr^S to exhaustion. A similar situation exists with anti-hr,^{B} which "prefers" RBCs from individuals with *Ce cis* genes to those from individuals with *ce cis* genes. The original "Bastiaan" anti-hr^B serum was believed to contain anti-C because of its preference for C+ RBCs, until it was found that this specificity could not be isolated by adsorption. In working with the sera from a series of individuals with highly exotic Rh phenotypes (Shabalala, Davis, Santiago, Ellington, and Fentry), Rosenfield[146] observed some reactions that were very similar to those of the "anti-E" in the eluate of the patient discussed in earlier paragraphs. Although these observations have never been published in full, they were mentioned briefly in a 1962 article by Rosenfield and coworkers.[147] In several of the sera studied, there were antibodies that showed very marked preferences for E or e. These antibodies were shown not to be anti-E or anti-e by adsorption studies with RBCs of appropriate phenotypes. It was shown that an antibody with a preference for E could be readily adsorbed with E+ e–, or E+ e+ RBCs, but that E–, e+ samples would eventually totally adsorb the antibody as well. In several instances the antibody makers were Hr–, so that their antibodies resembled the anti-Hr that is often made as an alloantibody by D– –/D– – or Dc–/Dc– individuals. Thus, Issitt and coworkers[127,128] feel that since autoanti-nl (i.e., autoantibody that reacts with all RBCs of common phenotypes but not –D– or Rh_{null} phenotypes) reacts similarly to alloanti-Hr, then the autoantibodies discussed above that appear to be anti-E may, in fact, be autoanti-Hr (anti-"Hr" or anti–"Hr-like"). We support this hypothesis. Data obtained from experiments on specificity of warm antibodies using the AutoAnalyzer would also seem to support this concept.[148]

Issitt and coworkers[128] also studied 48 autoantibodies with apparent "simple" anti-Rh specificity (anti-e, -E, -c, -D, -C, - Ce, -G) by means of multiple adsorption tests. They showed that 34 (70.8%) of these antibodies could be adsorbed by RBCs lacking the antigens the antibodies appeared to define. These autoantibodies that at first appeared to be directed against e, E, or c antigens, most often had anti-Hr or anti-Hr_0 specificity. Anti–"C-like" autoantibodies may represent autoanti-Rh34, rather than anti-Hr or anti-Hr_0. Issitt and coworkers[128] also comment that this new interpretation of the Rh-associated specificity does not change the philosophies (discussed in Chapter 10) for the selection of blood for transfusion. We would agree with this. If one believes (as we do) that a patient with an autoantibody showing some autoanti-E specificity should receive E– blood, then it makes no difference if we now call this autoantibody autoanti-Hr, anti-"Hr," anti-"E," or anti–"E-like." As E– RBCs are reacting so much more weakly than E+ RBCs (e.g., E– RBCs are sometimes negative by IAT), then we would expect these cells to survive better in vivo than more strongly reacting E+ RBCs. If one wishes to determine if the antibody (e.g., anti-E) is an alloantibody or autoantibody, the best way is to perform adsorptions with RBCs of different phenotypes (e.g., E– and E+ RBCs). An *alloanti*-E should be adsorbed only by E+ RBCs, and by not E– RBCs, whereas, as discussed previously, the autoanti-"E" will probably be adsorbed by E– as well as E+ RBCs.

*Auto*antibodies can also mimic *allo*antibodies: Many patients have now been described who have depressed antigens at the time they have autoantibody in their serum; sometimes the DAT is negative (but antibody can often be eluted from their RBCs). Thus, the autoantibody may appear like an alloantibody. Investigators have proved these are really autoantibodies by showing that when the hemolytic anemia is in remission and antibody is no longer detectable in the serum, the antigen strength returns to normal and the stored serum, taken previously during the hemolytic episode, will now react with the patient's RBCs. Some of the alloantibodies mimicking autoantibodies referred to above may also belong in this category because most patients' RBCs were not tested at different times for antigen strength. Growing numbers of specificities have been associated with this phenomenon; these include Rh,[127,128,130-133,145] LW,[134,136] Kell,[56-58,63,67,143] Ge,[51-54] AnWj,[137] Duffy,[138-140] Kidd,[76,81,141] En^a,[34] Co,[142] Sc1 and Sc3,[106,108] Lutheran,[143,144] and Lan.[144]

In 1996 Issitt and coworkers[149] studied apparent alloantibodies present in the sera of patients with autoantibodies. Nineteen of the 117 (16%) sera appeared to contain obvious alloantibodies without further testing (e.g., adsorptions). Seventy-five (77%) of the sera contained antibodies reacting with all RBCs tested. Forty-one of these sera were adsorbed with *autologous* RBCs, revealing the presence of apparent alloantibodies in 11 sera (27%); 69% of these were shown to be autoantibodies mimicking alloantibodies (i.e., adsorbed by "antigen-negative" RBCs). When 34 sera were adsorbed with *allogeneic* RBCs, 14 (41%) appeared to contain alloantibodies; only 19% of these appeared to be mimicking antibodies. Thus, only 33% (not 41% as first suspected) of patients' sera containing broadly reactive autoantibodies appeared to contain true alloantibodies. It is interesting to note the differences between adsorptions with autologous and allogeneic RBCs. Adsorption with allogeneic RBCs appeared to reveal more alloantibody specificity than adsorption with autologous RBCs. Also, apparent alloantibodies detected following adsorption with autologous RBCs were much more likely to be autoantibodies mimicking alloantibodies than when sera were adsorbed with allogeneic RBCs.

CHANGES IN SPECIFICITY OF AUTOANTIBODIES

We (unpublished observations), and others[150-152] have observed the specificity of warm autoantibodies to change during the course of a patient's disease. In our experience it has usually been a broadening of specificity. For instance, a patient will start with an autoantibody of "simple" Rh specificity and as the disease progresses the antibody will show more "nonspecific" characteristics until it reacts with all cells tested, even by IAT. Other authors have described other patterns. For instance, Beck and coworkers[150] described a patient whose autoantibody over a 5-year period changed from "nonspecific" to specific; furthermore, the specificity varied from anti-e to anti-c and anti-f. The authors wisely comment on the fact that the treatment the patient was receiving (prednisone and methotrexate) may have affected the specificity patterns seen. They suggest that particular clones of immunocytes may have been selectively destroyed or suppressed. We have also seen patients who first make a single *allo*antibody following transfusion, then make more *allo*antibodies, then eventually make *auto*antibodies (see Chapter 9).

SPECIFICITIES NOT ASSOCIATED WITH BLOOD GROUP ANTIGENS

There are an increasing number of observations relating to causes for positive DATs and reactions of serum antibodies with all, or most, RBCs including the patient's own RBCs, that are not associated with blood group antibodies. Table 7-11 lists these with appropriate references.

Optimal Reactions with Stored or "Old" RBCs

Since 1952, there have been reports in the literature of antibodies reacting better with stored RBCs than fresh RBCs.[153-158] These antibodies usually were cold autoagglutinins (see later), but sometimes reacted up to 37°C. Some of the patients having such antibodies had hemolytic anemia, but it was uncertain whether this was caused by the cold autoantibody reacting optimally with stored RBCs.

In 1989, we reported a patient with WAIHA associated with an autoantibody that reacted preferentially with stored RBCs.[158] The antibody showed similar characteristics to other antibodies described previously in that it reacted well with enzyme- and heat-treated RBCs. It also showed the characteristic "mixed-field" appearance described by Stratton and coworkers[154] and Ozer and Chaplin.[156] We separated "young" and "old" RBCs from fresh blood, by a capillary centrifugation method, and showed that the "stored RBC" antibody reacted preferentially with the older RBCs in fresh blood. This suggested to us that the target antigen might be similar, or identical, to the senescent cell antigen (SCA) described by Kay.[159] Kay[159] suggested that senescent cells are cleared from the circulation because they develop an SCA that reacts with naturally occurring IgG autoantibodies to SCA. These IgG-sensitized cells are then removed by macrophages. Kay[159] has characterized SCA biochemically; it is present on band 3 of the RBC membrane. We were able to demonstrate that the RBC autoantibody that reacted preferentially with stored and "old" RBCs could be inhibited in vitro with synthetic SCA that was kindly provided by Dr. Kay.[159] Thus, we believe that "stored" RBC antibodies are reacting against SCA and that the ubiquitous anti-SCA, which is usually present in very low levels, like the ubiquitous anti-I, can become pathogenic on occasions.

Gray and coworkers[160] found that reticulocytes have 60% of the D content of mature RBCs. They also showed that IgG autoantibodies eluted from the RBCs of patients with AIHA reacted weaker with reticulocytes than mature RBCs in four of five cases. Branch and coworkers[161] performed DATs on age-fractionated RBCs of 24 DAT+ patients. Seventy-nine percent of the DATs were stronger when the older RBC fraction was tested (type 1); 37% of the reticulocyte-enriched fractions had negative DATs. Twenty-one percent of the autoantibodies seemed to show no preference for old or young RBCs (type II). Branch and coworkers[161] suggested that type I warm autoantibodies might be recognizing an as yet unidentified RBC antigen, possibly a cryptantigen closely associated with the Rh peptide but not fully expressed on very young RBCs. They hypothesized that the type I autoantibody might represent augmented production of the physiological autoantibody responsible for clearing senescent RBCs. We would suggest that the antibody against stored RBCs (and older RBCs), that we showed was anti-SCA,[158] is identical to some of the type I autoantibodies[161] and that these are indeed directed against SCA.

Finally, Herron and coworkers[162] described an e+ patient with AIHA associated with a negative DAT but a strongly reacting IgM anti-e. Anti-e was eluted from the patient's RBCs. The anti-e reacted much weaker with the patient's RBCs than other e+ RBCs in vitro. The anti-e reacted preferentially with "older" RBCs when age-fractionated RBCs were tested. When the patient went into remission, the patient's RBCs reacted equally strongly as other e+ RBCs, with the patient's stored serum from the time of the hemolytic episode. The authors suggested that the patient's RBCs that survived destruction during the hemolytic episode were younger RBCs; they had less e antigen and thus, very little antibody on them, yielding a negative DAT but a reactive eluate.

TABLE 7-11. THE 37°C REACTIVE ANTIBODIES THAT REACT WITH ALL OR MOST RED BLOOD CELLS (RBCs), INCLUDING PATIENT'S OWN RBCs (IN VITRO AND IN VIVO) BUT ARE NOT DIRECTED AT BLOOD GROUP ANTIGENS

Antibody to	References
Older or stored RBCs	153–162
Younger RBCs	34, 163–166
RBC membrane proteins	167–173
Phospholipids	174–180
Ig idiotypes	181, 182

Optimal Reactions with Younger RBCs

When Branch and coworkers[161] performed DATs on age-fractionated RBCs from DAT+ patients, they found that none of the 24 autoantibodies they tested reacted better with younger (reticulocyte-rich fraction) RBCs than older RBCs. Nevertheless, there is some evidence that RBC autoantibodies sometimes react preferentially with targets on younger RBCs. Hedge and coworkers[163] reported on three patients with WAIHA who had low reticulocyte counts when they were most anemic and in whom no RBC autoantibodies could be detected by the DAT. They postulated that reticulocytes may be selectively destroyed if antibodies are directed against targets on young RBCs, thus giving rise to a population of cells whose target antigenic sites are poorly expressed (i.e., older RBCs). Conley and coworkers[164] reported on five cases of WAIHA with reticulocytopenia; all five had rapid-onset life-threatening anemia. Repeated aspiration and biopsy of the marrow revealed that it was hyperplastic and packed with erythroid cells showing a normal pattern of differentiation. Polychromatic RBCs were seen in marrow smears but none were observed in peripheral blood smears. Unlike the cases described by Hedge and coworkers[163] the DATs in all five cases were positive and autoantibodies were present in the sera. The eluate and serum of one of the patients were tested against reticulocyte-rich and reticulocyte-reduced RBCs. The autoantibody reacted weaker against the reticulocyte-reduced fraction than the reticulocyte-rich fraction. Reticulocyte-reduced RBCs sensitized with autoantibody reacted better in an in vitro monocyte phagocytic assay than reticulocyte-rich sensitized RBCs. Thus, there seemed no evidence for an antibody directed against a target present mainly on reticulocytes.

In 1983 Garratty and coworkers[34] described a case of pure red cell aplasia associated with a mimicking anti-En^a. It was suggested that the autoanti-En^a had destroyed a population of young RBCs in the marrow. Hauke and coworkers[165] described a patient with severe WAIHA, reticulocytopenia, RBC hyperplasia of the bone marrow, and a positive DAT (IgG and complement). The patient was found to have an autoantibody to early erythroid progenitors (BFU-E). It was unclear whether this was in addition to the antibody reacting with mature RBCs. Mangan and coworkers[166] described a similar case but provided much more data. The patient had first presented with AIHA and a 60% reticulocyte count. The IgG autoantibody on the RBCs was identified as anti-e. The patient responded to steroids. Two years later the patient presented again with severe anemia. The autoantibody now reacted with all RBCs tested except Rh_{null}, although an anti-e component could be demonstrated. The reticulocyte count ranged from 0.4% to 0.6%, and erythroid precursors were virtually absent from the bone marrow. The serum was found to contain a complement-dependent IgG inhibitor directed against CFU-E and BFU-E. The erythroid progenitor cell inhibitor was still present following adsorption of the serum with e+ RBCs, and was not present in an eluate from the patient's RBCs. These data strongly suggest that aplastic crises in some patients with AIHA can be due to autoantibodies directed against targets on erythroid progenitor cells. Davidyuk and coworkers[166a] reported that four of five patients with anti-phospholipid antibody syndrome had autoantibodies to immature RBCs. These antibodies inhibited the growth of hematopoietic precursor cells in vitro.

Miscellaneous Membrane Components as Targets for RBC-Bound Autoantibodies

IgG autoantibodies to RBC skeletal proteins have also been detected in human sera. Lutz and Wipf[167] detected autoantibodies to spectrin, actin, and band 6 in the sera from all 10 healthy donors that were tested. As these proteins are not present on the surface of the RBC membrane, one would think that RBC-bound IgG autoantibodies to such proteins would not be detected on normal RBCs. However, Wiener and coworkers[168] eluted IgG antispectrin from the RBCs of patients with β-thalassemia but not from the RBCs of patients with sickle cell anemia or normal donors. They suggested that this IgG may play a role in the increased rate of destruction of RBCs in thalassemic patients. Wakui and coworkers[169] recently described an autoantibody to RBC protein 4.1 in a patient with AIHA. This antibody was detected, together with "anti–En^a-like" and anti-S, in the patient's serum. It was unclear whether the anti-S was an autoantibody or alloantibody. Unfortunately, an eluate from the patient's RBCs was not tested for anti-protein 4.1 activity. An eluate prepared from S+ RBCs incubated with the patient's serum did not contain antiprotein 4.1.

In the section on mimicking antibodies, it was mentioned that antigens are sometimes depressed in AIHA when the autoantibody is first detected. This depression can be severe enough that the RBCs do not react with typing sera. Sometimes the patients have been shown to have RBC membrane abnormalities. Garratty and coworkers[34] described a case of AIHA and red cell aplasia associated with a "mimicking" autoanti-En^a where the patients RBCs reacted with some, but not all, anti-En^a. Examination of the RBC membrane by sodium dodecyl sulfate–polyacrylamide gel electrophoresis (SDS-PAGE) revealed only a slight reduction of glycophorin A. The RBCs from an En(a+) patient with an anti-En^{a}TS, which caused a fatal hemolytic transfusion reaction, showed greater abnormalities of the membrane.[170] The RBC membranes were shown to contain glycophorins B and C by SDS-PAGE with periodic acid–Schiff's base staining with weak staining of components in the regions corresponding to monomers and dimers of glycophorin A and heterologous dimers of glycophorins A and B. The nature of these components was not identified, but their presence suggested that the patient's RBCs expressed a previously undescribed glycophorin A variant. Several patients have been described with abnormalities of glycophorin. Beattie and Sigmund[51] reported a case of AIHA and aplasia, associated with autoanti-Ge. The RBCs of this patient showed an altered glycophorin C. Reid and coworkers[171] studied the immunochemical specificity of the target antigens reacting with autoanti-Ge from two patients with AIHA. One anti-Ge reacted with normal, but not with abnormal glycophorin C, associated with Ge– RBCs. This patient's RBCs had an alteration of glycophorin C with the other glycophorins being normal. The autoanti-Ge from the other patient was similar to alloanti-Ge3 in that it reacted with both glycophorins C and D from normal RBC membranes and with the abnormal glycophorin C found in RBCs from individuals with Ge– RBCs of the Yus type.

There have been other isolated reports of RBC membrane abnormalities associated with AIHA but these have not related to specific autoantibody specificity. Gomperts and coworkers[172] studied RBCs from nine cases of AIHA. RBC stroma was extracted using dilute acetic acid and the isolated protein electrophoresed on 8 M urea starch gel. Six of the nine cases showed the absence of one band and absence or decreased intensity of a second band. The pattern was the same as that observed when RBCs from hereditary spherocytosis were tested. The eluates from RBCs of the six cases with absent bands all showed definable "specificity" (e.g., anti-nl, -pdl, etc) but the remaining three were classified as "nonspecific." Kajii and coworkers[173] isolated a 12-kDa peptide from the RBCs of four patients with AIHA. This peptide could not be obtained from RBCs of 50 normal persons, or patients without AIHA. In one patient, with angioimmunoblastic lymphadenopathy and dysproteinemia (AILD), the peptide was still detectable following treatment, when the RBC autoantibodies had disappeared, but was no longer detectable when the patient's AILD was in complete remission, following chemotherapy.

Antibodies to Phospholipids

Antibodies to phospholipid (e.g., anticardiolipin) may attach to RBC membranes, leading to a positive DAT[174,175] and possibly AIHA.[166a,176-180] Hazeltine and coworkers[174] detected cardiolipin antibodies in 22% of patients with systemic lupus erythematosus (SLE). The presence of such antibodies in the serum was associated with a positive DAT. Analysis of eluates from the patient's RBCs and adsorption studies showed that some cardiolipin antibodies may react with phospholipid on RBC membranes. Win and coworkers[175] reported on positive DATs, associated with phospholipid antibodies, in blood donors. Sthoeger and coworkers[176] showed the presence of cardiolipin antibodies in the sera and eluates from RBCs of two SLE patients with AIHA. Following steroid treatment one patient went into remission, the DAT and IAT became negative, and cardiolipin antibodies were no longer detectable. The other patient remained DAT+, and cardiolipin antibodies were still detectable. The authors suggested that the cardiolipin antibodies may play a direct role in the pathogenesis of the AIHA. Cabral and coworkers[177] described a case of AIHA associated with high titer IgM cardiolipin antibodies. An interesting observation was that the cardiolipin antibodies bound more efficiently to stored RBCs than fresh RBCs; bromelin-treated RBCs reacted better than stored untreated RBCs. In contrast, Davidyuk and coworkers[166a] found that four of five autoantibodies from patients with anti-phospholipid antibody syndrome reacted better with immature RBCs.

Idiotypic Targets on RBC-Bound IgG Autoantibodies

Masouredis and coworkers[181] reported that eluates from DAT+ donors contained IgG antibodies to idiotypic determinants (anti-id) on the RBC-bound IgG autoantibody, in addition to RBC autoantibodies (see Figure 9-2 on page 321). Eight of 12 eluates prepared from the RBCs of DAT+ donors contained at least two populations of IgG autoantibodies. The first population reacted with RBCs by the IAT; this was the RBC autoantibody. The second population did not react with untreated RBCs but would directly agglutinate IgG (anti-D)-coated RBCs; this was the anti-id. In a later article, eluates from the RBCs of two patients with AIHA were shown to contain RBC autoantibody but no anti-id.[182] The antibodies were designated as anti-id by Masouredis and coworkers[182] because the autoantibody appeared to be directed against determinants on the Fab portion of IgG (only one antibody was studied), and the antibody would agglutinate RBCs coated with anti-D, but not antibodies of other specificities.

In 1999, Garratty reviewed specificities that have been reported to be associated with autoantibodies reacting optimally at 37°C.[183]

SPECIFICITIES ASSOCIATED WITH COLD AGGLUTININ SYNDROME

Nonspecific cold autoagglutinins were first reported by Mino in 1924.[184] The story of the unraveling of their specificity closely parallels the history of the Ii blood group antigens.

Three main groups of antigens recognized by human cold agglutinins (CAs) have been defined on a serological and biochemical basis. The first group consists of the Ii antigens. They are protease- and sialidase-resistant differentiation antigens. I antigen is fully expressed on adult and i antigen is fully expressed on fetal RBCs. Anti-i recognizes linear poly-*N*-acetyllactosamine or type 2 chains, which are converted into I antigens in the first year after birth by branching. The second group consists of the Pr and Sa antigens. They are not differentiation antigens on RBCs but are expressed in equal strength on adult and newborn RBCs. $Pr_{1,2,3}$ antigens are destroyed by protease and sialidase treatment of RBCs, whereas Pr_a is inactivated only by proteases. Anti-Pr and anti-Sa recognize the sialo-*O*-glycans of glycophorins. The third group consists of the Sia-l1, Sia-bl, and Sia-1b1 (formerly termed V_o, Fl, and Gd) antigens. They are susceptible to sialidase but are resistant to proteases on RBCs. Sia-l1 and Sia-b1 antigens are differentiation antigens created by sialyation of linear and branched type 2 chains, respectively. Sia-l1 and Sia-b1 resemble i and I antigens. Another antigen of this group, Sia-1bl, is not developmentally regulated, but is expressed in equal strength on adult and newborn RBCs. It is detected by anti–Sia-1bl CAs recognizing linear as well as branched sialylated type 2 chains.

Ii Blood Group Antigens and Antibodies

In 1956, Weiner and coworkers[185] studied an unusual patient with cold agglutinin syndrome (CAS) who had severe transfusion reactions, even if the donor blood was kept warm. They were energetic enough to screen RBCs from over 22,000 donors with the patient's serum, finding 5 to be compatible (4 blacks, 1 white). No correlation was found with the Lewis, Lutheran, Duffy, Kidd, P, Vel, or ABO systems. The authors concluded they were dealing with a new blood group specificity, which they designated I (to indicate its high degree of *individuality*). The antibody was thus anti-I, and the rare individuals whose RBCs were compatible with the serum (containing anti-I) were designated i, or "I-negative." Although RBCs from the five donors did not react at room temperature when untreated, they all reacted at 4°C and at room temperature when ficin-treated. A feature of Weiner's case that we find hard to understand is that the patient's own washed RBCs were not agglutinated by his own serum at room temperature, unless the RBCs were enzyme-treated; in fact, they reacted similarly to the so-called i donors!

In 1960 Jenkins and coworkers[186] found that 50 sera containing weak cold autoagglutinins that had previously been called "nonspecific cold agglutinins" had anti-I specificity; none of these donors had hemolytic anemia. Later in the same year, Marsh and Jenkins[187] and, in 1961, Marsh[188] described the first two examples of anti-i; antibodies that appeared to react antithetically to anti-I. Using anti-I and anti-i, Marsh was able to show that unlike other blood group systems so far described, cord RBCs from newborn babies were rich in i antigen and possessed very little I antigen. The I antigen slowly developed at the expense of i until at least 18 months of age, at which time adult status was reached. Adult RBCs normally are rich in I antigen but have only small amounts of i antigen present. Some adults are found to give intermediate reactions, I_{INT} (i.e., weaker I antigen). Rare adults are found whose RBCs have less I antigen and more i antigen than cord RBCs; these are the i adults. Marsh[188] suggested the following order of increasing strength of I: i_1, i_2, i_{cord}, I_{INT}, I; i_1 is usually associated with white individuals, and i_2 is usually associated with black individuals.

Although cord RBCs react much weaker than adult RBCs at all temperatures when tested with a low titer cold agglutinin, the results can be very confusing when a pathological high titer cold agglutinin is tested; very little difference in titer is noticed at 4°C, but the specificity becomes more obvious as the temperature is raised. Table 7-12 shows typical reactions of adult and cord RBCs with a pathological high titer anti-I. It should also be noted that various examples of cord RBCs can show marked differences in reactivity with some anti-I.

In 1970,[190] a powerful anti-I was described that was strongly inhibited by hydatid cyst fluid and inhibited to a varying extent by all of the 181 human saliva samples tested; previously, saliva had been reported not to inhibit anti-I.[191] Infants at birth and i adults were also found to have high concentrations of I substance in their saliva. This investigation suggested that I antibodies are of two kinds—those inhibitable by saliva and those not inhibited; this confirmed an earlier suggestion by Marsh who had termed the two

TABLE 7-12. REACTIONS OF A TYPICAL ANTI-I ASSOCIATED WITH COLD AGGLUTININ SYNDROME

	4°C		25°C		30°C	
Dilution of Patient's	Adult	Cord	Adult	Cord	Adult	Cord
2	4+	4+	4+	1+	1+	0
4	4+	4+	4+	1+	½+	0
8	4+	4+	3+	½+	0	0
16	4+	4+	3+	0	0	0
32	4+	4+	3+	0	0	0
64	4+	4+	2+	0	0	0
128	4+	3+	1+	0	0	0
256	3+	3+	½+	0	0	0
512	3+	2+	0	0	0	0
1024	2+	1+	0	0	0	0
2048	1+	0	0	0	0	0
4096	0	0	0	0	0	0

types Ia and Ib. Marsh and coworkers[191] found that human milk contained a high concentration of water-soluble I blood group substance. Tests with 24 different anti-I showed that, to a variable extent, all of them could be inhibited by milk and some could be inhibited by strong I secretor saliva. This susceptibility to inhibition was not related to titer, and the results suggested that qualitative differences in the antibody antigen reactions was responsible. In 1971, Marsh and coworkers[189] described two components of the I antigen, which they named I^F (fetal) and I^D (developed). The I^F component was found to be present on all human RBCs, including those of i_{cord}, i_{adult}, and also on rhesus monkey RBCs. The I^D component develops slowly on the RBCs before birth and, to a greater extent, 18 months after birth. Inhibition studies with human milk showed that strongly inhibitable anti-I were of the anti-I^D variety, but only a minority of such sera were inhibitable. Naturally occurring low titer cold autoagglutinins were found mainly to be anti-I^D, whereas the high titer cold autoagglutinins associated with AIHA were found commonly to contain anti-I^F, either alone or together with anti-I^D; rarely, anti-I^D was encountered exclusively. This suggested an explanation for the strong reaction of high titer anti-I associated with AIHA, with cord RBCs, which are rich in I^F but have very little, if any, I^D. Marsh and coworkers[189] also discussed the possible place of I^F and I^D in the development of the I antigen.

Dzierzkowa-Borodej and coworkers[192] suggested that the anti-I that are inhibitable are different than anti-I^D. Although they act similarly serologically, they can be differentiated by their capability to precipitate in gel at 4°C. Saliva, colostral IgA, and desialized glycoprotein from RBCs gave strong precipitin lines with inhibitable anti-I but not with other anti-I. They suggested that the inhibitable anti-I be called anti-I^S. In an extensive study on 12 anti-I cold autoantibodies (one of normal titer 32, the others ranging from 256 to 2×10^6), they found that only 4 of 12 sera demonstrated single specificity (1 anti-I^S, 3 anti-I^F) and that the others demonstrated two or more specificities (1 anti-I^D + anti-I^S, 1 anti-I^D + anti-I^F, 3 anti-I^D + anti-i, and 2 anti-I^D + anti-I^F + anti-I^S). These differences could not be easily determined by using I_{adult}, i_{cord}, and i_{adult} RBCs but became more obvious when the RBCs from a rare adult having only I^F were used (these RBCs failed to react with anti-I^D and anti-i but were agglutinated by anti-I^F). It is interesting to note that the same authors have shown that desialization of RBCs enhanced their agglutinability by anti-I^D and anti-I^S but had no effect on their reaction with anti-I^F.[193]

It has been clear over the years that autoanti-I can exist in two forms: (1) a low titer autoantibody occurring in almost all normal human serum as a naturally occurring cold agglutinin; reacting optimally at 0°C to 4°C; rarely acting above room temperature; and (2) a high titer autoantibody often associated with CAS; reacting optimally at 0°C to 4°C; and almost always reacting up to 30°C to 32°C and rarely reacting at 37°C, when saline-suspended RBCs are used (see Table 7-12). It is by far the most common antibody to be associated with CAS (both the chronic idiopathic cases and those secondary to *Mycoplasma pneumoniae* infection). In our own series, 49 of 54 cases (91%) were associated with anti-I. Other workers have reported similar findings. Anti-i is not commonly detected in normal serum as is anti-I but has been reported to be present in as high as 70% of sera from patients with infectious mononucleosis. When it is detected in other cases, it is often associated with diseases of the reticuloendothelial system. When it is present in high enough titer and its reactivity is of high thermal range, it can cause AIHA. Of 54 cases of CAS in our series, 4 (7.4%) were associated with anti-i. Although the clinical histories are very limited, there is a suggestion that one of the first two patients to be described as having anti-i had AIHA.[187] This patient came under investigation for suspected reticulosis and moderate anemia. An anti-i reacting to a titer of 256,000 with i_{adult} RBCs was present in his serum, reacting strongly at room temperature and weakly at 37°C. The anti-i only reacted to a titer of 4 to 16 with I_{adult} RBCs. Often, even strong anti-i (i.e., high titers against i_{adult} and i_{cord} RBCs) will not react or only react weakly at room temperature with normal adult RBCs, including the patient's own. Thus, hemolytic anemia is rare even when a powerful anti-i is present. Sometimes the i antigenic status of the patient's RBCs can be increased,[193,194] thus making the patient's RBCs more reactive with anti-i than normal adult RBCs. When performing cold agglutinin titers and thermal ranges, etc., it is always useful to include tests against the patient's own RBCs.

Since the original description of anti-i, other cases of CAS caused by anti-i have been described.[195-198]

Chemistry of Ii Antigens. Ii antigens are closely related to ABO, H, and Lewis blood group antigens. A number of antibodies have been described that will only react when I is present together with other antigens from the ABO, Hh, and Lewis systems (e.g., anti-IA, -IH, -iH, -IB, -IP, -IP_1, -iP_1, -I^TP_1, and anti-Le^bH). These antibodies appear to react with complex antigens distinct from the separate antigens, for example, anti-IB will only react with RBCs containing both I and B antigens, and not with RBCs containing I but not B or B but not I; the amount of IB on RBCs is not related to the amount of I or B on the RBCs,[199,200] thus appearing to be a completely separate "antigen." In 1971 Feizi and coworkers[201] analyzed the I-active antigen extracted from human milk. The sugar composition of this material closely resembled the chemistry associated with ABO blood group substances; however, its content of frucose was unusually low. In this respect, it resembled blood group precursor-like substances that had been isolated from human ovarian cyst fluid lacking ABO and Lewis substances.[202,203] Feizi and coworkers[201,204] suggested that I specificity was concealed in interior structures of the blood A, B, H, Le^a, and Le^b substances and may be exposed by stepwise periodate oxidation and Smith degradation of ABO and H substances. Thus, I substance would seem to be a precursor for the biosynthesis of H, A, and B. In a later study, the same workers studied 11 anti-I sera and found they could be divided into at least six groups based on their reactions with human milk, ovarian cyst fractions (containing "ABH" precursor blood group substances), degraded ABH substances, and hydatid cyst fluid. Four of five anti-i resembled each other, but the fifth differed in its reaction with hydatid cyst fluid and milk.

Burnie[195] and Cooper and coworkers[205] have shown that normal plasma can be shown to contain I and i substances in small quantities. Rosse and Lauf[206] extracted the antigens ("I") reacting with cold autoagglutinins from human RBCs, using *n*-butanol. A fascinating observation was made that although the antigen and antibody were not able to react at 37°C when the antigen was present in the intact RBC after solubilization, antigen and antibody reacted equally well at 37°C and 0°C. In addition, the amount of "I" antigen extracted from the RBCs of adult and newborns appeared to be about the same! In a previous study,[207] it had been suggested that the effect of temperature changes was not on the antibody but was rather on the antigen or the RBC membrane. This conclusion was based on the fact that the change in affinity of antibody for RBCs of newborn infants (i_{cord}) or of i_{adult} RBCs was very much greater than that for RBCs of normal adults. Because any effect on the antibody of change of temperature would have been the same in both situations, they concluded that a change in configuration of the antigen or the RBC surface must be responsible for the characteristic cold reactivity of the antigen–antibody interaction. They further concluded that their later experiments indicated that the reactivity of cold agglutinins only in the cold was due to an effect of cold on the RBC membrane, because the antigen–antibody reaction occurred as well at 37°C as at 0°C when the antigen was removed from the membrane. They suggested that at 37°C the antigen on the intact membrane may be "hidden," whereas at 0°C the antigen may become available for reaction with the antibody. Their studies led them to believe that the difference between "I" and "i" is largely a difference between the number of I antigenic sites. When the "affinity" of the antigen and antibody were increased by enzyme treatment of the RBCs or by incubation in the cold, the total amount of antibody fixed by both types of cells became nearly equal.

Gardas and Koscielak[208] isolated an I active substance from human RBCs by *n*-butanol extraction and found it to be identical to A, B, and H isolated antigens. The materials were sialic acid free and comprised about 90% carbohydrate, 7% to 7.5% of amino acids, and 2% of sphingosine. A, B, and H blood group activities were completely recovered in immune precipitates of appropriate water-soluble antigens with anti-I precipitating serum; on the contrary, I activity could be recovered form precipitates prepared with anti-A and -B precipitating sera. Thus, the water phase left after extraction of stroma with *n*-butanol comprises a single antigenic material in which all A, B, H, and I blood group activities are located on the same molecule. This conclusion offers an explanation for the anti-I that are influenced by ABH group of the test RBCs (e.g., anti-IH, -IA, -IB) in that the adjacent A, B, H, and I active structures may give rise to antibodies of mixed ABH and I specificity. The results obtained in this study would agree with Feizi and coworkers[201] and Marcus and coworkers[209] that terminal galactopyranosyl residues are part of the I structure. It is interesting to note that the isolated I and H blood group substances were easily adsorbed onto human RBCs in vitro and thus group Oi RBCs could easily be changed to OI RBCs. One finding contrasted with the finding of Rosse and Lauf[206] described earlier; isolated preparations of I active antigens precipitated only at 4°C and no reactions occurred at 37°C.

Red cell glycoproteins contain two kinds of oligosaccharide chains: (1) alkali-*labile* chains consisting of galactose, *N*-acetygalactosamine, and a large proportion of sialic acid; and (2) alkali-*stable* chains containing galactose, *N*-acetyglucosamine, mannose, and low amounts of sialic acid and fucose.[210-214] Aklali-*stable* chains are required for I activity, whereas MN activity depends on alkali-*labile* chains. Red cells contain one major glycoprotein (glycophorin) and a few minor ones. I activity has been reported to be associated with the minor glycoprotein by some workers[215] and glycophorin by others.[216] Lisowska and coworkers[193] tested three fractions of red cell glycoproteins obtained from Sepharose 4-B chromatography for I activity with 10 anti-I sera. Fraction 1 was further purified by separating ABHI-active substances from MN active sialoglycoprotein. This fraction had the greatest I activity and contained the lowest amount of alkali-labile obligosaccharide chains. The most abundant fraction (II), which was the major sialoglycoprotein of red cell membranes, showed no or only weak I activity, but I active glycopeptides could be isolated by digestion of fraction II with trypsin. The major product of digestion, sialoglycopeptide II T-2, showed I activity only after alkaline elimination of alkali-labile oligosaccharide chains. Fraction III showed weak I activity but was slightly stronger than fraction II. Fraction III showed less MN activity than fractions I and II.

Lisowska and coworkers[193] concluded that I active receptors were present in all fractions of the RBC glycoproteins they studied, but in some fractions they were "masked" and could be exposed by enzymatic and chemical degradation of glycoproteins. The I activity appeared to be associated with alkali-*stable* oligosaccharide chains. Sialic acid–rich alkali-*labile* oligosaccharides appeared to be responsible for the steric hindrance for the reaction between anti-I and some I antigens. The results were in favor of the concept that a unique I substance is *not* present on

RBCs but that I active receptors are located on different ABH or MN-active molecules, in a position less or more available for reaction with anti-I.

Several examples of ABO/I complex target antigens for nonpathogenic cold autoantibodies have been described (HI, Hi, IA, and IB). Two cases of CAS associated with autoanti-AI were described by McGinniss.[217,218] Postoway and coworkers[219] described a transient anti-IB in an A_2B patient that appeared to be the cause of the patient's AIHA; this antibody reacted to a titer of 2048 (at 4°C), and reacted up to 30°C with the patient's RBCs.

As the structure of ABH and Ii antigens became clear, it was no surprise that some antibodies appeared to react with ABH–Ii complex antigens. Wiener suggested that anti-I might be reacting against the "nucleus" of ABO, and he has been proven to be correct. Ii determinants are indeed internal structures of the ABH antigens. The Ii determinants are bound to glycolipids and glycoproteins in the RBC membrane; carrier molecules are band 3, the major intrinsic membrane protein and band 4.5 components. Only type 2 chains [Galβ(1→4)GlcNAcβ(1→3)Gal-R] generate Ii determinants on the RBC membranes. These type 2 sequences are the basic structures of glycolipids of the neolacto series. Ii antigens are built up by repeating *N*-acetyllactosamine units: Anti-i recognizes the linear chain and anti-I the branched chain. The branched chain is formed by adding a further lactosamine unit in (1→6) linkage to the penultimate galactose (Gal) of the linear chain. H substance is generated by substitution of the terminal Gal of the I structure, with Fucα(1→2). H substance serves as a precursor for A and B. The fine specificity of anti-I and anti-i will depend on the extent of the Ii structure that reacts with the specific antibody; many variations of the theme can be encountered, thus explaining the many subdivisions that have been made by serological testing (e.g., I^D, I^F, I^T, IH, IA, IB, iH, etc.).

"Cold" Autoantibody Specificities Other Than Anti-I and Anti-i

Specificities other than anti-I or anti-i are rare.[220] The most common specificity reacting with all human RBCs tested (adult and cord RBCs acting equally) was first popularly called, rather facetiously, anti–"not-I." Dr. Marsh, who christened it so, told us he was chagrined that the name ever appeared in print, and called it anti-SP_1 when the first extensive serological data on this antibody was published.[221]

Marsh and Jenkins[221] called the antibody anti-Sp_1 (species) as no human RBCs lacking the reacting antigen could be found but no RBCs from 25 other species reacted. The Sp_1 antigen showed a striking difference from I and i in that the Sp_1 antigen could be destroyed or markedly reduced by treating the RBC with proteolytic enzymes (trypsin, bromelin, papain, and ficin); both I and i give *enhanced* reactions following enzyme treatment. The antigen was found to be well developed at birth; the antibody was found to react better if the serum was at pH 6.5 or below (e.g., titer of 16 at pH 9.0 and 8000 at pH 6.2). In a series of 268 cold autoantibodies investigated, two were designated as anti-Sp_1. Both of these were high titer antibodies associated with AIHA; no examples of naturally occurring anti-Sp_1 were found in healthy individuals in the course of many thousand cold antibody investigations.

Independently, Roelcke[222] described an antibody called anti-HD (Heidelberg); this antibody appeared to be reacting with an antigen identical to Sp_1. In 1969, Roelcke published an extensive study showing heterogeneity of the HD (Sp_1) receptor.[223] HD_1 antigen could be demonstrated only on human RBCs, in contrast to the HD_2 antigen, which could be demonstrated on rat and guinea pig RBCs, as well as human RBCs. Neuraminidase and proteases inactivated both antigens. However, quantitative differences were observed; the HD_2 antigen showed more resistance to neuraminidase and proteases than HD_1.[223]

In 1970 Roelcke and Uhlenbruck[224] suggested replacing the terms "Sp" and "HD" with "Pr" (indicating the antigen inactivation by proteases). A complex heterogeneity has been discovered.[221-229] Pr_1 antibodies were originally classified according to their results with RBCs from humans and other animals. Pr_{1h} was said to be present only on human RBCs. Pr_{1d} was said to be present on RBCs from human and some animal species, including dogs. Pr_2 had a similar species distribution but in contrast to Pr_{1d}, was found to be increased on dog RBCs and not destroyed by protease treatment of dog RBCs. The anti-SP_1 described by Marsh and Jenkins is probably identical to anti-Pr_{1d} or -Pr_2 because SP_1 was found to be inactivated by neuraminidase and to be present on guinea pig RBCs. The RBCs of 24,150 humans, tested by Roelcke, were all found to have Pr_{1h} and Pr_2.

In 1971, a new determinant, Pr_a, was described.[229] Two IgG cold autoagglutinins causing transient hemolytic anemia were detected in children; they reacted with all RBCs tested (cord and adult RBCs reacted equally) and the reacting determinant was inactivated by proteolytic enzyme, but in contrast to Pr_1 and Pr_2, it was not inactivated by neuraminidase. It is easy to confuse anti-Pr_a with anti-En^aTS and anti-En^aFS (see earlier). Another determinant of the Pr system was also described in 1971, Pr_3.[228] A monoclonal IgM (kappa) antibody, associated with CAS, occurring after rubella infection, was shown to react as an anti-Pr, but was different than anti-Pr_1, -Pr_2, and -Pr_a. Pr_3 determinants are found on cat and sheep RBCs which lack Pr_1 and Pr_2 determinants. By carbodiimide treatment of human red cell glycoproteins, which causes intramolecular coupling of *N*-acetylneuraminic acid carboxyl group and nucleophilic centers of the glycoprotein backbone, Pr_3 antigen activity was greatly increased, whereas Pr_1 and Pr_2 were inactivated.

The Pr determinants are present on RBC glycophorins (e.g., glycophorin A). The O-glycosidically linked oligosaccharides of glycophorins are the Pr determinants. All fragments of glycophorin A carrying oligosaccharides are Pr_1-, Pr_2-, and Pr_3-inactive. The fine structure of the Pr antigenic site is unknown at present. Because En(a–) RBCs lack the major glycophorin, glycophorin A, they react very poorly, or not at all, with anti-Pr. As mentioned earlier, En(a–) RBCs adsorb anti-Pr; thus, glycophorins other than glycophorin A may carry some Pr. M^kM^k RBCs that lack glycophorins A and B do not react with anti-Pr, but adsorption and elution studies have not been performed.

Pr antibodies can now be classified biochemically.[220] Anti-Pr_{1h} and anti-Pr_{3h} react exclusively with human RBCs. Anti-Pr_{1d} and anti-Pr_{3d} react with human and dog RBCs. Pr_2 is not limited to human RBCs. Antibodies (anti-Pr^M and -Pr^N) acting like anti-Pr but showing a preference for RBCs of M or N phenotype, respectively, have been described.[220] Pr_1, Pr_2, and Pr_3 can be differentiated by simple biochemical procedures, using periodate-oxidized and carbodiimide-treated glycophorins. Pr_1 is inactivated by both procedures; Pr_2 is increased 100- to 200-fold by oxidation and is inactivated by carbodiimide treatment; Pr_3 is increased 100- to 200-fold by carbodiimide-treatment and is inactivated by oxidation. When characterizing 32 anti-Pr cold autoagglutinins, Roelcke[220] found 24 anti-Pr_{1h}, 3 anti-Pr_2, and 5 anti-Pr_3.

Several reports of anti-Pr cold autoantibodies associated with AIHA have appeared in the literature.[228-234] Three were unusual cases associated with anti-Pr_a. Curtis and coworkers[232] reported a life-threatening, DAT-negative acute hemolytic anemia associated with a non–complement-activating IgG1 monoclonal (kappa) cold autoantibody with anti-Pr_a specificity. Kadota and coworkers[233] reported a hemolytic anemia associated with a rubella infection and anti-Pr_a. Ramos and coworkers[234] reported a refractory immune hemolytic anemia asssciated with a high thermal amplitude, low affinity IgG anti-Pr_a cold autoantibody.

It is interesting that only five examples of IgA high titer cold autoagglutinins have been reported,[235-239] and four have been shown to be monoclonal (kappa) and have anti-Pr_1 specificity. Most anti-I associated with chronic CAS are IgM monoclonal (kappa) proteins, but rare examples of IgM (lambda) cold agglutinins have been reported.[225] Three of these were originally reported as having anti–"not-I" specificity, and one of them has since been identified as anti-Pr_1.[224] The restricted nature of anti-I cold agglutinins is not limited to their constant regions; their light chain variable regions are predominantly VKII subgroup, and their heavy chain variable regions are predominantly VHI subgroup.[240,241] Wang and coworkers[241] studied the amino acid sequence of the IgA cold agglutinin "Rob" that we had reported as having anti-Pr specificity in 1973.[237] They were able to define a new kappa chain variable region subgroup that was designated VKIV. Because the anti-Pr and anti-I cold agglutinins had variable region subgroups that clearly differed and because these specificities correspond to chemical differences in the RBC membrane, Wang and coworkers[241] suggested that their study illustrated a direct correlation between antibody specificity and the structure of the light and heavy chain variable regions. The case "Rob" that we described[237] had an interesting history. The patient was a 51-year-old white man whose major symptoms consisted of extreme sensitivity to the cold, as manifested by bluish discoloration of the extremities, ears, and face. With intense exposure to cold, his entire appearance was purplish, and his hands and, in particular, his feet became extremely painful. The diagnosis of cold agglutinin syndrome was not made until 21 years later. At this time, electrophoresis of his serum showed a monoclonal spike in the β globulin region, which was shown by immunoelectrophoresis to be IgA. The bone marrow was hypercellular and contained approximately 10% mature plasma cells. A diagnosis of multiple myeloma was considered, although the patient did not develop osteolytic bone lesions or urine protein abnormalities. Physical examination revealed no lymphadenopathy, splenomegaly, or hepatomegaly. Bone marrow examinations over the next 5 years showed an increase in plasma cells, and the serum IgA level rose to a concentration of 1.01 g%. His cold agglutinin titre was 16,000, reacting up to 35°C. The serum caused no hemolysis in vitro of normal or enzyme-treated RBCs. The antibody being IgA was incapable of activating complement; thus, although the patient had clinical signs due to the powerful cold autoagglutinin (e.g., acrocyanosis), no evidence of hemolytic anemia was ever detected.

Target Antigens (Gd, Fl, Vo, Li) That Are Sialidase Sensitive and Protease Resistant. Gd antigens are glycolipid dependent (Gd) and are fully expressed on adult and cord RBCs. They are created by sialyation of Ii glycolipid antigens.[220] The structure of the Gd determinant is NeuNAc(2→3)[Gal(1→4)GlcNAc(1 → $3)_n$]. Glycophorins are Gd inactive. The Gd major active ganglioside, sialylneolactotetraosylceramide, is increased in the RBC membranes of p individuals. It has been suggested that antibodies designated anti-p may be anti-Gd.[220]

Anti-Fl may be confused with anti-I as the Fl antigen is fully expressed only on I_{adult} RBCs; the antigen is poorly expressed on i_{cord} and i_{adult} RBCs. Anti-Fl differs from anti-I only in not reacting with sialidase-treated RBCs. The branched I active neolactosequence is the basic structure of the Fl antigen, but one or both branches are sialylated and NeuNAc is the immunodominant component.[220] I active sialoglycoproteins will inhibit antiFl.[220] Fl-like I antigens are membrane glycolipids and glycoproteins. O_h RBCs have very reduced reactivity with anti-Fl.[220]

Vo and Li are targets for cold autoagglutinins that are protease-resistant and fully expressed only on i_{cord} and i_{adult} RBCs; thus, anti-Vo and -Li may be confused with anti-i. Unlike i, Vo and Li are sialidase sensitive. Vo and Li differ in their susceptibility to sialidase treatment. Li is susceptible to sialidase on an intact surface, whereas Vo is susceptible to sialidase only after protease treatment. It has been suggested that Vo and Li are sialylated linear type 2 (neolacto) chains, NeuNAc(2→3)[Gal(1→4)Glc-Nac(1→3)], that is, sialylated i determinants.[220]

Target Antigens (Lud, Sa) That Are Sialidase-Sensitive and Partially Inactivated by Proteases. Another cold autoagglutinin, anti-Lud, may also be confused with anti-I and anti-Fl. Lud is fully expressed on I_{adult} but not on cord RBCs; thus, if only adult and cord RBCs are used, anti-I, -Fl, and -Lud give similar results. Unlike I and Fl, Lud is fully expressed on i_{adult} RBCs. Proteases partially inactivate Lud but do not inactivate I or Fl.[220] Thus, anti-Lud recognizes sialidase-sensitive antigens fully expressed only on adult RBCs. The structure of Lud is unknown at present.

The Sa antigens are sialidase sensitive but only partially inactivated by papain and do not react with glycoproteins obtained from papain-treated RBCs. The antigens are fully expressed on adult and cord RBCs. Glycophorin A carries Sa determinants. Like Pr_2 (see later), Sa antigens are gangliosides, but unlike Pr_2 they are restricted to the neolacto series.[220]

It is obvious from the above data that most reports of specificity of cold autoagglutinins being anti-I or anti-i are now suspect as these sera have not usually been tested with sialidase-treated RBCs. Indeed, this is a technical problem as most sera contain anti-T that may react with sialidase-treated RBCs. It is possible that sera designated as anti-I or anti-i may be found to contain anti-Gd, -Fl, -Vo, -Li, or -Lud, together with anti-I/i or even alone. This would parallel the discovery that anti-"dl" could contain, or be, anti-En^a or -Wr^b. As the epitopes for A, B, H, I, i, Gd, Fl, Vo, Li, and Lud are all on the same basic structure, and, similarly, M, N, En^a, Wr^b, and Pr are on the same structure (i.e., glycophorin A), it should be no surprise that interpretation of specificity, based on serological reactions, can be confusing and inaccurate.

Tables 7-13 and 7-14 show the serological characteristics of the antibodies discussed above.

Roelcke[220] has suggested a new terminology for Fl, Vo, and Gd. The antigens share several characteristics:

1. The antigens are differentiation antigens. Sia-b1 (formerly F1) is fully expressed only on adult RBCs. Sia-l1 (formerly Vo) is fully expressed only on newborn RBCs. As an exception, Sia-lb1 (formerly Gd) is expressed on adult and newborn RBCs in equal strength.
2. The antigens are present on the rare adult RBCs with the i phenotype (i adult RBCs) in equal strength as on newborn (i cord) RBCs. It can, therefore, be concluded that the structures responsible for Ii and Sia-1, -b, -1b antigens are related.
3. The antigens are inactivated by sialidase treatment of RBCs, indicating that NeuNAc, not involved in Ii antigenic determinants, serves as immunodominant component.

Anti-Sia-b1 (anti-Fl) may initially be mistaken for anti-I. Anti-Sia-l1 (anti-Vo) and anti-Sia-lb1 (anti-Gd) may initially be mistaken for anti-i (Table 7-15).

MISCELLANEOUS TARGETS FOR COLD AUTOANTIBODIES

Rare examples of anti-A and anti-B have been reported as cold and warm autoantibodies.[242] Three examples of autoanti-A and one example each of autoanti-IB and autoanti-B have been reported to be associated with CAS.[242-244] Sokol and coworkers[242]

TABLE 7-13. SEROLOGIC CHARACTERISTICS OF AUTOANTIBODIES THAT REACT WITH TARGET ANTIGENS THAT MAY BE AFFECTED BY PROTEASES OR SIALIDASES

Antibody	I_{adult}	i_{cord}	i_{adult}	I_{adult} PT	I_{adult} ST	I_{adult} En(a-)	I_{adult} Wr(b-)
Anti-I	+	↓	↓	↑	↑	+	+
-i	↓	+	+	↑*	↑*	↓	↓
-I^T	↓	+	↓	+	+	↓	↓
-Pr	+	+	+	0	0	0**	0
-Pr_a	+	+	+	0	+	0**	0
-Gd	+	+	+	+	0	+	+
-Fl	+	↓	↓	+	0	+	+
-Vo	↓	+	+	↑*	↓*	+	+
-Li	↓	+	+	+*	0*	+	+
-Lud	+	↓	+	↓	0	+	+
-Sa	+	+	+	↓	0	+	+
-En^a	+	+	+	0	+	0	0

PT, protease (papin or ficin) treated; +, antibody reacts; ↑, increased reaction compared with same RBCs untreated; ST, sialidase (neuraminidase) treated; 0, antibody does not react; ↓, decreased reaction; *, reactions apply to i_{cord} and i_{adult}, but not I_{adult} RBCs; **, antibody may be adsorbed/eluted by or from RBCs.

TABLE 7-14. TYPICAL REACTIONS OF ANTI-Pr SUBSPECIFICITIES§

	Antibody Directed Against							
Red Blood Cells	**Pr_{1h}**	**Pr_{1d}**	**Pr_2**	**Pr_{3h}**	**Pr_{3d}**	**Pr_a**	**Pr^M**	**Pr^N**
I_{adult}								
Untreated	+	+	+	+	+	+	+‡	+‖
Protease	0	0	0	0	0	0	0	0
Sialidase	0	0	0	0	0	+	0	0
i_{adult}								
Untreated	+	+	+	+	+	+	+‡	+‖
Protease	0	0	0	0	0	0	0	0
Sialidase	0	0	0	0	0	+	0	0
i_{cord}								
Untreated	+	+	+	+	+	+	+‡	+‖
Protease	0	0	0	0	0	0	0	0
Sialidase	0	0	0	0	0	+	0	0
Dog								
Untreated	0	+†	+	0	+	0		
Protease	0	V	E	0	0	0		
Sialidase	0	0	0	0	0	0		
Sheep	0	0	0	+	+			
Cat	0	0	0	+	+			
Guinea Pig	V	V	+	E				
Rat	V	V	V	V				
Rabbit¶	0	0	0	0				

+, Agglutination: V, variable reaction (i.e., some negative, some positive); in titration studies, results with red blood cells (RBCs) marked V usually react to a lower titer than those marked +; E, enhanced reaction; in titration studies, results with RBCs marked E usually react to higher titers than those marked +; blank spaces, no information available.
† Some anti-Pr_{1d} react only with dog RBCs.
‡ Reactions of all RBCs equal in tests at low (4°C) temperatures. Reactions of M+ RBCs stronger than those of M– RBCs in tests at higher (20°–25°C) temperatures.
§ The most usual reactions are shown.
‖ Similar to above except that preference is for N+ RBCs.
¶ RBCs from rabbits are useful in differential adsorption studies because they lack the Pr determinants but carry I and i.

reported six cases of autoanti-A detected in a 32-year period (4668 patients with autoantibodies studied). Three of the autoanti-A caused hemolytic anemia associated presumably with CAS. The autoanti-B was detected in a 52-year-old group B man who presented with numbness, tingling, and blue discoloration of fingers and toes when exposed to cold (acrocyanosis).[244] Later, the patient had slurring of speech and headaches; magnetic resonance angioplasty/magnetic resonance imaging showed mild small vessel brain disease. Hemolytic anemia was not apparent (hemoglobin/hematocrit = 13.1 g/dL/39.6%, total bilirubin = 1.9 mg/dL). An IgM kappa monoclonal protein was present. Regular plasmapheresis treatments were helpful in relieving clinical symptoms. The patient's RBCs were sensitized with IgM (3+), IgA (1+), and C3 (3+). The clinical laboratory reported a normal cold agglutinin titer of 2 (i.e., group O RBCs were used), but later the serum was shown to contain autoanti-B reacting to a titer of 8192 at 4°C and 16 at 30°C (nonreactive at 37°C) with allogeneic RBCs. DTT-treated autologous RBCs reacted to a titer of 8192 at 4°C and reacted at 30°C, in the presence of albumin. The antibody caused weak hemolysis of group B

TABLE 7-15. EXPRESSION OF SIA-B1, SIA-I1, SIA-IB1 ANTIGENS COMPARED WITH Ii ANTIGENS ON HUMAN UNTREATED AND ENZYME-TREATED RBCs

Antigen Designation		untr.	pap.	sial.	endo.	untr.	pap.	sial.	pap/sial	endo.	untr.
I		+	↑	↑	↓	↓				↓	↓
Sia-b1	F1	+	+	–	+	↓				↓	↓
i		↓				+	↑	↑	↑ –	+	+*
Sia-l1	Vo	↓				+	↑	+	– –	+	+*
Sia-lb1	Gd	+	+	–	+	+	+	–	– +	+	+

untr., untreated; pap., papain treated; sial., sialidase treated; endo., endo-β-galactosidase treated; pap./sal., sialidase treated after papainization; +, optimal reaction with untreated RBCs; ↑, reaction (slightly) increased; ↓, reaction markedly decreased; – no reaction; *, expressed as on adult RBCs.

enzyme-treated but not untreated RBCs. A heat eluate from the patient's RBCs reacted with group B enzyme-treated but not untreated RBCs. As the autoanti-B reacted up to 30°C in vitro, activated complement [in vitro (enzyme-treated B RBCs were hemolyzed) and in vivo (i.e., patient's RBCs were strongly sensitized with C3)], and the clinical symptoms indicated that the antibody was reacting in vivo, it was hard to understand why this patient did not have a more obvious hemolytic anemia.[244]

Anti-M and -N have been reported as pathogenic and nonpathogenic cold autoantibodies. Two cases of AIHA associated with high titer, high thermal amplitude autoanti-M[245,246] and one case of autoanti-N[247] have been reported. Many cases of nonpathogenic autoanti-M and -N have been detected[27]; these include autoanti-N in dialysis patients that may be induced by formalin.[27]

In 1980 the sera of two patients with CAS were found to contain antibodies of a new specificity.[248] These IgM autoagglutinins reacted equally well with I_{adult} and i_{adult} RBCs and weaker with cord RBCs; they reacted well with sialidase- and protease-treated RBCs. They appeared to react better at room temperature than at 37°C or 4°C. As they were inhibited by urine from Sd(a+) but not Sd(a–) individuals and did not appear to be anti-Sd^a, they were called anti-Sd^x.[248] They were later renamed anti-Rx; the inhibition with Sd(a+) urine was found to be a serologic artifact.[249] Severe AIHA, including a fatality, associated with autoanti-Rx, has been reported.[248,250,251] It is interesting to note that 12 cases were reported during the 1980 influenza epidemic in New York.[248-250]

Two "new" target antigens for cold autoantibodies were named Me and Ju by Salama and coworkers[252] and Göttsche and coworkers.[253] Anti-Me was detected in a patient with AIHA and Waldenström's macroglobulinemia. The antibody was IgM (kappa), of moderate titer (128 at 0°C), reacting up to 30°C with adult and cord RBCs. The antibody reacted better with protease- and sialidase-treated RBCs; papain-treated adult and cord RBCs were hemolyzed at 20°C and 37°C. The antibody was named anti-Me (milk-enhanced) because it gave greatly enhanced reactions in the presence of preheated human milk (titer of 1024 with milk versus 16 without milk at 20°C).[252] A cold autoantibody causing CAS was shown to have characteristics that seemed to exclude anti-I, -i, -Pr, -Gd, -Sa, -Vo, -Li, -Fl, -Lud, and -Me.[253] The antibody reacted equally well with adult and cord RBCs. The antigen reactivity was strongly diminished by sialidase (neuraminidase) treatment and to a lesser degree by protease (papain) treatment. The target antigen was named Ju.[253]

An interesting finding was that of Perrault, who found 10 examples of cold-reacting autoanti-LW in 45,000 donors, whose sera were screened using a low ionic strength Polybrene AutoAnalyzer system.[254] One of the antibodies was IgM, the others were thought to be IgG. The antibodies reacted well up to 20°C; a marked decrease in reactivity was noted at 22°C to 27°C; no reactions occurred at 37°C. One very unusual patient with an IgM autoanti-D that reacted optimally in the cold, but reacted up to 37°C, was described by Longster and Johnson.[255]

OPTIMAL REACTIONS WITH STORED OR "OLD" RBCs

In 1952 Brendemoen and coworkers[153] described a cold autoagglutinin that reacted with stored RBCs at 5°C and 15°C but not 37°C, and not with fresh RBCs at any temperature. No clinical data on the patient were given. Stratton[154] described a similar antibody, but this antibody reacted better at 37°C. In 1961 Jenkins and Marsh[155] described three patients with AIHA associated with autoagglutinins reacting with stored RBCs but not fresh RBCs. The serology of only one patient was reported in detail. The DAT was positive, due to complement sensitization. The autoagglutinin reacted equally well at 4°C, 18°C, and 37°C. The antibody would react with RBCs that had been enzyme- or heat (56°C)-treated. After the patients were treated with steroids the antibodies disappeared in two cases, and in one case the remaining antibody reacted only at low temperatures; the latter finding leads one to suspect this was a high thermal amplitude "cold" antibody rather than a "warm" autoantibody.

Ozer and Chaplin[156] studied an IgM monoclonal antibody, with similar specificity, in great detail. Their patient had macroglobulinemia and hemolytic anemia. The antibody had a cold agglutinin titer of 100,000 to 500,000 and reacted up to 37°C. Like Stratton and coworkers,[154] Ozer and Chaplin[156] noted that microscopically the agglutination gave a mixed-field appearance. Red cell survival studies were carried out using fresh and stored RBCs. Fresh RBCs survived normally and stored RBCs (mean storage period of 30.5 days) survived poorly (71% at 1 hour, 53% at 6 hours, 48% at 24 hours, 39% at 48 hours).

Beaumont and coworkers[256] described an antibody in a patient with macroglobulinemia, but no hemolytic anemia. This IgM antibody reacted with stored RBCs but not fresh RBCs, and also precipitated known low-density lipoprotein (LDL). It is of interest to note that LDL has been identified as an autoantigen in the AIHA of NZB mice.[257] Lightwood and Scott[258] reported a case of CAS, with high titer anti-I and anti-i, where an IgM antibody to stored RBCs developed 5 years after the initial diagnosis of AIHA. A cold autoantibody against stored RBCs was reported by Easton and coworkers[157] in a patient with mild hemolytic anemia, cirrhosis of the liver, and a false-positive test for syphilis.

As discussed for WAIHA, reticulocytopenia has also been observed in AIHA associated with "cold" autoantibodies.[259] In 1990 Kesmin and colleagues[260] presented a case of CAS where the high titer, high thermal amplitude cold agglutinin appeared to react preferentially with younger (i.e., reticulocyte-rich) RBCs. This was noticed because clumps on the peripheral blood smear appeared to be mainly polychromatic RBCs. Cold agglutinin titers/scores at 20°C with reticulocyte-rich RBCs were 32/54 and 8/34 with reticulocyte-reduced RBCs. Thus, the reactions did not reflect the presence or absence of a specific target antigen, but perhaps the presence of more antigen on younger RBCs.

AUTOANTIBODY SPECIFICITY ASSOCIATED WITH PAROXYSMAL COLD HEMOGLOBINURIA

In 1963 Levine and coworkers[261] reported that three sera from six patients with paroxysmal cold hemoglobinuria (PCH) failed to react with the rare Tj(a–) RBCs, but reacted with all other RBCs tested. Thus, Levine and coworkers[261] suggested the specificity of the autoantibodies in PCH was anti-P+P_1 (anti-Tj^a). Worlledge and Rousso[262] extended these findings by testing 11 patients with PCH, using the rare P^k RBCs in addition to p [Tj(a–)] RBCs (Levine and coworkers had mentioned in an addendum to their article that three of their sera tested did not react with P^k RBCs). All 11 sera reacted with P_1 and P_2 RBCs but not with p or P^k RBCs, which suggested a specificity similar to that of the anti-P naturally occurring in the rare P^k individuals. Other workers have also since reported cases of PCH with P specificity.[263-267]

Both von dem Borne and coworkers[268] and Ramos and coworkers[269] described cases of non-Hodgkin's lymphoma associated with an autoimmune hemolytic anemia that did not appear to be CAS but were not typical PCH; one autoantibody was a monoclonal IgM (kappa) anti-P, and the other was a mixture of anti-P and anti-I^TP cold hemolysins.

There are a few reports of other specificities said to be associated with PCH; these include single case reports of anti-p,[270] anti-HI,[271] anti-I,[272] anti–"Pr-like,"[273] and several anti-i.[274-276]

All cases of PCH we have encountered in the past 30 years were associated with anti-P specificity. Sokol and coworkers[277] found anti-P specificity in 27 of 30 patients with PCH; specificity was not clearly defined in the other three cases.

REFERENCES

1. Denys P, van den Broucke J: Anémie hémolytique acquise et réaction de Coombs. Arch Franc Pédiatr 1947;4:205.
2. Kuhns WJ, Wagley PF: Hemolytic anemia associated with atypical hemagglutinins. Ann Intern Med 1949;30:408.
3. Race RR, Sanger R, Selwyn JG: Possible deletion in human Rh chromosome: A serological and genetical study. Br J Exp Pathol 1951;32:124.
4. Weiner W, Battey DA, Cleghorn TE, et al: Serological findings in a case of haemolytic anaemia. Br Med J 1953;2:125.
5. Holländer L: Specificity of antibodies in acquired haemolytic anaemia. Experientia 1953;9:468.
6. Dacie JV: Serology of acquired haemolytic anaemia. Proceedings of 4th Congr Europ Soc Haemat, Amsterdam, 1953.
7. Dacie JV, Cutbush M: Specificity of auto-antibodies in acquired haemolytic anaemia. J Clin Pathol 1954;7:18.
8. Wiener A, Gordon EG, Gallop C: Studies on autoantibodies in human sera. J Immunol 1953;71:58.
9. Pirofsky B, Pratt K: The antigen in autoimmune hemolytic anemia. I. Reactivity of human autoantibodies and rhesus antibodies with primate and non-primate erythrocytes. Am J Clin Pathol 1966;45:75-81.
10. Dacie J: The Haemolytic Anaemias, 3rd ed. vol. 3, The Auto-Immune Haemolytic Anaemias. New York: Churchill Livingstone, 1992:161.
11. van Loghem JJ, van der Hart M: Varieties of specific auto-antibodies in acquired haemolytic anaemia. Vox Sang 1954;4:2.
12. Flückiger P, Ricci C, Usteri C: Zur Frage der Blutgruppensspezifität von Autoantikörpern. Acta Haematol 1955;13:53.
13. Dausett J, Colombani J, Jean RG, et al: The serology and prognosis of 128 cases of autoimmune hemolytic anemia. Blood 1954;14:1280.
14. Weiner W, Vos GH: Serology of acquired hemolytic anemias. Blood 1963;22:606–613.
15. Vos GH, Petz LD, Fudenberg HH: Specificity of acquired haemolytic anaemia autoantibodies and their serological characteristics. Br J Haematol 1970;19:57–66.
16. Vos GH, Petz LD, Fudenberg HH: Specificity and immunoglobulin characteristics of autoantibodies in acquired hemolytic anemia. J Immunol 1971;106:1172–1176.
17. Vos GH, Petz LD, Garratty G, Fudenberg HH: Autoantibodies in acquired hemolytic anemia with special reference to the LW system. Blood 1973;42:445–453.
18. Dacie JV, Worlledge SM: Auto-immune hemolytic anemias. Prog Hematol 1969;6:82–119.
19. Leddy JP, Peterson P, Yeaw MA, Bakemeier RF: Patterns of serologic specificity of human γG erythrocyte autoantibodies. J Immunol 1970;105:677–686.
20. Rosse WF: Fixation of the first component (C'1a) by human antibodies. J Clin Invest 1968;47:2430.
21. Sokol RJ, Hewitt S, Booker DJ, Bailey A: Red cell autoantibodies, multiple immunoglobulin classes, and autoimmune hemolysis. Transfusion 1990;30:714–717.
22. Dacie JV: Autoimmune hemolytic anemia. Arch Int Med 1975;135:1293.
23. Issitt PD, Pavone BG, Goldfinger D, et al: Anti-Wr^b, and other autoantibodies responsible for positive direct antiglobulin tests in 150 individuals. Br J Haematol 1976;34:5–18.
24. Celano MJ, Levine P: Anti-LW specificity in autoimmune acquired hemolytic anemia. Transfusion 1967;7:265–268.
25. Marsh WL, Reid ME, Scott EP: Autoantibodies of U blood group specificity in autoimmune haemolytic anaemia. Br J Haematol 1989;72:625.
26. Sistonen P, Tippett P: A "new" allele giving further insight into the LW blood group system. Vox Sang 1982;42:252–255.
27. Issitt PD, Anstee DJ: Applied blood group serology, 4th ed. Durham, NC: Montgomery Scientific Publications, 1998.
28. Eyster ME, Jenkins DE, Jr: IgG erythrocyte autoantibodies: Comparison of in vivo complement coating and in vitro "Rh" specificity. J Immunol 1970;105:221–226.
29. Nugent ME, Colledge KI, Marsh WL: Autoimmune hemolytic anemia caused by anti-U. Vox Sang 1971;20:519–525.
30. Schmidt PJ, Lostumbo MM, English CT, Hunter OB, Jr: Aberrant U blood group accompanying Rhnull. Transfusion 1967;7:33–34.
31. Worlledge SM: A classification of AIHA, based on clinical grounds and the use of antiglobulin sera specific for immunoglobulin class and various complement components, and its use in clinical practice. In Proceedings of the 25th Annual Meeting of the American Association of Blood Banks and the 13th Congress of the International Society for Blood Transfusion, 1972:43 (Abstr).
32. Goldfinger D, Zwicker H, Belkin GA, et al: An autoantibody with anti-Wr^b specificity in a patient with warm autoimmune hemolytic anemia. Transfusion 1975;15:351–352.
33. Bell CA, Zwicker H, Sacks HJ: Autoimmune hemolytic anemia: Routine serologic evaluation in a general hospital population. Am J Clin Pathol 1973;60:903–911.

34. Garratty G, Brunt D, Greenfield B, et al: An autoanti-En[a] mimicking an alloanti-En[a] associated with pure red cell aplasia. Transfusion 1983;33:408 (Abstr).
35. D'Orsogna DE, Heinz R, Wawryszczuk V, Loftis LL, Harrison CR: Severe autoimmune hemolytic anemia with anti-En[a] specificity in a four week old infant girl. Transfusion 1991;31:23S (Abstr).
36. Garratty G, Arndt P, Domen R, et al: Severe autoimmune hemolytic anemia associated with IgM warm autoantibodies directed against determinants on or associated with glycophorin A. Vox Sang 1997;72:124–130.
37. Dankbar DT, Pierce SR, Issitt PD, et al: Fatal intravascular hemolysis associated with autoanti-Wr[b]. Transfusion 1987;27:534 (Abstr).
38. Ainsworth BM, Fraser ID, Poole GD: Severe haemolytic anaemia due to anti-Wr[b]. In Book of Abstracts from the Joint Meeting of 20th Congress of International Society of Blood Transfusion/British Blood Transfusion Society, 1988:82.
39. Issitt PD, Combs MR, Allen J, et al: Anti-Di[b] as a red cell autoantibody. Transfusion 1996;36:802–804.
40. Sherburne B, Salamon JL, Shirey RS, et al: Warm autoimmune hemolytic anemia (AIHA) associated with IgG anti-Pr_{1h}. Transfusion 1987;27:535 (Abstr).
41. Dube VE, House RF, Jr, Moulds J, Polesky HB: Hemolytic anemia caused by autoanti-N. Am J Clin Pathol 1975;63:828–831.
42. Cohen DW, Garratty G, Morel P, Petz LD: Autoimmune hemolytic anemia associated with IgG autoanti-N. Transfusion 1979;19:329–331.
43. Combs MR, Telen MJ, Hall SE, Rosse WF: A case report: IgG autoanti-N as a cause of severe autoimmune hemolytic anemia. Immunohematology 1990;6:83.
44. Garratty G, Arndt P, Tsuneta R, Kanter M: Fatal hemolytic anemia associated with autoanti-N. Transfusion 1994;34:20S (Abstr).
45. Crosson JT, Moulds J, Comty CM, Polesky HF: A clinical study of anti-NDP in the sera of patients in a large repetitive hemodialysis program. Kidney Int 1976;10:463–470.
46. Fassbinder W, Frei U, Koch KM: Haemolysis due to formaldehyde-induced anti-N-like antibodies in haemodialysis patients. Klin Wochenschr 1979;57:673–679.
47. Johnson MH, Plett MJ, Conant CN, Worthington M: Autoimmune hemolytic anemia with anti-S specificity. Transfusion 1978;18:389 (Abstr).
48. Alessandrino EP, Costamagna L, Pagani A, Coronelli M: Late appearance of autoantibody anti-S in autoimmune hemolytic anemia. Transfusion 1984;24:369–370.
49. Domen RE, Clarke A: Case reports: Red blood cell autoantibodies mimicking alloantibodies. Immunohematology 1991;7:98.
50. Reynolds MV, Vengelen-Tyler V, Morel PA: Autoimmune hemolytic anemia associated with autoanti-Ge. Vox Sang 1981;41:61–67.
51. Beattie KM, Sigmund KE: A Ge-like autoantibody in the serum of a patient receiving gold therapy for rheumatoid arthritis. Transfusion 1987;27:54–57.
52. Gottsche B, SalamaA, Mueller-Eckhardt C: Autoimmune-hemolytic anemia associated with an IgA autoanti-Gerbich. Vox Sang 1990;58:211–214.
53. Poole J, Reid ME, Banks J, et al: Serological and immunochemical specificity of a human autoanti-Gerbich-like antibody. Vox Sang 1990;58:287–291.
54. Shulman IA, Vengelen-Tyler V, Thompson JC, et al: Autoanti-Ge associated with severe autoimmune hemolytic anemia. Vox Sang 1990;59:232–234.
55. Sererat T, Veidt D, Arndt PA, Garratty G: Warm autoimmune hemolytic anemia associated with autoanti-Ge. Immunohematology 1998;11:26.
56. Seyfried H, Gorska B, Maj S, et al: Apparent depression of antigens of the Kell blood group system associated with autoimmune acquired hemolytic anaemia. Vox Sang 1972;23:528–536.
57. Beck ML, Marsh WL, Pierce SR, et al: Auto-anti-Kp[b] associated with weakened antigenicity in the Kell blood group system: A second example. Transfusion 1979;19:197–202.
58. Garratty G, Sattler MS, Petz LD, Flannery EP: Immune hemolytic anemia associated with anti-Kell and a carrier state for chronic granulomatous disease. Blood Transfus Immunohaematol 1979;22:529.
59. Giblett ER, Klebanoff SJ, Pincus SH, et al: Kell phenotypes in chronic granulomatous disease: A potential transfusion hazard. Lancet 1971;i:1235–1236.
60. Marsh WL, Øyen R, Nichols ME, et al: Chronic granulomatous disease and the Kell blood groups. Br J Haematol 1975; 29:247–262.
61. Wilkinson SL, Vaithianathan T, Issitt PD: On the high incidence of anti-HL-A antibodies in anti-D typing reagents. Illustrated by a case of Matuhasi-Ogata phenomenon mimicking a "D with anti-D" situation. Transfusion 1974;14:27–33.
62. Issitt PD, Zellner DC, Rolih SD, Duckett JB: Autoantibodies mimicking alloantibodies. Transfusion 1977;17:531–538.
63. Viggiano E, Clary NL, Ballas SK: Autoanti-K antibody mimicking an alloantibody. Transfusion 1982;22:329–332.
64. Puig N, Carbonell F, Marty ML: Another example of mimicking anti-Kp[b] in a Kp(a+b-) patient. Vox Sang 1986;51:57–62.
65. Manny N, Levene C, Sela R, et al: Autoimmunity and the Kell blood groups: Autoanti-Kp[b] in a Kp(a+b–) patient. Vox Sang 1983;45:252–256.
66. Win N, Kaye T, Mir N, Damain-Willems C, Chatfield C: Autoimmune haemolytic anaemia in infancy with anti-Kp[b] specificity. Vox Sang 1996;71:187–188.
67. Marsh WL, DiNapoli J, Øyen R: Auto-immune hemolytic anemia caused by anti-K13. Vox Sang 1979;35:174–178.
68. Marsh WL, Oyen R, Alicea E, et al: Autoimmune hemolytic anemia and the Kell blood groups. Am J Hematol 1979;7:155–162.
69. Sabo B, Keeling MM, Winkler MA, McCreary J: Coexistence of a high frequency Kell-related autoantibody and alloanti-Kp[b] in a case of autoimmune disease (Abstr). In Book of Abstracts from the Joint Meeting of the 19th Congress of the International Society of Haematology/17th Congress of the International Society of Blood Transfusion, 1982:235.
70. Vengelen-Tyler V, Gonzalez B, Garratty G, et al: Acquired loss of red cell Kell antigens. Br J Haematol 1987;65:231–234.
71. Eveland D: AutoantiJs[b] enhanced by polyethylene glycol (Abstr). In Book of Abstracts from the ISBT/AABB Joint Congress. Arlington, VA: American Association of Blood Banks, 1990:156.
72. Holmes LD, Pierce SR, Beck M: Autoanti-Jk[a] in a healthy blood donor. Transfusion 1976;16:521.
73. Patten E, Beck CE, Scholl C, et al: Autoimmune hemolytic anemia with anti-Jk[a] specificity in a patient taking Aldomet. Transfusion 1977;17:517–520.
74. Guillausseau PJ, Wautier JL, Boizard B, et al: Une variété rare d'anémie hémolytique auto-immune: la spécificité anti-Jk[a]. Semin Hop Paris 1982;58:803.
75. Hoffman M, Berger MB, Menitove JE: Autoimmune hemolytic anemia due to autoanti-Jk[a]. Lab Med 1982;13:674.
76. Strikas R, Seifert MR, Lentino JR: Autoimmune hemolytic anemia and *Legionella pneumophilia* pneumonia. Ann Intern Med 1983;99:345.
77. Ciaffoni S, Ferro 1, Potenza R, Campo G: Evans's syndrome: A case of autoimmune thrombocytopenia and autoimmune hemolytic anemia caused by anti-Jk[a]. Haematologica 1987;72:245–247.
78. Sander RP, Hardy NM, van Meter SA: Anti-Jk[a] autoimmune hemolytic anemia in an infant. Transfusion 1987;27:58–60.
79. Ganly PS, Laffan MA, Owen 1, Hows JM: Auto-anti-Jk[a] in Evans's syndrome with negative direct antiglobulin test. Br J Haematol 1988;69:537–539.
80. Alpaugh K, Sysko-Stein L, Lusch C, et al: Autoanti-Jk[a] associated with hemolysis after transfusion with Jk(a+) RBCs. Lab Med 1989;20:682–684.
81. McGinniss MH, Leiberman R, Holland PV: The Jk[b] red cell antigen and gram-negative organisms. Transfusion 1979;19:663 (Abstr).
82. Ellisor SS, Reid ME, O'Day T, et al: Autoantibodies mimicking anti-Jk[b] plus anti-Jk3 associated with autoimmune hemolytic

anemia in a primipara who delivered an unaffected infant. Vox Sang 1983;45:53–59.
83. Grishaber JE, Cordle DG, Strauss RG: Development of alloanti-Jk[a] in a patient with hemolytic anemia due to autoanti-Jk[b]. J Clin Pathol 1992;98:542.
84. O'Day T: A second example of autoanti-Jk3. Transfusion 1987;27:442.
85. Issitt PD, Pavone BG, Frohlich JA, Mallory DM. Absence of autoanti-Jk3 as a component of anti-dl. Transfusion 1980; 20:733–736.
86. Issitt PD, Pavone BG. Critical re-examination of the specificity of auto-anti-Rh antibodies in patients with a positive direct antiglobulin test. Br J Haematol 1978;38:63.
87. van't Veer MB, van Wieringen PMV, van Leeuwen I, et al: A negative direct antiglobulin test with strong IgG red cell autoantibodies present in the serum of a patient with autoimmune haemolytic anaemia. Br J Haematol 1981;49:383–386.
88. Dickstein B, Kosanke J, Morris D, et al: Report of an autoantibody with mimicking allo anti-Fy[b] specificity. Transfusion 1998;38:37S (Abstr).
89. Szymanski I, Roberts PL, Rosenfield RE: Anti-A autoantibody with severe intravascular hemolysis. N Engl J Med 1976;294:995–996.
90. Parker AC, Willis G, Urbaniak SJ, Innes EM: Autoimmune haemolytic anaemia with anti-A autoantibody. Br Med J 1978;1:26.
91. Govoni M, Turbiani C, Menini C, Tomasi P: Anti-A autoantibody associated with immune hemolytic anemia. Vox Sang 1991;61:75.
92. McClelland WM, Bradley A, Morris TCM, et al: Auto-anti-B in a patient with acute leukaemia. Vox Sang 1981;41:231.
93. Atichartakarn V, Chiewsilp P, Ratanasirivanich P, Stabunswadgan S: Autoimmune hemolytic anemia due to anti-B autoantibody. Vox Sang 1985;49:301–303.
94. Kuipers EJ, van Imhoff GW, Hazenberg CAM Smit J: Anti-H IgM (Kappa) autoantibody mediated severe intravascular haemolysis associated with malignant lymphoma. Br J Haematol 1991;18:283–285.
95. Garratty G, Haffleigh B, Dalziel J, Petz LD: An IgG anti-I[T] detected in a Caucasian American. Transfusion 1972;12:325.
96. Booth PB, Jenkins WJ, Marsh WL: Anti-I[T]: A new antibody of the I blood-group system occurring in certain Melanesian sera. Br J Haematol 1966;12:341–344.
97. Garratty G, Petz LD, Wallerstein RO, Fudenberg HH: Autoimmune hemolytic anemia in Hodgkin's disease associated with anti-I [T]. Transfusion 1974;14:226–231.
98. Garratty G, Petz LD, Wallerstein RO, Fudenberg HH: Development of the I[T] antigen. Transfusion 1974;14:630.
99. Hafleigh EB, Wells RF, Grumet FC: Nonhemolytic IgG anti-I[T]. Transfusion 1978;18:592–597.
100. Levine AM, Thornton P, Forman SJ, et al: Positive Coombs test in Hodgkin's disease: Significance and implications. Blood 1980;55:607–611.
101. Freedman J, Newlands M, Johnson CA: Warm IgM anti-I[T] causing autoimmune haemolytic anaemia. Vox Sang 1977;32:135–112.
102. Szatoky A, van der Hart M: An auto-antibody anti-Vel. Vox Sang 1971;20:376–377.
103. Herron R, Hyde RD, Hillier SJ: The second example of an anti-Vel auto-antibody. Vox Sang 1979;36:179–181.
104. Ferrer Z, Cornwall S, Berger R, et al: A third example of haemolytic auto-anti-Vel. Blood Transfus Immunohaematol 1984;27:639.
105. Becton DL, Kinney TR: An infant girl with severe autoimmune hemolytic anemia: Apparent anti-Vel specificity. Vox Sang 1986;51:108–111.
106. McDowell MA, Stocker I, Nance S, Garratty G: Autoanti-Sc1 associated with autoimmune hemolytic anemia. Transfusion 1986;26:578 (Abstr).
107. Owen I, Chowdhury V, Reid ME, et al: Autoimmune hemolytic anemia associated with anti-Sc1. Transfusion 1992;32:173–176.
108. Peloquin P, Moulds M, Keenan J, Kennedy M: Anti-Sc3 as an apparent autoantibody in two patients. Transfusion 1989;29:49S (Abstr).
109. Yokoyama M, Eith DT, Bowman M: The first example of auto-anti-Xg[a]. Vox Sang 1967;12:138–139.
110. Marsh WL, Brown PJ, DiNapoli J, et al: Anti-Wj: An autoantibody that defines a high-incidence antigen modified by the *In(Lu)* gene. Transfusion 1983;23:128–130.
111. Fitzsimmons J, Caggiano V: Autoantibody to a high-frequency Lutheran antigen associated with immune hemolytic anemia and a hemolytic transfusion episode. Transfusion 1981;21:612 (Abstr).
112. Ward JM, Caggiano V: Clarification. Transfusion 1983;23:174.
113. van Alphen L, Poole J, Overbeeke M: The Anton blood group antigen is the erythrocyte receptor for *Haemophilus intuenzae.* FEMS Microbiol Lett 1986;37:69.
114. Denegri JF, Nanji AA, Sinclair M, Stillwell G: Autoimmune hemolytic anemia due to immunoglobulin G with anti-Sd[x] specificity. Acta Haematol 1983;69:19–22.
115. Sullivan CM, Kline WE, Rabin BI, et al: The first example of autoanti-Kx. Transfusion 1987;27:322–324.
116. Marsh WL, DiNapoli J, Oyen R, et al: "New" autoantibody specificity in autoimmune hemolytic anemia defined with RBCs treated with 2-aminoethylisothiouronium bromide and a dithiothreitol-papain solution. Transfusion 1985; 25:364–367.
117. Spielmann W: Spezifische autoantikörper bei hämolytischen Anämien. Klin Wschr 1956;34:248.
118. Meuli HC: Über blutgruppenspezifische antierythrocytäre Autoantikörper. Blut 1957;3:270.
119. Fudenberg HH, Rosenfield RE, Wasserman LR: Unusual specificity of auto-antibody in auto-immune hemolytic disease. J Mt Sinai Hosp 1958;25:324.
120. Dunsford I, Stapleton RR: In vitro absorption of the Rhesus antibody anti-D by Rhesus negative RBCs. Vox Sang 1959;4:406.
121. Matuhasi T: Plasma protein and antibody fractions observed from the serological point of view. In Proceedings of 15th General Assembly Japanese Medical Congress, Tokyo, Japan, 1959:80.
122. Ogata T, Matuhasi T: Problems of specific and cross reactivity of blood group antibodies. In Proceedings of 8th Congress of International Society of Blood Transfusion, Tokyo, Japan, 1960:208.
123. Ogata T, Matuhasi T: Further observations on the problems of specific and cross reactivity of blood group antibodies. Proc 9th Congr Int Soc Blood Transf, Mexico 1962:528 (Karger, Basel, New York 1964).
124. Svardel JM, Yarbro J, Yunis EJ: Ogata phenomenon explaining the unusual specificity in eluates from Coombs-positive cells sensitized by autogenous anti-I. Vox Sang 1967;13:472.
125. Allen FH, Jr, Issitt PD, Degnan TJ, et al: Further observations on the Matuhasi-Ogata phenomenon. Vox Sang 1969;16:47.
126. Bove JR, Holburn AM, Mollison PL: Non-specific binding of IgG to antibody-coated RBCs (the "Matuhasi-Ogata Phenomenon"). Immunology 1973;25:793–801.
127. Issitt PD, Pavone BG: Critical re-examination of the specificity of auto-anti-Rh antibodies in patients with a positive direct antiglobulin test. Br J Haematol 1978;38:63–70.
128. Issitt PD, Zellner DC, Rolih SD, Duckett JB: Autoantibodies mimicking alloantibodies. Transfusion 1977;17:531–538.
129. Issitt PD: Applied blood group serology, 3rd ed. Miami: Montgomery Scientific, 1985.
130. van't Veer MB, van Wieringen PMV, van Leeuwen I, et al: A negative direct antiglobulin test with strong IgG red cell autoantibodies present in the serum of a patient with autoimmune haemolytic anaemia. Br J Haematol 1982;52:537.
131. Issitt PD, Gruppo RA, Wilkinson SL, Issitt CH: Atypical presentation of acute phase, antibody-induced haemolytic anaemia in an infant. Br J Haematol 1982;52:537–541.
132. Issitt PD, Wilkinson SL, Gruppo RA: Depression of Rh antigen expression in antibody-induced haemolytic anaemia. Br J Haematol 1983;53:688.
133. Vengelen-Tyler V, Mogck N: Two cases of "hr[B]-like" autoantibodies appearing as alloantibodies. Transfusion 1991; 31:254–256.

134. Chown B, Kaita H, Lowen B, Lewis M: Transient production of anti-LW by LW-positive people. Transfusion 1971;11:220.
135. Perkins HA, Mcllroy M, Swanson J, Kadin M: Transient LW-negative red blood cells and anti-LW in a patient with Hodgkin's disease. Vox Sang 1977;33:299–303.
136. Komatsu F, Kajiwara M: Transient depression of LW^a antigen with coincident production of anti-LW^a repeated in relapses of malignant lymphoma. Transfus Med 1996;6:139.
137. Mannessier L, Rouger P, Johnson CL, et al: Acquired loss of red-cell Wj antigen in a patient with Hodgkin's disease. Vox Sang 1986;50:240–244.
138. van't Veer MB, van Leeuwen 1, Haas FJLM, et al: Red-cell auto-antibodies mimicking anti-Fy^b specificity. Vox Sang 1984;47:88–91.
139. Harris T: Two cases of autoantibodies that demonstrate mimicking specificity in the Duffy blood group system. Immunohematology 1990;6:87.
140. Dickstein B, Kosanke J, Morris D, et al: Report of an autoantibody with mimicking alloanti-Fy^b specificity. Transfusion 1998;38:37S (Abstr).
141. Issitt PD, Obarski G, Hartnett PL, Wren MR, Prewitt PL: Temporary suppression of Kidd system antigen expression accompanied by transient production of anti-Jk3. Transfusion 1990;30:46–50.
142. Moulds M, Strohm P, McDowell MA, et al: Autoantibody mimicking alloantibody in the Colton blood group system. Transfusion 1988;28:36S (Abstr).
143. Williamson LM, Poole J, Redman C, et al: Transient loss of proteins carrying Kell and Lutheran red cell antigens during consecutive relapses of autoimmune thrombocytopenia. Br J Haematol 1994;87:805–812.
144. Leger R, Garratty G, Vengelen-Tyler V: Sequential suppression of Lan and Lu^b antigens associated with mimicking anti-Lan and anti-Lu^b. Transfusion 1994;34:69S (Abstr).
145. Rand BP, Olson JD, Garratty G, et al: Coombs negative immune hemolytic anemia with anti-E occurring in the red blood cell eluate of an E-negative patient. Transfusion 1978;18:174–180.
146. Rosenfield RE: Unpublished observations 1974, cited by Issitt PD and Issitt CH in Applied blood group serology, 2nd ed., Spectra Biologicals, Oxnard, 1975.
147. Rosenfield RE, Allen FH Jr, Swisher SN, et al: A review of Rh serology and presentation of a new terminology. Transfusion 1962;2:287.
148. Lalezari P, Berens JA: Specificity and cross reactivity of cell-bound antibodies. Human Blood groups. 5th Int. Convoc Immunol, Buffalo, NY, 1976:44.
149. Issitt PD, Combs MR, Bumgarner DG, et al: Studies of antibodies in the sera of patients who have made red cell autoantibodies. Transfusion 1996;36:481–486.
150. Beck ML, Dixon J, Oberman HA: Variation of specificity of autoantibodies in autoimmune hemolytic anemia. Am J Clin Pathol 1971;56:475–478.
151. Bird GWG, Wingham J: Changes in specificity of erythrocyte autoagglutinins. Vox Sang 1972;22:364–365.
152. Gerbal A, Homberg JC, Rochant H, et al: Les autoanticorps d'anemies hemolytiques acquises. I. Analyse de 2234 observations. Nouv Rev Frank Haematol 1968;8:155.
153. Brendemoen OJ: A cold agglutinin specifically active against stored RBCs. Acta Pathol Microbiol Scand 1952;31:574.
154. Stratton F, Renton PH, Rawlinson VI: Serological difference between old and young cells. Lancet 1960;1:1388.
155. Jenkins WJ, Marsh WL: Autoimmune haemolytic anaemia. Lancet 1961;2:16.
156. Ozer FL, Chaplin H, Jr: Agglutination of stored erythrocytes by a human serum. Characterization of the serum factor and erythrocyte changes. J Clin Invest 1963;42:1735.
157. Easton JA, Priest CJ, Giles CM: An antibody against stored blood associated with cirrhosis of the liver and false-positive serological tests for syphilis. J Clin Pathol 1965;18:460.
158. Arndt P, O'Hoski P, McBride J, Garratty G: Autoimmune hemolytic anemia associated with an antibody reacting preferentially with "old" RBCs. Transfusion 1989;29:48S (Abstr).
159. Kay MMB: Senescent cell antigen: A red cell aging antigen. In Garratty G (ed): Red cell antigens and antibodies. Arlington, VA: American Association of Blood Banks, 1986:35.
160. Gray LS, Kleeman JE, Masouredis SP: Differential binding of IgG anti-D and IgG autoantibodies to reticulocytes and red blood cells. Br J Haematol 1983;55:335–345.
161. Branch DR, Shulman IA, Sy Siok Hian AL, Petz LD: Two distinct categories of warm autoantibody reactivity with age-fractionated RBCs. Blood 1984;63:177–180.
162. Herron R, Clark M, Smith DS: An autoantibody with activity dependent on red cell age in the serum of a patient with autoimmune haemolytic anaemia and a negative direct antiglobulin test. Vox Sang 1987;52:71–74.
163. Hedge UM, Gordon-Smith EC, Worlledge SM: Reticulocytopenia and "absence" of red cell autoantibodies in immune haemolytic anaemia. Br Med J 1977;2:1444–1447.
164. Conley CL, Lippman SM, Ness PM, et al: Autoimmune hemolytic anemia with reticulocytopenia and erythroid marrow. N Engl J Med 1982;306:281.
165. Hauke G, Fauser AA, Weber S, Maas D: Reticulocytopenia in severe autoimmune hemolytic anemia (AIHA) of the warm antibody type. Blut 1983;46:321–327.
166. Mangan KF, Besa EC, Shadduck RK, et al: Demonstration of two distinct antibodies in autoimmune hemolytic anemia with reticulocytopenia and red cell aplasia. Exp Hematol 1984;12:788–793.
166a. Davidyuk G, Goldsby RA, Dearden MT, Stec TC, Andrzejewski C: Autoantibodies to immature erythrocytes in patients with the anti-phospholipid antibody syndrome. Transfusion 2002;42:103S (Abstr).
167. Lutz HU, Wipf G: Naturally occurring autoantibodies to skeletal proteins from human red blood cells. J Immunol 1982;128:1695–1699.
168. Wiener E, Hughes-Jones NC, Irish WT, Wickramasinghe SN: Elution of antispectrin antibodies from RBCs in homozygous thalassaemia. Clin Exp Immunol 1986;63:680–686.
169. Wakui H, Imai H, Kobayashi R, et al: Autoantibody against erythrocyte protein 4.1 in a patient with autoimmune hemolytic anemia. Blood 1988;72:408–412.
170. Postoway N, Anstee DJ, Wortman M, Garratty G: A severe transfusion reaction associated with anti-En^aTS in a patient with an abnormal alpha-like red cell sialoglycoprotein. Transfusion 1988;28:77–80.
171. Reid ME, Vengelen-Tyler V, Shulman I, Reynolds MV: Immunochemical specificity of autoanti-Gerbich from two patients with autoimmune haemolytic anaemia and concomitant alteration in the red cell membrane sialoglycoprotein. Br J Haematol 1988;69:61–66.
172. Gomperts ED, Metz J, Zail SS: Red cell membrane protein in antibody-induced haemolytic anaemia. Br J Haematol 1973;25:421–428.
173. Kajii E, Ikemoto S, Ueki J, Miuras Y: Isolation of a peptide associated with autoimmune haemolytic anaemia from red cell membranes. Clin Exp Immunol 1988;73:406–409.
174. Hazeltine M, Rauch Y, Danoff D, et al: Antiphospholipid antibodies in systemic lupus erythematosus: Evidence of an association with positive Coombs' and hypocomplementemia. J Rheumatol 1988;15:80–86.
175. Win N, Islam SIAM, Peterkin MA, Walker ID: Positive direct antiglobulin test due to antiphospholipid antibodies in normal healthy blood donors. Vox Sang 1997;72:182–184.
176. Sthoeger Z, Sthoeger D, Green L, Geltner D: The role of anticardiolipin autoantibodies in the pathogenesis of autoimmune hemolytic anemia. Blood 1990;76(Suppl.):392a (Abstr).
177. Cabral AR, Cabiedes J, Alarcon-Segovia D: Hemolytic anemia related to an IgM autoantibody to phosphatidylcholine that binds in vitro to stored and to bromelain-treated human erythrocytes. J Autoimmun 1990;3:773–787.
178. Arvieux J, Schweizer B, Roussel B, Colomb MG: Autoimmune haemolytic anaemia due to anti-phospholipid antibodies. Vox Sang 1991;61:190–195.
179. Guzmán J, Cabral AR, Cabiedes J, Pita-Ramirez L, Alarcón-Segovia D: Antiphospholipid antibodies in patients with

idiopathic autoimmune haemolytic anaemia. Autoimmunity 1994;18:51–56.
180. Lang B, Straub RH, Weber S, et al: Elevated anticardiolipin antibodies in autoimmune haemolytic anaemia irrespective of underlying systemic lupus erythematosus. Lupus 1997; 6:652–655.
181. Masouredis SP, Branks MJ, Garratty G, Victoria EJ: Immunospecific red cell binding of iodine-125-labeled immunoglobulin G erythrocyte autoantibodies. J Lab Clin Med 1987;10:308–317.
182. Masouredis SP, Branks MJ, Victoria EJ: Antiidiotypic IgG cross reactive with Rh alloantibodies in red cell autoimmunity. Blood 1987;70:710–715.
183. Garratty G: Specificity of autoantibodies reacting optimally at 37°C. Immunohematology 1999;15:24–40.
184. Mino P: "La panemoagglutinina del sangue umane." Policlinico, Sez. prat. 1924;31:1355.
185. Wiener AS, Unger LJ, Cohen L, Feldman J: Type-specific cold auto-antibodies as a cause of acquired hemolytic anemia and hemolytic transfusion reactions: Biologic test with bovine RBCs. Ann Intern Med 1956;44:221.
186. Jenkins WJ, Marsh WL, Noades J, et al: The I antigen and antibody. Vox Sang 1960;5:97.
187. Marsh WL, Jenkins WJ: Anti-i: A new cold antibody. Nature 1960;188:753.
188. Marsh WL: Anti-i: A cold antibody defining the Ii relationship in human RBCs. Br J Haematol 1961;7:200.
189. Marsh WL, Nichols ME, Reid ME: The definition of two I antigen components. Vox Sang 1971;20:209–217.
190. Dzierzkowa-Borodej W, Seyfried H, Nichols M, et al: The recognition of water-soluble I blood group substance. Vox Sang 1970;18:222–234.
191. Marsh WL, Nichols ME, Allen FH: Inhibition of anti-I sera by human milk. Vox Sang 1970;18:149–154.
192. Dzierzkowa-Borodej W, Seyfried H, Lisowska E: Serological classification of anti-I sera. Vox Sang 1975;28:110–121.
193. Lisowska E, Dzierzkowa-Borodej W, Seyfried H, et al: Reactions of erythrocyte glycoproteins and their degradation products with various anti-I sera. Vox Sang 1975;28:122–132.
194. Giblett ER, Crookston MC: Agglutinability of RBCs by anti-i in patients with thalssaemia major and other haematological disorders. Nature 1964;201:1138.
195. Burnie K: Ii antigens and antibodies. Can J Med Technol 1973;35:5–7.
196. van Loghen JJ, Peetom F, van der hart M, et al: Serological and immunochemical studies in haemolytic anaemia with high-titre cold agglutinins. Vox Sang 1963;8:33.
197. Worlledge SM, Dacie JV: Haemolytic and other anaemias in infectious mononucleosis. In: Carter RL, Penman, (eds): Infectious mononucleosis. Oxford: Blackwell Scientific Publications, 1969.
198. Wilkinson LS, Petz LD, Garratty G: Reappraisal of the role of anti-i in haemolytic anaemia in infectious mononucleosis. Br J Haematol 1973;25:715–722.
199. Tegoli J, Harris JP, Issitt PD, et al: Anti-IB, an expected "new" antibody detecting a joint product of the I and B genes. Vox Sang 1967;13:144–157.
200. Morel P, Garratty G, Willbanks E: Another example of anti-IB. Vox Sang 1975;29:231–233.
201. Feizi T, Kabat EA, Vicari G, et al: Immunochemical studies on blood groups. XLVII. The I antigen complex-precursors in the A, B, H, Le^a and Le^b blood group system-hemagglutinin-inhibition studies. J Exp Med 1971;133:39–52.
202. Vicari G, Kabat EA: Immunochemical studies on blood groups. XLV. Structures and activitives of oligosaccharides produced by alkaline degradation of a blood group substance lacking A, B, H, Le^a and Le^b specificities. Biochemistry 1970;9:3414.
203. Watkins WM, Morgan WTJ: Possible genetical pathways of blood group mucopolysaccharides. Vox Sang 1959;4:97.
204. Feizi T, Kabat EA: Immunochemical studies on blood groups. LIV. Classification of anti-I and anti-i sera into groups based on reactivity patterns with various antigens related to the blood group A, B, H, Le^a, Le^b and precursor substances. J Exp Med 1972;135:1247–1258.
205. Cooper AG, Brown MC: Serum i antigen: A new human blood group glycoprotein. Biochem Biophys Res Commun 1973;55:297–304.
206. Rosse WF, Lauf PK: Reaction of cold agglutinins with I antigen solubilized from human RBCs. Blood 1970;36:777–784.
207. Rosse WF, Sherwood JB: Cold-reacting antibodies: Differences in the reaction of anti-I antibodies with adult and cord red blood cells. Blood 1970;36:28–42.
208. Gardas A, Koscielak J: I-active antigen of human erythrocyte membrane. Vox Sang 1974;26:227–237.
209. Marcus DM, Kabat EA, Rosenfield RE: The action of enzymes from clostridium tertium on the I antigenic determinant of human erythrocytes. J Exp Med 1963;118:175.
210. Adamany AM, Kathan RH: Isolation of a tetrasaccharide common to MM, NN and MN antigens. Biochem Biophys Res Commun 1969;37:171.
211. Lisowska E: The degradation of M and N blood group glycoproteins and glycopeptides with alkaline borohydride. Eur J Biochem 1969;10:574–579.
212. Thomas DB, Winzler RJ: Structural studies on human erythrocyte glycoproteins: Alkali-labile oligosaccharides. J Biol Chem 1969;244:5943–5946.
213. Thomas DB, Winzler RJ: Structure of glycoproteins of human erythrocytes: Alkali-stable oligosacharides. Biochem J 1971;124:55–59.
214. Dzierzkowa-Borodej W, Lisowska E, Seyfriedowa H: The activity of glycoproteins from erythrocytes and protein fractions from human colostrum towards anti-I antibodies. Life Sci 1970;9:111–120.
215. Hamaguchi H, Cleve H: Solubilization of human erythrocyte membrane glycoproteins and separation of the MN glycoprotein from a glycoprotein with I, S and A activity. Biochem Biophys Acta 1972;278:271–280.
216. Lau FO, Rosse WF: The reactivity of red blood cell membrane glycoprotein with cold-reacting antibodies. Clin Immunol Immunopathol 1975;4:1.
217. McGinniss MH, Binder RA, Kales AN, et al: Cold autoimmune hemolytic anemia with autoanti-AI specificity: ^{51}Chromium survival studies. Immunohematology 1987;3:20–22.
218. McGinniss MH: Auto-anti-AI in the serum of a patient with fatal autoimmune hemolytic anemia. Immunohematology 1987;3:232–234.
219. Postoway N, Garratty G, Guerra-Zevallos M: Transient autoimmune hemolytic anemia (AIHA) associated with an autoanti-IB in an A_2B individual. In Book of Abstracts from the ISBT/AABB Joint Congress. Arlington, VA: American Association of Blood Banks, 1990:27 (Abstr).
220. Roelcke D: Sialic acid-dependent red blood cell antigens. In Garratty G (ed): Immunobiology of transfusion medicine. New York: Dekker, 1994:69–95.
221. Marsh WL, Jenkins WJ: Anti-Sp_1: The recognition of a new cold autoantibody. Vox Sang 1968;15:177–186.
222. Roelcke D: A new serological specificity in cold antibodies of high titre: Anti-HD. Vox Sang 1969;16:76–79.
223. Roelcke D, Uhlenbruck G, Bauer K: A heterogeneity of the HD-receptor, demonstrable by HD-cold antibodies: HD_1/HD_2. Scand J Haematol 1969;6:280.
224. Roelcke D, Uhlenbruck G: Letter to the editor. Vox Sang 1970;18:478–479.
225. Roelcke D. Cold agglutinin: Antibodies and antigens. Clin Immunol Immunopathol 1974;2:266.
226. Roelcke D, Anstee DJ, Jungfer H, Nutzenadel W, Webb AJ: IgG-type cold agglutinins in children and corresponding antigens: Detection of a new Pr antigen: Pr_a. Vox Sang 1971;20: 218–229.
227. Roelcke D, Ebert W, Geisen HP: Anti-Pr_3: serological and immunochemical identification of a new anti-Pr subspecificity. Vox Sang 1976;30:122–133.
228. Dellagi K, Brouet JC, Schenmetzler C, Praloran V: Chronic hemolytic anemia due to a monoclonal IgG cold agglutinin with anti-Pr specificity. Blood 1981;57:189–191.

229. Roelcke D, Anstee DJ, Jungfer H, Nutzenadel W, Webb AJ: IgG-type cold agglutinins in children and corresponding antigens: Detection of a new Pr antigen: Pr_a. Vox Sang 1971; 120:218–229.
230. Meytes D, Adler M, Viraq I, Feigl D, Levene C: High-dose methylprednisolone in acute immune cold hemolysis. N Engl J Med 1985;312:318.
231. Northoff H, Martin A, Roelcke D: An IgG-monotypic anti-Pr_{1h} associated with fresh varicella infection. Eur J Haematol 19987;38:85–88.
232. Curtis BR, Lamon J, Roelcke D, Chaplin H: Life-threatening, antiglobulin test-negative, acute autoimmune hemolytic anemia due to a non-complement-activating IgG1 cold antibody with Pr_a specificity. Transfusion 1990;30:838–843.
233. Kadota Y, Fujinami S, Tagawa Y, et al: Haemolytic anaemia caused by anti-Pr^a following rubella infection. Transfus Med 1993;3:207.
234. Ramos RR, Curtis BR, Sadler JE, Eby CS, Chaplin H: Refractory immune hemolytic anemia with a high thermal amplitude, low affinity IgG anti-Pr_a cold autoantibody. Autoimmunity 1992;12:149–154.
235. Angevine CD, Andersen BR, Barnett EV: A cold agglutinin of the IgA class. J Immunol 1966;96:578–586.
236. Roelcke D, Dorow W: Besonderheiten der Reaktionswerte eines mit Plasmocytom-?A-Paraprotein identischen Kalteagglutinins. Klin Wschr 1968;46:126–131.
237. Garratty G, Petz LD, Brodsky I, et al: An IgA high-titer cold agglutinin with an unusual blood group specificity within the Pr complex. Vox Sang 1973;25:32–38.
238. Tonthat H, Rochant H, Henry A, et al: A new case of monoclonal IgA Kappa cold agglutinin with anti-Pr_1d specificity in a patient with persistent HB antigen cirrohosis. Vox Sang 1976;30:464–468.
239. Roelcke D: Specificity of IgA cold agglutinins: Anti-Pr_1. Eur J Immunol 1973;3:206–212.
240. Gergely J, Wang AC, Fudenberg HH: Chemical analyses of variable regions of heavy and light chains of cold agglutinins. Vox Sang 1973;24:432–440.
241. Wang AC, Fudenberg HH, Wells JV, et al: A new subgroup of the kappa chain variable region associated with anti-Pr cold agglutinins. Nat New Biol 1973;243:126–128.
242. Sokol RJ, Booker DJ, Stamps R, et al: Autoimmune haemolysis and red cell autoantibodies with ABO blood group specificity. Haematologia 1995;26:121–129.
243. Postoway N, Garratty G, Guerra-Zevallos M: Transient autoimmune hemolytic anemia (AIHA) associated with an autoanti-IB in an A_2B individual. In: Book of Abstracts from the ISBT/AABB Joint Congress, 1990:27 (Abstr).
244. Arndt P, Do J, Garratty G, et al: A high titer, high thermal amplitude autoanti-B associated with acrocyanosis but not obvious hemolytic anemia. Transfusion 2003;43:1133–1137 (Abstr).
245. Sangster JM, Kenwright MG, Walker MP, Pembroke AC: Anti blood group-M autoantibodies with livedo reticularis, Raynaud's phenomenon, and anaemia. J Clin Pathol 1979; 32:154–157.
246. Chapman J, Murphy MF, Waters AH: Chronic cold haemagglutinin disease due to an anti-M-like autoantibody. Vox Sang 1982;42:272–277.
247. Bowman HS, Marsh WL, Schumacher HR, et al: Autoanti-N immunohemolytic anemia in infectious mononucleosis. Am J Clin Pathol 1974;61:465–472.
248. Marsh WL, Johnson CL, Oyen R, Nichols ME, et al: Anti-Sd^x : A "new" auto-agglutinin related to the Sd^a blood group. Transfusion 1980;20:1.
249. Bass LS, Rao AH, Goldstein J, Marsh WL: The Sd^x antigen and antibody: biochemical studies on the inhibitory property of human urine. Vox Sang 1983;44:191–196.
250. Marsh WL, Johnson CL, DiNapoli J, et al: Immune hemolytic anemia caused by autoanti-Sd^x: A report on six cases (Abstr). Transfusion 1980;20:647.
251. O'Brien DA, Mullahy DE, Garvey MA, Jackson JF: Cold autoimmune haemolytic anaemia in a 3-year-old infant due to anti-Rx (previously anti-Sd^x). Clin Lab Haematol 1988; 10:105–108.
252. Salama A, Pralle H, Mueller-Eckhardt C: A new red blood cell cold autoantibody (anti-Me). Vox Sang 1985;49:277–284.
253. Götsche B, Salama A, Mueller-Eckhardt C: Autoimmune hemolytic anemia caused by a cold agglutinin with a new specificity (anti-Ju). Transfusion 1990;30:261–262.
254. Perrault R: "Cold" IgG autologous anti-LW. Vox Sang 1973;24:150–164.
255. Longster GH, Johnson E: IgM anti-D as auto-antibody in a case of "cold" autoimmune haemolytic anaemia. Vox Sang 1988;54:174–176.
256. Beaumont JL, Lorenzelli L, Delplanque B, et al: A new serum lipoprotein associated erythrocyte antigen which reacts with a monoclonal IgM. Vox Sang 1976;30:36–49.
257. Linder E, Edgington TS: Immunobiology of the autoantibody response. 11. The lipoprotein-associated soluble HB erythrocyte autoantigen of NZB mice. J Immunol 1973;110:53–62.
258. Lightwood AM, Scott GL: Autoimmune haemolytic anaemia due to red cell antibodies of different specificities in a patient with chronic hepatitis. Vox Sang 1973;24:331–336.
259. Cazzola M, Barosi G, Ascari E: Cold haemagglutinin disease with severe anaemia, reticulocytopenia and erythroid bone marrow. Scand J Haematol 1983;30:25.
260. Kosmin M, Tarantolo S, Arndt P, Garratty G: Cold agglutinin syndrome associated with an autoagglutinin reacting preferentially with young RBCs (Abstr). In Book of Abstracts from the ISBT/AABB Joint Congress. Arlington, VA: American Association of Blood Banks, 1990:86.
261. Levine P, Celano MJ, Falkowski F: The specificity of the antibody in paroxysmal cold hemoglobinuria (PCH). Transfusion 1963;3:278.
262. Worlledge SM, Rousso C: Studies on the serology of paroxysmal cold haemoglobinuria (PCH), with special reference to its relationship with the P blood group system. Vox Sang 1965;10:293.
263. Knapp T: The laboratory investigation of three cases of paroxysmal cold haemoglobinuria. Can J Med Tech 1964;26:172.
264. Vogel JM, Hellman M, Moloshok RE: Paroxysmal cold hemoglobinuria of nonsyphilitic etiology in two children. J Pediatr 1972;81:974–977.
265. Ries CA, Garratty G, Petz LD, et al: Paroxysmal cold hemoglobinuria: report of a case with an exceptionally high thermal range Donath-Landsteiner antibody. Blood 1971;38:491–499.
266. Bird GWG, Wingham J, Martin AJ, et al: Idiopathic nonsyphlitic paroxysmal cold haemoglobinuria in children. J Clin Pathol 1976;29:215–218.
267. Johnsen HE, Brostrøm K, Madsen M: Paroxysmal cold haemoglobinuria in children: 3 cases encountered within a period of 7 months. Scand J Haematol 1978;20:413.
268. von dem Borne AEG Kr, Mol JJ, Joustra-Maas N, et al: Autoimmune haemolytic anaemia with monoclonal IgM (K) anti-P cold autohaemolysins. Br J Haematol 1982;50:345–350.
269. Ramos RR, Curtis BR, Eby CS, Ratkin GA, Chaplin H: Fatal outcome in a patient with autoimmune hemolytic anemia associated with an IgM bithermic anti-I^TP. Transfusion 1994;34:427–431.
270. Engelfriet CP, Beckers D, von dem Borne AEG Kr, et al: Haemolysins probably recognizing the antigen p. Vox Sang 1971;23:176.
271. Weiner W: The specificity of the antibodies in acquired haemolytic anaemias. In: Proceedings of the Joint Meeting of the 10th Congress of the International Society of Haematology/l0th Congress of the International Society of Blood Transfusion 1964:24.
272. Shirey RS, Park K, Ness PM, et al: An anti-i biphasic hemolysin in chronic paroxysmal cold hemoglobinuria. Transfusion 1986;26:62–64.
273. Judd WJ, Wilkinson SL, Issitt PD, et al: Donath-Landsteiner hemolytic anemia due to an anti-Pr-like biphasic hemolysin. Transfuison 1986;26:423–425.
274. Bell CA, Zwicker H, Rosenbaum DL: Paroxysmal cold hemoglobinuria (PCH) following mycoplasma infection:

Possible Mechanisms for Methyldopa-Induced RBC Autoantibody Production

Because methyldopa-induced AIHA represents a human model for an important autoimmune disorder, Worlledge and colleagues[105] stated in 1966, "It is not too much to hope that the solution to the mechanism of antibody formation in patients on methyldopa will lead to a better understanding of the causation of AIHA and of autoimmune diseases in general." Unfortunately, this optimistic outlook has not been realized in its entirety, although a number of hypotheses have been presented and significant investigative work has been performed.

Several clinical and laboratory findings of methyldopa-induced AIHA are difficult to explain because they are inconsistent with the usual kinetics of antibody production in response to immunogens. For instance, the DAT usually does not become positive until the drug has been administered for 3 to 6 months, hemolytic anemia rarely occurs until 18 weeks after initiation of treatment, and the delay in onset of antibody production is not shortened when patients who previously gave positive DAT reactions are restarted on the drug—indicating that there is no anamnestic response on repeated administration of the drug.

In addition, the codevelopment of other autoantibodies (see the discussion that follows) strongly suggests a more generalized immune reaction than simply an alteration of the RBC membrane by the drug.

ALTERED AUTOANTIGENS

One hypothesis suggested that the drug alters normal RBC antigens in such a way that they are no longer recognized as self. Weigle[106] demonstrated that tolerance to antigens can be broken by injecting animals with self-antigens that have been altered minimally. For example, he produced thyroiditis and antibodies to native thyroglobulin by injecting rabbits with autologous thyroglobulin that had been picrylated or coupled with diazonium derivatives of sulfanilic acid.[106,107] Worlledge and coworkers,[105] in their original report in 1966, postulated that the drug or one of its metabolites might combine with the RBC membrane and alter Rh antigens in such a way as to lead to the development of autoantibodies by the patient's normal immune system. The delay in development of a positive DAT could be explained by the drug (or one of its metabolites) being incorporated into the RBCs at the normoblast or reticulocyte stage. Such RBCs would not necessarily have a reduced life span and would not reach the antibody-producing mechanism until at least 120 days had elapsed, thus explaining the delay in development of a positive DAT. As Worlledge[108] pointed out, however, this theory cannot explain the sometimes rapid reversal in the DAT after the drug is stopped, because it implies that there should be no significant change in the strength of the test for at least 3 months.

Also, binding of methyldopa to RBCs has not been demonstrated consistently. Although Green and coworkers[109,110] reported that methyldopa does bind to human RBC proteins, LoBuglio and Jandl[111] incubated 2-^{14}C-α-methyldopa with RBCs and concluded that they were unable to demonstrate binding of the labeled drug to the RBC membrane.

Finally, this theory does not explain the more general autoimmune phenomena that are often associated with methyldopa therapy, including antinuclear antibody production, chronic active hepatitis, and a lupus-like syndrome.[6,7,112-117]

Nevertheless, the hypothesis of alteration of RBC membrane antigens has its proponents, in part because of observations strengthening the suggestion that drugs might always bind to antigens on cell membranes even though such binding might be loose and difficult to demonstrate. Pertinent data were provided by Habibi,[118] who described patients who simultaneously developed drug-dependent antibodies and RBC autoantibodies both having specificity for the same well-defined blood group antigen. Habibi[118] pointed out that the simultaneous production of RBC autoantibodies and drug-dependent antibodies mimics the well-known hapten and carrier specificities commonly developed in experimental animals immunized by hapten-carrier conjugates. He speculated that because both antibodies shared the same membrane receptor, the formation of conjugates between drugs and the RBC membrane must be the initial step of most DIIHAs in humans. Mueller-Eckhardt and Salama[119] also have reported on numerous patients who simultaneously developed drug-dependent antibodies and drug-induced autoantibodies, some of which had the same specificity. They interpreted these findings to indicate that the drug most likely reacted with cell membranes and that two types of antibodies might be produced.[119] Drug-dependent antibodies could arise as a result of the production of a drug-dependent neoantigen that is composed of elements of both drug and cell membrane; drug-independent antibodies, which can arise simultaneously in a given patient, could be elicited by a subtle alteration of antigens as described by Weigle[106,107] in his classic experiments. The binding sites for these antibodies could be sufficiently similar to or could be composed of enough unaltered structures of normal blood cell membranes to support drug-independent binding to both the patient's cells and normal cells.[103,120] Such antibodies have the serologic characteristics of RBC autoantibodies, but we believe that they are formed as a result of mechanisms that are different from those of autoantibodies induced by drugs (e.g., methyldopa or other drugs mentioned in this section), which appear without the presence of drug-dependent antibodies.

EFFECTS ON THE CELLULAR IMMUNE SYSTEM

Dameshek[121] suggested that methyldopa could have a direct effect on the cellular immune system. He suggested that methyldopa produces an aberration in lymphocyte proliferation leading to the emergence of autoantibody-producing cells. This proposed mechanism is consistent with the prolonged period of time necessary to induce immunohematologic abnormalities in patients, even on repeated challenge with the drug.[108,122] Although a significant body of experimental work has been developed with regard to this proposed mechanism of autoantibody production, the studies have led to inconclusive results.

Kirtland and associates[123] measured cyclic AMP produced in vitro by lymphocytes from healthy donors after adding methyldopa, and by lymphocytes from patients who were receiving methyldopa. Significantly higher lymphocyte cyclic AMP concentrations were generated by both sets of lymphocytes compared with lymphocytes from healthy donors without methyldopa present. To measure the effect of methyldopa on suppressor cells, Kirtland and associates[123] used an assay of suppressor cell activity based on the finding that preincubation of lymphocytes before mitogen stimulation in culture leads to less IgG being generated by B cells. This is purportedly due to enhancement of suppressor T-cell activity after the in vitro preincubation phase.[123] Kirtland and associates[123] confirmed the results of Lipsky and colleagues[124] that less IgG was produced after preincubation of lymphocytes. They showed that if methyldopa was added during the preincubation phase, the inhibition of IgG generation during mitogen-stimulated culture was negated. The amount of IgG generated in vitro after adding methyldopa to the preincubation phase was significantly greater than the IgG generated without a preincubation phase. Similar differences were observed when lymphocytes from patients receiving methyldopa were compared with lymphocytes from healthy donors. These results were interpreted to show that methyldopa interfered with the normal function of suppressor T cells to moderate IgG autoantibody production by B cells. Using similar techniques to those used by Kirtland and associates,[123] Garratty and colleagues[125] confirmed the effect of preincubation on in vitro IgG generation by B cells reported by Lipsky and coworkers,[124] but they could not confirm the findings of Kirtland and associates[123] that methyldopa had any effect on suppressor functions, as defined by the in vitro production of IgG after a preincubation phase. Garratty and colleagues[125] agreed with the findings of Kirtland and associates[123] that methyldopa depressed the proliferative response of mononuclear cells to mitogen stimulation.

Procainamide also induces autoantibodies, including RBC autoantibodies.[126,127] The following hypotheses have been proposed for the induction of autoantibody production by procainamide:

1. It interacts with nucleoprotein to form a neoantigen.[128,129]
2. It acts as an adjuvant for polyclonal activation of autoantibody-producing clones.
3. It inhibits T-cell DNA methylation, inducing T-cell autoreactivity.[130]
4. It interferes with immunoregulation.[131-136]

The reported effects on cellular immune function conflict with one another, and the described effects were small, requiring relatively high concentrations of procainamide. Ochi and colleagues[137] showed that procainamide impaired generation of suppressor T-cell activity but that it exerted no enhancing effect on T-helper cell, B-cell, or macrophage activities. Some members of this same group later published findings that conflicted somewhat with their previous conclusions.[136,137] They found that patients on long-term procainamide therapy had normal numbers and ratios of helper and suppressor T cells and normal mitogen-induced suppressor cell activity. A significant reduction in mitogen-induced IgG secreting cells was attributed to a decrease in both T-helper and B-cell activity in 50% of the patients and to only a B-cell activity decrease in 25% of the patients. The authors suggested that the defects in B- and T-cell function could result from the ability of procainamide to inhibit membrane depolarization by a mechanism similar to that observed in the cardiac conduction system.[138] Procainamide could nonspecifically suppress lymphocyte function through the action of the hydrophobic parts of the molecule, analogous to the anesthetic effect of its analogue, procaine.[138]

Miller and Salem[134] found normal suppressor cell function in 14 patients receiving procainamide. Total in vitro IgG generation from their mitogen-stimulated lymphocytes was significantly increased, however, compared with healthy controls and patients with systemic lupus erythematosus (SLE). Separated T cells from patients taking procainamide did not affect in vitro suppressor function of T cells from healthy individuals. The authors postulated that procainamide induced autoantibodies by enhancing helper T-cell function rather than impairing suppression. DeBoccardo and associates[135] found that procainamide inhibited in vitro IgG secretion and generation of IgG plaque-forming cells. The drug inhibited differentiation of B cells to plasma cells rather than production and secretion of IgG. The authors postulated that procainamide inhibits mitogen-induced B-cell maturation to plasma cells by inhibiting production of cytokines by helper cells. These results contrasted with those reported by Ochi and colleagues,[137] but it should be pointed out that DeBoccardo and associates[135] used much higher concentrations of procainamide than those used by Ochi and colleagues,[137] which were within the usual therapeutic plasma range. Bluestein and coworkers[132] found a biphasic response when they studied the effect of different concentrations of procainamide on mitogen-induced lymphocyte proliferation. Marked suppression was observed at a high concentration of the drug, but at lower doses of the drug, enhanced proliferation was observed. The lower concentrations of procainamide were nearer those found in plasma following therapy. Garratty and colleagues[125] found that therapeutic levels (30 µg/mL) of procainamide did not significantly affect PHA-induced lymphocyte proliferation. This result did not agree with the results of Bluestein and coworkers[133] but agreed with those of Ochi and colleagues,[137] who reported that procainamide concentrations ranging from 10 µg/mL–40 µg/mL had no significant effect on PWM-induced proliferation as measured by tritiated thymidine incorporation. Using the assay described by Lipsky and associates[124] and Kirtland and coworkers,[123] Garratty and colleagues[125] found that procainamide did not affect suppressor cell activity. These results agree with those of Miller and Salem,[134] DeBoccardo and colleagues,[135] and Yu and Ziff[136] but do not agree with those of Ochi and coworkers.[137]

Newer Concepts of the Immune Response to Drugs Associated with Cytopenia

To explain why the sera of four patients with drug-induced IHA showed the characteristics associated with the "immune complex" and autoantibody mechanisms, Habibi[118] suggested a single mechanism. He suggested that after ingestion of a particular drug, the formation of both autoantibodies and drug-dependent antibodies could be explained by the well-known hapten and carrier specificities commonly developed in animals immunized with hapten-carrier conjugates. He suggested that formation of drug-cell conjugates must be the initial step of most drug-induced cytopenias, and that the rare incidence of this disorder is probably because only few individuals are capable either of coupling drugs to their cells in vivo to form efficient immunogens or of mounting an unusually strong immune response to such conjugates. Salama and colleagues[94] suggested a unifying concept that is basically similar to that of Ackroyd[30-34] and Habibi[118] regarding the proposed immune response to drugs. They suggested that the immune process is always initiated by a primary interaction of the drug and/or its metabolites with constituents of blood cell membranes. This interaction provides the composite antigenic structure, which provokes the production of two types of antibodies—drug-dependent and/or drug-independent. The specificity of drug-dependent antibodies is determined by elements of both drug and cell membrane (drug-dependent neo-antigen). These antibodies cannot bind sufficiently well to either drug or cell membrane alone. If one part is removed (e.g., by dialysis in vitro, by discontinuance of drug administration, or by subsequent excretion in vivo), the immune reaction subsides. The authors suggested that drug-independent antibodies could be elicited by a subtle alteration of the membrane by the drug, but their binding sites are sufficiently similar to (or are composed of enough unaltered structures of) normal cell membranes to support drug-independent binding to both the patient's cells and normal cells (drug-independent neo-antigen). Such antibodies behave like autoantibodies and cannot be distinguished from "true" autoantibodies (i.e., those associated with warm AIHA). Salama and colleagues[94] believe that only one hypothesis is necessary to explain all the phenomena we observe. They not only criticized the immune complex hypothesis but also criticized the concept of the drug-adsorption mechanism and the theory that some drugs (e.g., methyldopa and procainamide) cause autoantibody production by affecting the immune system directly.

It is tempting to draw cartoons as Habibi[118] and Garratty[103,120] did to illustrate how the immune complex, drug adsorption, and autoantibody mechanisms could be explained on the basis of classical hapten immunology (e.g., Fig. 8-6). These cartoons are based on the findings that in the haptenic response, antibodies can be made to the hapten (i.e., drug), the carrier (e.g., RBC membrane components), and/or a population of antibodies that could react with part hapten, part membrane. One could argue that a patient might make one or several populations of antibodies showing the different specificities. Thus, an antibody to the drug alone would react with drug-coated RBCs and be inhibited by the drug; this would be typical of penicillin antibodies or the "drug adsorption" mechanism. Antibodies to membrane components would appear only as autoantibodies. Antibodies directed to epitopes that are part drug/part membrane would require drug and RBCs to be present together before a reaction is observed. Because most of these drugs do not combine with RBCs efficiently enough to withstand in vitro washing, one cannot prepare drug-coated RBCs, and the only way of demonstrating such antibodies is to mix the patient's serum with drug and RBCs. This reaction is typical of the so-called immune complex mechanism, but if the foregoing concept is correct, the antibody is reacting with a neo-antigen that is formed when the drug binds loosely to cell membrane components, rather than drug immune complexes attaching to the cell. Extending the suggestions of Habibi[118] and Salama and Mueller-Eckhardt,[94] Garratty[103,120] suggested that sometimes the epitope inducing the immune response might be partially drug and partially membrane protein, but primarily membrane protein (see Fig. 8-6). In this case, the drug might not be needed to demonstrate the antibody in vitro, and the antibody might appear to be a drug-independent antibody (autoantibody).

The unifying hypothesis is attractive because it can be used to explain the Fab-dependent binding of the drug antibody, the specificity that is sometimes observed, and the serologic finding that suggests several mechanisms in one patient. When the antibody is made against part drug/part membrane, the proportions recognized as antigenic determinants will vary. For instance, one population of antibody molecules might be mainly antidrug, and another population might be mainly antibody directed at membrane proteins (as drug plus membrane proteins) (see Fig. 8-6).

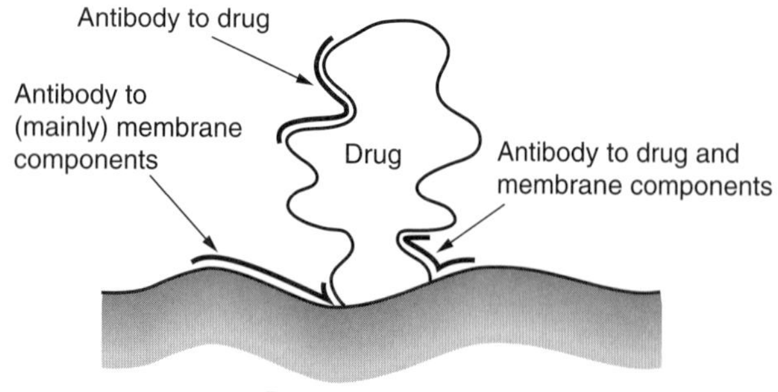

FIGURE 8-6. Proposed unifying hypothesis of drug-induced antibody reactions. The thicker, darker lines represent antigen-binding sites on the Fab region of the drug-induced antibody. Drugs (haptens) bind loosely (or firmly) to cell membranes, and antibodies can be made to (a) the drug (producing in vitro reactions typical of a drug adsorption [penicillin-type] reaction); (b) membrane components, or mainly membrane components (producing in vitro reactions typical of autoantibody); or (c) part-drug, part-membrane components (producing an in vitro reaction typical of the so-called immune complex mechanism). (From Garratty G: Target antigens for red-cell bound autoantibodies. In Nance SJ (ed): Clinical and basic science aspects of immunohematology. Arlington, VA: American Association of Blood Banks, 1991:33–72.)

Garratty[103,120] suggested that the membrane components composing the immunogen might contain specific, well-defined platelet or RBC antigens and that the "drug" antibody, therefore, will appear to have blood-group specificity. Because the proportion of membrane and drug antigenic determinants vary, one would expect to see a spectrum of serologic activity among different patients. Thus, patients said to have antibodies showing characteristics of the immune complex, drug adsorption, and autoantibody mechanisms could have three different antibody populations, but the serologic characteristics could be explained by a single mechanism.

Problems with the Unifying Hypothesis

The unifying hypothesis is based on classical hapten immunology studies performed by injecting into animals small MW substances that conjugated in vitro to heterologous proteins (e.g., albumin). In a review in which they propose a variation on the original immune complex hypothesis, Shulman and Reid[139] point out that when autologous or homologous protein (rather than heterologous protein) is used as a carrier, the complex is less immunogenic, and autoantibodies rarely develop. Thus, the claims that the "unifying" hypothesis is supported by classical hapten immunology is not strictly true, considering that all the situations we are discussing involve autologous protein carriers. As drug-induced IHA is so rare, it might be suggested that when we observe mixed serologic characteristics suggesting more than one mechanism, these could be rare examples that do not follow the usual hapten immunology and could be explained by the unifying hypothesis. We find it hard to accept that the unifying hypothesis explains autoantibodies induced by drugs such as methyldopa, fludarabine, and procainamide. Such drugs induce autoantibodies relatively commonly, and these are not seen together with antibodies showing characteristics of the immune complex or drug adsorption mechanism.

We believe that the drug-independent antibodies induced by drugs such as methyldopa, fludarabine, and procainamide are formed by a mechanism different from the mechanism illustrated in Figure 8-6. These drugs always lead to the development of autoantibodies and are never accompanied by drug-independent antibodies. In contrast, other drug-independent antibodies (e.g., nomifensine and the newer cephalosporins) almost always occur together with drug-dependent antibodies. This observation fits well with the concept (illustrated in Fig. 8-6) that several populations of antibodies are likely to be formed. Although it is possible for only one population to be formed in an individual patient, it is hard to accept that methyldopa, fludarabine, and procainamide always induce only a single population reacting primarily with membrane components. Although the findings of Garratty and colleagues[125] suggest that methyldopa and procainamide do not affect suppressor cell function as measured by Kirtland and associates,[123] we believe that these drugs do affect immune function in some way to allow proliferation of true autoantibody.

Shulman and Reid[139] have put forward a defense of the immune complex concept and have incorporated some aspects of the unifying hypothesis. They illustrate their article with several cartoons (Figs. 8-7 and 8-8) that combine elements of the original immune complex concept and the unifying hypothesis. They agree that drug antibodies (other than those related to penicillin) are induced by antigens formed when the drug binds loosely to the cell in vivo. They point out, however, that most experiments of hapten immunology have involved injecting animals with preconjugated hapten-protein complexes. Because drugs other than penicillin do not form covalent bonds rapidly with proteins in vivo, most drug antibodies are probably formed against metabolites of the original drug. These authors suggest that penicillin antibodies could react with preformed drug-cell complexes, but that antibodies to other drugs (e.g., quinidine/quinine) could react with drugs bound loosely to the cell membrane or with a drug that is not bound to cell membranes. In either case, one could say that a drug-antidrug immune complex is formed. To explain the Fab binding of drug antibody to the cell, Shulman and Reid[139] suggest that drug-immune complexes could attach to the cell by the weak attraction of the drug to the cell, or the antibody might bind to drug bound loosely to the cell. If the drug antibody also recognizes some membrane antigens (e.g., neo-antigens), then the binding of the complex to the membrane would be stronger. Finally, Shulman and Reid[139] suggest that conformational changes in the Fab portion of the drug antibody might occur after drug binding, and that such conformational changes might recognize membrane sites. Such interactions could convert a low-affinity reaction (i.e., antibody reacting with loosely bound drug) to a higher- (but still low-) affinity bimolecular association. If two of the drug

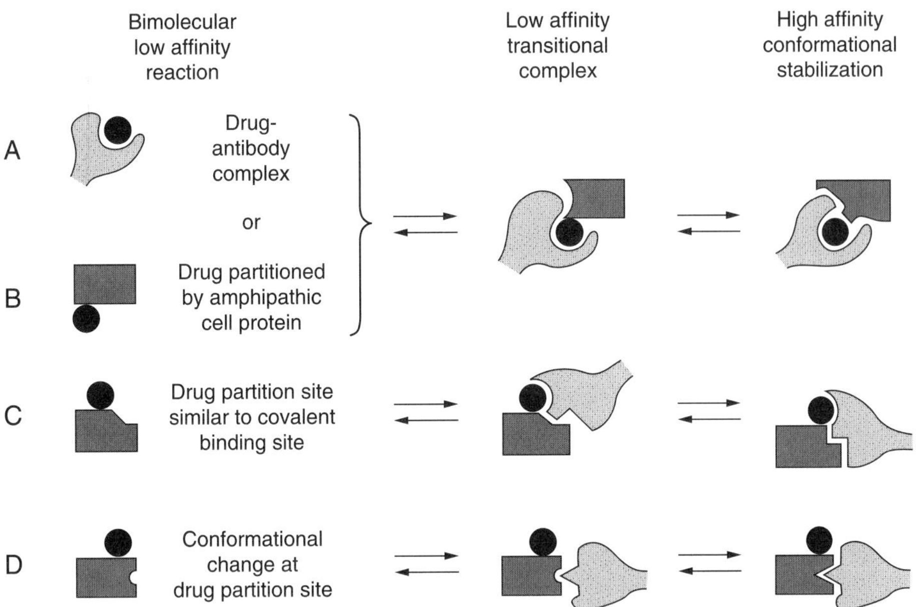

FIGURE 8-7. Possible rearrangements of transitional reactions leading to high affinity complexes. Note absence of covalent bond between drug and protein. (From Shulman NR, Reid DM: Mechanisms of drug-induced immunologically mediated cytopenias. Transfus Med Rev 1993;VII:215–229.)

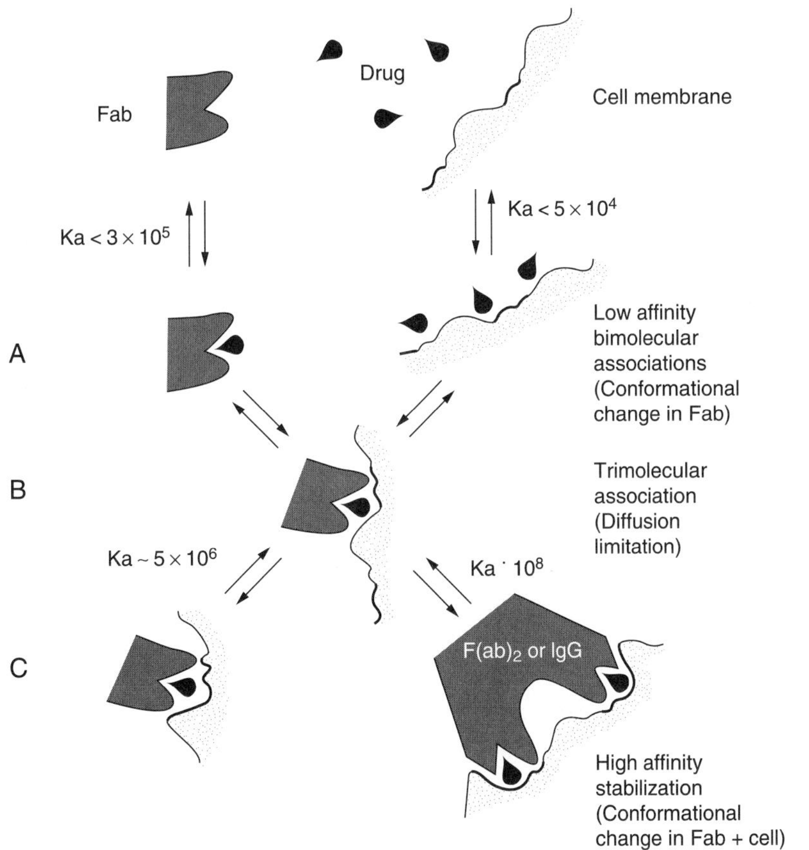

FIGURE 8-8. Possible changes in Fab and cell membrane protein leading to monovalent and divalent high-affinity complexes. (From Shulman NR, Reid DM: Mechanisms of drug-induced immunologically mediated cytopenias. Transfus Med Rev 1993;VII:215–229.)

antibody's Fab sites [$F(ab)_2$] are involved in the interaction, this process could convert a low-affinity monovalent reaction to a divalent high-affinity interaction (see Figs. 8-7 and 8-8).

SUGGESTED MECHANISMS OF DRUG-INDUCED HEMOLYTIC ANEMIA AND/OR POSITIVE DAT

Possible pathogenic mechanisms are closely related to the hypotheses discussed previously for the immune response to drugs. The cartoons used (e.g., Figs. 8-4, 8-6, 8-7, 8-8, and 8-9) reflect on both the suggested epitopes that are thought to stimulate drug antibodies and their reactions with drug and RBCs in vivo and in vitro.

Penicillin-Type Mechanism

This mechanism is the best understood and the least controversial; it has also been called the "hapten mechanism" and the "drug adsorption mechanism."[140] The term "hapten mechanism" implies that the hapten-like binding of penicillin to RBCs is essential for the drug to be immunogenic, as was postulated by Ackroyd.[30-34] There is no evidence, however, that RBC binding by penicillin is necessary for the drug to be immunogenic. Instead, the immunogenicity of penicillin could relate to its binding with plasma proteins, and hemolysis could result from the reaction of penicillin antibody with penicillin that has been adsorbed to the RBC membrane (this is why we termed it the "drug adsorption" mechanism[1,140]).

Some drugs (e.g., penicillins and cephalosporins) bond covalently to proteins (e.g., proteins on cell membranes) (see Table 8-2). When patients receive large enough doses (e.g., several million units of penicillin per day) of such a drug, the RBCs become coated with the drug, and any antibody the patient makes might attach to the drug on the RBCs (see Fig. 8-9). When these antibodies are IgG, the IgG/drug-coated RBCs could be removed by macrophages in the reticuloendothelial system in a similar way to RBCs coated with IgG RBC blood group auto- or alloantibodies (see Chapter 4).

Penicillin can be detected on the surface of the RBCs of most patients who are receiving high doses of the drug intravenously.[141-145] Using a rabbit penicillin antibody, Levine and Redmond[144] demonstrated penicillin on the RBCs of 30% of the patients taking 1.2–2.4 million units per day and on the RBCs of all patients taking 10 million units or more daily. This coating is not by itself injurious, but some patients develop a high-titer penicillin antibody that reacts with RBC-bound penicillin. Large doses of the drug appear to be necessary to coat RBCs sufficiently to furnish enough antigenic sites for reaction with penicillin antibody. Thus, the mechanism of cell sensitization and resultant hemolysis differs from those discussed previously; it appears to result from the coating of RBCs by penicillin during the administration of high doses of the drug, and from the reaction of penicillin antibodies with such drug-coated RBCs (see Fig. 8-9). The quantity of penicillin antibody sensitizing the RBC is related to the concentration of penicillin antigenic determinants on the RBC membrane, the plasma concentration of penicillin antibody, and the avidity of the antibody.

When sensitive techniques are used, penicillin antibodies can be detected in more than 90% of patients' sera. Most sera in the study by Levine and colleagues[37] contained IgM antibodies; the sera of approximately 16% of random patients and 38% of patients who had received penicillin recently contained IgG antibodies also. These antibodies were usually neutralized by BPO hapten. The antibodies associated with IHA due to penicillin are IgG, and these powerful antibodies are not easily neutralized by BPO hapten; inhibition is observed if dilutions of the high-titer penicillin antibody are used for the inhibition tests. The high incidence of penicillin antibodies detected in random patients (and in healthy individuals) is probably due to the continual exposure to penicillin in our modern environment.

Theoretically, antibodies to any of the drugs that bind firmly to RBCs (see Table 8-2) could cause a hemolytic anemia through a mechanism similar to

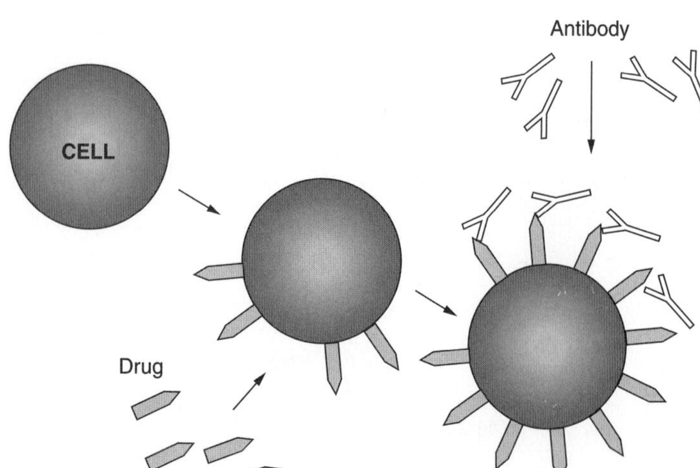

FIGURE 8-9. Mechanism of penicillin-induced DIIHA and/or positive DAT. Penicillin bonds to RBCs, and IgG penicillin antibody attaches to RBC-bound penicillin.

that described for penicillin. In practice, most such antibodies appear to cause hemolytic anemia through other or additional mechanisms. It could be that the classical penicillin mechanism is dependent on very large amounts of drug being given.

It is possible for penicillin antibodies to activate complement, and on rare occasions this process could be efficient enough to cause acute complement-mediated intravascular hemolysis.[146-148] This probably occurs in addition to the IgG-mediated destruction of RBCs by macrophages.

Table 8-4 shows the characteristic features of penicillin-induced hemolytic anemia.

TABLE 8-4. CHARACTERISTIC FEATURES OF PENICILLIN-INDUCED HEMOLYTIC ANEMIA

Hemolysis develops only in patients who are receiving large doses of penicillin intravenously (at least 10 million units daily in an adult for a week or longer).
Hemolytic anemia is less acute in onset than that caused by the immune complex mechanism, and it usually develops over a period of 7 to 10 days. Hemolysis can be life-threatening, however, if the etiology is not promptly diagnosed and if penicillin administration is continued.
The DAT is strongly positive due to RBC-bound IgG; about 45% of patients could have RBC-bound complement detected as well.
Antibody eluted from the patient's RBCs reacts with penicillin-treated RBCs but not with untreated RBCs.
A high-titer IgG penicillin antibody is present in the serum. Using a high-pH method to coat RBCs described later in this chapter, the titer is usually 1000 or greater.
Cessation of penicillin therapy is followed by complete recovery, although hemolysis of decreasing severity and a "mixed-field" positive DAT can persist for several weeks.
Other manifestations of penicillin allergy are not necessarily present.

Nonpenicillin-Type Mechanism ("Immune Complex" Mechanism)

Most of the drugs that have caused DIIHA do not covalently bind to RBCs, and one cannot prepare drug-coated RBCs in vitro to test for drug antibodies. As discussed in the section on the immune response to drugs, it is controversial how such drugs evoke an immune response, and it is equally controversial how the drug antibodies interact in vivo to cause cytopenia (e.g., hemolytic anemia). It is obvious that most of them, in contrast to penicillin-type antibodies, cause cytopenia by complement-mediated reactions. The hemolytic anemia is often acute, severe, and associated with hemoglobinemia and hemoglobinuria; many are associated with renal failure. Early work on drug-induced thrombocytopenia suggested that this group of drugs could sometimes evoke an antibody (often IgM) that binds efficiently to drug-forming immune complexes in vivo. These immune complexes would attach to platelets nonspecifically (or perhaps to the Fc receptor on platelets) and activate complement. It was suggested that only a small amount of drug (or immune complex) would be needed to activate complement and that the immune complexes would be able to move from cell to cell, activating complement, thus creating an efficient way of damaging many cells. This would be in contrast to the penicillin mechanism, where large amounts of drug are needed to coat enough RBCs to react efficiently with the IgG penicillin antibody. This mechanism has been called the immune complex mechanism (see Fig. 8-5) and also has been used to explain some types of DIIHA. The clinical and serologic findings associated with these types of antibodies certainly seem to fit with immune complex-mediated in vivo and in vitro reactions (Table 8-5).

Nevertheless, as discussed previously, the immune complex mechanism as originally described has been criticized strongly, and it has been suggested that it should be replaced by a mechanism that involves an interaction of the drug antibody against a neo-antigen. This neo-antigen could be a new antigen produced by a chemical change in the cell membrane induced by brief (i.e., noncovalent-binding) contact with the drug, or the new antigen could be a combination of part drug part membrane protein. The latter explanation is the basis of the unifying hypothesis discussed previously (see Fig. 8-6).

Regardless of which theoretic concept is correct, the laboratory and clinical findings associated with this group of drugs are quite distinct and contrast with the penicillin-type mechanism. Table 8-5 lists the characteristics of these drug-dependent antibodies.

Drug-Induced Nonimmunologic Adsorption of Protein onto RBCs

Some drugs appear to cause proteins to adsorb onto RBCs by a nonimmunologic mechanism, leading to a positive DAT. The first drug to be described as causing this effect was cephalothin.[149-151] Other cephalosporins might be capable of the same effect. Molthan and coworkers[149] reported that 81% of 31 patients receiving cephalothin had a positive DAT; Gralnick and associates[150] and Perkins and colleagues[151] reported the same finding in 40% of 20 patients and 38% of 143 patients, respectively. In an extensive study in 1971, Spath and coworkers[152,153] found that only 4% of 320 DATs performed on 97 patients receiving cephalothin were positive. They suggested the existence of several explanations for the difference between their results and those of other researchers.

TABLE 8-5. CHARACTERISTICS ASSOCIATED WITH DRUG-DEPENDENT ANTIBODIES OTHER THAN THE "PENICILLIN TYPE"

Patient need take only a small amount of the drug.
Acute complement-mediated hemolysis often occurs; 30%–50% of patients have associated renal failure.
The patient's RBCs are often sensitized with complement only, but RBC-bound IgG and/or IgM can be present.
Patient's serum reacts with RBCs in the presence of the drug and/or its metabolite. Antibodies are often IgM, but IgG antibodies can be present alone or together with IgM. Antibodies can cause hemolysis, agglutination, and/or sensitization of RBCs in the presence of drug.
After drug is stopped, hematological remission is usually rapid.

Nonimmunologic adsorption of proteins is usually suspected when most normal plasmas/sera react (e.g., by IAT) with drug-treated RBCs but eluates from the RBCs are nonreactive. After such findings, we usually confirm our suspicions by performing an antiglobulin test with an antihuman albumin that has been standardized for use with RBCs. The presence of RBC-bound albumin is strong evidence for nonimmunologic uptake of plasma proteins. IATs using antisera to other proteins are also often positive, as demonstrated by Spath and coworkers.[152]

Patient selection can influence the results greatly. The dosage and duration of therapy are likely to influence the incidence of positive reactions. The studies of Spath and coworkers[152] were carried out in consecutive unselected patients in a community hospital, and neither the mean daily cephalothin dosage (6.3 g), the mean duration of therapy (5.5 days), nor the incidence of renal insufficiency was high. The distribution of BUN levels in their patients was as follows: 80% normal levels, 12% in the range of 20–30 mg%, 4% between 30 mg% and 50 mg%, and 4% higher than 50 mg%. Three of the four patients with positive DATs in their series had elevated BUN levels. A greater incidence of positive DATs might logically be anticipated in referral centers or infectious disease units caring for more seriously ill patients. This might be especially true if a large percentage of patients studied have renal disease, as in the reports of Molthan and colleagues,[149] Gralnick and coworkers,[150] and Perkins and associates.[151] In addition, such patients could have a positive DAT unrelated to cephalothin therapy or because drug is not excreted efficiently, leading to high levels in the plasma. Gralnick and coworkers[150] and Perkins and associates[151] did not report results of pretreatment DATs and did not present specific immunologic data indicating that the positive DATs were caused by cephalosporin administration. Thus, in any series of patients and particularly among patients with renal disease, control series indicating the incidence of positive DAT in a similar group, pretreatment antiglobulin tests, or specific immunologic data in each patient (such as the elution of specific antibody from the patient's RBCs) are necessary before the positive DATs can be attributed to cephalosporin therapy.

The nature of the antiglobulin sera (AGS) could be of significance. To ensure that these results might be readily duplicated by others, Spath and coworkers[152] performed the initial antiglobulin tests with a readily available commercial polyclonal polyspecific AGS that had previously been evaluated and shown to possess potent anti-IgG and anti-C3. This AGS did not contain antialbumin, whereas some commercial AGS did have potent antialbumin. In vitro results indicated that albumin was absorbed readily onto cephalothin-treated RBCs and could be the cause of false-positive antiglobulin tests if an AGS rich in antialbumin was used. This could be another reason why Molthan and associates[149] or Gralnick and colleagues[150] found a higher percentage of positive DATs than did Spath and coworkers.[152]

Although Spath and coworkers[152] confirmed that cephalothin can cause nonimmunologic adsorption of protein, three of four patients with a positive DAT (but no hemolytic anemia) had demonstrable IgG anticephalothin on their RBCs. Thus, most of the positive DATs appeared to be due to an immune mechanism, although additional nonimmunologic uptake of protein was not excluded. In a companion paper, Spath and coworkers[153] studied optimal conditions for detecting cephalothin and penicillin antibodies. The studies confirmed earlier work indicating that penicillin binds optimally to RBCs at around pH 10. A penicillin antibody reacted to a titer of 200, 400, and 3200 with penicillin-coated RBCs prepared at a pH of 7.3, 8.2, and 10, respectively. A cephalothin antibody with a titer of 3200 showed no significant difference when RBCs were coated with cephalothin at pH 7.3, 8.2, or 10.[153]

Molthan and colleagues[149] and Gralnick and associates[150] suggested that the cephalothin-induced DATs were due to cephalothin-protein conjugates attaching to the RBCs and that antiglobulin sera reacted with RBC-bound protein. Spath and coworkers[152] showed quite conclusively that the suggestions of these other authors were not correct. Spath and coworkers[152] showed that washed cephalothin-treated RBCs adsorb a variety of proteins that react with antiglobulin sera (i.e., preformed cephalothin complexes are not necessary to obtain positive antiglobulin tests). In 1975, we suggested that cephalothin bonds (like penicillin) to the RBC membrane, but that unlike penicillin, cephalothin changes the RBC membrane, allowing proteins to attach to the membrane (Fig. 8-10).[140] It was not clear how the proteins attach to the modified membrane.

Petz and Branch[14] and Branch and associates[154] reported that some cephalosporins (cephalexin, cefazolin, cefamandole) did not cause nonimmunologic binding of protein to RBCs. They suggested that the nonimmunologic adsorption of protein might not occur because the RBC membrane is changed by the cephalosporin, and that cephalothin might bind to RBCs not through its β-lactam group but rather through acetoxymethylene and/or thiopene side chains.[154] An alternative suggestion was that RBCs might have a specific receptor site that remains active under mild acid conditions. If either of these events occurred, then perhaps the exposed β-lactam groups on cephalothin would be free to react with plasma proteins. This would explain why, under acid conditions, cephalothin still binds efficiently to RBCs (in contrast to penicillin), but the β-lactam ring is much less likely to undergo nucleophilic attack that would prevent binding of plasma proteins.[154] These authors also showed that nonspecific binding of proteins decreases as pH decreases. Ninety-seven percent of 133 normal sera reacted, by IAT, with RBCs coated with cephalothin at pH 8.5, but only four of 87 (4.6%) reacted weakly with RBCs coated with cephalothin at pH 6.0. It was suggested that at low pH, cephalothin

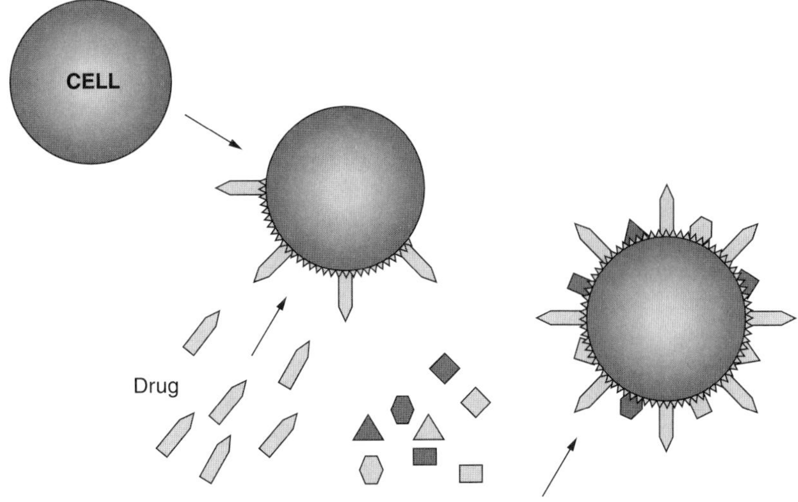

FIGURE 8-10. Nonimmunological adsorption of proteins onto RBCs. Drugs might change the RBC membrane so that many proteins attach to the membrane, leading to a positive DAT and, possibly, to DIIHA.

might still bind to RBCs (unlike penicillin), but that the β-lactam ring would be much less likely to undergo nucleophilic attack that would permit binding of proteins when the RBCs are incubated with serum or plasma.[14,149]

Garratty and Leger[155] were stimulated to defend the "membrane modification" concept of Garratty and Petz[140] because of two reports from 1968.[156,157] Sirchia and colleagues[156] and Ferrone and coworkers[157] showed that cephalothin-treated RBCs acted in some ways like RBCs from patients with paroxysmal nocturnal hemoglobinuria (PNH). The treated RBCs had enzymatic and metabolic activities similar to those of PNH RBCs and were similarly sensitive to the action of complement (e.g., cephalothin-treated RBCs gave a positive acidified-serum lysis test [Ham's Test]). It is now known that PNH RBCs have several membrane abnormalities.[158] For instance, phosphatidylinositol-glycan (GPI)-anchored proteins, which contain important complement control proteins (CD55 and CD59), are absent or markedly deficient in PNH RBCs. In 1995, Garratty and Leger[155] confirmed the findings of Sirchia and colleagues[156] and Ferrone and coworkers[157] and extended them by demonstrating (using flow cytometry) that RBCs treated with cephalothin and cefotetan had markedly decreased quantities of RBC membrane CD55 and CD58; CD59 was only slightly decreased. Thus, the RBC membrane changes were different from those demonstrated for PNH RBCs but proved the earlier suggestion by Garratty and Petz[140] that cephalsoporins modify the RBC membrane.

Other Drugs Causing Nonimmunologic Uptake of Protein onto RBCs

Jamin and associates[159] showed that diglycoaldehyde (INOX), an intravenous chemotherapeutic agent used to treat childhood malignancies, caused positive DATs in all eight patients receiving the drug. IgG and albumin were found to bind to human RBCs when they were incubated in vitro with normal plasma and INOX or with glutaraldehyde, which is similar in structure to INOX. In theory, any drug containing two or more aldehdye groups capable of reacting with proteins can produce a positive DAT. These could include the following: actinorhodine, aztreonam, citric acid, diglycoaldehyde, Evans blue, folic acid, glutamic acid, glutaraldehyde, glutaric acid, glycerol trinitrate (nitroglycerin), glyoxal, iodipamide (Chlorografin), maelic acid, menadiol sodium diphosphate (Synkayite), pamoic acid, penicillic acid, phthalic acid, picric acid, stibophen, sodium iodomethamate (Iodoxyl), terephthaldicarboxaldehyde, and terephthalic acid. Jamin and associates[160] also reported that suramin (a reverse transcriptase inhibitor that has been used in treating acquired immunodeficiency syndrome) caused in vitro adsorption of IgG onto RBCs associated with positive AGTs. No positive DATs have been reported after suramin administration.

Zeger and coworkers[161] showed that IgG could be adsorbed nonimmunologically onto RBCs treated in vitro with cisplatin, an anticancer chemotherapeutic agent. They also suggested that a positive DAT due to IgG and complement sensitization, which developed in a patient taking cisplatin, was due to nonimmunologic protein adsorption in vivo. The patient had a hemolytic anemia on presentation, but when rechallenged with the drug, the patient redeveloped a positive DAT but not a hemolytic anemia. Seven other patients have been reported to have cisplatin-induced HA.[160-166] Two drugs that are closely related to cisplatin—carboplatin and oxaliplatin—have also been reported as causing hemolytic anemia.[167-172] Oxaliplatin appears to cause positive DATs (and perhaps hemolytic anemia), due to oxaliplatin antibodies and/or nonimmunologic adsorption of protein onto the RBCs.[172] It is interesting that these drugs have been shown to cause nonspecific binding of protein onto RBCs in vitro, and that there are several cases of hemolytic anemia associated with this therapy. Unfortunately, many of these cases had poor serologic evaluations, and following the findings by Zeger and coworkers,[161] it has been assumed that the DATs could have been positive due to nonspecific binding of protein and that the hemolytic anemia might not have been associated with this. This assumption was supported by the knowledge that cephalothin was used commonly for more than 25 years with no cases of HA reported that were proved to be due to nonspecific binding of protein onto the RBCs.

In 1992, Lutz and Dzik[173] reported an analysis of the cause of all positive DATs at their institution in an 18-month period. They found that 45 of 189 positive DATs (23.8%) were associated with the use of Unasyn (Roerig Division, Pfizer Inc., New York, NY), an antibacterial combination of the semisynthetic antibiotic ampicillin sodium and the β-lactamase inhibitor sulbactam sodium. None of these patients had a HA. They also prospectively followed 59 patients with a negative DAT after receiving Unasyn.[173] Twenty-three of these patients (39%) developed a weakly positive DAT (microscopic to 1+ with an anti-IgG) after a median of 8.5 days of therapy (range, 3–15 days); there was no associated hemolytic anemia.

These results suggested that Unasyn caused positive DATs far more commonly than any other drug in present use. Up to that time, the drug most commonly causing positive DATs was methyldopa, with 10–36% of patients developing a positive DAT after 3–6 months of therapy, but methyldopa is no longer commonly used. Upon reviewing their records, Garratty and Arndt [174] found that they had studied four patients who developed positive DATs while on Unasyn or a similar drug, Timentin (a combination of the semisynthetic antibiotic ticarcillin disodium and the β-lactamase inhibitor clavulanate potassium; SmithKline Beecham Inc., Philadelphia, PA). The patients' sera, or eluates from their RBCs, had not reacted with RBCs in the presence of Unasyn or Timentin, but the patients' sera had reacted with Unasyn- or Timentin-treated RBCs by indirect antiglobulin test. As a control, drug-treated RBCs had always been tested with a pool of normal sera. The pooled normal sera control reacted with the drug-reacted RBCs equally well as the patients' sera, so the results with the patients' sera were initially interpreted as being insignificant (i.e., no drug antibodies detected).

The results of Lutz and Dzik[173] were reminiscent of earlier reports[149,150] of patients receiving cephalothin. Garratty and Arndt[174] wondered whether the reactions they had observed with normal sera and Unasyn-/Timentin-treated RBCs (results ignored at that time) might have been due to in vitro nonspecific uptake of protein onto the Unasyn- and Timentin-treated red cells, similar to what had been described with the cephalosporins, and whether this process might explain the high incidence of positive DATs observed by Lutz and Dzik.[173] Garratty and Arndt[174] also wondered whether Augmentin (SmithKline Beecham), an antibacterial combination of the semisynthetic antibiotic amoxicillin and the β-lacatamase inhibitor clavulanate potassium, would show similar serologic results. They found that the sera from their four patients did not react with RBCs in the presence of Unasyn or Timentin, but when drug-treated RBCs were tested, patients' sera and normal donor sera reacted equally by IAT.[174] After incubation in normal sera, RBCs treated with Unasyn, Timentin, Augmentin, sulbactam, and clavulanate reacted by IAT with a range of antiglobulin sera, including antihuman albumin (an index of nonimmunologic adsorption). RBCs treated with only ampicillin or amoxicillin were nonreactive.[174] Thus, it was concluded that the β-lactamase inhibitors sulbactam and clavulanate seem to cause nonimmunologic adsorption of protein onto RBCs in vitro and that this could be the cause of the high incidence of positive DATs. This study confirmed the findings of Williams and associates,[175] who in 1985 had shown that clavulanate could cause in vitro nonimmunologic adsorption of proteins onto human RBCs and was associated with positive DATs in patients taking drugs containing clavulanate (44% of patients developed a positive DAT).

Table 8-6 shows the drugs that are thought to cause nonimmunologic uptake of proteins onto RBCs. Table 8-7 shows the serologic characteristics associated with drug-induced nonimmunologic adsorption of proteins onto RBCs.

Nonimmunologic Uptake of Protein by RBCs as a Possible Cause of Hemolytic Anemia

Garratty and Arndt[174] further suggested that the nonimunologic uptake of protein (e.g., IgG) might lead to hemolytic anemia. Three of the four patients with positive DATs who had received clavulanate or sulbactam had an associated hemolytic anemia, and there was a temporal relationship to the drug therapy. A cause-and-effect relationship could not be proven, as no drug antibody was demonstrable. Broadberry and associates[176] showed that another β-lactamase inhibitor, tazobactam, could also be associated with a positive DAT and HA. They showed that

TABLE 8-6. DRUGS ASSOCIATED WITH NONIMMUNOLOGICAL ADSORPTION OF PROTEINS ONTO RBCS
cephalosporins
cisplatin/oxaliplatin
diglycoaldehyde (INOX)
suramin
sulbactam (contained in Unasyn)
clavulanate (contained in Augmentin and Timentin)
tazobactam (contained in Zosyn)

TABLE 8-7. CHARACTERISTICS ASSOCIATED WITH DRUG-INDUCED NONIMMUNOLOGICAL ADSORPTION OF PROTEINS ONTO RBCs

Patients have positive DAT but often do not have hemolytic anemia.
Positive DAT might be due to a multitude of proteins on RBC surface (e.g., IgG, IgM, IgA, C3, albumin).
Nonimmunological adsorption is suggested if the patient's RBCs react by a DAT using antialbumin (the antialbumin must be standardized for use with RBCs).
Eluate from patient's DAT+ RBCs is nonreactive with untreated or drug-treated RBCs, or in the presence of drug.
Patient's serum may react with drug-coated RBCs, but not with untreated RBCs in the presence of drug but normal donor sera show similar reactions. The strength of reactions might not be similar, as the serum IgG level can influence the nonimmunological uptake of protein.

there appeared to be a relationship with the plasma IgG level and the positive antiglobulin test. Their patient had a high gamma globulin level; it will be of interest, therefore, to attempt to correlate plasma IgG levels in future patients with hemolytic anemia suspected to be due to this mechanism. Arndt and Garratty[177] provided further data to support their hypothesis by showing that after in vitro incubation with clavulanate, sulbactam, or tazobactam, normal RBCs were phagocytosed by monocytes in a monocyte monolayer assay (MMA). This MMA has been pedigreed as an assay to predict in vivo RBC survival.[178,179] The MMA results were strongly positive, suggesting that RBCs coated with proteins by nonimmunologic means could have shortened RBC survival.

As discussed previously, the most convincing evidence to prove that a drug is the cause of a hemolytic anemia is to show that hemolytic anemia develops when the patient receives the drug again (accidentally or deliberately). This approach is obviously not usually possible, although it has been used to prove or disprove the role of the drug in the hemolytic process.[9,10,39,141] Although it has been argued that this is the most definitive proof to incriminate the drug in question, some of the early methyldopa data are of interest. Breckenridge and coworkers[9] reintroduced methyldopa in three patients whose methyldopa-induced positive DATs had become negative and found that only one of the three developed a positive DAT again. It is interesting to find, on once again reviewing the cisplatin publications, that six of the eight patients with cisplatin-associated hemolytic anemia were rechallenged with cisplatin following remission of the positive DATs and hemolytic anemia.[161-166] DATs became positive again in all cases, and three developed hemolytic anemia again. These data, together with the data reported in the foregoing discussion, cause us to question our previous assumptions that cisplatin (and other drugs that appear to cause only nonspecific uptake of proteins onto RBC membranes) cause positive DATs but not hemolytic anemia. We now believe that this could be a new mechanism for DIIHA.

SEROLOGIC AND CLINICAL FINDINGS ASSOCIATED WITH DIIHA

The serologic and clinical findings of DIIHA are associated with the previous discussion on the mechanisms thought to cause DIIHA. Regardless of the theoretic concepts, the serologic and clinical characteristics appear to fall into four distinct categories:

1. The penicillin-type drug-dependent antibodies
2. "Nonpenicillin"-type drug-dependent antibodies
3. Drug-independent (auto-) antibodies
4. Nonimmunologic adsorption of proteins onto RBCs

Most investigators would agree that drug antibodies can be classified either as drug independent (drug is not needed to demonstrate reactivity, i.e., autoantibodies) or as drug dependent (presence of drug is needed to demonstrate reactivity). We prefer to categorize the latter group into "penicillin-type" and "nonpencillin-type" antibodies. We do this because the serologic and clinical characteristics of these groups are so different (see Tables 8-4 and 8-5).

The penicillin-type drug-dependent antibody was said to react by a "drug adsorption" mechanism, implying that drug is adsorbed onto the RBC membrane and the drug antibody reacts with the drug-coated RBC. We see nothing wrong with continuing this terminology but could readily accept an alternative descriptive term to describe the mechanism. We do not like the term "hapten mechanism" because it could be applied to all drugs.

Whether we should continue to use the term "immune complex" mechanism to explain how drug-dependent antibodies other than pencillin react is open to debate. Some workers feel strongly that because of the recent criticisms of the theory, we should not continue to use the term. We have an intermediate view and feel that as no other theory has been proven to be correct, it is acceptable to use such terms as "the *so-called* immune complex mechanism," or to put the words "immune complex" in quotation marks to emphasize that it is not a proven fact. It is, of course, perfectly acceptable to use the terms immune complex "hypothesis"or "theory" without adulteration. It is difficult for us to completely reject that drug immune complexes sometimes form, as the serologic findings (e.g., very small amount of drug necessary for in vitro reactions; complement activation leading to lysis of RBCs in vitro) and clinical findings (acute intravascular hemolysis and sometimes renal failure following ingestion of very small quantities of drug) are so typical of immune complex–mediated reactions. We like many aspects of the unifying hypothesis, however.[118,119] Perhaps Shulman and Reid's[139] suggestions are a happy compromise because they appear to embrace the best of both approaches.

Drug-Dependent Antibodies

Drug-dependent antibodies appear to fall into two groups serologically: those that react with drug-coated RBCs (see Table 8-2), and those that are detected only when drugs, RBCs, and antibody are mixed. Of the drugs listed in Table 8-2, only the penicillins and sometimes cephalothin present with consistent characteristics that are different from most other drugs. Among patients receiving large doses of these drugs intravenously, 3–5% develop a positive DAT, and a small percentage of these develop IHA associated with IgG-mediated extravascular hemolysis. In contrast, the other drug-dependent drugs are usually associated with clinical symptoms more typical of immune-complex mediated disease (i.e., acute complement-mediated intravascular hemolysis, sometimes associated with renal failure).

PENICILLIN ANTIBODIES

Between 1959 and 1965, four patients were reported as having hemolytic anemia during penicillin administration, and also as having a positive DAT and penicillin antibodies in their sera. All these patients had serious systemic infection, however, and they also were receiving other drugs. For instance, Ley and colleagues[180] described a patient receiving 18 million units of penicillin daily who was found to have a positive DAT (no prior negative DATs had been recorded). On the seventh day of penicillin therapy, probenecid was added to the regimen, and at that time the hematocrit level began to fall. Despite blood transfusion the fall continued. Therapy with both penicillin and probenecid was then stopped; after further transfusions, the hematocrit level remained stable. The patient subsequently died; penicillin antibody was demonstrated in a sample of blood drawn on the day of death.

In 1966, Petz and Fudenberg[141] were the first to systematically study a case of penicillin-induced hemolytic anemia; they described a patient who developed hemolytic anemia during therapy with high doses of penicillin for suspected bacterial endocarditis (Fig. 8-11). Serologic tests revealed a strongly positive DAT with anti-IgG but negative reactions using an anti-"nongamma" reagent. In spite of the strongly positive DAT, no antibodies could be detected in the patient's serum or in an eluate from the patient's RBCs using standard serologic techniques. Using penicillin-coated RBCs, however, penicillin antibody was demonstrable in the serum by direct agglutination, by IAT, and in an eluate from the patient's RBCs. After the cessation of all drugs except prednisone, hemolysis persisted for about 3 weeks and then gradually resolved. The DAT became progressively weaker and was negative 6 weeks after cessation of the drug. Seven months later, the patient

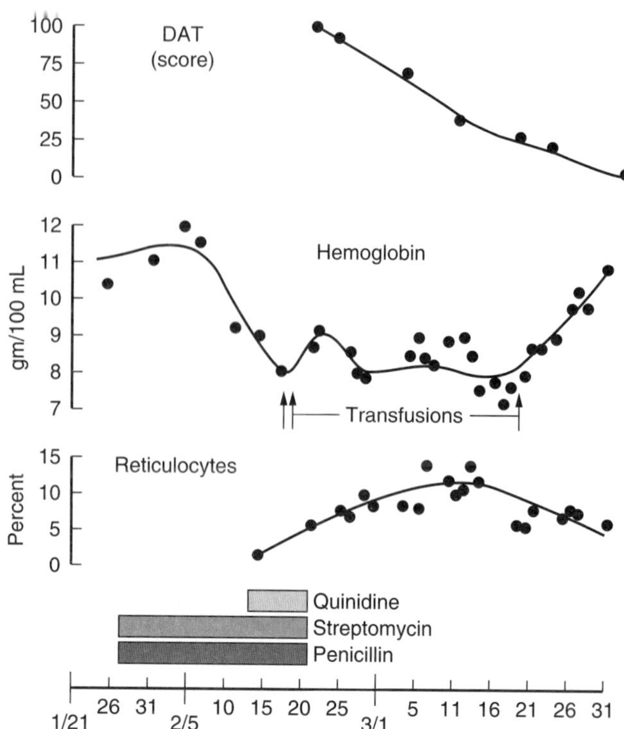

FIGURE 8-11. Course of a patient who developed immune hemolytic anemia while receiving intravenous penicillin for suspected bacterial endocarditis. The direct antiglobulin (Coombs') test was known to have been negative prior to initiation of penicillin therapy. (From Petz LD, Fudenberg HH: Coombs-positive hemolytic anemia caused by penicillin administration. N Engl J Med 1966;274:171–178.)

was challenged with penicillin at a time when there was no evidence of infection, to clarify the role of penicillin in production of hemolysis. All the original findings were reproduced (Fig. 8-12), thereby documenting the etiologic role of penicillin.

Further observations indicated that penicillin differed from drugs that had previously been described as causing thrombocytopenia or hemolytic anemia in that it was strongly bound to the RBC membrane in vitro in the absence of antibody. Indeed, when a serum containing penicillin antibody was tested against RBCs coated with penicillin, there was no decrease in titer even after the RBCs were washed 20–25 times with buffered saline; studies with tritium-labeled penicillin also indicated that penicillin was "firmly bound" to the RBCs.[141]

In approximately 3% of the patients who receive massive doses of intravenous penicillin, positive DATs will develop, but only a small percentage of these develop an obvious hemolytic anemia.[142,181] Levine[182] reported that 5–10% of patients receiving long-term, high-dose penicillin could develop mild hemolytic anemia that might not be noticed because of the underlying disease. The mechanism of the positive DAT and hemolytic anemia seems clear.[1,141] The drug is adsorbed to the RBCs, and the penicillin antibodies present in the patient's plasma react with the penicillin on the RBCs (see Fig. 8-9). The quantity of

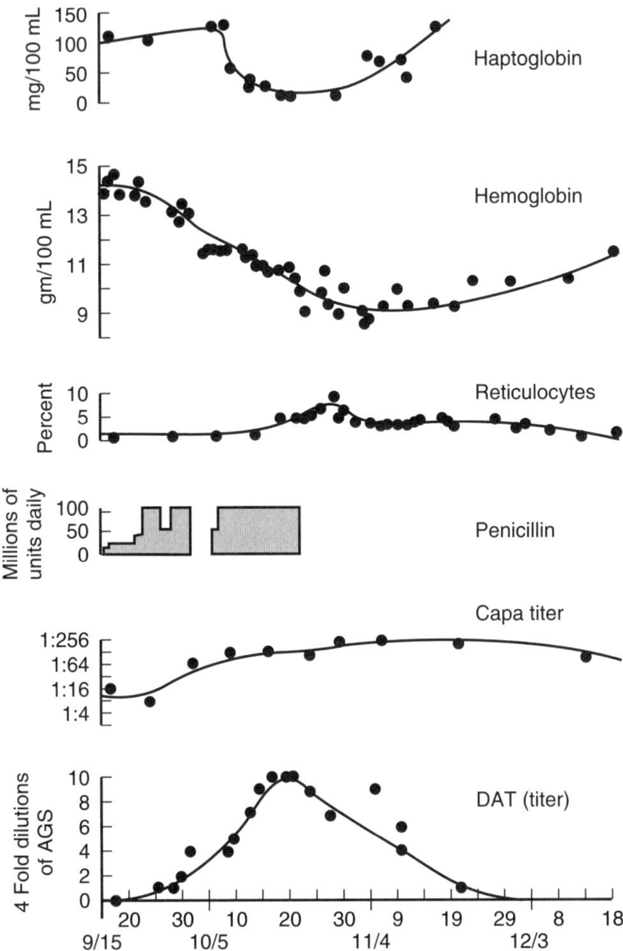

FIGURE 8-12. Documentation of etiologic role of penicillin in causation of immune hemolytic anemia. The patient is the same as in Figure 8-11 and a repeated administration of penicillin caused recurrence of all the original findings. (From Petz LD, Fudenberg HH: Coombs-positive hemolytic anemia caused by penicillin administration. N Engl J Med 1966;274:171–178.)

penicillin (BPO) antibody sensitizing the RBC is limited by the number of BPO haptenic groups on the cell, the plasma concentration of BPO-specific antibodies, and the avidity of the antibodies. Intravascular hemolysis rarely occurs; IgG-sensitized RBCs are removed extravascularly by the reticuloendothelial system in the same way as Rh (IgG) sensitized cells (see Chapter 4). It is interesting to note that although intravascular lysis rarely occurs, penicillin antibodies often hemolyze penicillin-coated RBCs in vitro (the hemolytic antibodies are always of low titer), and complement is detectable on 40% of the RBCs from patients with a positive DAT due to penicillin antibodies.[1]

Kerr and colleagues[146] described a patient whose RBCs reacted strongly with both anti-IgG and anti-complement antiglobulin sera, and they suggested that complement activation could contribute to immune hemolysis in some cases. In addition, we described a patient with penicillin-induced IHA who had intravascular hemolysis of life-threatening severity with hemoglobinemia and hemoglobinuria (Fig. 8-13).[147] Significant amounts of complement components C3 and C4 were detected on the patient's RBCs, in addition to the usual IgG antibody to penicillin. The patient's serum caused direct agglutination of penicillin-coated RBCs and reacted by IAT using anti-IgG, but not anti-C3. The penicillin-coated RBCs were not lysed in vitro, even in the presence of fresh complement. Complement fixation could be demonstrated, however, by incubating the patient's serum with normal serum and then measuring residual hemolytic complement activity. Similar complement fixation could also be demonstrated using serum from a patient with penicillin-induced serum sickness, but fixation could not be demonstrated with the serum of a patient with penicillin-induced hemolytic anemia without intravascular hemolysis, or with the sera of three people with relatively high titers of antibody to penicillin but without hemolytic anemia. The presence of complement components on the patient's RBCs and the finding that her serum fixed complement in vitro suggested that penicillin-antipenicillin immune complexes were present in her serum. We further suggested that RBC damage mediated by immune complexes might have augmented the noncomplement, IgG-mediated hemolysis that is usually seen in penicillin-induced IHA.[147] The unusual severity of hemolysis appeared to result from the high titer of antibody to penicillin (8000) and to participation of the complement system in hemolysis. Funicella and coworkers[148] reported a patient who was treated with ampicillin, oxacillin, and penicillin over an 11-day period. Hemolytic anemia ensued, and the DAT was positive with both anti-IgG and anti-C4/C3. The authors demonstrated the presence of immune complexes using a radiolabeled Clq-binding test, and they suggested that RBC destruction occurred both by the immune complex mechanism and the drug absorption mechanism (which they referred to as the "haptene type").

Our findings in 10 patients with penicillin-induced hemolytic anemia (which includes the patient with intravascular hemolysis described previously) indicate that in a majority of patients, the DAT is positive only with anti-IgG.[1] Four patients in our series and several patients reported by others, however, also had complement components on their RBCs.[1] Although these numbers are small, they suggest that hemolysis might be augmented by complement activation in a significant number of patients. This process might not be efficient enough to cause intravascular hemolysis but could enhance extravascular RBC destruction within the reticuloendothelial system (RES) (see Chapter 4).

One should appreciate that a positive DAT occurring during penicillin administration is not, in itself, an indication for cessation of the drug. Approximately 3% of patients receiving high doses of intravenous penicillin develop a positive DAT, but only a small

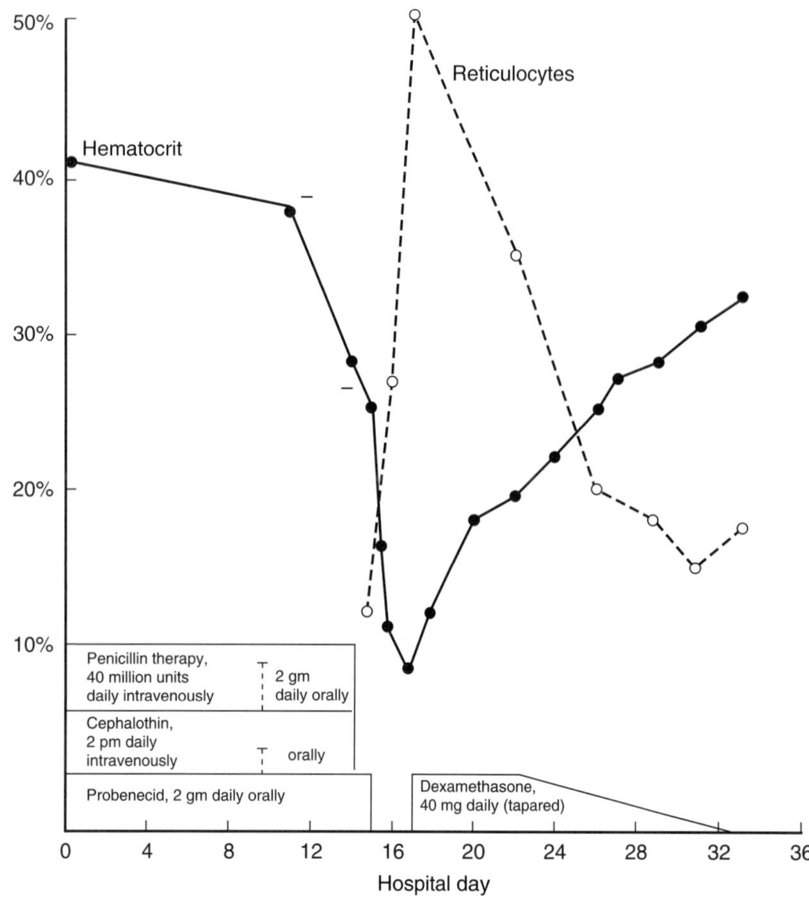

FIGURE 8-13. Clinical course of a patient with penicillin-induced hemolytic anemia with intravascular hemolysis of life-threatening severity. The patient's serum contained penicillin antibody to a titer of 8000, and her RBCs were sensitized with IgG, C3, and C4. She refused transfusion because of religious beliefs and was treated with oxygen, parenteral fluids, and corticosteroids. (From Reis CA, Rosenbaum TJ, Garratty G, et al: Penicillin-induced immune hemolytic anemia. JAMA 1975;233:432–435.)

percentage of these patients develop hemolytic anemia. Hemolysis might not ensue, even with continued administration of the drug.

There is no direct correlation between the presence of IgG and IgM penicillin hemagglutinating antibodies and allergic reactions, but high-titer IgG antibodies were found to occur more often in the allergic group.[182]

The clinical and laboratory features of penicillin-induced IHA are quite constant and are listed in Table 8-4.

Some of the cephalosporins (e.g., cephalothin and cefamandole) also caused drug-induced positive DATs and IHA by a mechanism that appeared the same as that for penicillin.[152,183-187] All of the patients with hemolytic anemia had RBCs sensitized with IgG antibodies to the appropriate cephalosporin, and their sera reacted with cephalosporin-coated RBCs; no intravascular hemolysis was observed. These results were in contrast to the more dramatic complement-mediated intravascular hemolysis associated with some of the newer second- and third-generation cephalosporins (to be discussed shortly).

DIIHA ASSOCIATED WITH PENICILLINS OTHER THAN PENICILLIN G

Penicillins (including semisynthetic products), other than penicillin G, that are used intravenously have caused positive DATs and IHA. Usually, the antibodies detected in the patients' sera react with RBCs coated with the putative penicillins (e.g., ampicillin, amoxicillin, piperacillin, and ticarcillin) and cross-react with penicillin-coated RBCs.[188-194] On rare occasions, this cross-reaction is not observed. Kroovand and associates[195] and Garratty and Brunt[196] reported on two patients who had positive DATs caused by nafcillin antibodies. The antibodies reacted with nafcillin-coated RBCs but not with penicillin-coated RBCs. The antibodies could be adsorbed with nafcillin- and methicillin-coated RBCs but not with penicillin-coated RBCs. Nafcillin and methicillin are the only penicillins that lack a CH group between the side chain and the β-lactam ring. Garratty and Brunt[196] suggested that the CH group in penicillin could sterically interfere with interaction of the nafcillin antibodies. This does not always occur, because we have encountered nafcillin and methicillin antibodies that react well with penicillin-coated RBCs.

On occasion, some penicillins yield unexpected serology. Arndt and coworkers[192] described two patients with cystic fibrosis who developed positive DATs and hemolytic anemia after 11–12 days of therapy with piperacillin or Zosyn (which contains piperacillin) and a β-lactamase inhibitor, tazobactam sodium. Both patients' sera were shown to contain piperacillin antibodies. One patient's serum contained an IgG complement activating antipiperacillin that did not react with piperacillin-coated RBCs but did react with untreated RBCs in the presence of piperacillin (i.e., "immune complex" method). The second patient's serum contained IgG + IgM complement-activating piperacillin antibodies that agglutinated piperacillin-coated RBCs and reacted with untreated RBCs in the presence of piperacillin. The latter patient died of severe intravascular hemolysis.

DRUG-DEPENDENT ANTIBODIES OTHER THAN "PENICILLIN TYPE" ("IMMUNE COMPLEX" MECHANISM)

This group of drug-dependent antibodies, which often is classified as of the "immune complex" mechanism type, includes the largest number of drugs, but many of them are represented by a single case report in the literature. Table 8-5 shows the clinical and serologic characteristics of this group.

The group is characterized by acute intravascular hemolysis, sometimes associated with renal failure. The patient's RBCs are often sensitized with only complement components (e.g., C3dg), but IgG is sometimes also present; on rare occasions only IgG is detected. The patient's serum reacts with RBCs in the presence of the drug and/or of a metabolite of the drug. Using drugs from this group, it is usually not possible to prepare drug-coated RBCs without using chemical coupling techniques (e.g., cross-linking reagents); thus, RBCs pretreated with drug do not react with the patient's serum.[197,198] The drug-dependent antibodies could be IgG and/or IgM; they almost always activate complement. In the presence of the drug, they can cause lysis, agglutination, and/or sensitization of RBCs detectable by the antiglobulin test. Enzyme-treated RBCs almost always react more strongly than untreated RBCs.

Drug-Independent Antibodies

Drug-independent antibodies appear as autoantibodies by serologic testing. That is to say, the antibodies are proven to be induced by a drug but react in vitro without drug being present. Table 8-8 lists drugs that have been reported to cause autoantibody production. It is difficult to prove that a particular drug is responsible for appearance of autoantibodies. As the antibodies react in vitro with RBCs in a way identical to non–drug-induced autoantibodies, they cannot be differentiated serologically. It is not acceptable to blame a drug just because a patient forms RBC autoantibodies after drug administration; this could be coincidental, and often is. If a patient forms autoantibodies after drug administration and hemolysis resolves after discontinuation of the drug, the evidence is better; but it still does not prove the drug caused the hemolysis; the two events could still be coincidental. Often, the patient is also treated with steroids, and remission might not be due to discontinuation of the drug. A good example of this is the cimetidine story discussed earlier in this chapter. Unfortunately, it is extremely difficult to perform such important confirmatory in vivo experiments as those performed by Petz and colleagues,[10] and such experiements could, in fact, be dangerous for a patient whose initial symptoms included acute intravascular hemolysis rather than only a positive DAT or milder extravascular RBC destruction.

TABLE 8-8. DRUGS THAT HAVE BEEN REPORTED TO INDUCE RBC DRUG-INDEPENDENT ANTIBODIES (I.E., AUTOANTIBODIES)

Group I[a]	Group II[c]
cladrabine	azapropazone
fludarabine	carbimazole
levodopa	ceftazidime
mefenamic acid	cefoxitin
methyldopa	cefotetan
procainamide	cefotaxime
catergen[b]	chlorinated hydrocarbons
chaparral[b]	diclofenac
chlordiazepoxide[b]	glafenine
cianidanol	latamoxef
cyclofenil[b]	nomifensine
diphenylhydantoin[b]	phenacetin
fenfluradime[b]	streptomycin
ibuprofen[b]	teniposide
interleukin-2[b]	tolmetin
methoin[b]	zomepirac
methysergide[b]	
rituximab[b]	

[a] These drugs have been reported to induce drug-independent antibodies only.
[b] More evidence is needed to prove that these drugs really can induce RBC autoantibodies.
[c] These drugs induce drug-independent antibodies together with drug dependent antibodies reacting by different mechanisms (see Table 8-3).

Table 8-8 divides the drugs into two groups: those that induce drug-independent antibodies alone and those that induce drug-independent antibodies together with drug-dependent antibodies. We believe that autoantibody production in the two groups could be induced by different mechanisms. The most thoroughly investigated drugs known to induce true autoantibodies are methyldopa and procainamide. In a 10-year period (1970–1980) studying immune hemolytic anemias, we reported that almost 70% of the DIIHAs we encountered were due to methyldopa (23% were due to penicillin).[1] Methyldopa was not used as much in the 1990s, and there are no reports on a large series similar to the one we reported in 1980[1] that would reflect on the incidence of methyldopa-induced hemolytic anemia in the 1990s. Suffice it to say that we have not had a case of methyldopa-induced hemolytic anemia referred to us in the last 10 years. Most of the cases of drug-induced AIHAs are associated with fludarabine (see the discussion later in the chapter). Nevertheless, it is worth discussing the characteristics of methyldopa-induced hemolytic anemia, as it is the prototype of AIHA associated with drugs and has been investigated more thoroughly than other drugs. Table 8-9 lists the characteristics associated with methyldopa-induced RBC autoantibodies.

There are two unanswered questions regarding methyldopa-induced autoantibodies:

1. Why do up to 15% of patients receiving methyldopa make autoantibodies to their own RBCs?
2. Why do only 0.5% of patients with a positive DAT due to methyldopa have hemolytic anemia?

van der Meulen and coworkers[199] suggested the existence of an in vivo hemolytic quantitative threshold. They used flow cytofluorometry to study 29 patients with positive DATs due to IgG1 autoantibodies; 17 of the patients had signs of overt hemolysis, and 12 had no obvious hemolysis. Twelve of the patients were receiving methyldopa; seven of these had overt hemolysis, while the other five had no hemolytic anemia. The authors were able to show a distinct difference in the number of IgG molecules on the RBCs of patients with and without AIHA. There appeared to be a "threshold"—a critical degree of sensitization—above which increased RBC destruction in vivo became apparent. Only two discrepant results were found, one in each group of patients; neither of these were patients taking methyldopa. van der Meulen and coworkers[199] concluded that the quantity of IgG1 autoantibody on the RBCs of DAT-positive patients taking methyldopa was the determining factor for in vivo hemolysis to occur. Garratty and Nance[200] also used flow cytometry to study 104 individuals with positive DATs, with and without AIHA, but they were unable to confirm this conclusion. They confirmed that flow cytometry was much better than the AGT (i.e., titration scores) for differentiating RBCs with different amounts of IgG on them, particularly when they were strongly sensitized (3+ to 4+). Although their results confirmed that the mean amount of RBC-bound IgG was always higher in patients with hemolytic anemia due to autoantibodies (idiopathic and methyldopa-induced) or alloantibodies (hemolytic disease of the newborn), compared with those without hemolytic anemia, they were unable to select a distinct "hemolytic threshold" to differentiate these groups. The range of RBC-bound IgG showed considerable overlap in each group of patients studied.

The differences between the conclusions of van der Meulen and coworkers[199] and Garratty and Nance[200] could not be explained by the subclass of the RBC-bound IgG. Garratty and Nance[200] studied a larger number of patients (104 vs. 29) covering a more diverse population of hemolytic anemias; 12 of the 17 cases of hemolytic anemia studied by van der Meulen and coworkers[199] were due to methyldopa, whereas the series of 28 patients with hemolytic anemia reported by Garratty and Nance[200] included 7 idiopathic cases, 8 methyldopa-induced cases, and 13 with hemolytic disease of the newborn. The conclusions of Garratty and Nance[200] that no definitive "hemolytic threshold" existed, were the same when the methyldopa-induced group was analyzed separately from the total group of hemolytic anemias. In conclusion, although we believe that there is good evidence to suggest that the amount of RBC-bound IgG is a major factor in determining the degree of in vivo RBC destruction, there are significant discrepancies between the amount of RBC-bound IgG and the degree of in vivo hemolysis seen in many cases.

TABLE 8-9. CHARACTERISTICS ASSOCIATED WITH METHYLDOPA-INDUCED RBC AUTOANTIBODIES

10%–30% of patients taking methyldopa develop RBC autoantibodies (i.e., positive DAT) within three to six months of therapy.
Incidence of positive DAT is dose dependent.
Only about 0.5% of patients develop hemolytic anemia.
Serological findings are similar to those associated with idiopathic AIHA, particularly those with only IgG on their RBCs:
- IgG autoantibody on RBCs (17% have weak C3 sensitization in addition to IgG)
- IgG autoantibody often present in serum
- Usually "Rh" specificity

Following cessation of drug therapy, the hemolytic anemia resolves quickly (usually within two weeks), but DAT might remain positive for up to two years.

Laboratory and Clinical Findings Associated with Methyldopa Administration

LABORATORY FINDINGS

Direct Antiglobulin Test. Carstairs and associates[201] performed serologic studies on 202 consecutive hypertensive patients receiving methyldopa and compared the results with those in 76 control patients who had never received methyldopa. Forty-one of the 202 patients (20%) had positive DATs, all of which were caused by coating of the RBCs with IgG only. None of the control patients had a positive DAT of the pure IgG type, but two had a positive test of non-IgG type. Of 65 patients taking 1 g methyldopa or less per day, 7 (11%) had a positive DAT; of 86 patients taking 1–2 g per day, 16 (19%) had a positive test; and of 51 patients taking more than 2 g per day, 18 (36%) had a positive DAT.

The development of a positive DAT usually occurs only after 3–6 months of treatment with the drug, although Hunter and colleagues[202] found that 11 of 26 patients with a positive DAT gave a positive reaction only after 3 or more years of therapy. This delay is not shortened when a patient who previously gave a positive test is restarted on the drug.[201,203-205]

The RBCs of patients with no evidence of hemolysis show varying degrees of reactivity in the DAT, whereas in patients who have overt hemolysis, the reaction is characteristically strongly positive.[1,6,205] In a series of 29 patients with methyldopa-induced hemolysis, the DAT was 2½+ to 4+ in all cases, with 66% of the patients having a 3½+ to 4+ reaction. Worlledge[205] reported that all patients with methyldopa-induced AIHA had a negative DAT using anti-C3, although we found that in four of 29 (14%) patients, the DAT was also weakly positive with anti-C3.[1]

Most patients taking methyldopa have little or no evidence of a shortened RBC survival. The incidence of hemolysis depends on the criteria used for the diagnosis, and minor degrees of hemolysis are probably not infrequent.[206] Six of the 202 patients taking methyldopa who were studied by Carstairs and colleagues[201] had reticulocyte counts between 3 and 6%, and one of four RBC survival studies performed on patients with a positive DAT showed a survival slightly less than normal. In a series of 572 patients on methyldopa therapy, two patients (0.3%) developed overt hemolytic anemia.[206] In a review of 1395 patients receiving methyldopa, 0.8% had overt hemolysis.[6]

Characteristics of the Autoantibody. IgG antibody can be eluted from the RBCs of patients with methyldopa-induced IHA and has been shown to be an autoantibody that reacts with normal RBCs without the addition of the drug.[206] The eluate can be reactive even in patients who have a positive DAT but do not have AIHA. Bakemeier and Leddy,[207] in a detailed study of one patient, showed that the eluted antibodies, although all IgG in type, had both kappa and lambda light chains and were of three distinct heavy chain subclasses. These findings are similar to those in idiopathic AIHA.

Lalezari and colleagues[208] used an antiglobulin test potentiated by polyvinylpyrrolidone (PVP) and detected IgG, IgM, and the first component of complement (Clq) on erythrocytes of eight patients who had hemolysis associated with methyldopa administration, but they found only IgG on the RBCs of three patients who did not have hemolysis. When the hemolyzing patients recovered, IgM and Clq were no longer detectable. These investigators proposed that high-affinity warm-reactive IgM antibodies (not the IgG antibodies) were primarily responsible for hemolysis. IgG and its subclasses were variably present on RBCs of all patients, regardless of hemolytic activity. Unfortunately, this finding has not been studied by other investigators.

Attempts to Demonstrate Specificity for Drug-Related Antigens. LoBuglio and Jandl[209] attempted to demonstrate specificity of the antibody for drug-related antigens by several methods. They incubated normal RBCs with methyldopa in concentrations of 1–5 mmol/L for 2 hours at 37°C and for 18 hours at 4°C; after subsequent incubation with the patients' sera, no agglutination or sensitization to antiglobulin serum took place. At higher concentrations of drug, serum proteins adsorbed nonspecifically to the RBCs, and there was no difference between patients' and control sera. Also, the mixture of methyldopa in concentrations of 1–5 mmol/L added to mixtures of normal RBCs and patients' sera did not induce a positive antiglobulin reaction. Inhibition tests were performed by adding methyldopa in concentrations of 0.1 to 10 mmol/L to sera or eluates, but this did not inhibit the activity of eluates toward normal RBCs or of serum activity toward enzyme-treated cells. The following metabolites or congeners of methyldopa yielded similar results:

- 1-(3,4-dihydroxyphenyl)-2-amino propanol
- D-2 methyl-3,4-dihydroxyphenylalanine hydrate
- L-2 methyl-3,4-dihydroxyphenylalanine hydrate
- R(-) l-(3,4-dihydroxylphenyl)-2-amino propane hydrochloride
- l-(3-methoxy-4-hydroxyphenyl)-2-amino propane hydrochloride
- l-(3-methoxy-4-hydroxyphenyl)-2-propanone
- (+)4-(2-amino propyl)-2-methoxyphenol hydrochloride

The results of inhibition and enhancement experiments were also reported by Worlledge.[108] They attempted to inhibit the antibodies in patients' sera by incubation with methyldopa or its derivatives, including methyldopa hydrochloride, D-α-methyldopamine hydrochloride, L-α-methyldopamine hydrochloride, and L-α-methyl-noradrenaline. Sera taken from three patients 3 hours after ingestion of 500 mg of methyldopa tablets was also tested as an inhibitor.

Additional experiments were performed in an attempt to enhance the activity of the serum autoantibody by using RBCs that had previously been incubated with methyldopa, its derivatives, or the serum of patients on methyldopa therapy.

None of the in vitro tests by LoBuglio and Jandl[209] or by Worlledge and colleagues[105] yielded positive results; both groups of investigators concluded that by none of the techniques available could it be established that methyldopa participated as antigen or hapten in sensitizing RBCs.

Specificity of Drug-Induced Autoantibodies. Worlledge[205] tested eluates from RBCs of 26 patients with methyldopa-induced hemolysis against two samples of Rh_{null} RBCs (one with abnormalities of the S, s, and U antigens and one without these abnormalities), two samples of U-negative RBCs, one sample of LW-negative RBCs, and RBCs of ordinary Rh genotypes. One third of the eluates showed some specificity for cells of ordinary Rh genotypes on dilution, and all but two eluates either did not react or yielded very weak reactions with both samples of Rh_{null} RBCs while reacting strongly with the other cells. The two eluates that seemed to react as well with Rh_{null} RBCs as with other RBCs were adsorbed with all the RBC samples. Adsorption with the Rh_{null} RBCs left an antibody that reacted only with the other RBCs and did not react with the Rh_{null} RBCs; adsorption with other RBCs removed all of the antibody. None of the eluates showed any anti-U or anti-LW specificity, and the antibodies in the serum reacted in a similar way.

Specificity for Rh antigens was confirmed by other investigators.[207,209] Bakemeier and Leddy[207] showed that at least four serologically separable antibodies were present: anti-c, anti-e, and two antibodies reacting with two defined antigens or groups of antigens absent from Rh_{null} RBCs. The most common specificity of autoantibody is against antigens of the Rh system. Much less commonly reported target antigens are Wr^b, Jk^a, and U.[210-212] The proportion of cases in which the antibody is directed against an antigen within the Rh system varies from 100% to 30%.[204,207] In some cases, the antibody has specificity for more than one antigen.[1,207]

Thus, it is remarkable that the antibodies not only react with normal RBCs but also show Rh specificity, and the pattern of specificity is similar to that of autoantibodies eluted from the RBCs or present in the serum of patients suffering from "idiopathic" AIHA of warm antibody type (see Chapter 7).

Reticuloendothelial Function. Branch and coworkers[213] and Gallagher and associates[214] studied monocytes and macrophages collected from the peripheral blood of patients receiving methyldopa and found that the circulating monocytes of the hemolyzing patients (but not of the nonhemolyzing patients) phagocytosed the DAT positive RBCs in vitro. Yust and colleagues[215] have reported similar findings. Other investigators have studied reticuloendothelial function in vivo by measuring the rate of clearance of radiolabeled autologous RBCs that have been heat damaged or sensitized by alloantibodies. Kelton[216] studied reticuloendothelial function in nine patients taking methyldopa. Five of the nine patients had a positive DAT. Only one patient had laboratory evidence of hemolysis. The patients without hemolysis had significantly impaired reticuloendothelial clearance. In contrast, the patient with hemolysis did not have impaired reticuloendothelial function. Kelton[216] suggested that the absence of hemolysis in many patients with methyldopa-induced autoantibodies could be caused by an impairment in reticuloendothelial function and, moreover, that the drug itself might be responsible for the impairment because abnormal reticuloendothelial function was found in patients taking the drug who had a negative DAT (Fig. 8-14).

CLINICAL FEATURES

Hemolytic anemia has been diagnosed as early as 18 weeks and as late as 4 years after the start of treatment with methyldopa.[217,218] Even though the incidence of a positive DAT increases with higher doses of the drug, there is no relation between the amount of methyldopa taken and the intensity of the anemia.[201] Eighteen of the 25 patients reported by Worlledge and colleagues[105] were taking 1 g or less of methyldopa per day. In some patients, the onset of hemolysis seemed to be acute, but in most it was insidious.

In 13 of the 25 cases (52%), enlargement of the liver and lymph nodes was absent but a variable degree of splenomegaly was present. In all anemic patients, the peripheral blood films showed spherocytosis and polychromasia and were indistinguishable from the films of other cases of AIHA of the warm antibody type.

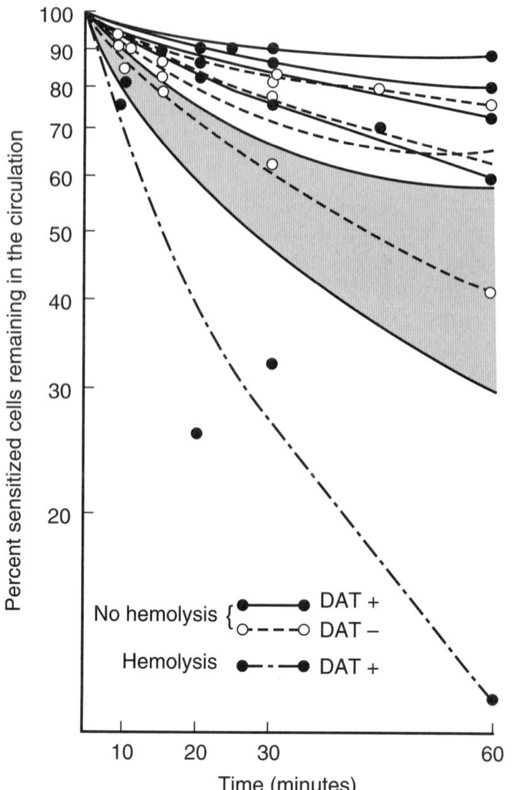

FIGURE 8-14. The clearence of IgG-sensitized Cr-labeled autologous RBCs in patients taking methyldopa. Four patients had positive DATs and no hemolysis (•—•), and four patients had negative DATs and no hemolysis (o---o). One patient had a positive DAT and hemolytic anemia (•---•). The hatched area represents the mean (±SD) clearance in 12 healthy controls. (Reprinted by permission of Kelton JG: Impaired reticuloendothelial function in patients treated with methyldopa. N Engl J Med 1985;313:596-600.)

DIAGNOSIS OF DRUG-INDUCED AIHA

There are no diagnostic serologic features of drug-induced AIHA that distinguish such cases from AIHA not caused by a drug. Thus, the diagnosis rests on the demonstration of characteristic serologic findings of AIHA of warm antibody type in a patient taking a drug known to cause AIHA. Resolution of hemolysis after discontinuing the drug strengthens the diagnosis, and recurrence of immunohematologic findings and hemolysis after restarting the drug confirms the diagnosis, but taking this step is ordinarily not appropriate. Although there are no diagnostic laboratory features, certain findings are particularly characteristic of methyldopa-induced AIHA and, if absent, would tend to exclude the diagnosis. If the DAT is negative or only weakly positive using anti-IgG or if no autoantibody is detected in the patient's serum, the diagnosis of methyldopa-induced AIHA is highly unlikely.[1,105,213]

BLOOD TRANSFUSION

The indications for blood transfusion and the methods appropriate for compatibility testing in patients with methyldopa-induced AIHA are the same as those for warm antibody AIHA not associated with methyldopa administration (see Chapter 10). Some patients who have a positive DAT caused by methyldopa but who do not have evidence of hemolysis might nevertheless have a positive IAT. Also, Worlledge[217] reported that a positive DAT is always accompanied by free IgG autoantibodies demonstrable with enzyme-treated RBCs. The presence of autoantibody in the patient's serum, especially when reactive by IAT, results in an incompatible cross-match test and makes difficult the detection of RBC alloantibodies. This problem can be circumvented by adsorbing the autoantibody from the serum using RBCs that do not adsorb alloantibodies from the patient's serum, that is, by performance of warm autoadsorption tests using autologous RBC or selected allogeneic RBC (see Chapter 10). It is reassuring that, if no alloantibodies are present and the patient has no laboratory evidence of hemolysis, transfused RBCs seem to survive normally even when both the DAT and IAT are positive.[219] Autologous blood for transfusion in patients who have a positive DAT and IAT but who do not have AIHA also may be used.[220,221]

Some patients receiving methyldopa and in need of blood transfusion might have a positive DAT but a negative IAT and no evidence of hemolysis. For these patients, the major cross-match test indicates compatibility, and transfused RBC can be expected to survive normally.

Laboratory and clinical features of methyldopa-induced AIHA are summarized in Table 8-9.

AIHA CAUSED BY DRUGS OTHER THAN METHYLDOPA

A number of drugs other than methyldopa have caused AIHA, as indicated in Table 8-8.

Purine Analogues

The most common drug by far to cause AIHA in current practice is a purine analogue, fludarabine.[222-246] A British group reported that 14 of 66 patients (21%) with chronic lymphocytic leukemia (CLL) developed AIHA following fludarabine therapy.[230,240] Another study from France found that 8 of 36 patients (22%) developed AIHA.[237] It is sometimes difficult to be confident that fludarabine caused the AIHA, as 10–20% of CLL patients are said to develop AIHA at some stage of their disease; 1.8–35% of CLL patients have been reported to develop positive DATs.[231] Data strongly implicating fludarabine administration as a cause of AIHA were reported by Diehl and Ketchum.[242] These authors reviewed reports indicating that 15 of 19 patients (79%) rechallenged with fludarabine experienced recurrence of the AIHA. Convincing data also came from a prospective randomized trial of cyclophosphamide, doxorubicin, and prednisone (CAP) vs. fludarabine in newly diagnosed or relapsed CLL patients.[243] In the fludarabine arm, 5% of the patients had autoimmune phenomena (2% AIHA, 2% ITP, 1% pure red cell aplasia), whereas no patients in the CAP arm had autoimmune phenomena.[243]

Di Raimondo and coworkers[224] found only five cases of AIHA among 112 CLL patients without preexisting HA who were treated with fludarabine; a further four patients had preexisting HA that deteriorated following treatment with fludarabine. Vick and associates[232] have described a case of "mixed-type" AIHA following the fifth cycle of fludarabine therapy. Myint and colleagues[226] reported that hemolysis occurred after a mean of four courses of fludarabine and that the hemolysis tended to be severe and to have an abrupt onset. The HA responded to steroid therapy (1 mg/kg). In some cases, it was possible to administer further fludarabine safely, but commonly, further courses exacerbated the hemolysis.

Some reports describe catastrophic hemolysis leading to a fatal outcome.[227,228] Such massive hemolysis appearing abruptly is not characteristic of AIHA occurring in CLL and is further evidence of the effect of fludarabine. An additional case of fatal AIHA was reported by Byrd and coworkers[225] in a patient who had recurrent fludarabine-associated AIHA and who was challenged with the adenosine deaminase inhibitor pentostatin, a potent immunosuppressant with no known fludarabine cross-reactivity. Orchard and associates[244] reported on a patient who had an episode of severe AIHA 19 weeks after the last of three courses of fludarabine; he did not respond to corticosteroids, but his hemoglobin returned to normal after a splenectomy. Three months later, at a time when his hemoglobin and platelet count were normal, he was treated with chlorambucil, 10 mg/day. After nine days of treatment, his hemoglobin was normal, but the next day he was admitted in a moribund state with a hemoglobin of 5.0 g/dL and evidence of severe hemolysis. Despite treatment with steroids, his hemoglobin fell further, and he died.

There are two reports of Evans's syndrome complicating fludarabine treatment for CLL. Shvidel and colleagues[245] described a patient who, after two cycles of fludarabine, developed AIHA and a drop in platelet count from normal levels to 12,000/μL. He recovered from Evans's syndrome after treatment with cyclosporine and prednisone. Sen and Kalaycio[246] reported on a 64-year-old woman who had a white count of 150,000/μL, a hemoglobin of 11 g/dL, and a platelet count of 250,000/μL. She was treated with two cycles of fludarabine, and 10 days later her DAT was positive, the white blood cell count was 14,000/μL, hemoglobin was 5.5 g/dL, and platelet count was 5000/μL. The patient improved during treatment with prednisone but ultimately required a splenectomy before entering into a durable remission of hemolysis with successful withdrawal of her corticosteroids.

Orchard and coworkers[244] summarized the association of AIHA and fludarabine as follows. AIHA is unlikely to occur in patients with de novo CLL who are being treated for the first time with fludarabine. Among patients who have been treated with multiple courses of alkylating agents, however, exposure to fludarabine triggers AIHA in about 20% of cases. The hemolysis is usually severe, difficult to treat, and can prove fatal. Autoimmune thrombocytopenia might also be present. After treatment with fludarabine, patients with AIHA are liable to relapse if they are reexposed to fludarabine, cladribine, or pentostatin. Also, other forms of potent immunosuppressive chemotherapy could cause a recurrence of fludarabine-induced AIHA, adding support to the hypothesis that effects on the cellular immune system are the basis for the development of AIHA in this setting.

AIHA has also been associated with 2-chlorodeoxyadenosine (cladribine). In one study, only two of 114 CLL patients (1.8%) with no AIHA before receiving cladribine developed AIHA after five and six courses of cladribine, respectively.[229] On the other hand, 23 patients had signs of AIHA before treatment with cladribine; the hemolytic anemia resolved completely for six patients and resolved partially for eight patients.[229] Chasty and coworkers[231] reported that four of 19 CLL patients (21%) treated with cladribine developed AIHA, which was the same incidence reported by the same group for fludarabine.[226] Hamblin and coworkers[235] reported that one patient with fludarbine-induced AIHA had severe hemolysis after receiving cladribine subsequently. They suggested that any purine analogue could lead to exacerbated hemolysis, and others have shown that even conventional chemotherapy (e.g., chlorambucil-based regimes) can exacerbate hemolysis.

Fludarabine is the 2-fluoro derivative of adenine avalinoside. The added fluoro group enables fludarabine to resist inactivation by adenosine deaminase, an enzyme found in high levels in lymphocytes.[241] The drug enters the cells in the form of fluoro-ara-A metabolite and is phosphorylated to a triphosphate that accumulates in cells and inhibits DNA and RNA synthesis.[241] It might also activate apoptosis. Fludarabine seems to exert an immunosuppressive effect on the CD4 subset of lymphocytes, thus leading to an impairment in the CD4/CD8 ratio, which could influence the induction or recurrence of RBC autoantibody.

Levodopa

Henry and associates[247] studied 80 patients with Parkinson's disease who received levodopa therapy and found three patients who developed a positive DAT caused by IgG sensitization after eight to 11 months of therapy, and an additional two patients with complement-coated RBCs. Eluates prepared from IgG-sensitized cells reacted strongly with all RBCs except Rh_{null} cells. None of the patients developed overt AIHA.

Joseph[248] reported that the incidence of a positive DAT was 9.5% among patients taking levodopa for longer than 90 days.

Gabor and Goldberg[249] reported a patient who developed AIHA after 4 years of therapy with levodopa. Six weeks after discontinuation of the drug, the hematologic values had returned to normal, and the DAT and IAT were negative. Five months following reinstitution of the drug, AIHA recurred and again resolved on discontinuation of the drug.

Anti-e specificity of levodopa-induced autoantibodies was reported by Lindstrom and coworkers[250] and by Bernstein,[251] and in the case reported by Territo and associates,[252] an eluate reacted with all RBCs except Rh_{null} cells.

Procainamide

Kleinman and colleagues[256] studied the prevalence of a positive DAT and IHA among 100 patients receiving procainamide and among 100 age- and sex-matched controls. There was a significant increase in the frequency of a positive DAT among patients receiving procainamide compared with controls; three patients had AIHA. The mean duration of procainamide administration was 23.8 months for the patients with positive DATs and 21.3 months for those with negative tests. Eluates were prepared from the RBCs of 18 patients with a positive DAT and gave positive results in 10 instances, including all three patients with hemolytic anemia. Seven of the 10 positive eluates were panagglutinins, and three showed Rh specificity, demonstrated by a lack of reactivity with Rh_{null} cells. In addition, there are multiple individual case reports of AIHA caused by procainamide.[253-255]

The presence of antinuclear factor (ANF) or clinical lupus syndrome was determined in 18 patients with a positive DAT.[253] The prevalence of ANF was 78%, which is similar to the rate previously reported for patients receiving procainamide. None of the three patients with hemolytic anemia had clinical evidence of drug-induced lupus, but two of the 15 without HA did have it.[253]

Nonsteroidal Anti-inflammatory Drugs

Immune hemolytic anemia has been reported following administration of nonsteroidal anti-inflammatory drugs (NSAIDs), but in many instances the serologic testing has been incomplete and the presence of RBC autoantibodies has not been documented well. In a detailed review in 1986, Sanford-Driscoll and Knodel[257] concluded that mefenamic acid caused HA by an autoimmune mechanism but that there was insufficient information concerning ibuprofen, sulindac, naproxen, tolmetin, and feprazone to assign specific mechanisms of immune hemolysis.

There have been multiple reports since that time,[258-273] but no convincing evidence that these drugs induce true autoantibodies. Many of the reports indicate that when autoantibodies are present, they are present together with drug-dependent antibodies.

In a number of instances, hemolysis associated with the administration of NSAIDs was part of a complex clinical picture involving multisystem organ failure with renal insufficiency, shock, and disseminated intravascular coagulation.[272,273]

Nomifensine

Nomifensine is an antidepressant drug that was used for about 8 years in Europe and for a much shorter time in the United States, having been withdrawn from sale worldwide in 1986 because of reports of side effects, which included numerous cases of immune hemolytic anemia. A variety of serologic reactions were reported, with most patients having drug-dependent antibodies and a syndrome of acute intravascular hemolysis as is typical of drugs reacting by the "immune complex" mechanism. There are multiple reports, however, of patients with nomifensine-induced immune hemolysis whose serum contained only RBC autoantibodies, some of which showed some Rh specificity.[274-276]

Alpha-Interferon

The occurrence of autoimmune disease among patients receiving alpha-interferon (α-IFN) therapy has been reported in several studies, and included among such side effects is the development of AIHA.[277-287]

The incidence of AIHA caused by α-IFN appears to be quite low. In a retrospective series of 11,241 consecutive patients with chronic viral hepatitis treated with α-IFN, Fattovich and colleagues[283] observed two cases of AIHA. Andriani and associates[278] observed nine patients over a ten-year period. Seven of the patients had been receiving α-IFN for a lymphoproliferative disorder, and two patients had chronic myelogenous leukemia. In all cases, the onset of hemolysis was acute and severe and was associated with a positive DAT. In five patients, the serum antibody was characterized and found to be a panagglutinin (IgG in four cases and IgA in one case). The interval between the start of α-IFN and AIHA varied from 1 day to 38 months. All patients recovered after discontinuation of the drug and treatment with prednisone. Fornaciari and coworkers[284] reported a patient in whom AIHA had occurred within one month after initiation of α-INF; after reintroduction of α-IFN 1 year leater, AIHA recurred within the same interval.

Other Drugs

Still other drugs may cause AIHA, for example, chlorpromazine, diphenylhydantoin, methoin, methysergide, chlordiazepoxide, interleukin-2, rituximab, and fenfluramine, although for these drugs the characterization of the responsible antibodies as RBC autoantibodies is less definite.

Cimetidine therapy has been reported to be associated with AIHA in one patient and with a case of hemolytic anemia with a negative DAT.[288,289] The authors of both reports express caution in implicating the drug, however. This caution was emphasized by Petz and associates.[10]

IMMUNE HEMOLYTIC ANEMIA AND/OR POSITIVE DATs ASSOCIATED WITH THE CEPHALOSPORINS

Cephalosporins differ from penicillins only in having a six-numbered dihydrothiazine ring instead of the five-nucleated thiazoldine ring, and in their side-chain groups (see Figs. 8-2 and 8-15). Thus, it is not surprising that the cephalosporins also have induced positive DATs, IHA, thrombocytopenia, and neutropenia. Nevertheless, cephalosporins were used for more than 25 years before immune cell destruction by the cephalosporins became a problem.

The cephalosporins have been grouped into "generations" on the basis of their spectrum of activity against gram-negative organisms.[290,291] First-generation cephalosporins were first used in the United States in 1964. Second-generation cephalosporins started to be used in 1976 (cefotetan was used from 1985), and third-generation cephalosporins came into common use in 1981 (ceftriaxone was used from 1984 onward). Table 8-10 lists the cephalosporins according to their generations and their respective proprietary names. In general, the pharmacologic properties of the cephalosporins are similar. Most are administered by parental injection, have a plasma half-life of approximately 1 to 2 hours, and are excreted unchanged from the body mainly via the urinary tract. Six of the cephalosporins (cephalexin, cefadroxil, cephradine, cefaclor, cefuroxime axetil, and cefixime) are used orally and are less likely to cause immune cytopenia because of the relatively lower dose used compared with those used intravenously.

Cephalosporin-Induced Positive DATs

In 1967, Molthan and colleagues[149] and Gralnick and coworkers[150] reported that 81% and 40%, respectively, of patients receiving cephalothin developed positive DATs. The patients were all quite ill and were receiving large doses of intravenous cephalothin (8–14 g/day and 2–8 g/day, respectively). Later workers found a much lower incidence of positive DATs. Petz[181] found that only 3% of 124 patients receiving an average dose of 6.3 g/day for an average of 5.5 days developed a positive DAT. Spath and coworkers[152] found that 4% of 97 patients receiving an average of 6.3 g/day for

USE OF CARBODIIMIDE TO COUPLE DRUGS TO RBCs[198,373]

Purpose of Test:
Carbodiimide is used to couple proteins and other compounds (e.g., drugs) with a variety of functional groups (i.e., carboxylic acids, amines, alcohols) to RBCs when the usual pH coupling method does not work.

Materials:

1. Carbodiimide: 1-ethyl-3-(3dimethyl-aminopropyl) carbodiimide HCl (stored frozen).
2. Drug to be coupled to RBCs.
3. Group O reagent RBCs, washed and resuspended to 50%.
4. Phosphate-buffered saline (PBS), pH 7.3.
5. 2% EDTA-PBS:
   2 g EDTA, tetrasodium salt in 100 mL PBS
   Adjust the pH to 7.2 with 1 N HCl
   Prepare this reagent ahead of time because it takes a while for the EDTA to go into solution; the reagent is to be used cold (4°C).

Procedure:

1. Dissolve 20 mg of drug in 3 mL PBS.
2. To a second tube, add 3 mL of PBS.
3. Add 0.1 mL of 50% washed RBCs to each tube.
4. Freshly prepare the carbodiimide solution: Dissolve 50 mg of carbodiimide in 1 mL deionized H_2O.
5. Add 0.5 mL carbodiimide solution to each tube.
6. Incubate at 4°C for 50 minutes.
7. Pour the carbodiimide mixtures into a 16 × 100 mm tube containing 5 mL of cold (4°C) EDTA-PBS.
8. Wash the RBCs three times in PBS.
9. Test the drug-carbodiimide–treated RBCs, the carbodiimide-treated RBCs, and untreated RBCs using the desired method.

Notes:

1. RBCs treated with carbodiimide without protein tend to stick to glass tubes, similar to glutaraldehyde-treated RBCs.
2. Use carbodiimide-treated RBCs as soon as possible after treatment. We have found that reactivity can weaken within hours of treatment.
3. When coupling a cephalosporin (or other drug known to cause nonspecific adsorption of protein) to RBCs using the carbodiimide method, include normal plasma/serum as a negative control for the test system.

DETECTION OF ANTIBODIES TO DRUGS BY THE IMMUNE COMPLEX METHOD

Materials:

1. Drug, 1 mg/mL in PBS (see "Preparation of Drug Solutions" procedure).
2. Phosphate-buffered saline (PBS), pH 7.3.
3. Fresh normal serum (source of complement [C]), thawed.
4. Pooled untreated and enzyme-treated group O RBCs (e.g., antigen detection RBCs), antigen negative if appropriate.
5. Polyspecific antihuman globulin serum; antiglobulin control cells.
6. 10 × 75-mm test tubes; 37°C incubator; serologic centrifuge; cell washer (optional).

Procedure:

1. Label two sets of 10 × 75-mm tubes for each drug to be tested: serum plus drug, serum plus PBS, serum plus C plus drug, serum plus C plus PBS, C plus drug, C plus PBS. Label 1 set of tubes "UT" (for untreated RBCs) and the other set of tubes "ET" (for enzyme-treated RBCs).
2. To each tube add two drops patient's serum, two drops fresh normal serum ("complement"), two drops drug solution, or two drops PBS as appropriate.
3. To the set labeled "UT," add one drop 6%–10% untreated RBCs. To the set labeled "ET," add one drop 6%–10% enzyme-treated RBCs.
4. Incubate both sets of tubes at 37°C for 1 to 2 hours with gentle periodic mixing.
5. Centrifuge and examine tests for hemolysis and agglutination. Record results.
6. Wash RBCs four times with PBS.
7. Add antiglobulin sera. Centrifuge and inspect for agglutination (examine all macroscopically negative tests microscopically). Record results.
8. Add antiglobulin control cells to all nonreactive tests. Centrifuge and inspect for agglutination. Record macroscopically positive results with a checkmark.

Quality Control:

1. The tubes with serum plus C plus PBS should normally be nonreactive. Reactivity in these control tubes can be compared with the appropriate test with drug solution. See interpretation.
2. The tubes with C plus drug and C plus PBS should be nonreactive. If positive and the patient's serum plus drug/PBS (without C in the test system) was noninformative, repeat the test with a new source of complement.

Interpretation:
Hemolysis, agglutination, or positive IATs might occur together or separately. A positive result for any of the patient's tests to which the drug was added, and a negative (or significantly weaker) result for the corresponding negative control tests (i.e., tubes in which PBS was substituted for drug and tubes with no patient's serum added) suggests the presence of an antibody to the drug being studied.

Examples of reactivity that might be seen and the interpretation are shown in Table 8-17:

Notes:

1. The decision regarding whether an eluate from the patient's RBCs should be tested by this method needs to be made on a case-by-case basis.
2. If positive test results are obtained, the antibody titer can be determined by preparing dilutions of the patient's serum in PBS (for agglutination and indirect antiglobulin test results) or in fresh normal serum (for hemolysis results) and testing those dilutions by the foregoing procedure. The titer is the reciprocal of the last dilution that reacts 1+.
3. If negative test results are obtained but the patient's clinical history warrants further evaluation, the following should be considered:
   a. Use of drug metabolites (ex vivo antigen), such as urine or serum from (an)other patient(s) taking the drug, instead of the drug solution; check previous publications for optimal source, timing of sample post drug ingestion, etc. Urine might need some processing (centrifuge to remove any precipitate/solid material, and check pH [see "Preparation of Drug Solutions" procedure, Note 4]).
   b. Use of different concentrations of drug (e.g., a saturated solution and dilutions of the drug).
   c. Wash for the antiglobulin test using a solution of drug (e.g., 10 mg drug in 500 mL of PBS) instead of PBS.

TABLE 8-17. INTERPRETATION OF RESULTS OF IMMUNE COMPLEX METHOD

Example	Serum ± C	37°C	IAT	Interpretation
1	+ drug	0	0	Negative (no drug antibody present)
	+ PBS	0	0	
2	+ drug	0	2+	Positive (drug antibody present)
	+ PBS	0	0	
3	+ drug	hemolysis +/− agglutination	1+	Positive (drug antibody present); weak auto- and/or alloantibody also present
	+ PBS	0	1+	
4	+ drug	0	1+	Negative (no drug antibody detected); weak auto- and/or alloantibody present (could miss weak drug antibody)
	+ PBS	0	1+	
5	+ drug	0	3+	Not interpretable due to presence of auto- and/or alloantibodies; test serum dilutions, adsorbed serum, and/or antigen-negative RBCs
	+ PBS	0	3+	

DETECTION OF ANTIBODIES TO CEFOTETAN

Procedure:

1. Prepare (see separate procedure) or thaw cefotetan-treated and untreated RBCs (at least eight to ten drops of a 3%–5% v/v suspension of each will be needed).
2. Prepare a 1 in 100 dilution of patient's serum/plasma in PBS (e.g., 0.01 mL serum/plasma plus 0.99 mL PBS, or one drop serum/plasma plus nine drops PBS, then one drop of the 1:10 dilution plus nine drops PBS).
3. For each sample to be tested, label two 10 × 75-mm test tubes: cefotetan-treated (CT) or untreated (UT). See sample worksheet.
4. Add two drops of patient's serum, patient's diluted serum, diluted positive control, PBS, eluate, or last wash to each of the two labeled tubes.
5. To the set of tubes labeled "CT," add one drop of 3%–5% (v/v) cefotetan-treated RBCs.
6. To the set of tubes labeled "UT," add one drop of 3%–5% (v/v) untreated RBCs.
7. Incubate 60 minutes at 37°C.
8. Centrifuge and examine tests for agglutination and/or hemolysis. Record results.
9. Wash four times with PBS.
10. Add AHG or anti-IgG to all tubes. Centrifuge and read for agglutination (check all macroscopically negative results microscopically). Record results.
11. Add AHG control cells to all nonreactive tests. Centrifuge and read. Record positive results with a checkmark.

Quality Control:

1. The positive control should be reactive with the cefotetan-treated RBCs and nonreactive with the untreated RBCs. The PBS-negative control should be nonreactive with the cefotetan-treated and untreated RBCs.
2. The positive plasma control, when diluted 1 in 100, should be strongly (3+ to 4+) reactive with the cefotetan-treated RBCs but nonreactive with the untreated RBCs. This expected reactivity provides a check for the stability of cefotetan-treated RBCs that have been stored frozen and the reactivity of antibody that might have been frozen-thawed multiple times. If the reactivity of the plasma is less than 3+ with cefotetan-treated RBCs (especially those that have been stored frozen), repeat the test with a fresh aliquot of control serum/plasma or with freshly treated RBCs.
3. A different positive control or a higher dilution of the plasma might not react as strongly with the cefotetan-treated RBCs.
4. Antiglobulin control cells should be macroscopically reactive.
5. Repeat the test if controls are not reacting as expected.

Interpretation:

1. A positive reaction of the patient's serum (i.e., undiluted serum = hemolysis, and/or the 1 in 100 dilution of serum/plasma = agglutination and/or positive antiglobulin test) or eluate with cefotetan-treated RBCs but not with untreated RBCs usually indicates the presence of an antibody to cefotetan (see Notes 1, 2). Reactions with the untreated RBCs could indicate the presence of alloantibod(y)(ies) or autoantibod(y)(ies) (see Notes 3, 4).
2. No reaction of the patient's serum and eluate with cefotetan-treated RBCs indicates that no cefotetan antibody is present.

Notes:

1. Sera/plasmas are diluted at least 1:100 to avoid the false-positive results (indirect antiglobulin test) seen when testing undiluted serum/plasma against cefotetan-treated RBCs. These false-positive tests are due to direct agglutination or nonimmunologic protein adsorption by the cefotetan-coated RBCs. There is usually not enough protein in serum diluted 1 in 100 or in an eluate to cause this problem.
2. The last-wash control can sometimes react with cefotetan-treated RBCs. If this reactivity is weaker than that of the eluate (i.e., eluate plus cefotetan-treated RBCs = 2+ to 3+, last wash plus cefotetantreated RBCs = w+), then the eluate can be interpreted as positive. If the reactivity of the eluate and last wash are similar, one can dilute both the eluate and last wash (e.g., 1 in 10 or 1 in 20 in PBS) and repeat the test; if the diluted eluate is reactive and the diluted last wash is nonreactive, then the eluate can be interpreted as positive. Fewer strongly positive (>1+) last washes were seen when RBCs were washed with LISS (vs. PBS) when the Gamma Elu-Kit II was used for eluate preparation.[352]
3. If the patient has alloantibod(y)(ies) or autoantibod(y)(ies) that react(s) with untreated RBCs even at the 1 in 100 dilution, prepare dilutions of the patient's serum (e.g., 1 in 500, 1 in 1000) and retest against untreated and cefotetan-treated RBCs. Antibodies to cefotetan typically have titers in the thousands; alloantibodies and autoantibodies should not be reactive to such high titers.[104]
4. About 30% of patients with antibodies to cefotetan also have drug-independent antibody that reacts with untreated RBCs.[104]
5. Antibodies to cefotetan usually also react by the "immune complex" method.[104]

DRUG (HAPTEN) INHIBITION[193]

Materials:

1. Drug solution, 10 mg/mL in PBS (see "Preparation of Drug Solutions" method).
2. Phosphate-buffered saline (PBS), pH 7.3.
3. Drug-treated RBCs (see method for "Preparation of Drug-Treated RBCs"), 3%–5% in PBS.
4. 37°C water bath/incubator; cell washer (optional); serologic centrifuge.
5. Antihuman globulin, polyspecific or anti-IgG; antiglobulin control cells.

Procedure:

1. Prepare a master serial dilution of the patient's serum in PBS, at least one tube past the titer endpoint. Prepare enough of each dilution for a PBS control and one drug test (e.g., 0.3 mL serum plus 0.3 mL PBS).
2. For each dilution to be tested, label two tubes (e.g., with dilution and "test" or "control").
3. Add 0.1 mL of each serum dilution to the two appropriate labeled tubes.
4. To the tubes labeled "test," add 0.1 mL of drug solution. Mix.
5. To the tubes labeled "control," add 0.1 mL of PBS. Mix.
6. Incubate 1 hour at 37°C.
7. Add one drop of 3%–5% drug-treated RBCs to all tubes. Mix.
8. Incubate 1 hour at 37°C.
9. Centrifuge and examine for agglutination. Record results. (This step is optional if the antibody is not an agglutinin.)
10. Wash RBCs four times with PBS.
11. Add two drops antihuman globulin serum.
12. Centrifuge and examine for agglutination.
13. Add one drop antiglobulin control cells to all negative tests.
14. Centrifuge and read for macroscopic agglutination. Record positive results with a checkmark.

Quality Control:

1. Dilutions of the patient's serum plus PBS should react with the drug-treated RBCs to a titer similar to the previously determined titer.
2. The antiglobulin control cells should be macroscopically reactive.
3. Repeat test if any controls do not react as expected.

Interpretation:

1. If the serum plus drug reacts to the same titer as the serum plus PBS, then no inhibition by that drug has occurred.
2. If the serum plus drug reacts to a lower titer than the serum plus PBS (a difference of at least two dilutions), then inhibition by the drug has occurred.
3. If the serum plus drug reacts to a higher titer than the serum plus PBS, then the drug antibody works preferentially by the "immune complex" method.

Notes:

1. IgG antibody is more difficult to "neutralize" than IgM antibody of the same titer.[145] A checkerboard approach can be used—dilutions of the patient's serum and different concentrations of the drug. Alternatively, a dilution of the patient's serum that reacts 2+ could be selected, and dilutions of drug could be added to that.

REFERENCES

1. Petz LD, Garratty G: Acquired Immune Hemolytic Anemias, 1st ed. New York: Churchill Livingstone, 1980.
2. Pirofsky B: Autoimmization and the autoimmune hemolytic anemias. Baltimore: Williams & Wilkins, 1969.
3. Snapper I, Marks D, Schwartz L, et al: Hemolytic anemia secondary to mesantoin. Ann Intern Med 1953;39:619.
4. Harris JW: Studies on the mechanism of a drug-induced hemolytic anemia. J Lab Clin Med 1956;47:760.
5. Dausset J, Contu L: Drug-induced haemolysis. Ann Rev Med 1967;18:55–70.
6. Worlledge SM: Immune drug-induced haemolytic anaemias. Sem Hematol 1969;6:181–200.
7. Garratty G: Current viewpoints on mechanisms causing drug-induced immune hemolytic anemia and/or positive direct antiglobulin tests. Immunohematology 1989;5:97.
8. George JN, Raskob GE, Shah SR, et al: Drug-induced thrombocytopenia: A systematic review of published case reports. Ann Intern Med 1998;129:886–890.
9. Breckenridge A, Dollery CT, Worlledge SM, et al: Positive direct coombs tests and antinuclear factor in patients treated with methyldopa. Lancet 1967;16:1265–1268.
10. Petz LD, Gitlin N, Grant K, et al: Cimetidine-induced hemolytic anemia: The fallacy of clinical associations. J Clin Gastroenterol 1983;5:405–409.
11. Landsteiner K: The Specificity of Serological Reactions (revised ed). Cambridge, MA: Harvard University Press, 1947:85.
12. Eisen HN, Carsten ME, Belman S: Studies of hypersensitivity to low molecular weight substances. III. The 2,4-dinitrophenyl group as a determinant in the precipitin reaction. J Immunol 1954;73:296.
13. Park BK, Coleman JW, Kitteringham NR: Drug disposition and drug hypersensitivity. Biochem Pharmacol 1987;36:581–590.
14. Petz LD, Branch DR: Drug-induced immune hemolytic anemia. In Chaplin H Jr (ed): Immune hemolytic anemias. New York: Churchill Livingstone, 1985:47–94.
15. De Weck AL: Low molecular weight antigens. In Sela M (ed): The Antigens, vol II. New York: Academic Press, 1974:142.
16. Plescia OJ, Palczuk NC, Braun W, et al: Antibodies to DNA and a synthetic polydeoxyribonucleotide produced by oligodexyribonucleotides. Science 1965;148:1102.
17. Plescia OJ, Palczuk NC, Cora-Figueroa E: Production of antibodies to soluble RNA (sRNA). Proc Natl Acad Sci USA 1965;54:1281–1285.
18. Kitteringham NR, Christie G, Coleman JW, et al: Drug-protein conjugates—XII. A study of the disposition, irreversible binding and immunogenicity of penicillin in the rat. Biochem Pharmacol 1987;36:601–608.

19. Kristofferson A, Ahlstedt S, Svard PO: Antigens in penicillin allergy. II. The influence of the number of penicilloyl residues on the antigenicity of macromolecules as determined by radioimmunoassay (RIA), passive cutaneous anaphylaxis (PCA) and antibody induction. Int Archs Allergy Appl Immun 1977;55:23–28.
20. Kitagawa M, Yagi Y, Pressman D: The heterogeneity of combining sites of antibodies as determined by specific immunoadsorbents. II. Comparison of elution patterns obtained with anti-P-azobenzoate antibodies by different kinds of immunoadsorbent and eluting hapten. J Immunol 1965;95:455–465.
21. De Weck AL: Studies on penicillin hypersensitivity. I. The specificity of rabbit "anti-penicillin" antibodies. Int Arch Allergy Appl Immunol 1962;21:20.
22. De Weck AL: Newer developments in penicillin immunochemistry. Int Arch Allergy Appl Immunol 1963;22:245.
23. Levine BB, Ovary Z: Studies on the mechanism of the formation of the penicillin antigen. III. The N-(D-alpha-benzylpenicilloyl) group as an antigenic determinant responsible for hypersensitivity to penicillin. G J Exp Med 1961;114:875.
24. Levine BB, Price VH. Studies on the immunological mechanisms of penicillin allergy. II. Antigenic specificities of allergic wheal-and-flare skin responses in patients with histories of penicillin allergy. Immunology 1964;7:542.
25. Levine BB, Redmond AP: Minor haptenic determinant-specific reagents of penicillin hypersensitivity in man. Int Arch Allergy Appl Immunol 1969;35:445–455.
26. Parker CW, De Weck AL, Kern M, et al: The preparation and some properties of penicillenic acid derivatives relevant to penicillin hypersensitivity. J Exp Med 1962;15:803.
27. Siegel BB, Levine BB: Antigenic specificities of skin-sensitizing antibodies in sera from patients with immediate systemic allergic reactions to penicillin. J Allergy 1964;35:488.
28. Thiel JA, Mitchell S, Parker CW: Specificity of hemagglutination reactions in human and experimental penicillin hypersensitivity. J Allergy 1964;35:399.
29. Garratty G: Immune cytopenia associated with antibiotics. Transfus Med Rev 1993;VII:255–267.
30. Ackroyd JF: The pathogenesis of thrombocytopenic purpura due to hypersensitivity to sedormid. Clin Sci 1949;7:249.
31. Ackroyd JF: The immunological basis of purpura due to drug hypersensitivity. Proc Royal Soc Med 1962;55:30.
32. Ackroyd JF, Rook AJ: Allergic drug reactions. In Gell PGH, Coombs RRA (eds): Clinical Aspects of Immunology, 2nd ed. Oxford: Blackwell Scientific, 1968:693.
33. Ackroyd JF: Immunological mechanisms in drug hypersensitivity. In Gell PGH, Coombs RRA, Lachmann PJ (eds): Clinical Aspects of Immunology, 3rd ed. Oxford: Blackwell Scientific, 1975:913.
34. Ackroyd JF: Drug-induced thrombocytopenia. Vox Sang 1983;45:257–259.
35. Ley AB, Harris JP, Brinkley M, et al: Circulating antibodies directed against penicillin. Science 1958;127:1118.
36. Watson KC, Joubert SM, Bennett MAE: Occurrence of haemagglutinating antibody to penicillin. Immunology 1960;3:1.
37. Levine BB, Redmond AP, Fellner MJ, et al: Penicillin allergy and the heterogeneous immune responses of man to benzylpenicillin. J Clin Invest 1966;45:1895–1906.
38. Dewdney JM: Immunology of the antibiotics. In Sela M (ed): The Antigens. New York: Academic Press, 1977:73–245.
39. Shaltiel S, Mizrahi R, Sela M: On the immunological properties of penicillins. Proc R Soc Lond B 1971;179:411–432.
40. Neftel KA: Effect of storage of penicillin-G solutions on sensitisation to penicillin-G after intravenous administration. Lancet 1982;1:986–988.
41. Neftel KA, Walti M, Schulthess HK, et al: Adverse reactions following intravenous penicillin-G relate to degradation of the drug in vitro. Klin Wochenschr 1984;62:25–29.
42. Miescher PA, Miescher A: Die sedormid-anaphylaxie. Schweiz Med Wochenschr 1952;82:1279.
43. Miescher PA, Gorstein F: Mechanisms of immunogenic platelet damage. In Johnson SA, Monto RW, Rebuck JW, Horn RC (eds): Blood Platelets. London: J & A Churchill, 1961:671.
44. Miescher PA, Pepper JJ: Drug-induced immunologic blood dyscrasias. In Miescher PA, Müller-Eberhard HJ (eds): Textbook of Immunopathology, 2nd ed. Philadelphia: WB Saunders, 1976:421.
45. Miescher PA, Pola W: Haematological effects of non-narcotic analgesics. Drugs 1986;32(Suppl. 4):90.
46. Shulman NR: Immunoreactions involving platelets. I. A steric and kinetic model for formation of a complex from a human antibody, quinidine as a haptene, and platelets; and for fixation of complement by the complex. J Exp Med 1958;107:665.
47. Shulman NR, Rall JE: Mechanism of blood cell destruction in individuals sensitized to foreign antigens. Trans Assoc Amer Physicians 1963;76:72.
48. Shulman N: Mechanism of blood cell damage by adsorption of antigen-antibody complexes. In Immunopathology, 3rd International Symposium, La Jolla, CA: Stuttgart: Schwabe, 1963:338.
49. Shulman NR: A mechanism of cell destruction in individuals sensitized to foreign antigens and its implications in autoimmunity. Ann Int Med 1964;60:506.
50. Neter E: Bacterial hemagglutination and hemolysis. Bacteriol Rev 1956;20:166–188.
51. Boyden SV, Anderson ME: Agglutination of normal erythrocytes in mixtures of antibody and antigen, and haemolysis in the presence of complement. Br J Exp Pathol 1955;36:162–170.
52. Miescher P, Cooper N: The fixation of soluble antigen-antibody complexes upon thrombocytes. Vox Sang 1960;5:138–142.
53. Dameshek W: Autoimmunity: Theoretical aspects. Part 1. Ann N Y Adac Sci 1965:124:6–28.
54. Cronin AE: The immunology of allergic drug reactions. PhD Thesis, University of Cambridge, 1965.
55. Salama A, Northoff H, Burkhardt H, et al: Carbimazole-induced immune haemolytic anaemia: Role of drug-red blood cell complexes for immunization. Brit J Haematol 1988; 68:479–482.
56. Christie DJ, Mullen PC, Aster RH: Fab-mediated binding of drug-dependent antibodies to platelets in quinidine- and quinine-induced thrombocytopenia. J Clin Invest 1985;75:310–314.
57. Smith ME, Reid DM, Jones CE, et al: Binding of quinine- and quinidine-dependent drug antibodies to platelets is mediated by the Fab domain of the immunoglobulin G and is not Fc dependent. J Clin Invest 1987;79:912–917.
58. Jordan JV, Smith ME, Reid DM, et al: A tolmetin-dependent antibody causing severe intravascular hemolysis binds to erythrocyte band 3 and requires only the $F(ab')_2$ domain to react [abstract]. Blood 1985;66(Suppl.):104a.
59. Shulman NR, Jones CE, Reid DM, et al: Evidence that drug, not a neoantigen, is the primary determinant of drug-dependent antibody reactions [abstract]. Blood 1993;82:268a.
60. Chong BH, Berndt MC, Koutts J, et al: Quinidine-induced thrombocytopenia and leukopenia: Demonstration and characterization of distinct antiplatelet and anti-leukocyte antibodies. Blood 1983;62:1218–1223.
61. Kunicki TJ, Johnson MM, Aster RH: Absence of the platelet-receptor for drug-dependent antibodies in the Bernard Soulier Syndrome. J Clin Invest 1978;62:716–719.
62. van Leeuwen EF, Engelfriet CP, von dem Borne AEG Jr: Studies on quinine- and quinidine-dependent antibodies against platelets and their reaction with platelets in the Bernard-Soulier syndrome. Brit J Haematol 1982;51:551–560.
63. Kunicki TJ, Russell N, Nurden AT, et al: Further studies of the human platelet receptor for quinine- and quinidine-dependent antibodies. J Immunol 1981;126:398–402.
64. Berndt MC, Chong BH, Bull HA, et al: Molecular characterization of quinine/quinidine drug-dependent antibody platelet interaction using monoclonal antibodies. Blood 1985;66:1292–1301.
65. Devine DV, Rosse WF: Identification of platelet proteins that bind alloantibodies and autoantibodies. Blood 1984;64:1240–1245.
66. Christie DJ, Mullen PC, Aster RH: Quinine- and quinidine platelet antibodies can react with GPIIb/IIIa. Brit J Haematol 1987;67:213–219.
67. Visentin GP, Newman PJ, Aster RH: Characteristics of quinine- and quinidine-induced antibodies specific for platelet glycoproteins IIb and IIIa. Blood 1991;77:2668–2676.

68. Christie DJ, Aster RH: Drug-antibody-platelet interaction in quinine- and quinidine-induced thrombocytopenia. J Clin Invest 1982;70:989–998.
69. Claas FHJ, Langerak J, van Rood JJ: Drug-induced antibodies with restricted specificity. Immunol Letters 1981;2:323.
70. Letona J, Barbolla L, Frieyro E, et al: Immune haemolytic anaemia and renal failure induced by streptomycin. Br J Haematol 1977;35:561–571.
71. Duran-Suarez JR, Martin-Vega C, Argelagues E, et al: Red cell I antigen as immune complex receptor in drug-induced hemolytic anemias. Vox Sang 1981;41:313–315.
72. Habibi B, Basty R, Chodez S, et al: Thiopental-related immune hemolytic anemia and renal failure. N Engl J Med 1985;312:353–355.
73. Salama A, Mueller-Eckhardt C: On the mechanisms of sensitization and attachment of antibodies to RBC in drug-induced immune hemolytic anemia. Blood 1987;69:1006–1010.
74. Sandvei P, Nordhagen R, Michaelsen TE, et al: Fluorouracil (5-FU) induced acute immune haemolytic anaemia. Br J Haematol 1987;65:357–359.
75. Pereira A, Sanz C, Cervantes F, et al: Immune hemolytic anemia and renal failure associated with rifampicin-dependent antibodies with anti-I specificity. Ann Hematol 1991;63:56–58.
76. Habibi B, Bretagne Y: Blood group antigens may be the receptors for specific drug-antibody complexes reacting with red blood cells. CR Acad Sc (D) (Paris) 1983;296:693.
77. Sosler SD, Behzad O, Garratty G, et al: Acute hemolytic anemia associated with a chlorpropamide-induced apparent auto anti-Jk^a. Transfusion 1984;24:206–209.
78. Beck ML: A fatty-acid dependent antibody with Rh specificity. In Book of Abstracts, ISBT/AABB Joint Congress. Arlington, VA: American Association of Blood Banks, 1972:6.
79. Dube VE, Zoes C, Adesman P: Caprylate-dependent autoanti-e.Vox Sang 1977;33:359–363.
80. Reviron M, Janvier D, Reviron J, et al: An anti-I cold autoagglutinin enhanced in the presence of sodium azide. Vox Sang 1984;46:211–216.
81. Halima D, Garratty G, Bueno R: An apparent anti-Jk^a reacting only in the presence of methyl esters of hydroxybenzoic acid. Transfusion 1982;22:521–524.
82. Judd WJ, Steiner EA, Cochran RK: Paraben-associated autoanti-Jk^a antibodies. Transfusion 1982;22:31–35.
83. Muirhead EE, Groves M, Guy R, et al: Acquired hemolytic anemia, exposure to insecticides and positive Coombs test dependent on insecticide preparations. Vox Sang 1959;4:277.
84. Hart MN, Mesara BW: Phenacetin antibody cross-reactive with autoimmune erythrocyte antibody. Am J Clin Pathol 1969;52:695–701.
85. Garratty G, Houston M, Petz LD, et al: Acute immune intravascular hemolysis due to hydrochlorothiazide. Am J Clin Pathol 1981;76:73–78.
86. Shulman IA, Arndt PA, McGehee W: Cefotaxime-induced immune hemolytic anemia due to antibodies reacting in vitro by more than one mechanism. Transfusion 1990;30:263–266.
87. Garratty G, Nance S, Lloyd M, et al: Fatal immune hemolytic anemia due to cefotetan. Transfusion 1992;32:269–271.
88. Shirey RS, Morton SJ, Lawton KB, et al: Fenoprofen-induced immune hemolysis: Difficulties in diagnosis and complications in compatibility testing. Am J Clin Pathol 1998;89: 410–414.
89. Florendo NT, MacFarland D, Painter M, et al: Streptomycin-specific antibody coincident with a developing warm autoantibody. Transfusion 1980;20:662–668.
90. Habibi B, Lopez M, Serdaru M, et al: Immune hemolytic anemia and renal failure due to teniposide. N Eng J Med 1982;306:1091–1093.
91. Bird GWG, Wingham J, Babb RG, et al: (1984). Azapropazone-associated antibodies. Vox Sang 1984;46:336–337.
92. Salama A, Mueller-Eckhardt C: Two types of nomifensine-induced immune haemolytic anaemias: Drug-dependent sensitization and/or autoimmunization. Br J Haematol 1986; 64:613–620.
93. Salama A, Mueller-Eckhardt C: Cianidanol and its metabolites bind tightly to red cells and are responsible for the production of auto- and/or drug-dependent antibodies against these cells. Br J Haematol 1987;66:263–266.
94. Salama A, Göttsche B, Mueller-Eckhardt C: Autoantibodies and drug- or metabolite-dependent antibodies in patients with diclofenac-induced immune haemolysis. Br J Haematol 1991;77:546–549.
95. Squires JE, Mintz PD, Clark S: Tolmetin-induced hemolysis. Transfusion 1985;25:410–413.
96. van Dijk BA, Rico PB, Hoitsma A, et al: Immune hemolytic anemia associated with tolmetin and suprofen. Transfusion 1989;29:638–641.
97. Schulenburg BJ, Beck ML, Pierce SR, et al: Immune hemolysis associated with Zomax^T [abstract]. Transfusion 1983;23:409.
98. Toy E, Nesbitt R, Savastano G, et al: Warm autoantibody following plasma apheresis, complicated by acute intravascular hemolysis associated with cefoxitin-dependent antibody resulting in fatality [abstract]. Transfusion 1989;29:51S.
99. Weitekamp LA, Johnson ST, Fueger JT, et al: Cefotetan-dependent immune hemolytic anemia due to a single antibody reacting with both drug coated and untreated red cells in the presence of drug. In Book of Book of Abstracts. ISBT/AABB Joint Congress. Arlington, VA: American Association of Blood Banks, 1990:33.
100. Wojcicki RE, Larson CJ, Pope ME, et al: (1990). Acute hemolytic anemia during cefotetan therapy. Book of Abstracts. ISBT/AABB Joint Congress. Arlington, VA: American Association of Blood Banks, 1990:33.
101. Chambers LA, Donovan LM, Kruskall MS: Ceftazidime-induced hemolysis in a patient with drug-dependent antibodies reactive by immune complex and drug adsorption mechanisms. Am J Clin Pathol 1991;95:393–396.
102. Gallagher MT, Schergen AK, Sokol-Anderson ML, et al: Severe immune mediated hemolytic anemia secondary to treatment with cefotetan. Transfusion 1992;32:266–268.
103. Garrratty G: Drug-induced immune hemolytic anemia. In Garratty G (ed): Immunobiology of transfusion medicine. New York: Dekker, 1994:523–551.
104. Arndt PA, Leger RM, Garratty G: Serology of antibodies to second- and third-generation cephalosporins associated with immune hemolytic anemia and/or positive direct antiglobulin tests. Transfusion 1999;39:11239–11246.
105. Worlledge SM, Carstairs KC, Dacie JV: Autoimmune haemolytic anaemia associated with alpha-methyldopa therapy. Lancet 1966;2:135–139.
106. Weigle WO: The induction of autoimmunity in rabbits following injection of heterologous or altered homologous thyroglobulin. J Exp Med 1965;121:289–308.
107. Weigle WO: The antibody response in rabbits to previously tolerated antigens. Ann N Y Acad Sci 1965;124:133–142.
108. Worlledge SM: Autoantibody formation associated with methyldopa (Aldomet) therapy. Br J Haematol 1979;15:5–8.
109. Green FA, Jung CY, Rampal A, et al: Alpha-methyldopa and the erythrocyte membrane. Clin Exp Immunol 1980;40:554–560.
110. Green FA, Jung CY, Hui H: Modulation of alphamethyldopa binding to the erythrocyte membrane by superoxide dismutase. Biochem Biophys Res Comm 1980;95:1037–1042.
111. LoBuglio AF, Jandl JH: The nature of the alphamethyldopa red-cell antibody. N Engl J Med 1967;276:658–665.
112. Sherman JD, Love DE, Harrington JF: Anemia, positive lupus and rheumatoid factors with methyldopa. Arch Intern Med 1967;120:321–326.
113. Harm M: LE cells and positive direct Coombs' test induced by methyldopa. Can Med Assoc J 68;99:277–280.
114. Mackay IR, Cowling DC, Hurley TH: Drug-induced autoimmune disease: Haemolytic anaemia and lupus cells after treatment with methyldopa. Med J Aust 1968;2:1047–1050.
115. Devereux S, Fisher DM, Foter BLT, et al: Factor VIII inhibitor and raised platelet IgG levels associatred with methyldopa therapy. Br J Haematol 1983;54:485–488.
116. Feltkamp TEW, Engelfriet CP, Van Loghem JJ: Autoantibodies and methyldopa. Lancet 1968;1:644.
117. Perry HM, Chaplin H, Carmody S, et al: Immunologic findings in patients receiving methyldopa: A prospective study. J Lab Clin Med 1971;78:905–917.

118. Habibi B: Drug induced red blood cell autoantibodies co-developed with drug specific antibodies causing haemolytic anaemias. Br J Haematol 1985;61:139–143.
119. Mueller-Eckhardt C, Salama A: Drug-induced immune cytopenias: A unifying pathogenetic concept with special emphasis on the role of drug metabolites. Transfus Med Rev 1990;4:69–77.
120. Garratty G: Target antigens for red-cell-bound autoantibodies. In Nance SJ (ed). Clinical and basic science aspects of immunohematology. Arlington, VA: American Association of Blood Banks, 1991:33–72.
121. Dameshek W: Alpha-methyldopa red-cell antibody: Cross-reaction or forbidden clones. N Engl J Med 1967;276:1382.
122. Petz LD, Fudenberg HH: Immunologic mechanisms in drug-induced cytopenias. Prog Hematol 1975;9:185–206.
123. Kirtland HH, Mohler DN, Horwitz DA: Methyldopa inhibition of suppressor-lymphocyte function. N Engl J Med 1980;302:825–832.
124. Lipsky PE, Ginsburg WW, Finkelman FD, et al: Control of human B lymphocyte responsiveness: Enhanced suppressor T cell activity after in vitro incubation. J Immunol 1978;120:902–910.
125. Garratty G, Arndt P, Prince HP, et al: The effect of methyldopa and procainamide on suppressor cell activity. Br J Haematol 1992;84:310–315.
126. Kleinman S, Nelson R, Smith L, et al: Positive direct antiglobulin tests and immune hemolytic anemia in patients receiving procainamide. N Engl J Med 1984;311:809–812.
127. Rubin RL: Autoimmune reactions induced by procainamide and hydralazine. In Kammüller ME, Bloksma N, Seinen W (eds): Autoimmunity and Toxicology. New York: Elsevier, 1989:119.
128. Blomgren SE, Condemi JJ, Vaughan JH: Procainamide-induced lupus erythematosus: Clinical and laboratory observations, Am J Med 1972;52:338–348.
129. Gold EF, Ben-Efraim S, Faivisewitz A, et al: Experimental studies on the mechanism of induction of anti-nuclear antibodies by procainamide. Clin Immunol Immunopathol 1977;7:176–186.
130. Schoen RT, Trentham DE: Drug-induced lupus: An adjuvant disease? Am J Med 1981;71:5–8.
131. Cornacchia E, Golbus J, Maybaum J, et al: Hydralazine and procainamide inhibit T cell DNA methylation and induce autoreactivity. J Immunol 1988;140:2197–2200.
132. Bluestein HG, Weisman MH, Zvaifler N, et al: Lymphocyte alteration by procainamide: Relation to drug-induced lupus erythematosus syndrome. Lancet 1979;2:816–819.
133. Bluestein HG, Redelman D, Zvaifler NJ: Procainamide-lymphocyte reactions. Arthr Rheum 1981;24:1019–1023.
134. Miller KB, Salem D: Immune regulatory abnormalties produced by procainamide. Am J Med 1982;73:487–492.
135. DeBoccardo G, Drayer D, Rubin AL, et al: Inhibition of pokeweed mitogen-induced B cell differentiation by compounds containing primary amine or hydrazine groups. Clin Exp Immunol 1985;59:69–76.
136. Yu C-L, Ziff M: Effects of long-term procainamide therapy on immunoglobulin synthesis. Arthr Rheum 1985;28:276–284.
137. Ochi T, Goldings EA, Lipsky PE, et al: Immunomodulatory effect of procainamide in man. J Clin Invest 1983;71:36–45.
138. Seeman P: The membrane actions of anesthetics and tranquilizers. Pharmacol Rev 1972;24:583–655.
139. Shulman NR, Reid DM: Mechanisms of drug-induced immunologically mediated cytopenias. Transfus Med Rev 1993;VII:215–229.
140. Garratty G, Petz LD: Drug-induced immune hemolytic anemia. Am J Med 1975;58:398–407.
141. Petz LD, Fudenberg HH: Coombs-positive hemolytic anemia caused by penicillin administration. N Engl J Med 1966; 274:171–178.
142. Abraham GN, Petz LD, Fudenberg HH: Immunohaematological cross-allergenicity between penicillin and cephalothin in humans. Clin Exptl Immunol 1968;3:343–357.
143. Croft JD, Swisher SN, Gilliland BC, et al: Coombs-test positivity induced by drugs: Mechanisms of immunologic reactions and red cell destruction. Ann Intern Med 1968;68:176–187.
144. Levine BB, Redmond A: Immunochemical mechanisms of penicillin induced Coombs positivity and hemolytic anemia in man. Int Arch Allergy Appl Immunol 1967;31:594–606.
145. White JM, Brown DL, Hepner GW, et al: Penicillin-induced haemolytic anaemia. Br Med J 1968;3:26–29.
146. Kerr RO, Cardamone J, Dalmasso AP, et al: Two mechanisms of erythrocyte destruction in penicillin-induced hemolytic anemia. N Eng J Med 1972;287:1322–1325.
147. Reis CA, Rosenbaum TJ, Garratty G, et al: Penicillin-induced immune hemolytic anemia. JAMA 1975;233:432–435.
148. Funicella T, Weinger RS, Moake JL, et al: Penicillin-induced immunohemolytic anemia associated with circulating immune complexes. Am J Hematol 1977;3:219–223.
149. Molthan L, Reidenberg MM, Eichman MF: Positive direct Coombs tests due to cephalothin. N Engl J Med 1967; 277:123–125.
150. Gralnick HR, Wright LD Jr, McGinniss MH: Coombs' positive reactions associated with sodium cephalothin therapy. JAMA 1967;199:135–136.
151. Perkins RL, Mengel CE, et al: Direct Coombs' test reactivity after cephalothin or cephaloridine in man and monkey. Proc Soc Exptl Biol Med 1968;129:397–401.
152. Spath P, Garratty G, Petz LD: Studies on the immune response to penicillin and cephalothin in humans. II. Immunohematologic reactions to cephalothin administration. J Immunol 1971;107:860–869.
153. Spath P, Garratty G, Petz L: Studies on the immune response to penicillin and cephalothin in humans. I. Optimal conditions for titration of hemagglutinating penicillin and cephalothin antibodies. J Immunol 1971;107:854–859.
154. Branch DR, Sy Siok Hian AL, Petz LD: Mechanism of nonimmunologic adsorption of proteins using cephalothin-coated red cells [abstract]. Transfusion 1985;24:415.
155. Garratty G, Leger R: Red cell membrane proteins (CD55 and CD58) are modified following treatment of RBCs with cephalosporins [abstract]. Blood 1995;86:68a.
156. Sirchia G, Murcuriali F, Ferrone S: Cephalothin-treated normal red cells: A new type of PNH-like cells. Experientia 1968;24:495–496.
157. Ferrone S, Zanella A, Mercuriali F, et al: Some enzymatic and metabolic activities of normal human erythrocytes treated in vitro with cephalothin. Eur J Pharmacol 1968;4:211–214.
158. Rosse WF: Phosphatidylinositol-linked proteins and paroxysmal nocturnal hemoglobinuria. Blood 1990;75:1595–1601.
159. Jamin D, Demers J, Shulman I, et al: An explanation for non-immunologic adsorption of proteins onto red blood cells. Blood 1986;67:993–996.
160. Jamin D, Shulman I, Lam HT, et al: Production of a positive direct antiglobulin test due to Suramin. Arch Pathol Lab Med 1986;112:898–900.
161. Zeger G, Smith L, McQuiston D, et al: Cisplatin-induced non-immunologic adsorption of immunoglobulin by red cells. Transfusion 1988;28:493–495.
162. Getaz EP, Beckley S, Fitzpatrick, J, et al: Cisplatin-induced hemolysis. N Engl J Med 1980;302:334–335.
163. Levi JA, Aroney RS, Dalley DN: Haemolytic anaemia after cisplatin treatment. Br Med J 1981;282:2003–2004.
164. Nguyen BV, Lichtiger B: Cisplatin-induced anemia. Cancer Treat Rep 1981;65:1121.
165. Cinollo G, Dini G, Franchini E, et al: Positive direct antiglobulin tests in a pediatric patient following high-dose cisplatin. Cancer Chemother Pharmacol 1988;21:85–86.
166. Weber JC, Couppie P, Maloisel F, et al: Anémie hémolytique au cisdiamino-dichloroplatinum. La Presse Médicale 1990;19: 526–527.
167. Marani TM, Trich MB, Armstrong KS, et al: Carboplatin-induced immune hemolytic anemia. Transfusion 1996;36: 1016–1018.
168. Desrame J, Broustet H, de Talilly PD, et al: Oxaliplatin-induced haemolytic anaemia. Lancet 1999;354:1179–1180.
169. Garufi C, Vaglio S, Brienza S, et al: Immunohemolytic anemia following oxaliplatin administration. Ann Oncol 2000;11:497.
170. Earle CC, Chen WY, Ryan DP, et al: Oxaliplatin-induced Evan's syndrome. Br J Cancer 2001;84:441.

171. Sørbye H, Bruserud Ø, Dahl O: Oxaliplatin-induced haematological emergency with an immediate severe thrombocytopenia and haemolysis. Acta Oncol 2001;40:882–883.
172. Arndt P, Garratty G: Positive direct antiglobulin tests associated with oxaliplatin can be caused by antibody and/or nonimmunological protein adsorption. Transfusion 2003 (in press).
173. Lutz P, Dzik W: Very high incidence of a positive direct antiglobulin test (+DAT) in patients receiving Unasyn® [abstract]. Transfusion 1992;32:23S.
174. Garratty G, Arndt PA: Positive direct antiglobulin tests and haemolytic anaemia following therapy with beta-lactamase inhibitor containing drugs may be associated with nonimmunologic adsorption of protein onto red blood cells. Br J Haematol 1998;100:777–783.
175. Williams ME, Thomas D, Harman CP, et al: Positive direct antiglobulin tests due to clavulanic acid. Antimicrob Agents Chemother 1985;27:125–127.
176. Broadberry RE, Farren TW, Kohler JA, et al: Haemolytic anaemia associated with tazobactam [abstract]. Vox Sang 2002;83(S2):227.
177. Arndt P, Garratty G: Can nonspecific protein coating of RBCs lead to increased RBC destruction? Drug-treated RBCs with positive antiglobulin tests due to nonspecific protein uptake give positive monocyte monolayer assays [abstract]. Transfusion 2000;40:29S.
178. Nance SJ, Arndt P, Garratty G: Predicting the clinical significance of red cell alloantibodies using a monocyte monolayer assay. Transfusion 1987;27:449–452.
179. Garratty G: Predicting the clinical significance of red cell antibodies with in vitro cellular assays. Transfus Med Rev 1990;IV:297–312.
180. Ley AB, Cahan A, Mayer K: Circulating antibody directed against penicillin. Bibl Haemat 1959;10:539.
181. Petz LD: Immunologic reaction of humans to cephalosporins. Postgraduate Med J 1971;47(Suppl.):64–69.
182. Levine BB: Immunologic mechanisms of penicillin allergy: A haptenic model system for the study of allergic diseases of man. N Engl J Med 1966;275:1115–1125.
183. Gralnick HR, McGinnis M, Elton W, et al: Hemolytic anemia associated with cephalothin. JAMA 1971;217:1193–1197.
184. Jeannet M, Bloch A, Dayer JM, et al: Cephalothin-induced immune hemolytic anemia. Acta Haemat 1976;55:109–117.
185. Rubin RN, Burka ER: Anti-cephalothin antibody and Coombs'-positive hemolytic anemia. Ann Int Med 1977;86: 64–65.
186. Moake JL, Butler CF, Hewell GM, et al: Hemolysis induced by cefazolin and cephalothin in a patient with penicillin sensitivity. Transfusion 1978;18:369–373.
187. Branch DR, Berkowitz LR, Becker RL, et al: Extravascular hemolysis following the administration of cefamandole. Am J Hematol 1985;18:213–219.
188. Thomson S, Williamson D: A case of ampicillin-induced haemolytic anemia. Canad J Med Tech 1974;36:228–229.
189. Bell CA, Zwicker H, Whitcomb M: Matuhasi-Ogata phenomenon involving anti-ampicillin. Transfusion 1978;18:244–249.
190. Gmür J, Wälti M, Neftel KA: Amoxicillin-induced immune hemolysis. Acta Haemat 1985;74:230–233.
191. Johnson ST, Weitekamp LA, Sauer DE, et al: Piperacillin-dependent antibody with relative e specificity reacting with drug treated red cells and untreated red cells in the presence of drug [abstract]. Transfusion 1994;34:20S.
192. Arndt PA, Garratty G, Hill J, et al: Two cases of immune haemolytic anaemia, associated with anti-piperacillin, detected by the "immune complex" method. Vox Sang 2002; 83:273–278.
193. Seldon MR, Bain B, Johnson CA, et al: Ticarcillin-induced immune haemolytic anaemia. Scand J Haematol 1982;28:459–460.
194. Arndt PA, Wolf CF, Kripas CT, et al: First example of an antibody to ticarcillin: A possible cause of hemolytic anemia [abstract]. Transfusion 1999;39:47S.
195. Kroovand S, Kirtland H, Issitt C: A positive direct antiglobulin test due to sodium nafcillin [abstract]. Transfusion 1977;17:682.
196. Garratty G, Brunt D: Difficulties in detecting nafcillin antibodies [abstract]. Transfusion 1983;23:409.
197. Orenstein AA, Yakulis V, Eipe J, et al: Immune hemolysis due to hydralazine. Ann Int Med 1977;86:450–451.
198. Petersen BH, Graham J: Immunologic cross-reactivity of cephalexin and penicillin. J Lab Clin Med 1974;83:860–870.
199. van der Meulen FW, de Bruin HG, Goosen PCM, et al: Quantitative aspects of the destruction of red cells sensitized with IgG1 autoantibodies: An application of flow cytofluorometry. Br J Haematol 1980;46:47–56.
200. Garratty G, Nance S: Correlation between in vivo hemolysis and the amount of red cell-bound IgG measured by flow cytometry. Transfusion 1990;30:617–621.
201. Carstairs KC, Breckenridge A, Dollery CT, et al: Incidence of a positive direct Coombs test in patients on α-methyldopa. Lancet 1966;ii:133–135.
202. Hunter E, Raik E, Gordon S, et al: Incidence of positive Coombs' test, LE cells and antinuclear factor in patients on alpha-methyldopa (Aldomet) therapy. Med J Aust 1971;2:810–812.
203. Dollery CT, Worlledge SM, Holbrow EJ, et al: Positive direct Coombs tests and antinuclear factor in patients treated with methyldopa. Lancet 1967;2:1265–1268.
204. Woodgate D, Feizi T: The direct antiglobulin (Coombs') test in hypertensive patients. Vox Sang 1967;12:273–278.
205. Worlledge SM: Immune drug-induced hemolytic anemias. Semin Hematol 1973;10:327–344.
206. Worlledge SM: Autoantibody formation associated with methyldopa (Aldomet) therapy. Br J Haematol 1979;16:5–8.
207. Bakemeier RF, Leddy JP: Erythrocyte autoantibody associated with alpha methyldopa: Heterogeneity of structure and specificity. Blood 1968;32:1–14.
208. Lalezari P, Louie JE, Fadlallah N: Serologic profile of alphamethyldopa-induced hemolytic anemia: Correlation between cell-bound IgM and hemolysis. Blood 1982;59:61–68.
209. LoBuglio AF, Jandl JH: The nature of the alpha methyldopa red-cell antibody. N Engl J Med1967;276:658–665.
210. Issitt PD, Pavone BG, Goldfinger D, et al: Anti-Wr^b and other autoantibodies responsible for positive direct antiglobulin test in 150 individuals. Br J Haematol 1976;34:5–18.
211. Patten E, Beck CE, Scholl C, et al: Autoimmune hemolytic anemia with anti-Jk^a specificity in a patient taking Aldomet. Transfusion 1977;17:517–520.
212. Kessey EC, Pierce S, Beck ML, et al: Alpha-methyldopa-induced hemolytic anemia involving autoantibody with U specificity [abstract]. Transfusion 1973;13:360.
213. Branch DR: Gallagher MT, Shulman IA, et al: Reticuloendothelial cell function in α-methyldopa-induced hemolytic anemia. Vox Sang 1983;45:278–287.
214. Gallagher MT, Branch DR, Mison A, et al: Evaluation of reticuloendothelial function in autoimmune hemolytic anemia using an in vitro assay of monocyte-macrophage interaction with erythrocytes. Exp Hematol 1983;11:82–89.
215. Yust I, Frisch B, Goldsher N: Antibody-dependent cell-mediated cytotoxicity and phagocytosis of autologous red blood cells in alphamethyldopa-induced haemolysis. Scand J Haematol 1986;36:211–216.
216. Kelton JG: Impaired reticuloendothelial function in patients treated with methyldopa. N Engl J Med 1985;313:596–600.
217. Worlledge S: Immune drug induced haemolytic anaemias. In Girdwood RH (ed): Blood disorders due to drugs and other agents. Amsterdam: Excerpta Medica, 1973:11–26.
218. Petz LD: Drug-induced immune haemolytic anaemia. Clin Haematol 1980;9:455–482.
219. Silvergleid AJ, Wells RF, Hafleigh EB, et al: Compatibility test using ^{51}chromium-labelled red blood cells in crossmatch positive patients. Transfusion 1978;18:8–14.
220. Snyder EL, Spivak M: Clinical and serological management of patients with methyldopa-induced positive antiglobulin tests. Transfusion 1979;19:313–316.
221. Parr GVS, Ballard JO: Autologous blood transfusion with methyldopa induced positive direct antiglobulin test. Transfusion 1980;20:119.
222. Bastion Y, Coiffier B, Dumontet C, et al: Severe autoimmune hemolytic anemia in two patients treated with fludarabine for chronic lymphocytic leukemia. Ann Oncol 1992;3:171–172.
223. Tosti S, Caruso R, D'Adamo F, et al: Severe autoimmune hemolytic anemia in a patient with chronic lymphocytic

leukemia responsive to fludarabine-based treatment. Ann Hematol 1992;65:238–239.
224. Di Raimondo F, Giustolisi R, Cacciola E, et al: Autoimmune hemolytic anemia in chronic lymphocytic leukemia patients treated with fludarabine. Leuk Lymph 1993;11:63–68.
225. Byrd JC, Hertler AA, Weiss RB, et al: Fatal recurrence of autoimmune anemia following pentostatin therapy in a patient with a history of fludarabine-associated hemolytic anemia. Ann Oncol 1995;6:730–731.
226. Myint H, Cooplestone JA, Orchard J, et al: Fludarabine-related autoimmune haemolytic anaemia in patients with chronic lymphocyte leukaemia. Br J Haematol 1995;91:341–344.
227. Tertian G, Cartron J, Bayle C, et al: Fatal intravascular autoimmune hemolytic anemia after fludarabine treatment for chronic lymphocyte leukemia. Hematol Clin Ther 1996;38:359–360.
228. Maclean R, Meiklejohn D, Soutar R: Fludarabine-related autoimmune haemolytic anaemia in patients with chronic lymphocytic leukaemia. Br J Haematol 1996;92:766–773.
229. Robak T, Blasiska-Morawiec M, Krykowski E, et al: Autoimmune haemolytic anaemia in patients with chronic lymphocytic leukaemia treated with 2-chlorodeoxyadenosine (cladribine). Eur J Haematol 1997;58:109–113.
230. Longo G: Fludarabine and autoimmune hemolytic anemia in chronic lymphocytic leukemia. Eur J Haematol 1997;59: 124–125.
231. Chasty RC, Myint H, Oscier DG, et al: Autoimmune haemolysis in patients with B-CLL treated with chlorodeoxtyadenosine (CDA). Leuk Lymph 1998;29:391–398.
232. Vick DJ, Byrd JC, Beal CL, et al: Mixed-typed autoimmune hemolytic anemia following fludarabine treatment in a patient with chronic lymphocytic leukemia/small cell lymphoma. Vox Sang 1998;74:122–126.
233. Gonzalez H, Leblond V, Azar N, et al: Severe autoimmune hemolytic anemia in eight patients treated with fludarabine. Hematol Cell Ther 1998;40:113–118.
234. Weiss RB, Freiman J, Kweder SL, et al: Hemolytic anemia after fludarabine therapy for chronic lymphocytic leukemia. J Clin Oncol 1998;16:1885–1889.
235. Hamblin TJ, Orchard JA, Myint H, et al: Fludarabine and hemolytic anemia in chronic lymphocytic leukemia. J Clin Oncol 1998;16:3209–3210.
236. Tetreault SA, Saven A: Delayed onset of autoimmune hemolytic anemia complicating cladribine therapy for Waldenstrom macroglobulinemia. Leuk Lymph 2000;37:125–130.
237. Mauro FR, Foa R, Cerretti R, et al: Autoimmune hemolytic anemia in chronic lymphocytic leukemia: Clinical, therapeutic, and prognostic features. Blood 2000;95:2786–2792.
238. Dighiero G, Travade P, Chevret S, et al: B-cell chronic lymphocytic leukemia: Present status and future directions. Blood 1991;78:1901–1914.
239. Bersagel DE: The chronic leukemias: A review of disease manifestations and the aim of therapy. Canadian Med Assoc J 1967;96:1615–1620.
240. Hamblin TJ, Oscier DG, Young BJ: Autoimmunity in chronic lymphocytic leukemia. J Clin Pathol 1986;39:713–716.
241. Astrow AB: Fludarabine in chronic leukemia. Lancet 1996; 347:1420–1421.
242. Diehl LF, Ketchum LH: Autoimmune disease and chronic lymphocytic leukemia: Autoimmune hemolytic anemia, pure red cell aplasia, and autoimmune thrombocytopenia. Semin Oncol 1998;25:80–97.
243. Johnson S, Smith AG, Loffler H, et al: Multicentre prospective randomized trial of fludarabine versus cyclophosphamide, doxorubicin, and prednisone (CAP) for treatment of advanced-stage chronic lymphocytic leukaemia. The French Cooperative Group on CLL: Lancet 1996;347:1432–1438.
244. Orchard J, Bolam S, Myint H, et al: In patients with lymphoic tumours recovering from the autoimmune complications of fludarabine, relapse may be triggered by conventional chemotherapy. Br J Haematol 1998;102:1112–1113.
245. Shvidel L, Shtarlid M, Klepfish A, et al: Evans syndrome complicating fludarabine treatment for advanced B-CLL. Br J Haematol 1997;99:706.
246. Sen K, Kalaycio M: Evans syndrome precipitated by fludarabine therapy in a case of CLL. Am J Hematol 1999;61:219.
247. Henry RE, Goldberg LS, Sturgeon P, et al: Serologic abnormalities associated with L-dopa therapy. Vox Sang 1971;20: 306–316.
248. Joseph C: Occurrence of positive Coombs test in patients treated with levodopa. N Engl J Med 1972;286:1401–1402.
249. Gabor EP, Goldberg LS: Levodopa induced Coombs positive haemolytic anaemia. Scand J Haematol 1973;11:201–203.
250. Lindstrom FD, Lieden G, Engstrom MS: Dose-related levodopa-induced haemolytic anaemia. Ann Intern Med 1977;86:298–300.
251. Bernstein RM: Reversible haemolytic anaemia after levodopa-carbidopa. Br Med J 1979;1:1461–1462.
252. Territo MC, Peters RW, Tanaka KR: Autoimmune hemolytic anemia due to levodopa therapy. JAMA 1973;226:1347–1348.
253. Jones GW, George TL, Bradley RD: Procainamide-induced hemolytic anemia. Transfusion 1978;18:224–227.
254. Kornberg A, Rachmilewitz E: Procainamide-induced hemolytic anemia in a patient with traumatic cardiac hemolytic anemia. Arch Intern Med 1981;141:1388.
255. Schifman RB, Garewal H, Shillington D: Reticulocytopenic. Coombs' positive anemia induced by procainamide. Am J Clin Pathol 1983;80:66–68.
256. Kleinman S, Nelson R, Smith L, et al: Positive direct antiglobulin tests and immune hemolytic anemia in patients receiving procainamide. N Engl J Med 1984;311:809–812.
257. Sanford-Driscoll M, Knodel LC: Induction of hemolytic anemia by nonsteroidal antiinflammatory drugs. Drug Intel Clin Pharm 1986;20:925–934.
258. Kramer MR, Levene C, Hershko C: Severe reversible autoimmune haemolytic anaemia and thrombocytopenia associated with diclofenac therapy. Scand J Haematol 1986;36:118–120.
259. Chan-Lam D, Thorburn AW, Chalmers EA, et al: Red cell antibodies and autoimmune haemolysis after treatment with azapropazone. Br Med J 1986;293:1474.
260. Salama A, Göttsche B, Mueller-Eckhardt C: Autoantibodies and drug- or metabolite-dependent antibodies in patients with diclofenac-induced immune haemolysis. Br J Haematol 1991;77:546–549.
261. Johnson ST, Fueger JT, Gottschall JL, et al: Ibuprofen-dependent antibody with Rh specificity reacting with untreated red cells in the presence of drug. Transfusion 1996;36:54S.
262. Laidlaw ST, Stamps R, Booker DJ, et al: Immune hemolytic anemia due to dicofenac. Immunohematology 1997;13:9–11.
263. Bougie D, Johnson ST, Weitekamp LA, et al: Sensitivity to a metabolite of diclofenac as a cause of acute immune hemolytic anemia. Blood 1997;90:407–413.
264. Madoz P, Muñiz-Diaz E, Martinez C, et al: Fatal immune hemolytic anemia induced by aceclofenac [abstract]. Transfusion 1997;37:36S.
265. van Dijk BA, Rico PB, Hoitsma A, et al: Immune hemolytic anemia associated with tolmetin and suprofen. Transfusion 1989;29:638–641.
266. Weitekamp LA, Johnson ST, Fueger JT, et al: A fatal case of tolmetin-induced hemolytic anemia with relative e specificity [abstract]. Transfusion 1991;31:52S.
267. McCall L, Owens M: Case report: Hemolytic anemia produced by tolmetin. Immunohematology 1992;8:17–18.
268. Weitekamp LA, Johnson ST, Fueger JT, et al: Sulindac-induced hemolytic anemia caused by antibody reacting with untreated red cells in the presence of drug [abstract]. Transfusion 1992;32:54S.
269. DeCoteau J, Reis MD, Pinkerton PH, et al: Positive antiglobulin test in association with sulindac: Involvement of the Rh factor. Vox Sang 1993;64:179–183.
270. Angeles ML, Reid ME, Yacob UA, et al: Sulindac-induced immune hemolytic anemia. Transfusion 1994;34:255–258.
271. Cunha PD, Lord RS, Johnson ST, et al: Immune hemolytic anemia caused by sensitivity to a metabolite of etodolac, a nonsteroidal anti-inflammatory drug. Transfusion 2000;40:663–668.
272. Guidry JB, Ogbum CL, Griffin EM: Fatal autoimmune hemolytic anemia associated with ibuprofen. JAMA 1979; 242:68–69.
273. Patmas MA, Willbom SL, Shankel SW: Acute multisystem toxicity associated with the use of nonsteroidal antiinflammatory drugs. Arch Intern Med 1984;144:519–521.

274. Prescott LF, Illingworth RN, Critchley JAJH, et al: Acute haemolysis and renal failure after nomifensine overdosage. Br Med J 1980;281:1392–1393.
275. Woodliff HJ, Wallace PF: Haemolytic anaemia caused by nomifensine. Med J Aust 1986;144:163.
276. Martlew VJ: Immune haemolytic anaemia and nomifensine treatment in north west England 1984–85: Report of six cases. J Clin Pathol 1986;39:1147–1150.
277. Conlon KC, Urba WJ, Smith JW, et al: Exacerbation of symptoms of autoimmune disease in patients receiving alpha-interferon therapy. Cancer 1990;65:2237–2242.
278. Andriani A, Bibas M, Callea V, et al: Autoimmune hemolytic anemia during alpha interferon treatment in nine patients with hematological diseases. Haematologica 1996;81: 258–260.
279. Landau A, Castera L, Buffet C, et al: Acute autoimmune hemolytic anemia during interferon-alpha therapy for chronic hepatitis C. Dig Dis Sci 1999;44:1366–1367.
280. Stavroyianni N, Stamatopoulos K, Viniou N, et al: Autoimmune hemolytic anemia during alpha-interferon treatmentin a patient with chronic myelogenous leukemia. Leuk Res 2001;25:1097–1098.
281. Akard LP, Hoffman R, Elias L, et al: Alpha-interferon and immune hemolytic anemia. Ann Intern Med 1986;105:306.
282. Radin AL, Buckley P, Duffy TP: Interferon therapy for agnogenic myeloid metaplasia complicated by immune hemolytic anemia. Hematol Pathol 1991;5:83–88.
283. Fattovich G, Giustina G, Favarato S, et al: A survey of adverse events in 11,241 patients with chronic viral hepatitis treated with alfa interferon. J Hepatol 1996;24:38–47.
284. Fornaciari G, Bassi C, Beltrami M, et al: Hemolytic anemia secondary to interferon treatment for chronic B hepatitis. J Clin Gastroenterol 1991;13:356–357.
285. Barbolla L, Paniagua C, Outeirino J, et al: Haemolytic anaemia to the alpha-interferon treatment: A proposed mechanism. Vox Sang 1993;65:156–157.
286. Sacchi S, Kantarjian H, O'Brien S, et al: Immune-mediated and unusual complications during interferon alfa therapy in chronic myelogenous leukemia. J Clin Oncol 1995;13: 2401–2407.
287. Ballester OF, Spiers ASD, Grattan J: Autoimmune hemolytic anemia (AIHA) accopanying treatment with alpha-intereferon (IFN) in a patient with chronic granulocytic leukemia (CGL). Blood 1989;74(Suppl.):352.
288. Rotoli B, Formisano S, Alfinito F: Autoimmune haemolytic anaemia associated with cimetidine. Lancet 1979;2:583.
289. Rate R, Bonnell M, Chervenak C, et al: Cimetidine and hematologic effects. Ann Intern Med 1979;91:795.
290. Donowitz GR, Mandell GL: Beta-lactam antibiotics. N Engl J Med 1988;318:490–500.
291. Petri WA: Penicililns, cephalosporins, and other β-lactam antibiotics. In Hardman JG, Limbird LE, Gilman AG (eds): Goodman & Gilman's The Pharmacological Basis of Therapeutics, 10th ed. New York: McGraw-Hill, 2001:1189–1218.
292. Ferrone S, Zanella A, Scalamogna M: Red cell metabolism in positive direct Coombs test after cephalothin therapy. Experientia 1971;27:194–195.
293. York PS, Landes RR, Seay LS: Coombs' positive reactions associated with cephaloridine therapy. JAMA 1968;206:1086.
294. Fass RJ, Perkins RL, Saslow S: Positive direct Coombs' tests associated with cephaloridine therapy. JAMA 1970;213:121–123.
295. Schwarz S, Gabl F, Huber H, et al: Positive direct antiglobulin (Coombs') test caused by cephalexin administration in humans. Vox Sang 1975;29:59–65.
296. van Winzum C: Clinical safety and tolerance of cefoxitin sodium: An overview. J Antimicrob Chemother 1978;4(Suppl. B):91–104.
297. Meyers BR: Comparative toxicities of third-generation cephalosporins. Am J Med 1985;79(Suppl. 2A):96–102.
298. Forbes CD, Mitchell R, Craig JA, et al: Acute intravascular haemolysis associated with cephalexin therapy. Postgrad Med J 1972;48:186–188.
299. Manoharan A, Kot T: Cephalexin-induced haemolytic anaemia. Med J Aust 1987;147:202.
300. DeTorres OH: Hemolytic anemia and pancytopenia induced by cefoxitin. Drug Intell Clin Pharm 1983;17:816–818.
301. Duran-Suarez JR, Trujillo J, Prat I, et al: Anti-cephalosporins and immune complexes. Transfusion 1982;22:541–542.
302. Salama A, Göttsche B, Schleffer T, et al: "Immune complex" mediated intravascular hemolysis due to IgM cephalosporin dependent antibody. Transfusion 1987;27:460–463.
303. Garratty G, Postoway N, Schwellenbach J, et al: A fatal case of ceftriaxone (Rocephin)-induced hemolytic anemia associated with intravascular immune hemolysis. Transfusion 1991;31: 176–179.
304. Ehmann WC: Cephalosporin-induced hemolysis: A case report and review of the literature. Am J Hematol 1992;40:121–125.
305. Chenoweth CE, Judd WJ, Steiner EA, Kauffman CA: Cefotetan-induced immune hemolytic anemia. Clin Infect Dis 1992;15:863–865.
306. Wagner BKJ, Heaton AH, Flink JR: Cefotetan disodium-induced hemolytic anemia. Ann Pharmacotherapy 1992;26: 199–200.
307. Dhawan M, Kiss JE, DiAddezzio NA, Triulzi DJ: Fatal cefotetan-induced immune hemolysis [abstract]. Blood 1993;82:582a.
308. Lo G, Higginbottom P: Ceftriaxone induced hemolytic anemia [abstract]. Transfusion 1993;33:25S.
309. Eckrich RJ, Fox S, Mallory D: Cefotetan-induced immune hemolytic anemia due to the drug-adsorption mechanism. Immunohematology 1994;10:51–54.
310. Peano GM, Menardi G, Quaranta L, et al: A rapidly fatal case of immune haemolytic anaemia due to cefotetan. Vox Sang 1994;66:84–85.
311. Ogburn JR, Knauss MA, Thapar K, et al: Cefotetan-induced immune hemolytic anemia (IHA) resulting from both drug adsorption and immune complex mechanisms [abstract]. Transfusion 1994;34:27S.
312. Mohammed S, Knoll S, vanAmburg A III, Mennes PA: Cefotetan-induced hemolytic anemia causing severe hypophosphatemia. Am J Hematol 1994;46:369–370.
313. Bernini JC, Mustafa MM, Sutor LJ, Buchanan GR: Fatal hemolysis induced by ceftriaxone in a child with sickle cell anemia. J Pediatr 1995;126:813–815.
314. Lascari AD, Amyot K: Fatal hemolysis caused by ceftriaxone. J Pediatr 1995;126:816–817.
315. Borgna-Pignatti C, Bezzi TM, Reverberi R: Fatal ceftriaxone-induced hemolysis in a child with acquired immunodeficiency syndrome. Ped Infec Dis J 1995;14:1116–1117.
316. Scimeca PG, Weinblatt ME, Boxer R: Hemolysis after treatment with ceftriaxone. J Pediat 1996;128:163.
317. Moallem HJ, Garratty G, Wakeham M, et al: Ceftriaxone-related fatal hemolysis in an adolescent with perinatally acquired human immunodeficiency virus infection. J Pediatrics 1998; 133:279–281.
318. Longo F, Hastier P, Buckley MJM, et al: Acute hepatitis, autoimmune hemolytic anemia, and erythroblastocytopenia induced by ceftriaxone. Am J Gastroenterol 1998;93:836–837.
319. Garratty G, Leger RM, Arndt PA: Severe immune hemolytic anemia associated with prophylactic use of cefotetan in obstetric and gynecologic procedures. Am J Obstet Gynecol 1999;9:337–342.
320. Maraspin V, Lotric-Furlan S, Strle F: Ceftriaxone-associated hemolysis. Wien Klin Wochenschr 1999;111(9):368–370.
321. Meyer O, Hackstein H, Hoppe B, et al: Fatal immune haemolysis due to a degradation product of ceftriaxone. Br J Haematol 1999;105:1084–1085.
322. Badon SJ, Cable RG: Hemolysis due to cefotetan [abstract]. Transfusion 1999;39:42S.
323. Johnson ST, Fueger JT, Gottschall JL: Cefotetan-dependent antibody cross-reacting with ceftriaxone treated RBCs [abstract]. Transfusion 1999;39:81S.
324. Shammo JM, Calhoun B, Mauer AM, et al: First two cases of immune hemolytic anemia associated with ceftizoxime. Transfusion 1999;39:838–844.
325. Endoh T, Yagihashi A, Sasaki M, Watanabe N: Ceftizoxime-induced hemolysis due to immune complexes: Case report and the epitope responsible for immune complex-mediated hemolysis. Transfusion 1999;39:306–309.

326. Punar M, Özsü H, Eraksoy H, et al: An adult case of fatal hemolysis induced by ceftriaxone. Clin Microbiol Infect 1999;5:585–586.
327. Viner Y, Hashkes PJ, Yakubova R, et al: Severe hemolysis induced by ceftriaxone in a child with sickle cell anemia. Pediatr Infect Dis J 2000;19(1):83–85.
328. Stroncek D, Proctor JL, Johnson J: Drug-induced hemolysis: cefotetan-dependent hemolytic anemia mimicking an acute intravascular immune transfusion reaction. Am J Hematol 2000;64:67–70.
329. Naylor CS, Steele L, Hsi R, Margolin M, Goldfinger D: Cefotetan-induced hemolysis associated with antibiotic prophylaxis for cesarean delivery. Am J Obst Gynecol 2000;182:1427–1428.
330. Moes GS, MacPherson BR: Cefotetan-induced hemolytic anemia: A case report and review of the literature. Arch Pathol Lab Med 2000;124(a):1344–1346.
331. Marques MB, Carr KD, Brumfield CG, Huang ST: A pregnant patient with sickle cell disease and cefotetan-induced immune hemolysis. Lab Med 2000;31(10):541–543.
332. Seltsam A, Salama A: Ceftriaxone-induced immune haemolysis: Two case reports and a concise review of the literature. Intensive Care Med 2000;26:1390–1394.
333. Ray EK, Warkentin TE, O'Hoski PL, Gregor P: Delayed onset of life-threatening immune hemolysis after perioperative antimicrobial prophylaxis with cefotetan. Can J Surg 2000;43:461–462.
334. Falezza GC, Piccoli PL, Franchini M, Gandini G, Aprili G: Ceftriaxone-induced hemolysis in an adult [letter]. Transfusion 2000;40:1543–1545.
335. Malaponte G, Arcidiacono C, Mazzarino C, et al: Cephalosporin-induced hemolytic anemia in a Sicilian child. Hematology 2000;5:327–334.
336. Calhoun BW, Junsanto T, DeTolve Donoghue M, Naureckas E, Baron JM, Baron BW: Ceftizoxime-induced hemolysis secondary to combined drug adsorption and immune-complex mechanisms. Transfusion 2001;41:893–897.
337. Chai L, Pomper GJ, Ross RL, Neal ZM, Champion MH, Snyder EL: Severe hemolytic anemia and liver damage induced by prophylactic use of cefotetan [abstract]. Transfusion 2001; 41(Suppl. 1):58S.
338. Fueger JT, Bell JA, Gottschall JL, Johnson ST: Ceftazidime-dependent antibody reacting with untreated red cells in the presence of drug [abstract]. Transfusion 2001;41(Suppl. 1):104S.
339. Citak A, Garratty G, Ücsel R, et al: Ceftriaxone-induced haemolytic anaemia in a child with no immune deficiency or haematological disease. J Pediatr Child Health 2002;38: 209–210.
340. Afenyi-Annan AN, Judd WJ: Cefotetan induced immune-mediated hemolysis complicated by thrombocytopenia: alloimmune or thrombotic? [abstract] Transfusion 2002;52:46S.
341. Kim S, Song KS, Kim HO, et al: Ceftriaxone induced immune hemolytic anemia: Detection of drug-dependent antibody by ex-vivo antigen in urine. Yonsei Med J 2002;43:391–394.
342. Arndt P: Practical aspects of investigating drug-induced immune hemolytic anemia due to cefotetan or ceftriaxone—a case study approach. Immunohematology 2002;18:27–32.
343. Viraraghavan R, Chakravarty AG, Soreth J: Cefotetan-induced haemolytic anaemia: A review of 85 cases. Adv Drug React Toxicol Rev 2002;21:101–107.
344. Eastlund T, Mulrooney D, Neglia J, et al: Self-limited immune hemolysis in a child after six days of ceftriaxone therapy [abstract]. Transfusion 2002;42:96S.
345. Bateman ST, Hu E, Lane C, et al: Antibody to ceftriaxone in HIV pediatric patients and potential implications for RBC hemolysis [abstract]. Blood 2002;100(11):48b.
346. Ferrone S, Mercuriali F, Scalamogna M: Cephalothin positive direct Coombs test: Relationship to serum immunoglobulin concentration. Experientia 1971;27:193–194.
347. Garratty G: Laboratory investigation of drug-induced immune hemolytic anemia and/or positive direct antiglobulin tests. Washington, DC: American Association of Blood Banks, 1980:1–30.
348. Kosakai N, Miyakawa C: Fundamental studies on the positive Coomb's tests due to cephalosporins. Postgrad Med J 1970; 46(Suppl.):107–109.
349. Mine Y, Nishida M, Goto S, et al: Studies on direct Coombs reaction by cefazolin in vitro. J Antibiotics 1970;23:575–580.
350. Garratty G, Arndt P, Nance S: Nonimmunological adsorption of proteins onto red cells treated with second and third generation cephalosporins [abstract]. Transfusion 1994;34:69S.
351. Arndt P, Garratty G: Is severe immune hemolytic anemia, following a single dose of cefotetan, associated with the presence of "naturally-occurring" anti-cefotetan? [abstract] Transfusion 2001;41:24S.
352. Arndt PA, Leger RM, Garratty G: Reactivity of "last wash" elution controls in investigations of cefotetan antibodies [abstract]. Transfusion 1999;39:47S.
353. Leger RM, Arndt PA, Ciesielski DJ, et al: False-positive eluate reactivity due to the low-ionic wash solution used with commercial acid-elution kits. Transfusion 1998;38:565–572.
354. Hamilton-Miller JMT, Abraham EP: Specificities of haemagglutinating antibodies evoked by members of the cephalosporin C family and benzylpenicillin. Biochem J 1971;123:183–190.
355. Delafuente JC, Panush RS, Caldwell JR: Penicillin and cephalosporin immunogenicity in man. Ann Allergy 1979;43:337–340.
356. Novalbos A, Sastre J, Cuesta J, et al: Lack of allergic cross-reactivity to cephalosporins among patients allergic to penicillins. Clin Exp Allergy 2001;31:438–444.
357. Cerney A, Pichler W: Allergy to antibacterials: the problem with beta-lactams and sulfonamides. Pharmacoepidemiol Drug Saf 1998;7:S23–S36.
358. Abraham NC, Petz LD, Fudenberg HH: Cephalothin hypersensitivity associated with anti-cephalothin antibodies. Int Arc Allergy Appl Immunol 1968;34:65–74.
359. Petz LD: Immunologic cross-reactivity between penicillin and cephalosporins: A review. J Infect Dis 1978;137(Suppl.): S74–S79.
360. Arndt PA, Garratty G: Cross-reactivity of cefotetan and ceftriaxone antibodies, associated with hemolytic anemia, with other cephalosporins and penicillin. Am J Clin Pathol 2002;118:256–262.
361. Toy PTCY, Chin CA, Reid ME, et al: Factors associated with positive direct antiglobulin tests in pretransfusion patients: A case-control study. Vox Sang 1985;49:215–220.
362. Heddle NM, Kelton JG, Turchyn KL, et al: Hypergammaglobulinemia can be associated with a positive direct antiglobulin test, a nonreactive eluate, and no evidence of hemolysis. Transfusion 1988;28:29–33.
363. Garratty G: The significance of IgG on the red cell surface. Transfus Med Rev 1987;1:47–57.
364. Brown JL: Incomplete labeling of pharmaceuticals: a list of "inactive" ingredients. N Engl J Med 1983;309:439–441.
365. Law IP, Wickman CJ, Harrison BR: Coombs'-positive hemolytic anemia and ibuprofen. Southern Med J 1979;72:707–710.
366. O'Neil MJ, ed. The Merck Index: An Encyclopedia of Chemicals, Drugs, and Biologicals. Whitehouse Station, NJ: Merck Research Laboratories, 2001.
367. Physicians' desk reference, 57th ed. Oradell, NJ: Medical Economics, 2003.
368. Curtis BR, McFarland JG, Aster RH: Enhanced detection of antibodies (DDAb) responsible for drug-induced thrombocytopenia (DITP) [abstract]. Transfusion 1993;33:77S.
369. Osbourne SE, Johnson ST, Weitekamp LA, et al: Enhanced detection of drug-dependent antibodies reacting with untreated red blood cells in the presence of drug [abstract]. Transfusion 1994;34:20S.
370. Arndt P, Garratty G: Use of albumin solutions for solubilizing certain drugs can decrease binding of drugs to RBCs [abstract]. Transfusion 2002;42:105S.
371. Wong KY, Boose GM, Issitt CH: Erythromycin-induced hemolytic anemia. J Pediatr 1981;98:647–649.
372. Nance SJ, Ladisch W, Williamson TL: Erythromycin-induced immune hemolytic anemia. Vox Sang 1988;55:233–236.
373. Johnson HM, Brenner K, Hall HE: The use of a water-soluble carbodiimide as a coupling reagent in the passive hemagglutination test. J Immunol 1966;97:791–796.

CHAPTER 9

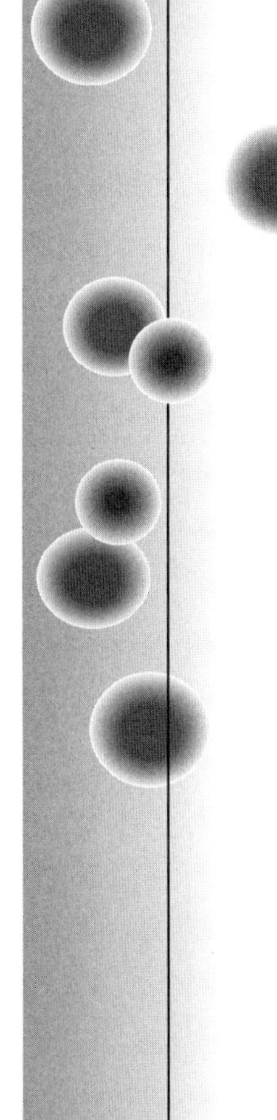

Unusual Aspects of Acquired Immune Hemolytic Anemias

A. Autoimmune Hemolytic Anemia with a Negative Direct Antiglobulin Test (DAT)

Patients with acquired hemolytic anemia whose red blood cells (RBCs) do not react with antiglobulin serum (AGS) have been reported by numerous investigators. In some instances, the hemolysis is clearly not antibody-induced; examples include hemolytic anemia caused by oxidant drugs in patients with glucose 6-phosphate dehydrogenase deficiency, mechanical hemolytic anemias, paroxysmal nocturnal hemoglobinuria, and so on. In other patients, however, extensive evaluation fails to reveal a nonimmunologic etiology, and clinical findings are suggestive of AIHA associated with warm autoantibodies (WAIHA). That is, these patients destroy transfused normal compatible RBCs at a rate approximating destruction of their own RBCs, thus indicating an extrinsic mechanism for RBC destruction. In addition, they usually respond to steroid therapy and/or splenectomy as do patients with more typical serologic findings of AIHA. For many such patients, evidence supporting the hypothesis that these are indeed WAIHAs can be obtained by using techniques that are more sensitive than standard serologic procedures.

INCIDENCE OF DAT-NEGATIVE WAIHA

The exact incidence of WAIHA with a negative DAT is not known. Evans and Weiser[1] described four patients with negative DATs who were clinically similar to 37 other patients with serologic abnormalities indicative of AIHA. Dacie[2] so noted persistently negative DATs among some patients who otherwise appeared to have WAIHA. Worlledge and Blajchman[3] reported 10 (3%) similar cases in their series of 333 cases consisting of all types of AIHA; in 8 of these cases, survival of ^{51}Cr-tagged compatible normal RBCs was shortened. Chaplin[4] reported that 2% to 4% of patients with AIHA have a negative DAT. Boccardi and colleagues[5] reported that 11 of 98 patients (11%) who appeared to have AIHA had negative DATs.

During a 10-year period during which we studied 347 patients with definite AIHA (244 were WAIHA), we encountered 27 other patients who appeared to have WAIHA but had negative routine DATs.[6] This represented about 10% of the patients with WAIHA and 7% of all the patients with acquired immune hemolytic anemias we encountered during that period. Sometimes, small amounts of RBC-bound IgG could be detected by methods more sensitive than the antiglobulin test (AGT). Sometimes, the phenomenon appeared to be associated with the presence of low-affinity IgG autoantibodies that eluted from the RBCs during the in vitro washing of the RBCs, and sometimes the RBC-bound autoantibody was IgA or IgM, which was not detectable by AGS routinely used for the DAT.

RELATIONSHIP OF ANTIBODY CONCENTRATION TO RATE OF HEMOLYSIS

The inability to demonstrate autoantibodies on the RBCs of some patients with AIHA seems to sometimes result from the concentration of antibody being too low for detection by the routine DAT. This was first suggested by Gilliland and coworkers.[7-9] That such small concentrations of IgG autoantibody are capable of producing RBC destruction is supported by observations with alloantibodies. Mollison and Hughes-Jones[10] studied the clearance of Rh-positive RBCs by low concentrations of Rh antibody. They injected anti-Rh(D) into an Rh-negative person and followed the injection by ^{51}Cr-tagged Rh(D)-positive RBCs, demonstrating that when RBCs were coated with about 10 molecules of antibody per RBC, their T_{50} survival was approximately 100 hours. They also demonstrated that the lowest concentration of antibody capable of bringing about RBC destruction in vivo was about 1/50th of the lowest concentration detectable by the indirect antiglobulin test (IAT) in vitro. This finding, however, must not be taken to mean that all antibodies have the same degree of potency with regard to their ability to cause RBC destruction in vivo. Indeed, ample data indicate that the ability of autoantibodies to produce RBC destruction varies. Although hemolytic anemia occurs in some patients who have low concentrations of antibody on their RBCs, other patients have mild or no RBC destruction with a strongly positive DAT (see Chapter 4). Constantoulakis and associates[11] demonstrated that the rate of hemolysis depends more on the characteristics of the individual antibody than on the antibody concentration. Although wide variations of antibody concentration per RBC and hemolytic activity are observed among patients, in the individual patient with AIHA the rate of RBC destruction is generally related to the concentration of RBC-bound antibody[12,13] (also see Chapter 4).

If the theory of Gilliland and colleagues[7-9] is correct, we must accept the notion that macrophages can interact with RBCs sensitized with less than 200 IgG molecules per RBC. Not only do they have to interact, but the interaction must be efficient enough to cause a hemolytic anemia. If senescent RBCs are removed by an immune mechanism, there must be a delicate balance between the amount of IgG causing normal daily RBC destruction and the amount causing DAT-negative AIHA (see Fig. 9-1).[14-16] IgG is thought to be present on the RBCs of most individuals. Most investigators reporting on the quantity of IgG on normal RBCs calculate the amount of IgG per RBC (5–90 [mean of 39] molecules of IgG per RBC) as if it were spread evenly among all the RBCs.[17,18] If the IgG present on normal RBCs is an autoantibody to senescent cell antigen (SCA) and appears predominantly on older RBCs (see later in this chapter), then the calculations used by Merry and associates[17] and Jeje and coworkers,[18] which yielded similar results of about 30–40 IgG molecules per RBC in the total RBC population, might be incorrect. Their results could also be interpreted to mean that the oldest RBCs (i.e., approximately 1% of the total RBC population) might have several thousand IgG molecules per RBC. This would certainly explain why these older RBCs react efficiently with macrophages, whereas it is hard to explain why RBCs with 30–40 IgG molecules would be phagocytosed.

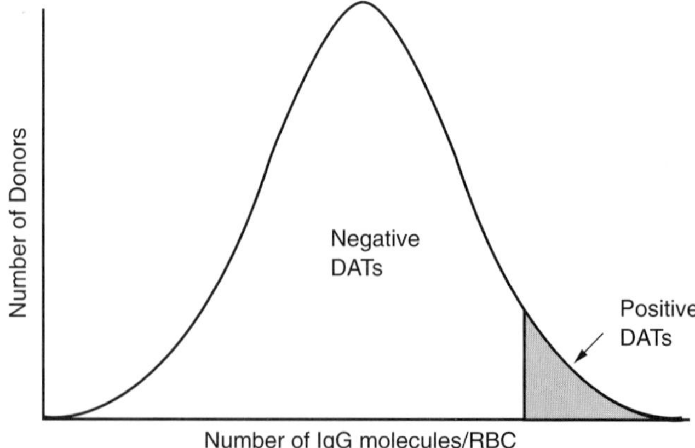

FIGURE 9-1. The expected Gaussian distribution of naturally occurring RBC-bound IgG. Do the positive DATs found in normal donors represent the outer limit of this distribution? (From Garratty G: Effect of cell-bound proteins on the in vivo survival of circulating blood cells. Gerontology 1991;37:68–94.)

The RBC-bound IgG of most healthy individuals is not detectable by the DAT. As mentioned previously, this is probably a quantitative effect (Table 9-1 and

TABLE 9-1. THE STRENGTH OF THE ANTIGLOBULIN TEST USING RED CELLS COATED WITH VARYING CONCENTRATIONS OF IgG AS DETERMINED BY THE COMPLEMENT FIXING ANTIBODY CONSUMPTION TEST. (A SINGLE ANTI-IgG ANTIGLOBULIN SERUM WAS USED AT OPTIONAL DILUTION.)

RBCs Sensitized In Vitro with Anti-RhD)	
Antiglobulin Test	**IgG Molecules per RBC**
Negative	<25–120
½+	120
1+	200
2+	300–500
3+, 4+	>500

Fig. 9-1). Even if the older RBCs have amounts of IgG (i.e., >120 molecules/RBC) that should be detectable by the AGT, they would be too minor a population to form agglutinates readily visible under the conditions by which the routine AGT is performed. We do not know whether the RBC-bound IgG detectable by the DAT in approximately one in 1400 seemingly healthy blood donors represents the upper end of the quantitative range typical of the normal gaussian distribution of RBC-bound IgG (Fig. 9-1), or whether it suggests autoantibodies to SCA or a different population of IgG molecules.[14-16] We do not know whether there is any relationship between the pathogenicity of certain IgG autoantibodies and increased amounts of RBC-bound SCA autoantibody, or whether pathogenic autoantibodies are always of a different specificity. There is some evidence that SCA autoantibody can be pathogenic at times (see Chapter 7).

The situation can be even more complicated than that described in the foregoing discussion. Masouredis and colleagues[19] showed that the IgG eluted from the RBCs of DAT-positive, seemingly healthy blood donors was composed of at least two antibody populations. The first was an IgG autoantibody directed at RBC antigens; the second was an IgG autoanti-idiotype, directed against the RBC-bound IgG autoantibody (Fig. 9-2). The same group also showed that the RBC-bound IgG anti-idiotype did not appear to be present in eluates prepared from the RBCs of DAT-positive patients with AIHA.[20] Masouredis and associates[19,20] suggested that the IgG autoanti-idiotype could play a role in protecting the IgG-sensitized RBCs in normal donors from being destroyed at an abnormal rate, thus preventing AIHA in DAT-positive donors.

SENSITIVITY OF THE DAT

The concentration of IgG antibody on the RBCs that is required for a positive DAT is quite variable. The characteristics of the RBCs, the RBC antibody, and the AGS

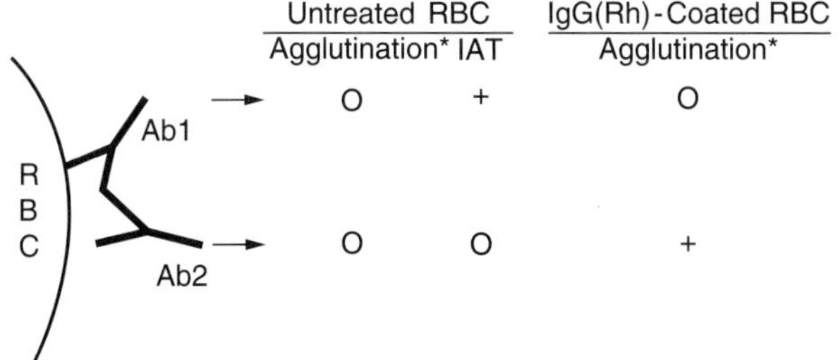

FIGURE 9-2. Eluates from RBCs of DAT-positive blood donors contained two antibody populations: Ab1 and Ab2. Ab1 was the RBC autoantibody that reacted with untreated RBCs by IAT but did not agglutinate them or IgG(Rh)-coated RBCs. Ab2 was an IgG autoantibody to an epitope on the IgG RBC autoantibody (said to be anti-idiotype). Ab2 did not react with untreated RBCs but directly aggultinated Ig(Rh)-coated RBCs. (*Agglutination= agglutination at 37°C.) (From Garratty G: Autoimmune hemolytic anemia. In Garratty G (ed): Immunolobiology of Transfusion Medicine. New York: Dekker, 1994:493–521.)

are important variables. Gilliland and coworkers[7-9] reported that the RBCs of some patients with 150 molecules of IgG per cell were agglutinated by AGS, while RBCs from other patients were not agglutinated even though they were sensitized with 700 molecules per RBC. Petz and Garratty[6] reported similar results. Dupuy and colleagues[21] observed weak agglutination of RBCs coated with 100 molecules of anti-Rh(D) per RBC by some AGS; with other AGS, however, 10–20 times more RBC-bound antibody was required for agglutination. Other observers, using RBCs coated with either IgG anti-A or anti-Rh(D), have observed minimally detectable agglutination by AGS, with antibody concentrations ranging from 100 to 500 molecules per RBC.[22,23]

Results carried out in our laboratory with RBCs sensitized in vitro with anti-Rh(D) are shown in Table 9-1. Negative AGT results were obtained with RBCs coated with fewer than 120 molecules per RBC. Progressively stronger reactions occurred with higher concentrations of IgG. The concentration of IgG on the RBCs was determined using the complement-fixing antibody consumption test described later in this chapter.

MEASUREMENT OF SMALL AMOUNTS OF RBC-BOUND IgG

Small amounts of IgG RBC-bound autoantibodies can be measured by techniques not available in most laboratories. These include the complement fixation antibody consumption (CFAC) test, the radiolabeled anti-IgG test, the enzyme-linked antiglobulin test (ELAT), and flow cytometry.[6-9,24-47]

Gilliland and coworkers[8] reported that the RBCs of five of six patients with acquired hemolytic anemia and a persistently negative DAT were found to have abnormal quantities of IgG as measured by the CFAC test. The amount of IgG per RBC ranged from 70 to 434 molecules, compared with 35 or fewer molecules of IgG per RBC found on the RBCs of normal persons. RBCs of patients with other types of hemolytic anemia had fewer than 35 molecules per RBC. These included RBCs of two patients with chronic hemolytic anemia due to cold agglutinins, two patients with paroxysmal nocturnal hemoglobinuria (PNH), two with hereditary spherocytosis, and one with burr cells related to chronic liver disease. In patients who had abnormal concentrations of IgG on their RBCs, eluates prepared from 50–200 mL of blood and concentrated to a final volume of 1 mL reacted in the IAT. Eluates prepared from RBCs of normal subjects or from subjects with other types of hemolytic anemia were nonreactive. Further evidence that the IgG in the RBC eluates had antibody characteristics was shown by their specificities. Three of the eluates reacted with RBCs of common Rh phenotypes but did not react with Rh_{null} RBCs, thus reflecting the diversity of specificity seen in patients with AIHA and positive DATs (see Chapter 7). One of the six patients with acquired hemolytic anemia had a normal concentration of IgG on her RBCs as measured by the CFAC test, and no IgG, IgA, or IgM RBC antibodies could be identified in a concentrated eluate prepared from 200 mL of blood. Further, no free antibody was detected in her serum; however, survival of transfused normal compatible RBCs was greatly shortened.

Gilliland[9] extended these findings by reporting on an additional nine patients. The amount of IgG per RBC in these patients ranged from 76 to 350 molecules. Six of the nine responded to corticosteroid therapy, one did not improve, one died of chronic lymphocytic leukemia before results of therapy could be assessed, and one patient was lost to follow-up. The patient who showed no improvement had the same quantity of IgG on his RBCs three weeks later. Follow-up quantitative RBC antibody data were obtained for some of the patients who responded to therapy, and these data revealed a decrease in the amount of antibody per RBC.

We performed 82 CFAC tests on 59 subjects who were healthy or who had disorders other than idiopathic acquired hemolytic anemia.[6] In addition, we studied 27 patients who were referred to our laboratory with a diagnosis of acquired hemolytic anemia with a negative DAT.[6] Results in the former group of patients are summarized in Table 9-2. Of 54 studies on 31 normal subjects, only one was positive—that is, only one indicated more than 25 molecules of IgG per RBC. Of 11 patients with hereditary spherocytosis, one CFAC test was positive in a patient who also had Hodgkin's disease. Tests in one patient with pyruvate kinase deficiency and two with Gilbert syndrome with mild reticulocytosis were negative, as were tests for three patients who had had splenectomy for a myeloproliferative disorder. Only one of 11 patients with mild hemolysis associated with the presence of a prosthetic heart valve had a positive CFAC test.

Our experience with 27 patients who were referred to our laboratory with a diagnosis of acquired hemolytic anemia with a negative DAT are summarized in Table 9-3.[6] Although the DAT was negative in all cases in the referral laboratory, we were able to detect complement sensitization of the patients' RBCs in 11 (41%) instances, using an anti-C3 containing a potent anti-C3d that was prepared in our laboratory. In most of these instances, the antiglobulin test was only weakly positive. Also, in one instance, we obtained a weakly positive reaction using an anti-IgG made in our laboratory.

TABLE 9-2. COMPLEMENT FIXING ANTIBODY CONSUMPTION TEST IN NORMAL SUBJECTS AND IN PATIENTS WITH DISORDERS OTHER THAN IDIOPATHIC ACQUIRED HEMOLYTIC ANEMIA

Diagnosis	Number of Studies	Number with >25 Molecules of IgG/RBC
Normal persons	54	1
Hereditary spherocytosis	11	1*
Pyruvate kinase deficiency	1	0
Gilbert syndrome	2	0
Postsplenectomy	3	0
Mechanical hemolytic anemia (prosthetic heart valves)	11	1

* Patient also had Hodgkin's disease.

Autoantibodies were detected in the serum or eluate in 11 of 27 patients (41%). For some patients, eluates prepared from several mL of RBCs and concentrated two to five times resulted in a positive reaction. Most often, the autoantibody was detected in the serum using enzyme-treated RBCs.

The CFAC test revealed more than 25 molecules of IgG per RBC in all patients and between 100 and 300 molecules of IgG per RBC in 15 of the 27 cases (56%).[6] In five instances, more than 400 molecules of IgG per RBC were detected; this result includes one extraordinary case of a patient with recurrent episodes of brisk hemolysis (see Patient 1), in whom 1400 molecules of IgG per RBC were found in spite of a negative DAT.

Information concerning response to therapy was available for 17 patients, and follow-up CFAC tests were performed for seven of these.[6] Six of these patients revealed marked clinical improvement in response to steroids or splenectomy. The subsequent CFAC test revealed fewer than 25 molecules of IgG per RBC for five patients, but in one patient, 228 molecules of IgG were present after therapy (compared with 173 prior to therapy) in spite of clinical improvement. One patient who did not improve as a result of treatment with steroids and splenectomy had 180 molecules of IgG per RBC before therapy and 607 when retested 2 years later. Twenty-two of the patients had no associated disorder and were diagnosed as having idiopathic AIHA, although one of these had a history of idiopathic thrombocytopenic purpura. Five patients had active associated disease. Spherocytes were noted on the peripheral blood film of seven patients, although this information is not indicated in the table. This finding suggests that the interaction of antibody-coated RBCs with the cells of the reticuloendothelial system (see Chapter 4) occurred in spite of the small numbers of IgG molecules present on the RBCs.

While accumulating this experience, we also observed five patients who were referred with a diagnosis of idiopathic acquired hemolytic anemia despite a negative DAT and in whom the CFAC test indicated that the patients' RBCs were coated with fewer than 25 molecules of IgG per RBC (the lower limit of sensitivity of the test in our laboratory).[6] In four of these patients, C3d was detectable on the patients' cells by the DAT, but in none were autoantibodies detectable in the serum or eluate. Whether these patients' hemolytic anemia was also immunologically mediated is conjectural.

The following case reports illustrate the value of sensitive serologic tests and the CFAC test in evaluating patients with acquired hemolytic anemia with a negative DAT.

TABLE 9-3. WARM ANTIBODY AUTOIMMUNE HEMOLYTIC ANEMIC WITH A NEGATIVE DIRECT ANTIGLOBULIN TEST

				Test for Autoantibody						
				Serum		Eluate	CFAC Test:			
	DAT in Referral Laboratory	DAT in Authors' Laboratory			Enzyme Treated		IgG Molecules per RBC			Associated
		IgG	C3d	IAT	RBC	IAT	(Normal ≤ 25)	Therapy	Course	Disease
1	Neg	Neg	1½+	Neg	Neg	Neg	144	None	Improved	
2	Neg	Neg	2+	Neg	Neg	Neg	>400			History of ITP
3	Neg	Neg	Neg	Neg	Neg	NT	126			Wiskott-Aldrich
4	Neg	Neg	1+	Neg	3½+	Neg	251	Steroids	Improved	
5	Neg	Neg	Neg	Neg	Neg	Neg	93			
6	Neg	Neg	Neg	Neg	Neg	NT	59	Steroids	Improved	
7	Neg	Neg	1+	Neg	1½+	Neg	234			
8	Neg	½+	½+	½+	3½+	Neg	126			
9	Neg	Neg	Neg	Neg	Neg	Neg	>400	Steroids	Improved	
10	Neg	Neg	Neg	Neg	½+	Neg	166			
11	Neg	Neg	½+	2+	3½+	½+	173	Steroids	Improved	
12	Neg	Neg	1+	Neg	Neg	NT	339			
13	Neg	Neg	Neg	Neg	3+	Neg	243	Steroids	Persistent hemolysis: expired	Chronic persistent hepatitis
14	Neg	Neg	Neg	Neg	Neg	Neg	54	Steroids	Unchanged	Metastatic carcinoma: microangiopathic hemolytic anemia
15	Neg	Neg	Neg	1+	Neg	NT	128	Steroids	Improved	
16	Neg	Neg	Neg	Neg	Neg	2+	185	Steroids	Improved	
17	Neg	Neg	Neg	Neg	Neg	Neg	70	Steroids	Unchanged	TTP
18	Neg	Neg	Neg	Neg	Neg	NT	>400	Steroids	Improved	
19	Neg	Neg	Neg	Neg	Neg	½+	95	Steroids	Improved	
20	Neg	Neg	1+	Neg	Neg	NT	122			Carcinoma of ovary
21	Neg	Neg	Neg	Neg	Neg	Neg	127			
22	Neg	Neg	Neg	½+	Neg	Neg	290	Steroids	Improved	
23	Neg	Neg	Neg	NT	NT	NT	59			
24	Neg	Neg	3+	Neg	2+	1+	1400	Splenectomy	Long term remission	
25	Neg	Neg	2½+	Neg	Lysis	1½+	138	Splenic irradiation	Marked temporary improvement	
26	Neg	Neg	½+	Neg	Neg	Neg	180	Prednisone and splenectomy	Unchanged	
27	Neg	Neg	Neg	Neg	Neg	Neg	640	Steroids	Rapid improvement	

Neg = Negative
NT = Not tested
ITP = Idiopatnic thrombocytopenic purpura
TTP = Thrombotic thrombocytopenic purpura

PATIENT 1: A 12-year history of episodic acquired hemolytic anemia with a negative DAT.[6] A 49-year-old male had a 12-year history of recurrent episodes of hemolytic anemia. He developed malaise, fatigue, gastrointestinal symptoms, jaundice, and dark urine. An acute hemolytic anemia was diagnosed, and there was no evidence of precipitating events. The hemolysis resolved spontaneously without therapy, and over the next 2 years, the patient had recurrent episodes at approximately 60–90 day intervals. The episodes gradually decreased in severity, and 2 years later, he was free of symptoms. Six years later, he developed recurrent attacks consisting of progressive weakness, darkening of the urine, malaise, pallor, and (by the fourth or fifth day) jaundice and symptoms of anemia. The nadir of hemoglobin depression was generally in the range of 5–7 g/dL and occurred 7–10 days after the onset of symptoms. Reticulocytopenia (1% or less) was present during the period of progressive fall in hemoglobin, usually continuing for about 72 hours after reaching the nadir. Leukopenia and thrombocytopenia also occurred, with the white cell count dropping to about 2000/μL with a normal differential and the platelets falling to about 80,000/μL. Then followed a progressive reticulocytosis to a value of about 20% over the succeeding 7–10 days and complete recovery at the end of approximately 3 weeks. At that time, the patient's hemoglobin was in the range of 14 g/dL, and the reticulocyte count, white cell count, and platelet count were normal. These episodes continued to recur at 60–90 day intervals for the next 4 years, during which time numerous studies were undertaken.

The patient was questioned repeatedly about any environmental factor relating to occupation or hobbies that might be of significance in precipitating attacks, but none could be identified. There was no history of drug ingestion. Physical examination was remarkable for the presence of mild tachycardia and icterus during episodes of marked anemia. In addition, he had persistent splenomegaly, the edge of the spleen usually palpable 4 cm below the left costal margin.

Laboratory data revealed characteristic findings of hemolysis during periods of progressive anemia. In a typical episode, the total bilirubin was 1.6 mg/dL with 0.3 mg direct reacting, haptoglobin absent, LDH 90, and urine hemosiderin weakly positive. The RBC morphology was essentially normal, although an occasional target cell and rare spherocytes were present. A bone marrow aspirate performed at a point of maximum anemia revealed intense erythroid hyperplasia with some megaloblastoid features. A repeat bone marrow study performed during a phase of remission revealed some residual erythroid hyperplasia that was normoblastic. An RBC survival study using ^{51}Cr-labeled RBCs was begun near the onset of an episode of hemolysis. The curve initially began with a steady exponential fall revealing a halftime of 17 days (normal = 25 to 35 days). Suddenly, on the 11th day of the study, the chromium disappearance became markedly accelerated with a halftime of 3 days. Excessive splenic sequestration was noted. Another RBC survival study was begun when the patient's hematocrit reached 12.5%. During the study, his hematocrit level rose to 24% on the 10th day and to 38% on the 17th day. The disappearance curve of the radioactive chromium was within normal limits.

Extensive diagnostic studies to determine the cause of the hemolysis were unproductive. Tests performed included the DAT, Ham's acid serum test, the sucrose hemolysis test, osmotic fragility before and after incubation at 37°C for 24 hours, hemoglobin electrophoresis, quantitation of hemoglobins A and E, isopropanol and heat tests for unstable hemoglobins, and biochemical measurement (RBC G-6PD, 6-phosphogluconic hydrogenase, hexokinase, pvruvate kinase, aldolase, catalase, pyruvate, and lactate).

Prednisone at a dose of 80 mg per day was given at the onset of symptoms. This regimen had no significant effect on the progression of the hemolytic episode. The patient was also treated with folic acid without effect. Transfusions were given during his first episode of hemolysis, but thereafter the patient learned to tolerate symptoms in spite of striking drops in hemoglobin. When his disease became progressively more severe 12 years later, however, he was given 2 units of RBCs during each of two successive hemolytic episodes after his hemoglobin had dropped to 3.5 g/dL.

When referred for immunohematologic evaluation 1 year later, his DAT was negative with anti-IgG but moderately strongly positive with anti-C. His serum contained an antibody that reacted equally with all enzyme-treated RBCs of a panel. An alloantibody (anti-Wr^a) was also detectable by IAT. An eluate prepared from the patient's RBCs contained a weak antibody without evident specificity. In spite of the negative DAT using anti-IgG, the CFAC test revealed a surprising value of 1400 molecules of IgG per RBC at a time when the patient's hemoglobin was 5.9 g/dL. A repeat test in January 1979, when the hemoglobin was 13.6 g/dL, revealed 396 molecules of IgG per RBC.

A splenectomy was performed. The spleen weighed 1164 g and revealed congestion of the red pulp, follicular center hyperplasia, and abundant iron. Subsequently (13 years after his first hemolytic episode), the patient was asymptomatic and had no further hemolytic episodes during a 3-year follow-up period. His hemoglobin was 17.2 g/dL, hematocrit was 51.4%, white cell count was 11,200/μL, platelet count was 329,000/μL, and reticulocytes were 1.7%. A repeat CFAC test performed 6 months after splenectomy revealed fewer than 25 molecules of IgG per RBC. Three years later, the CFAC test revealed 240 molecules of IgG per RBC; his DAT was negative with anti-IgG and anti-C3, and no antibody was detected in his serum or in a RBC eluate.

Comment: This patient had a long history of recurrent attacks of hemolysis without evident cause. Attacks occurred every 60–90 days, and his hemoglobin fell to as low as 3.5 g/dL. Immunohematologic evaluation (including the use of the CFAC test) revealed evidence of WAIHA. The patient responded to splenectomy with complete cessation of episodes of hemolysis, and follow-up immunohematologic evaluations revealed significant improvement.

PATIENT 2: **Acquired hemolytic anemia with a negative DAT with anti-E, occurring in the RBC eluate of an E-negative patient.[44]** A previously untransfused 20-year-old male presented with a 7-day history of malaise, fatigue, jaundice, dark urine, and splenomegaly. Hemolytic anemia was indicated by a hemoglobin of 8.7 g/dL, reticulocyte count 8%, lactic dehydrogenase 389 IU/L, bilirubin 4.3 mg/dL (direct 0.1 mg/dL), and undetectable serum haptoglobin. Tests for nonimmunologic causes of hemolytic anemia were negative. The DAT was repeatedly negative with polyspecific, anti-IgG, -IgA, and -IgM antisera. The patient's serum contained a weak anti-I, and anti-E strongly reactive as determined by IAT, and an antibody reactive against all RBCs tested. The latter antibody reacted weakly by the IAT but strongly against enzyme-treated RBCs (titer 160). Eluates from the patient's RBCs reacted only with E+ RBCs. The patient was E-negative. He was treated for WAIHA with high doses of prednisone. By the

12th day, his response allowed the medication to be tapered, and by 1 month from the onset of treatment, laboratory studies had returned to normal. The DAT remained negative; following recovery, however, anti-E could not be eluted from the RBCs. Anti-E remained in his serum, and the titer of the enzyme-reactive antibody had decreased to 16. It was suggested that the anti-E–like antibody represented autoanti-Hr preferentially reacting with E+ RBCs (see Chapter 7).

Our experience has indicated that when IgG antibody is present in an eluate prepared from RBCs, the CFAC test is always abnormal. Thus, we performed the assay only on RBCs obtained 5 days following remission, at which time the eluate was nonreactive. The CFAC revealed normal findings (<25 molecules IgG/RBC).

Ganly and associates[45] described a similar case with an anti-Jk^a eluted from a Jk(a–) DAT-negative patient with Evans's syndrome. Later, the patient's DAT became positive, and the patient's RBCs at that time were found to be Jk(a+). The specificities in these two cases are similar to the mimicking antibodies discussed in Chapter 7.

PATIENT 3: WAIHA erroneously diagnosed as cold agglutinin syndrome. A 17-year-old male was admitted to the hospital for evaluation of severe hemolytic anemia. Physical examination revealed an icteric young man in no acute distress. The spleen was palpable 2 cm below the left costal margin. The hemoglobin was 7.6 g/dL, reticulocytes 10.8%, white cell count 7600/μL, serum bilirubin 7.2 mg/dL (0.8 direct reacting), urine hemoglobin 4+, and the mono spot test negative. The peripheral blood film revealed anisocytosis, polychromasia, and numerous spherocytes. The patient required transfusion of 10 units of blood in a 10-day period to maintain a hematocrit level of about 25%. The DAT was negative. The only free antibody detectable in his serum was a cold agglutinin with anti-I specificity that had a maximum titer of 512 at 4°C and demonstrated weak reactivity up to 22°C. The Donath-Landsteiner test was negative. A diagnosis of atypical cold agglutinin syndrome was made, and the patient was treated by keeping the temperature of his room at 37°C. Brisk hemolysis continued, however. He received 16 additional units of RBCs during the next month without his hematocrit level rising above 30%.

Studies on blood referred to our laboratory revealed the DAT was negative using anti-IgG, -IgA, -IgM, and anti-C3. No warm autoantibodies were detected in the serum by IAT or by agglutination of enzyme-treated RBCs. A cold agglutinin was present to a titer of 8 at 4°C in saline; it did not cause agglutination in saline or albumin at 25°C. The CFAC test revealed more than 400 molecules of IgG per RBC. The patient was subsequently treated with therapy appropriate for WAIHA and had a partial response to steroids, but he subsequently required splenectomy before achieving remission.

PATIENT 4: Relapsing AIHA in pregnancy in a patient with a negative DAT.[46] This interesting case is discussed in detail in the section on AIHA During Pregnancy on page 348.

The CFAC Test in Patients with Sickle Cell Disease (SCD) and Other Hemoglobinopathies

In extending our studies to include a representative sample of other nonimmune hemolytic anemias, we performed CFAC tests on RBCs from patients with a variety of congenital hemolytic anemias.[6,47] Table 9-4 shows the results. Rather surprisingly, we found that 39 of 62 patients (63%) who were homozygous for hemoglobin S had a mean of 195 (median of 290) and a maximum of 890 molecules of IgG per RBC; these patients would have fit our criteria for DAT-negative WAIHA.

The patients ranged in age from 11 months to 30 years, the hemoglobin from 6.0 to 11.1 g/dL, and the reticulocytes from 0.8% to 20%. We observed no significant correlations between the number of IgG molecules on patients' RBCs and the severity of their anemias, the incidence of painful sickle cell crisis, the reticulocyte counts, or blood transfusion histories. RBC survival studies were not performed.

Eluates were made from the RBCs of 23 of the 29 patients with SCD who had increased numbers of IgG molecules per RBC. Although only small volumes of RBCs were generally available for preparing eluates, six of the 23 eluates (26%) demonstrated antibody activity against normal RBCs by the IAT. In each case,

TABLE 9-4. RESULTS OF CFAC TESTS ON NORMAL PERSONS AND PATIENTS

Diagnosis	Number of Subjects Tested	Number of Patients with Positive Results*
Normal persons	42	1
Hemolytic anemias		
Hereditary spherocytosis	11	1
Pyruvate kinase deficiency	1	0
Mechanical hemolytic anemia (prosthetic heart valves)	11	1
Hemoglobin abnormalities		
Sickle cell anemia (S–S)	62	39
Sickle cell disease (S–C, S–D, S/β-thalassemia)	14	8
Sickle cell trait (A-S)	57	7
β-thalassemia major	6	5

* A positive result indicates >25 molecules of IgG/red cell.
From Petz LD, Yam P, Wilkinson L, Garratty G, Lubin B, Mentzer W: Increased IgG molecules bound to the surface of red blood cells of patients with sickle cells anemia. Blood 1984;64:301–304.

specificity tests revealed no definite specificity, thus suggesting autoantibody activity.

One patient's case history (Patient 5) illustrates the possible significance of these studies.

PATIENT 5: The patient was a 24-year-old female with SCD who had received multiple transfusions during childhood, although in the past 4 years she had received only 3 units of RBCs, which had been administered 6 months previously. Her hematocrit level was 18%, and her reticulocyte count was 18.1%. She was admitted to the hospital for an elective cholecystectomy, and the decision was made to transfuse her until her hematocrit level was about 36% in an attempt to reduce her anesthetic risk. Her DAT was negative, but a CFAC test done at the onset of the transfusions revealed 533 molecules of IgG per RBC, and a RBC eluate was weakly reactive with no definable specificity. She was known to have had allo-anti-M and anti-C in the past, as well as multiple HLA antibodies, and she was therefore transfused with leukocyte-poor M–, C–RBCs, even though anti-M and anti-C were not detectable at this time.

After transfusion of 8 units of leukocyte-poor RBCs over a 4-day period, her hematocrit level reached 36.8%. Two days later, she began to have shaking chills, abdominal pain, and fever, and she experienced a life-threatening hemolytic reaction, with her hematocrit level dropping to 13% in 48 hours and ultimately reaching a low of 7.4%. The serum hemoglobin reached 283 mg/dL, and she had hemoglobinuria and hemosiderinuria. She also suffered a hyporegenerative crisis, with a reticulocyte count of 0.

A DAT was negative. Repeat screening of her serum for alloantibodies revealed negative results except for very weak reactions with enzyme-treated cells, with no antibody specificity defined. She was treated with high doses of corticosteroids and two additional units of leukocyte-poor packed RBCs, and she gradually improved to a hematocrit level of 19.8%.

This patient's course was consistent with that of a delayed transfusion reaction, although there were no detectable alloantibodies. Our data offer a possible alternative explanation in that autoimmunization might have played a key role.

Autoimmunization was suggested by the presence of 533 molecules of IgG on the patient's RBCs at the onset of transfusions, by an RBC eluate that was weakly reactive by the IAT, and by the response to corticosteroids. It is possible that the transfusions stimulated the further production of autoantibodies, which also reacted with the donor RBCs to cause a transient AIHA. The lack of strongly reactive serologic abnormalities usually found in AIHA could be analogous to the cases of AIHA with a negative DAT described previously.

The suggestion that an augmentation of autoantibody production could be of significance in this clinical setting is strengthened by reports of numerous investigators concerning the production of autoantibodies after immunization with RBCs. This is reviewed in detail in the section later in this chapter regarding the development of autoantibodies and autoimmune hemolytic anemia following transfusion. In addition, Constantoulakis and associates[11] suggested that above a certain level ("hemolytic threshold"), minute increases of RBC-bound antibody induce pronounced effects on RBC survival. These authors emphasized that an acute, explosive hemolytic crisis in a patient with an otherwise chronic, compensated AIHA could result from a relatively small increment in antibody production, and that this increase in antibody production would not be detected by conventional serologic tests. The patient's hyporegenerative crisis could also be immunologically mediated, as there is ample precedent for reticulocytopenia as part of the presentation for an acute AIHA (see Chapter 3, page 69).

In addition to 98 SCD patients, we used the CFAC assay to test RBCs from 59 patients with sickle cell trait, 11 patients with hemoglobin S-C, nine patients with thalassemia syndrome (including heterozygous and homozygous thalassemia), and patients doubly heterozygous for sickle cell hemoglobin and thalassemia.[47] Ten patients with sickle cell trait (17%) yielded abnormal results. Six patients had more than 250 molecules of IgG per RBC on at least one occasion. Of the five patients in whom repeat samples were obtained, only one patient was found to have consistently abnormal results. Six of the 11 patients with hemoglobin S-C had increased numbers of IgG molecules per RBC, as did six of the nine patients with thalassemia syndromes.

There are some interesting findings related to the IgG on normal RBCs and RBCs of patients with SCD. Kay[48] has suggested that as RBCs age, they develop an SCA, and such RBCs can take up IgG autoantibody, leading to removal of the older RBCs by macrophages in the RES (see associated literature reviewed by Garratty).[14] Green and colleagues[49] confirmed other researchers' findings that the amount of IgG was greater on old than on younger RBCs when RBCs are separated by density. They also reported similar findings when SCD patients were studied; older sickle cells contained two to three times more RBC-bound IgG than younger sickle cells. Green and associates[50] went on to determine that irreversibly sickled cells (ISC) formed in vivo alterations in the topography of the membrane proteins on the external RBC surface that would cause preferential in vivo binding of autologous IgG. Using flow cytometry, they demonstrated a nonuniform distribution of RBCs within each density-separated RBC fraction exhibiting fluorescence as a result of labeling with FITC-conjugated anti-IgG. Each RBC fraction contained at least three distinct subpopulations:

1. A weakly fluorescent subpopulation, representing most of the RBCs in the dense (older) population, and considered to be IgG negative
2. A comparatively small subpopulation representing 1% to 12% of total RBCs, that were coated with IgG

3. A small (<1%) subpopulation that showed very bright fluorescence, indicating comparatively larger amounts of RBC-bound IgG

The researchers proposed the following role for RBC-bound IgG in the transformation of the reversible sickle cell (RSC) to ISC: Immunoglobulin molecules bind rapidly to high-affinity membrane proteins that emerge sequentially as the cell undergoes successive sickling-desickling cycles in vivo; IgG binding cross-links and inhibits the regression of the newly emerged surface proteins into the lipid layer. If the IgG binding proteins are also transmembrane proteins attached to the membrane cytoskeleton, cross-linking by surface-bound IgG (even 200–300 molecules per RBC) could inhibit the return of the membrane skeleton to the discoid shape (e.g., after a critical number of sickling-desickling cycles), producing RBCs fixed in the ISC morphology. The researchers also suggested that it was possible that at least part of the RBC-bound IgG (measured in this study for the most dense ISC-enriched sickle RBC fractions) was the senescent RBC autoantibody, as demonstrated for normal RBCs.[48] Because investigations have shown that sickle RBCs must be chronologically younger (life span in vivo, 10–40 days compared with normal RBCs [life span ~120 days]), their findings suggest the possibility that transformations of sickle RBCs to the ISC morphology could be associated with rapid RBC aging in vivo.[50]

Hebbel and Miller[51] showed that RBCs from SCD patients were excessively susceptible to phagocytosis. They reported that SCD RBCs were 1.03–6.85 times more adherent to macrophages than normal RBCs and that the degree of adherence correlated significantly with irreversibly sickled cell counts and hematologic values reflecting hemolysis rate. SCD RBCs spontaneously generate twice the normal amounts of dialdehyde byproducts of lipid peroxidation (i.e., malondialdehyde [MDA]), and MDA treatment of normal RBCs significantly enhances their phagocytosis. Hebbel and Miller[51] suggested the possibility that appearance of the SCA on old normal RBCs represents modification of the membrane by MDA. This report prompted Solanki[52] to look for evidence of in vivo erythrophagocytosis (Ep) in SCD patients. He examined blood smears of 27 patients and found 10 (37%) to show Ep (i.e., 1 to 6/1000 white blood cells or 1 to 10/100 monocytes). No Ep was seen in the blood smear of 25 normal controls or nine splenectomized subjects. The mean hematocrit value of the Ep(+) patients was significantly lower than that of the Ep(–) SCD patients.

Galili and coworkers,[53] using a modified AGT based on the high affinity between the Fc portion of RBC-bound IgG and the Fc receptor on the myeloid cell K-562, also found increased levels of IgG on RBCs from thalassemias. Immunoglobulin was found on the RBCs of 73 out of 80 patients (90%) with thalassemia. The immunoglobulin on the thalassemic RBCs belonged to the IgG class and was said to be autoreactive. Elution studies using various carbohydrates and thermal stripping indicated that at least a proportion of the IgG molecules found on the thalassemic RBCs were specifically reactive, with terminal galactosyl residues on the RBC membrane. IgG antibodies with similar reactivity were also demonstrated in normal human serum. These IgG natural antigalactosyl antibodies in normal sera could bind to IgG-depleted thalassemic RBCs. Thalassemic RBCs and normal senescent RBCs had been described previously as having reduced amounts of membrane sialic acid. Galili and colleagues[53] suggested that the IgG galactosyl antibodies interact with newly exposed galactosyl residues underlying the sialic acid residues, and that such interaction could lead to the shortened life span of thalassemic RBCs and result in sequestration of normal RBCs by the RES.

The foregoing findings suggest that there could be an immune component of the increased RBC destruction in SCD and possibly also in thalassemia.

Could Positive Sensitive Assays for RBC-Bound IgG (e.g., ELAT Results) Be Due to Nonspecific Uptake of IgG Rather Than Autoantibody?

Toy and coworkers[54] and Heddle and associates[55] found that RBCs with positive DATs yielding nonreactive eluates commonly were associated with levels of gamma globulin at the higher end of the normal range or hypergammaglobulinemia; this suggested that IgG was bound nonspecifically to the RBC membrane. Thus, it would seem essential that any interpretation of assays for RBC-bound IgG in suspected DAT-negative AIHA be related to serum globulin levels. Garratty and Arndt[56] measured the serum IgG levels in 48 patients who were thought to have DAT-negative AIHA and had positive sensitive test results (i.e., a positive ELAT, a positive direct Polybrene test, and/or a reactive concentrated eluate). Results were compared with a control group of 52 patients with a similar suspected diagnosis but yielding negative ELAT, Polybrene, and eluate results. The serum IgG levels were divided into four arbitrary groups of 0–600, 601–1200, 1201–1800, and greater than 1801 mg/dL. Within the first three groups (0–1800 mg/dL), there was no correlation between increasing levels of serum IgG and detection of increased RBC-bound IgG by sensitive tests. Two patients had serum IgG levels above 1800 mg/dL; the IgG of one patient was 1950 mg/dL and of the other, 3000 mg/dL. Both of these patients appeared to have increased RBC-bound IgG, as indicated by positive sensitive tests; it is possible that these results were due to nonspecific uptake of IgG onto the RBCs.

Thus, there appeared to be no correlation between positive direct ELATs, direct Polybrene tests, or reactive concentrated eluates and serum IgG levels among patients with normal (even up to 1800 mg/dL) IgG levels.[56] We think it reasonable to continue assuming that we are detecting IgG autoantibody rather than nonspecifically bound IgG on the RBCs of these patients. When rare patients with DAT-negative AIHA and hypergammaglobulinemia (such as the latter two patients just mentioned) are encountered, it is always possible that positive sensitive test results could reflect nonspecific uptake rather than autoantibody. Thus, to improve the accuracy of the interpretation, we would recommend that hematologists relate the serum IgG level to the results of sensitive tests for RBC-bound IgG. In patients with hypergammaglobulinemia, positive results of tests that are more sensitive than the antiglobulin test would have to be suspected to be unreliable.

Does Quantity of RBC-Bound IgG Always Explain the Phenomenon? Do Qualitative Factors Play a Role?

Some findings suggest that the explanation for DAT-negative AIHA is not simply quantitative and that it could represent a qualitative defect of the sensitivity of the routine DAT. Gilliland and associates[8,9] and the current authors[6] found that some patients classified as having DAT-negative AIHA had far more than 200 IgG molecules per RBC. For example, five of the 27 patients in our series had more than 400 IgG molecules per RBC when measured by the CFAC test (see Table 9-3). IgG sensitization to this degree should be easily detectable by the AGT; indeed, more than 400 molecules would usually yield >3+ DAT reactions.

Garratty[15] reported data supporting suspicions that the explanation might not be totally quantitative. Figure 9-3 shows examples of RBCs tested by ELAT. The triangles represent the optical density results obtained on the RBCs of 12 patients suspected of having DAT-negative AIHA; the circles represent the mean optical density readings (ODs) obtained on the RBCs from six normal donors tested at the same time the patients' RBCs were tested. The patients with hemolytic anemia obviously have increased amounts of RBC-bound IgG compared with normal donors, but it is hard to be convinced that this represents a purely quantitative difference.

When using ELAT, positive controls of IgG- (anti-D) sensitized RBCs are always tested; Garratty[15] noticed that the ODs on these controls, with obvious positive IATs, were often less than the ODs on some DAT-negative patients. The ½+, 1+, and 2+ results in Figure 9-3 represent the IAT results of RBCs that were sensitized with anti-D in vitro and yielded similar ODs to the DAT-negative patients, which are represented by the triangle next to the plus (+) signs. Thus, it is a mystery why the RBC-bound IgG on the RBCs of the patients with hemolytic anemia was not detected by the AGT, when anti-D sensitized cells with similar ELAT results yielded obvious positive IATs.

The results suggest something other than a simple quantitative reason for the detection of RBC-bound IgG in the presence of a negative DAT. The answer cannot be differences in the AGS, as Petz and Garratty[6] used the same anti-IgG for the CFAC tests that was used for the DATs. It is possible that the RBC-bound IgG could be oriented in such a way on the RBC membrane that the anti-IgG could not bridge between adjacent RBCs to cause agglutination, and that this IgG would be detected by assays that are not dependent on agglutination (e.g., the CFAC test or ELAT). This might occur if the IgG was not bound to the RBC by its Fab portion (i.e., if it was not an antibody directed against RBC antigen).

Engelfriet and colleagues[57] suggested that DAT-negative AIHA could be due to small amounts of RBC-bound IgG3 autoantibody. In vitro experiments suggested that about 500–1000 IgG1 molecules per RBC were needed for in vitro interactions with peripheral

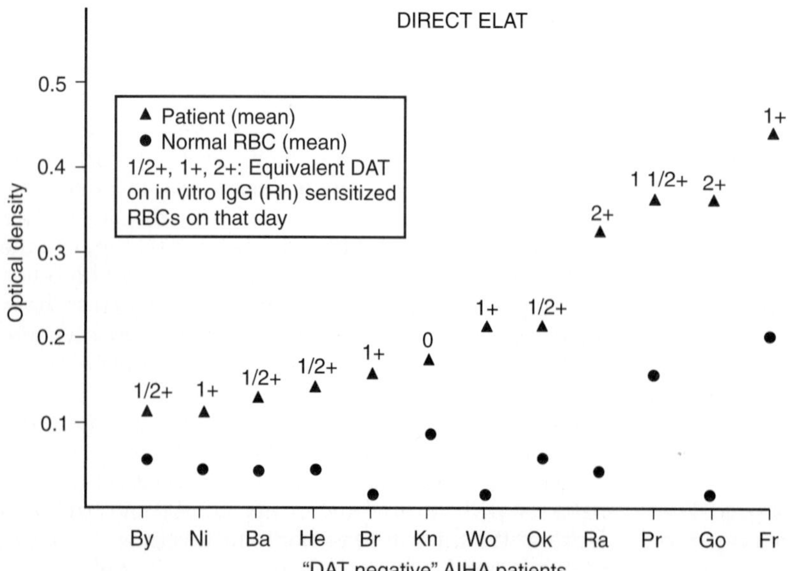

FIGURE 9-3. Comparison of enzyme-linked antiglobulin test results on RBCs from patients with "DAT-negative" AIHA (▲), normal donors (•) (mean OD of 6 donors), and D + RBCs sensitized in vitro with dilutions of anti-D and giving the same OD readings as the RBCs from the "DAT-negative" patients tested on the same day. The results of the indirect antiglobulin tests of the anti-D sensitized RBCs are graded from 0 to 2 +. (From Garratty G: Factors affecting the pathogenicity of red cell auto- and alloantibodies. In Nance SJ (ed): Immune Destruction of Red Blood Cells. Arlington, Va: American Association of Blood Banks, 1989: 109–169.)

blood monocytes, but only 100 to 150 IgG3 molecules per RBC were necessary for similar interactions.[57,58] It should be emphasized that these experiments used peripheral blood monocytes and that smaller numbers of IgG molecules could yield similar interactions with macrophages, which are more active than monocytes.

Engelfriet and colleagues[57] used dilutions of IgG1 and IgG3 to sensitize RBCs in vitro; the sensitized RBCs were tested by AGT and a monocyte antibody-dependent cellular cytotoxicity (ADCC) assay. They found that cytotoxic damage of IgG1-sensitized RBCs occurred only when the AGT was positive, but that RBCs sensitized with two dilutions of IgG3 anti-D yielding negative AGTs were cytotoxically damaged. Zupanska and coworkers[58] also showed that RBCs sensitized in vitro with IgG3 anti-D (but not IgG1 anti-D) sometimes adhered to monocytes in an in vitro monocyte monolayer assay (MMA) when the DAT on those RBCs was negative. Thus, it is possible that the difference between normal RBC destruction by naturally occurring IgG autoantibodies and the abnormal destruction associated with DAT-negative AIHA could be qualitative as well as (or instead of) quantitative. It would be of great interest to know whether the IgG antibody to the RBC senescence antigen (see Chapter 4) is always IgG1, which would suggest that subclass difference could be more important than the subtle quantitative differences.

DAT-NEGATIVE AIHA ASSOCIATED WITH LOW-AFFINITY IgG AUTOANTIBODIES

When the routine DAT is performed, the patient's RBCs are washed three to four times in large volumes of saline at room temperature (RT). Sometimes, because cold autoagglutinins are noted, the RBCs are washed with 37°C saline. We have encountered rare patients in whom a DAT that is negative or weakly positive becomes strongly positive when the routine procedure is processed under different conditions.

Garratty and associates[41,59,60] studied 22 patients with AIHA who were associated with low-affinity autoantibodies; 17 of these patients were referred because of suspected DAT-negative AIHA. Eleven of the 22 (including 6 of 17 referred as DAT-negative AIHA) patients had a positive DAT if the RBCs were washed with saline at RT, but the DATs were negative in 8 of 11 patients when the RBCs were washed at 37°C. RBC-bound IgG was detected on all 22 patients when the RBCs were washed with ice-cold (0–4°C) saline and/or low ionic-strength saline (LISS). When the RBCs were washed with cold saline or LISS, they were always tested with 10% albumin (as a negative control), in parallel with the antiglobulin sera, to control against cold autoagglutinins causing the positive test result. When RBCs from some of these patients were washed and allowed to stand at RT for 20–160 minutes before performing the DAT, all DATs were much weaker or negative. When 22 random DAT-positive RBC samples were subjected to the same conditions, DAT titration scores appeared similar to those of the RBCs that were tested immediately following washing; none of the positive DATs became negative.

Sokol and coworkers[61] described two patients with suspected AIHA who had negative routine DATs. Their DATs were positive when the patients' RBCs were washed with saline at 4°C. In one case, the DAT was also positive by a column agglutination technique (ID gel from DiaMed-AG, Cressier sur Morat, Switzerland). Eluates from the patients' RBCs were reactive if eluates were prepared from RBCs washed at 4°C.

Lai and colleagues[62] described a patient with hemolytic anemia who had a negative routine DAT but whose DAT was 4+ when the RBCs were washed with saline at 4°C. The DAT was also positive when tested by column agglutination techniques (CAT).

Johnson and Bandouveres[63] described a 6-month-old infant with a severe hemolytic anemia (hemoglobin of 4 g/dL). The routine DAT was negative. The DAT was 3+ after the patient's RBCs were washed with 4°C LISS. An eluate from the patient's RBCs reacted at 3+, showing anti-Pr specificity. The patient's serum contained an IgG anti-Pr detectable only by IAT using 4°C LISS for the washing phase.

We believe that low-affinity antibodies can sometimes cause technical problems in obtaining an accurate DAT result; they might possibly cause a false-negative IAT in addition to a false-negative DAT. Low-affinity autoantibodies (and possibly alloantibodies) may be dissociated from the RBCs by the process of washing for the DAT (and probably for the IAT). This loss of antibody occurs more frequently when the RBCs are washed at 37°C (note that 6 of 17 patients referred as DAT negative AIHA were DAT positive when the DAT was performed using the routine method using RT saline). The referring hospitals usually had used a "prewarm" procedure.[41,59,60]

It is of interest to add that some of the cases that we have encountered that were associated with low-affinity autoantibodies have had quite severe hemolytic anemias. This fact does not seem to agree with early published work that RBCs sensitized with high-affinity antibody are destroyed much more efficiently than those sensitized with low-affinity antibodies (see also Chapter 4).[15,41,64]

Schwartz and Costea[64] performed the only published experiments relating alloantibody affinity to in vivo RBC destruction. They studied three examples of anti-D with different affinities for D+ RBCs. They expressed the antibody affinity in terms of the amount of time it took for in vitro spontaneous elution of 50% of the RBC-bound anti-D. The elution times (ET) were 160 minutes, 100 minutes, and 40 minutes, respectively, for the three anti-D. RBC survival studies were carried out on ^{51}Cr-labeled RBCs sensitized with these three anti-D. Figure 9-4 shows the results. There was an inverse relationship between RBC survival and ET; that is, the RBCs coated with anti-D of the highest

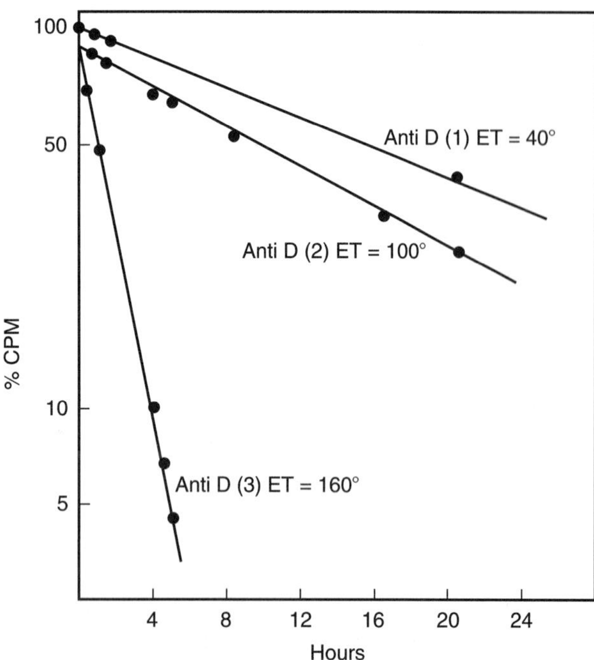

FIGURE 9-4. The effect of antibody affinity on RBC survival: The ordinate and abscissa indicate the in vivo RBC survival of D + ^{51}Cr-labeled RBCs sensitized with three anti-D, of different affinity, in terms of ^{51}Cr counts (% CPM) and collection time of samples tested, respectively. ET refers to "elution time," which is the time required for 50% of the sensitizing antibody to dissociate from the RBCs In vitro. Thus, short elution time indicates a low avidity antibody [e.g., anti-D (1)], and a long elution time indicates an antibody with higher affinity [e.g., anti-D (3)]. (From Schwartz RS, Costea N: Autoimmune hemolytic anemia: Clinical correlations and biological implications. Semin Hematol 1966;3:2–26.)

affinity (longest ET) had a shorter survival than the RBCs coated with anti-D of lower affinity (shorter ET). Although equilibrium constants were not calculated, one would expect that the ET, as measured in these experiments, should correlate with the equilibrium constants of the antibodies. These experiments were carried out in 1966, and it is surprising that there are no other good data in humans relating antibody affinity to the degree of RBC destruction; this relationship would appear to be an important factor.

Garratty[15] suggested that one explanation might be that the low-affinity antibodies that were detected might not have been the major cause of the severe hemolysis in the patients discussed previously. High-affinity antibodies might have been present and, being of higher affinity, would have reacted with the patient's RBCs first, leaving predominantly lower-affinity antibodies in the plasma. If most of the RBCs sensitized with the high-affinity antibody were removed by the mononuclear phagocyte system, the only RBCs left circulating might be those sensitized with low-affinity autoantibodies. This is a good example of where the results of our in vitro tests might not correlate with the clinical course observed in actual patients. In contrast to the early experiments using human antibodies, a more recent publication showed that low-affinity autoantibodies in a mouse model had high pathogenic potential.[65]

Although low-affinity antibodies appear to be uncommon, the foregoing results emphasize that when we wash RBCs, we are creating conditions very different from those found in vivo. The antiglobulin test must be performed immediately following washing of the RBCs. If RBCs are washed at 37°C, one should remember that some antiglobulin tests could be weaker or even negative when low-affinity antibodies are present; on rare occasions, even RBCs washed at RT might yield false weak positive or negative antiglobulin tests.

DAT-NEGATIVE AIHA ASSOCIATED WITH RBC-BOUND IgA AND IgM

Routine polyspecific AGSs are not standardized to react with IgA- or IgM-sensitized RBCs; they are required only to detect IgG and C3 (C3d). Most of the polyclonal polyspecific AGS used routinely for DATs do contain anti-IgA, but they sometimes react only following the 5- to 10-minute incubation period recommended by the manufacturers to enhance anti-C3 reactivity.[66] Anti-IgA and anti-IgM that are standardized for the DAT are not readily available. One can standardize immunological reagents, but as agglutination is far more sensitive than many immunological procedures, great care must be taken to avoid specificity problems with heterophile antibodies and anti-light chain cross-reactivity (see Chapter 6). Anti-IgM does not work well with the DAT, even when a reagent that is potent by other criteria is used.[6] We (and others) have been quite successful detecting RBC-bound IgA and IgM using flow cytometry.[41,42,67-70]

On rare occasions, WAIHA can be associated with IgA and IgM autoantibodies without the presence of IgG. For the reasons just discussed, they can sometimes present as DAT-negative AIHA.

WAIHA Associated with IgA Autoantibodies

The clinical and hematological features of patients with AIHA associated with IgA autoantibodies are very similar to those of patients whose AIHA is associated with warm IgG autoantibodies.[66,70-83] Patients with both types of AIHA also respond to the same therapy (i.e., steroids and/or splenectomy). Macrophages were originally said not to have (or to have very inefficient) receptors for IgA, but increasing evidence suggested that IgA sometimes participates in phagocytosis and ADCC.[84-87] A human Fc receptor (FcαR) for IgA has been cloned.[84] The monoclonal antibody used to isolate the clone is capable of inhibiting any binding of IgA and phagocytosis of IgA-coated targets.[88]

Clark and associates[75] studied the mechanism of hemolysis in a patient whose WAIHA was associated with an IgA autoantibody. The patient pursued a clinical course (spherocytosis, splenic sequestration of red cells, response to corticosteroids, and splenectomy) very similar to that of individuals with WAIHA associated with IgG autoantibodies, which suggests that the mechanism of hemolysis might be similar to that occurring in WAIHA associated with IgG autoantibodies. An eluate from the patient's RBCs was shown to react by ADCC toward sensitized RBCs that appeared to be IgA dependent. The ADCC-promoting effect of the eluate was blocked by a solid-phase anti-IgA immunosorbent and by fluid-phase normal IgA, and the effect was dependent on the dose of IgA eluate used to sensitize RBCs. The patient's eluate promoted phagocytosis of sensitized RBCs by normal mononuclear phagocytes. Both ADCC and phagocytosis promoted by the patient's eluate were complement independent. The eluate failed to produce complement-mediated hemolysis, and complement components could not be detected on sensitized RBCs either in vitro or in vivo. Taken together, these observations suggested a possible mechanism for what appeared, clinically, in this patient to be a WAIHA mediated by IgA—a complement-independent interaction of IgA-coated RBCs with the patient's mononuclear phagocytes.

Salama and colleagues[78] studied a 6-year-old patient with AIHA who had a strongly positive DAT due predominately to IgA, although small amounts of RBC-bound IgG were also detected; no RBC-bound C3 was detected. This patient had severe hemolysis associated with an upper respiratory tract infection. Evidence was presented that C3-independent intravascular immune hemolysis had occurred through "reactive hemolysis" (see the section on bystander immune cytolysis later in this chapter). Reactive hemolysis involved C3-independent binding of C5b-9 complexes in addition to IgA (and IgG), but no C3. Salama and colleagues[78] pointed out that several reports of AIHA associated with IgA autoantibodies appeared to have signs of intravascular lysis and that perhaps reactive lysis might play a role in the hemolytic process.

WAIHA Associated with IgM Autoantibodies

IgM warm autoantibodies might agglutinate untreated and/or enzyme-treated RBCs, hemolyze untreated and/or enzyme-treated RBCs, and/or sensitize RBCs so that IgM and/or complement is detectable by the DAT.[67-69,89-92] The routine DAT is sometimes negative in patients with warm IgM warm autoantibodies, however.

Some authors have detected IgM on the RBCs of patients who have AIHA but a negative routine DAT.[67-69,89-92] This IgM was sometimes detectable by the DAT using anti-IgM, and sometimes detectable only by more sensitive procedures. Garratty and colleagues[69] found that four of 41 (10%) cases of WAIHA associated with IgM autoantibodies had a negative DAT when routine AGS (anti-IgG and anti-C3) were used; IgM was detectable on the RBCs of two of these four patients using flow cytometry. Sokol and coworkers[34] studied 219 patients suspected of having AIHA. DAT and ELAT results were the same in 61 patients; in 43 cases, the ELAT detected additional immunoglobulin classes; in 33 cases, the DAT showed only RBC-bound C3 (C3d), but ELAT showed RBC-bound IgM in 16 (50%) of these. In five of 16 cases, the DAT was negative and the ELAT detected RBC-bound IgM. Kay and associates[89] and Szymanski and colleagues[92] detected low molecular weight (monomeric) IgM on patients' RBCs.

It is still controversial whether IgM non–complement-activating antibodies can cause immune RBC destruction, and if they do, how this is possible, as macrophages are said to lack IgM receptors. Schreiber and Frank[93,94] injected a strain of guinea pig, genetically deficient in C4, with ^{51}Cr-labeled IgM sensitized RBCs (it should be noted that these RBCs were sensitized with relatively small numbers of IgM molecules) and showed that the RBCs survived normally. Later, similar experiments in humans with complement deficiencies yielded similar results.[95] IgM anti-M, anti-D, and anti-c have been reported as a cause of increased RBC destruction; it was suggested that RBC agglutinates might become trapped in small blood vessels and eventually suffer metabolic damage.[96,97] Mollison[98,99] reviewed his earlier data and reported that he could not be confident that the IgM anti-M studied in 1958[96] did not activate complement. He also could not exclude the possibility that some IgG anti-D had been present, in addition to the IgM anti-D, in the serum reported in 1971.[97] He had no good explanation for the increased destruction of the RBCs that were seemingly sensitized only by IgM anti-c.[97] In this case, ^{51}Cr-labeled c+ RBCs were almost totally cleared in the liver, which suggested complement-mediated destruction rather than IgG-mediated destruction, but no in vitro complement sensitization was observed.[99]

Thus, there would seem to be very little experimental evidence that RBC-bound IgM alone can cause increased RBC destruction. Nevertheless, there are reports of cases of AIHA that appear to be associated with non–complement-binding IgM antibodies. Salama and Mueller-Eckhardt[100] reported on 12 children (eight of whom were infants) with relatively severe AIHA associated with non–complement-binding IgM autoantibodies. The routine DATs were negative in 11 cases and positive due to RBC-bound C3d in one case. All patients were shown to have RBC-bound IgM when a radioimmune assay was used; two cases also had IgA and/or IgG detected by this assay. An unusual finding with these patients was that no antibodies were detected in the patients' sera either by conventional serology or the radioimmune assay. Eluates from RBCs of all 11 patients were nonreactive by conventional serology, but two reacted with anti-IgM by the radioimmune assay.

(For a further discussion of AIHA associated with warm IgM autoantibodies, see Chapter 5.)

SEROLOGICAL AIDS IN DIAGNOSING DAT-NEGATIVE AIHA

The sensitive assays discussed previously for detecting RBC-bound IgG below the threshold of the DAT are sometimes called by hematologists "Super Coombs' tests." These assays are tedious to standardize and perform; they often take most of a working day to obtain a result. Their predictive value is not good. Garratty and colleagues[40,41] reported that less than one third of DAT-negative patients suspected of having WAIHA have increased amounts of RBC-bound IgG detected by such assays (Table 9-5). These assays are not available in many laboratories in the United States; even in our own laboratory, we rarely employ them. Our routine approach now is to employ serological tests, such as the ones listed later in this chapter; methods are given in more detail in Chapter 6.

Direct Antiglobulin Tests

We sometimes find that a DAT reported as negative by a referring hospital is weakly positive, with routine reagents, when tested by experienced technologists in our reference or research laboratories. In one study, Garratty and coworkers[40] found that 10% of DATs reported as negative by referring hospitals were positive when tested in their research laboratory. The false-negative results obtained by the hospital sometimes occurred because the hospital unnecessarily washed the patient's RBCs at 37°C; loss of RBC-bound, low-affinity IgG warm autoantibodies is greater when RBCs are washed at 37°C.[41,59,60]

Washing Patient's RBCs in Room Temperature LISS or Cold (0–4°C) Saline or LISS

To retain low-affinity RBC-bound autoantibodies during the washing phase, in addition to using the routine RT wash, we wash the patient's RBCs with cold LISS or saline. Careful controls are necessary to ensure that false-positive DATs are not caused by cold autoagglutinins (see Chapter 6). If cold agglutinins are a problem with a 0–4°C wash, then washing with RT LISS could be a compromise.

TABLE 9-5. COMPARISON OF TESTS USED FOR DETECTING RBC-BOUND IgG WHEN DAT IS NEGATIVE

Test	No. of Patients	No./% Positive
Flow cytometry	70	15/21
Direct Polybrene	205	38/19
Direct ELAT	201	32/16
Direct PEG	160	16/10
Concentrated eluate	162	15/9
DAT using cold saline washes	209	7/3
MMA	105	4/4

From Garratty G: Autoimmune hemolytic anemia. In Garratty G (ed): Immunolobiology of Transfusion Medicine. New York: Dekker, 1994: 493–521.

Using Column Agglutination Tests (CAT) for DAT

CATs (e.g., gel test) sometimes yield a positive DAT on RBCs that are DAT negative by routine tube methods.[62,101-103] This could be because no washing of RBCs is involved; thus, low-affinity autoantibodies that would be lost during the wash phase used in the tube method can be detected.

Using Special Antiglobulin Sera

We test patients' RBCs with anti-IgA and anti-IgM that have been standardized for use with RBCs (see Chapter 6). We also use an anti-C3 that is known to be rich in anti-C3d.

Direct Polybrene Test

We have found that one of the most useful serological tests for detecting RBC-bound IgG that is undetectable by routine DAT is the direct Polybrene test (see Chapter 6 for details of performing the test).[28,40,41,104] Normal RBCs aggregate when added to Polybrene in a low-ionic strength milieu. This aggregation can be dispersed by adding sodium citrate and mixing gently. If RBCs are coated with IgG added to Polybrene and centrifuged, they agglutinate, and this agglutination is not dispersed by sodium citrate. If agglutination is not observed at this stage, RBC-bound IgG can sometimes be detected by washing the RBCs and adding anti-IgG. Such a test can detect RBC-bound IgG that is not detectable by routine DAT. Garratty and colleagues[28,40] found the direct Polybrene test to be almost as sensitive as flow cytometry and more sensitive than ELAT (which is equivalent to the CFAC test) for detecting RBC-bound IgG (see Table 9-5). The method we use is described in detail in Chapter 6. Owen and Hows[105] and Rubino and associates,[106] using a slight variation of the procedure given in Chapter 6, also found the direct Polybrene test useful.

If Polybrene is not available, a polyethylene glycol (PEG) DAT can be used, but Garratty and colleagues[40] and Rubino and coworkers[106] did not find this as sensitive as the Polybrene test.

Detection of Autoantibody in Eluates

Gilliland and associates[8] found that they could demonstrate that IgG autoantibody was present on the RBCs of six of six patients with DAT-negative AIHA if they tested concentrated eluates prepared from the patients' RBCs. Eluates (three cycles) were prepared from 50–200 mL of a patient's RBCs and then concentrated to 1 mL. The eluates reacted strongly by the routine IAT. It is not often possible or practical to use this approach, but we also have found that eluates prepared by a routine method from 3–5 mL of a patient's RBCs will sometimes react (see Table 9-5).[6,28,40-41] We found that a two- to fivefold concentration yielded more positive reactions (we used Minicon filters [Amicon Corporation, Lexington, MA] to concentrate the eluates).

Detection of IgG Autoantibodies in Patients' Sera

Sometimes IgG autoantibodies are readily detectable in the patient's sera when the DAT is negative.[6,107-109] These autoantibodies are usually potentiator dependent, only being detectable with the use of enzyme-treated RBCs, in the presence of PEG, or by using CATs. The results might indicate the presence of low-affinity antibodies that are lost from the patient's RBCs during the washing phase of the IAT, or transient depression of antigens on patients' RBCs[108,109] (see also Chapter 7).

Table 9-6 summarizes the laboratory tests we perform to evaluate a patient referred to our laboratory for DAT-negative AIHA.

CORRELATIONS WITH IN VITRO FUNCTIONAL CELLULAR ASSAYS

The first report we know of applying cellular assays to investigate DAT-negative AIHA is that of Parker and coworkers[110] in 1972. These investigators used an erythrophagocytosis assay, in which a patient's washed RBCs were added to mouse macrophages. The assay was strongly positive in a patient who was DAT negative but appeared to have AIHA. van der Meulen and colleagues[111] also applied an RBC adherence assay to study RBCs from patients with AIHA. RBCs from 42 patients with positive DATs were added to monocytes in vitro, and RBC adherence occurred with RBCs from all 22 patients who had AIHA; no adherence was noted with RBCs from 20 patients without increased RBC destruction. Galili and associates[112] used an assay measuring adherence of patients' RBCs, following incubation in antiglobulin serum, to a K-562 erythro-myeloid cell line. Six of six DAT-negative patients suspected of having AIHA gave positive results with this assay.

Nance and Garratty[113] used an MMA that measured both RBC adherence and phagocytosis. RBCs from 174 normal donors with negative DATs had a mean total reactivity (MTR) of adherence and phagocytosis of 0.3%. RBCs from 45 normal donors with positive DATs (mean of 2+) had an MTR of 0.6%. They had definitive clinical and laboratory data on 44 of 70 DAT-positive patients tested. Twenty-five of the 44 had no evidence of hemolysis at the time of testing and had an MTR of 3.8%, whereas the 19 with AIHA had an MTR of 11.4%. The MTR of RBCs from 19 other patients with DAT-negative AIHA were within two standard deviations of the normal range. The MMA results correlated perfectly with the presence of AIHA, except in one patient with AIHA and a 2+ DAT, whose RBCs yielded 0% reactivity in the MMA. The MTR of DAT-positive patients with AIHA was three times greater than that of DAT-positive patients without AIHA, 19 times greater than that of DAT-positive normal donors, and 42 times greater than that of DAT-negative normal donors. Later results by the same laboratory found that RBCs from only four of 105 patients with DAT-negative AIHA reacted by the MMA (see Table 9-5).[40]

Gallagher and associates[114] also found a good correlation with their assay and AIHA. RBCs from all 18 DAT-positive patients with AIHA adhered or were phagocytosed by monocytes. RBCs from all 10 DAT-positive patients without AIHA were not significantly phagocytosed, but four of the 10 showed increased adherence to monocytes. This led Gallagher and associates[114] to use only phagocytosis as an index of clinical significance in future studies. The same reasearchers also studied 11 patients with DAT-negative AIHA. RBCs from seven of the 11 patients yielded significantly elevated results; however, three of these results were significantly elevated only if autologous monocytes were used. Of the seven patients showing significant reactions, six had a weakly positive DAT using C3d; it is unclear whether this influenced the reactions.

TABLE 9-6. FURTHER TESTING OF RBCs FROM PATIENTS WHO HAVE A NEGATIVE DAT AND SUSPECTED AIHA

1. Repeat DAT. If referral laboratory washed RBCs at 37°C, it is important to use RT washing when the DAT is repeated.
2. DAT using anti-IgA and IgM in addition to anti-IgG and anti-C3; it is important that the anti-C3 contain potent anti-C3d activity.
3. If DAT is still negative, repeat DAT using RBCs washed with 4°C saline or, preferably, 4°C LISS (controls to exclude false-positive results due to cold auto-agglutinins are essential—see Chapter 6).
4. Direct Polybrene test (see Chapter 6 for details).
5. Additional serological tests that might be useful include a DAT using CAT (e.g., gel columns); IAT using patient's serum and/or an eluate from the patient's RBCs, tested against enzyme-treated RBCs or in the presence of PEG.
6. If serological tests are nonproductive, a DAT using flow cytometry (or one of the other sensitive assays discussed earlier) can be used.

Brojer and coworkers[115] also found a good correlation with their monocyte assays and in vivo hemolysis in DAT-positive patients. The same group found that the number of RBC-bound IgG molecules generally correlated with the presence of phagocytosis and the degree of anemia, but there were exceptions.[116] Phagocytosis was always observed when there were more than 2000 IgG molecules per RBC. In patients having less than 700 IgG molecules per RBC, the interaction with monocytes was observed only if IgG3 was present on the RBCs; the minimum number of IgG3 molecules per RBC initiating phagocytosis was 150–640, in contrast to RBCs with IgG1 sensitization where 1250 to 4020 molecules were needed. They found no differences in reactivity when comparing autologous monocytes with homologous monocytes from patients with AIHA.[116]

Using a mononuclear phagocyte assay, Herron and colleagues[117] found a good correlation with AIHA but failed to detect RBC-bound IgG on three DAT-negative patients suspected of having AIHA.

In summary, although on occasion we have obtained a positive result (sometimes with only autologous monocytes), in many cases the MMA was noninformative. We no longer use the MMA routinely in our workup of DAT-negative AIHA.

Could DAT-Negative AIHA Be Due to an Antibody-Independent, Cell-Mediated, Cytotoxicity Mechanism?

In 1981, Garratty[118] suggested the possibility that natural killer (NK) cells might recognize foreign determinants on RBCs and cause alloimmune or autoimmune hemolytic anemia by antibody-independent cell-mediated cellular cytotoxicity. As six of 22 patients with hemolytic transfusion reactions and no demonstrable antibodies had chronic lymphatic leukemia, this author tried to demonstrate NK cell activity by one chronic lymphatic leukemia patient's mononuclear cells against putative donor RBCs; the experiment was unsuccessful.

Gilsanz and colleagues[119] reported success in demonstrating NK cell activity against autologous RBCs in a patient with DAT-negative AIHA. A 65-year-old patient with a 5-year history of asymptomatic large granular lymphocytic leukemia developed hemolytic anemia. She had a hemoglobin of 97 g/L and an increased reticulocyte count (6%); the bilirubin was 1.4 mg/dL and lactate dehydrogenase (LDH) was 350 IU/L; serum haptoglobins were absent. The peripheral blood smear showed marked spherocytosis; splenomegaly was found by ultrasonography. DATs were repeatedly negative. The large granular lymphocyte count was 6.0×10^9/L; the NK phenotype was CD2+, CD3–, CD16+, CD38+, CD57+. No coexisting disease or hemolytic triggering factors were found. She did not improve with prednisone (20 mg/day) and had to be transfused twice for symptomatic anemia. The response to transfusions was good.

To assess a possible role for NK cells in the hemolysis, a cytotoxicity assay was designed.[119] NK cells were obtained by density gradient and purified. Cytotoxicity was measured by a ^{51}Cr-specific release assay using autologous RBCs and ABO-identical allogeneic RBCs as targets. The resulting hemolysis was expressed as a percentage of the mean release, corrected for spontaneous release. Autologous RBCs (but not allogeneic RBCs) were lysed in vitro by the patient's NK cells, either in the presence or absence of serum, which indicated that a direct lytic mechanism was effected by the proliferating and activated NK cells. The patient was started on treatment with cyclophosphamide. After 1 month, the anemia improved, and 2 months later, NK blood cell counts and spleen size normalized. Thereafter, the patient's NK cells failed to show any lytic activity against autologous RBCs in the cytotoxicity assay. It was suggested that NK cell activation and cytotoxicity could have contributed to the hemolytic anemia in this patient with large granular lymphocytic leukemia.[119]

THERAPY AND COURSE

Patients with acquired hemolytic anemia who have a negative DAT without evidence for a nonimmune cause of the hemolysis, but who do have abnormal numbers of IgG molecules on their RBCs, should be treated similarly to patients who have more characteristic findings of WAIHA (see Chapter 11). The variable responses to therapy indicated in Table 9-3 and described previously are similar to these observed in patients who present with a positive DAT and typical serologic findings of WAIHA. Gilliland[9] has also demonstrated that, in many patients, a reduction of cell-bound IgG antibody can be documented after remission induced by corticosteroids or splenectomy. Other patients, however, develop a well-compensated hemolytic anemia with little change in the abnormal quantity of IgG per RBC. Gilliland further indicated that some patients who originally presented with AIHA with a positive DAT, once given corticosteroids therapy, have shown a reduction of RBC-bound IgG antibody to levels that are still elevated, but below detection by routine antiglobulin testing.[9] The quantity of IgG antibody in some of these patients remained at these low levels for several years, whereas in others, the quantity of IgG per RBC increased, and hemolytic anemia recurred after therapy with steroids was decreased or stopped. In still other patients, the quantity of IgG per RBC fell to the range observed on normal RBCs, and therapy was discontinued without an increase of RBC-bound antibody or exacerbation of hemolytic disease.

PCH is much more commonly reported among children than among adults; in some series, it makes up a significant percentage of patients.[200-202] Indeed, Sokol and colleagues[199] reported that a Donath-Landsteiner antibody was found in 17 of 42 of their patients (40%) (see Table 9-10).

A number of cases with unusual serological findings have been reported. For example, Friedmann and coworkers[216] reported a 9-year-old girl with Evans's syndrome who had high-titer, high thermal amplitude (37°C) complete IgM autoantibody. Despite aggressive management, the patient ultimately died of complications of her disease. Such a clinical course is consistent with the dismal prognosis among adults with similar warm-reactive IgM autoantibodies.[217-220] Issitt and colleagues[109] described a case of WAIHA in which marked depression of RBC Rh antigen expression resulted in the patient presenting with severe anemia but a negative DAT. Unlike two previously reported cases cited by these researchers, in which the diagnosis of AIHA was established before the DAT became negative, the authors' patient presented with negative serological findings during his first episode of anemia. Win and associates[221] reported an infant with AIHA who had an autoantibody with anti-Kp^b specificity.

Hemoglobinuria is much more common in children than in adults, which is due partly to the more frequent occurrence of PCH. Hemoglobinuria occurred in all 17 patients reported by Sokol and associates[199] who had Donath-Landsteiner antibodies, but it also occurred in patients with cold agglutinins and in mixed-type AIHA. (PCH is discussed in more detail in Chapter 5.)

AIHA OCCURRING AT A VERY EARLY AGE

Sokol and associates[199] reported that their youngest patient was 3 months old. Other reports, however, include patients with AIHA occurring at even earlier ages,[197,204,212,222,223] including one patient who was diagnosed at the age of 2 weeks.[224] Erler and coworkers[225] described an infant who was found to have a positive DAT at birth without evidence of maternal alloantibodies or autoantibodies. No antibody was found in the infant's serum, and he had no evidence of hemolysis, but an eluate from his RBCs contained an IgG panagglutinin. The DAT was still positive 6 weeks after birth but was negative at 6 months of age. The authors suggested that autoantibody production had occurred in utero.

Hadnagy[226] provided a brief report of a child whose AIHA dated from birth and had continued for 13 years at the time of publication. The child was born severely jaundiced in 1976 and was exchange-transfused on the third day after birth. There was no evidence of fetomaternal incompatibility, and there were no unexpected antibodies in the mother's serum. The infant's DAT was positive at birth and remained positive in 1977 and 1978, and evidences of hemolysis were still present. The RBC count was 2.2–2.3 million/mm^3, reticulocytes were 13.8%–23.4%, and spherocytes were found on the peripheral blood film. The autoantibody was of the warm type and possibly of anti-e specificity. The child was treated with corticosteroids and responded well; the DAT became negative, only to become positive again when corticosteroids were reduced. Splenectomy at age 3.5 years resulted in significant improvement, although evidence of hemolysis was still present in 1989.

Management

Habibi and colleagues[197] reported that corticosteroid therapy seemed to be effective frequently, but it was often difficult to exclude the possibility of spontaneous remission, especially in acute cases. Patients who respond to steroids frequently demonstrate a significant decrease in hemolysis within 10 days of diagnosis. Splenectomy was performed for 16 patients who showed corticosteroid resistance or dependence with severe side effects. Eight patients were fully cured of hemolysis, although positive serologic findings remained in three of these; moderate improvement occurred in four patients, and four others were not evaluable. The efficacy of immunosuppressive agents was estimated in seven patients who had been given regular and sufficient doses for periods of longer than 4 months. Four patients were judged to have benefited with development of compensated hemolysis and reduced corticosteroid dosage.

Sokol and associates[199] stated that corticosteroids and blood transfusion were the mainstays of treatment and that splenectomy was performed on only four patients who had hemolysis that was not controlled by the initial therapy. "Spectacular responses" occurred in three of the four cases, but in the fourth patient (who also had thrombocytopenia), hemolysis recurred 1 year later. Similarly, Buchanan and colleagues[198] reported beneficial effects among three of four patients who underwent a splenectomy.

On the other hand, Heisel and Ortega[204] and Johnson and Abildgaard[227] reported poor results with splenectomy, which was used as a therapy for patients with chronic AIHA not responsive to corticosteroids. Five patients underwent splenectomy, and in no case was this treatment associated with complete resolution of the disease.[204] Three of these patients died within 1 year, all with evidence of sepsis (see Chapter 11 for a detailed discussion of overwhelming post-splenectomy infection, or OPSI).

Olcay and coworkers[213] described a 4-month-old patient with AIHA and reticulocytopenia who did not respond to corticosteroid therapy of 7 days' duration but was successfully treated when a combination of immunosuppressive therapies (cyclophosphamide, 6-

mercaotppurine, and IVIG) were added to the corticosteroids. In contrast, Heisel and Ortega[204] reported poor results for seven patients with chronic disease who were steroid dependent and were treated with immunosuppressive therapy that included azathioprine, cyclophosphamide, 6-mercaptopurine, hydrochloroquine sulfate, and chlorambucil. Only one complete remission was observed among these patients. Duru and associates[209] treated two patients with cyclosporine without benefit.

Anecdotal case reports have indicated success using high-dose intravenous immunoglobulin therapy. Sasaki and coworkers[228] reported a 7-week-old male infant with WAIHA who had normal levels of serum IgG, IgA, and IgM and normal concentrations of whole complement, C3, and C4. He was treated with RBC transfusions and prednisolone (3 mg/kg/day) or methylprednisolone (1.5 mg/kg/day). After 15 weeks, his hemoglobin was less than 5 g/dL, and during the therapy he had pneumonia, a subcutaneous abscess, and sepsis. On day 110, he began a course of IVIG at a dose of 0.4 g/kg for 5 days. At that time, corticosteroid therapy was switched from methylprednisolone to betamethasone. The hemoglobin level improved rapidly, and the DAT became negative. Six months later, he was well, the hemoglobin was 13.0 g/dL, reticulocytes were 5%, and the DAT was negative even though betamethasone had gradually been withdrawn.

Otheo and colleagues[229] reported a 4-year-old child with Evans's syndrome who presented with a hemoglobin level of 5.2 g/dL, reticulocytes 20%, and platelets 55,000/μL. The DAT was positive with anti-IgG but negative with anticomplement serum. A nonspecific IgG RBC autoantibody was demonstrated, as were antiplatelet antibodies. Initial treatment included IVIG at a dose of 800 mg/kg/day for 5 days and transfusions of RBCs. The hemoglobin and platelet counts rapidly reached normal values, and the reticulocyte count was 2.7% 5 weeks after IVIG. The patient was given maintenance doses of IVIG (800 mg/kg) every 2 weeks for 8 months, although there was no longer any trace of autoantibody by the fifth month. Eighteen months later, the patient still had normal hematological values.

The successful use of plasma exchange has also been reported. McConnell and colleagues[230] described the course of a boy aged 2 years and 10 months, who was admitted with a hemoglobin level of 5.1 g/dL, a reticulocyte count of 0.7%; hemoglobin in the urine in the absence of RBCs, DAT positive for C3, IAT positive for a Donath-Landsteiner antibody (anti-P), and a cold reactive antibody with anti-IH specificity. Bone marrow aspiration revealed marked erythroid hypoplasia and phagocytosis of RBCs by macrophages. He was treated with 2 mg/kg/day of prednisone and transfusions, but his hemoglobin concentration fell progressively to a nadir of 2.9 g/dL, hemoglobinuria worsened during transfusions, and the reticulocytopenia persisted. The steroid dose was increased to 6 mg/kg/day, additional RBC transfusions were administered, and 36 hours after admission, the authors began plasma exchange. They initially used plasma as the replacement, but prior to completion of the exchange, one unit of RBCs was infused instead of plasma. The patient remained clinically stable during the next 2 days and after a final transfusion was discharged on oral prednisone with a hematocrit of 32% and a reticulocyte count of 1.5%. After an additional week of treatment, prednisone was discontinued, and there was no recurrence of hemolysis or detectable antibody after 1 year of follow-up. The authors suggested that plasma exchange could be indicated for selected patients with fulminant AIHA who cannot be stabilized with steroid and transfusion therapy alone.

PROGNOSIS

There is a wide range of mortality rates among various reported series of cases. Most authors indicate that many cases are acute and transient, but that there is a significant mortality rate among patients with chronic illness, especially if this related to an underlying disorder.

In the series of Habibi and coworkers,[197] 80% of the patients had acute, transient disease with no deaths, but there was an 11.2% mortality among chronic cases. These patients generally had associated disorders and inherent complications at the time of death: thrombocytopenia and cerebral hemorrhage, malignant varicella, septicemia, cytomegalovirus infection, marrow aplasia, and immune deficiency disease.

Poschmann and Fischer[231] reported that the mortality rate of patients with AIHA appears to be considerably lower among children than among adults. In their review of the literature, they found that the mortality among children was 10%–28%, whereas in adults, it was 28%–70%.

Zupanska and associates[196] stated that, although the prognosis in AIHA is generally good, about 10% of their children died. In no case, however, was death due directly to severe anemia. The children died from uncontrollable bleeding caused by thrombocytopenia, uremia, or the accompanying disease (e.g., SLE).

Carapella de Luca and colleagues[205] reported that eight of their 29 patients (28%) died—two as a direct consequence of acute hemolysis. These two deaths occurred 1 and 20 days, respectively, after diagnosis of AIHA was made.

Sokol and coworkers[199] found that recovery was rapid and that complete recovery occurred in 83% of their 42 patients, usually within 6 months. Two patients died—one from profound hemolysis shortly after admission and the other of miliary tuberculosis.

Heisel and Ortega[204] reported a mortality rate of 25% among their 16 patients with chronic AIHA.

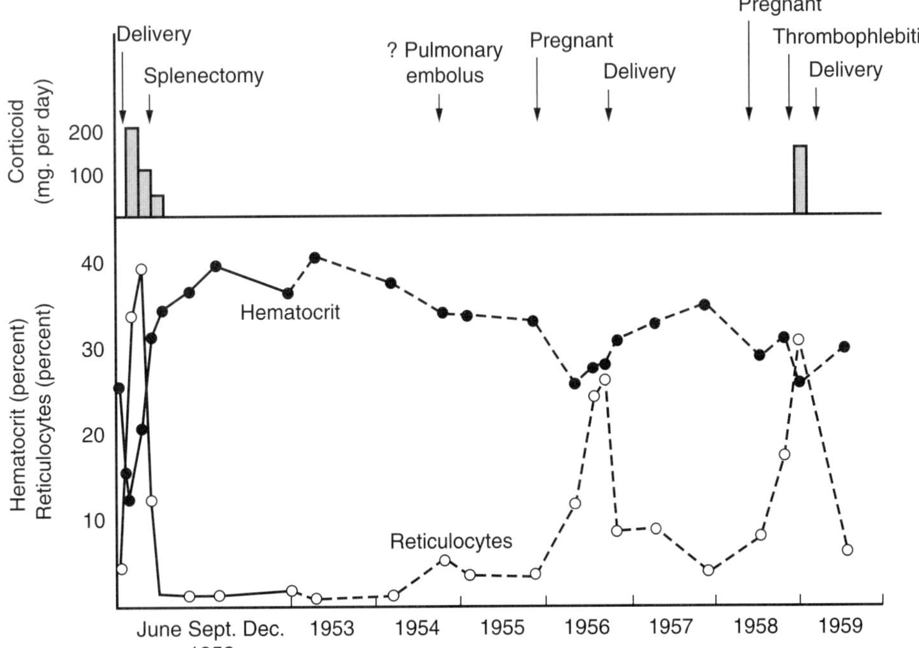

FIGURE 9-6. Clinical course of idiopathic AIHA in 25-year-old female through repeated pregnancies. (From Swisher SN: Acquired hemolytic disease. Postgrad Med 1966;40:378–386.)

D. Autoimmune Hemolytic Anemia During Pregnancy

Because AIHA commonly occurs in young women, it is not surprising that there are reports of AIHA during pregnancy. Coincidence alone, however, does not fully explain the coexistence of these two conditions, as pregnancy has definite effects on the course of AIHA. Swisher[232] described a patient with idiopathic AIHA, whose degree of hemolysis was increased with each of three pregnancies and remitted with each parturition (Fig. 9-6). Similarly, Benraad and associates[233] described a woman who developed AIHA during her first pregnancy; during her second pregnancy, AIHA developed once again. Also, Sokol and colleagues[234] found that AIHA was at least four times more frequent during pregnancy as in the nonpregnant female population, and concluded that it is most unlikely that the association of AIHA with pregnancy is a mere coincidence. Hoppe and coworkers[235] reported an increase in autoimmunization against RBCs during pregnancy, and Buyon[236] pointed out that there is also a significant effect of pregnancy on other autoimmune diseases.

The clinical findings vary widely among patients, with most women responding well to therapy and delivering a fetus with minimal or no evidence of hemolysis. Anemia in some patients can be so severe as to threaten the patient's life, however, and maternal red cell autosensitization also can induce fetal hemolysis, requiring management as for hemolytic disease of the newborn (see Chapter 13). Accordingly, close observation throughout pregnancy and appropriate therapy are critical to a successful outcome.[234,237]

Serologic findings are those of WAIHA in a large majority of patients, although some reports have included patients with cold antibodies[234,238] or with both warm and cold antibodies.[237,239]

MATERNAL FINDINGS

Chaplin and associates[237] reviewed reports of 19 pregnancies with presumed AIHA. All patients had unequivocal evidence of acquired hemolysis, but evidence of an autoimmune etiology was often incomplete. The DAT on maternal cells was positive in seven patients, negative in five, and not performed in seven. Four of the five mothers with a negative DAT were treated with corticosteroids, and all improved.

The hazard to maternal survival was often extremely serious. In nine patients, the hemoglobin fell below 5 g/dL, and in another eight instances, hemoglobin values were in the range of 5–8 g/dL. Leukopenia was present in four pregnancies and thrombocytopenia in three. Vigorous transfusion therapy, high doses of corticosteroids, and/or early induction of labor were employed as life-saving measures for critically ill patients.

Particularly significant is the observation that hemolysis worsened as the pregnancy progressed in 18 of the 19 patients. Complete or partial remissions of hemolysis occurred in 16 patients within 3 months after delivery. The two patients who did not improve subsequently were diagnosed as having SLE.

Sokol and colleagues[234] reported much less serious clinical findings for 20 pregnant patients with RBC autoantibodies. The researchers indicated that autosensitization occurred in one in 50,000 pregnancies, although only seven of the patients in their report had hemolytic anemia. The serological abnormalities in all cases were discovered during pregnancy. Most patients had warm autoantibodies, although three had cold antibodies, and both warm and cold antibodies were found in one patient. The clinical presentation varied from severe hemolytic anemia (lowest hemoglobin between 5 g/dL and 8 g/dL) to merely finding serological abnormalities in otherwise well patients. Treatment of AIHA with corticosteroids was necessary in only three patients in whom the hemolysis was severe. Eight of the patients had 11 further pregnancies, and all remained asymptomatic, although some had weak red cell autoantibodies and one patient had active disease. The authors concluded that the risks associated with AIHA occurring in pregnancy were less than thought previously provided that the mother received treatment promptly.

The severity of clinical findings among the patients reported on by Issaragrisil and Kruatrachue[240] are intermediate between the findings described by Chaplin and colleagues[237] and Sokol and coworkers.[234] They described 14 cases, which they divided into two groups. Group one consisted of four patients who were diagnosed during pregnancy, and group two consisted of 10 patients who became pregnant during the remission period of previously diagnosed AIHA.

All four patients in group one were first found to have AIHA when they were in the third trimester of pregnancy—at term in two cases and in the seventh month in the other two. The two cases that were not diagnosed until term had been seen earlier in pregnancy and found to have normal hemoglobin levels at that time. Three patients were treated with corticosteroids without improvement in their hemoglobin values which, prior to delivery, ranged from 3.7 g/dL to 7.4 g/dL. After deliveries, three patients responded well to cortocosteroid therapy, but one patient with SLE had hemoglobin levels that waxed and waned between 6.5 g/dL and 8.0 g/dL.

In contrast to the patients in group one, seven of 10 patients in group two presented during the first trimester of pregnancy with a falling hemoglobin, including three cases in which anemia was detected during the first month. Except for the anemia, the first trimester was uneventful, although one patient had a therapeutic abortion for reasons unrelated to hemolysis. A second phase of anemia occurred more abruptly somewhere between the third and fourth months of gestation, however. Severe anemia developed in three patients (hemoglobin 4.0–4.7 g/dL), and moderate anemia occurred in four patients (hemoglobin 6.7–7.9 g/dL). In two other patients, the lowest hemoglobin values were 9.7 g/dL and 11.7 g/dL.

OUTCOME OF PREGNANCIES

Four of the 19 pregnancies reviewed by Chaplin and coworkers[237] resulted in the delivery of a stillborn premature infant, and a fifth premature infant died of bronchopneumonia 48 hours after birth. No hematologic data were reported on these five infants, and none were described as having pallor, jaundice, or hydrops. All of the infants, however, were born to mothers with severe anemia (hemoglobin <5 g/dL), which suggests that fetal death was related more to the critical maternal state than to autoantibody-induced hemolytic disease of the newborn. Accordingly, the authors advocated a policy of frequent adjustment of corticosteroid dosage during pregnancy in an effort to maintain the patient's hemoglobin above 10 g/dL.

Among the four patients in group one in the report of Issaragrisil and Kreuatrachue,[240] there were three spontaneous deliveries (with normal infants in two of the cases) and one stillbirth. The fourth patient, who had SLE, developed toxemia of pregnancy, and her hemoglobin level declined from 7.1 g/dL to 3.7 g/dL within 5 days in spite of receiving prednisolone, 60 mg/day. Labor was therefore induced for this patient. The mother delivered a low-birth-weight infant; both mother and child survived.

Of six patients in group two who developed hemoglobin values below or equal to 6.7 g/dL, spontaneous abortion occurred in three patients, and therapeutic abortion was performed for two patients because of a lack of response to prednisolone therapy. One patient had a spontaneous delivery. After termination of the pregnancies, the mothers' hemoglobin levels responded well to glucocorticoid therapy.

Only five pregnancies in this group continued into the third trimester. Anemia in two patients responded well to prednisolone (40 mg/day), and one patient did not need corticosteroid therapy. These pregnancies resulted in spontaneous deliveries with normal infants. A cesarean section was performed in one case due to severe preeclampsia and fetal distress; both mother and child survived. One patient, who had SLE and nephrotic syndrome, had a spontaneous abortion followed by acute renal failure and later died.

It should be noted that corticosteroid therapy for the patients reported on by Issaragrisil and Kruatrachue[240] generally was started only after significant anemia occurred. Patients were not treated at a time when obvious hemolytic anemia was present if the hemoglobin was in the range of 9.0 g/dL. Indeed, some patients were not treated with corticosteroids at hemoglobin values 6.7–7.4 g/dL. Although such hemoglobin values are generally well tolerated, perhaps more favorable outcomes would have occurred if an attempt had been made to cause remissions in the patients' hemolysis before the sharp drops in hemoglobin occurred later in their pregnancies. This is in keeping with the suggestions of Chaplin and colleauges[237] and Sokol and coworkers.[234]

NEONATAL HEMOLYSIS

Hemolytic disease of the newborn, usually mild but occasionally requiring therapy, has been reported among infants born to mothers with AIHA. In some but not all instances, there is documentation of an immune pathogenesis of the hemolysis caused by the maternal autoantibody traversing the placenta. Lawe[241] reported on a 25-year-old woman with apparently inactive Hodgkin's disease who developed fulminant AIHA in the 37th week of pregnancy. The baby required four exchange transfusions for hyperbilirubinemia. The same IgG antibody was found in mother and infant. In the case reported by Bauman and Rubin,[242] the mother had a strongly positive DAT, and both her serum and an eluate from her RBCs contained a broadly reactive autoantibody. The newborn had a positive DAT and a compensated hemolytic process in the first week of life. The infant's hemoglobin fell to a low of 9.7 g/dL, but no specific therapy was required. Vedovini and Benedetti[243] reported a case of AIHA that developed during the last month of pregnancy and resulted in hemolysis in the newborn, which was treated with steroids and blood transfusions. The mother did not receive steroids until after delivery. In the report of Sokol and associates[234] concerning seven patients with AIHA, three infants were mildly affected with hemolytic disease due to the maternal autoantibodies crossing the placenta, but no treatment was needed.

In other reports, however, the immune etiology of the newborn's hemolysis is not clear. For example, Burt and Prichard[244] described an infant who required two exchange transfusions during the first 26 hours of life to control hyperbilirubinemia. Both the mother and infant had negative DATs and IATs; however, the authors suggested that the diagnosis could have been WAIHA because of the clinical setting and because there was improvement in the hemolytic process in the mother following splenectomy. The blood type of both mother and infant was group A, Rh positive, and there was no evidence of maternal alloimunization.

Soderhjelm[245] reported an infant who became severely anemic and jaundiced in the fourth week of life and seemed to respond to therapy with corticosteroids. Seip[246] described an infant who was severely anemic (hemoglobin 2.5 g/dL; reticulocytes 22%) and leukopenic (WBC 1800/μL) at 2 months of age and required multiple transfusions. The mother, who had SLE, also had leukopenia during pregnancy. Although the anemia in both infants was attributed to placentally transferred IgG autoantibody, the infants had negative or equivocal DATs.

A number of cases of Evans's syndrome in pregnancy have been reported.[247,249] Passi and associates[249] reported on a patient who presented with a hemoglobin of 7.7 g/dL and a platelet count of 36,000/μL. After treatment with corticosteroids, her hemoglobin improved to 10.2 g/dL, and the platelets varied between 60,000 and 80,000/μL. She delivered a 2.6-kg male infant at 37 weeks of gestation, and at birth, the infant's hemoglobin was 15.8 g/dL and the DAT and IAT were negative. Nevertheless, at 2 months, the hemoglobin had dropped to 8.6 g/dL, and there were spherocytes along with anisocytosis, poikilocytosis, and broken cells on the peripheral smear. Although no antibodies were demonstrated in the infant's serum or on his RBCs, the authors attributed the drop in hemoglobin to placental transfer of maternal autoantibodies.

INFANTS WITHOUT HEMOLYSIS

In spite of the rather significant complications of pregnancy involving the mothers in the series reported by Issaragrisil and Kruatrachue,[240] there was no evidence of hemolysis in any of the infants. In the review of Chaplin and colleagues,[237] hematological characterization of the infants was inadequate for evaluation in 16 of the 19 pregnancies. Nevertheless, 11 infants were inferred as normal because no hematologic abnormalities were noted, even though the mothers had "brisk hemolysis" during the latter months of pregnancy. Sacks and coworkers[250] also point out that severe maternal hemolytic anemia does not necessarily correlate with neonatal outcome. These authors reported a patient with a positive DAT and IgG autoantibody in her serum who nonetheless maintained a hemoglobin above 13 g/dL without treatment. The neonate also had a positive DAT and IAT but no evidence of hemolytic disease.

In addition, a number of other case reports of well-documented AIHA in pregnancy indicate that the newborns were healthy with no evidence of hemolysis.[233,248,251-254] In all of these cases—including one case of Evans's syndrome[248] and one report of WAIHA in two successive pregnancies—the mothers were treated successfully with corticosteroids during pregnancy.[233]

HEMOLYTIC ANEMIA OF PREGNANCY WITH A NEGATIVE DIRECT ANTIGLOBULIN TEST AND FREQUENT RECURRENCES

In addition to the cases already cited, there are other reports of hemolytic anemia in pregnancy in which the DAT is negative and the cause of the hemolysis is uncertain.[251,255-260]

Kumar and associates[260] reported on a patient who developed severe life-threatening hemolytic anemia during the last trimester of three successive pregnancies, with spontaneous recovery 11–12 weeks postpartum after each pregnancy. She remained normal during the entire nongravid state. Extensive investigations were performed to find the cause of the hemolysis, but none was documented. In particular, the DAT was negative; there were no RBC antibodies; tests for congenital hemolytic anemias were negative in the patient and her family; the blood film was normal; and no RBC membrane abnormalities could be found. Corticosteroids and high-dose IVIG were ineffective, and she was treated with blood transfusions. The authors commented that this was the only example of its kind that came to their attention among 55,000 deliveries conducted over the course of a decade in their hospital.

Starksen and colleagues[258] reviewed cases of unexplained hemolytic anemia during 19 pregnancies in 12 women. They described striking anemia beginning in the first (38%) or second (38%) trimester, resolving within 5 months after delivery (18 of 19 patients, 95%) and recurring in a subsequent pregnancy (six of 12 patients [50%]). Corticosteroid treatment, when employed, has resulted in a uniformly favorable response.[251,256,258]

Transient hemolysis was present in four of 19 (22%) infants. In a number of instances, detailed hematologic evaluations have been carried out, which excluded folate deficiency, hemoglobinopathies, red blood cell enzymopathies, hereditary spherocytosis, PNH, PCH, and SLE.[251,257,258] An extracorpuscular abnormality seems to be present, as a number of case reports document that transfused RBCs did not survive normally.[256,261,262]

Yam and colleagues[251] studied a patient with hemolytic anemia of pregnancy with a negative DAT and applied the CFAC test in an effort to document an immune pathogenesis (Patient 7) (Fig. 9-7).

PATIENT 7: The patient was a 34-year-old woman who had had seven previous pregnancies. She had a single blood count during her seventh pregnancy; the hematocrit level was 29% and reticulocytes were 6.7%; a single hematocrit level of 39% was available from her records in the non-gravid state. On referral, during the second trimester of her eighth pregnancy, her hemoglobin level was 9.6 g/dL, the hematocrit level 28% and the reticulocyte count 10.3%. She had a hemolytic anemia as manifested by persistent anemia (hematocrit 24–27%) and reticulocytosis (6.3–10.3%) (Fig. 9-7).

The patient's DAT was negative throughout her pregnancy using polyspecific antiglobulin serum and multiple dilutions of monospecific anti-IgG, -C3, and -C4, and no antibody was detected in her serum or in an eluate from her red cells. Hereditary spherocytosis was suspected because her blood film revealed a moderate number of spherocytes, but six of her seven children were examined, and none showed evidence of spherocytes. The peripheral blood films, hematocrits, and reticulocyte counts were normal in all six children, thus making hereditary spherocytosis unlikely.

A CFAC test performed on the patient's blood revealed 212 molecules of IgG per red cell (normal <25) (Table 9-12). The patient was treated with 50 mg of prednisone daily during the last 12 weeks of her pregnancy, which caused an increase in her hematocrit from 24% to 27% to 31% with a reticulocyte count of 7.5% (Fig. 9-7). After parturition, the prednisone was gradually decreased and then discontinued. The CFAC test performed 2 weeks postpartum revealed a significant reduction in RBC sensitization. At that time, only 53 molecules of IgG per RBC were present. The baby was anemic at birth, with a hemoglobin of 12.2 g/dL. The CFAC test on a cord blood sample revealed 250 molecules of IgG per RBC. The infant did not require therapy, and 14 days later only 25 molecules of IgG per RBC were detectable (Table 9-12).

TABLE 9-12. COMPLEMENT FIXING ANTIGLOBULIN CONSUMPTION TEST IN A PATIENT WITH RELAPSING HEMOLYTIC ANEMIA OF PREGNANCY AND A NEGATIVE DIRECT ANTIGLOBULIN TEST

	Molecules of IgG/RBC	
	Prepartum	**Postpartum**
Mother	212	53
Newborn	—	250 (cord blood) <25 (14 days postpartum)

From Yam P, Wilkinson L, Petz LD, Garratty G: Studies on hemolytic anemia in pregnancy with evidence for autoimmunization in a patient with a negative direct antiglobulin (Coombs') test. Am J Hematol 1980;8:23–29.

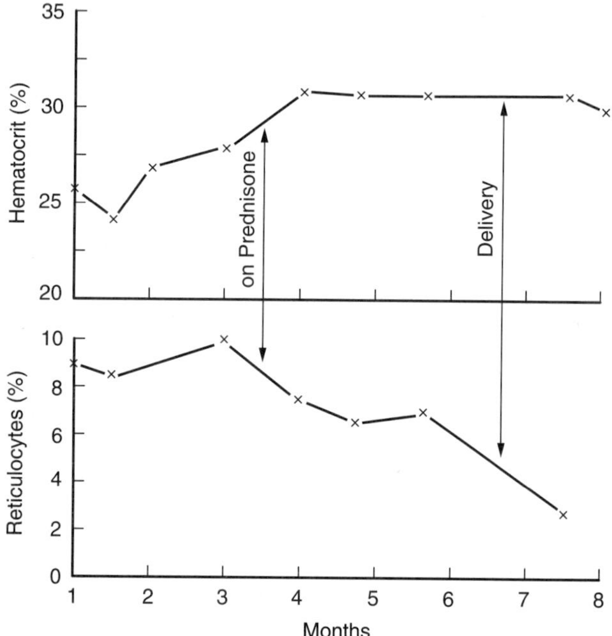

FIGURE 9-7. The clinical course of a patient with relapsing hemolytic anemia of pregnancy with a negative direct antiglobulin test. Hemolytic anemia was evident prior to the initiation of therapy with prednisone, as manifested by anemia with reticulocytosis. The anemia resolved, but reticulocytosis persisted during prednisone therapy until the delivery of the patient's baby. Thereafter, the reticulocytosis subsided and prednisone therapy was gradually withdrawn (see text). (From Yam P, Wilkinson L, Petz LD, Garratty G: Studies on hemolytic anemia in pregnancy with evidence for autoimmunization in a patient with a negative direct antiglobulin (Coombs') test. Am J Hematol 1980;8:23–29.)

Starksen and colleagues[258] reported on a patient whose CFAC test during pregnancy revealed a result at the upper limit of normal (40 molecules IgG per red blood cell, with an abnormal range reported by that laboratory as >40 molecules of IgG per RBC). Other techniques used to document a possible immune mechanism for the hemolysis were a five-times concentrated ether eluate reacted against enzyme treated RBCs and an enzyme-linked antiglobulin test for cell-bound IgG. The results of both these tests were negative.

Kumar and coworkers[260] summarized reported cases of DAT-negative hemolytic anemia of pregnancy as follows: In most cases, the hemolytic anemia occurs during the last trimester of pregnancy, although in some cases hemolysis is noted in the first and second trimesters. Most commonly, its first occurrence is noted in the primigravida state, but instances of hemolysis first occurring in the fifth and seventh pregnancies have been reported. Most patients show spontaneous reversal to normalcy within 2 months postpartum, although hemolysis can persist up to the fifth month after delivery. The majority of patients have a single recurrence in a subsequent pregnancy, but relapsing hemolysis has been reported in as many as three to five successive pregnancies. The anemia is usually severe and even life threatening. Most often, it requires support with blood transfusions. Bjornson and associates[259] had to transfuse their patient with a total of 121 units of blood for relapsing hemolytic anemia in five successive pregnancies. Corticosteroids and IVIG have been reported to be of value but not confirmed to be universally effective. The majority of infants born to mothers with this type of hemolytic anemia show evidence of transient hemolysis lasting for 1 to 2 months.

Although extensive investigations have not documented the cause of hemolysis, several findings suggest the possibility of an immune mechanism. There are no documented intracorpuscular defects, transfused RBCs have a shortened survival time,[256,262] corticosteroids and IVIG are often effective, and hemolysis occurs in some neonates.[259,263]

MANAGEMENT

The potential seriousness of AIHA in pregnancy, particularly in inadequately treated patients, justifies very close observation throughout pregnancy of any patient known to have a history of AIHA or who is discovered to have AIHA while pregnant. Antenatal hematologic evaluation appears indicated every two weeks until the eighth month of pregnancy and weekly thereafter until delivery. Such evaluations should include as a minimum a blood count and a reticulocyte count. Changes in the strength of the DAT and IAT might offer additional information, although there no data are available on the correlation of autoantibody titers and the severity of autoantibody-induced hemolytic disease of the newborn.

Patients with evident hemolysis should be treated with corticosteroid therapy in doses adequate to maintain a hemoglobin level above 10 g/dL. This is true both for patients with characteristic serological findings of AIHA and for patients with hemolytic anemia with a negative DAT. There are no reports of autoantibody-mediated hemolytic disease of the newborn requiring exchange transfusion in mothers whose AIHA is well controlled with corticosteroids during pregnancy. Although the incidence of hemolytic disease of the newborn requiring therapy is low, amniocentesis appears indicated in the presence of brisk hemolysis, which is mediated by an IgG autoantibody.[237,251] Some authors have reported early termination of pregnancy in instances in which corticosteroids were not effective in controlling hemolysis. In contrast to alloantibody-induced hemolytic disease of the newborn, early termination of pregnancy has been primarily for unrelenting maternal anemia but would be reasonable if amniocentesis indicates high fetal risk (see Chapter 13).

For patients who do not respond to corticosteroids and who have brisk hemolysis with severe anemia, additional or alternative therapeutic measures should be considered.

THE EFFECTS OF IMMUNOSUPPRESSIVE DRUGS DURING PREGNANCY

Although the use of corticosteroids and other immunosuppressive drugs during pregnancy causes significant concerns, there is an extensive medical literature regarding the use of these drugs during pregnancy in other autoimmune diseases (Table 9-13).[264,265] Immunosuppressive drugs other than corticosteroids seem not to have been used for treatment of AIHA in pregnant patients, but they could be reasonable therapeutic alternatives when the risk of severe anemia unresponsive to corticosteroids appears to be greater than the risk of the use of immunosuppressive drugs.

Corticosteroids

Controlled studies comparing corticosteroid-treated and nontreated patients during pregnancy have failed to show an increased incidence of birth defects,[266] and a National Institutes of Health consensus opinion indicates that antenatal corticosteroid therapy reduces morbidity in preterm infants with little or no effect on long-term physical or psychologic development and only a questionable increase in perinatal infection in both the mother and her neonate.[267] Accordingly, corticosteroids are the most widely used immunosuppressive drugs in pregnancy and are probably the safest. Nevertheless, significant risks include premature rupture of the membranes, intrauterine growth retardation, and accentuation of several pregnancy-induced maternal complications, including hypertension, gestational diabetes, osteoporosis, and osteonecrosis.[264]

Azathioprine

Most large-scale studies of transplant patients have demonstrated that azathioprine is fairly well tolerated

TABLE 9-13. SUMMARY OF TOXICITIES OF IMMUNOSUPPRESSIVE AGENTS IN ANIMALS AND HUMANS

	Animals		Humans		
Drug	**Embryotoxic**	**Fetal**	**Maternal**	**Fetal**	**Breast-feeding**
Glucocorticoids	No	Cleft palate Aggressive behavior	Premature rupture of membranes Hypertension Glucose intolerance Osteoporosis Osteonecrosis	Small for gestational-age offspring Adrenal hypoplasia Promotes lung maturity Cleft palate* Stillbirth*	Crosses into breast milk at low concentration, well tolerated
Chlorambucil	Yes	Small for gestational-age offspring Skeletal abnormalities Renal agenesis	†	Small for gestational-age offspring Skeletal abnormalities Renal agenesis	Contraindicated*
Cyclophosphamide	Yes	Small for gestational-age offspring Skeletal abnormalities Cleft palate Exophthalmos Decreased fertility	Decreased fertility in males and females	Small for gestational-age offspring Limb abnormalities Coronary artery agenesis Late onset tumors in offspring*	Contraindicated
Azathioprine	Yes	Skeletal abnormalities Cleft palate Decreased thymic development and hematopoiesis	†	Diminished fertility in offspring*	Contraindicated‡
6-mercaptopurine	Yes	Cleft palate	†	Small for gestational-age offspring Prematurity Intrauterine growth retardation Cleft palate	†
Methotrexate	Yes	Skeletal abnormalities Cleft palate	†	Embryotoxic Skeletal abnormalities Facial abnormalities	Contraindicated‡
Cyclosporin A	Yes	Renal tubular cell damage	Renal insufficiency	Spontaneous abortions Decreased lymphocyte subsets	Contraindicated
Intravenous immunoglobulin	†	†	†	Small for gestational-age offspring Autoantibodies	†

* Theoretical risk, or case reports only.
† No information available.
‡ Conflicting information.
From Bermas BL, Hill JA: Effects of immunosuppressive drugs during pregnancy. Arthritis Rheum 1995;38:1722–1732. Reprinted by permission of Wiley-Liss, Inc., a subsidiary of John Wiley & Sons, Inc.

during pregnancy. There have been isolated reports of immunoglobulin deficiency, chromosomal abnormalities, and malformations, but it is not clear whether the rate of these events is significantly greater than that seen in a healthy obstetric population. Another unanswered question is whether treatment of mothers with azathioprine during pregnancy will affect the germ-cell lines of offspring and therefore affect the future fertility of those offspring. In cases where immunosuppression is necessary during pregnancy, however (e.g., transplant recipients, severe autoimmune disease), Bermans and Hill[264] suggest that azathioprine could be a reasonable drug of choice. Janssen and Genta[265] are more cautious and state that the drug should be reserved for pregnant women whose (rheumatic) diseases are severe or life threatening.

Cyclosporine

Cyclosporine's lack of bone marrow toxicity and its low carcinogenic potential make this medication an appealing alternative for patients who do not respond to more conventional immunosuppressive therapies.[264] There are increasing data on offspring exposed to cyclosporine in utero because more and more female transplant recipients survive to childbearing age. In one series, 154 pregnancies were evaluated in renal transplant recipients treated with cyclosporine in addition to other immunosuppressive agents (prednisone and azathioprine).[268] Overall, complications among newborns were slightly lower than complications observed among patients treated with other immunosuppressive agents, and no malformations were seen. Other investigators, however, reported a high rate of spontaneous abortion and preterm labor in women treated with cyclosporine and prednisone during pregnancy.[269] Renal function in children has been reported to be normal.[270] Whether there will be long-term immunomodulatory effects on offspring who have been exposed to cyclosporine in utero is unknown.

Bermas and Hill[264] suggest that cyclosporine can be used successfully in pregnancy, whereas Janssen and Genta[265] state that, in general, the drug is contraindicated during pregnancy.

Other Drugs

Drugs such as chlorambucil, cyclophosphamide, 6-mercaptopurine, and methotrexate should generally be avoided during pregnancy.[264] High-dose intravenous immunoglobulin (IVIG) could be a reasonable treatment, although it is not entirely benign, as there have been case reports of hemolytic disease of the newborn severe enough to require exchange transfusion after the mother received IVIG during pregnancy.[271]

Conclusions

One must keep in mind that much of the literature on the use of immunosuppressive drugs during pregnancy has been developed from reports of patients who have received a transplant, and in these cases, immunosuppressive therapy is essential. These drugs, other than corticosteroids, will be necessary in only very unusual instances in the management of AIHA. Bermas and Hill[264] provide treatment recommendations during pregnancy for patients with autoimmune disease and transplant recipients (Table 9-14). The evidence suggests that corticosteroids, azathiporine, cyclosporine, and IVIG might be tolerated, but methotrexate, chlorambucil, 6-mercaptopruine, and cyclosporine should be avoided.

TABLE 9-14. PROPOSED TREATMENT RECOMMENDATIONS DURING PREGNANCY FOR PATIENTS WITH AUTOIMMUNE DISEASE*

Mild Disease	Moderate-Severe Disease	Life-threatening
No treatment	Steroids	Steroids—high dose
Steroids—low dose	Cyclosporin A	Cyclosporine
	Azathioprine	Azathioprine
		Cyclophosphamide†

* Methotrexate, chlorambucil, and 6-mercaptopurine should be avoided.
† Life-threatening illness with no alternative treatment.
Modified from Bermas BL, Hill JA: Effects of immunosuppressive drugs during pregnancy. Arthritis Rheum 1995;38:1722–1732. Reprinted by permission of Wiley-Liss, Inc., a subsidiary of John Wiley & Sons, Inc.

THE ROLE OF SPLENECTOMY

Although splenectomy is an effective measure for AIHA, we are not aware of it having been performed for this indication during pregnancy. Only rarely will splenectomy become necessary, but consideration should be given to this option if it appears that maternal benefits outweigh the increased risk for fetal death.

Several authors, in discussing therapy of idiopathic thrombocytopenic purpura (ITP), have advised against splenectomy in pregnancy, citing a maternal mortality rate of 10% and a high neonatal mortality rate due to premature labor.[272-274] Nevertheless, splenectomy has been performed successfully during pregnancy for patients with ITP and for thrombocytopenia associated with the antiphospholipid syndrome.[275-279] The technique of laparoscopic splenectomy has been used by some.[278,279] Gottlieb and colleagues[275] state that for patients with ITP, splenectomy during pregnancy should be carried out on maternal indication if there is poor or no response to medical treatment, or if medical treatment is hazardous to the mother. They further state that strong warnings against surgical treatment during pregnancy should be revised because of improvements in surgical technique and care of the premature infant.

For patients who develop severe AIHA that is poorly responsive to corticosteroids during pregnancy, an elective postpartum splenectomy should be considered as a means of preventing recurrent problems in a subsequent pregnancy.[251]

E. Familial Autoimmune Hemolytic Anemia

There is a rather significant body of medical literature regarding the occurrence of AIHA in more than one member of a family (Table 9-15).[280-304] Among reported cases of familial AIHA are four sets of twins, of which three sets were reported as being identical.[293,300,305,306] On the other hand, Dacie[263] followed a patient for 20 years after the diagnosis of AIHA had been made, and during this time her twin remained free from the disease. McLeod and associates[303] reported the clinical course of three siblings, all of whom had Evans's syndrome in childhood.

Even more common are reports of family members of patients with AIHA who have been afflicted with another type of autoimmune disease. There are many reports of patients with AIHA in whose family one or more members suffer from an immunologically mediated disorder other than AIHA.[263] Pirofsky[289,290] reported that one or more relatives of eight of 43 (19%) of his patients had suffered from a wide range of probable or possible autoimmune disorders, including glomerulonephritis, pernicious anemia, Stevens-Johnson syndrome, rheumatoid arthritis, SLE, and

TABLE 9-15. OCCURRENCES OF AIHA IN MORE THAN ONE MEMBER OF A FAMILY

Relationship and Age at Onset (Years, Except Where Stated)	Reference
Mother (61) and daughter (23)	280
Mother (72) and son (33)	281, 282
Two sisters (18 and 14)	283
Sister (55) and brother (38); a further sister (35) possibly affected	284
Two children had "symptoms of acquired hemolytic anemia" "Two brothers developed autoimmune hemolytic anemia"	285
Mother (40) and daughter (8)	286
Sister (57) and brother (who had died earlier of AIHA and lymphosarcoma)	287
Sister (3 months) and two brothers (3 and 4 months)	288
Two sisters (66 and 49) and brother (48)	289, 290
Two sisters (4 and 12)	291
Brother (14) and sister (19); also paternal aunt	292
Identical twin girls (1 and 2½)	293
Mother and daughter (12)	294
Sister (40) and brother (62)	295
Brother (20) and two sisters (17 and 15)	296
Two sisters (66 and 62)	297
Two sisters (68 and 60)	298
Mother and son (14)	299
Twin brothers (21 and 23)	300
Two sisters (71 and 73)	301
Two families with two affected sisters (7 months and 6, and 12 months and 9 months)	302
Three siblings with Evans's Syndrome	303

Modified from Conley CL, Savarese DM: Biologic false-positive serologic tests for syphilis and other serologic abnormalities in autoimmune hemolytic anemia and thrombocytopenic purpura. Medicine (Baltimore) 1989;68:67–84.

thrombocytopenic purpura. Conley[307] found an even higher incidence of autoimmune disorders among family members: 14 of 33 patients (42%) had family members known to have an immunologically mediated disorder similar to those listed by Pirofsky or from a lymphoma or leukemia. Conley and Savarese[298] reviewed the occurrence of other autoimmune and lymphoproliferative disorders among patients with AIHA and emphasized the frequent association of abnormal serological reactions and abnormalities in the levels of serum immunoglobulins.

The development of AIHA and the finding of other manifestations of autoimmunity among family members of numerous patients suggests that a fortuitous relationship is unlikely. It is more probable that genetic factors play an etiologic role. The nature of the genetic mechanism, however, is unknown. Conley and Saverese[298] suggested that an abnormality of cells of the immune system, often genetically determined, could predispose to serologic changes, immune deficiency, autoimmune diseases, and neoplasia.

F. Cardiac Surgery and Cold Autoantibodies

Development of hemolysis in patients with cold agglutinins of high thermal amplitude, or exacerbation of the rate of hemolysis in patients with cold agglutinin syndrome (CAS), are risks of cardiac surgery under conditions of hypothermia. There is also the potential for intracoronary hemagglutination with inadequate distribution of cardioplegic solutions, thrombosis, embolism, ischemia, or infarction.[308-311] When measures have been taken to avoid the hematologic and cardiac consequences of exposure to cold in patients with cold agglutinins, the reported results have been excellent.[312]

ADVERSE EVENTS

Although complications are not common, there are well-documented events precipitated by cold during surgery among patients with cold agglutinins of high thermal amplitude. Bedrosian and Simel[313] reported a patient with well-compensated chronic CAS who had an acute "life-threatening" hemolytic crisis during an elective herniorrhaphy in a cool (20°C) operating room. The patient's hematocrit decreased from 36% to a low of 12.6%. The cold agglutinin was an anti-I with a titer of 51,200 against adult (I) RBC at 4°C in albumin and a titer of 100 at 30°C.

Wertlake and colleagues[314] attributed hemolysis that began during cardiac surgery under hypothermia to an anti-HI cold agglutinin that destroyed A_2B donor RBCs in an A_1B patient. Preoperatively, the hematocrit was 45%, but it dropped progressively to a level of 30% on the fifth day after surgery and did not begin to rise until day 15 despite a reticulocytosis. The cause of the hemolysis was somewhat uncertain, however, because the direct Coombs' test was consistently negative, and the thermal amplitude of the antibody was elevated only transiently to a level of 22°C on the sixth day after surgery.

Izzat and coworkers[311] reported a case in which agglutination of RBCs occurred within 1 minute of initiation of antegrade cold blood cardioplegia at 10°C and led to embolization in the coronary microcirculation. After the multiple agglutinates were noted, a coronary sinus cannula was inserted through the right atrium, and continuous retrograde cold crystalloid cardioplegia was infused. Agglutinates were noted to

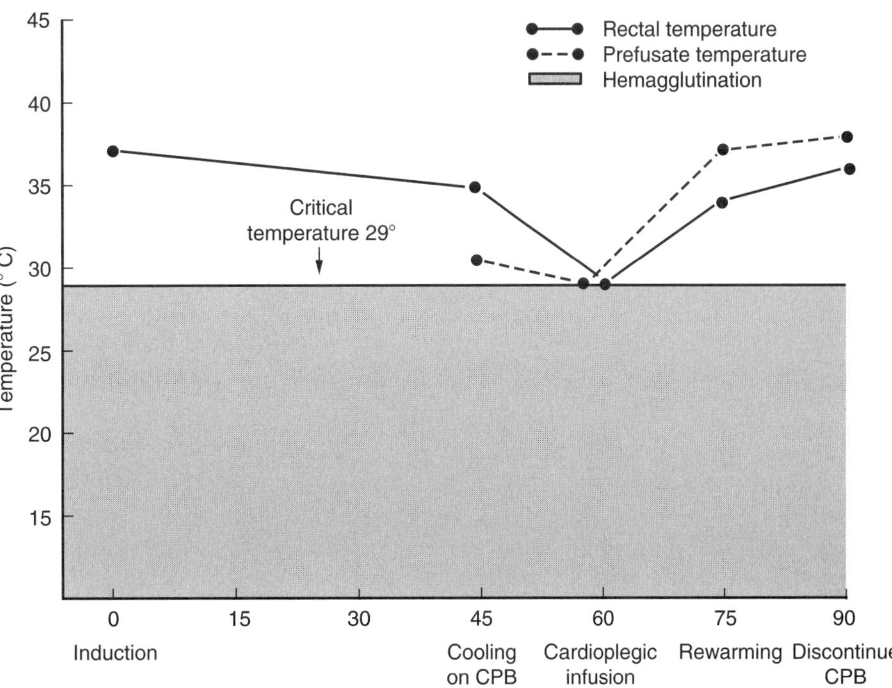

FIGURE 9-8. Clinical determination of critical temperature for hemagglutination (29°C) (CPB, cardiopulmonary bypass). (From Diaz JH, Cooper ES, Ochsner JL: Cardiac surgery in patients with cold autoimmune diseases. Anesth Analg 1984;63:349–352.)

flush back from the coronary arteries into the aortic root. Nevertheless, the patient did not show any signs of cardiac damage postoperatively.

Diaz and associates[315] observed large RBC agglutinates within the coronary vessels and the coronary sinus when a patient's rectal temperature decreased from 36°C to 30°C during cardiopulmonary bypass. This led to the diagnosis of previously unsuspected CAS. They stated that the most important principle in the immediate management of unanticipated cold hemagglutination is the early determination and maintenance of body temperature above that highest temperature (critical temperature) at which the cold antibody reacts (Fig. 9-8).

Bracken and colleagues[316] described cardiopulmonary bypass performed on two patients who had cold agglutinins that had gone undetected prior to surgery. In one patient, a 67-year-old male, the red cells in the cardioplegia heat exchanger were clumped and separated from the plasma, and the patient developed hemoglobinuria. On the evening of surgery, the patient was noted to have a cold, pulseless left leg and underwent a bedside revascularization procedure. He died of hemodynamic compromise on the second day after surgery. The authors commented that it is not clear whether cold agglutinins were directly related to the terminal event.

Holman and coworkers[317] reported on a patient who developed intracoronary agglutination of the blood cardioplegia solution. The patient was a 69-year-old male with severe pulmonary dysfunction and class IV angina pectoris who was referred for bypass grafting of a proximal stenosis of the anterior descending artery. During surgery, the heart was arrested using a 4°C blood cardioplegia solution, and agglutinated blood was found when the anterior descending artery was incised. Postcardioplegia reperfusion of the heart was begun with a blood cardioplegia solution delivered at 37°C under controlled conditions of flow and pressure. Postoperatively, there was no grossly evident hemolysis and no evidence for myocardial necrosis. The patient's convalescence was uneventful. It should be noted that the patient's cold agglutinin was an anti-I that had an agglutination titer of 256 at 4°C and a titer of 4 at 24°C but did not react at 30°C or 37°C. The fact that the cold agglutinin was of low thermal amplitude might have mitigated against the development of complications.

Stalker[318] reported that clumps of agglutinated RBCs can plug the microcirculation and cause myocardial necrosis, and Davidsohn and associates[319] reported hepatic infarcts in mice injected with anti-RBC serum.

Shahian and colleagues[308] stated that cold-mediated RBC agglutination within the coronary microcirculation might lead to inadequate distribution of cardioplegic solution, poor myocardial protection, and perioperative infarction. They cautioned that unless cold antibodies are identified prior to surgery or by the surgeon or perfusionist during bypass, such sequelae of microscopic RBC agglutinates may be attributable to other causes. Indeed, the numerous other causes of hemolysis during cardiopulmonary bypass, including mechanical trauma, will likely be considered before testing for the presence of cold agglutinins with a high thermal amplitude.[320]

Although not related to surgery, other instances of exacerbation of CAS with exposure to cold have been reported. Niejadlik and Lozner[321] described a patient who developed acute, severe hemolysis after being placed on a cooling mattress. The patient was a 51-year-old white female who was hospitalized with fever and right lower lobe pneumonia. Her hematocrit on admission was 44%, but after being placed on a cooling mattress, signs of intravascular hemolysis developed with marked hemoglobinuria, and her hematocrit decreased to a low of 16%. *Mycoplasma pneumoniae* infection was documented, and cold agglutinins were present at a titer of 25 at 4°C, a titer of 32 at room temperature, and a titer of 8 at 37°C.

Colmers and Snavely[322] reported on a patient with primary atypical pneumonia and cold agglutinin syndrome with a cold agglutinin titer of 1280 whose hemoglobin decreased from 7.5 g/dL to 4.5 g/dL overnight following three general body sponges using iced alcohol. The drop in hemoglobin was accompanied by passage of dark-brown urine. After recovery from her pneumonia and hemolysis, the authors performed an experiment in which the patient's right arm was immersed for 15 minutes in ice-cold water containing pieces of ice. A blood specimen was drawn immediately before immersion of the arm, then 15 minutes after cessation of immersion and at 15-minute intervals thereafter. The control and the 120-minute serums were completely free from any trace of hemoglobin on gross visual inspection. The 30-minute specimen was markedly hemolyzed, and the 45-minute specimen showed somewhat less marked hemolysis, as determined visually and by spectral analysis. The patient did not develop hemoglobinuria, a fact which suggests that the systemic hemoglobinemia did not reach a sufficient concentration to appear in the urine.

IDENTIFICATION OF PATIENTS AT RISK

Because cold agglutinins can be detected in the sera of almost all individuals, the critical problem is to decide which characteristics of a given patient's cold agglutinin would warrant special precautions during surgery. This question cannot be answered precisely, but special precautions would seem important when a patient has a cold antibody-induced AIHA. Although cold-reactive antibodies are not routinely characterized in detail in the blood transfusion service, if the antibodies have a high enough thermal amplitude to cause AIHA, they will ordinarily be noticed during routine compatibility test procedures. Also, for patients who have hemolytic anemia, one would hope that a diagnosis of CAS would have been made prior to surgery on the basis of clinical and laboratory findings (see Chapters 2, 5, and 6).

For patients without hemolytic anemia, the thermal amplitude of the antibody (the highest temperature at which agglutination occurs) is probably the best guide to possible complications during surgery. The thermal amplitude can be determined in the hospital's transfusion service (see Chapter 6), and this procedure should be carried out whenever strong autoagglutination occurs at room temperature. Antibodies that are reactive at temperatures of 30°C or higher are capable of causing hemolysis (see Chapter 5), and special precautions would seem to be warranted during hypothermia, even though the manifestations of hemolysis might be minimal to none prior to exposure to cold.

In some cases, autoagglutination will first be noticed in the operating room.[311,315-317,323] Indeed, Dake and coworkers[323] and Bracken and colleagues[316] have recommended that observation of the blood cardioplegia system for agglutination before cardioplegia administration and systemic cooling be a routine part of the perfusion checklist.

PATIENTS WITH COLD AGGLUTININS WHO DO NOT APPEAR TO BE AT RISK

Normal persons may have cold agglutinins that react at 4°C with a titer of 32 or less and with a thermal amplitude of less than 20°C. Although cold agglutinins reactive up to room temperature (~20°C) might seem to be of potential significance during hypothermic surgical procedures, there is an impressive lack of reports of complications caused by such antibodies, even though they are quite common.[324] Indeed, there is general agreement that patients with low-titer, low-thermal amplitude antibodies can undergo operation without any change in routine management plan.[325] The thermal amplitude of the cold agglutinin is of particular significance as indicated by the data of Bracken and colleagues,[316] who reported on 19 patients who had cold agglutinins with titers of 64–512 at 4°C; the researchers found that only three of these patients had cold agglutinins that reacted at 25°C. Moore and associates[326] stated that patients with titers of 32 or lower at 4°C and no detectable agglutination at 28°C or lower tolerated hypothermia well. Moore, however, studied only five patients who had strongly positive agglutination in the cold, and only one had an antibody that reacted at temperatures as high as 23°C.

Nydegger and colleagues[327] reported on a 51-year-old male who needed a liver transplant and who had a cold agglutinin titer of 32 at 4°C, reacting with undiluted plasma at temperatures up to 30°C. The authors were concerned because the orthotopic liver transplant still is cool from preservation when placed into the recipient. No intra- or perioperative complications occurred, however.

AuBuchon and associates[320] studied 16 patients undergoing hypothermic extracorporeal circulation. They found that total extracorporeal circulation time had a significant correlation with a rise in hemoglobin during the procedure, but no correlation was noted between the extent of hemolysis and the presence of cold-reacting autoantibodies that were present in 12 patients at temperatures of 22°C or below.

That patients with abnormal cold agglutinin titers requiring special management in hypothermic surgery are unusual is indicated by the data of Bracken and

TABLE 9-16. TITER AND THERMAL AMPLITUDE OF COLD AGGLUTININS IN 19 ADULT PATIENTS HAVING CARDIOPULMONARY BYPASS SURGERY

Patient No.	Age	Sex	Titer	Highest Temperature Agglutination Observed*
1	51	F	64	4°C
2	54	M	512	4°C
3	67	M	256	+ at 4°C, minimal at 25°
4	62	F	128	4°C
5	73	F	256	4°C
6	77	M	256	4°C
7	59	M	128	4°C
8	77	F	64	4°C
9	65	M	512	4°C
10	42	F	64	4°C
11	69	F	128	4°C
12	53	F	128	4°C
13	58	M	512	4°C
14	58	M	128	4°C
15	23	M	64	4°C
16	77	F	256	25°C
17	76	M	64	4°C
18	53	M	64	25°C
19	77	F	64	4°C

* Agglutination test performed only at 4°C, 25°C, and 37°C
From Bracken CA, Gurkowski MA, Naples JJ, et al: Case 6—1993. Cardiopulmonary bypass in two patients with previously undetected cold agglutinins. J Cardiothorac Vasc Anesth 1993;7:743–749.

TABLE 9-17. RESULTS OF COLD AGGLUTININ TITERS IN ADULT PATIENTS HAVING CARDIOPULMONARY BYPASS SURGERY

	No. of Patients
Surgeries requiring CPB	969
Preoperative CA titers performed	504
Patients with titers ≥ 64	19
Patients with agglutination at >4°C	3
Change in management of case	4
Change in management clearly of benefit	1
Complications related to CA	1

Modified from Bracken CA, Gurkowski MA, Naples JJ, et al: Case 6—1993. Cardiopulmonary bypass in two patients with previously undetected cold agglutinins. J Cardiothorac Vasc Anesth 1993;7:743–749.

colleagues.[316] They reviewed their data regarding adult patients seen over a 1-year period. Only 19 0f 504 patients had a titer of 64 or greater (Table 9-16), and of these, agglutination occurred at 25°C in only three patients (tests were preformed at 4°C, 25°C, and 37°C only) (Table 9-17).

MANAGEMENT

Hematologists, transfusion medicine specialists, and cardiovascular surgeons who identify patients at risk should collaborate to develop a protocol for management. It is prudent to do this in advance of need, especially as cold agglutinins might not be detected prior to surgery in some patients.[311,315,316,323] A plethora of published accounts (including several reviews) have recommended various approaches to management of patients who require cardiac surgery and who have cold autoantibodies.[308,309,311,313,315-317,323,325,326,328-345]

Reported techniques of cardioplegic management include warm ischemic arrest (simple aortic cross-clamping), warm blood cardioplegia, and the use of a combination of warm and cold crystalloid cardioplegia.[345] In general, cold blood cardioplegia is not appropriate, as one would expect significant agglutination in the coronary circulation. The alternative is to use crystalloid hypothermic cardioplegic protection. To avoid the exposure of blood to hypothermic solution in the coronary system, warm crystalloid cardioplegia can be used to flush the coronary circulation clear of blood; this is then followed by cold crystalloid cardioplegia to induce myocardial hypothermia. Toward the end of the procedure, the heart may be rewarmed by warm crystalloid cardioplegia before the cross-clamp is removed.

More recently, continuous warm blood cardioplegia,[346–349] which can be delivered antegradely[337,350,351] or retrogradely,[339–341] has been employed. This procedure obviates the need for hypothermia and is recommended by a number of authors in this setting.[325,339,343,352]

THE ROLE OF PLASMA EXCHANGE IN PREPARATION FOR SURGERY

Plasma exchange has been used as adjunctive therapy for some patients.[309,328,340,342] This procedure requires special techniques, however, as it must be performed at temperatures above the cold agglutinin's thermal amplitude to avoid in vitro cold agglutination.[328,336,353] Also, the procedure is not reliably effective[340,354,355] (see also Chapter 11).

Klein and colleauges[328] used plasma exchange before surgery for a patient with an anti-I cold agglutinin. The antibody reacted strongly with RBCs at 15°C, 22°C, and after papain treatment at 37°C; in addition, it agglutinated several panel RBCs in saline at 30°C and occasionally reacted with saline-suspended RBCs at 37°C. The titer at 22°C was reduced by plasma exchange from 4 to 1. During surgery, body temperature was lowered with the core temperature of 29°C as measured with an esophageal sensor. There were no adverse effects during or after hypothermia. These authors point out that they could not be sure that difficulties would have developed had plasma exchange not been performed.

Beebe and coworkers[340] described a case in which plasma exchange was only minimally effective. Beginning 10 days before surgery, the patient received plasmapheresis every other day for five total treatments, with each treatment exchanging 1.25 plasma volumes with an equal volume of 5% albumin. The cold agglutinin titer decreased from 4096 to 512 the day before surgery, but on the morning of surgery, the cold agglutinin had rebounded to a titer of 1024. The patient had chronic CAS but was managed throughout surgery for splenectomy and cholecystectomy by intraoperative forced air convection warming; esophageal and peripheral temperatures were maintained above 37°C throughout surgery, and she did not have an exacerbation of her hemolysis.

In the case reported by Park and Weiss,[309] the patient had a cold agglutinin titer of 10,000 at 4°C and 5000 at 20°C but did not have evidence of hemolysis. Plasmapheresis was performed 1 day before surgery and produced "an eightfold reduction in titers." Body temperature was maintained above 35°C throughout coronary artery bypass grafting, which was performed during a 72-minute normothermic cardiopulmonary bypass at 36°C–37°C. No ventricular fibrillation occurred, and no hemolysis, hemagglutination, myocardial infarction, or organ damage resulted.

Zoppi and associates[342] reported on a 53-year-old male with abnormally elevated cold agglutinins who was treated by two one-volume plasma exchanges. There was a reduction of the titer of the cold agglutinins against group O RBC at 4°C from 128 to 32, but the titers of 8 at 30°C and of 2 at 37°C were not affected. The surgery was successful, and the patient was discharged on the 16th day after surgery.

G. Differentiating Delayed Hemolytic Transfusion Reactions from Autoimmune Hemolytic Anemia

Delayed hemolytic transfusion reactions (DHTRs) are a recognized risk of blood transfusion. The reaction is caused by the reappearance of an antibody that presumably was first stimulated by pregnancy or a previous transfusion. Unlike immediate transfusion reactions, which are usually caused by human error, delayed reactions are usually not avoidable.[356-361] Because hemolysis is delayed in onset (typically 3 to 14 days after transfusion), the relationship of hemolytic anemia to prior transfusion might not be suspected, and a diagnosis of AIHA might seem more appropriate.

As in any patient with the acute onset of hemolysis, findings can include fever, pallor, jaundice, hemoglobinemia, hemoglobinuria, and, rarely, disseminated intravascular coagulation or renal failure.[356,362-364] Further, laboratory tests are likely to reveal the presence of a positive DAT and IAT, spherocytosis, and reticulocytosis. If multiple alloantibodies or an alloantibody against a high-incidence antigen is formed, the findings can be difficult to differentiate from AIHA. The diagnostic problem is compounded by the fact that, in some cases, AIHA might actually develop as a consequence of blood transfusion (see the segment of this chapter regarding AIHA following transfusion). Indeed, therapy with corticosteroids for suspected AIHA has been instituted[365,366] or contemplated in some reported cases of DHTRs before the correct diagnosis was made.[364,367]

A characteristic example of a patient who had a DHTR simulating AIHA was reported by Croucher and colleagues.[365] They described a patient with vaginal bleeding who was transfused with 10 units of blood over a period of 8 days. Despite the arrest of hemorrhage, her hemoglobin level continued to fall. The patient was found to be pale and jaundiced; her urine was dark and contained "urobilin" but did not contain hemoglobin or bile. The spleen was just palpable. Her hemoglobin, which had been 8.5 g/dL at the time that hemorrhage ceased, dropped to about 6 g/dL. At that time, her reticulocyte count was 13%, and it subsequently rose to a peak of 24%. The blood film showed small agglutinates, many spherocytes, and some myelocytes and normoblasts. The serum bilirubin was 4.5 mg/dL, and serum haptoglobin was absent. The DAT was strongly positive. The patient's serum reacted with her own RBCs and with samples from more than 30 donors and thus appeared to have a nonspecific autoantibody; however, careful serologic studies documented the presence of anti-Fy^a, anti-Ce, and anti-e, and the patient's hemolytic anemia resolved without therapy. The DAT rapidly weakened and became negative 10 days after the last transfusion, but the IAT remained strongly positive throughout hospitalization.

DIAGNOSTIC AIDS

As mentioned in Chapters 5 and 6, a presumptive diagnosis of WAIHA may be entertained for a patient who has not been transfused during the previous 3 months, has an acquired hemolytic anemia with a positive DAT, does not have a cold agglutinin of high thermal amplitude, has not been taking drugs known to cause immune-mediated hemolysis (see Chapter 8), and has a warm antibody with broad reactivity in the serum or RBC eluate. Such a presumptive diagnosis tends to be correct because if donor RBCs no longer remain in the patient's circulation, alloantibodies cannot be causing the acquired immune hemolytic anemia. One should note, however, that a DAT can persist for at least 3 to 4 months following a DHTR (see Chapter 14). Even if the patient has not been transfused over the previous 3 months, we recommend further tests to characterize the patient's RBC antibody(ies) to avoid diagnostic error and to have results of specificity tests available should transfusion become necessary.

If a patient has been transfused within recent weeks, such additional testing is mandatory to distinguish between a DHTR and AIHA. The following measures will afford important clues.

Comparison of DAT and IAT

A simple observation that could yield valuable information is the comparison of the strength of the DAT and IAT. As is stressed in Chapter 10, the DAT is almost always stronger than the IAT in WAIHA. It appears that autoantibody is largely adsorbed onto the patient's RBCs, and only when the RBCs are heavily coated does one find a large amount of antibody in the serum. In contrast, strongly reactive alloantibodies might be present in a patient's serum, but this finding cannot result in a strongly positive DAT unless large numbers of transfused RBCs of appropriate antigenic type are present. Thus, the presence of a weakly positive DAT in association with a strongly positive IAT is presumptive evidence for the presence of an alloantibody. These findings are therefore highly suggestive of a DHTR. Further, even if the DAT is strongly positive at the time of initial evaluation, it can soon become weaker in subsequent tests as a result of the destruction of the transfused RBCs, as was true in the case from Croucher and colleagues that was described previously. This is true even though the DAT might remain weakly positive for several months following a DHTR. In contrast, a rapid diminution in the strength of the DAT would not be expected in AIHA except as a result of treatment, as would be the case with the use of corticosteroids, immunosuppressive drugs, or splenectomy.

Antibody Specificity

An important means of differentiating AIHA from a DHTR relates to the specificity of the antibody(ies) present in the serum and in an RBC eluate. Some antibodies that commonly cause DHTR reactions have not been found or have been reported only rarely as autoantibodies in AIHA. Examples are anti-K and anti-Fy[a], which are encountered frequently in published cases of DHTRs.[356,362,363,368,369] Many autoantibodies in warm antibody AIHA demonstrate specificity within the Rh system, but even here, a distinction between autoantibodies and alloantibodies with Rh specificity is often possible. Whereas alloantibodies demonstrate truly specific reactions and give clearly negative reactions with cells lacking the appropriate antigen, autoantibodies commonly demonstrate "relative specificity." That is, autoantibodies that are described as having specificity within the Rh system react more strongly or to a higher titer against RBCs bearing a particular Rh antigen, but they will nevertheless react with RBCs lacking that antigen. Thus, a truly specific Rh antibody strongly suggests that it is an alloantibody, whereas an antibody demonstrating "relative specificity" is characteristic of autoantibody. On the other hand, a mixture of an Rh alloantibody and an autoantibody reacting equally but less strongly with all normal RBCs will appear similar to an autoantibody. A differentiation of these two possibilities would be difficult except by using the patient's pretransfusion RBCs for cell typing or for the warm autoadsorption test, or by using the allogeneic adsorption test (see Chapter 10).

A further clue to the differentiation of autoantibodies and alloantibodies having Rh specificity is the specificity itself. That is, anti-e is a rare cause of a DHTR, but it is the most frequently described autoantibody specificity.[362] In contrast, anti-E is the most common Rh alloantibody responsible for DHTRs, but it is a relatively unusual autoantibody.[362,368] Again, if pretransfusion RBCs are still available, it is possible to use them to distinguish alloantibody from autoantibody with certainty.

If the antibody shows a defined specificity, the patient's RBCs should be tested for the relevant antigen. If it is an autoantibody, the patient's RBCs should possess the antigen. It is not always easy to determine the patient's phenotype, as DAT+ RBCs are difficult to phenotype and because transfused RBCs may be present. Chapter 6 describes some methods that help in phenotyping DAT+ RBCs. If transfused RBCs are present, several methods are available for determining the phenotype of only the patient's RBCs:

1. One method depends on separating the younger RBCs (e.g., reticulocytes are presumed to be the patient's own RBCs).[370-375]
2. Another method utilizes flow cytometry.[376-378] We believe that this method is much more reliable than the reticulocyte method.
3. A recent approach is to use DNA typing.[379-381]

Additional Approaches

If the recipient's DAT was known to be negative prior to transfusion, or if the recipient's RBCs are still available for the performance of the DAT and it is demonstrated to be negative, this can be valuable information. An abrupt change in the DAT from negative to positive is strong evidence that the patient has a DHTR rather than AIHA.

If it is possible to test the donor units of blood, this procedure can be of significance if an antibody having specificity that could be either an alloantibody or an autoantibody is detected (anti-E, for example). If, by chance, none of the donor units contains the E antigen, AIHA or an alloantibody-induced HTR caused by an undetected antibody must be considered.

Thus, with careful serologic testing, it is possible to distinguish a DHTR from AIHA in almost all cases. If pretransfusion RBCs are not available (as, unfortunately, is usually the case), and if the patient has an alloantibody or mixture of alloantibodies with a broad range of reactivity, the distinction could be difficult.

A final note of caution is that the acquired immune hemolytic anemia might be neither a DHTR nor AIHA but instead could be drug-induced immune hemolytic anemia. In particular, cephalosporin drugs are used frequently in association with surgical procedures that could require transfusion. In this setting, abrupt onset of a positive DAT and hemolysis could be misinterpreted as a DHTR or the sudden onset of AIHA. This topic is discussed in detail in Chapter 8.

H. Bystander Immune Hemolysis

THE CONCEPT OF BYSTANDER IMMUNE CYTOLYSIS

Immune lysis of blood cells may occur in situations in which accepted immunologic principles would not lead one to expect hemolysis of the cells that are being destroyed. The following examples may be cited:

1. When an RBC alloantibody causes destruction of transfused RBCs in a hemolytic transfusion reaction, one would not expect hemolysis of the patient's own RBCs.
2. When ABO antibodies are produced by the donor's lymphocytes following hematopoietic cell transplantation and cause hemolysis of the patient's RBCs, one would not expect that transfused group O RBCs would be hemolyzed. (See the section on passenger lymphocyte syndrome in Chapter 12.)
3. When a person who has been transfused or who has been pregnant develops an alloantibody against the HPA-1a antigen (Pl^{A1}) on platelets, one would not expect that lysis of the patient's own HPA-1a-negative platelets would occur following a subsequent transfusion.
4. When a patient is infected with malaria parasites that enter RBCs and cause their disruption, one would not expect immune lysis of RBCs that are not infected.
5. When a patient develops an immune reaction to a drug, a vaccination, or a micro-organism, one does not expect the development of immune hemolytic anemia.
6. When a patient receives a blood transfusion, one does not expect the development of autoimmune hemolytic anemia.

In the foregoing examples, an alloimmune stimulation results in an antibody that apparently causes lysis of the patient's own RBCs. In many instances, the only RBC antibody detected is directed against RBC antigens not intrinsic to the patient's RBCs. In other instances, alloimmunization leads to the development of autoantibodies. We suggest that such examples of immune cell lysis be grouped under the heading of *bystander immune cytolysis*. Accordingly, we have developed the following definition to encompass these occurrences.

Definition of Bystander Immune Cytolysis

Bystander immune cytolysis may be defined as immune destruction of cells by antibody directed against an antigen that is not an unmodified intrinsic component of the cell membrane.[382,383] We also apply the term *bystander immune cytolysis* when autoimmune hemolytic anemia occurs following exposure to alloantigens.

A BRIEF HISTORY OF THE DEVELOPMENT OF THE CONCEPT OF BYSTANDER IMMUNE CYTOLYSIS

In 1965, Dameshek[384] described instances in which an exogenous factor (e.g., bacterial infection) caused an immune response leading to an antigen-antibody reaction on a cell, or which resulted in injury to the cell via the development of immune complexes. He referred to cells involved in such reactions as "innocent bystander" cells. He emphasized that these reactions involved exogenous antigens leading to the development of endogenous disease and distinguished such reactions from true autoimmune disorders. Instead, he considered these reactions to be temporary "allergic" reactions.

Subsequently, a number of studies have investigated possible mechanisms for bystander immune cytolysis and, more recently, additional clinical settings in which bystander immune cytolysis occurs have been recognized.[382,383,385]

Complement-Mediated Lysis of "Bystander Cells"

In the 1960s and early 1970s, several groups of investigators described a form of RBC cell lysis differentiated from classical complement-mediated hemolysis by its occurrence in the absence of antibody on the cells.[386-391] That is, RBCs are lysed by complement even though they are not involved in an antigen-antibody reaction. These investigators demonstrated that activated complement components ($\overline{C567}$) were generated by an immune reaction and that the activated components could attach to normal RBC membranes, which are then lysed in the presence of late-reacting complement components. Thus, the hemolysis results from activation of complement components at one site, which leads to the lysis of normal cells at a distance. The term most commonly used to describe this mechanism was "reactive hemolysis." In these studies, the early-reacting components of complement (C1, C4, C2, and C3) were not required for the reaction. RBCs from patients with PNH were exceptionally susceptible to this mode of hemolysis,[392,393] although hemolysis of normal human RBCs also occurred.[389]

Subsequently, Salama and Mueller-Eckhardt[193] and Ness and associates[394] reported that autologous RBCs were sensitized by complement during many DHTRs. That is, DHTRs caused by antibodies to transfused RBCs resulted in sensitization by complement components of autologous RBCs that did not contain the antigen to which the causative antibody was directed. Because C3 was detected on the patients' RBCs, complement sensitization of the autologous cells occurred by a mechanism that is different from classical reactive hemolysis. In neither study was an effort made to determine whether autologous RBCs had a shortened life span during the DHTRs.

Lack of Frequent Clinical Reports of Bystander Immune Hemolysis. Although complement-mediated bystander lysis was described in detail in experimental studies, instances of bystander immune hemolysis in clinical medicine were not well documented. Yachnin and Ruthenberg[392] suggested that the hemolysis in patients with PNH—especially the bouts of worsened hemolysis occurring during acute infections—might occur by this mechanism. They also suggested that such a mechanism might explain the pathogenesis of other DAT-positive acquired immune hemolytic anemias wherein complement but not antibody could be demonstrated on the patients' RBCs. In addition, there were isolated reports, often incompletely documented, of the destruction of autologous RBCs during DHTRs.[131,395-397] Because so few clinical reports suggesting bystander hemolysis were available, there was little interest in the phenomenon.

The Passenger Lymphocyte Syndrome and Bystander Immune Hemolysis. Our interest in bystander immune cytolysis was stimulated by observations of an extraordinary group of patients who developed the passenger lymphocyte syndrome following minor ABO-incompatible bone marrow transplantation using matched-unrelated donors (see Chapter 12).[398]

Hemolysis in the passenger lymphocyte syndrome is generally attributed to destruction of the patient's incompatible RBCs by donor-derived anti-A and/or anti-B produced from "passenger" immunocompetent donor lymphocytes that are infused with the marrow product. In three such patients whom we described, however, transfusion requirements for group O RBCs during the hemolytic episode clearly indicated that the amount of hemolysis that occurred was far in excess of what could be explained on the basis of hemolysis of the patients' RBCs alone.[398] The total RBC volumes of the patients at the onset of hemolysis were estimated as being between 1592 mL and 2039 mL, whereas approximately 4680 mL of washed group O RBCs (26 units) had to be transfused in the subsequent 15 days to maintain a reasonable hemoglobin level. (These data are presented in detail in Chapter 12.) As the patients were not bleeding, these findings provided compelling evidence that transfused group O RBCs were also hemolyzed. All of the patients developed strongly reactive anti-A or anti-B as is characteristic of the passenger lymphocyte syndrome, and no other antibodies were detected in their sera or in eluates from their RBCs. Because anti-A and anti-B were the only RBC antibodies present, yet group O RBCs were also hemolyzed, we suggested that this was an example of bystander immune hemolysis, in which the anti-A and anti-B indirectly caused the hemolysis of the group O RBCs, perhaps through a mechanism such as reactive hemolysis.

These cases stimulated us to review and extend the concept of bystander immune cytolysis.[382] In so doing, numerous other clinical examples were identified, and a number of potential mechanisms were proposed.

TABLE 9-18. CLINICAL SETTINGS IN WHICH BYSTANDER IMMUNE CYTOLYSIS COULD OCCUR

1. The passenger lymphocyte syndrome, especially in association with minor ABO-incompatible marrow transplants.
2. The sickle cell hemolytic transfusion reaction syndrome.
3. Severe hemolytic transfusion reactions.
4. Posttransfusion purpura.
5. Immune hemolytic associated with infectious agents.
6. Paroxysmal nocturnal hemoglobinuria.
7. Drug-induced immune hemolytic anemia.
8. AIHA following transfusion.
9. AIHA following vaccination.

CLINICAL SETTINGS IN WHICH BYSTANDER IMMUNE CYTOLYSIS MAY OCCUR

Bystander cytolysis could play an important role in immune lysis in a number of clinical entities (Table 9-18).

The Passenger Lymphocyte Syndrome. The passenger lymphocyte syndrome is reviewed briefly above and in more detail in Chapter 12. In addition to the patients previously cited who were reported by Gajewski and colleagues,[398] there have been a number of other reports of severe hemolysis in this setting, some of which strongly suggest the hemolysis of transfused group O RBCs in addition to the patients' own ABO-incompatible RBCs.[399-405] These cases provide strong evidence for bystander immune hemolysis, as serologic studies have revealed only antibodies against the patient's own group A or B RBCs, yet large volumes of transfused group O RBCs are hemolyzed as well.

The sickle cell hemolytic transfusion reaction syndrome is described in Chapter 14. A prominent feature of the syndrome is the fact that the patient's hemoglobin level following transfusion can be significantly lower than was present prior to transfusion, thereby suggesting that, in addition to hemolysis of the transfused RBCs, the patient's own RBCs are involved in the hemolytic reaction. The analysis is complicated by the fact that a shortened RBC survival time is an invariable finding in SCD, and by the fact that reticulocytopenia frequently occurs during the DHTR.[406] Nevertheless, a frequently proposed mechanism for the profound drop in hemoglobin that often occurs in this setting is an increased rate of destruction of the patient's own RBCs ("hyperhemolysis").[382,406-410] Briefly stated, the patient's own RBCs are affected by the immune lysis of allogeneic RBC. Although "hyperhemolysis" is most often described among patients with SCD who have DHTRs, similar findings have been described among patients with thalassemia.[411]

Because "hyperhemolysis" resulting in a lower hemoglobin level following transfusion than that prior to transfusion has been reported following DHTRs in patients with two forms of hereditary hemolytic anemia, one wonders whether a similar occurrence might not sometimes follow DHTRs in patients with acquired hemolytic anemias.[383]

Severe hemolytic transfusion reactions in which the patients' own RBCs are also hemolyzed have been described infrequently. Polesky and Bove[131] described a 72-year-old female who was hospitalized because of severe anemia. On the patient's fourth hospital day, an RBC survival study using her own ^{51}Cr-labeled RBCs was started because she had a positive DAT and a nonspecific cold autoantibody with a wide thermal amplitude and had recently had a febrile transfusion reaction. Twelve days after the ^{51}Cr-labeled RBC survival study was started, 300 mL of washed RBCs were transfused. No symptoms occurred during the transfusion, but about 1 hour later, the patient voided 145 mL port wine–colored urine. Hemoglobinuria and hemoglobinemia were documented, and her hematocrit, which had been stable at 18%–19% for 12 days, was 11% on the day after transfusion. She developed anuria and increasing jaundice and expired 3 days later.

The RBC survival study demonstrated that 28% of the patient's own RBCs were acutely hemolyzed. It is also probable that all of the transfused RBCs were hemolyzed. The DHTR was attributed to an anti-Jk^a that had been obscured by the presence of the autoantibody and was ultimately detected after the patient's death. The authors suggested that the autoantibody was the most probable cause of the hemolysis of the patients' own RBCs during the DHTR. They also cited two similar cases,[395,396] but added that these cases had not been documented in detail.

Wiener[397] described a patient whose hemoglobin dropped from 6 g/dL to 2.7 g/dL following transfusion of 500 mL of blood that was subsequently determined to be incompatible. Signs and symptoms of hemolysis were present, and there was no evidence of blood loss. Accordingly, he concluded that transfusions of incompatible blood could initiate some mechanism that causes destruction of the patient's own RBCs in addition to causing lysis of the donor's RBCs.

Greene and Khan[412] described a 62-year-old female whose pretransfusion testing demonstrated alloanti-c. During surgery, 5 units of c-negative RBCs were transfused, and 10 days later her hemoglobin plummeted to 4.9 g/dL—a 9.6 g/dL drop. Serologic studies indicated a DHTR due to alloanti-s, -Fy^a, and -Jk^b. The authors pointed out that the drop in hemoglobin was greater than could be attributed to lysis of the transfused RBCs only and stated that it was evident that autologous RBCs were being hemolyzed as well. They indicated that anti-Jk^b might fix complement and concluded that complement activation occurring during the DHTR resulted in lysis of innocent bystander (autologous) RBCs.

Post-transfusion purpura (PTP) is characterized by sudden onset of severe thrombocytopenia approximately 1 week following transfusion of blood or blood fractions containing platelet material.[413,414] At the time thrombocytopenia develops, an antibody against an alloantigen on transfused platelets is present in the patient's serum. The alloantibody, usually anti-HPA-1a (anti-Pl^{A1}), develops as a result of prior transfusion or pregnancy but appears to result in destruction of the patient's HPA-1a-negative platelets. The mechanism of thrombocytopenia has remained enigmatic because the patient's platelets after recovery are invariably nonreactive with alloantibody that is present during the acute phase of PTP.[415]

Several hypotheses have been proposed.[416] Soluble HPA-1a antigen on platelet membrane microparticles is present in blood products[417] and might adsorb to the patient's platelets, providing target antigen.[418,419] A second hypothesis is that immune complexes of soluble HPA-1a antigen and anti-HPA-1a alloantibodies mediate autologous platelet destruction.[413,420] A third hypothesis is that an autoantibody forms in parallel with the alloantibody, recognizing a conserved structural determinant adjacent to the specific antigen polymorphic site, and that this antibody then destroys autologous platelets.[421]

AIHA associated with infectious agents might develop by a number of mechanisms that are reviewed in another segment of this chapter (see the section on AIHA and infectious agents). These cases of AIHA are further examples of bystander immune hemolysis.

Paroxysmal nocturnal hemoglobinuria (PNH) is a disorder in which RBCs are particularly sensitive to the action of complement. Bystander immune hemolysis has been thought to contribute to at least some episodes of hemolysis.[422]

There are several abnormalities of PNH RBC membranes that modulate complement, especially decay accelerating factor (DAF, CD55) and the membrane inhibitor of reactive lysis (MIRL, CD59). It appears that absence of the CD59 antigen plays the most critical role in the complement sensitivity of PNH RBCs. Inherited deficiency of DAF is not associated with clinical hemolysis, whereas a hereditary deficiency of CD59 is associated with PNH. Restoration of CD59 in vitro corrects the complement sensitivity of RBCs more completely than restoration of DAF, and PNH can occur in the absence of DAF deficiency.[422]

Yachnin and Ruthenberg[392] emphasized that their experiments with PNH RBCs indicated that production of the RBC membrane damage by complement did not involve an antigen-antibody reaction specific for the RBCs that were lysed. They suggested that the well-known propensity of patients with PNH to be worsened by bouts of intercurrent infection might be related to immune interactions between antibody and the invading agent or its products that nonspecifically ("indifferently") activate the complement system. Rosse[423] and Nakakuma and coworkers[424,425] have made similar suggestions.

Sirchia and colleagues[426] demonstrated that when PNH RBCs were incubated in vitro with leukocytes and a fresh, unacidified serum containing an antileukocyte antibody, hemolysis was observed, and the intensity of lysis varied according to the number of leukocytes used. These researchers stated that their findings supported a previous suggestion made by Dacie[427] that DHTRs that have been reported in some PNH patients[428-435] might be caused by the interaction between transfused leukocytes and leukocyte antibodies in the patients' sera. Indeed, washed RBCs[431,436] or white-cell poor RBCs[426,437] have been recommended for transfusion of patients with PNH to avoid DHTRs. Other investigators, however, have suggested that this might not be necessary[438] provided that group-specific blood products are transfused.[439]

Drug-induced immune hemolytic anemia is reviewed in depth in Chapter 8. A number of mechanisms have been proposed by which the development of an immune response to a drug results in hemolysis. As indicated previously, the resultant antibodies are not directed against unmodified intrinsic RBC antigens; they therefore satisfy our definition of bystander immune hemolysis.

Autoimmune hemolytic anemia following transfusion is an example of an alloimmune stimulus resulting in autoimmune hemolysis. Because the patient's own RBCs are hemolyzed as a result of an alloimmune response, we include this as an example of bystander immune hemolysis. This topic is reviewed in another segment of this chapter (see the section on development of RBC autoantibodies and AIHA following transfusion).

Autoimmune Hemolytic Anemia Following Vaccination. This topic is reviewed in Chapter 3.

POSSIBLE MECHANISMS OF BYSTANDER IMMUNE CYTOLYSIS

A number of possible mechanisms have been proposed as the basis for bystander immune cytolysis (Table 9-19) and are detailed in the following paragraphs.[382]

Complement-Mediated Lysis of Unsensitized Cells

Reactive Hemolysis. Thompson and Rowe[386] described a novel mechanism of cell lysis, and further experimental data were published by Thompson and Lachmann[387] and Lachmann and Thompson.[388] As indicated previously, they described a form of RBC lysis (which they termed *reactive lysis*) in which cells are lysed by complement even though they are not involved in an antigen-antibody reaction. They emphasized that this is a mechanism by which complement activation at one site can lyse normal cells at a distance.[388] Other in vitro test systems demonstrated complement activation by somewhat different mechanisms that also resulted in sensitization of bystander cells.[193,394,440]

Experimental Data. Thompson and Rowe[386] suspended antibody-sensitized sheep RBCs in agarose gel and placed human serum as a source of complement in wells cut in the gel. In addition to zones of hemolysis surrounding the wells, they observed linear zones of hemolysis beyond the initial hemolytic zones. They referred to the latter zones of hemolysis as reactive hemolysis because they appeared as a result of the interaction of factors from different sera, although it became apparent during their investigation that both factors could be obtained from the same serum. They further determined that sensitization of the cells by antibody was not necessary for reactive hemolysis and that sheep, rabbit, or human RBCs could be lysed in this system. Hemolysis also occurred even when EDTA was incorporated into the plate, thus excluding the sequential activation of RBC surface-bound complement components.

Reactive hemolysis was demonstrable following "activation" of certain sera by agents known to activate complement, such as antibody-coated bacteria and zymosan. Some activation procedures were especially effective in producing the lytic factors that caused reactive hemolysis, and the authors suggested that hemolysis was particularly likely to occur in circumstances in which serum inhibitors of complement were not effective.

Lachman and Thompson[388] demonstrated that the complement factor generated by activation of serum that was responsible for reactive hemolysis was $C\overline{567}$ (a complex of complement factors 5, 6, and 7). This complex is formed by the complexing of C7 with $C\overline{56}$, the latter being formed in the fluid phase after immune activation. The investigators demonstrated that $C\overline{567}$ can attach to normal RBC membranes, which are then lysed in the presence of C8 and C9. $C\overline{567}$ can only be generated in a minority of sera, generally those from patients in the "acute phase" of inflammation. They determined that much more $C\overline{567}$ is bound to cells when it is generated in solution rather than at the complement fixation site (i.e., the cell membrane in an antigen-antibody reaction), and they suggested that this is due to the fact that there could be a much greater area of membrane available in the former case. They confirmed that the earlier-reacting components of complement (C1, C4, C2, and C3) are not required for the reaction, although activation of C3 by the classical immune hemolytic sequence utilizing C1, C4, and C2 can also be used to generate $C\overline{56}$. Although it is convenient to carry out reactive

TABLE 9-19. POSSIBLE MECHANISMS OF BYSTANDER IMMUNE CYTOLYSIS

1. Complement mediated lysis of unsensitized cells.
   a. Reactive hemolysis
   b. Complement activation by mechanisms other than reactive hemolysis.
2. Immune reactions against antigens adsorbed from plasma.
3. Adsorption of antigen-antibody complexes.
4. Modification of cellular antigens by drugs.
5. Development of RBC autoantibodies as a result of alloimmunization.

hemolysis in immunodiffusion plates, the reaction works equally well in the test tube.

Götze and Muller-Eberhard[389] also described mechanisms of cell lysis by complement that were entirely independent of antibody and that did not require binding of the first four complement components to the target-cell surface. The actual attack of the target cell begins with the attachment of C5, C6, and C7. The binding reaction is catalyzed by $C\overline{423}$, an enzyme that might be formed in cell-free solution. $C\overline{423}$ might effect binding of $C\overline{567}$ by acting from the fluid phase or from the surface of another cell to which it is bound specifically. The resulting cells are susceptible to lysis by C8 and C9. Transfer of $C\overline{567}$ from the site of activation on one cell to the site of binding on another cell is distinct from any other known transfer phenomenon of complement components. The authors stated that this mechanism might underline the phenomenon of reactive hemolysis reported by Thompson and Lachmann.[387] They also pointed out that PNH cells were exceptionally susceptible to this mode of hemolysis.

Yachnin and Ruthenberg[392] and Yachnin[393] previously had described fluid phase activation of complement resulting in the lysis of normal human RBCs and of the RBCs from patients with PNH. They pointed out that the demonstration that cells can suffer damage and destruction by the complement system without the mediation of specific anticell antibody suggests that autoimmune mechanisms need not necessarily be invoked to explain the presence of complement components on cells. At the time of these earlier studies, the components of complement causing the reaction were not as well defined, and these authors did not use the term *reactive lysis*, although subsequent researchers have commented that the underlying mechanisms seem similar.[382,385]

Other investigators also described various basic aspects of the reaction mechanism of reactive hemolysis.[390,391] Goldman and colleagues[390] reported that when the average numbers of $C\overline{567}$ sites per RBC generated in the presence of optimal C7 were plotted as a function of $C\overline{56}$ input, linear responses were obtained, indicating that a single competent $C\overline{567}$ site on a RBC membrane is sufficient to prepare the cell for lysis by C8 and C9.

Gocke[441] reported a similar system involving in vitro damage to platelets by the complement system, which is initiated by an antigen-antibody system in which the antigen is not an integral part of the platelet.

Complement Activation by Mechanisms Other Than Reactive Hemolysis. Salama and Mueller-Eckhardt[193] performed detailed serologic studies on 26 patients with DHTRs and found a positive DAT due to C3d in all cases. The antiglobulin reactions were not of the "mixed-field" type, which indicated that all of the patients' RBCs were coated with complement. The authors concluded that complement is activated regularly in DHTRs and binds to both autologous RBCs and the transfused cells. These researchers suggested that the autologous RBCs could become sensitized with complement components because of cross-reactivity of alloantibodies with autologous RBCs, or as a result of fluid-phase complement activation. A later report by Ness and coworkers[394] also described sensitization of autologous RBCs in DHTRs. Because C3 was detected on the patients' RBCs, complement sensitization of the autologous cells occurred by a mechanism that is different from that of classical reactive hemolysis.

Although Götze and Muller-Eberhard[389] had failed to demonstrate C3 binding after activation of complement at the surface of an adjacent cell, Salama and Mueller-Eckhardt[440] presented evidence that C3 can indeed be attached to bystander human RBCs if complement is activated either through the classical pathway or through the alternative pathway.

The Role of Complement-Mediated Lysis of Unsensitized Cells as a Mechanism for Bystander Immune Cytolysis. PNH is a disorder in which such a mechanism would seem likely because of the markedly increased sensitivity of the RBCs in this disorder to lysis by complement. Increased sensitivity to complement-mediated lysis has also been demonstrated in RBCs from patients with sickle cell anemia,[442] suggesting that this mechanism might contribute to "hyperhemolysis" in the sickle cell hemolytic transfusion reaction syndrome. Further, this mechanism might be operative in patients who have immune hemolysis caused by ABO blood group antibodies, as these antibodies regularly cause activation of complement. This could occur during the passenger lymphocyte syndrome following ABO-incompatible hematopoietic cell transplantation, or during HTRs caused by anti-A or anti-B.

Immune Reactions Against Antigens Adsorbed from Plasma by RBCs

Adsorption of A and B Antigens. Because A and B antigens can be demonstrated in plasma,[443-445] one possible explanation for the hemolysis of transfused group O RBCs in patients with the passenger lymphocyte syndrome caused by anti-A or anti-B is the adsorption of the A or B antigen onto the transfused RBC. This could allow for hemolysis by the strongly reactive anti-A and anti-B produced by the passenger lymphocytes in the donor stem cell product. This scenario could be more likely in patients who are secretors than in patients who are nonsecretors because "nonsecretors" secrete very small amounts of A or B according to their ABO group.[443,446]

There is a significant body of data indicating adsorption of A and B antigens onto group O RBCs following transfusion, after ABO-incompatible hematopoietic cell transplantation, or in congenital blood group chimeras. Renton and Hancock[447] observed that when group O RBCs are transfused to group A or group B recipients, they can acquire small amounts of A or B substance. The uptake of antigen is best demonstrated by using certain group O sera and to a lesser extent with group A and B sera. This phenomenon has been illustrated well by Crookston and Tilley[443] in a patient who was

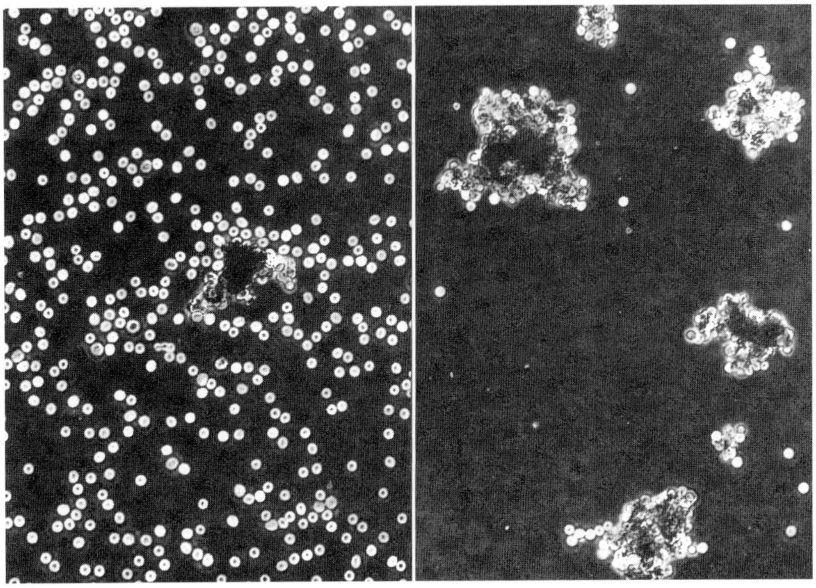

FIGURE 9-9. In both pictures, the red cells are from the same suspension of a patient's blood (16% A, 84% O). On the left, the cells are tested with anti-A serum. On the right, the cells are tested with anti-A,B (group O) serum.[58] (From Szymanski IO, Tilley CA, Crookston MC, Greenwalt TJ, Good RA: Lewis substances in a human marrow-transplantation chimaera. Lancet 1: 396, 1971. Reprinted with permission from Elsevier.)

blood group chimera and had 16% group A_1 RBCs and 84% group O RBCs (Fig. 9-9). On the left, the RBCs are tested with anti-A serum; on the right, they are tested with anti-A,B (group O) serum. (This degree of agglutination is much stronger than typically occurs after transfusion of group O RBCs to a group A patient.) Other investigators also have reported that group O RBCs in blood group chimeras who are genetically group A are agglutinated by group O sera.[448-450]

Although routine ABO blood grouping following ABO-incompatible marrow transplantation generally indicates conversion to donor type, we have observed weakly positive agglutination reactions a year or longer after marrow transplantation using anti-A,B sera when testing RBCs from patients who had been group A prior to transplantation with a group O marrow.[382] Also, Crookston and Tilley[443] reported on three patients who were tested about two years after receiving a bone marrow transplant from a group O donor. In two group A_1, Le(a-b+) recipients, the grafted group O RBCs reacted strongly with anti-A,B sera. In a group A_1, Le(a+b-) recipient, the grafted group O RBCs reacted weakly with anti-A,B sera. Further, Maeda and coworkers[451] found positive DAT reactions and could elute anti-B from the RBCs of a patient who had been group B and had received a transplant from a group A person. They suggested that the most likely explanation was that anti-B was produced by the donor marrow and reacted with B antigen adsorbed from the patient's plasma onto the group B RBCs produced by the transplanted stem cells.

As reviewed in Chapter 12, Arndt and associates[452] used flow cytometry to demonstrate that the recipient's RBCs following hematopoietic cell transplantation of group A or B patients with group O stem cells were uniformly coated with A or B substance. These findings are consistent with the concept of adsorption of group A and B substance rather than a mixture of group A and O RBCs.

Adsorption of Other Antigens from Plasma. One of the mechanisms proposed for lysis of HPLA-1a negative platelets in patients with anti-HPA-1a is the adsorption to the patient's platelets of soluble HPA-1a antigen, thereby providing target antigen. A similar mechanism could account for bystander immune hemolysis associated with infectious agents. Further, in some instances, drug administration might cause adsorption of drug antigens to the RBC membrane, with lysis mediated by antidrug antibody.

Adsorption of Antigen-Antibody Complexes

Another mechanism that could account for the hemolysis of group O RBCs in minor ABO-mismatched transplant patients is the adsorption of antigen-antibody complexes. It is possible that the anti-A or anti-B produced by the passenger lymphocytes reacts with A or B antigen in the plasma and that these antigen-antibody complexes are adsorbed by the transfused group O RBCs. Further, destruction of antigen-negative cells as a result of adsorption of antigen-antibody complexes has been proposed as a possible mechanism responsible in some instances of drug-induced immune hemolysis, and in the destruction of HPA-1a negative platelets in post-transfusion purpura. Also, in infectious diseases, antibody-antigen complexes specifically related to the infectious agent might coat the RBC, which then act as an "innocent bystander." Similarly, parasite antigen-antibody immune complexes likely contribute to the pathogenesis of the anemia in *falciparum* malaria. In some autoimmune disorders, particularly SLE, immune complexes frequently are detected in the patient's plasma and could contribute to the frequent finding of hemolysis in these patients. Further, several groups of investigators have indicated that immune complexes could play an important role in removing transfused platelets from the circulation.[453-456]

Modification of Cellular Antigens by Drugs

The possible mechanisms by which the administration of drugs might cause immune hemolysis are reviewed in Chapter 8. Prominent among the proposed mechanisms is the development of antibodies that are directed against cellular antigens modified by the drug.

Development of RBC Autoantibodies as a Result of Alloimmunization

AIHA following transfusion is an example of alloimmunization leading to an autoimmune reaction[457] (and see Section B of this chapter). The mechanism by which this occurs is uncertain, but other possible examples include the development of AIHA associated with infection and vaccination. These topics are reviewed in Chapter 3.

Lack of Specificity of Alloantibodies ("Cross-Reacting" Alloantibodies)

There is evidence that alloantibodies are not as exquisitely specific as appears to be the case in routine serologic reactions.[385] The work of Marks and colleagues,[458] Ouwehand and coworkers,[459] Thompson and associates,[460] and Barker and Elson[461] at the molecular level suggests that perhaps all alloantibodies are capable of reacting, under some circumstances, with RBCs lacking the putative antigens.

Salama and Mueller-Eckhardt[193] and Ness and associates[394,462] have suggested that one possible mechanism involved in the sensitization of autologous RBCs with complement during a HTR could be the presence of "cross-reacting" alloantibodies. In two patients with DHTRs, Salama and Mueller-Eckhardt[193] were able to adsorb alloanti-E from the serum with E-negative RBCs. This lack of definitive specificity could also be the explanation for "mimicking antibodies"[154–156] (i.e., alloantibodies that react with antigen-negative RBCs).[385]

Morrison and Mollison[464] suggested that in cases of PTP, a weaker cross-reacting antibody (which they referred to as an *autoantibody*) is formed, in addition to the allo-HPA-1a, and that it is this weaker antibody that reacts with the HPA-1a-negative platelets.

The lack of definitive specificity of alloantibodies might explain the presence of complement components on autologous RBCs more than 100 days after the reaction, as has been reported by Salama and Mueller-Eckhardt[193] and by Ness and associates.[394,462] The presence of cross-reacting alloantibodies could be the explanation for some instances of bystander immune cytolysis.

REFERENCES

1. Evans RS, Weiser RS: The serology of autoimmune hemolytic disease: Observations on forty-one patients. Arch Intern Med 1957;100:371–399.
2. Dacie JV: Auto-immune haemolytic anaemia (AIHA): Warm-antibody syndromes VI: Coombs-negative (DAT-negative) haemolytic anaemia; positive direct antiglobulin tests in normal subjects and in hospital patients; polyagglutinability and haemolytic anaemia. In The Haemolytic Anaemias, 3rd ed. Vol. 3, The Autoimmune Haemolytic Anaemias. New York: Churchill Livingstone, 1992:183–209.
3. Worlledge SM, Blajchman MA: The autoimmune haemolytic anaemias. Br J Haematol 1972;23(S):61–69.
4. Chaplin H, Jr: Clinical usefulness of specific antiglobulin reagents in autoimmune hemolytic anemias. Progr Hematol 1973;8:25–49.
5. Boccardi V, Girelli G, Perricone R, Ciccone F, Romoli P, Isacchi G: Coombs-negative autoimmune hemolytic anemia: Report of 11 cases. Haematologica 1978;63:301–310.
6. Petz LD, Garratty G: Acquired Immune Hemolytic Anemias, 1st ed. New York: Churchill Livingstone, 1980.
7. Gilliland BC, Leddy JP, Vaughan JH: The detection of cell-bound antibody on complement-coated human red cells. J Clin Invest 1970;49:898–906.
8. Gilliland BC, Baxter E, Evans RS: Red-cell antibodies in acquired hemolytic anemia with negative antiglobulin serum tests. N Engl J Med 1971;285:252–256.
9. Gilliland BC: Coombs-negative immune hemolytic anemia. Seminars Hematol 1976;13:267–275.
10. Mollison PL, Hughes-Jones NC: Clearance of Rh-positive red cells by low concentrations of Rh antibody. Immunology 1967;12:63–73.
11. Constatoulakis M, Costea N, Schwartz RS, Dameshek W: Quantitative studies of the effect of red blood cell sensitization in vitro hemolysis. J Clin Invest 1963;42:1790–1801.
12. Jandl JH, Kaplan ME: The destruction of red cells by antibodies in man. III: Quantitative factors influencing the patterns of hemolysis in vivo. J Clin Invest 1960;39:1145.
13. Garratty G, Nance SJ: Correlation between in vivo hemolysis and the amount of red cell-bound IgG measured by flow cytometry. Transfusion 1990;30:617–621.
14. Garratty G: Effect of cell-bound proteins on the in vivo survival of circulating blood cells. Gerontology 1991;37:68–94.
15. Garratty G: Factors affecting the pathogenicity of red cell auto- and alloantibodies. In Nance SJ (ed): Immune Destruction of Red Blood Cells. Arlington, VA: American Association of Blood Banks, 1989:109–169.
16. Garratty G: The significance of IgG on the red cell surface. Transfus Med Rev 1987;1:47–57.
17. Merry AH, Thomson EE, Rawlinson VI, Stratton F: A quantitative antiglobulin test for IgG for use in blood transfusion serology. Clin Lab Haematol 1982;4:393–402.
18. Jeje MO, Blajchman MA, Steeves K, Horsewood P, Kelton JG: Quantitation of red cell-associated IgG using an immunoradiometric assay. Transfusion 1984;24:473–476.
19. Masouredis SP, Branks MJ, Victoria EJ: Antiidiotypic IgG crossreactive with Rh alloantibodies in red cell autoimmunity. Blood 1987;70:710–715.
20. Masouredis SP, Branks MJ, Garratty G, Victoria EJ: Immunospecific red cell binding of iodine 125-labeled immunoglobulin G erythrocyte autoantibodies. J Lab Clin Med 1987;110:308–317.
21. Dupuy ME, Elliot M, Masouredis SP: Relationship between red cell bound antibody and agglutination in the antiglobulin reaction. Vox Sang 1964;9:40–44.
22. Hughes-Jones NC, Polley MJ, Telford R, et al: Optimal conditions for detecting blood group antibodies by the antiglobulin test. Vox Sang 1964;9:385–395.
23. Romano EL, Hughes-Jones NC, Mollison PL: Direct antiglobulin reaction in ABO-haemolytic disease of the newborn. Br Med J 1973;1:524–526.
24. Schmitz N, Djibey I, Kretschmer V, Mahn I, Mueller-Eckhardt C: Assessment of red cell autoantibodies in autoimmune hemolytic anemia of warm type by a radioactive anti-IgG test. Vox Sang 1981;41:224–230.
25. Yam P, Petz LD, Spath P: Detection of IgG sensitization of red cells with 125I staphylococcal protein A. Am J Hematol 1982; 12:337–346.

26. Salama A, Mueller-Eckhardt C, Bhakdi S: A two-stage immunoradiometric assay with 125I-staphylococcal protein A for the detection of antibodies and complement on human blood cells. Vox Sang 1985;48:239–245.
27. Nilsson EK, Loof L, Nilsson UR, Nilsson B: Development of an immunoassay for the detection of minute amounts of IgG-coated erythrocytes in whole blood and its application for the assessment of Fc-mediated clearance of anti-D-coated erythrocytes in vivo. Vox Sang 1989;57:188–192.
28. Garratty G, Postoway N, Nance S, et al: The detection of IgG on the red cells of "Coombs-negative" autoimmune hemolytic anemias [abstract]. Transfusion 1982;22: 430.
29. Bodensteiner D, Brown P, Skikne B, Plapp F: The enzyme-linked immunosorbent assay: Accurate detection of red blood cell antibodies in autoimmune hemolytic anemia. Am J Clin Pathol 1983;79:182–185.
30. Hasselbalch H, Berild D, Hansen OP: Red-cell sensitization in myelofibrosis. Scand J Haematol 1984;32:179–182.
31. Leach M: A direct enzyme-linked antiglobulin test for detection of red cell autoantibodies in auto-immune haemolytic anaemia. Med Lab Sci 1984;41:232–237.
32. Hansen OP, Hansen TM, Jans H, Hippe E: Red blood cell membrane-bound IgG: Demonstration of antibodies in patients with autoimmune haemolytic anaemia and immune complexes in patients with rheumatic diseases. Clin Lab Haematol 1984;6:341–349.
33. Postoway N, Nance SJ, Garratty G: Variables affecting the enzyme-linked antiglobulin test when detecting and quantitating IgG red cell antibodies. Med Lab Sci 1985;42:11–19.
34. Sokol RJ, Hewitt S, Booker DJ, Stamps R: Enzyme linked direct antiglobulin tests in patients with autoimmune haemolysis. J Clin Pathol 1985;38:912–914.
35. Sokol RJ, Hewitt S, Booker DJ, Stamps RL: Small quantities of erythrocyte bound immunoglobulins and autoimmune haemolysis. J Clin Pathol 1987;40:254–257.
36. Howard PR, MacPherson B: An antiglobulin consumption ELAT technique for the detection of red cell antibodies. J Med Technol 1987;4:218–222.
37. Gutgsell NS, Issitt PD, Tomasulo PA, et al: Use of the direct enzyme-linked antiglobulin test (ELAT) in patients with unexplained anemia [abstract]. Transfusion 1988;28:36S.
38. Tomasulo PA, Issitt PD, Gutgsell NS, et al: Predictive value of the direct enzyme-linked antiglobulin test (ELAT) in patients with unexplained anemia [abstract]. London, Proceedings of the 20th Congress of the International Society of Blood Transfusion, 1988:121.
39. Kiruba R, Han P: Quantitation of red cell-bound immunoglobulin and complement using enzyme-linked antiglobulin consumption assay. Transfusion 1988;28:519–524.
40. Garratty G, Postoway N, Nance S, Arndt P: Detection of IgG on red cells of patients with suspected direct antiglobulin test negative autoimmune hemolytic anemia (AIHA) [abstract]. Book of Abstracts of the ISBT/AABB Joint Congress, Los Angeles, 1990: 87.
41. Garratty G: Autoimmune hemolytic anemia. In Garratty G (ed): Immunolobiology of Transfusion Medicine. New York: Dekker, 1994:493–521.
42. Garratty G, Arndt P: Applications of flow cytofluorometry to transfusion science. Transfusion 1995;35:157–178.
43. Wang Z, Shi J, Zhou Y, Ruan C: Detection of red blood cell-bound immunoglobulin G by flow cytometry and its application in the diagnosis of autoimmune hemolytic anemia. Int J Hematol 2001;73:188–193.
44. Rand BP, Olson JD, Garratty G, Petz LD: Coombs' negative immune hemolytic anemia with anti-E occurring in the red blood cell eluate of an E-negative patient. Transfusion 1978;18:174–180.
45. Ganly PS, Laffan MA, Owen I, Hows JM: Auto-anti-Jka in Evans' syndrome with negative direct antiglobulin test. Br J Haematol 1988;69:537–539.
46. Yam P, Wilkinson L, Petz LD, Garratty G: Studies on hemolytic anemia in pregnancy with evidence for autoimmunization in a patient with a negative direct antiglobulin (Coombs') test. Am J Hematol 1980;8:23–29.
47. Petz LD, Yam P, Wilkinson L, Garratty G, Lubin B, Mentzer W: Increased IgG molecules bound to the surface of red blood cells of patients with sickle cell anemia. Blood 1984; 64:301–304.
48. Kay MM: Aging of cell membrane molecules leads to appearance of an aging antigen and removal of senescent cells. Gerontology 1985;31:215–235.
49. Green GA, Rehn MM, Kalra VK: Cell-bound autologous immunoglobulin in erythrocyte subpopulations from patients with sickle cell disease. Blood 1985;65:1127–1133.
50. Green GA, Kalra VK: Sickling-induced binding of immunoglobulin to sickle erythrocytes. Blood 1988;71:636–639.
51. Hebbel RP, Miller WJ: Phagocytosis of sickle erythrocytes: Immunologic and oxidative determinants of hemolytic anemia. Blood 1984;64:733–741.
52. Solanki DL: Erythrophagocytosis in vivo in sickle cell anemia. Am J Hematol 1985;20:353–357.
53. Galili U, Korkesh A, Kahane I, Rachmilewitz EA: Demonstration of a natural antigalactosyl IgG antibody on thalassemic red blood cells. Blood 1983;61:1258–1264.
54. Toy PT, Chin CA, Reid ME, Burns MA: Factors associated with positive direct antiglobulin tests in pretransfusion patients: A case-control study. Vox Sang 1985;49:215–220.
55. Heddle NM, Kelton JG, Turchyn KL, Ali MA: Hypergammaglobulinemia can be associated with a positive direct antiglobulin test, a nonreactive eluate, and no evidence of hemolysis. Transfusion 1988;28:29–33.
56. Garratty G, Arndt P: Is there a correlation with RBC-bound IgG detected by sensitive assays, such as the enzyme-linked antiglobulin test (ELAT), and serum levels of IgG? [abstract] Transfusion 1987;27:545.
57. Engelfriet CP, von dem Borne AEG, Beckers D, et al: Immune destruction of red cells. In Bell CA (ed): A Seminar on Immune-Mediated Cell Destruction. Washington, DC: American Association of Blood Banks, 1981:93–130.
58. Zupanska B, Brojer E, Maslanka K, Hallberg T: A comparison between Fc receptors for IgG1 and IgG3 on human monocytes and lymphocytes using anti-Rh antibodies. Vox Sang 1985;49:67–76.
59. Garratty G, Arndt P, Nance S, et al: Low affinity autoantibodies—A cause of false negative direct antiglobulin tests [abstract]. Book of Abstracts of the ISBT/AABB Joint Congress, 1990:87.
60. Garratty G: Low affinity autoantibodies—A cause of false negative direct antiglobulin tests. Transfus Today 1991; 12:3–4.
61. Sokol RJ, Booker DJ, Stamps R, et al: Direct Coombs test-negative autoimmune hemolytic anemia and low-affinity IgG class antibodies. Immunohem 1997;13:115–118.
62. Lai M, Rumi C, D'Onofrio G, et al: Clinically significant autoimmune hemolytic anemia with a negative direct antiglobulin test by routine tube test and positive by column agglutination method. Immumnohematology 2002;18:109–113.
63. Johnson ST, Bandouveres S: DAT negative autoimmune hemolytic anemia due to low affinity IgG warm-reactive anti-Pr in an infant [abstract]. Transfusion 2002;42:20S.
64. Schwartz RS, Costea N: Autoimmune hemolytic anemia: Clinical correlations and biological implications. Semin Hematol 1966;3:2–26.
65. Fossati-Jimack L, Reininger L, Chicheportiche Y, et al: High pathogenic potential of low-affinity autoantibodies in experimental autoimmune hemolytic anemia. J Exp Med 1999;190:1689–1696.
66. Sturgeon P, Smith LE, Chun HMT, Hurvitz CH, Garratty G, Goldfinger D: Autoimmune hemolytic anemia associated exclusively with IgA of Rh specificity. Transfusion 1979; 19:324–328.
67. Arndt P, Garratty G: Use of flow cytometry for detection of IgM on RBCs showing spontaneous agglutination [abstract]. Transfusion 1994;34:68S.
68. Garratty G, Arndt P, Domen R, et al: Severe autoimmune hemolytic anemia associated with IgM warm autoantibodies directed against determinants on or associated with glycophorin A. Vox Sang 1997;72:124–130.

69. Garratty G, Arndt P, Leger R: Serological findings in autoimmune hemolytic anemia associated with IgM warm autoantibodies [abstract]. Blood 2001;98:61a.
70. Talano J-AM, Johnson ST, Friedman KD, et al: Serologic characteristics of three cses of IgA mediated autoimmune hemolytic anemia (AIHA) confirmed by flow cytometry [abstract]. Blood 2002;100:283a.
71. Wager O, Haltia K, Rasanen JA, Vuopio P: Five cases of positive antiglobulin test involving IgA warm type autoantibody. Ann Clin Res 1971;3:76–85.
72. Stratton F, Rawlinson VI, Chapman SA, Pengelly CD, Jennings RC: Acquired hemolytic anemia associated with IgA anti-e. Transfusion 1972;12:157–161.
73. Suzuki S, Amano T, Mitsunaga M, Yagyu F, Ofuji T: Autoimmune hemolytic anemia associated with IgA autoantibody. Clin Immunol Immunopathol 1981;21:247–256.
74. Wolf CF, Wolf DJ, Peterson P, Brandstetter RD, Hansen DE: Autoimmune hemolytic anemia with predominance of IgA autoantibody. Transfusion 1982;22:238–240.
75. Clark DA, Dessypris EN, Jenkins DE, Jr, Krantz SB: Acquired immune hemolytic anemia associated with IgA erythrocyte coating: Investigation of hemolytic mechanisms. Blood 1984;64:1000–1005.
76. Kowal-Vern A, Jacobson P, Okuno T, Blank J: Negative direct antiglobulin test in autoimmune hemolytic anemia. Am J Pediatr Hematol Oncol 1986;8:349–351.
77. Reusser P, Osterwalder B, Burri H, Speck B: Autoimmune hemolytic anemia associated with IgA—Diagnostic and therapeutic aspects in a case with long-term follow-up. Acta Haematol 1987;77:53–56.
78. Salama A, Bhakdi S, Mueller-Eckhardt C: Evidence suggesting the occurrence of C3-independent intravascular immune hemolysis. Reactive hemolysis in vivo. Transfusion 1987;27:49–53.
79. Gottsche B, Salama A, Mueller-Eckhardt C: Autoimmune hemolytic anemia associated with an IgA autoanti-Gerbich. Vox Sang 1990;58:211–214.
80. Girelli G, Perrone MP, Adorno G, et al: A second example of hemolysis due to IgA autoantibody with anti-e specificity. Haematologica 1990;75:182–183.
81. Sokol RJ, Booker DJ, Stamps R, Booth JR, Hook V: IgA red cell autoantibodies and autoimmune hemolysis. Transfusion 1997;37:175–181.
82. Janvier D, Sellami F, Missud F, et al: Severe autoimmune hemolytic anemia caused by a warm IgA autoantibody directed against the third loop of band 3 (RBC anion-exchange protein 1). Transfusion 2002;42:1547–1552.
83. Bardill B, Mengis C, Tschopp M, Wuillemin WA: Severe IgA-mediated auto-immune haemolytic anaemia in a 48-yr-old woman. Eur J Haematol 2003;70:60–63.
84. Fanger MW, Goldstine SN, Shen L: Cytofluorographic analysis of receptors for IgA on human polymorphonuclear cells and monocytes and the correlation of receptor expression with phagocytosis. Mol Immunol 1983;20:1019–1027.
85. Shen L, Maliszewski CR, Rigby WF, Fanger MW: IgA-mediated effector function of HL-60 cells following treatment with calcitriol. Mol Immunol 1986;23:611–618.
86. Yeaman GR, Kerr MA: Opsonization of yeast by human serum IgA anti-mannan antibodies and phagocytosis by human polymorphonuclear leucocytes. Clin Exp Immunol 1987;68:200–208.
87. Shen L, Fanger MW: Secretory IgA antibodies synergize with IgG in promoting ADCC by human polymorphonuclear cells, monocytes, and lymphocytes. Cell Immunol 1981;59: 75–81.
88. Maliszewski CR, March CJ, Schoenborn MA, Gimpel S, Shen L: Expression cloning of a human Fc receptor for IgA. J Exp Med 1990;172:1665–1672.
89. Kay NE, Douglas SD, Mond JJ, Flier JS, Kochwa S, Rosenfield RE: Hemolytic anemia with serum and erythrocyte-bound low-molecular-weight IgM. Clin Immunol Immunopathol 1975;4:216–225.
90. Schanfield MS, Pisciotta A, Libnock J: Seven cases of hemolytic anemia associated with warm IgM autoantibodies [abstract]. Transfusion 1978;18:623.
91. Garratty G, Brunt D, Greenfield B, et al: An auto anti-Ena mimicking an allo anti-Ena associated with pure red cell aplasia [abstract]. Transfusion 1983;23:408.
92. Szymanski IO, Huff SR, Selbovitz LG, Sherwood GK: Erythrocyte sensitization with monomeric IgM in a patient with hemolytic anemia. Am J Hematol 1984;17:71–77.
93. Schreiber AD, Frank MM: Role of antibody and complement in the immune clearance and destruction of erythrocytes. I: In vivo effects of IgG and IgM complement-fixing sites. J Clin Invest 1972;51:575–582.
94. Schreiber AD, Frank MM: Role of antibody and complement in the immune clearance and destruction of erythrocytes. II: Molecular nature of IgG and IgM complement-fixing sites and effects of their interaction with serum. J Clin Invest 1972; 51:583–589.
95. Atkinson JP, Frank MM: Studies on the in vivo effects of antibody. Interaction of IgM antibody and complement in the immune clearance and destruction of erythrocytes in man. J Clin Invest 1974;54:339–348.
96. Cutbush M, Mollison PL: Relation between characteristics of blood-group antibodies in vitro and associated patterns of red cell destruction in vivo. Br J Haematol 1958;4:115–137.
97. Holburn AM, Frame M, Hughes-Jones NC, Mollison PL: Some biological effects of IgM anti-Rh (D). Immunology 1971; 20:681–691.
98. Mollison PL: Blood Transfusion in Clinical Medicine, 8th ed. Oxford: Blackwell Scientific Publications, 1987.
99. Mollison PL: Survival curves of incompatible red cells: An analytical review [Review]: Transfusion 1986;26:43–50.
100. Salama A, Mueller-Eckhardt C: Autoimmune haemolytic anaemia in childhood associated with non-complement binding IgM autoantibodies. Br J Haematol 1987;65:67–71.
101. Fabijanska-Mitek J, Namirska-Krzton H, Seyfried H: The value of gel test and ELAT in autoimmune haemolytic anaemia. Clin Lab Haematol 1995;17:311–316.
102. Kroll H, Salama A, Berghofer H, et al: The direct antiglobulin test: Clinical significance and prospective comparison of column agglutination technology, gel test and tube test in 163 patients [abstract]. Vox Sanguinis 1994;67(S2):65.
103. Sajur J, Fournier Y, Sheridan B: Comparison of gel and tube techniques for direct antiglobulin tests [abstract]. Transfusion 1997;37:27S.
104. Petz LD, Branch DR: Serological tests for the diagnosis of immune hemolytic anemias. In McMillan R (ed): Methods in Haematology: Immune Cytopenias. New York: Churchill Livingstone, 1983:9–48.
105. Owen I, Hows J: Evaluation of the manual hexadimethrine bromide (Polybrene) technique in the investigation of autoimmune hemolytic anemia. Transfusion 1990;30:814–818.
106. Rubino M, Kavitsky DM, Nance S: Serologic testing in autoimmune hemolytic anemia (AIHA) with negative direct antiglobulin test (DAT) [abstract]. Transfusion 2002;42:104S.
107. Garratty G, Petz LD: Acquired hemolytic anemia associated with negative direct antiglobulin tests but enzyme reactive autoantibodies in the serum [abstract]. Book of Abstracts of the 24th Annual Meeting of the American Association of Blood Banks, 1971:83.
108. van't Veer MB, van Wieringen PM, van L, I, Overbeeke MA, dem Borne AE, Engelfriet CP: A negative direct antiglobulin test with strong IgG red cell autoantibodies present in the serum of a patient with autoimmune haemolytic anaemia. Br J Haematol 1981;49:383–386.
109. Issitt PD, Gruppo RA, Wilkinson SL, Issitt CH: Atypical presentation of acute phase, antibody-induced haemolytic anaemia in an infant. Br J Haematol 1982;52:537–543.
110. Parker AC, Habeshaw J, Cleland JF: The demonstration of a "plasmatic factor" in a case of Coombs' negative haemolytic anaemia. Scand J Haematol 1972;9:318–321.
111. van der Meulen FW, van der Hart M, Fleer A, Von dem Borne AE, Engelfriet CP, Van Loghem JJ: The role of adherence to human mononuclear phagocytes in the destruction of red cells sensitized with non-complement binding IgG antibodies. Br J Haematol 1978;38:541–549.

112. Galili U, Manny N, Izak G: EA rosette formation: A simple means to increase sensitivity of the antiglobulin test in patients with anti red cell antibodies. Br J Haematol 1981; 47:227–233.
113. Nance S, Garratty G: Correlations between an in vitro monocyte monolayer assay and autoimmune hemolytic anemia (AIHA) [abstract]. Transfusion 1982;22:410.
114. Gallagher MT, Branch DR, Mison A, Petz LD: Evaluation of reticuloendothelial function in autoimmune hemolytic anemia using an in vitro assay of monocyte-macrophage interaction with erythrocytes. Exp Hematol 1983;11:82–89.
115. Brojer E, Zupanska B, Michalewska B: Adherence to human monocytes of red cells from autoimmune haemolytic anaemia and red cells sensitized with alloantibodies. Haematologia (Budapest) 1982;15:135–145.
116. Zupanska B, Brojer E, Thomson EE, Merry AH, Seyfried H: Monocyte-erythrocyte interaction in autoimmune haemolytic anaemia in relation to the number of erythrocyte-bound IgG molecules and subclass specificity of autoantibodies. Vox Sang 1987;52:212–218.
117. Herron R, Clark M, Young D, Smith DS: Correlation of mononuclear phagocyte assay results and in vivo haemolytic rate in subjects with a positive direct antiglobulin test. Clin Lab Haematol 1986;8:199–207.
118. Garratty G: Basic mechanisms of in vivo cell destruction. In Bell CA (ed): A Seminar on Immune-Mediated Cell Destruction. Bethesda, Md: American Association of Blood Banks, 1981:1–28.
119. Gilsanz F, De La SJ, Molto L, Alvarez-Mon M: Hemolytic anemia in chronic large granular lymphocytic leukemia of natural killer cells: Cytotoxicity of natural killer cells against autologous red cells is associated with hemolysis. Transfusion 1996;36:463–466.
120. Rous P, Robertson OH: Free antigen and antibody circulating together in large amounts (hemagglutinin and agglutinogen in the blood of transfused rabbits). J Exp Med 1918;27:509–517.
121. Ovary Z, Spiegelman J: The production of "cold autoagglutinins" in the rabbit as a consequence of immunization with isologous erythrocytes. Ann N Y Acad Sci 1965;124:147–153.
122. Zmijewski CM: The production of erythrocyte autoantibodies in chimpanzees. J Exp Med 1965;121:657.
123. Liu CK, Evans RS: Production of positive antiglobulin serum test in rabbits by intraperitoneal injection of homologous blood. Proc Soc Exp Biol Med 1952;79:194.
124. Cox KO, Keast D: Erythrocyte autoantibodies induced in mice immunized with rat erythrocytes. Immunology 1973;25:531–539.
125. Cox KO, Keast D: Autoimmune haemolytic anaemia induced in mice immunized with rat erythrocytes. Clin Exp Immunol 1974;17:319–327.
126. Naysmith JD, Ortega-Pierres MG, Elson CJ: Rat erythrocyte-induced anti-erythrocyte autoantibody production and control in normal mice. Immunol Rev 1981;55:55–87.
127. Gengozian N, McLaughlin CL: Actively induced platelet-bound IgG associated with thrombocytopenia in the marmoset. Blood 1978;51:1197–1210.
128. Gengozian N, Annostby D: Antibodies selectively reactive to autologous and host-type platelets are obtained following interspecies immunizations in marmosets. Clin Exp Immunol 1981;43:128–134.
129. Dameshek W, Levine P: Isoimmunization with Rh factor in acquired hemolytic anemia. N Engl J Med 1943;228:641–644.
130. Allen FH: Proceedings of the 8th Congress of the International Society of Blood Transfusion 1960:359.
131. Polesky HF, Bove JR: A fatal hemolytic transfusion reaction with acute autohemolysis. Transfusion 1964;4:285–292.
132. Fudenberg HH, Rosenfield RE, Wasserman LR: Unusual specificity of autoantibody in autoimmune hemolytic anemia. J Mt Sinai Hosp 1958;25:324.
133. Chown B, Kaita H, Lowen B, Lewis M: Transient production of anti-LW by LW-positive people. Transfusion 1971;11:220–222.
134. Cook IA: Primary rhesus immunization of male volunteers. Brit J Haemat 1971;20:369–375.
135. Beard ME, Pemberton J, Blagdon J, Jenkins WF: Rh immunization following incompatible blood transfusion and a possible long-term complication of anti-D immunoglobulin therapy. J Med Genet 1971;8:317–320.
136. Lalezari P, Talleyrand NP, Wenz B, Schoenfeld ME, Tippett P: Development of direct antiglobulin reaction accompanying alloimmunization in a patient with Rhd (D, category III) phenotype. Vox Sang 1975;28:19–24.
137. Worlledge SM: The interpretation of a positive direct antiglobulin test. Brit J Haemat 1978;39:157–162.
138. Chaplin H Jr, Zarkowsky HS: Combined sickle cell disease and autoimmune hemolytic anemia. Arch Intern Med 1981;141:1091–1093.
139. Sosler SD, Perkins JT, Saporito C, Unger P, Koshy M: Severe autoimmune hemolytic anemia induced by transfusion in two alloimmunized patients with sickle cell disease [abstract]. Transfusion 1989;29:49S.
140. Argiolu F, Diana G, Arnone M, Batzella MG, Piras P, Cao A: High-dose intravenous immunoglobulin in the management of autoimmune hemolytic anemia complicating thalassemia major. Acta Haematol 1990;83:65–68.
141. Chan D, Poole GD, Binney M, Hamon MD, Copplestone JA, Prentice AG: Severe intravascular hemolysis due to autoantibodies stimulated by blood transfusion. Immunohematology 1996;12:80–83.
142. Zumberg MS, Procter JL, Lottenberg R, Kitchens CS, Klein HG: Autoantibody formation in the alloimmunized red blood cell recipient: Clinical and laboratory implications. Arch Intern Med 2001;161:285–290.
143. Szymanski IO, Smith VC: Red Blood Cell (RBC) autoimmunity in alloimmunized patients: Clinical observations [abstract]. Blood 2001;98:111b.
144. Mohn JF, Lambert RM, Bowman HS, et al: Experimental production in man of autoantibodies with Rh specificity. Ann NY Acad Sci 1965;124:477.
145. Mohn JF, Bowman HS, Lambert RM, Brason FW: The formation of Rh specific autoantibodies in experimental isoimmune hemolytic anemia in man. Tenth Congress of the International Society for Blood Transfusion, Stockholm, 1964.
146. Wodzinski MA, Collin RC, Booker DJ, Stamps R, Bellamy JD, Sokol RJ: Delayed hemollytic transfusion reaction and paroxysmal cold hemoglobinuria: An unusual association. Immunohematology, 1997;13:54.
147. Castellino SM, Combs MR, Zimmerman SA, Issitt PD, Ware RE: Erythrocyte autoantibodies in paediatric patients with sickle cell disease receiving transfusion therapy: Frequency, characteristics and significance. Br J Haematol 1999; 104:189–194.
148. Singer ST, Wu V, Mignacca R, Kuypers FA, Morel P, Vichinsky EP: Alloimmunization and erythrocyte autoimmunization in transfusion-dependent thalassemia patients of predominantly asian descent. Blood 2000;96:3369–3373.
149. Aygun B, Padmanabhan S, Paley C, Chandrasekaran V: Clinical significance of RBC alloantibodies and autoantibodies in sickle cell patients who received transfusions. Transfusion 2002;42:37–43.
150. Kaminski ER, Hows JM, Goldman JM, Batchelor JR: Lymphocytes from multi-transfused patients exhibit cytotoxicity against autologous cells. Br J Haematol 1992;81:23–26.
151. Paglieroni TG, Ward J, Holland PV: Changes in peripheral blood CD5 (Bla) B-cell populations and autoantibodies following blood transfusion. Transfusion 1995;35:189–198.
152. Marks JD, Ouwehand WH, Bye JM, et al: Human antibody fragments specific for human blood group antigens from a phage display library. Biotechnology (N Y): 1993;11:1145–1149.
153. Ouwehand WH, Bye JM, Gorick BD, et al: The humoral immune response against blood group antigens at the molecular level. Vox Sang 1994;67(Suppl 3):7–12.
154. Issitt PD, Zellner DC, Rolih SD, Duckett JB: Autoantibodies mimicking alloantibodies. Transfusion 1977;17:531–538.
155. Issitt PD, Pavone BG: Critical re-examination of the specificity of auto-anti-Rh antibodies in patients with a positive direct antiglobulin test. Br J Haematol 1978;38:63–74.

156. Issitt PD, Anstee DJ: Applied Blood Group Serology, 4th ed. Miami, FL: Montgomery Scientific, 1998.
157. Garratty G: Specificity of autoantibodies reacting optimally at 37°C. Immunohematology 1999;15:24–40.
158. Thompson KM, Sutherland J, Barden G, et al: Human monoclonal antibodies specific for blood group antigens demonstrate multispecific properties characteristic of natural autoantibodies. Immunology 1992;76:146–157.
159. Barker RN, Elson CJ: Multiple self epitopes on the Rhesus polypeptides stimulate immunologically ignorant human T cells in vitro. Eur J Immunol 1994;24:1578–1582.
160. Barker RN, Hall AM, Standen GR, Jones J, Elson CJ: Identification of T-cell epitopes on the Rhesus polypeptides in autoimmune hemolytic anemia. Blood 1997;90:2701–2715.
161. Petrakis N, Politis G: Prolonged survival of viable, mitotically competent mononuclear leukocytes in stored whole blood. New Engl J Med 1962;267:286.
162. Turner JH, Hutchinson DL, Petricciani J: Cytogenetic and growth characteristics of human lymphocytes derived from stored donor blood packs. Scand J Haematol 1971;8:169–176.
163. McCullough J, Yunis EJ, Benson SJ, Quie PG: Effect of blood-bank storage on leucocyte function. Lancet 1969; 2:1333–1337.
164. Schechter GP, Soehnlen F, McFarland W: Lymphocyte response to blood transfusion in man. N Engl J Med 1972; 287:1169–1173.
165. Schechter GP, Whang-Peng J, McFarland W: Circulation of donor lymphocytes after blood transfusion in man. Blood 1977;49:651–656.
166. Adams PT, Davenport RD, Reardon DA, Roth MS: Detection of circulating donor white blood cells in patients receiving multiple transfusions. Blood 1992;80:551–555.
167. Houbiers JGA, Niewwenhuys C, Brand A: Chimerism after blood transfusion: PCR applied as a detection technique [abstract]. Vox Sanguinis 1994;67(Suppl 2):24.
168. Lee TH, Donegan E, Slichter S, Busch MP: Transient increase in circulating donor leukocytes after allogeneic transfusions in immunocompetent recipients compatible with donor cell proliferation. Blood 1995;85:1207–1214.
169. Hutchinson DL, Turner JH, Schlesinger ER: Persistence of donor cells in neonates after fetal and exchange transfusion. Am J Obstet Gynecol 1971;109:281–284.
170. Shapiro M: Familial autohemolytic anemia and runting syndrome with Rh-o-specific autoantibody. Transfusion 1967; 7:281–296.
171. Fudenberg HH, Solomon A: "Acquired agammaglobulinemia" with autoimmune hemolytic disease: Graft-versus-host reaction? Vox Sang 1961;6:68.
172. Hobbs JR, Russell A, Worlledge SM: Dysgammaglobulinaemia type IV C. Clin Exp Immunol 1967;2:589–599.
173. Schaller J, Davis SD, Ching YC, Lagunoff D, Williams CP, Wedgwood RJ: Hypergammaglobulinaemia, antibody deficiency, autoimmune haemolytic anaemia, and nephritis in an infant with a familial lymphopenic immune defect. Lancet 1966;2:825–829.
174. Lee TH, Reed W, Mangawang-Montalvo L, Watson J, Busch MP: Donor WBCs can persist and transiently mediate immunologic function in a murine transfusion model: Effects of irradiation, storage, and histocompatibility. Transfusion 2001;41:637–642.
175. Goodarzi MO, Lee TH, Pallavicini MG, Donegan EA, Busch MP: Unusual kinetics of white cell clearance in transfused mice. Transfusion 1995;35:145–149.
176. Lee TH, Paglieroni T, Ohto H, Holland PV, Busch MP: Survival of donor leukocyte subpopulations in immunocompetent transfusion recipients: Frequent long-term microchimerism in severe trauma patients. Blood 1999;93:3127–3139.
177. Nelson JL: Microchimerism and scleroderma. Curr Rheumatol Rep 1999;1:15–21.
178. Nelson JL: Microchimerism: Implications for autoimmune disease. Lupus 1999;8:370–374.
179. Famularo G, De Simone C: Systemic sclerosis from autoimmunity to alloimmunity. South Med J 1999;92:472–476.
180. Bianchi DW: Fetal cells in the mother: From genetic diagnosis to diseases associated with fetal cell microchimerism. Eur J Obstet Gynecol Reprod Biol 2000;92:103–108.
181. Tyndall A, Fassas A, Passweg J, et al: Autologous haematopoietic stem cell transplants for autoimmune disease—Feasibility and transplant-related mortality. Autoimmune Disease and Lymphoma Working Parties of the European Group for Blood and Marrow Transplantation, the European League Against Rheumatism and the International Stem Cell Project for Autoimmune Disease. Bone Marrow Transplant 1999;24: 729–734.
182. Johnson KL, McAlindon TE, Mulcahy E, Bianchi DW: Microchimerism in a female patient with systemic lupus erythematosus. Arthritis Rheum 2001;44:2107–2111.
183. Nelson JL: Pregnancy and microchimerism in autoimmune disease: Protector or insurgent? Arthritis Rheum 2002;46: 291–297.
184. Nelson JL: Microchimerism: Incidental byproduct of pregnancy or active participant in human health? Trends Mol Med 2002;8:109–113.
185. Nelson JL: Microchimerism and human autoimmune diseases. Lupus 2002;11:651–654.
186. Johnson KL, Samura O, Nelson JL, McDonnell M, Bianchi DW: Significant fetal cell microchimerism in a nontransfused woman with hepatitis C: Evidence of long-term survival and expansion. Hepatology 2002;36:1295–1297.
187. Nelson JL: Microchimerism: Expanding new horizon in human health or incidental remnant of pregnancy? Lancet 2001;358:2011–2012.
188. Nelson JL: HLA relationships of pregnancy, microchimerism and autoimmune disease. J Reprod Immunol 2001;52:77–84.
189. Nelson JL: Microchimerism and HLA relationships of pregnancy: Implications for autoimmune diseases. Curr Rheumatol Rep 2001;3:222–229.
190. Johnson KL, Nelson JL, Furst DE, et al: Fetal cell microchimerism in tissue from multiple sites in women with systemic sclerosis. Arthritis Rheum 2001;44:1848–1854.
191. Reed AM, Picornell YJ, Harwood A, Kredich DW: Chimerism in children with juvenile dermatomyositis. Lancet 2000;356:2156–2157.
192. Ishikura H, Endo J, Saito Y, et al: Graft-versus-host antibody reaction causing a delayed hemolytic anemia after blood transfusion. [letter]. Blood 1993;82:3222–3223.
193. Salama A, Mueller-Eckhardt C: Delayed hemolytic transfusion reactions. Evidence for complement activation involving allogeneic and autologous red cells. Transfusion 1984;24:188–193.
194. Ness PM, Shirey RS, Thoman SK, Buck SA: The differentiation of delayed serologic and delayed hemolytic transfusion reactions: Incidence, long-term serologic findings, and clinical significance. Transfusion 1990;30:688–693.
195. Dzik WH: Microchimerism after transfusion: The spectrum from GVHD to alloimmunization. Transfus Sci 1995;16:107–108.
196. Zupanska B, Lawkowicz W, Gorska B, et al: Autoimmune haemolytic anaemia in children. Br J Haematol 1976;34:511–520.
197. Habibi B, Homberg JC, Schaison G, Salmon C: Autoimmune hemolytic anemia in children: A review of 80 cases. Am J Med 1974;56:61–69.
198. Buchanan GR, Boxer LA, Nathan DG: The acute and transient nature of idiopathic immune hemolytic anemia in childhood. J Pediatr 1976;88:780–783.
199. Sokol RJ, Hewitt S, Stamps BK, Hitchen PA: Autoimmune haemolysis in childhood and adolescence. Acta Haematol 1984;72:245–257.
200. Heddle NM: Acute paroxysmal cold hemoglobinuria. Transfus Med Rev 1989;3:219–229.
201. Gottsche B, Salama A, Mueller-Eckhardt C: Donath-Landsteiner autoimmune hemolytic anemia in children: A study of 22 cases. Vox Sang 1990;58:281–286.
202. Nordhagen R, Stensvold K, Winsnes A, Skyberg D, Storen A: Paroxysmal cold haemoglobinuria: The most frequent acute autoimmune haemolytic anaemia in children? Acta Paediatr Scand 1984;73:258–262.

203. Gurgey A, Yenicesu I, Kanra T, et al: Autoimmune hemolytic anemia with warm antibodies in children: Retrospective analysis of 51 cases. Turk J Pediatr 1999;41:467–471.
204. Heisel MA, Ortega JA: Factors influencing prognosis in childhood autoimmune hemolytic anemia. Am J Pediatr Hematol Oncol 1983;5:147–152.
205. Carapella de Luca E, Casadei AM, di Piero G, Midulla M, Bisdomini C, Purpura M: Auto-immune haemolytic anaemia in childhood: Follow-up in 29 cases. Vox Sang 1979;36:13–20.
206. Ammann AJ, Hong R: Selective IgA deficiency: Presentation of 30 cases and a review of the literature. Medicine (Baltimore) 1971;50:223–236.
207. Miescher PA, Tucci A, Beris P, Favre H: Autoimmune hemolytic anemia and/or thrombocytopenia associated with lupus parameters. Semin Hematol 1992;29:13–17.
208. Kalmanti M, Polychronopoulou S: Autoimmune hemolytic anemia as an initial symptom in childhood Hodgkin's disease. Pediatr Hematol Oncol 1992;9:393–395.
209. Duru F, Gurgey A, Cetin M, Kanra T, Altay C: Chronic autoimmune hemolytic anemia in children: A report of four patients. J Med 1994;25:231–240.
210. Perez-Atayde AR, Sirlin SM, Jonas M: Coombs-positive autoimmune hemolytic anemia and postinfantile giant cell hepatitis in children. Pediatr Pathol 1994;14:69–77.
211. Bernard O, Hadchouel M, Scotto J, Odievre M, Alagille D: Severe giant cell hepatitis with autoimmune hemolytic anemia in early childhood. J Pediatr 1981;99:704–711.
212. Miyazaki S, Nakayama K, Akabane T, et al: Follow-up study of 34 children with autoimmune hemolytic anemia. Nippon Ketsueki Gakkai Zasshi 1983;46:6–10.
213. Olcay L, Duzova A, Gumruk F: A warm antibody mediated acute hemolytic anemia with reticulocytopenia in a four-month-old girl requiring immunosuppressive therapy. Turk J Pediatr 1999;41:239–244.
214. Liesveld JL, Rowe JM, Lichtman MA: Variability of the erythropoietic response in autoimmune hemolytic anemia: Analysis of 109 cases. Blood 1987;69:820–826.
215. Zuelzer WW, Mastrangelo R, Stulberg CS, Poulik MD, Page RH, Thompson RI: Autoimmune hemolytic anemia. Natural history and viral-immunologic interactions in childhood. Am J Med 1970;49:80–93.
216. Friedmann AM, King KE, Shirey RS, Resar LM, Casella JF: Fatal autoimmune hemolytic anemia in a child due to warm-reactive immunoglobulin M antibody. J Pediatr Hematol Oncol 1998;20:502–505.
217. McCann EL, Shirey RS, Kickler TS, Ness PM: IgM autoagglutinins in warm autoimmune hemolytic anemia: A poor prognostic feature. Acta Haematol 1992;88:120–125.
218. Shirey RS, Kickler TS, Bell W, Little B, Smith B, Ness PM: Fatal immune hemolytic anemia and hepatic failure associated with a warm-reacting IgM autoantibody. Vox Sang 1987;52:219–222.
219. Waterbury L, Parnes H, Katz RS: Fatal warm antibody autoimmune hemolysis with marked erythrocyte autoagglutination and liver necrosis. South Med J 1986;79:646–647.
220. Freedman J, Wright J, Lim FC, Garvey MB: Hemolytic warm IgM autoagglutinins in autoimmune hemolytic anemia. Transfusion 1987;27:464–467.
221. Win N, Kaye T, Mir N, Damain-Willems C, Chatfield C: Autoimmune haemolytic anaemia in infancy with anti-Kpb specificity. Vox Sang 1996;71:187–188.
222. Ritz ND, Haber A: Autoimmune hemolytic anemia in a 6 week old child. J Pediatr 1962;61:904–910.
223. Oski FA, Abelson NM: Autoimmune hemolytic anemia in an infant. Report of a case treated unsuccessfully with thymectomy. J Pediatr 1965;67:752–758.
224. Bakx CJA, van Loghem JJ: Acquired hemolytic anemia in a newborn. Vox Sang 1953;42:79.
225. Erler BS, Smith L, McQuiston D, Pepkowitz SH, Goldfinger D: Red cell autoantibody production in utero: A case report. Transfusion 1994;34:72–74.
226. Hadnagy C: Severe chronic autoimmune haemolytic anaemia presenting haemolytic disease of the newborn. Lancet 1989; ii:749.
227. Johnson CA, Abildgaard CF: Treatment of idiopathic autoimmune hemolytic anemia in children. Review and report of two fatal cases in infancy. Acta Paediatr Scand 1976; 65:375–379.
228. Sasaki H, Akutagawa H, Kuwakado K, Uemura M, Emi I: High-dose intravenous IgG therapy in a seven-week-old infant with chronic autoimmune hemolytic anemia. Am J Hematol 1987;25:215–218.
229. Otheo E, Maldonado MS, Munoz A, Hernandez-Jodra M: High-dose intravenous immunoglobulin as single therapy in a child with autoimmune hemolytic anemia. Pediatr Hematol Oncol 1997;14:487–490.
230. McConnell ME, Atchison JA, Kohaut E, Castleberry RP: Successful use of plasma exchange in a child with refractory immune hemolytic anemia. Am J Pediatr Hematol Oncol 1987;9:158–160.
231. Poschmann A, Fischer K: Autoimmune haemolytic anaemia: Recent advances in pathogenesis, diagnosis and treatment. Eur J Pediatr 1985;143:258–260.
232. Swisher SN: Acquired hemolytic disease. Postgrad Med 1966;40:378–386.
233. Benraad CE, Scheerder HA, Overbeeke MA: Autoimmune haemolytic anaemia during pregnancy. Eur J Obstet Gynecol Reprod Biol 1994;55:209–211.
234. Sokol RJ, Hewitt S, Stamps BK: Erythrocyte autoantibodies, autoimmune haemolysis and pregnancy. Vox Sang 1982;43:169–176.
235. Hoppe B, Stibbe W, Bielefeld A, Pruss A, Salama A: Increased RBC autoantibody production in pregnancy. Transfusion 2001;41:1559–1561.
236. Buyon JP: The effects of pregnancy on autoimmune diseases. J Leukoc Biol 1998;63:281–287.
237. Chaplin H, Jr, Cohen R, Bloomberg G, Kaplan HJ, Moore JA, Dorner I: Pregnancy and idiopathic autoimmune haemolytic anaemia: A prospective study during 6 months gestation and 3 months post-partum. Brit J Haemat 1973;24:219–229.
238. Quinlivan WL, Goldberg S: Autoimmune hemolytic anemia of the cold antibody type associated with pregnancy. Am J Obstet Gynecol 1967;98:1102–1104.
239. Jain S, Agarwal S, Dash SC, Grewal KS: Autoimmune hemolytic anaemia and foetal loss. J Assoc Physicians India 1977;25:765–766.
240. Issaragrisil S, Kruatrachue M: An association of pregnancy and autoimmune haemolytic anaemia. Scand J Haematol 1983;31:63–68.
241. Lawe JE: Successful exchange transfusion of an infant for AIHA developing late in mother's pregnancy. Transfusion 1982;22:66–68.
242. Baumann R, Rubin H: Autoimmune hemolytic anemia during pregnancy with hemolytic disease in the newborn. Blood 1973;41:293–297.
243. Vedovini F, Benedetti PA: Anemia emolitica da autoanticorpi materni. Riv Clin Pediatr 1963;72:339.
244. Burt RL, Prichard RW: Acquired hemolytic anemia in pregnancy: Report of a case. Obstet Gynecol 1957;90:444.
245. Soderhjelm L: Non-spherocytic haemolytic anaemia in mother and new-born infant. Acta Paediatrica 1959;48(Suppl. 117):34.
246. Seip M: Systemic lupus erythematosus in pregnancy with haemolytic anaemia, leucopenia and thrombocytopenia in the mother and her newborn infant. Arch Dis Child 1960;35:364.
247. Letts HW, Kredentser B: Thrombocytopenia, hemolytic anemia, and two pregnancies: Report of a case. Am J Clin Pathol 1968;49:481–486.
248. Silverstein MN, Aaro LA, Kempers RD: Evans' syndrome and pregnancy. Am J Med Sci 1966;252:206–211.
249. Passi GR, Kriplani A, Pati HP, Choudhry VP: Isoimmune hemolysis in an infant due to maternal Evans' syndrome. Indian J Pediatr 1997;64:893–895.
250. Sacks DA, Platt LD, Johnson CS: Autoimmune hemolytic disease during pregnancy. Am J Obstet Gynecol 1981;140:942–946.
251. Yam P, Wilkinson L, Petz LD, Garratty G: Studies on hemolytic anemia in pregnancy with evidence for autoimmunization in a patient with a negative direct antiglobulin (Coombs') test. Am J Hematol 1980;8:23–29.

252. Ng SC, Wong KK, Raman S, Bosco J: Autoimmune haemolytic anaemia in pregnancy: A case report. Eur J Obstet Gynecol Reprod Biol 1990;37:83–85.
253. Tsai YC, Chang JM, Chang JC, Changahien CC, Chen PH, Jeng TT: Idiopathic autoimmune hemolytic anemia during pregnancy. J Formos Med Assoc 1994;93:328–331.
254. de Groot AW: A pregnant woman with hemolytic anemia [in Dutch]. Ned Tijdschr Verloskd Gynaecol 1969;69:283–286.
255. Eldor A, Yatziv S, Hershko C: Relapsing Coombs-negative haemolytic anaemia in pregnancy with haemolytic disease in the newborn. Br Med J 1975;4:625.
256. Hershko C, Berrebi A, Resnitzky P, Eldor A: Relapsing haemolytic anaemia of pregnancy with negative antiglobulin reaction. Scand J Haematol 1976;16:135–140.
257. Goodall HB, Ho-Yen DO, Clark DM, Thomson MA, Browning MC, Crowder AM: Haemolytic anaemia of pregnancy. Scand J Haematol 1979;22:185–191.
258. Starksen NF, Bell WR, Kickler TS: Unexplained hemolytic anemia associated with pregnancy. Am J Obstet Gynecol 1983;146:617–622.
259. Bjornsson S, Brennand JE, Calder AA, et al: Unexplained haemolytic anaemia in successive pregnancies with negative direct antiglobulin test and response to high dose i.v. IgG. Br J Obstet Gynaecol 1994;101:75–77.
260. Kumar R, Advani AR, Sharan J, Basharutallah MS, Al Lumai AS: Pregnancy induced hemolytic anemia: An unexplained entity. Ann Hematol 2001;80:623–626.
261. Craig GA, Turner RL: A case of symptomatic haemolytic anaemia in pregnancy. Br Med J 1955;i:1003–1005.
262. Jankelowitz T, Eckerling B, Joshua H: A case of acquired haemolytic anaemia associated with pregnancy. S Afr Med J 1976;34:911–913.
263. Dacie JV: Auto-immune haemolytic anaemia (AIHA): Warm-antibody syndromes I: "idiopathic" types: history and clinical features. In The Haemolytic Anaemias, 3rd ed.,Vol. 3, The Auto-Immune Haemolytic Anaemias. New York: Churchill Livingstone, 1992:6–53.
264. Bermas BL, Hill JA: Effects of immunosuppressive drugs during pregnancy. Arthritis Rheum 1995;38:1722–1732.
265. Janssen NM, Genta MS: The effects of immunosuppressive and anti-inflammatory medications on fertility, pregnancy, and lactation. Arch Intern Med 2000;160:610–619.
266. Schatz M, Patterson R, Zeitz S, O'Rourke J, Melam H: Corticosteroid therapy for the pregnant asthmatic patient. JAMA 1975;233:804–807.
267. NIH Consensus Development Panel on the Effect of Corticosteroids for Fetal Maturation on Perinatal Outcomes. Effect of corticosteroids for fetal maturation on perinatal outcomes. JAMA 1995;273:413–418.
268. Armenti VT, Ahlswede KM, Ahlswede BA, Jarrell BE, Moritz MJ, Burke JF: National transplantation Pregnancy Registry—Outcomes of 154 pregnancies in cyclosporine-treated female kidney transplant recipients. Transplantation 1994;57:502–506.
269. Haugen G, Fauchald P, Sodal G, Leivestad T, Moe N: Pregnancy outcome in renal allograft recipients in Norway: The importance of immunosuppressive drug regimen and health status before pregnancy. Acta Obstet Gynecol Scand 1994;73:541–546.
270. Shaheen FA, al-Sulaiman MH, al-Khader AA: Long-term nephrotoxicity after exposure to cyclosporine in utero. Transplantation 1993;56:224–225.
271. Potter M, Stockley R, Storry J, Slade R: ABO alloimmunisation after intravenous immunoglobulin infusion. Lancet 1988; 1:932–933.
272. Letsky EA, Warwick R: Hematological Problems. In James PK, Steer PJ, Weiner CP, Gonik B (eds): High Risk Pregnancy: Management Options. London: WB Saunders, 1996:359–372.
273. Sipes SL, Weiner C: Coagulation Disorders in Pregnancy. In Reece EA, Hobbins JC, Mahoney MJ, Petrie RH (eds): Medicine of the Fetus and Mother. Philadelphia: JB Lippincott, 1992:1111–1138.
274. Letsky EA: Coagulation Defects. In de Swiet M (ed): Medical Disorders in Obstetric Practice. Oxford: Blackwell Science, 1989:104–165.
275. Gottlieb P, Axelsson O, Bakos O, Rastad J: Splenectomy during pregnancy: An option in the treatment of autoimmune thrombocytopenic purpura. Br J Obstet Gynaecol 1999;106: 373–375.
276. Sendag F, Kazandi M, Terek MC: Splenectomy combined with cesarean section in a patient with severe immunological thrombocytopenic purpura refractory to medical therapy. J Obstet Gynaecol Res 2001;27:85–88.
277. Iwase K, Higaki J, Yoon HE, et al: Hand-assisted laparoscopic splenectomy for idiopathic thrombocytopenic purpura during pregnancy. Surg Laparosc Endosc Percutan Tech 2001;11:53–56.
278. Burrows R: Splenectomy during pregnancy: An option in treatment of autoimmune thrombocytopenic purpura. Br J Obstet Gynaecol 1999;106:1330–1331.
279. Hardwick RH, Slade RR, Smith PA, Thompson MH: Laparoscopic splenectomy in pregnancy. J Laparoendosc Adv Surg Tech A 1999;9:439–440.
280. Kissmeyer-Nielsen FS, Grent-Hansen K, Kieler J: Immuno-hemolytic anemia with familial occurrence. Acta Med Scand 1952;144:35–39.
281. Fialkow PJ, Fudenberg HH, Epstein WV: "Acquired" antibody hemolytic anemia and familial aberrations in gamma globulins. Amer J Med 1964;36:188–199.
282. Olanoff LS, Fudenberg HH: Familial autoimmunity: Twenty years later. J Clin Lab Immunol 1983;11:105–111.
283. Hennemann HH, Krause H: Chronische Thrombozytopenie (Morbus Werlhof) und erworbene hamolytische Anamie bei zwei Schwestern. Dtsch med Wschr 1964;89:1161–1166.
284. Dobbs CE: Familial auto-immune hemolytic anemia. Arch Intern Med 1965;116:273–276.
285. Loghem-Langereis E, Peetoom F, van der HM, Van Loghem JJ, Bosch E, Goudsmit R: The occurrence of gammaglobulin/anti-gammaglobulin complexes in a patient suffering from hypogammaglobulinaemia and haemolytic anaemia. Bibl Haematol 1965;23:55–61.
286. Cordova MS, Baez-Villasenor J, Mendez JJ, Campos E: Acquired hemolytic anemia with positive antiglobulin Coombs' test) in mother and daughter. Arch Intern Med 1966;117:692–695.
287. Schwartz RS, Costea N: Autoimmune hemolytic anemia: Clinical correlations and biological implications. Semin Hematol 1966;3:2–26.
288. Shapiro M: Familial autohemolytic anemia and runting syndrome with Rh-o-specific autoantibody. Transfusion 1967;7:281–296.
289. Pirofsky B: Autoimmunization and the Autoimmune Hemolytic Anemias. Baltimore, Md: Williams & Wilkins, 1969.
290. Pirofsky B: Hereditary aspects of autoimmune hemolytic anemia; a retrospective analysis. Vox Sang 1968;14:334–347.
291. Seip M, Harboe M, Cyvin K: Chronic autoimmune hemolytic anemia in childhood with cold antibodies, aplastic crises, and familial occurrence. Acta Paediatr Scand 1969;58:275–280.
292. Pollock JG, Fenton E, Barrett KE: Familial autoimmune haemolytic anaemia associated with rheumatoid arthritis and pernicious anaemia. Br J Haematol 1970;18:171–182.
293. Zuelzer WW, Mastrangelo R, Stulberg CS, Poulik MD, Page RH, Thompson RI: Autoimmune hemolytic anemia. Natural history and viral-immunologic interactions in childhood. Am J Med 1970;49:80–93.
294. Blajchman MA, Hui YT, Jopnes TE, Luke KH: Familial autoimmune hemolytic anemia with an autoantibody demonstrating U specificity [abstract]. Program of the 24th Annual Meeting of the American Association of Blood Banks, 1971:82.
295. Dacie JV, Worlledge SM: Auto-allergic blood diseases. In Gell PGH, Coombs RRA, Lachmann PJ (eds): Clinical Aspects of Immunology. Oxford: Blackwell Scientific, 1975:1149–1182.
296. Roth P, Morell A, Hunziker HR, Gehri P, Bucher U: Familial autoimmune hemolytic animia (AIHA) with negative Coombs test, lymphocytopenia and hypogammaglobulinemia [in German]. Schweiz Med Wochenschr 1975;105:1584–1585.
297. Toolis F, Parker AC, White A, Urbaniak S: Familial autoimmune haemolytic anaemia. Br Med J 1977;1:1392.

298. Conley CL, Savarese DM: Biologic false-positive serologic tests for syphilis and other serologic abnormalities in autoimmune hemolytic anemia and thrombocytopenic purpura. Medicine (Baltimore) 1989;68:67–84.
299. Reynolds MV, Vengelen-Tyler V, Morel PA: Autoimmune hemolytic anemia associated with autoanti-Ge. Vox Sang 1981;41:61–67.
300. Perez-Mateo M, Tascon A: Idiopathic autoimmune hemolytic anemia in twins [in Spanish]. Med Clin (Barc) 1982;79:476.
301. Boling EP, Wen J, Reveille JD, Bias WB, Chused TM, Arnett FC: Primary Sjogren's syndrome and autoimmune hemolytic anemia in sisters: A family study. Am J Med 1983;74:1066–1071.
302. Horowitz SD, Borcherding W, Hong R: Autoimmune hemolytic anemia as a manifestation of T-suppressor-cell deficiency. Clin Immunol Immunopathol 1984;33:313–323.
303. McLeod AG, Pai M, Carter RF, Squire J, Barr RD: Familial Evans syndrome: A report of an affected sibship. J Pediatr Hematol Oncol 1999;21:244–247.
304. Lippman SM, Arnett FC, Conley CL, Ness PM, Meyers DA, Bias WB: Genetic factors predisposing to autoimmune diseases: Autoimmune hemolytic anemia, chronic thrombocytopenic purpura, and systemic lupus erythematosus. Am J Med 1982;73:827–840.
305. Schmid FR: Pirofsky, editor. 1969 [personal communication].
306. Habibi B, Homberg JC, Schaison G, Salmon C: Autoimmune hemolytic anemia in children: A review of 80 cases. Am J Med 1974;56:61–69.
307. Conley CL: Immunologic precursors of autoimmune hematologic disorders: Autoimmune hematologic disorders: Autoimmune hemolytic anemia and thrombocytopenic purpura. Johns Hopkins Med J 1981;149:101–109.
308. Shahian DM, Wallach SR, Bern MM: Open heart surgery in patients with cold-reactive proteins. Surg Clin North Am 1985;65:315–322.
309. Park JV, Weiss CI: Cardiopulmonary bypass and myocardial protection: Management problems in cardiac surgical patients with cold autoimmune disease [review]. Anesth Analg 1988;67:75–78.
310. Menasche P, Subayi JB, Piwnica A: Retrograde coronary sinus cardioplegia for aortic valve operations: A clinical report on 500 patients. Ann Thorac Surg 1990;49:556–563.
311. Izzat MB, Rajesh PB, Smith GH: Use of retrograde cold crystalloid cardioplegia in a patient with unexpected cold agglutination. Ann Thorac Surg 1993;56:1395–1397.
312. Shulman IA, Petz LD: Red cell compatibility testing: Clinical significance and laboratory methods. In Petz LD, Swisher SN, Kleinman S, Spence RK, Strauss RG (eds): Clinical Practice of Transfusion Medicine, 3rd ed. New York: Churchill Livingstone, 1996:199–244.
313. Bedrosian CL, Simel DL: Cold hemagglutinin disease in the operating room. South Med J 1987;80:466–471.
314. Wertlake PT, McGinniss MH, Schmidt PJ: Cold antibody and persistent intravascular hemolysis after surgery under hypothermia. Transfusion 1969;9(2):70–73.
315. Diaz JH, Cooper ES, Ochsner JL: Cardiac surgery in patients with cold autoimmune diseases. Anesth Analg 1984;63:349–352.
316. Bracken CA, Gurkowski MA, Naples JJ, et al: Case 6—1993. Cardiopulmonary bypass in two patients with previously undetected cold agglutinins. J Cardiothorac Vasc Anesth 1993;7:743–749.
317. Holman WL, Smith SH, Edwards R, Huang ST: Agglutination of blood cardioplegia by cold-reacting autoantibodies. Ann Thorac Surg 1991;51:833–835.
318. Stalker AL: Intravascular erythrocyte aggregation. Bibl Anat 1964;4:108–111.
319. Davidsohn I, Lee CL, Takahashi T: Hepatic infarcts in mice injected with anti-erythrocytic serum. Arch Pathol 1963;76: 398–403.
320. AuBuchon JP, Scofan BA, Davey RJ: Hemolysis during extracorporeal circulation: Signifiance of cold-reactive auto-antibodies and mechanical trauma [abstract]. Blood 1983;65:42a.
321. Niejadlik DC, Lozner EL: Cooling mattress induced acute hemolytic anemia. Transfusion 1974;14:145–147.
322. Colmers RA, Snavely JG: Acute hemolytic anemia in primary atypical pneumonia produced by exposure and chilling. N Engl J Med 1947;237:505–510.
323. Dake SB, Johnston MF, Brueggeman P, Barner HB: Detection of cold hemagglutination in a blood cardioplegia unit before systemic cooling of a patient with unsuspected cold agglutinin disease. Ann Thorac Surg 1989;47:914–915.
324. Schmidt PJ: Cold agglutinins and hypothermia [letter]. Arch Intern Med 1985;145:578–579.
325. Agarwal SK, Ghosh PK, Gupta D: Cardiac surgery and cold-reactive proteins. Ann Thorac Surg 1995;60:1143–1150.
326. Moore RA, Geller EA, Mathews ES, Botros SB, Jose AB, Clark DL: The effect of hypothermic cardiopulmonary bypass on patients with low- titer, nonspecific cold agglutinins. Ann Thorac Surg 1984;37:233–238.
327. Nydegger U, Hardegger T, Tobler A, Rieder H, Cerniak A, Lammle B: Cold agglutinin syndrome and liver transplantation. Vox Sang 1994;67:85.
328. Klein HG, Faltz LL, McIntosh CL, Appelbaum FR, Deisseroth AB, Holland PV: Surgical hypothermia in a patient with a cold agglutinin: Management by plasma exchange. Transfusion 1980;20:354–357.
329. Williams AC: Cold agglutinins: Cause for concern? Anaesthesia 1980;35:887–889.
330. Berreklouw E, Moulijn AC, Pegels JG, Meijne NG: Myocardial protection with cold cardioplegia in a patient with cold autoagglutinins and hemolysins. Ann Thorac Surg 1982;33:521–522.
331. Blumberg N, Hicks G, Woll J, et al: Successful cardiac bypass surgery in the presence of a potent cold agglutinin without plasma exchange [letter]. Transfusion 1983;23:363.
332. Diaz JH, Cooper ES, Ochsner JL: Cold hemagglutination pathophysiology: Evaluation and management of patients undergoing cardiac surgery with induced hypothermia. Arch Intern Med 1983;144:1639–1641.
333. Landymore R: Cold agglutinins and coronary artery bypass grafting. Ann Thorac Surg 1983;35:472.
334. Landymore R, Isom W, Barlam B: Management of patients with cold agglutinins who require open-heart surgery. Can J Surg 1983;26:79–80.
335. Leach AB, Van Hasselt GL, Edwards JC: Cold agglutinins and deep hypothermia. Anaesthesia 1983;38:140–143.
336. Andrzejewski C, Jr, Gault E, Briggs M, Silberstein L: Benefit of a 37 degree C extracorporeal circuit in plasma exchange therapy for selected cases with cold agglutinin disease. J Clin Apheresis 1988;4:13–17.
337. Paccagnella A, Simini G, Nieri A, Da Col U, Frugoni C, Valfre C: Cardiopulmonary bypass and cold agglutinin. J Thorac Cardiovasc Surg 1988;95:543.
338. Lee MC, Chang CH, Hsieh MJ: Use of a total wash-out method in an open heart operation. Ann Thorac Surg 1989;47:57–58.
339. Aoki A, Kay GL, Zubiate P, Ruggio J, Kay JH: Cardiac operation without hypothermia for the patient with cold agglutinin. Chest 1993;104:1627–1629.
340. Beebe DS, Bergen L, Palahniuk RJ: Anesthetic management of a patient with severe cold agglutinin hemolytic anemia utilizing forced air warming. Anesth Analg 1993;76:1144–1146.
341. Hearnsberger J, Ziomek S, Tobler G, Maxson T, VanDevanter S, Harrell JE, Jr: Management of cold agglutinemia with warm heart surgical intervention: A case report. J Thorac Cardiovasc Surg 1993;106:756–757.
342. Zoppi M, Oppliger R, Althaus U, Nydegger U: Reduction of plasma cold agglutinin titers by means of plasmapheresis to prepare a patient for coronary bypass surgery. Infusionsther Transfusionsmed 1993;20:19–22.
343. Mastrogiovanni G, Masiello P, Iesu S, Senese I, Di Benedetto G: Management of cold agglutinemia with intermittent warm blood cardioplegia and normothermia. Ann Thorac Surg 1996; 62:317.
344. Onoe M, Magara T, Yamamoto Y: Cardiac operation for a patient with autoimmune hemolytic anemia with warm-reactive antibodies. Ann Thorac Surg 2001;71:351–352.
345. Ko W, Isom OW: Cardiopulmonary bypass procedures in patients with cold-reactive hemagglutination: A case report

and a literature review. J Cardiovasc Surg (Torino) 1996;37: 623–626.
346. Lichtenstein SV, Salerno TA, Slutsky AS: Pro: Warm continuous cardioplegia is preferable to intermittent hypothermic cardioplegia for myocardial protection during cardiopulmonary bypass. J Cardiothorac Anesth 1990;4:279–281.
347. Salerno TA, Houck JP, Barrozo CA, et al: Retrograde continuous warm blood cardioplegia: A new concept in myocardial protection. Ann Thorac Surg 1991;51:245–247.
348. Lichtenstein SV, Ashe KA, el Dalati H, Cusimano RJ, Panos A, Slutsky AS: Warm heart surgery. J Thorac Cardiovasc Surg 1991;101:269–274.
349. Roe BB: Warm blood cardioplegia: Back to square one. Ann Thorac Surg 1993;55:330–331.
350. Muehrcke DD, Torchiana DF: Warm heart surgery in patients with cold autoimmune disorders. Ann Thorac Surg 1993; 55:532–533.
351. Gokhale AG, Suhasini T, Saraswati V, Chandrasekhar N, Rajagopal P: Cold agglutinins and warm heart surgery. J Thorac Cardiovasc Surg 1993;105:557.
352. Donatelli F, Mariani MA, Triggiani M, Pocar M, Santoro F, Grossi A: Warm heart surgery in cold haemagglutinin disease. Cardiovasc Surg 1995;3:191–192.
353. Taft EG, Propp RP, Sullivan SA: Plasma exchange for cold agglutinin hemolytic anemia. Transfusion 1977;17:173–176.
354. Rodenhuis S, Maas A, Hazenberg CA, Das PC, Nieweg HO: Inefficacy of plasma exchange in cold agglutinin hemolytic anemia—A case study. Vox Sang 1985;49:20–25.
355. Shumak KH, Rock GA: Therapeutic plasma exchange. N Engl J Med 1984;310:762–771.
356. Pineda AA, Brzica SM, Jr, Taswell HF: Hemolytic transfusion reaction. Recent experience in a large blood bank. Mayo Clin Proc 1978;53:378–390.
357. Myhre BA: Fatalities from blood transfusion. JAMA 1980;244:1333–1335.
358. Honig CL, Bove JR: Transfusion-associated fatalities: Review of Bureau of Biologics reports 1976–1978. Transfusion 1980;20:653–661.
359. Sazama K: Reports of 355 transfusion-associated deaths: 1976 through 1985. Transfusion 1990;30:583–590.
360. Linden JV, Kaplan HS: Transfusion errors: Causes and effects. [review]. Transfus Med Rev 1994;8:169–183.
361. Williamson L, Cohen H, Love E, Jones H, Todd A, Soldan K: The Serious Hazards of Transfusion (SHOT) initiative: The UK approach to haemovigilance. Vox Sang 2000;78(Suppl. 2): 291–295.
362. Croucher BEE: Differential diagnosis of delayed hemolytic transfusion reaction. In Bell CA (ed): A Seminar on Laboratory Management of Hemolysis. Washington, DC: American Association of Blood Banks, 1979:151–160.
363. Blood Transfusion in Clinical Medicine, 10th ed., Mollison PL, Engelfriet CP, Contreras M (ed). Oxford: Blackwell Science, 1997.
364. Holland PV, Wallerstein RO: Delayed hemolytic transfusion reaction with acute renal failure. JAMA 1968;204:1007–1008.
365. Croucher BEE, Crookston MC, Crookston JH: Delayed haemolytic transfusion reactions simulating auto-immune haemolytic anaemia. Vox Sang 1967;12:32.
366. Thomson S, Johnstone M: Delayed haemolytic transfusion reaction due to anti Jk a and anti M. Can J Med Technol 1972;34:159–161.
367. Rothman IK, Alter HJ, Strewler GJ: Delayed overt hemolytic transfusion reaction due to anti-U antibody. Transfusion 1976;16:357–360.
368. Pineda AA, Taswell HF, Brzica SM, Jr: Delayed Hemolytic Transfusion reaction. An immunologic hazard of blood transfusion. Transfusion 1978;18:1–7.
369. Redman M, Regan F, Contreras M: A prospective study of the incidence of red cell alloimmunisation following transfusion. Vox Sang 1996;71:216–220.
370. Constantoulakis M, Kay HEM: Observations on the centrifugal segregation of young erythrocytes: A possible method of genotying the transfused patient. J Clin Path 1963;12:312.
371. Renton PH, Hancock JA: A simple method of separating erythrocytes of different ages. Vox Sang 1964;9:183.
372. Branch DR, Hian AL, Carlson F, Maslow WC, Petz LD: Erythrocyte age-fractionation using a Percoll-Renografin density gradient: Application to autologous red cell antigen determinations in recently transfused patients. Am J Clin Pathol 1983;80:453–458.
373. Technical Manual, 14th ed. Brecher, M (ed). Bethesda, Md: American Association of Blood Banks, 2002.
374. Reid ME, Toy PT: Simplified method for recovery of autologous red blood cells from transfused patients. Am J Clin Pathol 1983;79:364–366.
375. Vengelen-Tyler V, Gonzales B: Reticulocyte rich RBCs will give weak reactions with many blood typing antisera [abstract]. Transfusion 1985;25:476.
376. Garratty G, Arndt PA: Applications of flow cytofluorometry to red blood cell immunology. Cytometry 1999;38:259–267.
377. Griffin GD, Lippert LE, Dow NS, Berger TA, Hickman MR, Salata KF: A flow cytometric method for phenotyping recipient red cells following transfusion. Transfusion 1994;34:233–237.
378. Wagner F: Identification of recipient Rh phenotype in a chronically transfused child by two-colour immunofluorescence. Transfus Med 1994;4:205–208.
379. Wenk RE, Chiafari PA: DNA typing of recipient blood after massive transfusion. Transfusion 1997;37:1108–1110.
380. Reid ME, Rios M, Powell VI, Charles-Pierre D, Malavade V: DNA from blood samples can be used to genotype patients who have recently received a transfusion. Transfusion 2000;40:48–53.
381. Castilho L, Rios M, Pellegrino J, Rodrigues A, Costa FF: Blood group genotyping for the management of patients with "warm" antibody-induced hemolytic anemia (WAIHA) [abstract]. Blood 2001;98:62a.
382. Petz LD: The expanding boundaries of transfusion medicine. In Nance SJ (ed): Clinical and Basic Science Aspects of Immunohematology. Arlington, VA: American Association of Blood Banks, 1991:73–113.
383. Petz LD: Blood transfusion in hemolytic anemias. Immunohematology 1999;15:15–23.
384. Dameshek W: Autoimmunity: Theoretical aspects. Ann N Y Acad Sci 1965;124:6–28.
385. Garratty G: Novel Mechanisms for Immune Destruction of Circulating Autologous Cells. In Silberstein LE (ed): Autoimmune Disorders of Blood. Bethesda, Md: American Association of Blood Banks, 1996:79–114.
386. Thompson RA, Rowe DS: Reactive haemolysis—A distinctive form of red cell lysis. Immunology 1968;14:745–762.
387. Thompson RA, Lachmann PJ: Reactive lysis: The complement-mediated lysis of unsensitized cells. I: The characterization of the indicator factor and its identification as C7. J Exp Med 1970;131:629–641.
388. Lachmann PJ, Thompson RA: Reactive lysis: The complement-mediated lysis of unsensitized cells. II: The characterization of activated reactor as C56 and the participation of C8 and C9. J Exp Med 1970;131:643–657.
389. Götze O, Muller-Eberhard HJ: Lysis of erythrocytes by complement in the absence of antibody. J Exp Med 1970;132:898–915.
390. Goldman JN, Ruddy S, Austen KF: Reaction mechanisms of nascent C567 (reactive lysis). I: Reaction characteristics for production of EC567 and lysis by C8 and C9. J Immunol 1972;109:353–359.
391. McLeod BC, Baker P, Gewurz H. Studies on the inhibition of C56-initiated lysis (reactive lysis). II: C567-INH—An inhibitor of the C567 trimolecular complex of complement. Int Arch Allergy Appl Immunol 1974;47:623–632.
392. Yachnin S, Ruthenberg JM: The initiation and enhancement of human red cell lysis by activators of the first component of complement and by first component esterase; studies using normal red cells and red cells from patients with paroxysmal nocturnal hemoglobinuria. J Clin Invest 1965;44:518–534.
393. Yachnin S: The hemolysis of red cells from patients with paroxysmal nocturnal hemoglobinuria by partially purified subcomponents of the third complement component. J Clin Invest 1965;44:1534–1546.
394. Ness PM, Shirey RS, Thoman SK, Buck SA: The differentiation of delayed serologic and delayed hemolytic transfusion reac-

tions: Incidence, long-term serologic findings, and clinical significance. Transfusion 1990;30:688–693.
395. Dameshek W, Levine P: Isoimmunization with Rh factor in acquired hemolytic anemia. N Engl J Med 1943;228:641–644.
396. Allen FH: Proceedings of the 8th Congress of the International Society of Blood Transfusion, 1960:359.
397. Weiner AS: Hemolytic reactions following transfusions of blood of the homologous group. Arch Pathol 1941;32:227–250.
398. Gajewski JL, Petz LD, Calhoun L, et al: Hemolysis of transfused group O red blood cells in minor ABO-incompatible unrelated-donor bone marrow transplants in patients receiving cyclosporine without posttransplant methotrexate. Blood 1992;79:3076–3085.
399. Greeno EW, Perry EH, Ilstrup SJ, Weisdorf DJ: Exchange transfusion the hard way: Massive hemolysis following transplantation of bone marrow with minor ABO incompatibility. Transfusion 1996;36:71–74.
400. Herzog P, Korinkova P, Stambergova M, Lukasova M: Auto anti-A1 and auto anti-NA1 after bone marrow transplantation. Folia Haematol Int Mag Klin Morphol Blutforsch 1987;114:874–880.
401. Toren A, Dacosta Y, Manny N, et al: Passenger B-lymphocyte-induced severe hemolytic disease after allogeneic peripheral blood stem cell transplantation. Blood 1996;87:843–844.
402. Oziel-Taieb S, Faucher-Barbey C, Chabannon C, et al: Early and fatal immune haemolysis after so-called "minor" ABO-incompatible peripheral blood stem cell allotransplantation. Bone Marrow Transplant 1997;19:1155–1156.
403. Bolan CD, Childs RW, Procter JL, Barrett AJ, Leitman SF: Massive immune haemolysis after allogeneic peripheral blood stem cell transplantation with minor ABO incompatibility. Br J Haematol 2001;112:787–795.
404. Tiplady CW, Fitzgerald JM, Jackson GH, Conn JS, Proctor SJ: Massive haemolysis in a group A recipient of a group O peripheral blood stem cell allogeneic transplant. Transfus Med 2001;11:455–458.
405. Worel N, Greinix HT, Keil F, et al: Severe immune hemolysis after minor ABO-incompatible allogeneic peripheral blood stem cell transplantation occurs more frequently after non-myeloablative than myeloablative conditioning. Transfusion 2002;42:1293–1301.
406. Petz LD, Calhoun L, Shulman IA, Johnson C, Herron RM: The sickle cell hemolytic transfusion reaction syndrome. Transfusion 1997;37:382–392.
407. King KE, Shirey RS, Lankiewicz MW, Young-Ramsaran J, Ness PM: Delayed hemolytic transfusion reactions in sickle cell disease: Simultaneous destruction of recipients' red cells. Transfusion 1997;37:376–381.
408. Reed W, Walker P, Haddix T, Perkins HA: Acute anemic events in sickle cell disease. Transfusion 2000;40:267–273.
409. Garratty G: Severe reactions associated with transfusion of patients with sickle cell disease. Transfusion 1997;37:357–361.
410. Win N, Doughty H, Telfer P, Wild BJ, Pearson TC: Hyperhemolytic transfusion reaction in sickle cell disease. Transfusion 2001;41:323–328.
411. Sirchia G, Morelati F, Rebulla P: The sickle cell hemolytic transfusion reaction syndrome [letter]. Transfusion 1997; 37:1098–1099.
412. Greene D, Khan S: A phenomenon of delayed hemolytic transfusion reaction [abstract]. Transfusion 1991;31:23S. 1991.
413. Shulman NR: Posttransfusion purpura: Clinical features and the mechanism of platelet destruction. In Nance ST (ed): Clinical and Basic Science Aspects of Immunohematology. Arlington, VA: American Association of Blood Banks, 1991:137–154.
414. Mueller-Eckhardt C: Post-transfusion purpura. Br J Haematol 1986;64:419–424.
415. Lau P, Sholtis CM, Aster RH: Post-transfusion purpura: An enigma of alloimmunization. Am J Hematol 1980;9:331–336.
416. George JN, Rizvi MA: Thrombocytopenia. In Beutler E, Lichtman MA, Coller BS, Kipps TJ, Seligsohn U (eds): Williams' Hematology, 6th ed. New York: McGraw-Hill, 2001:1495–1539.
417. George JN, Pickett EB, Heinz R: Platelet membrane microparticles in blood bank fresh frozen plasma and cryoprecipitate. Blood 1986;68:307–309.
418. Kickler TS, Ness PM, Herman JH, Bell WR: Studies on the pathophysiology of posttransfusion purpura. Blood 1986;68:347–350.
419. Dieleman LA, Brand A, Claas FH, van de KC, Witvliet M, Giphart MJ: Acquired Zwa antigen on Zwa negative platelets demonstrated by western blotting. Br J Haematol 1989; 72:539–542.
420. McCrae KR, Herman JH: Posttransfusion purpura: Two unusual cases and a literature review. Am J Hematol 1996;52:205–211.
421. Bussel JB, Zabusky MR, Berkowitz RL, McFarland JG: Fetal alloimmune thrombocytopenia. N Engl J Med 1997;337:22–26.
422. Beutler E: Paroxysmal nocturnal hemoglobinuria. In Beutler E, Lichtman MA, Coller BS, Kipps TJ, Seligsohn U (eds): Williams' Hematology, 6th ed. New York: McGraw-Hill, 2001:419–424.
423. Rosse WF: Paroxysmal nocturnal hemoglobinuria: The biochemical defects and the clinical syndrome [review]. Blood Rev 1989;3:192–200.
424. Nakakuma H: Mechanism of intravascular hemolysis in paroxysmal nocturnal hemoglobinuria (PNH). Am J Hematol 1996;53:22–29.
425. Nakakuma H, Hidaka M, Nagakura S, et al: Expression of cryptantigen Th on paroxysmal nocturnal hemoglobinuria erythrocytes in association with a hemolytic exacerbation. J Clin Invest 1995;96:201–206.
426. Sirchia G, Ferrone S, Mercuriali F: Leukocyte antigen-antibody reaction and lysis of paroxysmal nocturnal hemoglobinuria erythrocytes. Blood 1970;36:334–336.
427. Dacie JV: Clinicopathological Conference: A fatal case of paroxysmal haemoglobinuria demonstrated at the Postgraduate Medical School of London. Br Med J 1959;2:559.
428. Crosby WH, Stefanini M: Pathogenesis of the plasma transfusion reaction with especial reference to the blood coagulation system. J Lab Clin Med 1952;40:374–386.
429. Dameshek W, Neber J: Transfusion reactions to a plasma constituent of whole blood: Their pathogenesis and treatment by washed red blood cell transfusions. Blood 1950;5:129–147.
430. Crosby WH, Dameshek W: Paroxysmal nocturnal hemoglobinuria: The mechanism of hemolysis and its relation to the coagulation mechanism. Blood 1950;5:822–842.
431. Dacie JV, Firth D: Blood transfusion in nocturnal haemoglobinuria. Br Med J 1943;1:626–628.
432. Heffernan CK, Jaswon N: A case of paroxysmal nocturnal haemoglobinuria associated with secondary haemochromatosis, a lower nephron nephrosis, and a megaloblastic anaemia. J Clin Pathol 1955;8:211–217.
433. Heitzman EJ, Campbell JS, Stefanini M: Paroxysmal nocturnal hemoglobinuria with hemosiderin nephrosis. Am J Clin Path 1953;23:975–986.
434. Baranett EC, Dunlop JB, Pullar TH: Chronic haemolytic anaemia with paroxysmal haemoglobinuria (Marchiafava syndrome). Report of a case improved by splenectomy. N Z Med J 1951;50:39–43.
435. Hirsch J, Ungar B, Robinson JS: Paroxysmal nocturnal haemoglobinuria: An acquired dyshaemopoiesis. Austral Ann Med 1964;13:24–31.
436. Dacie JV: Transfusion of saline-washed red cells in nocturnal haemoglobinuria (Machiafava-Micheli disease). Clin Sci 1948;7:65–75.
437. Sirchia S, Zanella A: Transfusion of PNH patients. Transfusion 1990;30:479.
438. Rosse WF: Paroxysmal nocturnal hemoglobinuria as a molecular disease. Medicine (Baltimore) 1997;76:63–93.
439. Brecher ME, Taswell HF: Paroxysmal nocturnal hemoglobinuria and the transfusion of washed red cells. A myth revisited. Transfusion 1989;29:681–685.
440. Salama A, Mueller-Eckhardt C: Binding of fluid phase C3b to nonsensitized bystander human red cells: A model for in vivo effects of complement activation on blood cells. Transfusion 1985;25:528–534.
441. Gocke DJ: In vitro studies of the plasma requirement in platelet damage by an unrelated antigen-antibody reaction. Fed Proc 1964;23:404.
442. Test ST, Woolworth VS: Defective regulation of complement by the sickle erythrocyte: Evidence for a defect in control of membrane attack complex formation. Blood 1994;83:842–852.

basis of these results. For example, if the patient is R_1R_1, K-negative, Jk(a-), Jk(b+), one may simply adsorb with ZZAP-treated RBCs that are R_1R_1 and Jk(a-). It could be less labor intensive to determine the Rh, Kell, and Kidd system phenotypes of the patient and to minimize the number of RBCs used for adsorptions than to routinely use multiple samples of RBC for adsorptions. But because phenotyping for all relevant antigens might not be feasible for a patient who has a positive DAT, it is prudent to have available a supply of the three examples of RBCs previously suggested, which can be used for adsorption regardless of the patient's RBC phenotype.

Autoantibody Specificity

Defining the specificity of the autoantibody[73,74] is not as important as excluding the presence of alloantibodies, but if time allows and if blood lacking the putative antigens can be found expeditiously, it might promote the survival of transfused RBCs. If the autoantibody shows a well-defined specificity (e.g., anti-e), compatible blood should be obtained unless this would delay transfusion significantly.

AUTOANTIBODIES WITH RH SPECIFICITY OR "RELATIVE SPECIFICITY"

Serologists are frequently vague regarding the criteria used to report an autoantibody as having Rh specificity. Most warm autoantibodies react with all RBCs of common Rh phenotypes, but they might fail to react with gene deletion cells, such as Rh_{null} cells. Other autoantibodies react with all RBCs tested but react to a higher titer or score against RBCs bearing a particular Rh antigen. In either case, the autoantibody is usually said to have Rh specificity without distinguishing such reactions from each other or from the clear-cut specificity of Rh alloantibodies, wherein cells lacking the appropriate antigen yield strictly negative reactions. We will use the term *relative specificity* to refer to antibodies that react with all normal RBCs bearing common Rh antigens but react consistently to a higher titer or score against RBCs containing one or another Rh antigen.

Tests for determining "relative specificity" of autoantibody should be performed if time allows, as RBCs lacking the more strongly reactive antigen survive significantly better than RBCs that do contain it. The dilution technique may be used for determining Rh-relative specificity. In essence, one need only titrate the patient's serum or eluate against R_1R_1, R_2R_2, and rr RBCs. Table 10-8 shows results of an eluate that would be interpreted as showing "relative specificity" against the e antigen. Such reactions should be confirmed by testing against several examples of RBCs with and without the appropriate antigen before making clinical decisions based on the "relative specificity" of the autoantibody.

SIGNIFICANCE OF AUTOANTIBODY SPECIFICITY

Several investigators have studied the in vivo survival of RBCs of varying Rh phenotypes among patients who have warm autoantibodies with Rh "specificity." In most instances, detailed serologic data are not given, and the autoantibodies are likely to have demonstrated "relative specificity."

Mollison[75,76] described a case in which survival of the patient's own e-positive RBCs was shortened markedly, whereas transfused e-negative RBCs survived almost normally. The patient's serum contained an autoantibody that reacted preferentially with e+ RBCs (Fig. 10-1).

Salmon[77] described two patients who had anti-e and anti-nl autoantibodies. In the first case, the T_{50} of ^{51}Cr-labeled RBCs was 23 days for -D-/-D- RBCs (e-, nl-), 24 days for cDE/cDE RBCs (e-, nl+), and 12.5 days for cde/cde RBCs (e+, nl+). In the second case, the T_{50} was 14 days for cDE/cDE RBCs but only 4 days for CDe/cde RBCs.

von dem Borne and colleagues[78] reported on a patient who had autoanti-e and anti-nl antibodies. The ^{51}Cr half-time of CDe/CDe RBCs was 1.9 days, and that of cDE/cDE RBCs was 4.0 days.

In Höllander's patient, the autoantibodies had anti-D specificity; whereas cde/cde blood survived for at least 31 days, CDe/cde blood survived for only 3 days.[79] In Crowley and Bouroncle's patient, two autoantibodies—anti-D and anti-E—were present, and cde/cde cells survived normally.[80] In the patient of Wiener, Gordon and Russow,[81] the autoantibody reacted to highest titers with cells containing the rh' (C) factor; when transfused with blood lacking this

TABLE 10-8. ELUATE SHOWING ANTI-E "RELATIVE SPECIFICITY"

	Dilutions of Eluate							
	2	4	8	16	32	64	128	256
rr(cde/cde)	4+	3+	3+	2+	2+	1+	0	0
R_1R_1(CDe/CDe)	4+	3+	3+	2+	2+	1+	0	0
R_2R_2(cDE/cDE)	3+	2+	1+	0	0	0	0	0

Agglutination reactions are graded as 1+ to 4+.

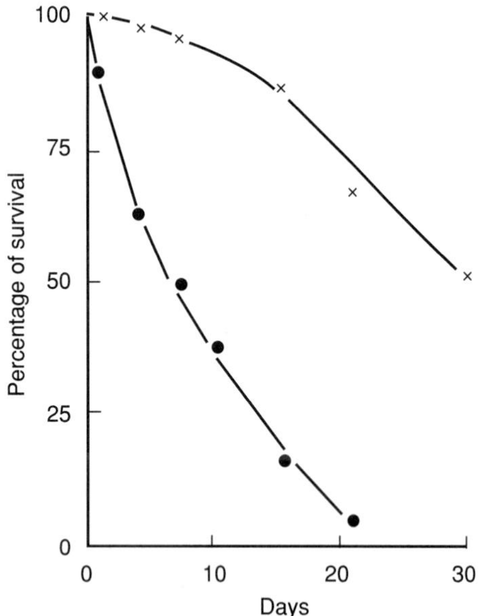

FIGURE 10-1. Survival, in a ddccee patient with autoimmune haemolytic anaemia of e+ (DCCee) red cells (•), estimated by differential agglutination, and of e− (DccEE) cells (×), estimated by ^{51}Cr-labeling and corrected for Cr elution. The patient's serum contained an autoantibody reacting preferentially with e+ cells. (From Mollison PL: Measurement of survival and destruction of red cells in haemolytic syndromes. Brit Med Bull 1959;15:59.)

factor, the patient made a complete and lasting recovery. Previously, she had been treated with randomly selected Rh-positive donors and had failed to improve. Ley, Mayer, and Harris's[82] patient was group 0 cde/cde. RBCs of phenotype cDE/cDE survived normally (^{51}Cr T_{50} = 25 days), but cde/cde cells survived even less well than the patient's own cells (^{51}Cr T_{50} 5 days and 13–14 days, respectively).

Hogman, Killander and Sjolin's case was a 13-year-old child of phenotype CDe/CDe who had formed autoanti-e antibody and an apparent "nonspecific" component.[83] The latter component did not appear to be of much importance, as cDE/cDE RBCs survived normally.

Bell and coworkers[84] mentioned one patient with anti-e who tolerated two e-negative units with the expected rise and maintenance of hemoglobin levels. No further details are given.

Habibi and associates[29] transfused cDE/cDE RBCs to six patients with autoantibodies of e, ce, or Ce specificities. The blood "proved normally efficient in vivo," but two of six homozygous e+ patients developed anti-E.

Although the preceding data are scanty, we feel that if an autoantibody demonstrates "relative specificity" (e.g., if the titer against RBCs containing the e antigen is consistently two tubes higher than when tested against cells lacking the e antigen), it is preferable to avoid transfusion of blood containing the antigen in question, even though this could involve the deliberate administration of RBCs containing Rh antigens that the patient lacks. An exception to this course is generally made if it would be necessary to give D-positive blood to a D-negative patient.

In contrast to our approach, some immunohematologists recommend ignoring the specificity of the autoantibody. This recommendation is based on two considerations. First, the evidence indicating good survival related to autoantibody "relative specificity" is not extensive. Indeed, in some reports no difference in survival in vivo can be demonstrated,[85] and in others, the benefit has been minimal.[78] In other instances, good survival of donor blood lacking the more reactive antigen has not been shown to be due to the autoantibody specificity, as survival of transfused RBCs containing the more reactive antigen has not been studied.[29,80,83,84] Second, if one transfuses RBCs that lack an antigen with which an autoantibody reacts, one might need to use RBCs containing an antigen not found on the patient's own RBCs, thus causing the potential for alloimmunization. This does not seem to be a critical argument, as typing for Rh antigens other than the D antigen is not part of routine blood transfusion practice. Such a precaution might be warranted, however, as some data suggest that patients with AIHA have an increased incidence of development of RBC alloantibodies after transfusion (see the earlier section on the incidence of alloantibodies in patients with AIHA who require transfusion).

"LEAST INCOMPATIBLE UNITS"

The term *least incompatible unit* is not an official term in transfusion medicine and is not defined in the medical literature.[86] It appears to mean the selection of a unit of blood that gives weaker reactions in the compatibility test than other incompatible units. That is, one may perform cross-match tests using a number of donor units that are ABO- and Rh-matched with the patient and then select the one that reacts least strongly. The rationale for using "least incompatible" units appears to be that the stronger reactions could be caused by an alloantibody. The use of this term apparently lingers on from the days before effective and practical serologic tests were devised for the identification of alloantibodies in the presence of autoantibodies that react with all RBCs.

Selecting "least incompatible" units must not be considered an acceptable alternative to the techniques described earlier in this chapter for selecting donor units for transfusion. Reliance on "least incompatible" units instead of performance of appropriate serologic studies is a dangerous practice and should be abandoned, except in extremely urgent settings when time to perform adequate serologic tests is insufficient.

Some transfusion services appear to use the term "least incompatible unit" in another context. They select donor units for transfusion after adequately accounting for RBC alloantibodies or select units on the basis of extended phenotyping. Nevertheless, any unit selected is incompatible with the patient's autoantibody. Transfusion services might choose to cross-match the selected units with the patient's serum, although all such cross-matches are incompatible. Choosing the "least incompatible unit" from among those that have been selected might provide a level of comfort to the transfusion service personnel and can do no harm, but this provides no known benefit to the patient. Some variability in reactivity caused by an autoantibody can be expected to occur when a number of units are cross-matched with the patient's serum; this phenomenon is due simply to the limitations of precision of serologic reactions.

The term "least incompatible" unit should be placed in the garbage heap of serologic terminology. It is not defined in transfusion medicine nomenclature; it is undoubtedly used differently by various transfusion services; its use does not convey information regarding the extent of compatibility testing performed; and finally, the term implies that this is an acceptable alternative to adequate serologic evaluation prior to transfusion of patients with AIHA.[86]

AUTOIMMUNE HEMOLYTIC ANEMIA WITHOUT SERUM AUTOANTIBODY

In contrast to the previously described problems frequently encountered among patients with AIHA, it should also be pointed out that in some patients, the autoantibody does not interfere with compatibility testing. This is true because the autoantibody might be undetectable in the patient's serum (apparently because it is entirely adsorbed onto the patient's RBCs) or is detectable only by techniques more sensitive than are used in routine compatibility tests. Even though the donor blood appears to be compatible, the transfused RBCs cannot be expected to survive normally. Indeed, Mollison[71] has stated that in all those conditions in which a hemolytic anemia is due to some extrinsic mechanism rather than to any intrinsic RBC defect, transfused normal RBCs are expected to undergo accelerated destruction.

Selection of Blood: Summary

With regard to selection of blood for transfusion to patients with WAIHA, we feel that it is most important to determine the extended RBC phenotype of the patient, to save some of the patient's RBCs for future warm autoadsorption tests, to compare the strength of the DAT and IAT, to test for antibody specificity using a routine RBC panel, and to perform the warm autoadsorption test. In a recently transfused patient, an allogeneic adsorption test should replace the warm autoadsorption test unless pretransfusion RBCs are available. If time allows, one may also test for autoantibody specificity (e.g., Rh "relative specificity"). Table 10-9 summarizes our recommendations.

The Optimal Frequency of Tests for Alloantibodies in a Patient with AIHA Who Is Transfused Repeatedly

The question frequently arises as to how often a search for alloantibodies using adsorption procedures must be performed in a patient with AIHA who is being transfused repeatedly. As pointed out by Leger and Garratty,[53] patients who have autoantibodies should receive the same protection from hemolytic transfusion

TABLE 10-9. SUMMARY OF METHODS USED IN SELECTION OF BLOOD FOR TRANSFUSION TO PATIENTS WITH WARM ANTIBODY AUTOIMMUNE HEMOLYTIC ANEMIA*

A. Patient not recently transfused (within previous 3 months)
  1. Determine patient's ABO and Rh phenotype.
  2. Determine the patient's extended RBC phenotype (e.g., K, Jk^a, Jk^b, Fy^a, Fy^b, S), if feasible.
  3. Compare strength of DAT and IAT. If IAT is stronger, the presence of an alloantibody is highly suspected.
  4. Test patient's serum against a panel. If an alloantibody causes stronger reactions than the autoantibody, the alloantibody specificity might be evident.
  5. Obtain RBCs for autoadsorption tests; save as many RBCs as practical in anticoagulant or in frozen state for use in subsequent warm autoadsorption tests, should repeated transfusions be required.
  6. Perform autoadsorptions for detection of alloantibodies.
  7. If RBCs are not available for the autoadsorption test, perform allogeneic adsorptions for detection of alloantibodies.
  8. If the IAT is strongly reactive and adsorptions are not possible (lack of time or lack of autologous or allogeneic RBCs), prepare a dilution of the patient's serum that reacts about 1+ by IAT and test against a panel.

B. Patient recently transfused (within previous 3 months)
  1. Pretransfusion RBCs are available for warm autoadsorption test.
    a) Follow steps 1–5, above (accurate determination of the patient's RBC phenotype could be difficult or impossible)
    b) Perform warm autoadsorption for detection of alloantibodies, using pretransfusion RBCs.
  2. Pretransfusion RBCs are not available for warm autoadsorption test.
    a) Follow steps 1–4, above (accurate determination of patient's RBC phenotype could be difficult or impossible)
    b) Perform allogeneic adsorptions for detection of alloantibodies or, if extended RBC phenotype of the patient is known, one may use phenotypically matched RBC units, if available. Using partially matched units (e.g., units matched for Rh and K) will provide only partial safety (see text).

* If a patient has never been transfused or pregnant, it is highly unlikely that clinically significant alloantibodies are present.
Testing the patient's autoantibody for specificity could provide additional benefit (see text).

reactions as other patients. In particular, the American Association of Blood Banks' Standards indicate that if a patient has received a transfusion or been pregnant within the preceding 3 months, the sample must be obtained from the patient within 3 days of the scheduled transfusion.[87] Indeed, Shulman and colleagues[88] have published data indicating that 13 of 60 retrospectively studied patients developed newly detectable antibodies within 83 hours of a sample reported to be negative for the new antibody. Thus, after a patient with autoantibodies receives a transfusion, compatibility test procedures, including adsorption studies, should be performed on samples obtained within 3 days of subsequent transfusions.

The Use of Phenotypically Matched RBCs for Transfusion

As the frequent performance of adsorptions is labor intensive, there is a never-ending search for less technically demanding but safe approaches to providing blood for patients with AIHA. Some investigators suggest the transfusion of RBCs that are prophylactically antigen matched (PAM) with the patient's, rather than performing adsorption studies to detect and identify alloantibodies.[89] Providing phenotypically matched RBCs can provide a significant measure of safety,[90] but some caveats and precautions should be noted.

Performing an autoadsoption provides protection against the presence of antibodies against high-incidence antigens, whereas providing blood selected on the basis of the patient's phenotype or by the alloadsorption technique does not. Therefore, autoadsorption should be considered a preferable approach when feasible.

To provide adequate safety, the patient's extended phenotype must be determined (D, C, E, c, e, K, Jk^a, Jk^b, Fy^a, Fy^b, S, and s antigens), and all donor units must be matched with the patient's. If the patient's RBCs can be phenotyped for all of these antigens, and if the blood supplier can provide units that are negative for all of these antigens not present on the patient's RBC, this method of selecting blood would appear to be about as safe as using an allogeneic adsorption procedure. Although performing an extended phenotype is a labor-intensive and expensive procedure, it need be done only once per patient, and the information can be used for all subsequent transfusions. This might not be a significant advantage, however, as data from the Los Angeles Red Cross (LARC) Reference Laboratory (unpublished) shows that only 90 of 418 patients (22%) needed more than the initial set of adsorptions, evidently because the patients responded to therapy and repeated transfusions were not required. Further, one must keep in mind that even in the most skilled hands, extended phenotyping of RBCs that have a strongly positive direct antiglobulin test might not be possible. Indeed, Shirey and coworkers[89] could not obtain a reliable phenotype from 40% of their patients, and in these cases, adsorption procedures were necessary for alloantibody detection and identification.

Data from the LARC Reference Laboratory[91] suggests that the use of phenotypically matched RBCs prevents most of the alloantibody-induced hemolytic transfusion reactions that potentially would occur in patients with AIHA. Table 10-10 shows the specificities of 202 alloantibodies detected in the sera of 418 patients with AIHA. Anti-E was by far the most common alloantibody detected, being twice as common as the next most common specificity, anti-K. The next most common group included anti-C, $-Fy^a$, $-Jk^a$, and anti-c, in that order. A third group of alloantibodies—anti-Jk^b, -S, -D, -e, "HTLA", -M, -V, $-Js^a$, $-C^w$,

TABLE 10-10. ALLOANTIBODY SPECIFICITIES OF 202 ANTIBODY-CONTAINING SERA FROM 418 AIHA PATIENTS

Specificity*	*n*	Percentage Present in Antibody-Containing Sera	Percentage Present in Total AIHA Patients
Anti-E	92	46	22
-K	45	22	10.8
-C	36	18	8.7
$-Fy^a$	30	15	7.8
$-Jk^a$	21	10	5.0
-c	20	10	4.8
$-Jk^b$	19	9.4	4.6
-S	17	8.4	4.0
-D	14	7	3.4
-e	10	5	2.4
"HTLA"	9	4.5	2.2
-M	9	4.5	2.2
-V	8	4	1.9
$-Js^a$	7	3	1.7
$-C^w$	7	3	1.7
$-Le^a$	7	3	1.7
$-Wr^a$	5	2.5	1.2
-s	4	2	1.0
-rhi	4	2	1.0

* Other specificities detetected in only 1 or 2 sera included anti-Kp^a, -VS, $-P_1$, -Ch, -G, -N, $-Di^a$, -Ce, $-KnMc^a$, -U, $-Lu^a$, -Lu14, -He, $-Xg^a$, -Mit, $-Fy^5$.
From Garratty G, Petz LD: Approaches to selecting blood for transfusion to patients with auto-immune hemolytic anemia. Transfusion 2002;42:1390–1392.

Le^a, -Wr^a, -s, and –rh$_i$—were present in 1% to 10% of the alloantibody containing sera. A fourth group of various specificities was associated with only one or two of the patients. Approximately 40% of the sera contained alloantibody of only a single specificity; 30% contained two specificities; and 16% contained three specificities. Approximately 10% of the alloantibody-containing sera contained alloantibodies of four or more specificities.

Providing PAM RBCs might present a significant problem for hospitals and smaller blood suppliers. The phenotypes of the 12 patients who received PAM RBCs (listed in Table 2 of Shirey and associates[89]) range from 0.0002 to 0.09 (mean = 0.04), meaning that 51,000–65,000, or a total of 76,300 random units would have to be screened to obtain the 149 PAM RBCs that were transfused to these patients. Even if the frequency of the rarest of the phenotypes, E–, K–, Fy(a–b–), S– (patient #9, who was probably African American) is removed from the calculation (as this phenotype could be obtained more easily by screening African Americans), 51–6714, or a total of 11,306 random donors would have to be screened to obtain the 136 PAM RBCs transfused to 11 patients.[91] Nevertheless, Lau and colleagues[90] have suggested that, with the use of a sophisticated computer program, it is feasible and cost effective in a relatively homogeneous population in Hong Kong to obtain phenotype-matched blood for all patients without need for pretransfusion antibody screening.

Partial phenotyping (e.g., for Rh, K and Jk^a antigens) would not provide protection against alloimmunization by antigens of other blood group systems that can cause hemolytic transfusion reactions, and therefore, it would not preclude the necessity of pretransfusion adsorption studies.[71,92,93] Determining the partial genotype of patients' RBCs using DNA technology might be helpful in identifying at least some RBC antigens (see the earlier discussion of red cell phenotyping and genotyping).

Whether implementation of this approach is feasible and cost effective at many blood centers has not been determined. If the intention is to place emphasis on providing phenotype-matched units, one must determine that the blood supplier could provide such units reliably, and one must recognize that adsorption studies will be required in cases in which a patient's RBCs cannot be phenotyped and/or when the blood supplier cannot provide matched units.

COMPATIBILITY TESTING IN COLD-ANTIBODY AIHAs

Cold Agglutinin Syndrome

PERFORMING COMPATIBILITY TESTING AT 37°C USING SALINE-SUSPENDED RBCs

There are several approaches to compatibility testing for patients with CAS. One method is to perform the compatibility test strictly at 37°C and to use only saline-suspended RBCs (i.e., without potentiators). Cold agglutinins from only 7% of patients with cold agglutinin syndrome react at 37°C using saline-suspended RBCs, although we found positive reactions in 30% of cases in albumin media.[94,95] If positive reactions occur at 37°C with saline-suspended RBCs, one must first suspect faulty technique. If cells and serum are not prewarmed before mixing, if centrifugation is performed at a temperature lower than 37°C, or if the initial washes of the cells after incubation do not use saline at 37°C, reactions can occur within seconds. Even if direct agglutination is not evident, complement might be bound by the antibody reactivity and result in a positive IAT using polyspecific antiglobulin serum (one molecule of IgM antibody might bind several hundred molecules of complement). This reaction may be circumvented by using anti-IgG antiglobulin serum.

The advantages of this method are that time-consuming autoadsorptions of the patient's serum are not necessary and that the method can be used even if the patient has recently received a transfusion.

Several disadvantages are also apparent. First, it is obvious that RBC alloantibodies reacting at temperatures lower than 37°C will not be detected. This finding is of little consequence, as alloantibodies that do not react in vitro at temperatures less than 37°C are rarely, if ever, clinically significant. Indeed, the Standards for Blood Banks and Transfusion Services of the American Association of Blood Banks does not require a room temperature incubation phase of the crossmatch but instead states that methods for testing for unexpected antibodies "shall include 37°C incubation preceding an antiglobulin test using reagent RBCs that are not pooled."[87]

It is also true that potentiator-dependent antibodies will be missed, but here, again, the risk is minimal because such antibodies are quite unusual.[96] Because compatibility testing at 37°C is quicker than other methods, it can be used even if the patient has recently received a transfusion, and because it results in a low risk of missing clinically significant alloantibodies, we believe it is the method of choice. Attention to certain technical details is crucial, however, to be certain that one is truly working strictly at 37°C.

One must validate that procedures are actually being carried out strictly at 37°C. A heated centrifuge or a centrifuge in a 37°C warm room may be used, a centrifuge may be placed in an incubator, or the tubes may be placed in centrifuge cups containing warm water. Samples transferred from a 37°C water bath and centrifuged immediately at room temperature drop by approximately 7–8°C after only one minute of centrifugation. One must be aware that, if one uses saline at 40–45°C, the temperature will drop by a few degrees when it enters a test tube and by a few more degrees when centrifuging is in progress. A few simple experiments are all that is required to determine the appropriate conditions.

COLD AUTOADSORPTION AND ALLOGENEIC ADSORPTION

An alternative approach is to adsorb the cold autoantibody from the patient's serum before performing the compatibility test. If facilities are not available to work strictly at 37°C, one or two cold autoadsorptions will frequently remove enough of the cold agglutinin so that compatibility tests can be performed with less stringent control of the incubation temperature. It is interesting that cold autoadsorptions remove antibody reactive at 30–37°C before all antibody reactive at 4°C is adsorbed, thus making compatibility testing feasible without adhering strictly to 37°C temperatures.

Even if the transfusion service can work strictly at 37°C, cold autoadsorptions might be necessary in the small percentage of patients whose antibody is reactive at 37°C, even in saline. If a patient has a very high-titer cold agglutinin, one should not attempt to remove all of the antibody by adsorption. Doing so would require multiple adsorptions even when enzyme-treated RBCs are being used and is not necessary. Table 10-11 shows the results of autoadsorbing a serum with a cold-agglutinin titer of 2048 (saline) and 8096 (albumin). After three adsorptions for one-half hour each at 4°C using the patient's papainized RBCs, the serum still reacted strongly (4+ with undiluted serum) at room temperature (25°C), but it no longer reacted at 37°C.

In recently transfused patients, allogeneic adsorption studies can be performed as for warm-antibody AIHA. This is rarely necessary if compatibility tests are carried out as described previously.

OTHER METHODS

An alternative approach to compatibility testing is to adsorb the serum with rabbit erythrocyte stroma, which can be used to adsorb anti-I and –IH[40] but might also remove clinically significant alloantibodies (notably anti-B, -D, -E, and others).[97]

Still another approach to compatibility testing in cold agglutinin syndrome is to inactivate the IgM cold agglutinin with 2-mercaptoethanol (2ME) or DTT.[98,99]

Pirofsky and Rosner[100] described the use of DTT at a concentration of 0.01 M in a rapid 15-minute, 37°C incubation test system. Dialysis was not required. They reported that this procedure caused at least a fourfold or greater decrease in IgM antibody titers without affecting the activity of IgG antibodies.

Olson and associates[101] used DTT in a concentration of 0.01 M, added equal volumes to test sera, and incubated for 30 minutes at 37°C. Thirty sera that contained RBC antibodies reactive by the IAT showed virtually no alteration in activity after DTT treatment, while 20 sera containing cold-reactive RBC antibodies showed almost total elimination of activity. However, none of the cold-reactive antibodies tested were pathologic high-titer cold agglutinins from patients with CAS.

Freedman and colleagues[102] reviewed the optimal conditions for the use of sulphydryl compounds in dissociating RBC antibodies. They noted that incubation at 37°C with 0.2 M 2ME provided the best conditions for inactivating IgM antibodies. Incubation still failed to inactivate completely the extremely potent autoanti-I (titer of 1,024,000) that was used, however. False-positive reactions in the IAT using anti-IgG or anticomplement antiglobulin serum were obtained consistently when sera that had been treated with 2ME were not subsequently dialyzed. Although in many cases dialysis for as short as 30 minutes was sufficient, in others overnight dialysis was found to be necessary. Incubation of serum with DTT produced a slower effect than did incubation with 2-mercaptoethanol, and incubation for 2.5 hours was necessary to reduce the anti-I titer from 1,024,000 to 1024.

Using either reagent, IgM alloantibodies will, of course, be inactivated in addition to the cold autoagglutinins. Other disadvantages are that blood bank technologists are often unfamiliar with the use of such reagents, and both reagents can inactivate or diminish complement activity.

TRANSFUSION OF ADULT-i RBCs

Some investigators have suggested that adult-i RBCs be used for transfusion of patients with cold agglutinin

TABLE 10-11. ABSORPTION OF COLD AGGLUTININ BY PATIENT'S OWN RBCs AT 4°C

	Titer against Adult OI RBCs					
	4°C		25°C		37°C	
	Saline	Albumin	Saline	Albumin	Saline	Albumin
Unadsorbed	2048	8098	1024	8098	0	32
Absorbed × 1	1024	2048	256	1024	0	16
Absorbed × 2	256	256	128	256	0	8
Absorbed × 3	128	128	16	64	0	0

syndrome who have anti-I autoantibodies. van Loghem and associates[103] studied the survival of I and i RBCs labeled with ^{51}Cr in one patient with chronic CAS. They demonstrated normal survival for the i donor RBCs with greatly shortened survival of both the patient's I RBCs and donor I RBCs. Woll and coworkers[104] reported one patient with transient CAS who responded to transfusion of warmed, freeze-thawed adult-i RBCs. These researchers did not test the survival of adult I RBCs, however. Bell and colleagues[84] reported unfavorable experiences transfusing two patients with CAS with adult-i RBCs. Two adult-i units given to a patient with strong anti-I survived for approximately the same period of time (i.e., 3 to 4 days) as several adult-I units given subsequently. In a second patient with anti-I, no elevation of hematocrit was noted after transfusion of two units of adult-i blood. These authors suggested that the minimal I antigen present on adult-i RBCs seemed sufficient to render them biologically incompatible.

Our own experience indicates that transfusion of adult-I RBCs to patients with chronic CAS usually results in an appropriate rise in hemoglobin. Unusual patients might fail to respond to transfusion of adult-I RBCs, but a majority of available data indicate that the use of adult-i cells is not a solution to the problem. In patients with chronic CAS, the repeated use of i RBCs is certainly not feasible because of their extreme rarity.

Paroxysmal Cold Hemoglobinuria

Transfusion of compatible blood for patients with paroxysmal cold hemoglobinuria (PCH) might be possible if the rare p or P^k cells are available through a rare donor file. Although the routine cross-match test could appear to be compatible with other RBCs because the antibody reacts only in the cold (usually <15°C), there are some suggestions that p or P^k RBCs will survive better.[22,105]

Rausen and colleagues[22] reported on two children with PCH who were severely anemic. The first patient, a 4-year-old boy with blood type A_1, was transfused with two 100-mL aliquots of frozen-thawed RBCs from a compatible type O, Tj(a-) donor 5 days after the sudden onset of hemolytic anemia. The blood was administered at room temperature, and the hematocrit level rose from 11% to 19% following the transfusions. Although the hematocrit had been expected to reach 28%, the authors determined that the post-transfusion blood contained fewer than 5% type A RBCs and therefore concluded that the lack of an appropriate rise in the hematocrit was because the patient's own cells were rapidly being hemolyzed. Within 2 more days, hemoglobinuria subsided, and the patient's hemoglobin rose progressively.

The second child, a 2½-year-old boy with blood type AB, was treated with intravenously administered hydrocortisone on the first day of hospitalization, and subsequently he was transfused with 100 mL of type AB RBCs that were incompatible with the Donath-Landsteiner antibody. The hematocrit temporarily improved from 13.5% to 20% but decreased over the next 36 hours to 11.5%. A second incompatible transfusion of 130 mL again resulted in a temporary rise in hematocrit to 24.5% but with a drop to 15% over the next 36 hours. The urine then abruptly became clear and at this point, 100 mL of frozen-thawed RBCs from a compatible type O, Tj(a-) donor were transfused through a warming coil adjusted to 37°C. Following this transfusion, the hematocrit rose to 20%, and the patient's hemolytic anemia stabilized and then gradually resolved. The authors state that these were the first recorded cases of successful compatible transfusion therapy in PCH. One should note, however, that both patients' hemolysis spontaneously subsided soon after the transfusions of compatible blood and that one cannot determine the comparative efficacy of the compatible and incompatible transfusions from the data provided.

Sabio and associates[105] reported on a 4½-year-old girl with PCH who was transfused twice with ABO/Rh (D)-compatible, P+-incompatible RBCs. These transfusions only worsened the patient's hemoglobinuria without increasing the hemoglobin concentration significantly. Transfusion with RBC of the rare p phenotype was attempted successfully with a rise in hemoglobin and amelioration of symptoms. The patient was also treated with 2 mg/kg prednisone "without any effect" following the first transfusions.

Nordhagen and colleagues[106] reported on four children with acute PCH who required transfusion in spite of aggressive therapy with corticosteroids. One patient received three transfusions of P-positive blood during the first 3 days of hospitalization. One week later, the patient became febrile again, with increasing hemolysis and a hemoglobin that dropped from 7.3 to 4.6 g/dL. He was given another transfusion on the 10th day and the last on the 14th day. The last transfusion consisted of washed, P-negative (pp) erythrocytes, after which the patient's condition stabilized.

Patients are likely to require transfusion before RBCs of the p phenotype are available. Generally, transfusion of RBCs of common P types should be provided, as patients with PCH often have severe hemolysis, and waiting for availability of p or P^k RBC is likely to delay a needed transfusion. Successful transfusion of patients with PCH has been reported by numerous authors and, almost certainly, the transfusions were of P-positive blood.[33,106-112]

Although there are some reports of Donath-Landsteiner antibodies having other specificities, these are extraordinarily rare (see Chapter 5).

OPTIMAL VOLUME OF BLOOD TO BE TRANSFUSED

The optimal volume of blood to be transfused to patients with AIHA varies with the clinical setting. In patients who have severe hemolysis but who might require transfusion only temporarily until therapy becomes effective, the transfusion of modest volumes of RBCs just sufficient to maintain a tolerable hematocrit level appears advisable. In patients with severe anemia, however, there is a tendency to transfuse large volumes of blood to restore the hemoglobin and hematocrit to near-normal levels quickly. This approach can lead to tragic consequences.

Indeed, Rosenfield and Jagathambal[37] point out that the salutary effect of just 100 mL of packed RBCs can be quite remarkable when given to a patient with cardiopulmonary embarrassment from anemia. They suggest that 100 mL may be given as needed (perhaps twice daily, depending on the severity of hemolysis) and that there is generally no need to increase the hemoglobin even to a level of 8 g/dL. The aim of such transfusions is to supply just enough RBCs to prevent hypoxemia while avoiding dangerous reactions resulting from overtransfusion.

Complications of Aggressive Transfusion Therapy in Patients with AIHA

VOLUME OVERLOAD

The dangers of overtransfusion among patients with AIHA are several. If the anemia is very severe (hematocrit 10–15%, hemoglobin 3.5–5.0 g/dL), and especially if the patient is elderly or if cardiac reserve might be reduced, transfusion can overload the circulation easily and precipitate cardiac failure. In slowly developing anemia, total blood will not be as severely reduced as are hemoglobin and hematocrit values, so that even modest volumes of transfused RBCs will result in hypervolemia. Not only should the total volume that is transfused be kept modest but RBCs should also be administered slowly, the total volume transfused not exceeding 1 mL/kg/hour. One must look for evidence of congestive heart failure during and following the transfusion—particularly elevated venous pressure and the presence of rales on auscultation of the chest. Cardiac failure after the administration of as little as 200 mL of RBCs can develop up to 6 to 12 hours later and can be fatal. Although diuretics are of value and probably should be given to patients with diminished cardiac reserve, responses vary, and their administration must not replace close clinical observation of the patient.

POST-TRANSFUSION HEMOGLOBINEMIA, HEMOGLOBINURIA, AND DISSEMINATED INTRAVASCULAR COAGULATION

An additional danger for patients with AIHA relates to the fact that the kinetics of RBC destruction always describe an exponential curve of decay, indicating that the number of cells removed in a unit of time is a percentage of the number of cells present at the start of this time interval.[37] Thus, the more cells present at zero time, the greater the absolute number of RBCs that will be destroyed in the unit time span. Indeed, Chaplin[113] indicates that the most common cause of post-transfusion hemoglobinuria in AIHA might not be alloantibody-induced hemolysis but rather the quantitative effect of transfusion in increasing the RBC mass subjected to ongoing autoantibody-mediated destruction. Such marked post-transfusion hemoglobinemia and hemoglobinuria have the potential for a significant degree of associated morbidity and possibly, mortality. Indeed, Gürgey and coworkers[114] pointed out that two children who were treated with exchange transfusions died of profound hemolysis shortly after the procedure (although Heidemann and colleagues[115] reported successful exchange transfusion in one patient).

Patients undergoing severe post-transfusion intravascular hemolysis can develop disseminated intravascular coagulation (DIC), possibly as a result of procoagulant substances present in RBC lysates.[36,116] These potential problems emphasize the need for restraint in the volume of blood transfused per transfusion episode to patients with AIHA.

CASE SUMMARIES

An example of such a complication of transfusion therapy was reported by Bilgrami and associates.[116] They described a patient who was infected with human immunodeficiency virus (HIV) who had severe AIHA. His hemoglobin was 2.9 g/dL; hematocrit, 8%; corrected reticulocyte count, 1.2%; white cell count, 12,500/µL; platelet count, 101,000/µL; total bilirubin, 3 mg/dL; direct bilirubin, 0.7 mg/dL; lactate dehydrogenase, 1902 U/L; prothrombin time, 11.8 seconds (normal 11–13 seconds); and partial thromboplastin time 20.8 seconds (normal, 25–35 seconds). The urine was grossly red but with no intact RBCs. The peripheral smear demonstrated spherocytes, polychromasia, and nucleated RBCs. The DAT was positive using polyspecific AGS, anti-IgG, and anti-C3. "Least incompatible" (w+ to 2+) units were selected for transfusion using differentially adsorbed sera for cross-matching. Before transfusion, immune complexes were detected in the serum by several techniques.

The patient underwent aggressive transfusion, receiving 8 units of packed RBCs over the course of 24 hours, as shown in Figure 10-2. The patient was transfused to a hematocrit level of greater than 25%. Signs of DIC developed, however, with the platelet count demonstrating a progressive decline and the prothrombin time and partial thromboplastin times showing an upward trend within 24 hours. One-half hour before the patient's death, the following laboratory results were obtained: prothrombin time, 16.8 seconds; partial thromboplastin time, 81 seconds; serum fibrinogen, 130 mg/dL (normal, 150–400 mg/dL); thrombin time, 45 seconds (control, 16.5 seconds); fibrin degradation products titer, greater than 40 mg/mL; and D-dimer, greater than 1 µg/mL. A diagnosis of DIC was made. The patient became hypotensive shortly thereafter and could not be resuscitated.

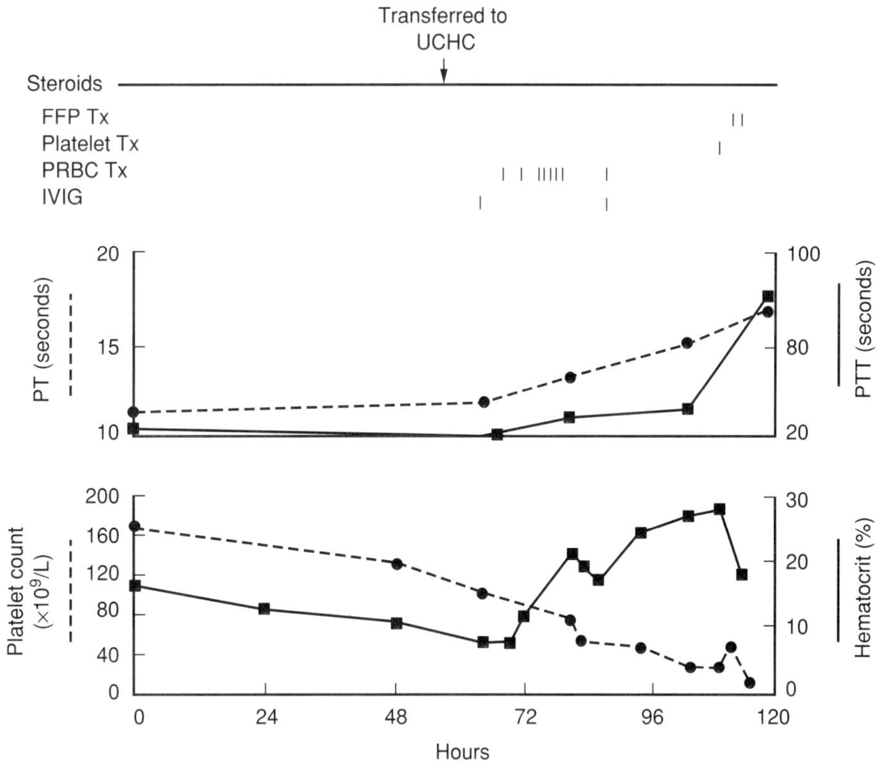

FIGURE 10-2. Clinical course of AIHA and DIC in a patient with HIV infection PT, prothrombin time; PTT, partial thromboplastin time; PRBC, packed red blood cell; FFP, fresh-frozen plasma; Tx, transfusion; UCHC, University of Connecticut Health Center. (From Bilgrami S, Cable R, Pisciotto P, Rowland F, Greenberg B: Fatal disseminated intravascular coagulation and pulmonary thrombosis following blood transfusion in a patient with severe autoimmune hemolytic anemia and human immunodeficiency virus infection. Transfusion 1994;34:248–252.)

The autopsy demonstrated widespread multiple pulmonary thrombi. There was widespread thrombosis of small arterioles of both lungs. Some of the thrombi had begun to organize and others were very acute, a presentation most consistent with the formation of thrombi in situ rather than secondary to thromboembolic disease. The extensive pulmonary thrombi resulted in acute right ventricular failure, which was the immediate cause of death. The authors pointed out that less aggressive transfusion therapy would have sufficed to meet the patient's tissue oxygen needs and concluded that the most likely etiology of the patient's DIC was the aggressive transfusion therapy. They concluded that their case illustrates the need to consider the possibility of serious transfusion complications for patients with AIHA (even when alloantibodies have been excluded) and underscores the value of the judicious use of transfusion for specific indications in this group of patients.[5]

Additional examples of unfavorable outcomes of transfusion are indicated in the following two case summaries (Patient 1, Patient 2), which were supplied by Dr. Hugh Chaplin, Jr (Chaplin H Jr, personal communication).

PATIENT 1: A 34-year-old white gravida-1, para-1, with relapsing primary autoimmune hemolytic anemia for 4 months, was admitted to the hospital with a hemoglobin level of 5.0 g/dL; reticulocytes of 16%; DAT strongly positive for C3d, moderately positive for IgM, and negative for IgG; and all crossmatches deemed "incompatible." Despite high-dose therapy with corticosteroids, she required 1 to 2 units of packed RBCs daily to maintain her hemoglobin level at 4.5 to 6.0 g/dL. She experienced increasingly severe hemoglobinemia and hemoglobinuria associated with transfusions, clearing within a few hours. No alloantibodies were demonstrable. On the 10th hospital day, a splenectomy was performed without benefit. On the 12th hospital day, several hours following a transfusion, she developed acute respiratory distress followed by cardiopulmonary arrest, which did not respond to resuscitative measures. Autopsy revealed a single large para-aortic lymph node diagnosed as plasmacytoid malignant lymphoma; death was attributed to multiple fresh small pulmonary emboli.

PATIENT 2: A 56-year-old white female, never previously pregnant or transfused, was semistuporous at the time of admission to the hospital. She had a hemoglobin level of 1.6 g/dL; hematocrit level 6.2%; reticulocytes 19%; DAT strongly positive for C3d, moderately positive for IgG, and weakly positive for IgM; and all crossmatches "incompatible." She was given corticosteroids and 3 units of packed group O, Rh-negative RBCs and developed fever and striking hemoglobinemia and hemoglobinuria, which improved over the ensuing 3 hours. Her state of consciousness improved, and the hemoglobin level rose transiently to 5.7 g/dL but was declining rapidly when she developed severe respiratory distress followed by cardiopulmonary arrest, which did not respond to resuscitation. At autopsy, no underlying cause for the AIHA was found; death was attributed to multiple fresh small pulmonary emboli.

Saif and coworkers[117] reported a complication of transfusion in a patient with HIV-associated AIHA. Following transfusion of 1 unit of RBCs, the patient developed a pulmonary embolism. The authors cited two other reports of thromboembolism in patients with HIV-associated AIHA[118,119] and also cited the case of Bilgrami and associates (reviewed previously), although the latter case described DIC rather than thromboembolism.

These complications of transfusion patients with AIHA are not common, as emphasized by Salama and associates,[27] who found no instances of a definite increase in signs of hemolysis among 53 patients with AIHA who received blood transfusions. Nevertheless, for patients with AIHA, RBCs must be transfused cautiously and for appropriate indications.[5]

IN VIVO COMPATIBILITY TESTING

In vivo compatibility testing has been advocated by some and is based on testing the survival of an aliquot of RBCs from a unit that has been selected for transfusion.[56,120] Although such tests are potentially of value in determining the clinical significance of some alloantibodies in patients without AIHA, we feel that such studies are of limited value for patients with AIHA and should never be considered a substitute for meticulous serologic evaluation and detailed compatibility testing. This is particularly true because the original use of in vivo survival studies in patients with AIHA occurred at a time when less effective methods were available for the detection of RBC alloantibodies in such patients. Using the modern compatibility tests described previously, little is to be gained from in vivo survival studies.

Some investigators have measured the survival of an aliquot of RBCS using ^{51}Cr-tagged cells.[120,121] In this procedure, 0.5 to 1 mL of RBCs from a donor unit are labeled with ^{51}Cr. If the amount of radioactivity in the plasma, both at 10 and 60 minutes, does not exceed 5% of the radioactivity injected, and if RBC survival at 60 minutes is not less than 70%, the expectation was that donor RBCs could be transfused with minimum hazard.[71,121] The potential value of this procedure according to available data is that an acceptable result in an in vivo compatibility test seems to preclude the possibility of an immediate symptomatic hemolytic reaction when cells from the whole unit subsequently are transfused.[120-122] If the in vivo test is performed after detailed compatibility testing using modern techniques, however, and if it demonstrates short survival of the test cells, it is difficult to understand what should be done next to select a unit of RBC different from the one used for the in vivo test.

Indeed, Meyer and colleagues[123] presented data on 11 patients with AIHA who had an in vivo survival of ^{51}Cr-tagged donor red blood cells of less than 70% in 1 hour but who nevertheless required transfusion. Only one of these patients had a complication directly attributable to the transfusion.[123] Also, Mollison[124] points out that the survival of a small volume of incompatible RBCs might be different from the survival of a larger volume of the same RBCs. Data are not available to determine the rate of destruction of a test dose of RBCs that would predict an acute symptomatic hemolytic reaction.

Also, the results of an in vivo compatibility test could impart a false sense of security, as only a small percentage of transfused RBCs might survive in the 16 to 24 hours following acceptable results in an in vivo survival study.[120,125]

For example, Silvergleid and coworkers[120] described patients with WAIHA who had adequate 1-hour RBC survival of a test dose of RBCs and who did not evidence an acute transfusion reaction, but who had short survival of the transfused RBCs in subsequent hours. One such patient had a pretransfusion hematocrit level of 10.5%, a post-transfusion hematocrit level of 20.6%, but a hematocrit level of only 10% just 16 hours after transfusion. Another patient with PCH had a 1-hour survival of Tj (a+) RBCs of 87%, but only 53% of the radiolabeled cells survived to 48 hours after transfusion. Still another patient with an alloantibody (anti-Jk^b) had 94% survival of tagged cells at 1 hour but only 10% survival at 24 hours after transfusion. Similar data were reported by Peters and associates,[125] who described a patient with anti-Lu^b; survival of radiolabeled Lu(b+) RBCs was 84.4% at 1 hour but only 48% at 5 hours and 8.5% at 24 hours after transfusion.

At the present time, in vivo compatibility tests using radiolabeled RBC seem to be rarely, if ever, performed in clinical services on patients with AIHA.

An alternative method for determining in vivo survival of transfused RBCs in a patient with AIHA is to infuse over a period of 20–30 minutes an aliquot containing 20–30 mL of RBCs from the unit to be transfused. The patient is observed for symptoms of a hemolytic transfusion reaction, and a blood sample is obtained after the infusion of the "test dose" to look for hemoglobinemia (and urine, if available, is observed for hemoglobinuria). The intravascular lysis of as little as 5 mL of RBCs will raise the plasma hemoglobin concentration of an adult by about 50 mg/100 mL, an amount easily detected by visual inspection.[113] One merely needs to obtain an anticoagulated specimen of blood, centrifuge it, and visually compare it to the plasma obtained prior to the infusion. Absence of hemoglobinemia and hemoglobinuria suggests that an acute hemolytic transfusion reaction will not occur with infusion of the entire unit of blood.

One benefit of this technique is that the test requires evaluation of the patient's status during the early phase of a transfusion. Close observation of the patient is critical, although it obviously should be carried out in any case. As a modification of this procedure, one can merely transfuse slowly until the equivalent of about 20–30 mL of RBCs have been infused, and then obtain a blood sample for visual inspection of the plasma. One need not stop the transfusion if the patient remains asymptomatic.

An acute hemolytic transfusion serious enough to cause immediate hemoglobinemia is not likely to occur except as a result of ABO incompatibility. Thus, little information, if any, is provided about the presence of other alloantibodies that have the potential to cause a hemolytic transfusion reaction. Even if no immediate adverse effects are noted, the survival of the full unit is not likely to be better than that of the patient's own RBCs.

More important, if a careful serologic study has been done using the techniques and principles already described to select the best possible blood for transfusion, and if an in vivo test nevertheless demonstrates a very short RBC survival, there is no logical way to select an alternative unit. Certainly, a patient should never be denied a needed transfusion because laboratory data (whether from a compatibility test or from an RBC survival study) suggest that the transfused blood will not survive well. If the patient requires transfusion, such incompatible blood must still be given in the hope of obtaining temporary benefit.

In conclusion, we feel that the significance of in vivo survival studies with respect to transfusion of patients with AIHA has been overemphasized.

THE USE OF WARM BLOOD FOR PATIENTS WITH COLD AGGLUTININ SYNDROME AND PAROXYSMAL COLD HEMOGLOBINURIA

Eminent authorities offer sharply differing opinions concerning the need for warm blood when transfusing patients with CAS. Dacie[33] states that properly crossmatched blood can probably be transfused with safety if run in at a slow drip rate, in which case there is probably no need to attempt to warm it above room temperature. By contrast, Rosenfield and Jagathambol[37] state that patients with cold agglutinin disease must receive warmed blood. Mollison and colleagues[71] state that blood should be warmed before transfusion to patients with cold agglutinin syndrome, and they also recommend that the patient be kept warm. Wallace[126] comments that hemolytic reactions are unlikely, provided that the donor blood is warmed to body temperature and the recipient is kept warm. As is evident, the question has not been studied in much depth, and no RBC survival studies are available comparing survival of blood transfused at various temperatures.

With regard to PCH, Rausen[22] does report that even compatible Tj(a-) blood needs to be warmed to 37°C before transfusion. Wallace[126] states that transfusion of RBCs of the common P groups is unlikely to precipitate an acute hemolytic transfusion reaction in PCH provided that the blood is warmed to 37°C and the patient is maintained at a warm temperature. Johnsen and coworkers[107] reported the results of transfusion of 150 mL of prewarmed, packed RBCs (P-positive) to an 18-month-old boy with PCH. The transfusion was followed by a temperature rise and passage of red-colored urine. The hemoglobin improved from 4.7 g/dL to 12.4 g/dL and remained at that level.

In the absence of extensive data, logic must prevail. Our experience in CAS has been consistent with Dacie's view, although in some instances we have empirically used an in-line blood warmer for seriously ill patients. The use of an in-line blood warmer would appear indicated if the patient has either severe PCH or florid CAS. It is also logical to keep the patient warm, even if the efficacy of such a maneuver has not been proven.

If blood is to be warmed, it must be done properly. Unmonitored or uncontrolled heating of blood is extremely dangerous and should not be attempted. RBCs heated too much are rapidly destroyed in vivo and can be lethal.[37] Very efficient in-line blood warmers are available that are simple, efficient, and safe to use. Guidelines for the use of blood warming devices have been published.[127]

THE USE OF RBC SUBSTITUTES

Considerable progress has been made in the development of RBC substitutes, and the availability of O_2-carrying therapeutic agents for clinical use could affect the practice of transfusion medicine.[25,26,128-132]

Mullon and associates[26] described the use of a polymerized bovine hemoglobin in a patient with severe AIHA. The patient had life-threatening AIHA that was refractory to treatment with high doses of glucocorticoids, plasmapheresis, splenectomy, and intravenous immune globulin. To maintain a hematocrit greater than 12% and a hemoglobin level greater than 4.0 g/dL, as many as 8 units of RBC per day were needed; she received a total of 53 units of RBCs before initiation of therapy with the hemoglobin solution. During RBC transfusions, the patient developed symptoms attributed to acute hemolysis, including fever, nausea, and back pain. Ischemic changes were present in the electrocardiogram when the hemoglobin was at a level of about 4.0 g/dL.

A total of 11 units of a sterile solution of gluteraldehyde-polymerized bovine hemoglobin were transfused over a 7-day period. Five units were administered in response to clinical evidence of ischemia, three as part of volume resuscitation during an episode of septic shock, and three to maintain the total hemoglobin level above 4 g/dL. This therapy resulted in relief of ischemia, and no clinically important adverse hemodynamic responses occurred. She received further treatment for her AIHA with cyclophosphamide and developed profound neutropenia, gram-negative septic shock, and gram-negative pelvic osteomyelitis. Subsequent immunosuppressive

Indeed, a significant number of patients with WAIHA have had favorable responses to splenectomy in spite of ^{51}Cr sequestration studies that predicted a therapeutic failure. For example, Allgood and Chaplin[13] reported a good response to splenectomy in four of seven patients who failed to show evidence for splenic sequestration. Parker and associates[87] studied 12 patients and found that three of seven patients with spleen-to-liver ratios of less than 2.5 had a good result from splenectomy, while two of five patients with ratios greater than 2.5 had a poor response. They concluded that surface counting measurements are not reliable indicators of the outcome of splenectomy. Ben-Bassat and colleagues[83] reported that in three out of five patients, the response to splenectomy was contrary to that expected from sequestration studies.

Zupanska and coworkers[11] reported the results of splenectomy in comparison with the spleno-hepatic index and also in comparison with spleen weight (Fig. 11-2).[11] These authors concluded that there was no correlation between postsplenectomy results and spleen-to-liver radioactivity ratios. Discrepant results also have been reported by other investigators, and Crosby[93] succinctly concludes that the test gives false-positive and false-negative results, which vitiate its value.[63,68,90]

Therefore, clinical findings rather than ^{51}Cr sequestration studies should indicate the advisability of performing splenectomy.[12,13,78,93-95] The operation need not be considered if satisfactory remission results from corticosteroid administration. If corticosteroids yield unsatisfactory results, the options are few: splenectomy, immunosuppressive drugs, and a variety of miscellaneous therapies that will be reviewed shortly. The favorable results of splenectomy are more impressive than those of any of the alternatives, and although a splenic sequestration study might predict a higher probability of response than would be true for a randomly selected patient, a good clinical response frequently occurs in spite of prediction of failure by the isotope study. In cases in which the indications for splenectomy are not compelling (e.g., an incomplete remission maintained on less than 15 mg of prednisone per day, or patients with relative contraindications to splenectomy), the sequestration study might be of some value in arriving at a decision. Among those who require 10–15 mg per day or more of prednisone for adequate control of hemolysis, however, no patient should be denied the possible beneficial results of splenectomy on the basis of a ^{51}Cr splenic sequestration study.

Serologic Tests as a Predictor of Efficacy of Splenectomy. A number of investigators have attempted to correlate the results of splenectomy with the presurgical serologic findings in cases of warm antibody AIHA. Zupanska and colleagues[11] stated that excellent results were more frequent in patients who had no complement on their RBCs. The authors added, however, that the number of cases is too small to form firm conclusions.

Similarly, neither the strength of the DAT nor the presence or absence of antibody in the serum have been of predictive value. Although the quantity of surface antibody has been shown under experimental conditions to be an important determinant of red cell destruction, this is not measured reliably in quantitative terms by the antiglobulin test.[26,96] In 1976, Bowdler[79] suggested that if techniques of investigation would become more available regarding both the qualitative and quantitative characteristics of immunoglobulin bound to the RBC surface, it would reasonably be anticipated that decisions about splenectomy would become more precise. This potential has not been realized in the more than a quarter-century since his remarks were published.

ADVERSE EFFECTS OF SPLENECTOMY

Surgical Morbidity and Mortality. The mortality and morbidity associated with splenectomy vary greatly, depending on the underlying disease for which

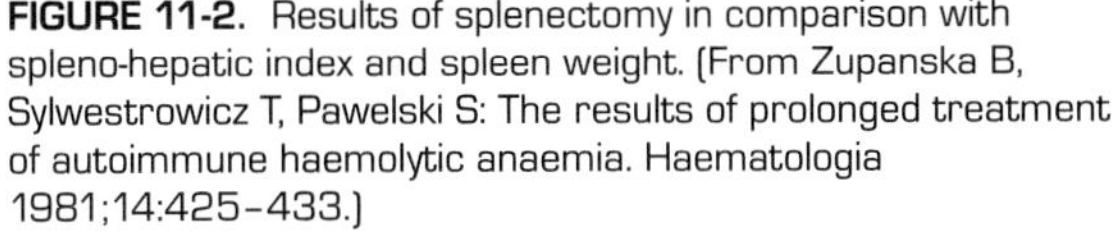

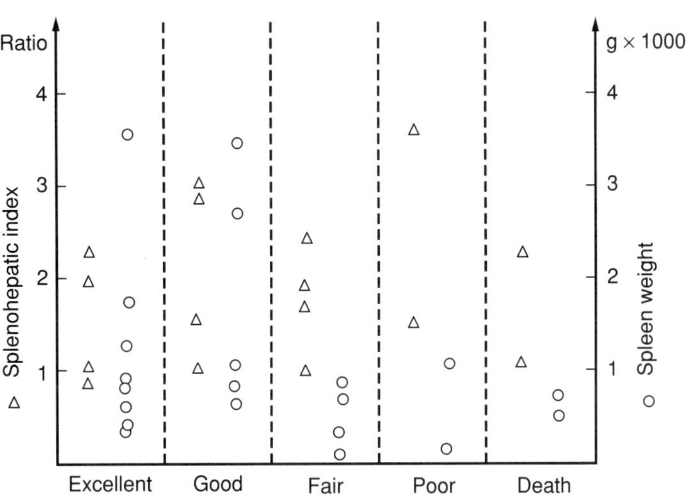

FIGURE 11-2. Results of splenectomy in comparison with spleno-hepatic index and spleen weight. (From Zupanska B, Sylwestrowicz T, Pawelski S: The results of prolonged treatment of autoimmune haemolytic anaemia. Haematologia 1981;14:425–433.)

the operation is performed. Thus, Schwartz and associates[66,97] reported on a series of 200 splenectomies for hematologic disorders in which a 7% mortality occurred during the immediate hospitalization. All deaths, however, occurred in patients with idiopathic thrombocytopenic purpura, thrombotic thrombocytopenic purpura, lymphomas, or leukemias. The immediate cause of death was usually cerebral hemorrhage caused by severe thrombocytopenia. In good risk patients who underwent elective splenectomy, no deaths occurred. Similar experience with almost identical mortality rates has been reported in other large series.[98-100]

Postoperative morbidity occurred in 18% of the patients reported on by Schwartz and colleagues.[66] The most frequent complication is that of left lower lobe atelectasis. Wound complications, septicemia, and development of subphrenic hematoma and abscess occurred almost exclusively in patients with myeloid metaplasia or hematologic malignancies with significant bleeding from the splenic bed.

Overwhelming Postsplenectomy Infection (OPSI). Morris and Bullock in 1919[101,102] were first to predict that removal of the spleen would result in an increased susceptibility to infection. King and Schumacher[103] reported in 1952 on five cases of fulminant sepsis in splenectomized infants with hereditary spherocytosis. In 1957, Smith and colleagues[104] presented his data on postsplenectomy infection in patients with thalassemia, and in 1960, Lucas and Krivit[105] published data on overwhelming infection in children following splenectomy. It was not until the 1970s, however, that a distinct syndrome became well defined and accepted, largely as a result of reviews by Singer[106] in 1973 and Krivit[102,107] in 1977 and 1979. Subsequently, a large body of data has accumulated concerning the incidence, prognosis, prevention, and management of this entity, and the syndrome of overwhelming postsplenectomy infection has been anointed with its own acronym, OPSI. Despite the large number of published cases, however, insufficient data exist to determine the true incidence, exact nature of infection, risk factors, and the contribution of underlying conditions.[108]

Clinical Findings. The initial prodrome may be mild and nonspecific, with flulike symptoms that include fever, malaise, myalgias, headache, vomiting, diarrhea, and abdominal pain.[109] The presence of gastrointestinal symptoms should never prevent the attending physician from entertaining a possible diagnosis of OPSI. Although meningitis or pneumonia accompanies OPSI in approximately 50% of cases, in many patients there is no obvious site of bacterial colonization. When sufficient detail has been reported in the literature, many patients will have had true rigors for a day or two before receiving definitive medical management.

This prodrome may be followed by rapid evolution to full-blown bacteremic septic shock accompanied by hypotension, anuria, and clinical evidence of disseminated intravascular coagulation, thus making this syndrome a true medical emergency. Severe hypoglycemia might also be present. The subsequent clinical course often mirrors that of the Waterhouse-Friderichsen syndrome, with bilateral adrenal hemorrhages noted at autopsy. Peripheral gangrene requiring amputations has been reported in survivors, secondary to the combination of hypotension and disseminated intravascular coagulation.

Despite appropriate antibiotics and intensive therapeutic intervention, the overall mortality in older published studies for established cases of OPSI varied from 50% to 70%.[108,110-112] More recent information suggests that when informed patients seek medical attention promptly, mortality could be reduced to the range of 10%.[109] Of those patients who die, more than 50% die within the first 48 hours of hospital admission. Among patients who survive, other sequelae have included deafness associated with either meningitis or mastoid osteomyelitis, and aortic insufficiency secondary to endocarditis.[110]

Responsible Organisms. Most instances of serious infection are due to encapsulated bacteria, such as *Pneumococcus* (*Streptococcus pneumoniae*). Other, less common organisms include *Haemophilus influenzae*, *Neisseria meningitides*, and *Escherichia coli*. Additional organisms that may cause OPSI include, but are not limited to, *Plasmodia* (malaria), *Babesia*, and *Capnocytophaga canimorsus* (an organism acquired from animal bites).

Incidence and Risk Factors. The precise incidence of OPSI remains controversial, and published estimates vary considerably.[109] Lynch and Kapila[108] reviewed all published series and, in 1996, indicated that the lifetime risk for OPSI was 5%. Children less than 15 years of age have a greater overall risk of OPSI (0.13%–8.1%) compared with adults (0.28%–1.9%). In one retrospective review of 5902 postsplenectomy patients studied between 1952 and 1987, the incidence of OPSI was 4.4% in children under 16 years and 0.9% in adults.[113] Another study calculated the risk of sepsis as 0.73 per 1000 person-years after splenectomy for hereditary spherocytosis.[114] Schwartz and coworkers[115] estimated the risk of fulminant infection as reasonably low—in the range of one case per 500 person-years of observation. The overall cumulative risk of infection severe enough to require hospitalization, however, was 33% by the end of a 10-year follow-up. Cullingford and associates[116] reported that the incidence of overwhelming infection after splenectomy was only 0.04 per 100 person years.

Most of the published data antedate the widespread availability of the pneumococcal and *Haemophilis influenzae* vaccines, so current rates could be lower. For instance, a Danish study found that the incidence of pneumococcal infection in splenectomized children decreased dramatically following the introduction of the pneumococcal vaccine and the promotion of early penicillin therapy for febrile episodes.[117]

In addition to age, major factors relating to risk include the reason for splenectomy and the subsequent time interval from splenectomy. Patients with thalassemia or sickle cell disorders and patients with lymphomas are at greatest risk.[108] Although most infections occur within the first 2 years after splenectomy, 33% of postsplenectomy pneumococcal infections and 42% of OPSI occurred more than 5 years after splenectomy.[108] The data of Waghorn and Mayon-White[118] indicate that OPSI occurs at any age and that it does not necessarily occur within the first few years after splenectomy (Table 11-8). OPSI has been reported as late as 59 years after splenectomy.[118]

Clinical and Laboratory Diagnostic Testing. Initial diagnosis must rely on a high index of clinical suspicion for any febrile presentation in a splenectomized patient, because aggressive early management is thought to be critical. Diagnostic work-up should never delay the initiation of empiric antibiotic therapy.

A quick and often helpful initial test is the examination of the peripheral blood smear and buffy coat for the presence of bacteria. Visualization of organisms on the peripheral smear suggests a quantitative bacteremia of greater than 10^6 micro-organisms/mL (10^4 or more greater than the usual bacteremia), which contributes greatly to morbidity and mortality.[108]

Blood cultures are usually positive within 24 hours and should be performed to identify the pathogen and guide subsequent therapy. Cultures should also be obtained from other sites, and lumbar puncture should be performed, especially in infants and children. Standard laboratory tests and appropriate x-ray studies are indicated, and the possibility of disseminated intravascular coagulation and septic shock should be anticipated.[109]

TABLE 11-8. SPLENECTOMY IN OPSI CASES

Ages of OPSI Cases

Age Group	No. of Cases (Total = 42)
<2 years	1
2–19 years	0
20–29 years	5
30–39 years	10
40–49 years	10
50–59 years	7
60–69 years	4
70–79 years	4
80–89 years	1

Time Interval from Splenectomy to OPSI

Time Interval	No. of Cases (Total = 40)*
<3 months	2
1–4 years	2
5–9 years	3
10–19 years	15
20–29 years	8
30–39 years	6
40–49 years	1
>50 years	2
Unknown	1

* Child with congenital asplenia and adult with severe splenic atrophy not included.
Modified from Waghorn DJ, Mayon-White RT: A study of 42 episodes of overwhelming postsplenectomy infection: Is current guidance for asplenic individuals being followed? J Infect 1997;35:289–294.

Managing Patients with OPSI. Although there is currently no proof that early treatment prevents incipient bacteremia from progressing to full-blown OPSI, the literature does support improved survival from an aggressive approach.[111] Possible choices of empiric antimicrobial agents useful fo the initial treatment of OPSI are included in Table 11-9.[109] Intravenous penicillin therapy generally has been superseded by broad-spectrum antibiotic therapy active against penicillin-resistant pneumococci, β-lactamase–producing *H. influenzae,* and other possible organisms that are not normally penicillin sensitive. Expert opinion from an infectious disease specialist should be sought urgently. Aggressive supportive care is necessary, including appropriate evaluation and any necessary management of disseminated intravascular coagulation and septic shock. The use of high-dose corticosteroids remains controversial but has not been demonstrated to be of benefit.[108]

Preventive Strategies. Education, immunoprophylaxis, and chemoprophylaxis are all considered important in the prevention of OPSI (Table 11-10).[119]

Patient education is a mandatory strategy in attempting to prevent OPSI. Unfortunately, studies have shown that 11%–50% of postsplenectomy patients remain unaware of their increased risk for serious infection or of the appropriate health precautions that should be undertaken.[109] Published guidelines regarding immunizations suggest that pneumococcal vaccine should be given a minimum of 2 weeks before elective splenectomy to ensure an optimal antibody response. If this is not practicable, the patient should be immunized as soon as possible after recovery from the operation. Reimmunization of asplenic patients is recommended every 5 to 10 years. Although there is a paucity of data showing clear clinical efficacy in asplenic patients, it is encouraging to note that in one reported series of asplenic hematology patients, only four episodes of pneumococcal septicemia/meningitis were observed in more 200 vaccinated individuals within a 13-year period, and in all four episodes, the infecting capsular type was not included in the vaccine.[120]

H. Influenza type B vaccine is also generally recommended for all patients who have not already received it.[121] The overall efficacy and utility of this vaccine is less clear than for pneumococcal vaccine, however, as most adults already have antibody and many infections involve non–type B strains.[109] The need for reimmunization is unclear.

The efficacy and importance of meningoccoccal vaccination in splenectomized individuals is unknown, although it is often recommended.[108,109] The current meningococcal vaccine covers types A, C, W135, and Y but misses other pathogenic strains.[109]

TABLE 11-9. EMPIRIC TREATMENT FOR SUSPECTED OVERWHELMING POSTSPLENECTOMY INFECTION

Drug	Adult Dose[a]	Pediatric Dose[a]
Cefotaxime	2 g IV every 8 hr	25–50 mg/kg IV every 6 hr
Ceftriaxone	2 g IV every 12–24 hr	50 mg/kg IV every 12 hr
+/− Gentamycin[b]	5–7 mg/kg IV every 24 hr	2.5 mg/kg IV every 8 hr
or		
+/− Ciprofloxacin[b,c]	400 mg IV every 12 hr	
+/− Vancomycin[d]	1–1.5 g IV every 12 hr	30 mg/kg IV every 12 hr

[a] Doses are for normal renal function and should be adjusted if creatinine clearance is reduced.
[b] Gentamycin or ciprofloxacin may be added if an enteric or urologic source of infection is suspected.
[c] Ciprofloxacin is not indicated for children.
[d] Vancomycin should be added when pneumococcus with high-level penicillin resistance is likely.
From Brigden ML, Pattullo AL: Prevention and management of overwhelming postsplenectomy infection—An update. Crit Care Med 1999;27:836–842.

Immunity appears to diminish over the course of a few years, suggesting a requirement for frequent boosters.

Influenza vaccine is recommended yearly and might be of particular value to asplenic patients by reducing the risk of secondary bacterial infection.[119]

The American Advisory Committee on Immunization Practices also recommends *Neisseria meningitides* vaccine.[122]

Most authorities recommend antibiotic prophylaxis for asplenic patients. Some recommend that lifelong prophylactic antibiotics should be offered in all cases—especially in the first 2 years after splenectomy—for all children up to age 16 and when there is underlying impaired immune function.[119] Traditionally, a single daily dose of penicillin or amoxicillin has constituted the regimen of choice. With the development of resistant organisms, however, antibiotics with broader activity have increasingly been utilized.[109]

TABLE 11-10. GUIDELINES FOR PREVENTION OF OPSI

- All splenectomized patients and those with functional hyposplenism should receive pneumococcal immunization (*a*, *b*).
- Documentation, communication, and reimmunization require attention (*a*, *b*).
- Patients not previously immunized should receive *Haemophilus influenzae* type b vaccine (*a*, *b*).
- Meningococcal immunization is not routinely recommended (*b*).
- Influenza immunization may be beneficial (*b*).
- Lifelong prophylactic antibiotics are recommended (oral phenoxymethylpenicillin or an alternative) (*a*, *b*).
- Asplenic patients are at risk of severe malaria (*a*).
- Animal and tick bites could be dangerous (*a*).
- Patients should be given a leaflet and a card to alert health professionals to their risk of overwhelming infection (*a*, *b*).
- Patients developing infection despite measures must be given a systemic antibiotic and urgently admitted to hospital (*a*, *b*).

a = Based on published evidence.
b = Expert opinion.
nb: There are no randomized controlled trials or case-controlled studies on this issue.
From Working Party of the British Committee for Standards in Haematology Clinical Haematology Task Force: Guidelines for the prevention and treatment of infection in patients with an absent or dysfunctional spleen. Br Med J 1996; 312:430–434. Reprinted with permission of the BMJ Publishing Group.

In contrast, Flegg[121] suggests that beyond 5 years postoperatively in adulthood, by which time the risks of overwhelming infection are much reduced, prophylaxis should be reserved for only the most vulnerable subgroups, that is, those with malignant or hematological disease.

Perhaps the biggest problem in managing postsplenectomy patients is the lack of implementation of the foregoing preventive strategies. Waghorn and Mayon-White[118] reported 42 cases of OPSI. They found that pneumococcal infection had caused at least 37 of the 42 episodes, but only 12 patients had received pneumococcal vaccine. They concluded that much more needs to be done to ensure that asplenic patients are warned of the risks of infection and provided with appropriate prophylactic measures. Similarly, Deodhar and colleagues[123] reported that among 184 patients who had had a splenectomy during a 12-year period, 58% had not received advice or prophylaxis against infection and only 36% had received pneumococcal vaccination.

In addition, for patients not allergic to penicillin, a supply of amoxycillin should be kept available, and the patient should be instructed in immediate self-medication should symptoms of fever, malaise, or shivering develop. Others recommend cefotaxime or ceftriaxone as empiric treatment for symptomatic patients who have been taking antibiotic prophylaxis.[109] In any case, the patient should also seek immediate medical help.

Thrombocytosis. An additional potential complication of splenectomy is the development of postsplenectomy thrombocytosis and thromboembolism. Splenectomy is usually followed by a mild, symptomless thrombocytosis that reaches a peak at about the end of the second week and gradually subsides within 3 months.[124] Occasionally, however, postsplenectomy thrombocytosis persists. Hirsh and Dacie[124] studied the postsplenectomy platelet count in patients suffering from various types of anemia and in hematologically normal persons. Persistent postsplenectomy thrombocytosis was noted in all patients with continuing anemia after splenectomy, and the height of the persistent thrombocytosis was closely related to the severity of the anemia ($P < 0.001$). No such relationship existed between the platelet count and hemoglobin level in a comparable group of patients who had not been subjected to splenectomy. Visudhiphan and coworkers[125] also found a significant negative correlation between hemoglobin level and platelet count following splenectomy (Fig. 11-3).[125] Hirsh and Dacie[124] suggested that in the presence of active hemopoiesis, anemia stimulates both thrombopoiesis and erythropoiesis, but that increased thrombopoiesis does not result in persistent thrombocytosis unless the spleen is removed. They indicated that the persistence of thrombocytosis after splenectomy can usually be predicted; this happens when anemia continues after splenectomy in association with active hemopoiesis.

Hirsh and Dacie[124] also pointed out that postsplenectomy thromboembolism in association with postsplenectomy thrombocytosis has been reported after splenectomy, and they reported on five patients in whom this complication occurred out of 80 patients who had undergone splenectomy for hematologic disease. Four of the five patients had congenital hemolytic anemias, but none of the patients in their series had an acquired immune hemolytic anemia. The authors were careful to point out that many other patients in their series had comparable increases in the postsplenectomy platelet count, which had been maintained for many years without development of thromboembolism.

Indeed, a relationship between postsplenectomy thrombocytosis and the incidence of thromboembolism is not always found. Boxer[126] reported an incidence of thromboembolic complications of 3.9% with increased platelet counts, compared with 1.3% in patients who did not have thrombocytosis following splenectomy (the difference was not statistically significant). On the other hand, Traetow[127] reported a 6% incidence of thromboembolism in 223 patients with postsplenectomy thrombocytosis, compared with 0.4% in 250 patients with postoperative platelet counts of less than 400,000/µL. Both of these groups noted that if the platelet count was greater than 1,000,000/µL, there was no further increase in thromboembolic risk.

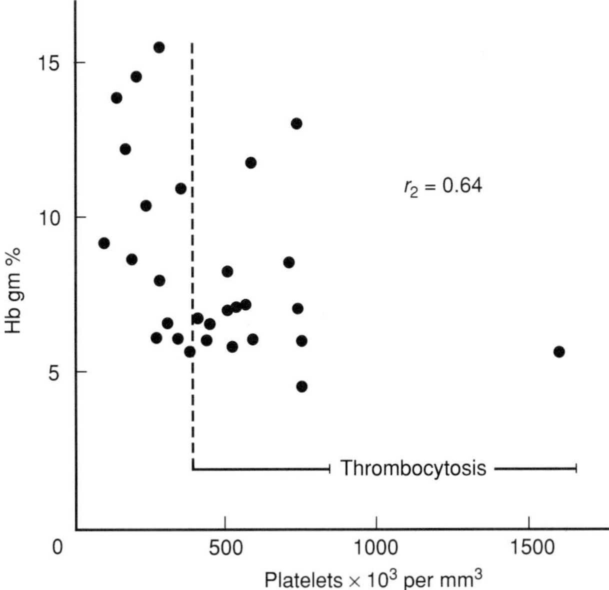

FIGURE 11-3. The correlation between hemoglobin level (g/dL) and platelet count in 29 splenectomized subjects. (From Visudhiphan S, Ketsa-Ard K, Piankijagum A, Tumliang S: Blood coagulation and platelet profiles in persistent post-splenectomy thrombocytosis: The relationship to thromboembolism. Biomed Pharmacother 1985;39:264–271.)

Coon and colleagues[128] studied 86 patients who underwent elective splenectomy and detected deep vein thrombosis in five patients by using labeled fibrinogen and dye phlebography. In none of these five patients, however did an elevation in platelet count to 600,000/µL develop before or at the time of development of the thrombosis. None of 21 other patients who had a rise in platelet count to greater than 1,000,000/µL had evidence of venous thrombosis.

Clearly, other factors are important in the etiology of postsplenectomy thromboembolic complications.[129] A number of authors have indicated that the thromboembolic risk is highest among patients with hypersplenism and myeloprolifertive disorders such as chronic myelogenous leukemia, agnogenic myeloid metaplasia, and polycythemia vera.[129,130] Some authors found no substsantial increase in thromboembolic risk in patients without myeloproliferative disease.[126,131]

Bensinger and coworkers[132] reported on four patients (none of whom had AIHA) who developed hemorrhagic complications associated with "spectacular" thrombocytosis postsplenectomy. Therapy with melphalan (L-phenylalanine mustard) effectively controlled the abnormal thrombocytosis and the clinical evidence of disease.

Coon and colleagues[128] concluded that there was no need for the routine administration of prophylactic antithrombotic therapy in patients in whom postsplenectomy thrombocytosis develops.

Thus, patients who have undergone splenectomy for AIHA may develop thrombocytosis if anemia persists, but there are no clear indications for treatment unless hemorrhagic or thromboembolic phenomena occur.

ABNORMAL LABORATORY TESTS FOLLOWING SPLENECTOMY

Pseudohyperkalemia may be encountered following splenectomy as a result of the in vitro release of intracellular potassium from platelets during clotting.[133-135] This can be avoided by using heparinized tubes with plasma separated without delay.

The reduction or absence of normal splenic function can be recognized by certain hematologic changes.[136,137] Some of these are nonspecific, such as a slight to moderate increase in the white cell count and platelet count.

Findings of Howell-Jolly bodies, pitted erythrocytes, and target cells in the blood smear, however, are of greater diagnostic significance. For reasons that still remain unknown, the red cell surface area is increased after splenectomy, causing buckling and target cell formation.[138] Nuclear fragments that normally are removed in the spleen are present in circulating red cells and are termed *Howell-Jolly bodies*.[138] They are almost always present in the asplenic state, but only 1 of 100 to 1 of 1000 RBCs is affected. A sensitive indication of hyposplenism is the appearance of pits or pocks on the cell surface.[138a,b,139] They consist of submembraneous vacuoles and can be seen only in wet preparations of RBCs using direct interference-contrast microscopy.[139]

Oxidative drugs may produce Heinz bodies even in normal individuals, but those RBC inclusions are removed effectively by the spleen. After splenectomy, they may be observed in supravital-stained blood films. Nucleated RBCs, on the other hand, are seen only rarely on blood films after splenectomy, except in patients with hemolytic disorders, in whom their number may increase dramatically.[136]

Mature circulating RBCs containing persistent granules of nonheme iron are called siderocytes, while nucleated red cells bearing iron-containing inclusions are designated sideroblasts. In both cases, the iron-containing particles are known as siderotic granules. Siderocytes are best demonstrated with the Prussian blue staining technique and are not detectable on ordinary Wright-Giemsa–stained blood smears. A few siderocytes can be found in the blood of an asplenic but otherwise normal person, whereas substantial numbers may be found in asplenic individuals with an underlying hematologic disease such as sideroblastic or Heinz-body anemia.[137]

Splenic Irradiation

Splenic irradiation can be an effective modality in controlling AIHA and is utilized most often when patients are too ill for splenectomy.[140] Markus and Forfar[141] described a 73-year-old male with AIHA unresponsive to corticosteroids, whose condition precluded splenectomy. A course of splenic irradiation was given, and his hemoglobin concentration subsequently rose to normal.

Immunosuppressive Drugs

Since the publication of the first edition of this book,[1] there have been remarkable advances in the development of immunosuppressive drugs. Indeed, the discipline of human organ transplantation has made major strides because of significantly more effective immunosuppressive drug regimens, and they have been used increasingly for management of autoimmune diseases.[142,143]

The new millennium seems to have inspired a number of comprehensive reviews that provide a wealth of information regarding the various drugs, their mechanisms of action, pharmacokinetics, effectiveness, and adverse effects.[142,144-146] Unfortunately, however, the literature regarding the appropriate use of these drugs in the treatment of AIHA is meager and consists largely of anecdotal case reports.

EARLY REPORTS

Dacie[6] has reviewed the early medical literature regarding the development and use of immunosuppressive alkylating and antimetabolite drugs for the therapy for warm antibody AIHA. Some of the more informative of these early reports include that of Schwartz and Dameshek,[147] who reported the results of the use of antimetabolites in 14 patients. This series included six idiopathic cases, two associated with systemic lupus erythematosus (SLE), and single cases associated with myxedema, hepatitis, chronic lymphocytic leukemia, Dilantin ingestion, virus infection, and rheumatoid arthritis. Two patients were treated exclusively with immunosuppressive drugs. Nine of the 14 patients experienced a beneficial effect of therapy with either 6-mercaptopurine or thioguanine at a dosage of 2.5 mg/kg. Of nine patients who were prior steroid failures, four had good responses, and one had a partial response to cytotoxic therapy.

Taylor[148] reported on a patient with AIHA and possible Hodgkin's disease who failed to respond to corticosteroids and splenectomy. Over the next 6 years, remissions of the hemolytic state were induced with triethylene melamine, chlorambucil, and cyclophosphamide.

Hitzig and Massimo[149] treated three children with AIHA with azathioprine at a dosage of 2.5 mg/kg in combination with steroid therapy. In one patient there was a complete response, and two experienced a partial response that permitted the reduction of steroid dosage.

Habibi and colleagues[70] treated seven children with AIHA with azathioprine, four of whom obtained good responses.

Worlledge[150] reported that 6 of 14 patients treated with 75–200 mg of azathioprine daily had a good response, and 1 patient had a partial response. The duration of treatment ranged from 4 months to 6 years.

Skinner and Schwartz[151,152] reviewed 42 reported cases of warm antibody AIHA. Most of the patients were treated with a combination of azathioprine and corticosteroids, and in many cases splenectomy was performed before the azathioprine had been instituted. All patients seemed to have failed to respond to corticosteroid treatment. Twenty of the 42 patients (48%) were said to have improved with immunosuppressive therapy. Unfortunately, no objective criteria for improvement were listed in many cases, and the response was often merely described as "beneficial."

A similar analysis of the literature by Mueller-Eckhardt and Kretschmer[153] reported a 45% incidence of "good" response in 66 patients with AIHA treated with cytotoxic drugs.

Johnson and Abildgaard[154] reviewed the literature relating to pediatric patients and described two additional cases. In all, 9 of 17 patients (53%) showed improvement. Eight of the nine children who improved received azathioprine as one of their immunosuppressive agents, but at least four children who failed to improve also had received this drug.

SUBSEQUENT REPORTS

Moyo and associates[155] studied high-dose cyclophosphamide (50 mg/kg ideal body weight per day intravenously for 4 days) without stem cell rescue in nine patients with severe refractory AIHA. The patients had not responded to a median of three (range, 1–7) other treatments. The median time to reach an absolute neutrophil count of 500/µL or greater was 16 days (range, 12–18 days). Six patients achieved complete remission, and none relapsed after a median follow-up of 15 months (range, 4–29 months). Three patients achieved and continued in partial remission. The therapy was well tolerated.

Zupanska and coworkers[11] reported that of 80 idiopathic and secondary AIHA patients originally treated with prednisone, 43 needed additional treatment with azathioprine or cyclophosphamide; 26 of these (60.5%) responded favorably.

Worlledge[10] summarized her experience with the use of azathioprine as follows: 15 patients had been treated for 3.5 months to 2.5 years; six patients had responded well, two had responded partially, and six had failed to respond. One patient presented with signs of Hodgkin's disease after 2.5 years of treatment; one patient developed leukopenia; none became thrombocytopenic.

Heisel and Ortega[156] reported that seven children with chronic AIHA who were steroid dependent had been treated with immunosuppressive drugs; only one had achieved a complete remission.

Panceri and colleagues[147] reported the case of a 5-month-old boy with a life-threatening AIHA that was unresponsive to therapy with steroids, high-dose immunoglobulin, azathioprine, and splenectomy. Despite these therapies, the patient's condition worsened, his hemoglobin level remained below 4 g/dL, and he required two to three blood transfusions daily. Immunosuppression was increased by giving high-dose methylprednisolone (40 mg/kg/day) followed by high-dose cyclophosphamide (10 mg/kg/day for 10 days). The child showed a striking, sudden improvement starting on the fifth day of high-dose cyclophosphamide therapy, followed by complete recovery. No major long-term complications were observed.

Silva and coworkers[157] reported two patients with severe AIHA who had failed multiple treatment modalities and subsequently were treated with synchronization of cyclophosphamide and plasma exchange.

VINCA ALKALOIDS

The therapeutic effects of vinca alkaloids in AIHA have not been investigated systematically.[158] There have been some anecdotal reports of benefit after the use of vinblastine and vincristine, however.[159,160] Vincristine was generally given as part of a multiple-drug regimen, often to patients with underlying lymphoproliferative disorders.[161-163]

Dovat and associates[164] reported an 8-month-old male with X-linked lymphoproliferative disease who underwent an unrelated, partially matched (with major mismatch at DR locus) cord blood stem cell transplant. Four months following the transplant, he developed immune thrombocytopenia with hemolytic anemia (Evans's syndrome). He received multiple courses of intravenous immunoglobulin, anti-Rh D immunoglobulin, a pulse of high-dose corticosteroids, and cyclosporine with some improvement of hemolytic anemia, but no improvement of the thrombocytopenia. Addition of vincristine resulted in long-term resolution of thrombocytopenia and anemia. No major toxicity was observed during treatment.

INDICATIONS AND THERAPEUTIC REGIMENS

On the basis of the preceding reports, immunosuppressive drugs appear to be beneficial in some patients with WAIHA. Most clinicians suggest their use after both corticosteroids and splenectomy have failed to produce an adequate remission, and if it is further demonstrated that an adequate remission is not possible using small doses of prednisone after splenectomy.[165] Immunosuppressive drugs may be used instead of splenectomy, however, if contraindications to surgery exist, but many physicians opt first for the use of other, less toxic measures.

Several authors have recommended regimens for the administration of immunosuppressive drugs to patients with AIHA.[2,165-168] These regimens have been designed arbitrarily and are quite similar. Azathioprine in a dose of 1–2 mg/kg/day or cyclophosphamide (1.5–2 mg/kg/day) can be used to initiate cytotoxic drug therapy. If corticosteroids have been responsible for an incomplete remission prior to the initiation of therapy with immunosuppressive drugs, they should be continued until signs of hematologic improvement occur, at which time they should be reduced gradually in dosage and discontinued if possible. Murphy and LoBuglio[166] recommend continuing immunosuppressive drug therapy at the initial dosage for 6 months in those who respond, although this is evidently an empiric recommendation, and a shorter period of time may be chosen. It is possible that, for adults, maintenance doses of 25 mg every other day or even twice weekly might suffice.

In patients who do not respond after 4 weeks of therapy, the alternative drug can be substituted, or the dose of the drug used initially can be increased by increments of 25 mg/day every 2 weeks until a response or limiting side effects occur. Particularly important adverse effects are gastrointestinal intolerance and evidence of marrow depression as manifested by leukopenia, thrombocytopenia, or increasing anemia with reticulocytopenia. Additional adverse effects of cyclophosphamide are hemorrhagic cystitis, alopecia, and adverse effects on the reproductive system. Blood counts should be obtained weekly during the first month of therapy and for a similar period of time after each dose increase. Thereafter, blood counts should be performed biweekly for several months and, if they become stable, monthly thereafter.

If a therapeutic response occurs while the patient is being maintained at full dosage but hemolysis reappears during decrease of the cytotoxic agent, full doses should be reinstituted for several additional months. If the relapse occurs after the patient has been in remission for some time after all drugs have been withdrawn, a trial of corticosteroids alone has a chance of success and may be considered before proceeding to additional cytotoxic therapy.[166]

ADVERSE EFFECTS

Although some adverse effects of immunosuppressive drug therapy have already been mentioned, a more complete discussion of possible complications is warranted.

Infection. There is little doubt that the major immediate complication of cytotoxic drug therapy is infection. It is also noteworthy that most patients, at the dose levels recommended in the preceding paragraphs, seem to do well over extended periods without apparent trouble from exogenous organisms. Specifically, pyogenic organisms do not seem to cause an unexpected amount of disease in these patients provided that the granulocyte count is maintained at adequate levels. Granulocytopenia of less than 1000 polymorphonuclear leukocytes/µL is much more likely to result in disseminated pyogenic infection that is unresponsive to antibiotics.

Even without the presence of leukopenia, several classes of agents can give trouble. Herpes zoster is very common but usually heals uneventfully. Dissemination of herpes zoster virus has been recognized, with death from this organism; deaths from chickenpox pneumonia and systemic measles have also been reported. Rarer viral agents apparently also produce major illnesses in the immunosuppressed patient.

Other organisms that cause "intracellular infections" are organisms to which cellular immunity appears to be of more importance to the host's defenses than is circulating antibody. Mycotic and mycobacterial infections are in this group.

Virtually all the fungi have been seen to disseminate under cytotoxic therapy, usually with a fatal outcome. Infections with fungi that are ordinarily not of great pathogenetic significance for man, such as *Nocardia* or *Aspergillus*, have been shown to be a hazard for the cytotoxic-treated patient. The same is true of a number of bacterial organisms: *Listeria, Herellea, Serratia,* and the like.

To summarize, the most important immediate problem for patients taking cytostatic drugs is infection from a great variety of organisms, some common and some exotic.

Impaired Fertility. Immunosuppressive drugs can affect conception, pregnancy, fetal development, and lactation.[169] An important risk of some of these medications is that of sterilization.[169] In treating nonmalignant disease of various types, there are substantial chances for long-term remission, periods when procreation could be of the utmost concern to the patient. These potential side effects represent serious problems, which must be dealt with in discussing the use of the medications, especially with youthful patients.

Teratogenic Side Reactions. All drugs affecting nucleic acid and protein metabolism exhibit teratogenicity in animals. The doses necessary to trigger this effect vary greatly from compound to compound, and with the same compound from species to species, considerations that make it difficult to extrapolate conclusions from animals to humans. Men should be apprised of the possibility of teratogenicity, and women must be informed of the risks of congenital malformations and must use effective methods of contraception.[169] Cytotoxic drugs may be used after the first trimester to treat life-threatening disease, although this would seem to rarely be necessary in patients with AIHA.[169]

Neoplasia. One of the most difficult of all problems related to cytotoxic agents is the potential threat of neoplasia, perhaps first becoming apparent only years after initial exposure to a drug.[170-173] The increased prevalence of neoplasia in the immunosuppressed patient after organ transplantation is an unequivocal fact. Admittedly, this information cannot necessarily be extended to cover those patients whose diseases require more modest doses of cytotoxic drugs.

The explanation for the development of malignant disease in patients treated with cytotoxic drugs is not clear. The most commonly expressed view is that, in their immunosuppressed state, immune surveillance is defective and that mutant or perhaps virus-transformed cells that would be promptly destroyed in a normal person are instead permitted to survive and multiply.

NEWER AGENTS

Cyclosporine. Cyclosporine has had a major effect on human organ transplantation since its approval in 1983.[146] It is a potent immunosuppressive drug, reflecting its ability to block the transcription of cytokine genes in activated T cells,[174] and it has been used for therapy of a variety of autoimmune diseases.[175] A number of reports attest to its effectiveness in patients with AIHA.

Emilia and coworkers[176] used cyclosporine therapy for three patients with AIHA and one with Evans's syndrome. All patients had resistant, life-threatening hemolysis and were refractory to previous treatments. The treatment protocol was as follows: Cyclosporine was begun at an initial total dose of 5 mg/kg/day and administered twice daily for 6 days, after which the dose was reduced to 3 mg/kg/day and continued with slight changes to maintain a serum level between 200 and 400 ng/mL. To increase cyclosporine blood concentration, low-dose prednisone (5 mg/day) was added also.[177]

All three patients with AIHA achieved a complete response, and the patient with Evans's syndrome responded partially. All patients required continued cyclosporine administration to maintain remission. Adverse effects included a slight elevation of creatinine level but no persistent nephrotoxicity. Hypertension requiring drug therapy was always resolved with dose adjustments. The simultaneous administration of grapefruit juice enabled a 25% reduction of the drug dose.[178,179] An adverse effect of chlorambucil was seen in one patient, leading to a dramatic decrease of cyclosporine levels.[180] The authors suggest that cyclosporine should be recommended for refractory patients because it shows long-term efficacy and safety and is able to maintain remission at low doses without significant side effects. They further suggest that its use be considered before immunosuppressive chemotherapy to avoid myelotoxicity or mutagenic effects.

Dundar and associates[181] reported a patient with Evans's syndrome who was refractory to conventional and high-dose methylprednisolone treatment and to splenectomy. The patient experienced excellent benefit from cyclosporine; his hematological values were completely normal at the 12th month of therapy, without any side effect from the drug.

Hershko and colleagues[182] reported results of cyclosporine treatment in two patients with AIHA and one with Evans's syndrome. All three were responsive initially to standard corticosteroid treatment but relapsed despite continued therapy. All improved significantly following the introduction of cyclosporine. Follow-up was a maximum of 8 months at the time of the report.

Rackoff and Manno[183] described the clinical course of a 6-year-old child with severe Evans's syndrome who had experienced life-threatening episodes of hemolysis despite the use of multiple therapeutic modalities. Cyclosporine was given at a dose of 10 mg/kg/day divided into two doses on alternate days. The hemoglobin and platelet counts both improved, and it was possible to reduce the patient's prednisone dose from 2 mg/kg/day to as low as 1 mg/kg every other day. With this regimen, the patient had less severe hemolytic anemia, was less thrombocytopenic, and had fewer hospitalizations. At the time of the report, the patient had completed almost 2 years of alternate-day cyclosporine and prednisone therapy, with minimal toxic effects attributable to cyclosporine.

Some authors have reported that cyclosporine, when used to treat patients with AIHA associated with B-cell chronic lymphocytic leukemia, not only controled the hemolysis but also reduced the leukemic mass.[184] In contrast, Emilia and colleagues[185] treated a patient with B-cell chronic lymphocytic leukemia who had repeated episodes of AIHA that were resistant to therapy, which included high-dose prednisone, cyclophosphamide, antilymphocyte globulin, and splenectomy. As a result of cyclosporine treatment, the patient's hemoglobin level improved rapidly and was maintained at a normal level. After a 5-month decrease of the white blood count with a reduction of lymph node size, however, the chronic lymphocytic leukemia progressed with an increasing WBC count and lymph node enlargement.

A number of reports of failure of cyclosporine therapy in AIHA also exist.[186-188]

When cyclosporine is used to treat patients with autoimmune disease, the potential for toxicity—particularly nephrotoxicity—during long-term use is a significant concern. Because patients are at risk for irreversible and perhaps progressive changes in renal structure, one must consider the risk-benefit ratio carefully before deciding whether to treat them with cyclosporine.[175]

Mycophenolate Mofetil. Mycophenolate mofetil has a potent cytostatic effect on lymphocytes; this is the principal mechanism by which the drug exerts immunosuppressive effects.[189,190] The FDA has approved marketing of the drug for prevention of rejection in patients with allogeneic renal transplants.[191] It prolongs allograft survival and reverses graft rejection; it has also been used to treat rheumatoid arthritis and psoriasis. Nephrotoxicity and overt hepatotoxicity have not been reported, but the drug could be linked to bone marrow suppression and certain malignancies.[191]

Zimmer-Molsberger and coworkers[192] used mycophenolate mofetil as second-line treatment for two patients with severe AIHA, both of whom had been treated with 2-chlorodesoxyadenosine (2-CDA) for B-cell lymphocytic leukemia. Both patients had been treated unsuccessfully for hemolysis with oral prednisolone therapy. One patient had an excellent response to mycophenolate mofetil, which resulted in the cessation of blood transfusion support and a hemoglobin level of greater than 12 g/dL for more than 32 weeks. The other patient, who developed insulin-dependent diabetes and varicella zoster infection while on prednisolone, was able to discontinue corticosteroid therapy. His response was incomplete, but he did develop a decreased transfusion requirement.

Howard and colleagues[193] reported the use of mycophenolate mofetil in four patients with AIHA and six with idiopathic thrombocytopenic purpura (ITP). All four patients with AIHA showed a complete or good partial response to treatment.

Rituximab. Rituximab (Rituxan) is a genetically engineered chimeric murine/human monoclonal antibody designed to target the CD20 antigen.[194,195] CD20 expression is restricted to B-cell precursors and mature B cells and is not found on uncommitted hematopoietic precursor stem cells, plasma cells, dendritic cells, or other normal tissues. The drug is highly effective for in vivo B-cell depletion, with B-lymphocytes becoming undetectable in peripheral blood after a single infusion and recovering only 6 to 9 months after discontinuation of treatment.[196] The antibody was introduced for the treatment of B-cell lymphomas.[196-199] Rituximab has also been used in the treatment of immune thrombocytopenia[200,201] and AIHA in an attempt to decrease the number of platelet or anti-RBC antibody-producing B cells. Experience with the drug is accumulating rapidly; many anecdotal experiences and a few rather small series of patients have been reported.[201a]

The drug represents an appealing and promising treatment modality for patients with the most severe and/or refractory forms of AIHA. In refractory or chronic disease, the use of rituximab is attractive because it could reduce or avoid some side effects of prolonged therapy with corticosteroids and other immunosuppressive drugs. Serious adverse effects have also been reported, however (see the discussion that follows).

Clinical Effectiveness. Lee and associates[202] reported the results of rituximab treatment of six patients with AIHA. Three patients had cold agglutinin syndrome, and three had WAIHA. Low-grade lymphoma was diagnosed in three subjects. Prior therapy consisted of steroids, chemotherapy, splenectomy, and plasmapheresis, with disease duration ranging from 3 months to 20 years. Rituximab (375 mg/m^2) was administered once weekly for 4 weeks. One patient received six infusions of rituximab. Of five evaluable patients, all had complete hematological responses as indicated by the hemoglobin and hematocrit values. One subject was retreated with rituximab after 5 months, with continued response for an additional 10 months. The duration of response ranged between 4 months and 2.7 years. The authors stated that no unusual toxicity or complications occurred as a result of the treatment.

Grossi and colleagues[203] treated five patients with autoimmune hematologic disorders with rituximab. Three patients had ITP, and two subjects had ITP plus AIHA (Evans's syndrome). The patients were refractory to steroids, high-dose IgG, splenectomy, and immunosuppressive treatments that included cytotoxic agents. Platelet counts increased and remained stable in one patient with ITP plus AIHA after 6 months, although further therapy was required. A decrease in hemoglobin was noted in another patient with ITP plus AIHA who did not respond to therapy and subsequently expired. No improvement of platelet count was observed in the remaining patients.

Rai and coworkers[204] reported treatment with a combination of rituximab, cyclophosphamide, and dexamethasone in eight patients with chronic lymphocytic leukemia who had AIHA. All subjects responded to therapy, with one patient achieving a normal hemoglobin level. The median duration of response was reported as greater than 12 months, with one patient experiencing a relapse after 11 months.

Ahrens and associates[205] described a 68-year-old man with an 8-year history of AIHA refractory to treatment with prednisolone, azathioprine, cyclophosphamide, mycophenolate-mofetil, and pulsed high-dose dexamethasone. Rituximab was given once a week for 4 weeks, with baseline therapy consisting of prednisolone, 15 mg/day (Fig. 11-4). CD19-positive cells in the peripheral blood decreased from 4% to undetectable levels and remained below 0.05% of the lymphocytes. Although the DAT remained positive, hemolysis decreased during the 6 months of observation after treatment, and his hemoglobin rose from 8.4 to 12.3 g/dL. Although the reticulocyte count remained elevated and the haptoglobin value remained low, the patient became largely asymptomatic.

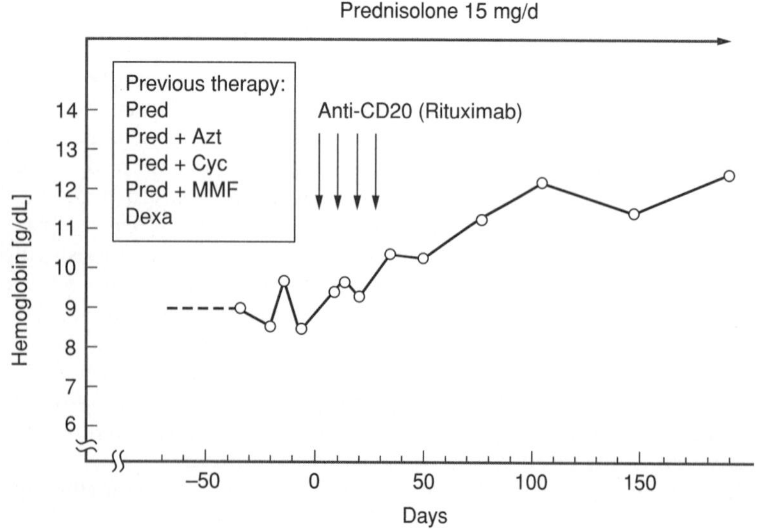

FIGURE 11-4. Hemoglobin concentration after rituximab application (4 × 375 mg/m^2) in a patient with refractory autoimmune haemolytic anaemia. Pred, prednisolone; Azt, azathioprine 2 mg/kg/d; Cyc, cyclophosphamide 1–3 mg/kg/d; MMF, mycophenolate mofetil 2 g/d; Dexa, dexamethasone 40 mg (once). (From Ahrens N, Kingreen D, Seltsam A, Salama A: Treatment of refractory autoimmune haemolytic anaemia with anti-CD20 (rituximab). Br J Haematol 2001;114:244–245.)

Seipelt and colleagues[206] reported a 65-year-old male with CLL and Evans's syndrome. Therapy with cyclophosphamide, vincristine, and prednisone lead to an improvement of hemolysis, but the patient remained thrombocytopenic. Subsequently, lymphocytes increased to 135,000/µL, and cyclophosphamide 3 g/m^2 was given without effect on the peripheral lymphocyte count. At this stage, therapy with rituximab (375 mg/m^2 four times weekly) was initiated. The platelet count normalized within 1 week after the first dose of rituxuimab, and the lymphocyte count dropped within 2 months to 11,000/µL.

Circulating CD19 and CD20 cells were no longer detectable within 2 weeks of treatment, and B cells did not reappear in blood until 5 to 9 months after the last treatment. Normal counts were then reached within the following month in all patients. Immunoglobulin concentrations in serum fell below normal values for age during the same period. Five patients were kept on prophylactic intravenous immunoglobulin replacement for 9 to 10 months after the last rituximab infusion. Normal hemoglobin concentrations and reticulocyte counts of fewer than 100 × 10^9/L were achieved in all cases within 4 months; these levels persisted until the last follow-up, 15–22 months after the start of rituximab. Coombs tests became negative, and associated autoimmune features resolved within 12 weeks.

Rituximab's effectiveness was not limited to the period of profound B-cell depletion, as no patient relapsed thereafter within a 5- to 14-month follow-up. The authors concluded that the optimal number of rituximab infusions required to be effective still remains to be determined. They suggested that a reduction to one or two injections—which would limit the duration of the B-cell deficiency—would be worth assessing.

Perrotta and colleagues[207] reported an 18-year-old girl with SLE and life-threatening AIHA that did not respond to steroids, intravenous immunoglobulin, or cyclosporin A. Rituximab was given weekly at 375 mg/m^2 for two doses. The drug was well tolerated, and the patient experienced no adverse effects. Her hemolytic disorder ameliorated markedly, with a progressive increase of hemoglobin levels, starting a few days after therapy. The patient remained disease-free 7 months later.

Chemnitz and coworkers[208] reported a 63-year-old female with chronic lymphocyte leukemia who developed AIHA that was unresponsive to corticosteroids and three cycles of chemotherapy with cyclophosphamide. She was treated subsequently with rituximab (375 mg/m^2 intravenously for 4 weeks). The patient's condition improved rapidly, transfusions were no longer needed, and prednisone was reduced to 10 mg per day.

McMahon and associates[209] described a 16-year-old boy with AIHA who repeatedly relapsed after aggressive therapy over a period of about 8 years. Treatment included corticosteroids, IVIG, azathioprine, vincristine, splenectomy, cyclosporine, plasmapheresis, antithymocyte globulin, and transfusions. Subsequent treatment with two courses of rituximab, each consisting of four doses of 375 mg/m^2 at weekly intervals, led to complete remission, which was sustained for 19 months at the time of the report.

Seeliger and colleagues[210] reported the clinical course of a 6-year-old boy with refractory AIHA. Due to failure of conventional immunosuppressive therapy, an autologous peripheral blood stem cell transplantation was performed. He showed a partial response, with a reduced demand for RBC transfusions. Due to persistence of the hemolytic process, however, he was started on rituximab therapy on the 40th day after transplantation. Following two doses of rituximab, the patient improved rapidly and developed a sustained complete response. After 10 months, hemolysis recurred and again responded to rituximab therapy without the necessity for RBC transfusions. Some 15 months after initial antibody treatment, however, the patient developed a second relapse, which was now refractory to rituximab therapy, although CD20+ B lymphocytes were cleared from the peripheral blood. The authors concluded that rituximab and autologous peripheral blood stem cell transplantation are important, though not curative, elements in the treatment of patients with severe AIHA who are refractory to conventional immunosuppressive therapy.

Further favorable results of rituximab therapy for warm antibody AIHA have been reported by a number of other investigators,[211-213] including a report of one patient with mixed warm and cold AIHA.[214] Also see the section on cold agglutinin syndrome later in this chapter.

Rituximab in Young Children. Quartier and colleagues[215] reported the effectiveness of rituximab in six children with severe AIHA that was refractory to prednisone therapy that included pulsed intravenous methylprednisolone or to combination therapy with immunosuppressive drugs, and (in two cases) to splenectomy. Four rituximab infusions were given intravenously at a dose of 375 mg/m^2 once a week. Patients three and five received eight additional infusions at the same dose over the course of 14 weeks. Results are illustrated in Figure 11-5.

Ng and coworkers[216] reported the case of an 8-week-old infant with fulminant AIHA refractory to conventional therapy. Massive hemolysis resulted in cardiac decompensation and acute renal failure, which necessitated mechanical ventilation and peritoneal dialysis. Rituximab halted progression of the hemolytic process, but the patient died of acute viral pneumonia and disseminated fungal infection.

Zecca and associates[196] described the case of an 18-month-old child with immune-mediated pure red cell aplasia and AIHA refractory to first- and second-line immunosuppressive therapy, who was successfully treated with rituximab. The authors used replacement therapy with intravenous immunoglobulins, as the

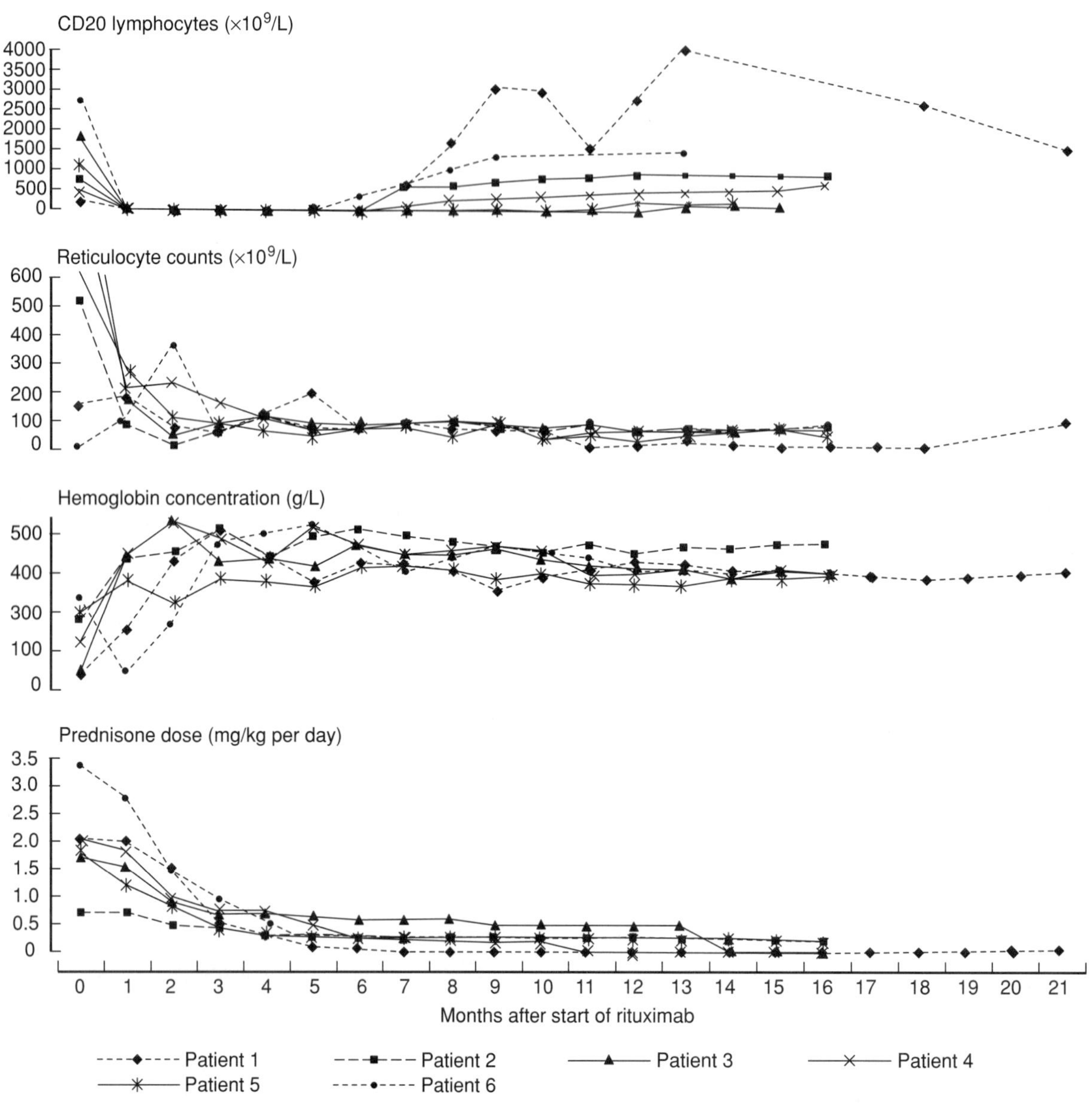

FIGURE 11-5. Changes in biological variables and prednisone treatment during rituximab therapy. (From Quartier P, Brethon B, Philippet P, Landman-Parker J, Le Deist F, Fischer A: Treatment of childhood autoimmune haemolytic anaemia with rituximab. Lancet 2001;358:1511–1513.)

reduction of B-cell numbers can be expected to reduce serum levels of IgM and IgG, leading to a possible risk of infectious complications.

Subsequently, Zecca and colleagues[217] reported the results of the use of rituximab for the treatment of 15 patients with AIHA resistant to conventional treatment. All patients had previously received two or more courses of immunosuppressive therapy; two patients had undergone splenectomy. After completing treatment, all children received intravenous immunoglobulin for 6 months. With a median follow-up of 13 months, 13 patients (87%) responded. Median hemoglobin levels increased from 7.7 g/dL to a 20-month post-treatment level of 11.8 g/dL; reticulocyte counts decreased; and an increase in platelet count was observed in patients with concomitant thrombocytopenia (Evans's syndrome). Three responder patients had relapse 7, 8, and 10 months, respectively, after rituximab infusion. All three children received a second course of rituximab, again achieving disease remission. The authors concluded that rituximab is both safe and effective in reducing or even abolishing hemolysis in children with AIHA and that a sustained response can be achieved in the majority of cases.

Hongeng and colleagues[218] reported on a 37-month-old boy who had β-thalassemia major and who underwent unrelated T-cell–nondepleted bone marrow transplantation. On day 180 after the transplantation, a diagnosis of AIHA was made, and it proved to be refractory to corticosteroids and IVIG therapy. After two doses of rituximab, hemolysis decreased and remained so during 3 months of observation (hemoglobin improved from 5 g/dL to 10 g/dL), and corticoseroids were tapered and discontinued in 1 month after the second infusion.

Although these results in young children are encouraging, a note of caution was sounded by Matthews[219] because there have been scattered reports of opportunistic infections following rituximab therapy for pediatric patients. *Pneumocystis carinii* and varicella pneumonia were reported by Motto and coworkers,[220] and enteroviral meningoencephalitis associated with particularly prolonged B-cell depletion was reported by Quartier and associates.[221] Matthews[219] recommended longer-term study of the impact of rituximab-induced B-cell depletion with larger numbers of patients to better define the risk-benefit ratio in the treatment of autoimmune disorders.

Adverse Effects. The toxicity of ribuximab in patients with non–Hodgkin's lymphoma has been reviewed in detail.[222,223] Most adverse effects are mild to moderate and can be managed effectively with premedication, supportive care, and adjusted infusion rates.[223] Nevertheless, for the 36,000 patients treated with rituximab since its product launch in 1998 through mid-1999, a total of 675 medically confirmed adverse reaction reports were received worldwide, and 494 of these reactions (73%) were classified as serious according to criteria defined by the International Congress for Harmonization.[222] The postmarketing surveillance database includes reports of 18 deaths that were judged to be caused by infusion-related adverse reactions similar in type to those commonly reported during early clinical trials. The infusion-related symptom complex consists of fever and chills or rigors, which occur in the majority of patients during the first rituximab infusion. Other frequent infusion-related symptoms included nausea, urticaria, fatigue, headache, pruritus, bronchospasm, dyspnea, the sensation of tongue or throat swelling, rhinitis, vomiting, hypotension, flushing, and pain at disease sites. Serious cardiopulmonary infusion reactions culminating in death have been reported to occur in approximately 0.04%–0.07% of patients. The tumor lysis syndrome has been reported within 12–24 hours after the first antibody infusion and is estimated to occur in 0.04%–0.05% of patients. Major risk factors include high numbers of circulating malignant lymphoma cells, pulmonary infiltrates or lymphoma involvement, and prior cardiovascular disease. There are two reports of hemolytic anemia and one occurrence of transient aplastic anemia following rituximab therapy.

In May 2001 the manufacturer distributed updated safety information, which indicated that there have been 20 postmarketing reports of severe mucocutaneous reactions associated with the use of rituximab in an estimated 100,000 patients since product launch. Eight of these cases resulted in fatal outcomes. The onset of the reaction in the reported cases has varied from 1 to 13 weeks following rituximab exposure. Patients experiencing a severe mucocutaneous reaction should not receive any further infusions and should seek prompt medical evaluation.

Huhn and colleagues[224] described a 65-year-old patient who, 10 hours after the first dose of rituximab, developed multiorgan failure with renal failure, elevation of serum potassium to 6.6 mM, acidosis, and, finally, cardiac arrest.

Since recovery of B-lymphocytes after administration of rituximab has been described as starting after 6 to 9 months and being completed only after 12 months, a significant decline in IgM and IgG serum levels can be expected, and the possibility of infectious complications is a concern.[207,225] There have been several reports of such complications, and this has led some physicians to give replacement therapy with intravenous immunoglobulin.[207,217,226-228]

Rituximab has also been reported to cause severe worsening of mild AIHA in a patient with B-cell CLL.[229] The patient was a 64-year-old male who had progressive disease, for which he had received several courses of standard therapy. Subsequently, rituximab was administered for 4 consecutive weeks. Before rituximab administration, the patient had evidence of mild hemolysis (hemoglobin 11.9 g/dL), but just after the fourth administration of the drug, the hemoglobin level dropped to 4.6 g/dL, the reticulocyte count was 23%, LDH and bilirubin levels were increased, and the haptoglobin level was reduced. The DAT was found positive due to IgG (3+) and complement (weak), and the hemolysis responded quickly to prednisone therapy. The authors suggested that massive destruction of CD20-positive cells by rituximab might create an important liberation of cytokines (especially IL-6), leading to the overexpression of antierythrocyte autoreactive plasmacytes (which were CD20-negative).

Danazol. A possible efficacy of danazol, an attenuated androgen, has been reported among patients with AIHA.[230-237] Ahn[231] has reported results of treatment of 28 patients. Excellent or good responses were obtained in 77% of patients with idiopathic AIHA and in 60% with secondary disease. When the drug was discontinued after 1 year or more of therapy, lasting, unmaintained remissions of up to 5 years were often observed. The side effects of danazol are generally much less serious than those of glucocortocoids, which can often be tapered or discontinued completely.

Pignon and colleagues[234] reported the results of treatment of 17 adult patients with WAIHA. For 10 patients, danazol (600–800 mg daily) was used, with prednisone (1 mg/kg/day) as first-line therapy. Among these patients, there were eight excellent responses and two failures. The mean follow-up for responding patients was 21 months. A second group of patients included five who were initially treated with prednisone and who relapsed, and two patients with refractory AIHA who had failed to respond to various therapies, including splenectomy and immunosuppressive therapy. In this group, an excellent response was observed in three of the five patients who had relapsed after initial prednisone therapy. One partial response and one failure were observed in the two refractory AIHA patients. Manoharan[232] reported that five patients with AIHA responded to danazol therapy and that three had a complete response.

Cervera and associates[235] reported on three patients with SLE and coexisting AIHA who were treated with danazol. The hemolysis was unresponsive to prednisone, which was used at a dose of 1 mg/kg/day or higher for at least 1 month. One of the patients had had a prior splenectomy. Danazol was commenced at 200 mg/day and was added to the corticosteroid therapy. Dosage was increased stepwise by 200 mg daily every 4 weeks, with a maximum dose of 1200 mg/day. When the hemolysis had resolved for at least 1 month, treatment with corticosteroids was tapered, and treatment with danazol continued. If patients had sustained remissions with danazol or experienced side effects, the doses were gradually reduced to 200–400 mg/day. Two patients, including the patient with a prior splenectomy, had excellent responses lasting for 25 and 42 months, respectively, at the time of the report, and they were able to taper glucocorticoid therapy significantly. The third patient responded well but developed jaundice, hepatomegaly, and splenomegaly, necessitating discontinuation of the drug after 41 months of treatment. After withdrawal of danazol, signs and symptoms of hepatic disease disappeared, and the patient had a relapse of hemolytic anemia. The authors state that danazol was well tolerated by most patients, although undesirable effects severe enough to necessitate discontinuation of the drug have been reported. These include weight gain, dizziness, rash, pseudotumor cerebri, hepatic adenoma, cholestatic hepatitis, and thrombocytopenia.

Chan and Sack[236] reported on one patient with SLE and severe AIHA that did not respond to therapy with corticosteroids, splenectomy, azathioprine, chlorambucil, and intravenous immunoglobulin (IVIG). The patient responded to danazol, with maintenance of her hemoglobin and reductions in her transfusion and corticosteroid requirements.

There seems to have been a decrease in interest in danazol as therapy for AIHA, as indicated by the fact that, with the exception of the study by Cervera and associates,[235] no articles emphasizing its use have been published in the last decade.

Complement Inhibitors. Complement is an important effector system of host defense. It consists of more than 35 proteins, which in their native state either circulate as serum-soluble components of the blood or are associated with cellular membranes.[238] A focal point of regulation of complement activity is at the level of C3/C5 convertases. Regulation occurs through the action of a number of plasma proteins, all of which are members of the complement activation (RCA) gene cluster on human chromosome 1q32 and share a common 60–70 amino-acid short consensus repeat (SCR).[239] An excellent review of complement has been published (also see Chapter 4).[240,241]

A number of strategies for inhibiting complement have been devised, including the therapeutic use of soluble recombinant proteins derived from the RCA family, the transfer of native RCA proteins from exogenously administered RBCs, and the overexpression of native complement regulators, which has been achieved by culturing normal cells ex vivo followed by reimplantation.[242] As the half-lives of the inhibitors are short, the limited clinical trials that have been undertaken have been done in disease states in which complement activation is well demarcated, as in reperfusion injury of the allograft in lung transplantation. In the case of chronic diseases such as SLE and AIHA, the study and use of recombinant complement inhibitors is not yet a reality.[239]

Kirschfink[243] pointed out that with increasing evidence that complement activation significantly contributes to the pathogenesis of a large number of inflammatory diseases, strategies that interfere with its deleterious action have become a major focus in pharmacological research (Fig. 11-6). Endogenous soluble complement inhibitors (C1 inhibitor, recombinant soluble complement receptor 1, antibodies) blocking key proteins of the cascade reaction, neutralizing the action of the complement-derived anaphylatoxin C5a, or interfering with complement receptor 3 (CR3, CD18/11b)-mediated adhesion of inflammatory cells to the vascular endothelium have been tested successfully in various animal models in recent years. Promising results consequently led to clinical trials.

Basta[244] has suggested that the mechanism of the therapeutic effect of high-dose IVIG (see later discussion) could be interference with the complement system. This conclusion is based on the results obtained in animal models of complement-mediated pathology, in vitro complement assays, and studies on related human diseases.

Yazdanbakhsh and colleagues[245] assessed the ability of a human recombinant soluble form of complement receptor 1 (sCR1) to inhibit complement-mediated RBC destruction in vitro and in vivo. Treatment with sCR1 increased the survival of transfused human group A RBCs by 50% in the circulation of mice with preexisting anti-A for 2 hours after transfusion, reduced intravascular hemolysis, and lowered the levels of complement deposition (C3 and C4), but not IgG or IgM, on the transfused cells by 100-fold. The authors suggested that their data highlight a potential use of CR-1–based inhibitors for prevention of complement-dependent immune hemolysis.

Intravenous Immunoglobulin. The efficacy of IVIG treatment of autoimmune thrombocytopenia and neutropenia suggested that it might also be beneficial for treatment of AIHA. IVIG is frequently used as a second-line therapy for AIHA for patients who do not respond to corticosteroids. The choice of IVIG is in part

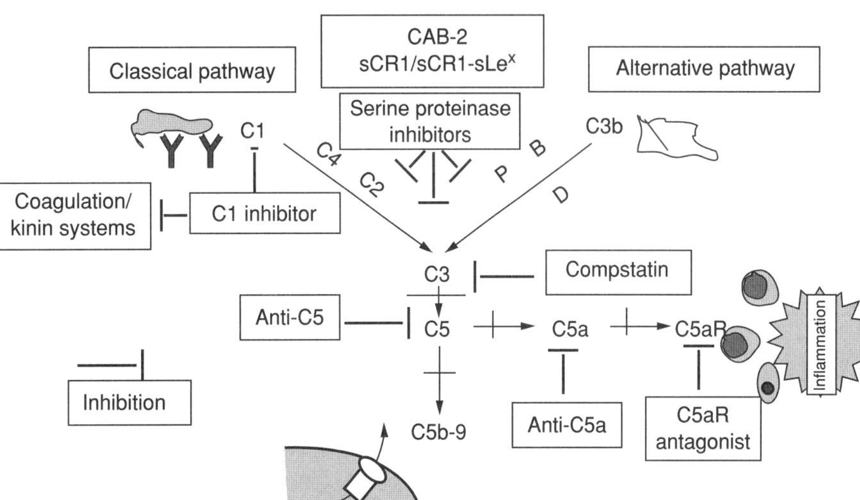

FIGURE 11-6. Complement as a target in antiphlogistic therapy. Complement activation, potentially leading to severe inflammation, can be blocked by the administration of either physiological regulatory proteins, blocking antibodies, receptor antagonists, RNA aptamers, serine proteinase inhibitors, or intravenous application of high-dose immunoglobulins. (From Kirschfink M: Targeting complement in therapy. Immunol Rev 2001;180:177–189.)

because of its relatively low incidence of adverse effects compared with other treatment options. Its effectiveness is rather disappointing, however, and it is quite expensive.

Mechanisms of Action. Numerous mechanisms of action have been postulated regarding the immunoregulatory effects of IVIG.[246-248] Some of these are listed in Table 11-11 and are illustrated in Figure 11-7. They include the following:

1. Antigen-specific suppression through antimicrobial antibodies or antiautoantigen antibodies.
2. Immunomodulatory effects that could be mediated by inhibition of phagocytosis by blocking Fc receptors, or by effects on B-cell activation and changes in T-cell distribution and function, in part related to anti–T-cell receptor antibodies. Also, modulation of the immune system by idiotypic antibodies could play a critical role in the establishment of long-term remission for patients with autoimmune disorders.[249] Idiotypic antibodies can
   a. Neutralize an autoantibody, preventing the binding of the autoantibody to its antigen and facilitating the clearance of the autoantibody
   b. Downregulate the B-cell receptor for a specific antigen, thereby decreasing the autoantibody production
   c. Exert effects mediated through regulatory T cells
3. Other effects of IVIG could be a membrane stabilizing and an immune complex solubilizing effect.
4. Finally, inhibition of deposition of early complement activation products (C4b, C3b) onto target surfaces has been suggested as a mechanism of action.[246]

Masson[250] and Yu and Lennon[251] have suggested that acceleration of the rate of IgG catabolism is the most plausible unifying explanation for the beneficial action of high doses of exogenous IgG in antibody-mediated autoimmune disorders. Such a process would eliminate individual IgG molecules in direct proportion to their relative concentration in plasma (Fig. 11-8). Bleeker and colleagues[252] reported experimental data supporting such a mechanism and concluded that a single high dose of IVIG induces a relatively small but long-lasting reduction of autoantibody levels by accelerated IgG clearance. This mechanism can fully explain, as the sole mechanism, the gradual decrease in autoantibody levels observed in several patient studies. In some clinical studies, however, larger or more rapid effects have been observed that cannot be explained by accelerated clearance. Hence, IVIG also can reduce autoantibody levels through mechanisms such as down-regulation of antibody production or neutralization by anti-idiotypic antibodies.

TABLE 11-11. IMMUNOREGULATORY EFFECTS OF IMMUNE GLOBULIN

Fc receptors
Blockade of Fc receptors on macrophages and effector cells
Induction of antibody-dependent cellular cytotoxicity
Induction of inhibitory Fcγ receptor IIB
Inflammation
Attenuation of complement-mediated damage
Decrease in immune-complex-mediated inflammation
Induction of anti-inflammatory cytokines
Inhibition of activation of endothelial cells
Neutralization of microbial toxins
Reduction in corticosteroid requirements
B cells and antibodies
Control of emergent bone marrow B-cell repertoires
Negative signaling through Fcγ receptors
Selective down-regulation and up-regulation of antibody production
Neutralization of circulating antoantibodies by anti-idiotypes
T cells
Regulation of the production of helper-T-cell cytokines
Neutralization of T-cell superantigens
Cell growth
Inhibition of lymphocyte proliferation
Regulation of apoptosis

From Kazatchkine MD, Kaveri SV: Immunomodulation of autoimmune and inflammatory diseases with intravenous immune globulin. N Engl J Med 2001;345:747–755.

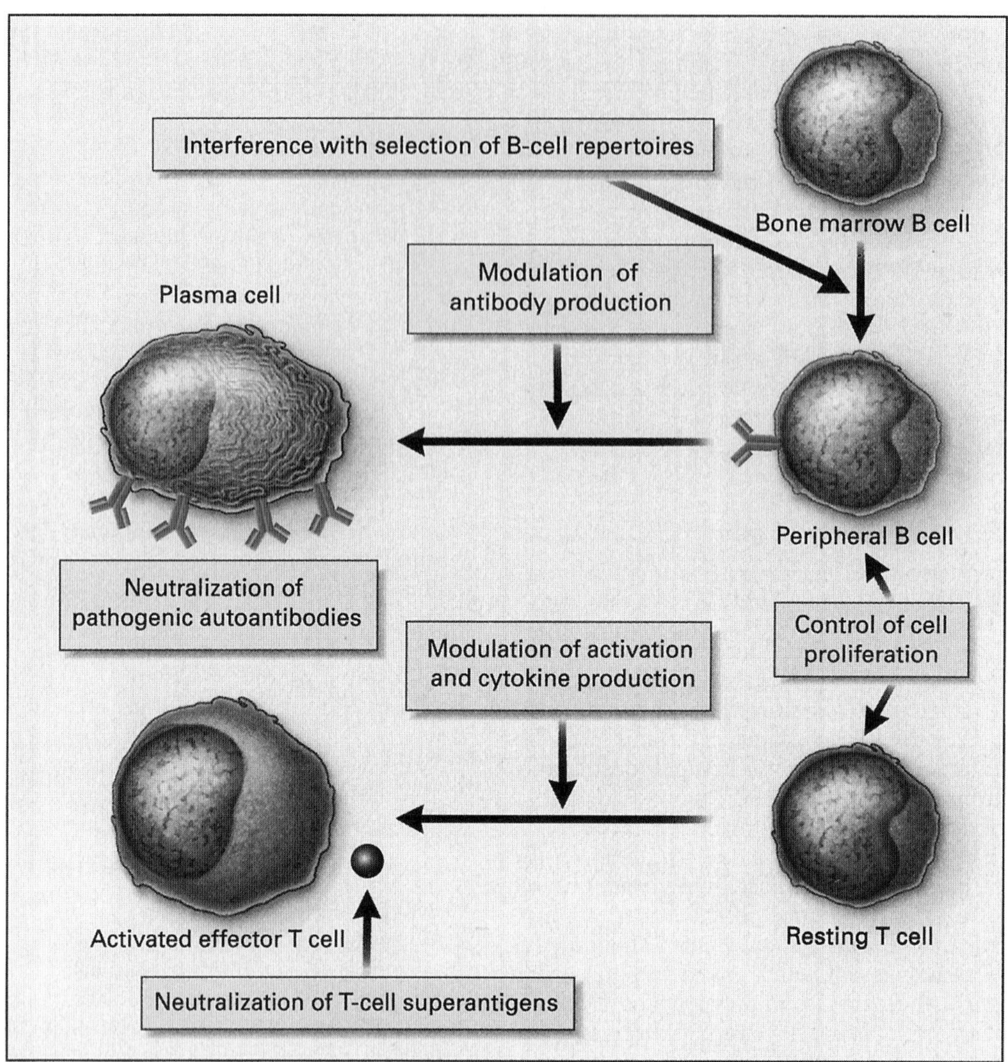

FIGURE 11-7. Immunomodulatory effects of immune globulin on B cells and T cells. Arrows indicate the sites targeted for the effect of immune globulin. Immune globulin interferes with the selection of B-cell repertoires, down-regulates or up-regulates antibody production, neutralizes pathogenic autoantibodies and T-cell superantigens, modulates the activation and function of the effector T cells and the production by CD4 T cells of cytokines mediated by type 1 and type 2 helper T cells, and controls cell growth. (From Kazatchkine MD, Kaveri SV: Immunomodulation of autoimmune and inflammatory diseases with intravenous immune globulin. N Engl J Med 2001;345:747–755.)

A novel mechanism for the effectiveness of IVIG in AIHA was suggested by Mueller-Eckhardt and coworkers.[253,254] These investigators suggested that IVIG administration causes coating of RBC by IgG and that such IgG-coated RBC are phagocytosed by the cells of the mononuclear phagocyte system (MPS). The consequent saturation of the MPS would result in a decrease in phagocytosis of antibody-coated platelets and would explain why IVIG is generally effective in immune thrombocytopenia. In AIHA, however, the MPS capacity might already be exhausted by autoantibody-coated RBC, thus explaining the relative ineffectiveness of IVIG in treatment of AIHA.

Clinical Results. Although IVIG is probably used frequently in the treatment of AIHA, published reports of its effectiveness or lack thereof are surprisingly scanty. In 1993, Flores and associates[255] pointed out that no previous publication included results in as many as ten cases, and only one study reported more than five. These authors conducted pilot studies at three institutions, enrolling a total of 37 patients, and combined these results with a review of 36 cases reported in the literature. This remains the largest study of the effectiveness of IVIG in AIHA.

All patients reported by Flores and associates[255] had WAIHA. Their report reviewed results in a very heterogenous group of patients. There were 62 adults and 11 children; 34 of the patients had idiopathic AIHA, and 26 patients had an associated chronic lymphocytic leukemia or lymphoma. Other patients had immunodeficiencies, AIDS, or connective tissue disease. All but four patients either had received prior prednisone therapy or were receiving it concurrently. Indeed, it was because most patients showed

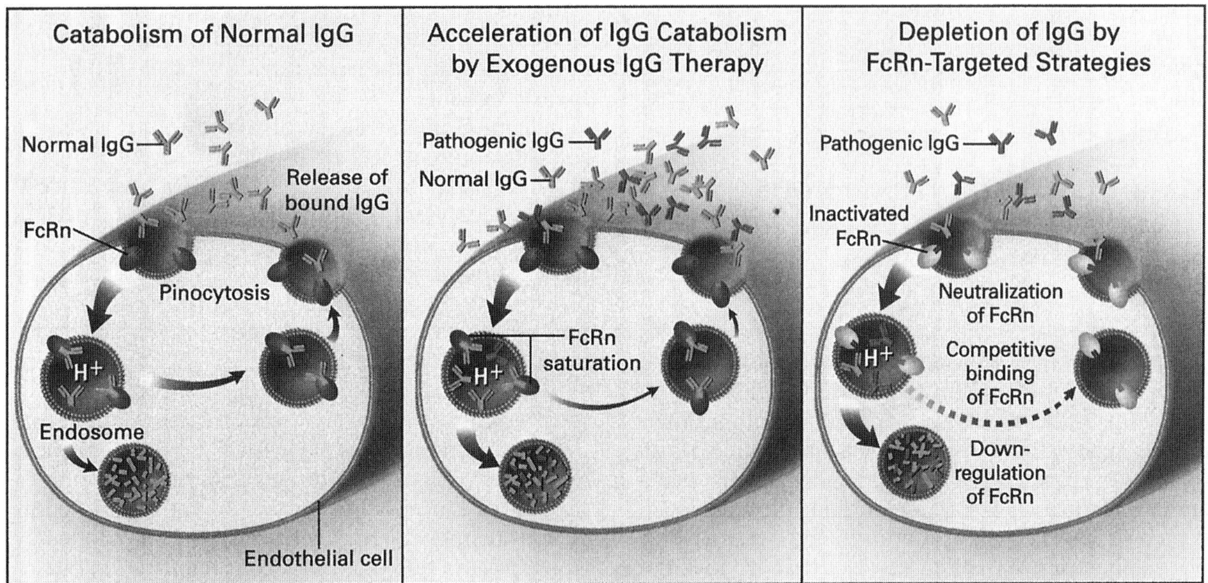

FIGURE 11-8. Regulation of catabolism of IgG by FcRn, a specialized intracellular Fc receptor. (From Yu Z, Lennon VA: Mechanism of intravenous immune globulin therapy in antibody-mediated autoimmune diseases. N Engl J Med 1999;340:227–228. Copyright © 1999 Massachusetts Medical Society. All rights reserved.)

little or no response after 2 or more weeks of initial corticosteroid therapy that they received a trial of IVIG therapy. Some patients had also received immunosuppressive agents or plasmapheresis or had had a splenectomy. Patients in the published reports received 0.4–2 g/kg/day for 2 to 5 days; most received 0.4–0.5 g/kg/day for 5 days. The authors' patients received either 0.5 g/kg/day for 5 days or 1 g/kg/day for 5 to 7 days.

The authors used liberal criteria for a response. They defined a "Type I response" as an increase of hemoglobin of 2 or more g/dL within 10 days of initiation of treatment with IVIG, regardless of the final hemoglobin level. A "Type II response" was defined as fulfillment of the criteria of a Type I response plus achievement of a peak hemoglobin value of 10 g/dL or greater. Data regarding hemoglobin levels were not available for all patients in the literature.

Of the 62 evaluable cases, only nine (14.8%) had a Type II response (Table 11-12).[255] Type I responses occurred in 25 of 62 patients (40.3%) (all Type II responses also qualified as Type I responses and were included in the Type I response total). A significant shortcoming of the report is the lack of follow-up information. The authors' only comment about the duration of response is that "the hemoglobin remained elevated for three or more weeks in most cases."

Contrary to previous reports,[256] higher doses of IVIG (5 g/kg) could not be shown to increase the response rate. There was a strong correlation of a low pretreatment hemoglobin level with treatment response (Table 11-13).[255] Thirteen patients had a pretreatment hemoglobin level of 6 g/dL or lower, and 12 of these (92%) showed a Type I response. Four of these 13 patients were among the 9 in the entire study with a Type II response. The presence of hepatomegaly was the second strongest predictor of treatment response.

The authors point out that the response rate for IVIG compares unfavorably with the efficacy of other treatment modalities for AIHA, including corticosteroids and splenectomy. They suggest that high-dose IVIG be recommended only as adjunctive therapy for selected cases, such as for children in whom the toxic effects of chronic high-dose corticosteroids and immunosuppressive agents could be especially frequent and severe. No mention was made of the expense of high-dose IVIG, which is considerable.

Subsequently, Ratko and colleagues[257,258] published the results of a consensus conference developed by a University Hospital Consortium Expert Panel, which considered off-label uses of IVIG preparations available in the United States. All English-language review articles ($n = 201$) and original reports ($n = 1904$) were evaluated, and extracted data were reviewed by an expert panel. At the time of publication of the detailed

TABLE 11-12. RESPONSE OF AIHA CASES TO IVIG TREATMENT

Overall response rate	29/73 = 39.7%
Response rate in literature cases	17/36 = 47.2%
Response rate in combined pilot studies	12/37 = 32.4%
Response rate in pediatric cases	6/11 = 54.5%
Type I response rate	25/62 = 40.3%[a]
Type II response rate	9/61 = 14.8%

[a] Eleven of seventy three patients were literature cases with no specific data available. All Type II responses also qualify as Type I responses (see text for definitions) and are included in the Type I response total.

From Flores G, Cunningham-Rundles C, Newland AC, Bussel JB: Efficacy of intravenous immunoglobulin in the treatment of autoimmune hemolytic anemia: Results in 73 patients. Am J Hematol 1993;44:237–242.

TABLE 11-13. RELATIONSHIP BETWEEN THE PRETREATMENT HEMOGLOBIN LEVEL (EXPRESSED IN GRAMS PER DECILITER) AND RESPONSE TO IVIG THERAPY IN PATIENTS WITH AIHA

Hemoglobin Level	Type I Response	Type II Response	No Response
≤6.0	12/13 = 92.3%	4/13 = 30.8%	1/13 = 7.7%
6.1–7.0	4/9 = 44.4%	1/9 = 11.1%	5/9 = 55.6%
7.1–8.0	2/10 = 20.0%	0/10 = 0	8/10 = 80.0%
8.1–9.0	4/12 = 33.3%	3/12 = 25.0%	8/12 = 66.7%
≥9.1	2/16 = 12.5%	1/16 = 6.3%	14/16 = 87.5%

From Flores G, Cunningham-Rundles C, Newland AC, Bussel JB: Efficacy of intravenous immunoglobulin in the treatment of autoimmune hemolytic anemia: Results in 73 patients. Am J Hematol 1993;44:237–242.

proceedings in 1999, the effectiveness of IVIG had been evaluated in a total of 77 patients with AIHA.[258] All 18 reports were either case studies or series or open, uncontrolled trials. All of the reports were summarized in tabular form, including information on the number of patients, dosage, and the responses observed. Patients received initial total IVIG doses ranging from 2 g/kg to 7 g/kg and maintenance infusions for as long as 4 years. A positive response, signified by a hemoglobin concentration increasing into the normal range, occurred in 40 patients (52%). In contrast to the report by Flores and colleagues,[255] data were not supplied concerning the pretreatment hemoglobin level. Most IVIG recipients had WAIHA refractory to other therapies, including corticosteroids, cytotoxic drugs, and splenectomy. Although some patients experienced sustained responses to IVIG treatment, many required maintenance doses. No clinically significant adverse events related to IVIG infusion were reported in these studies. The report concludes by stating that it is difficult to evaluate the clinical value of IVIG therapy for AIHA adequately, primarily because no data from randomized, comparative trials are available. The routine use of IVIG is therefore not recommended. It could have a role in treating patients with WAIHA that does not respond to corticosteroids or splenectomy, or in treating patients in whom corticosteroids or splenectomy are contraindicated.

A further consensus panel was convened in 2000 to evaluate and define the therapeutic areas in which IVIG has demonstrated effectiveness. AIHA was not mentioned in the report of this panel.[259]

Selected Case Reports. Besa[260] reported eight patients with WAIHA in association with a lymphoproliferative disorder. Seven patients had chronic lymphocytic leukemia, and one had Hodgkin's disease. An additional patient with non–Hodgkin's lymphoma had AIHA caused by an IgM cold antibody. IVIG therapy was given at a dose of 0.4 g/kg/day for five doses, followed by maintenance therapy every 21–28 days if evidence of recurrence was noted. Hematocrit levels of patients with WAIHA stabilized, followed by a gradual improvement at 21 days after IVIG without steroids. Treatment with steroids resulted in faster and higher increments in hematocrit levels. Patients did not have any episodes of AIHA from 6 months to as long as 4 years while receiving IVIG at 3-week intervals. The patient with IgM-mediated AIHA was not benefited by IVIG therapy.

Leickly and Buckley[261] reported reversal of AIHA with IVIG treatment at a dose of 450 mg/kg/day for 5 days in a patient with common variable immunodeficiency. At the time of publication, the remission had been maintained for 34 months by single doses of 100–200 mg/kg at 4-week intervals or whenever the hemoglobin level fell or the reticulocyte count increased.

Most reports of IVIG indicate its use in conjunction with other therapy, especially corticosteroids. In contrast, Otheo and colleagues[262] reported the successful treatment of high-dose IVIG when used as a single therapy in a 4-year-old child with AIHA. The patient's hemoglobin was 5.2 g/dL, hematocrit was 13.9%, reticulocytes were 20%, and platelets were 55,000/µL. The DAT was positive with anti-IgG but not anticomplement antibody; the IAT was positive without clear specificity. IVIG was begun at 800 mg/kg/day for 5 days. Hemoglobin and platelet counts reached normal values rapidly, and the reticulocyte count was 2.7% on the fifth week after IVIG. A maintenance dose of 800 mg/kg was given every 2 weeks for 8 months. There was no trace of IgG autoantibody at the fifth month, and 18 months later, he still had normal hematological values.

Successful treatment of AIHA with IVIG has been reported in a patient with AIDS,[263] in a patient with refractory and life-threatening AIHA in a man with the primary antiphospholipid syndrome,[264] and in four patients with thalassemia major who had a large increase in blood consumption following the development of RBC autoantibodies.[265]

A number of reports fail to show any significant effect of IVIG in AIHA.[253,254,266,267]

Adverse Effects. No clinically significant adverse events related to IVIG infusion in patients with AIHA were reported in the comprehensive reviews just cited.[255,257,258] Adverse effects have been reported in other publications, however.

The risk of transmitting infectious agents accompanies the use of almost any blood-derived pharmaceutical preparation. The steps used in preparing the IVIG products available in the United States, however, practically eliminate the risk of transmitting HIV, HBV, and HCV. Although an outbreak of hepatitis C in 1994 was attributed to IVIG, the manufacturing process has since been changed, and the Centers for Disease Control and Prevention (CDC) states that IVIG products should now contain essentially no risk of HCV transmission.[258]

Adverse effects, which are generally mild, can occur in 1% to 10% of IVIG recipients.[268,269] These reactions may include back or chest pain or sensation of chest heaviness, chills, fever, headache, malaise, myalgia, nausea, vomiting, or renal damage. Sherer and colleagues[270] reported that 36% of patients had at least one adverse effect, but that these effects were usually mild and transient. Patients who develop adverse effects during the first treatment course may be at increased risk of adverse effects during the subsequent course.

In one retrospective study, aseptic meningitis with severe headache was reported in about 11% of patients who received high-dose IVIG therapy for various autoimmune diseases.[271] This complication was more frequent among patients with a history of migraine headaches and occurred regardless of the product type or infusion rate. Most adverse effects are associated with rapid infusion and usually resolve with temporary discontinuation or reduction in infusion rate.

Acute renal failure was recognized as an adverse effect of IVIG therapy in 1987.[272] Since then, it has emerged as an important complication, and there is a plethora of relevant reports.[272-282] As of 1998, the FDA had received a total of 120 reports of adverse renal events (acute renal failure and renal insufficiency) associated with high-dose IVIG therapy.[281] On review of these case reports, 90% of the patients had received sucrose-containing IVIG, 56% had diabetes mellitus, and 26% had pretreatment renal impairment. All renal adverse events occurred in the first 7 days following administration of IVIG therapy.

Acute renal failure, including fatal cases, has been reported predominantly in association with higher doses of preparations containing sucrose that were used during consecutive days.[273] This finding led to recommendations to ensure that patients are adequately hydrated, to consider the risk of sucrose-containing preparations in patients with risk factors for renal insufficiency, to limit the rate at which sucrose-containing preparations are infused, and to monitor renal function in patients receiving IVIG.[274]

Levy and Pusey[280] studied the incidence of renal impairment in an unselected cohort of patients receiving two different preparations of IVIG over the course of 20 months. A total of 287 courses of IVIG were administered to 119 patients for a variety of indications. Eight patients showed deterioration in renal function (6.7%), and in two patients (1.7%), no renal recovery occurred. There were no significant differences in patient characteristics, dose, or preparation of IVIG administered to those patients with or without changes in serum creatinine. There was no association between the amount of sucrose in the IVIG and the development of renal failure. The researchers concluded that IVIG is associated with renal impairment which could be irreversible, with a maximum incidence of 6.7%.

Twelve cases of IVIG-related thrombosis have been reported in the literature.[283-290] Adverse events were myocardial infarctions, strokes, spinal cord ischemia, and deep venous thrombosis of the leg or arm. Most of these events developed during or immediately after IVIG infusion. The pathogenesis of the thrombotic events has been attributed to IVIG-induced platelet activation and increases in plasma viscosity.[283] There is a dose-dependent increase in plasma viscosity with increasing plasma immunoglobulin concentration. Reinhart and Berchtold[287] reported a more than fourfold increase in plasma immunoglobulin concentration after IVIG therapy, which was accompanied by an increase in plasma viscosity from a mean of 1.26 cP to 1.54 cP (reference value < 1.40 cP). This effect lasted up to 5 days after treatment. Two studies have shown an increase in the incidence of fatal hepatic veno-occlusive disease when IVIG is used prophylactically to prevent transplant-related infections.[291,292]

Patients most at risk for thrombosis are the elderly; patients with a history of vascular disease, thrombosis, or acquired or inherited thrombophilic disorders; and patients with prolonged periods of immobilization.[283] For these patients, IVIG can be infused at a slower rate (8 to 12 hours), and high-dose infusion (400 mg/kg to 1 g/kg/day) should be avoided. IVIG should also be used with caution for patients who have high levels of serum monoclonal protein and concomitant hyperviscosity.

Rizk and associates[293] reported on a 23-year-old, 91-kg male with multifocal motor neuropathy who developed transfusion-related acute lung injury (TRALI) 6 hours after receiving 90 g of IVIG over the course of 3 hours. Prior to the IVIG infusion, he received hydrocortisone (60 mg), diphenhydramine (25 mg), and famotidine (20 mg), all given intravenously, and acetaminophen (650 mg), given orally. Four hours after the IVIG infusion, he became increasingly dyspneic and coughed up pink, frothy sputum. Chest x-ray revealed bilateral interstitial and alveolar infiltrates consistent with noncardiogenic pulmonary edema or adult respiratory distress syndrome. He recovered spontaneously with only bed rest and nasal oxygen. TRALI is thought to be caused by infusion of a blood component or derivative containing granulocyte- or HLA antibody, a biologically active lipid, or a cytokine that activates adherent, primed granulocytes resulting in damage to pulmonary endothelium.[293] Antibody to granulocytes was detected in the IVIG product by indirect granulocyte immunofluorescence assay, and the authors propose that transfusion of a large quantity of granulocyte antibody precipitated TRALI in their patient.

IVIG has also been implicated in episodes of immune hemolysis (see Chapter 12).

Plasma Exchange

Plasma exchange has been used in the therapy of a wide variety of disorders, particularly those associated with a well-documented or suspected immunologic pathogenesis.[294-298] This therapy would seem logical for IgM-mediated hemolytic anemias, as IgM resides exclusively within the plasma compartment and therefore can be expected to be removed efficiently by the exchange process. IgG, which is distributed almost equally between the intravascular and extravascular spaces, is less efficiently removed and quickly re-equilibrates to fill the void created by removal of the patient's plasma. Nevertheless, therapeutic successes and failures have been reported for both warm and cold antibody AIHA.

Published results generally consist of case reports of small numbers of patients, and the results have been inconsistent. Further, concomitant therapy with steroids and immunosuppressive agents often obscures the contribution of plasma exchange to the outcome. In a number of cases, the AIHA seems to stabilize, but other acutely ill patients have not improved. Finally, favorable effects are generally short-lived.

Branda and colleagues[299] reported on a patient who developed WAIHA while convalescing from a viral illness. The patient was treated on one occasion only with 3000 mL plasma exchange followed by transfusions of 2 units of whole blood. The hemoglobin that had been rapidly falling stabilized, and an autoanti-e antibody, which had a titer of two before exchange, became negative. The patient recovered from the hemolytic anemia without further therapy.

Patten and Reuter[300] reported benefit from plasma exchange in a 45-year-old woman with Evans's syndrome. Before plasma exchange, the patient's hematocrit level could not be raised above 10% despite 8 units of red cells administered over a 4-day period. After plasma exchange, the hematocrit level rose to 29%, the platelet count rose from 14,500 to 222,000/mL, and the transfusion requirements declined to only 2 units of red cells over the next 37 days. The patient subsequently had a severe exacerbation of hemolysis that did not respond to plasma exchange, however, and she expired.

Rosenfield and Jagathambal[301] commented that plasmapheresis has not been useful in their experience for patients with WAIHA.

Garelli and colleagues[302] described a patient with a hyperacute hemolytic crisis treated by combined plasmapheresis and exchange transfusion. Immediately afterwards, the hemoglobin level rose from 2.6 g/dL to 9.8 g/dL. The DAT became weakly positive, and the hemolytic crisis subsided. Thereafter, the clinical and laboratory picture stabilized.

Bernstein and colleagues[303] reported on a 17-year-old boy with fulminating acute hemolysis of 3 weeks' duration that was unresponsive to massive doses of corticosteroids (up to 10 mg/kg/day) and splenectomy. He required 20 units of RBCs over a 14-day period to maintain a hemoglobin concentration above 4 g/dL. A splenectomy was performed, but there was a rapid fall in hemoglobin concentration in the first 4 days after surgery. Plasma exchange was performed, with 8.5 liters of plasma removed and replaced with 5% albumin. A second exchange was carried out 10 days later, and he was started on azathioprine at a dose of 2 mg/kg/day; prednisone was also continued. After the second exchange, his hemoglobin stabilized, and it was eventually found possible to withdraw both prednisone and azathioprine. The authors suggested that plasma exchange could be indicated for acute reversal of severe hemolysis while other therapies are taking effect. In this way, plasma exchange has advantages over other therapies that might take days or weeks to become effective.

A similar approach that combines plasma exchanges with immunosuppressive agents has been recommended. Silva and coworkers[157] reported treatment of a patient with AIHA using a protocol of synchronized plasma exchange and cyctotoxic drug therapy originally developed for treatment of patients with severe SLE.[304] A 46-year-old female had recurrent episodes of WAIHA that was not responsive to a wide variety of therapies (splenectomy, corticosteroids, IVIG, vincristine, azathioprine, danazol, cyclosporin, erythropoietin, and 10 plasma perfusions over staphylococcal protein A). Combined therapy was begun with three one-volume plasma exchanges followed by intravenous cyclophosphamide on the third day. Subsequently, cyclophosphamide and prednisone were given orally in tapering doses. This regimen quickly produced remarkable improvement, and by day 51 after starting the combined therapy, the patient had no evidence of AIHA. The authors suggest that the favorable outcome might have been caused by the enhanced cytotoxic effect of cyclophosphamide on proliferating lymphocytes participating in the antibody rebound phenomena, a suppression of B lymphocytes with daily cyclophosphamide/prednisone therapy, and/or formation of anti-idiotypic antibodies. The relative effectiveness of plasma exchanges and the immunosuppressive drugs in the outcome of therapy with this protocol is not clear.

Somewhat similarly, Hughes and Toogood[305] used plasma exchange as a prelude to the administration of high-dose IVIG. In so doing, they achieved a complete remission in a patient with refractory AIHA.

Silberstein and Berkman[306] reported results in two patients with WAIHA. One patient's initial treatment consisted of corticosteroids and transfusions, to which plasma exchange therapy was added shortly after admission. The patient improved and subsequently required intermittent treatment with corticosteroids. The second patient was treated with corticosteroids for 9 days prior to initiation of plasma exchanges. Transfusion requirements decreased, but parameters indicating hemolysis showed only mild improvement. RBC survival studies revealed no improvement attributable to the plasma exchanges.

In 1993, McLeod and coworkers[298] reviewed 17 cases of WAIHA treated with plasma exchange.[306-311] In a number of cases, plasma exchange seemed to stabilize the disease in patients who had entered a period of fulminant hemolysis; however, other acutely ill patients seemed not to have improved.

McConnell and colleagues[312] described favorable results in a 34-month-old child (see Chapter 9). McCarthy and associates[313] reported the smallest infant (7.5 kg) to receive intensive plasma exchange therapy (52 procedures) as treatment for AIHA. Although the patient's clinical course was prolonged and complicated by cytomegalovirus infection with spontaneous perforation of the colon, his recovery was eventually complete. Because of his small size, calcium gluconate was added to replacement fluids, and calcium levels were monitored closely. The apheresis machine and tubing were routinely primed with RBCs, and fresh-frozen plasma (FFP) was substituted for 5% albumin during the second half of all procedures to maintain adequate levels of procoagulants. The patient had remained healthy for 2 years at the time of publication.

Shehata and coworkers[314] performed an extensive review of randomized controlled trials published between 1976 through 1999 in which therapeutic apheresis was used for numerous indications. AIHA was not mentioned in this review. In a summary of current indication categories endorsed by the AABB and the American Society for Apheresis, plasma exchange for AIHA is listed as a category III indication, meaning: "Therapeutic apheresis is not clearly indicated based on insufficient evidence, conflicting results, or inability to document a favorable risk-to-benefit ratio. Applications in this category may represent heroic or last-ditch efforts on behalf of a patient."[315]

Hematopoietic Stem Cell Transplantation

The majority of autoimmune diseases are controlled more or less satisfactorily by conventional therapeutic manipulation of the immune system, but there is a hard core of refractory, relapsing, treatment-resistant autoimmune diseases for which the term *malignant autoimmunity* has appropriately been proposed.[316,317] The concept of using intense immunosuppression followed by allogeneic or autologous human stem cells to treat autoimmune diseases is based on encouraging results in experimental animals, serendipitous cases of patients with both autoimmune disease and malignancies who were allotransplanted for the latter, and phase I/II trials in various disease states.[318-320] Van Bekkum[323] reported that more than 500 patients have been treated with autologous stem cells for severe refractory autoimmune diseases. Indeed, Burt and colleagues[324] reported that, by percentage of transplantations performed, autoimmune diseases are the most rapidly expanding indication for stem cell transplantation. These authors concluded, however, that further improvements in the efficacy and safety of both autologous and allogeneic stem cell transplantation procedures need to be developed, and larger cohorts of patients need to be studied to assess the full benefits of stem cell transplantation as a most promising new armamentarium for the treatment of autoimmune diseases.

RESULTS IN ANIMAL MODELS

In 1974, Morton and Siegel[325] transferred murine SLE to irradiated BALB/C mice by transplanting whole marrow from NZB mice. This adoptive transfer with marrow grafts was subsequently confirmed for many autoimmune diseases in animals, including murine models of SLE, the antiphospholipid syndrome, insulin-dependent diabetes mellitus, experimental autoimmune encephalomyelitis, and adjuvant arthritis.[326,327]

The same experimental autoimmune diseases that have been transmitted by transplantation have been cured by transplants from healthy animals.[319] A putative graft-versus-autoimmunity effect is supported by experiments showing that allogeneic chimerism achieved using a sublethal radiation conditioning regimen followed by allogeneic transplantation can prevent the onset of diabetes and even reverse preexisting insulitis in nonobese diabetic mice, whereas the same radiation protocol without allogeneic human stem cells was insufficient.[328] Both allogeneic and autologous bone marrow transplants have been shown to be capable of preventing or treating autoimmune disease in experimental animal models.[329]

Van Bekkum[323] reviewed the experimental basis of hematopoietic stem cell transplantation for the treatment of autoimmune diseases. He points out that the discovery that autologous bone marrow transplantation (BMT) is equally effective as allogeneic BMT in inducing complete remissions in rats with experimental autoimmune diseases cleared the way for clinical application. Actually, the experiments with syngeneic BMT were included because of the (mistaken) assumption that they would serve as negative controls.

RESOLUTION OF AIHA AFTER ALLOGENEIC STEM CELL TRANSPLANTATION

A 5-year-old boy affected from infancy by relapsing, life-threatening Evans's syndrome was transplanted successfully with HLA-identical sibling cord blood.[330] There was total disappearance of autoantibodies, but the patient died of acute liver failure 9 months after transplantation. Another patient with Evans's syndrome developed 100% donor hematopoiesis, no graft-vs.-host disease (GVHD), and a complete hematologic and immunologic remission, which had persisted for 5 months at the time of reporting.[319]

De Stefano and coworkers[331] reported on a patient with thalassemia intermedia and immune-mediated hemolytic anemia who relapsed 7 weeks after an autologous lymphocyte-depleted peripheral blood stem cell transplant. A complete remission, which had lasted 18 months at the time of publication, was obtained with allogeneic bone marrow transplantation from an HLA-matched, unrelated donor. The authors suggested that a graft-versus-autoimmunity effect could have been important in the eradication of the patient's autoaggressive lymphocytes.

Oyama and colleagues[331a] reported on a 28-year-old male with Evans's syndrome that was refractory to multiple interventions. He developed life-threatening complications and was treated with an allogeneic hematopoietic cell transplant from his HLA-matched sister. This resulted in complete clinical and serologic remission of the immune-mediated hemolytic anemia and thrombocytopenia, which had persisted for more than 30 months at the time of the report. The clinical course after transplantation was complicated, however, by drug-related thrombotic thrombocytopeic purpura, chronic extensive GVHD, and immune suppression-related opportunistic infections.

Marmont and associates[332] reported on a 21-year-old male with refractory Evans's syndrome (predominantly thrombocytopenic) who was treated with an allogeneic reduced-intensity bone marrow transplant from his HLA-identical sister. He had an initial dramatic platelet peak, but while still evidencing mixed chimerism he again became progressively thrombocytopenic. He finally remitted following five donor lymphocyte infusions and remained in complete clinical and biological remission for 2 years after transplantation. The authors state that evidence is accumulating that a graft-vs.-autoimmunity effect exists, consisting most probably in the substitution of normal T, B, and lymphoid progenitor cells for the autoimmune clones of the patient's immune system. A role for graft-vs.-autoimmunity was also demonstrated by Hinterberger and coworkers,[333] who reviewed reports of hematopoietic cell transplants for autoimmune diseases published between June 1977 and September 2001. They found that freedom of relapse was superior after allogeneic transplantation compared with autologous transplants ($P = 0.0002$). These data suggest that a graft-vs.-autoimmunity effect after allogeneic hematopoietic cell transplantation mediates elimination of autoimmunity.

AUTOLOGOUS TRANSPLANTS FOR AUTOIMMUNE DISEASE

Although one hesitates to use the oxymoron "autologous transplant," it is a commonly used term in the literature of transplantation and refers to high-dose marrow ablative therapy followed by rescue with autologous hematopoietic stem cells. Such "transplants" from marrow or from peripheral blood are much more commonly used than allogeneic hematopoietic cell transplants to treat autoimmune disease because of the greater safety of autologous procedures, although transplant-related mortality has been higher (8.6%) than initially anticipated (1–3%).[334] Some centers, however, have performed autologous transplantation on more than 70 autoimmune patients with no transplant-related mortality.[334] Possible reasons for center differences include the diseases transplanted, selection or exclusion criteria, and intensity of immune-suppressive preparative regimens.

It has been postulated that if immunosuppressive regimens can eliminate or effectively reduce the level of autoreactive T and B cells, then regeneration of de novo immunity even in the autologous setting could bypass the initial breakdown of self-tolerance and ensure prolonged disease remission.[334]

Although autologous transplants have been performed mainly for neurologic conditions such as multiple sclerosis[335] and for rheumatologic conditions,[336] a smaller group of patients with refractory hematological autoimmune diseases also have undergone the procedure.[319,337,338] Paillard and colleagues[339] reported on a case of a child with severe AIHA who did not respond to conventional treatments but was cured with an autologous peripheral blood CD34+ cell transplantation. No further RBC transfusions were required beyond day 16 after the autograft. At 20 months after autograft, the patient was in complete hematological remission.

SLE, a disorder frequently complicated by immune cytopenias, is becoming a major target for autologous transplants.[319,340,341] Musso and coworkers[341] reported on a 19-year-old female with a 6-year history of SLE with secondary antiphospholipid syndrome who later developed refractory Evans's syndrome. She was treated with an autologous hematopoietic cell transplant, and 8 months later she had normal blood counts, although with persistent low-titer direct antiglobulin and antinuclear antibody tests. Anti-double stranded DNA, lupus anticoagulant tests, and anticardiolipin tests were negative.

In one patient with SLE and non–Hodgkin's lymphoma, the lymphoma did not relapse, but autoimmune thrombocytopenic purpura supervened. The autoimmune disease thus appeared more refractory than the neoplasia.[342] A similar sequence occurred in the case of a patient with Sjögren's syndrome and lymphoma; complete remission of the lymphoma occurred, but thrombocytopenia and vasculitis recurred 2 months after transplantation.[343]

Intense Immunosuppression without Human Stem Cell Rescue for Treatment of Autoimmune Disease

A novel approach to circumventing the problem of reinfusing autoreactive lymphocytes is to give an immunoablative regimen that spares early hematopoietic precursors, obviating the need for an autograft.[344-347] Brodsky and associates[344] found that immunoablative doses of cyclophosphamide, without stem cell rescue, can induce durable complete remissions (median follow-up >10 years) in the majority of patients with severe aplastic anemia. This approach has subsequently been extended to a spectrum of severe autoimmune diseases including Felty's syndrome, autoimmune thrombocytopenic purpura, Evans's syndrome, SLE, chronic inflammatory demyelinating polyneuropathy,[346,348,349] and paraneoplastic pemphigus.[347]

years, with an expected recurrence-free proportion of 83% at 5 years after the initial episode of hemolysis (Fig. 11-11).[436]

Because AIHA so commonly occurs as an initial manifestation of SLE, the authors suggested that testing for antinuclear antibodies and other lupus-related autoantibodies is warranted for patients who present with AIHA.[436] Patients with SLE who present with AIHA, when compared with controls with other types of anemia at the onset of SLE, had an increased risk of renal involvement, thrombocytopenia, and (possibly) thrombotic episodes during follow-up.

The older medical literature contains a number of reports of favorable responses of AIHA to splenectomy without adversely affecting the course of the underlying SLE.[445-450] For example, Sarles and Levin[445] reported on three patients with AIHA and SLE in whom hematologic improvement did not occur during treatment with steroids but did ensue following splenectomy. On the other hand, Rivero and colleagues[451] found that the operation produced only short-term benefit in the management of hemocytopenic episodes in SLE and stated that it seems warranted only as an emergency procedure for patients unresponsive to medical treatment.

It is not certain whether AIHA portends a more benign or a more severe prognosis for patients with SLE. Two reports have indicated that AIHA was associated with increased mortality in univariate analyses, although multivariate analyses did not indicate hemolytic anemia as an independent predictor of mortality.[441,452] Other studies either found no association of AIHA with adverse outcomes or suggested that it could be associated with a more benign course.[440]

Patients with AIHA and SLE were more likely to have IgG anticardiolipin antibodies than patients with SLE who had other causes of anemia.[436] Anticardiolipin antibodies are found in the sera of patients with SLE, primary antiphospholipid antibody syndrome, and several other diseases.[442,443] Patients with AIHA who fulfill the criteria of SLE could represent an intermediate group of patients who have some manifestations of the anticardiolipin syndrome (e.g., thromboses).[436] Some investigators have reported that anticardiolipin antibodies act as anti-RBC autoantibodies in SLE patients with active hemolysis and have identified these antibodies to be mostly of the IgG isotype.[454]

Hodgkin's Disease

AIHA among patients with Hodgkin's disease is quite unusual, with a reported association of 1.7–2.7%.[455,456] Accordingly, there are no large studies of the effectiveness of various approaches to therapy.

A detailed description of results of therapy among nine patients with Hodgkin's disease and WAIHA has been reported by Eisner and associates.[456] All patients responded well to various forms of management, including corticosteroids, splenectomy, and splenic irradiation. DATs became negative before death in all of the patients who died of disseminated disease, and AIHA was not present in the terminal stages of the disease.

Levine and colleagues[457] reported that splenectomy or corticosteroids plus vincristine were effective in slowing the hemolytic process for two patients, but neither of these therapeutic modalities resulted in conversion to a negative DAT; however, definitive chemotherapy for the underlying Hodgkin's disease in these patients (and in a third who received no other therapy for AIHA) resulted in a disappearance of the positive DAT. Numerous other authors also have reported that effective therapy for the treatment of Hodgkin's disease results in resolution of the AIHA.[161,455,458-462]

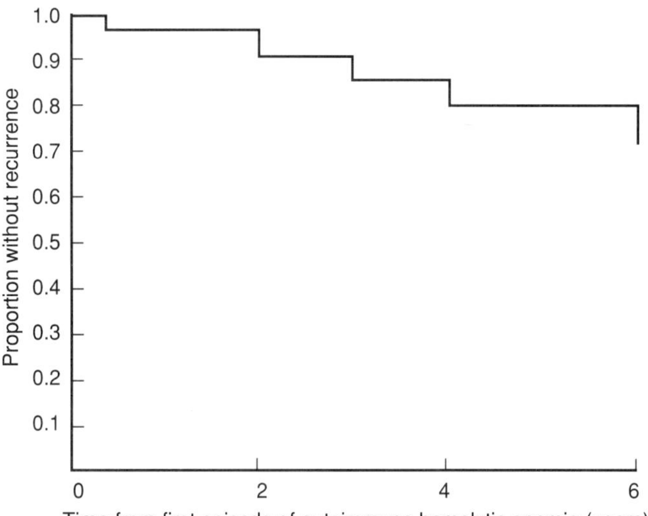

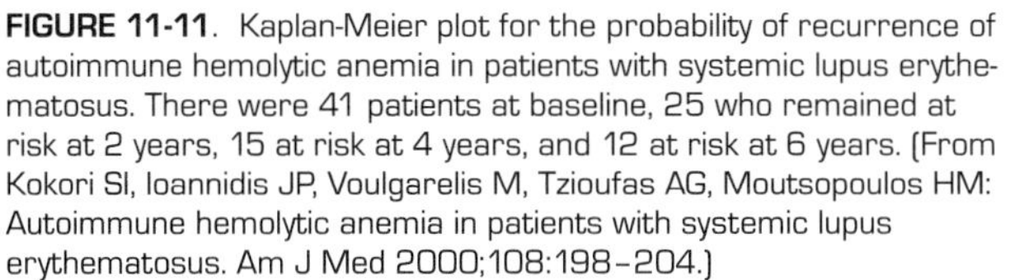
FIGURE 11-11. Kaplan-Meier plot for the probability of recurrence of autoimmune hemolytic anemia in patients with systemic lupus erythematosus. There were 41 patients at baseline, 25 who remained at risk at 2 years, 15 at risk at 4 years, and 12 at risk at 6 years. (From Kokori SI, Ioannidis JP, Voulgarelis M, Tzioufas AG, Moutsopoulos HM: Autoimmune hemolytic anemia in patients with systemic lupus erythematosus. Am J Med 2000;108:198–204.)

Non–Hodgkin's Lymphoma and other Lymphoproliferative Disorders

Economopoulos and associates[463] found that, among 370 patients with non–Hodgkin's lymphoma, 23 (6.2%) had AIHA. There were 19 cases of WAIHA (5.1%) and 4 (1.1%) with CAS. They reported results of therapy for the four patients with CAS and concluded that a combination of alkylating agents with corticosteroids or even more intensive chemotherapy (in cases with aggressive clinical behavior) appears to be the treatment of choice.

Cases of PCH also have been reported in association with non–Hodgkin's lymphoma; combination chemotherapy for the lymphoma caused a remission in both the lymphoma and the AIHA.[464,465]

There are only a few reports of the association between hairy cell leukemia and WAIHA.[466] Mainwaring and colleagues[467] reported two patients with fatal CAS complicating hairy cell leukemia. One patient died before therapy could be started, and the other patient was unresponsive to intravenous methylprednisolone and cyclophsophamide, plasma exchanges, interferon, IVIG, and oral cyclosporine.

Cesana and coworkers[468] reported a patient with hairy cell leukemia and AIHA who was treated with prednisone yielding temporary improvement of the hemolysis. Subsequent treatment with interferon-α resulted in resolution of both the AIHA and the hairy cell leukemia. The AIHA relapsed during temporary interferon-α withdrawal. The authors commented that although the safety of interferon-α in hairy cell leukemia–related immune hemolysis needs further confirmation, the case stresses the importance of treating the underlying disease in secondary forms of AIHA, even if the appropriate drug is contraindicated per se for AIHA.

Cohen and associates[469] reported a patient with refractory and transfusion-dependent CAS secondary to an indolent B-cell lymphoma. She was treated with rituximab (four weekly injections) and achieved complete remission with a significant improvement in hemolysis and also became transfusion independent with a follow-up of more than 1 year.

Mori and colleagues[470] reported a case of lymphoplasmacytoid lymphoma associated with a monoclonal IgM, who also had CAS and thrombocytopenia. He became refractory to prednisolone and combination chemotherapy and was therefore treated with rituximab. The CAS ameliorated, and the serum level of IgM decreased in association with the disappearance of lymphoma cells and the clonal rearrangement of the Ig heavy chains in the bone marrow.

Carcinoma

AIHA occurs more frequently among patients with carcinoma than can be accounted for by chance alone.[471] A number of studies have indicated that removal of the tumor led to remission of the AIHA, which relapsed with the appearance of metastases.[12,472-478] If therapy directed against the underlying tumor is ineffective in resolving the hemolysis, the AIHA should be treated independently according to the principles already reviewed.

Mycoplasma Pneumoniae Infections and Infectious Mononucleosis

In some forms of secondary AIHAs, a spontaneous remission can be predicted confidently (e.g., hemolytic anemias associated with *Mycoplasma pneumoniae* infections and infectious mononucleosis). Cold antibodies with a high thermal maximum are always present with the former and often present with the latter, so that keeping the patient warm is a logical and uniformly recommended therapeutic maneuver.[481-484] For patients with severe anemia, the hospital room should be warmed to as high a temperature as is tolerable, and mittens and warm slippers should be worn as well. One group even resorted to the use of a NASA space suit to provide constant warmth for a rare patient with profound disease.[485,485a] These measures prevent acute exacerbations that result from exposure to cold, although more severely affected patients—whose disease is perhaps associated with antibodies of particularly high thermal amplitude—might have continued hemolysis and progressively more severe anemia even while being kept as warm as possible. Therefore, close observation and consideration of additional therapy are warranted.

Several reports attest to the effectiveness of corticosteroid therapy in CAS associated with *M. pneumoniae* infection.[486-488] As pointed out by Chu and associates,[486] however, hemolytic anemia due to cold agglutinins in patients with *M. pneumoniae* infection is self-limited, so that the contribution of the corticosteroid therapy to recovery is difficult to ascertain. Nevertheless, it is difficult to resist the temptation to give corticosteroids, as complications are minimal in a short-term illness.

Specific antimicrobial agents for *M. pneumonie* have been recommended.[484] Indeed, antibiotics have produced more impressive results than corticosteroids for those patients who still have evidence of unresolved pneumonia at the time of development of hemolytic anemia,[489] but in many cases, the infection will have resolved before the onset of the hemolytic anemia.[481]

Corticosteroids have been reported to be of distinct value in the management of patients with hemolytic anemia associated with infectious mononucleosis.[486,490-493] Tonkin and colleagues[493] reported three patients with severe acute hemolytic anemia. In one patient, steroids were not used, and the hemolysis resolved spontaneoulsy over the course of 7 weeks. The two other patients were treated with corticosteroids and demonstrated marked improvement within a week. Keyloun and Grace[492] reported a patient who was started on therapy with corticosteroids after 2 weeks of illness; prompt improvement was noted, with defervescence of the patient's fever, relief of airway obstruction caused by lymphoid enlargement, a general feeling of well-being, and improvement in the hematocrit level. A less dramatic effect of corticosterold therapy was noted by Bowman and coworkers.[490] In their patient, therapy with 60 mg of prednisone resulted in the stabilization of the hematocrit level at 22%, but there was no improvement for the subsequent 9 days. In spite of the reported effectiveness of corticosteroids, many patients do not require them, as early spontaneous recovery can be expected with confidence.[482,494]

Geurs and associates[308] reported success of plasmapheresis in a patient with corticosteroid-resistant hemolysis in infectious mononucleosis. The patient was febrile for 3 weeks and had continuing signs of hemolysis in spite of corticosteroid and antibiotic therapies. Finally, plasmapheresis was started, and there was a marked and sustained improvement of her laboratory values.

A SUMMARY OF THERAPEUTIC PRINCIPLES IN THE MANAGEMENT OF PATIENTS WITH AUTOIMMUNE HEMOLYTIC ANEMIA

Idiopathic Warm Antibody Autoimmune Hemolytic Anemia

1. Initial therapy should be prednisone at a dose of 1.0–1.5 mg/kg/day (or an equivalent dose of another corticosteroid drug).
2. Higher doses of corticosteroids may be tried, but the potential benefits vs. the potential adverse effects of high-dose corticosteroid therapy are not well defined.
3. Responses are often rapid, and it is unusual for improvement to become evident after 3 weeks of therapy.
4. For patients who respond to treatment, tapering of steroid dosage should begin after the hematocit level reaches 30% and should be carried out slowly over a period of months.
5. If more than 10 mg of prednisone per day (or, at most, 15 mg prednisone per day) is required to maintain an adequate remission (hematocrit level >30%), therapy with corticosteroids should be considered to have failed. Alternative approaches to management should be initiated because of the very significant adverse effects of long-term corticosteroid therapy, even at moderate doses. A common therapeutic error is the prolonged administration of prednisone (i.e., longer than 4 to 6 months) at a dose of over 15 mg per day to maintain a partial remission.
6. Intravenous immunoglobulin and plasma exchange have modest benefits that are generally of short duration. Data regarding the effectiveness of danazol is sparse in the recent medical literature. The adverse effects of these therapies are minimal, and consequently they are frequently used as temporizing measures.
7. Splenectomy should be considered if the response to corticosteroids is inadequate, because splenectomy carries the potential for complete and long-term remission, and available data suggest that it achieves this aim in more than 50% of patients. The decision to perform a splenectomy should not be delayed until adverse effects of corticosteroids become evident but instead should be made early enough to prevent the emergence of such problems. Ordinarily, this means making a decision within weeks or a few months of diagnosis for cases not responding to other therapies.
8. The major adverse effect of splenectomy is OPSI. Education, immunoprophylaxis, and chemoprophylaxis for OPSI must be a perpetual part of management of patients in whom splenectomy has been performed.
9. Immunosuppressive and cytotoxic drugs have had modest benefits and have significant adverse effects but could be necessary for patients refractory to other forms of therapy.
10. A rapidly increasing number of reports suggest a role for newer immunosuppressive drugs, especially cyclosporine and rituximab.
11. Hematopoietic stem cell transplantation is being attempted for some autoimmune diseases but is presently experimental.
12. Blood transfusion should be performed when necessary, even though the compatibility test might reveal gross incompatibility of all units. Special compatibility test procedures are necessary prior to selection of the most appropriate unit for transfusion (see Chapter 10).

Idiopathic Cold Agglutinin Syndrome

1. Exposure to cold should be avoided; this may be the only therapy necessary even though a chronic hemolytic anemia might persist.
2. The patient should be encouraged to tolerate the presence of mild or moderate symptoms of anemia because of the high risk-to-benefit ratio of therapeutic maneuvers that have been used for this disorder.
3. Chlorambucil (or cyclophosphamide) produces benefit for a minority of patients and should be tried if significant symptoms of anemia are present.

4. Patients who have anemia with intolerable symptoms and who do not respond to chlorambucil are probably best managed by a chronic program of transfusion.
5. Corticosteroids are generally ineffective for this disorder. In a few patients, high doses might cause some benefit, but the hazards of prolonged corticosteroid therapy usually greatly outweigh the benefits. The degree of improvement must justify the considerable long-term risks.
6. Plasma exchange offers a modest degree of temporary benefit to some patients. The procedure is complicated by autoagglutination at room temperature.
7. Splenectomy is generally ineffective, although a few reports of success have been published, particularly for patients with atypical serologic findings that include the presence of warm hemolysins.
8. Anecdotal reports suggest that rituximab, fludarabine, and interferon could be of benefit for some patients.
9. Other therapies are of unproven value.

Paroxysmal Cold Hemoglobinuria

1. Most patients with this disorder have an acute and transient hemolytic anemia, so that often only supportive care is necessary. Frequent monitoring of the patient's hematologic status is necessary because the hemoglobin and hematocrit can drop precipitously. Meticulous attention should be given to keeping the patient warm.
2. The severity of hemolysis could dictate the need for blood transfusion (see Chapter 10).
3. A short course of corticosteroid therapy is warranted empirically if hemolysis is severe.
4. If signs of an infection are present, appropriate antibiotics should be provided.
5. In the rare patient with chronic paroxysmal cold hemoglobinuria, very limited data suggest that splenectomy might be of benefit.

Secondary Autoimmune Hemolytic Anemias

1. In patients with AIHA secondary to chronic lymphocytic leukemia, the hemolysis often responds well to corticosteroids. Alternative forms of therapy that have been used include cyclosporine, chlorambucil, fludarabine, 2-chlorodeoxyadenosine, IVIG, and splenectomy. Infections represent the main cause of morbidity and mortality related to treatment of the immune hemolysis.
2. Hemolysis associated with SLE generally responds well to therapy described for idiopathic WAIHA.
3. The most effective therapy for AIHA in patients with lymphomas is treatment of the underlying disorder.
4. Cold agglutinin syndrome associated with *M. pneumoniae* infection should be treated by keeping the patient warm and administering antibiotics if signs of infection are still present. The effectiveness of corticosteroids is uncertain.
5. Hemolytic anemia associated with infectious mononucleosis should be treated with corticosteroids unless the anemia is mild. If cold reactive antibodies with high thermal maximum are demonstrated, the patient should be kept warm.

REFERENCES

1. Petz LD, Garratty G: Acquired Immune Hemolytic Anemias, 1st ed. New York: Churchill Livingstone, 1980.
2. Petz LD: Treatment of autoimmune hemolytic anemias. Curr Opin Hematol 2001;8:411–416.
3. Domen RE: An overview of immune hemolytic anemias. Cleve Clin J Med 1998;65:89–99.
4. Jandl JH: Textbook of Hematology, 2nd ed. Boston: Little, Brown, 1996
5. Boumpas DT, Chrousos GP, Wilder RL, Cupps TR, Balow JE: Glucocorticoid therapy for immune-mediated diseases: Basic and clincal correlates. Ann Intern Med 1993;119:1198–1208.
6. Dacie JV: Auto-immune haemolytic anaemias (AIHA): Treatment. In The Haemolytic Anaemias, 3rd ed. vol. 3. The Auto-Immune Haemolytic Anaemias. New York: Churchill Livingstone, 1992:452–520.
7. Engelfriet CP, Overbeeke MA, van dem Borne AE: Autoimmune hemolytic anemia. Semin Hematol 1992;29:3–12.
8. Rosse WF: Clinical Immunohematology: Basic Concepts and Clinical Applications. Boston: Blackwell Scientific, 1990.
9. Gibson J: Autoimmune hemolytic anemia: Current concepts. Aust N Z J Med 1988;18:625–637.
10. Worlledge S: Immune Haemolytic Anaemias. In Hardisty RM, Weatherall DJ (eds): Blood and Its Disorders. Oxford: Blackwell Scientific, 1982:479–513.
11. Zupanska B, Sylwestrowicz T, Pawelski S: The results of prolonged treatment of autoimmune haemolytic anaemia. Haematologia 1981;14:425–433.
12. Pirofsky B: Autoimmunization and the Autoimmune Hemolytic Anemias. Baltimore: Williams & Wilkins, 1969.
13. Allgood JW, Chaplin H Jr: Idiopathic acquired autoimmune hemolytic anemia: A review of forty-seven cases treated from 1955 through 1965. Am J Med 1967;43:254–273.
14. Eyster ME, Jenkins DE Jr: Erythrocyte coating substances in patients with positive direct antiglobulin reactions: Correlation of gamma-G globulin and complement coating with underlying diseases, overt hemolysis and response to therapy. Am J Med 1969;46:360–371.
15. Dameshek W, Komninos ZD: The present status of treatment of autoimmune hemolytic anemia with ACTH and cortisone. Blood 1956;11:648
16. Dacie JV: The Haemolytic Anaemias. Part II. Auto-Immune Haemolytic Anaemias, 2nd ed. London: J&A Churchill, 1962.
17. Horster JA: Die Korticosteroid-Behandlung Hematologische und Verwandter Erkrankungen. Stuttgart: Georg Theime Verlag, 1961.
18. Ozsoylu S: High dose intravenous methylprednisolone (HIVMP) in hematologic disorders. Hematol Rev 1990;4:197–207.
19. Ozsoylu S: Megadose methylprednisolone for Evans syndrome. Pediatr Hematol Oncol 2000;17:725–726.
20. Meyer O, Stahl D, Beckhove P, Huhn D, Salama A: Pulsed high-dose dexamethasone in chronic autoimmune haemolytic anaemia of warm type. Br J Haematol 1997;98:860–862.
21. Meytes D, Adler M, Viraq I, Feigl D, Levene C: High-dose methylprednisolone in acute immune cold hemolysis. N Engl J Med 1985;312:318.
22. Hari P, Srivastava RN: Pulse corticosteroid therapy with methylprednisolone or dexamethasone. Indian J Pediatr 1998;65:557–560.
23. Leddy JP, Swisher SN: Acquired Immune Hemolytic Disorders (Including Drug-Induced Immune Hemolytic

Anemia). In Samter M (ed): Immunologic Diseases. Boston: Little, Brown, 1978:1187.
24. Nordoy A, Neset G: Splenectomy in hematologic diseases. Acta Med Scand 1968;183:117–126.
25. Lester RS, Knowles SR, Shear NH: The risks of systemic corticosteroid use. Dermatol Clin 1998;16:277–288.
26. Rosse WF: Quantitative immunology of immune hemolytic anemia. II. The relationship of cell-bound antibody to hemolysis and the effect of treatment. J Clin Invest 1971;50:734.
27. Evans RS: Autoantibodies in hematologic disorders. Stamf Med Bull 1955;13:152–166.
28. Chaplin H Jr: Clinical usefulness of specific antiglobulin reagents in autoimmune hemolytic anemias. Progr Hematol 1973;8:25–49.
29. Chaplin H, Avioli LV: Grand rounds: Autoimmune hemolytic anemia. Arch Int Med 1977;137:346–351.
30. Frank MM, Schreiber AD, Atkinson JP, Jaffe CJ: Pathophysiology of immune hemolytic anemia. Ann Int Med 1977; 87:210–222.
31. Kay NE, Douglas SD: Monocyte-erythrocyte interaction in vitro in immune hemolytic anemias. Blood 1977;50:889–897.
32. Stanbury RM, Graham EM: Systemic corticosteroid therapy—Side effects and their management. Br J Ophthalmol 1998;82:704–708.
33. Bialas MC, Routledge PA: Adverse effects of corticosteroids. Adverse Drug React Toxicol Rev 1998;17:227–235.
34. Dequeker J: NSAIDs/corticosteroids—Primum non nocere. Adv Exp Med Biol 1999;455:319–325.
35. Caldwell JR, Furst DE: The efficacy and safety of low-dose corticosteroids for rheumatoid arthritis. Semin Arthritis Rheum 1991;21:1–11.
36. Recommendations for the prevention and treatment of glucocorticoid-induced osteoporosis: 2001 update. American College of Rheumatology Ad Hoc Committee on Glucocoritcoid-Induced Osteoporosis. Arthritis Rheum 2001;44: 1496–1503.
37. Stuck AE, Minder CE, Frey FJ: Risk of infectious complications in patients taking glucocorticosteroids. Rev Infect Dis 1989;11:954–963.
38. Piper JM, Ray WA, Daugherty JR, Griffin MR: Corticosteroid use and peptic ulcer disease: Role of nonsteroidal anti-inflammatory drugs. Ann Intern Med 1991;114:735–740.
39. Luo JC, Chang FY, Lin HY, et al: The potential risk factors leading to peptic ulcer formation in autoimmune disease patients receiving corticosteroid treatment. Aliment Pharmacol Ther 2002;16:1241–1248.
40. Katkhouda N, Mavor E: Laparoscopic splenectomy. Surg Clin North Am 2000;80:1285–1297.
41. Schlinkert RT, Teotia SS: Laparoscopic splenectomy. Arch Surg 1999;134:99–103.
42. Katkhouda N, Hurwitz MB, Rivera RT, et al: Laparoscopic splenectomy: Outcome and efficacy in 103 consecutive patients. Ann Surg 1998;228:568–578.
43. Delaitre B, Pitre J: Laparoscopic splenectomy versus open splenectomy: A comparative study. Hepatogastroenterology 1997;44:45–49.
44. Friedman RL, Hiatt JR, Korman JL, Facklis K, Cymerman J, Phillips EH: Laparoscopic or open splenectomy for hematologic disease: Which approach is superior? J Am Coll Surg 1997;185:49–54.
45. Caprotti R, Porta G, Franciosi C, et al: Laparoscopic splenectomy for hematological disorders: Our experience in adult and pediatric patients. Int Surg 1998;83:303–307.
46. Stephens BJ, Justice JL, Sloan DA, Yoder JA: Elective laparoscopic splenectomy for hematologic disorders. Am Surg 1997;63:700–703.
47. Rosen M, Brody F, Walsh RM, Tarnoff M, Malm J, Ponsky J: Outcome of laparoscopic splenectomy based on hematologic indication. Surg Endosc 2002;16:272–279.
48. Katkhouda N, Manhas S, Umbach TW, Kaiser AM: Laparoscopic splenectomy. J Laparoendosc Adv Surg Tech A 2001;11:383–390.
49. Tanoue K, Okita K, Akahoshi T, et al: Laparoscopic splenectomy for hematologic diseases. Surgery 2002;131(1 Suppl.):S318–S323.
50. Antonelli G: Effeti della splenectomia di una particolare forma di ittero emolitico acquisto con anemia a tuipo perniciouso. Polyclinico (med) 1913;13:193–222.
51. Eppinger H: Die Hepato-Lienallen Erkrankungen. Berlin: Julius Springer, 1920.
52. Dameshek W, Schwartz SO: Acute hemolytic anemia (acquired hemolytic icterus, acute type). Medicine 1940;19:231–327.
53. Dameshek W: The management of acute hemolytic anemia and the hemolytic crisis. Clinics 1943;2:118.
54. Stickney JM, Heck FJ: Primary nonfamilial hemolytic anemia. Blood 1948;3:431.
55. Robson HN: Medical aspects of splenectomy. Edinb Med J 1949;56:381.
56. Welch CS, Dameshek W: Splenectomy in blood dyscrasias. New Engl J Med 1950;242:601.
57. Dreyfus B, Dausset J, Vidal G: Etude clinque et hematologique de douze cas d'anemie hemolytique acquise avec auto-anticorps. Rev Hemat 1951;6:349.
58. Learmonth J: The surgery of the spleen. Br Med J 1951;2:67.
59. Chertkow G, Dacie JV: Results of splenectomy in autoimmune haemolytic anaemia. Br J Haematol 1956;2:237.
60. Young LE, Miller G, Swisher SN: The treatment of hemolytic disorders. J Chronic Dis 1957;6:307.
61. Crosby WH, Rappaport H: Autoimmune hemolytic anemia. 1. Analysis of hematologic observations with particular reference to their prognostic value; a survey of 57 cases. Blood 1957;12:42.
62. Dausset J, Colombani JL: The serology and the prognosis of 128 cases of autoimmune hemolytic anemia. Blood 1959;14:1280.
63. Goldberg A: Radiochromium in the selection of patients with haemolytic anaemia for splenectomy. Lancet 1966;1:109.
64. Kinlough RL, Bennett RC, Lander H: The place of splenectomy in haematological disorders: The value of ^{51}Cr techniques. Med J Aust 1966;22:1022–1027.
65. Mappes G, Fischer J: Experience with splenectomy in hematologic diseases. Dtsch Med Wochenschr 1969;94:584–589.
66. Schwartz SI, Bernard RP, Adams JT, Bauman AW: Splenectomy for hematologic disorders. Arch Surg 1970;101:338–347.
67. Devlin HB, Evans DS, Birkhead JS: Elective splenectomy for primary hematologic and splenic disease. Surg Gynecol Obstet 1970;131:273–276.
68. Ahuja S LSSL: Value of surface counting in predicting response to splenectomy in haemolytic anaemia. J Clin Pathol 1972;25:467.
69. Christensen BE: The pattern of erythrocyte sequestration in immunohaemolysis: Effects of prednisone treatment and splenectomy. Scand J Haematol 1973;10:120–129.
70. Habibi B, Homberg JC, Schaison G, Salmon C: Autoimmune hemolytic anemia in children: A review of 80 cases. Am J Med 1974;56:61–69.
71. Ikkala E, Kivilaakso E, Hastbacka J: Splenectomy in blood diseases: A report of 80 cases. Ann Clin Res 1974;6:290–299.
72. Coon WW: Splenectomy in the treatment of hemolytic anemia. Arch Surg 1985;120:625–628.
73. Wilhelm MC, Jones RE, McGehee R, Mitchener JS, Sandusky WR, Hess CE: Splenectomy in hematologic disorders: The ever-changing indications. Ann Surg 1988;207:581–589.
74. Ly B, Albrechtsen D: Therapeutic splenectomy in hematologic disorders: Effects and complications in 221 adult patients. Acta Med Scand 1981;209:21–29.
75. Akpek G, McAneny D, Weintraub L: Comparative response to splenectomy in Coombs-positive autoimmune hemolytic anemia with or without associated disease. Am J Hematol 1999;61:98–102.
76. Karpatkin S, Strick N, Siskind GW: Detection of splenic antiplatelet antibody synthesis in idiopathic autoimmune thrombocytopenic purpura (ATP). Br J Haematol 1972;23: 167–176.
77. McMillan R, Longmire RL, Yelenosky R, Donnell RL, Armstrong S: Quantitation of platelet-binding IgG produced

in vitro by spleens from patients with idiopathic thrombocytopenic purpura. N Engl J Med 1974;291:812–817.
78. Bowdler AJ: The spleen and hemolytic disorders. Clinics Haematol 1975;4:231.
79. Bowdler AJ: The role of the spleen and splenectomy in autoimmune hemolytic disease. Semin Hematol 1976;13:335–348.
80. Hughes-Jones NC, Szul L: Determination of the sites of red-cell destruction using ^{51}Cr-labeled cells. Br J Haematol 1957;3:320.
81. Jandl JH, Greenberg MS, Yonemoto RH, Castle WB: Clinical determination of the sites of red cell sequestration in hemolytic anemias. J Clin Invest 1956;35:842.
82. Jandl JH, Jones AR, Castle WB: The destruction of red cells by antibodies in man. I. Observations of the sequestration and lysis of red cells altered by immune mechanisms. J Clin Invest 1957;36:1428.
83. Ben-Bassat I, Seligsohn U, Leiba H, Leef F, Chaitchik S, Ramot B: Sequestration studies with chromium-51 labelled red cells as criteria for splenectomy. Israel J Med Sci 1967;3:832.
84. Lewis SM, Szur L, Dacie JV: The pattern of erythrocyte destruction in haemolytic anaemia, as studied with radioactive chromium. British Journal of Haematology 1960;6:122.
85. McCurdy PR, Rath CE: Splenectomy in hemolytic anemia: Results predicted by body scanning after injection of Cr^{51}-tagged red cells. New Engl J Med 1958;259:459.
86. Najean Y, Cacchione R, Dresch C, Rain JD: Methods of evaluating the sequestration site of red cells labelled with ^{51}Cr: A review of 96 cases. Br J Haematol 1975;29:495–510.
87. Parker AC, MacPherson AIS, Richmond J: Value of radiochromium investigation in autoimmune haemolytic anaemia. Br Med J 1977;1:208.
88. Schloesser LL, Korst DR, Clatanoff DV, Schilling RF: Radioactivity over the spleen and liver following transfusion of chromium ^{51}-labelled erythrocytes in hemolytic anemia. J Clin Invest 1957;36:1470.
89. Szur L: Surface counting in the assessment of sites of red cell destruction. Brit J Haemat 1970;18:591.
90. Veeger W, Woldring MG, VanRood JJ, et al: The value of the determination of the site of red cell sequestration in hemolytic anemia as a prediction test for splenectomy. Acta Med Scand 1962;171:507.
91. Williams ED, Szur L, Glass HI, Lewis SM, Pettit JE, Ahuja S: Measurement of red cell destruction in the spleen. J Lab Clin Med 1974;84:134–146.
92. Nightingale D, Prankerd TA, Richards JD, Thompson D: Splenectomy in anaemia. Q J Med 1972;41:261–267.
93. Crosby WH: Splenectomy in hematologic disorders. New Engl J Med 1972;286:1252.
94. Dacie JV, Worlledge SM: Auto-immune hemolytic anemias. In Brown EB, Moore CV (eds): Progress in Hematology. New York: Grune and Stratton, 1969:82–120.
95. Pirofsky B: Immune haemolytic disease: The autoimmune haemolytic anaemias. Clin Haematol 1975;4:167.
96. Rosse WF: Quantitative immunology of immune hemolytic anemia. I. The fixation of C1 by autoimmune antibody and heterologous anti-IgG antibody. J Clin Invest 1971;50:727.
97. Schwartz SI, Adams JT, Bauman AW: Splenectomy for hematologic disorders. Curr Probl Surg 1971;1–57.
98. DeWeese MS, Coller FA: Splenectomy for hematologic disorders. West J Surg 1959;67:129.
99. Sandusky WR, Leavell BS, Benjamin BI: Splenectomy: Indications and results in hematologic disorders. Ann Surg 1964;159:695–710.
100. Sedgwick CE, Hume AH: Elective splenectomy: An analysis of 220 operations. Ann Surg 1960;151:163.
101. Morris DH, Bullock FD: The importance of the spleen in resistance to infection. Ann Surg 1919;70:513.
102. Krivit W, Giebink GS, Leonard A: Overwhelming postplenectomy infection. Surg Clin North Am 1979;59:223–233.
103. King H, Schumacher HB: Splenic studies. I. Susceptibility to infection after splenectomy performed in infancy. Am Surg 1952;136:239.
104. Smith CH, Erlandson ME, Schulman I, et al: Hazards of severe infections in splenectomized infants and children. Am J Med 1957;22:380.
105. Lucas RV, Krivit W: Overwhelming infection in children following splenectomy. J Peds 1960;57:185.
106. Singer DB: Postsplenectomy Sepsis. In Rosenberg HS, Bolande RP (eds): Perspectives on Pediatric Pathology. Chicago: Year Book, 1973:285.
107. Krivit W: Overwhelming postsplenectomy infection. Am J Hematol 1977;2:193–201.
108. Lynch AM, Kapila R: Overwhelming postsplenectomy infection. Infect Dis Clin North Am 1996;10:693–707.
109. Brigden ML, Pattullo AL: Prevention and management of overwhelming postsplenectomy infection—An update. Crit Care Med 1999;27:836–842.
110. Styrt B: Infection associated with asplenia: Risks, mechanisms, and prevention. Am J Med 1990;88(5N):33N-42N.
111. Green JB, Shackford SR, Sise MJ, Fridlund P: Late septic complications in adults following splenectomy for trauma: A prospective analysis in 144 patients. J Trauma 1986;26:999–1004.
112. Brigden ML: Overwhelming postsplenectomy infection still a problem. West J Med 1992;157:440–443.
113. Holdsworth RJ, Irving AD, Cuschieri A: Postsplenectomy sepsis and its mortality rate: Actual versus perceived risks. Br J Surg 1991;78:1031–1038.
114. Schilling RF: Estimating the risk for sepsis after splenectomy in hereditary spherocytosis. Ann Intern Med 1995;122:187–188.
115. Schwartz PE, Sterioff S, Mucha P, Melton LJ III, Offord KP: Postsplenectomy sepsis and mortality in adults. JAMA 1982;248:2279–2283.
116. Cullingford GL, Watkins DN, Watts AD, Mallon DF: Severe late postsplenectomy infection. Br J Surg 1991;78:716–721.
117. Konradsen HB, Henrichsen J: Pneumococcal infections in splenectomized children are preventable. Acta Paediatr Scand 1991;80:423–427.
118. Waghorn DJ, Mayon-White RT: A study of 42 episodes of overwhelming post-splenectomy infection: Is current guidance for asplenic individuals being followed? J Infect 1997;35:289–294.
119. Working Party of the British Committee for Standards in Haematology Clinical Haematology Task Force: Guidelines for the prevention and treatment of infection in patients with an absent or dysfunctional spleen. Br Med J 1996;312:430–434.
120. Fielding AK: Prophylaxis against late infection following splenectomy and bone marrow transplant. Blood Rev 1994;8:179–191.
121. Flegg PJ: Long term management after splenectomy. Br Med J 1994;308:131.
122. Advisory Committee on Immunization Practices: Recommendations of the Advisory Committee on Immunization Practices (ACIP): Use of vaccines and immune globulins in persons with altered immunocompetence. MMWR 1993;42:1–18.
123. Deodhar HA, Marshall RJ, Barnes JN: Increased risk of sepsis after splenectomy. Br Med J 1993;307:1408–1409.
124. Hirsh J, Dacie JV: Persistent post-splenectomy thrombocytosis and thrombo-embolism: A consequence of continuing anaemia. Br J Haematol 1966;12:44–53.
125. Visudhiphan S, Ketsa-Ard K, Piankijagum A, Tumliang S: Blood coagulation and platelet profiles in persistent post-splenectomy thrombocytosis: The relationship to thromboembolism. Biomed Pharmacother 1985;39:264–271.
126. Boxer MA, Braun J, Ellman L: Thromboembolic risk of post-splenectomy thrombocytosis. Arch Surg 1978;113:808–809.
127. Traetow WD, Fabri PJ, Carey LC: Changing indications for splenectomy. 30 years' experience. Arch Surg 1980;115:447–451.
128. Coon WW, Penner J, Clagett P, Eos N: Deep venous thrombosis and postsplenectomy thrombocytosis. Arch Surg 1978;113:429–431.
129. Ellison EC, Fabri PJ: Complications of splenectomy. Etiology, prevention, and management. Surg Clin North Am 1983;63:1313–1330.
130. Chaffanjon PC, Brichon PY, Ranchoup Y, Gressin R, Sotto JJ: Portal vein thrombosis following splenectomy for hematologic disease: Prospective study with Doppler color flow imaging. World J Surg 1998;22:1082–1086.
131. Hayes DM, Spurr CL, Histoff LW, et al: Post splenectomy thrombocsytosis. Ann Intern Med 1963;58:259–267.

132. Bensinger TA, Logue GL, Rundles RW: Hemorrhagic thrombocythemia; control of postsplenectomy thrombocytosis with melphalan. Blood 1970;36:61–69.
133. Gluch L, Khouri JM: Pseudohyperkalaemia after splenectomy: Pitfall for the unwary. Med J Aust 1994;161:509–510.
134. Parker NE, Jacobs P: Pseudohyperkalaemia—A cause of diagnostic confusion. S Afr Med J 1981;60:973–974.
135. Ho AM, Woo JC, Kelton JG, Chiu L: Spurious hyperkalaemia associated with severe thrombocytosis and leukocytosis. Can J Anaesth 1991;38:613–615.
136. Erslev AJ: Hypersplenism and hyposplenism. In Beutler E, Lichtman MA, Coller BS, Kipps TJ, Seligsohn U (eds): Williams Hematology. New York: McGraw-Hill, 2001:683–687.
137. Pearson HA: Red-cell "rubbish" as a key to splenic function. Lab Mgmt 1982;(September):25–33.
138. Corazza GR, Ginaldi L, Zoli G, Frisoni M, Lalli G, Gasbarrini G, et al: Howell-Jolly body counting as a measure of splenic function: A reassessment. Clin Lab Haematol 1990;12:269–275.
138a. Holroyde CP, Oski FA, Gardner FH: The "pocked" erythrocyte: Red-cell surface alterations in reticuloendothelial immaturity of the neonate. N Engl J Med 1969;281:516–520.
138b. Reinhart WH, Chien S: Red cell vacuoles: Their size and distribution under normal conditions and after splenectomy. Am J Hematol 1988;27:265–271.
139. Zago MA, Covas DT, Figueiredo MS, Bottura C: Red cell pits appear preferentially in old cells after splenectomy. Acta Haematol 1986;76:54–56.
140. Diehl LF, Ketchum LH: Autoimmune disease and chronic lymphocytic leukemia: Autoimmune hemolytic anemia, pure red cell aplasia, and autoimmune thrombocytopenia. Semin Oncol 1998;25:80–97.
141. Markus H, Forfar JC: Splenic irradiation in treating warm autoimmune haemolytic anaemia. Br Med J (Clin Res Ed) 1986;293:839–840.
142. Fathy N, Furst DE: Combination therapy for autoimmune diseases: The rheumatoid arthritis model. Springer Semin Immunopathol 2001;23:5–26.
143. Moroni G, Della Casa AO, Ponticelli C: Combination treatment in autoimmune diseases: Systemic lupus erythematosus. Springer Semin Immunopathol 2001;23:75–89.
144. Ciancio G, Burke GW, Miller J: Current treatment practice in immunosuppression. Expert Opin Pharmacother 2000;1:1307–1330.
145. Allison AC: Immunosuppressive drugs: The first 50 years and a glance forward. Immunopharmacology 2000;47:63–83.
146. Gonin JM: Maintenance immunosuppression: New agents and persistent dilemmas. Adv Ren Replace Ther 2000;7:95–116.
147. Schwartz R, Dameshek W: The treatment of autoimmune hemolytic anemia with 6–mercaptopurine and thioguanine. Blood 1962;19:483.
148. Taylor L: Idiopathic autoimmune hemolytic anemia: Response of a patient to repeated courses of alkylating agents. Am J Med 1963;35:130.
149. Hitzig WH, Massimo L: Treatment of autoimmune hemolytic anemia in children with azathioprine (imuran). Blood 1966;28:840–850.
150. Worlledge S: Immune Haemolytic Anemias. In Hardisty RM, Weatherall DJ (eds): Blood and Its Disorders. Oxford: Blackwell, 1974:714.
151. Skinner MD, Schwartz RS: Immunosuppressive therapy. 1. N Engl J Med 1972;287:221–227.
152. Skinner MD, Schwartz RS: Immunosuppressive therapy. 2. N Engl J Med 1972;287:281–286.
153. Mueller-Eckhardt CH, Kretschmer V: Immunosuppressive Therapy in Blood Diseases. New York: Schwabe, 1972:85.
154. Johnson CA, Abildgaard CF: Treatment of idiopathic autoimmune hemolytic anemia in children: Review and report of two fatal cases in infancy. Acta Paediatr Scand 1976;65:375–379.
155. Moyo VM, Smith D, Brodsky I, Crilley P, Jones RJ, Brodsky RA: High-dose cyclophosphamide for refractory autoimmune hemolytic anemia. Blood 2002;100:704–706.
156. Heisel MA, Ortega JA: Factors influencing prognosis in childhood autoimmune hemolytic anemia. Am J Pediatr Hematol Oncol 1983;5:147–152.
157. Silva VA, Seder RH, Weintraub LR: Synchronization of plasma exchange and cyclophosphamide in severe and refractory autoimmune hemolytic anemia. J Clin Apheresis 1994;9:120–123.
158. Ahn YS, Harrington WJ, Byrnes JJ, Pall L, McCrainie J: Treatment of autoimmune hemolytic anemia with Vinca-loaded platelets. JAMA 1983;249:2189–2194.
159. Gertz MA, Petitt RM, Pineda AA, Wick MR, Burgstaler EA: Vinblastine-loaded platelets for autoimmune hemolytic anemia. Ann Intern Med 1981;95:325–326.
160. Medellin PL, Patten E, Weiss GB: Vinblastine for autoimmune hemolytic anemia. Ann Intern Med 1982;96:123.
161. Brady-West DC, Thame J, West W: Autoimmune haemolytic anaemia, immune thrombocytopenia, and leucopenia: An unusual presentation of Hodgkin's disease. West Indian Med J 1997;46:95–96.
162. Vaiopoulos G, Kyriakou D, Papadaki H, Fessas P, Eliopoulos GD: Multiple myeloma associated with autoimmune hemolytic anemia. Haematologica 1994;79:262–264.
163. Majumdar G, Brown S, Slater NG, Singh AK: Clinical spectrum of autoimmune haemolytic anaemia in patients with chronic lymphocytic leukaemia. Leuk Lymphoma 1993;9:149–151.
164. Dovat S, Roberts RL, Wakim M, Stiehm ER, Feig SA: Immune thrombocytopenia after umbilical cord progenitor cell transplant: Response to vincristine. Bone Marrow Transplant 1999;24:321–323.
165. Shastri KA, Logue GL: Autoimmune Hemolytic Anemia. In Conn HF (ed): Current Therapy. Philadelphia: WB Saunders, 1997:352–355.
166. Murphy S, LoBuglio AF: Drug therapy of autoimmune hemolytic anemia. Semin Hematol 1976;13:323–334.
167. Petz LD: Hemolytic Anemias-Immune. In Conn HF (ed): Current Therapy. Philadelphia: WB Saunders, 1977:256–260.
168. Rosse WF, Logue GL: Immune hemolytic anemias. Mod Treat 1971;8:379–401.
169. Janssen NM, Genta MS: The effects of immunosuppressive and anti-inflammatory medications on fertility, pregnancy, and lactation. Arch Intern Med 2000;160:610–619.
170. Leone G, Voso MT, Sica S, Morosetti R, Pagano L: Therapy related leukemias: Susceptibility, prevention and treatment. Leuk Lymphoma 2001;41:255–276.
171. Kyle R: Second malignancies associated with chemotherapic agents. Semin Oncol 1982;9:133.
172. Park D, Koeffler P: Therapy related myelodysplastic syndromes. Sem Hematol 1996;33:256–273.
173. Feig SA: Second malignant neoplasms after successful treatment of childhood cancers. Blood Cells Mol Dis 2001;27:662–666.
174. Matsuda S, Koyasu S: Mechanisms of action of cyclosporine. Immunopharmacology 2000;47:119–125.
175. Fathman CG, Myers BD: Cyclosporine therapy for autoimmune disease. N Engl J Med 1992;326:1693–1695.
176. Emilia G, Messora C, Longo G, Bertesi M: Long-term salvage treatment by cyclosporin in refractory autoimmune haematological disorders. Br J Haematol 1996;93:341–344.
177. Kahan BD: Cyclosporine. N Engl J Med 1989;321:1725–1738.
178. Yee GC, Stanley DL, Pessa LJ, et al: Effect of grapefruit juice on blood cyclosporin concentration. Lancet 1995;345:955–956.
179. Kane GC, Lipsky JJ: Drug-grapefruit juice interactions. Mayo Clin Proc 2000;75:933–942.
180. Emilia G, Messora C: Interaction between cyclosporin and chlorambucil. Eur J Haematol 1993;51:179.
181. Dundar S, Ozdemir O, Ozcebe O: Cyclosporin in steroid-resistant auto-immune haemolytic anaemia. Acta Haematol 1991;86:200–202.
182. Hershko C, Sonnenblick M, Ashkenazi J: Control of steroid-resistant autoimmune haemolytic anaemia by cyclosporine. Br J Haematol 1990;76:436–437.
183. Rackoff WR, Manno CS: Treatment of refractory Evans syndrome with alternate-day cyclosporine and prednisone. Am J Pediatr Hematol Oncol 1994;16:156–159.
184. Ruess-Borst MA, Waller HD, Muller CA: Successful treatment of steroid-resistant hemolysis in chronic lymphocytic leukemia with cyclosporine A. Am J Hematol 1994;46:375–376.

185. Emilia G, Messora C, Bensi L: The use of cyclosporin-A in the treatment of B-chronic lymphocytic leukemia. Leukemia 1995;9:357–359.
186. Ferrara F, Copia C, Annunziata M, et al: Complete remission of refractory anemia following a single high dose of cyclophosphamide. Ann Hematol 1999;78:87–88.
187. Friedmann AM, King KE, Shirey RS, Resar LM, Casella JF: Fatal autoimmune hemolytic anemia in a child due to warm-reactive immunoglobulin M antibody. J Pediatr Hematol Oncol 1998;20:502–505.
188. Duru F, Gurgey A, Cetin M, Kanra T, Altay C: Chronic autoimmune hemolytic anemia in children: A report of four patients. J Med 1994;25:231–240.
189. Allison AC, Eugui EM: Mycophenolate mofetil and its mechanisms of action. Immunopharmacology 2000;47:85–118.
190. Gregoor PJHS, van Gelder T, Weimar W: Mycophenolate mofetil, Cellcept, a new immunosuppressive drug with great potential in internal medicine. Neth J Med 2000;57: 233–246.
191. Hood KA, Zarembski DG: Mycophenolate mofetil: A unique immunosuppressive agent. Am J Health Syst Pharm 1997; 54:285–294.
192. Zimmer-Molsberger B, Knauf W, Thiel E: Mycophenolate mofetil for severe autoimmune haemolytic anemia. Lancet 1997;350:1003–1004.
193. Howard J, Hoffbrand AV, Prentice HG, Mehta A: Mycophenolate mofetil for the treatment of refractory auto-immune haemolytic anaemia and auto-immune thrombocytopenia purpura. Br J Haematol 2002;117:712–715.
194. Maloney DG, Smith B, Rose A: Rituximab: Mechanism of action and resistance. Semin Oncol 2002;29(1 Suppl. 2):2–9.
195. Grillo-Lopez AJ, Hedrick E, Rashford M, Benyunes M: Rituximab: Ongoing and future clinical development. Semin Oncol 2002;29(1 Suppl. 2):105–112.
196. Zecca M, De Stefano P, Nobili B, Locatelli F: Anti-CD20 monoclonal antibody for the treatment of severe, immune-mediated, pure red cell aplasia and hemolytic anemia. Blood 2001;97:3995–3997.
197. Coiffier B, Haioun C, Ketterer N, et al: Rituximab (anti-CD20 monoclonal antibody) for the treatment of patients with relapsing or refractory aggressive lymphoma: a multicenter phase II study. Blood 1998;92:1927–1932.
198. Leget GA, Czuczman MS: Use of rituximab, the new FDA-approved antibody. Curr Opin Oncol 1998;10:548–551.
199. Byrd JC, Waselenko JK, Maneatis TJ, et al: Rituximab therapy in hematologic malignancy patients with circulating blood tumor cells: Association with increased infusion-related side effects and rapid blood tumor clearance. J Clin Oncol 1999;17:791–795.
200. Ratanatharathorn V, Carson E, Reynolds C, et al: Anti-CD20 chimeric monoclonal antibody treatment of refractory immune-mediated thrombocytopenia in a patient with chronic graft-versus-host disease. Ann Intern Med 2000;133: 275–279.
201. Stasi R, Pagano A, Stipa E, Amadori S: Rituximab chimeric anti-CD20 monoclonal antibody treatment for adults with chronic idiopathic thrombocytopenic purpura. Blood 2001;98: 952–957.
201a. Kakaiya R: New therapy with anti-CD20 antibody (Rituximab) for autoimmune hemolytic anemia. Blood Therapies in Medicine 2003;3:91–96.
202. Lee E, Zamkoff KW, Gentile TC, Zimrin A: Rituxan in the treatment of auto-immune hemolytic anemia (AIHA) [abstract]. Blood 2000;96:596–597.
203. Grossi A, Santini V, Longo G, Balestri F, Rossi-Ferrini P, Morfini M: Treatment with anti-CD20 antibodies of patients with autoimmune thrombocytopenia with or without hemolytic anemia; worsening in hemoglobin level [abstract]. Blood 2000;96:523.
204. Rai KR, Gupta NK, Janson D, Patel DV, Ahmed I, Kavuru S: Rituximab, cyclophosphamide and decadron combination is highly effective in auto-immune hemolytic anemia associated with chronic lymphocytic leukemia [abstract]. Blood 2000; 96:754–755.
205. Ahrens N, Kingreen D, Seltsam A, Salama A: Treatment of refractory autoimmune haemolytic anaemia with anti-CD20 (rituximab). Br J Haematol 2001;114:244–245.
206. Seipelt G, Bohme A, Koschmieder S, Hoelzer D: Effective treatment with rituximab in a patient with refractory prolymphocytoid transformed B-chronic lymphocytic leukemia and Evans syndrome. Ann Hematol 2001;80:170–173.
207. Perrotta S, Locatelli F, La Manna A, Cennamo L, De Stefano P, Nobili B: Anti-CD20 monoclonal antibody (Rituximab) for life-threatening autoimmune haemolytic anaemia in a patient with systemic lupus erythematosus. Br J Haematol 2002;116: 465–467.
208. Chemnitz J, Draube A, Diehl V, Wolf J: Successful treatment of steroid and cyclophosphamide-resistant hemolysis in chronic lymphocytic leukemia with rituximab. Am J Hematol 2002;69:232–233.
209. McMahon C, Babu L, Hodgson A, Hayat A, Connell NO, Smith OP: Childhood refractory autoimmune haemolytic anaemia: Is there a role for anti-CD20 therapy (rituximab)? Br J Haematol 2002;117:480–483.
210. Seeliger S, Baumann M, Mohr M, Jurgens H, Frosch M, Vormoor J: Autologous peripheral blood stem cell transplantation and anti-B-cell directed immunotherapy for refractory auto-immune haemolytic anaemia. Eur J Pediatr 2001;160: 492–496.
211. Schiller G, Tillisch J, Rosen P: Use of anti-CD20 monoclonal antibody for the treatment of Evans syndrome and monoclonal gammopathy/neuropathy syndrome [abstract]. Blood 1999;94(Suppl. 1):3536.
212. Zompi S, Tulliez M, Conti F, et al: Rituximab (anti-CD20 monoclonal antibody) for the treatment of patients with clonal lymphoproliferative disorders after orthotopic liver transplantation: A report of three cases. J Hepatol 2000;32:521–527.
213. Abdel-Raheem MM, Potti A, Kobrinsky N: Severe Evans's syndrome secondary to interleukin-2 therapy: Treatment with chimeric monoclonal anti-CD20 antibody. Ann Hematol 2001;80:543–545.
214. Morselli M, Luppi M, Potenza L, et al: Mixed warm and cold autoimmune hemolytic anemia: complete recovery after 2 courses of rituximab treatment. Blood 2002;99:3478–3479.
215. Quartier P, Brethon B, Philippet P, Landman-Parker J, Le Deist F, Fischer A: Treatment of childhood autoimmune haemolytic anaemia with rituximab. Lancet 2001;358:1511–1513.
216. Ng PC, Lee KK, Lo AF, Li CK, Fok TF: Anti B cell targeted immunotherapy for treatment of refractory autoimmune haemolytic anaemia in a young infant. Arch Dis Child 2003;88:337–339.
217. Zecca M, Nobili B, Ramenghi U, et al: Rituximab for the treatment of refractory autoimmune hemolytic anemia in children. Blood 2003;101:3857–3861.
218. Hongeng S, Tardtong P, Worapongpaiboon S, Ungkanont A, Jootar S: Successful treatment of refractory autoimmune haemolytic anaemia in a post-unrelated bone marrow transplant paediatric patient with rituximab. Bone Marrow Transplant 2002;29:871–872.
219. Matthews DC: Ribuximab in the very young: Benefits in AIHA, at what risk? Blood 2003;101:3761.
220. Motto DG, Williams JA, Boxer LA: Rituximab for refractory childhood autoimmune hemolytic anemia. Isr Med Assoc J 2002;4:1006–1008.
221. Quartier P, Tournilhac O, Archimbaud C, et al: Enteroviral meningoencephalitis after anti-CD20 (rituximab) treatment. Clin Infect Dis 2003;36:e47–e49.
222. Kunkel L, Wong A, Maneatis T, et al: Optimizing the use of rituximab for treatment of B-cell non-Hodgkin's lymphoma: A benefit-risk update. Semin Oncol 2000;27(Suppl. 12):53–61.
223. Wood AM: Rituximab: An innovative therapy for non-Hodgkin's lymphoma. Am J Health Syst Pharm 2001;58:215–229.
224. Huhn D, von Schilling C, Wilhelm M, et al: Rituximab therapy of patients with B-cell chronic lymphocytic leukemia. Blood 2001;98:1326–1331.
225. Reff ME, Carner K, Chambers KS, Chinn PC, Leonard JE, Raab R, et al: Depletion of B cells in vivo by a chimeric

mouse human monoclonal antibody to CD20. Blood 1994;83: 435–445.
226. Sharma VR, Fleming DR, Slone SP: Pure red cell aplasia due to parvovirus B19 in a patient treated with rituximab. Blood 2000;96:1184–1186.
227. Dervite I, Hober D, Morel P: Acute hepatitis B in a patient with antibodies to hepatitis B surface antigen who was receiving rituximab. N Engl J Med 2001;344:68–69.
228. Goldberg SL, Pecora AL, Alter RS, Kroll MS, Rowley SD, Waintraub SE, et al: Unusual viral infections (progressive multifocal leukoencephalopathy and cytomegalovirus disease) after high-dose chemotherapy with autologous blood stem cell rescue and peritransplantation rituximab. Blood 2002;99:1486–1488.
229. Jourdan E, Topart D, Richard B, Jourdan J, Sotto A: Severe autoimmune hemolytic anemia following rituximab therapy in a patient with a lymphoproliferative disorder. Leuk Lymphoma 2003;44:889–890.
230. Ahn YS, Harrington WJ, Mylvaganam R, Ayub J, Pall LM: Danazol therapy for autoimmune hemolytic anemia. Ann Intern Med 1985;102:298–301.
231. Ahn YS: Efficacy of danazol in hematologic disorders. Acta Haematol 1990;84:122–129.
232. Manoharan A: Danazol therapy in patients with immune cytopenias. Aust N Z J Med 1987;17:613–614.
233. Tan AM, Lou J, Cheng HK: Danazol for treatment of refractory autoimmune hemolytic anaemia. Ann Acad Med Singapore 1989;18:707–709.
234. Pignon JM, Poirson E, Rochant H: Danazol in autoimmune haemolytic anaemia. Br J Haematol 1993;83:343–345.
235. Cervera H, Jara LJ, Pizarro S, Enkerlin HL, Fernandez M, Medina F, et al: Danazol for systemic lupus erythematosus with refractory autoimmune thrombocytopenia or Evans' syndrome. J Rheumatol 1995;22:1867–1871.
236. Chan AC, Sack K: Danazol therapy in autoimmune hemolytic anemia associated with systemic lupus erythematosus. J Rheumatol 1991;18:280–282.
237. Lugassy G, Reitblatt T, Ducach A, Oren S: Severe autoimmune hemolytic anemia with cold agglutinin and sclerodermic features—Favorable response to danazol. Ann Hematol 1993;67:143–144.
238. Narayana SVL, Babu YS, Volanakis JE: Inhibition of Complement Serine Proteases as a Therapeutic Strategy. In Lambris JD, Holers VM (eda): Contemporary Immunology: Therapeutic Interventions in the Complement System. Totowa, NJ: Homana Press, 2000:57–74.
239. Quigg RJ: Modulation of disease using recombinant human endogenous complement inhibitors. In Lambris JD, Holers VM (eds): Contemporary Immunology: Therapeutic Interventions in the Complement System. Totowa, NJ: Homana Press, 2000:155–170.
240. Walport MJ: Complement: First of two parts. N Engl J Med 2001;344:1058–1066.
241. Walport MJ: Complement: Second of two parts. N Engl J Med 2001;344:1140–1144.
242. Sahu A, Lambris JD: Complement inhibitors: A resurgent concept in anti-inflammatory therapeutics. Immunopharmacology 2000;49:133–148.
243. Kirschfink M: Targeting complement in therapy. Immunol Rev 2001;180:177–189.
244. Basta M: Modulation of complement-mediated immune damage by intravenous immune globulin. Clin Exp Immunol 1996;104(Suppl. 1):21–25.
245. Yazdanbakhsh K, Kang S, Tamasauskas D, Sung D, Scaradavou A: Complement receptor 1 inhibitors for prevention of immune-mediated red cell destruction: Potential use in transfusion therapy. Blood 2003;101:5046–5052.
246. Bjorkholm M: Intravenous immunoglobulin treatment in cytopenic haematological disorders. J Intern Med 1993;234:119–126.
247. Kazatchkine MD, Kaveri SV: Immunomodulation of autoimmune and inflammatory diseases with intravenous immune globulin. N Engl J Med 2001;345:747–755.
248. Reilly MP, McKenzie SE: Mechanisms of action of IVIg: physiology of Fc receptors. Vox Sang 2002;83(Suppl. 1):57–63.
249. Dwyer JM: Manipulating the immune system with immune globulin. N Engl J Med 1992;326:107–116.
250. Masson PL: Elimination of infectious antigens and increase of IgG catabolism as possible modes of action of IVIg. J Autoimmun 1993;6:683–689.
251. Yu Z, Lennon VA: Mechanism of intravenous immune globulin therapy in antibody-mediated autoimmune diseases. N Engl J Med 1999;340:227–228.
252. Bleeker WK, Teeling JL, Hack CE: Accelerated autoantibody clearance by intravenous immunoglobulin therapy: Studies in experimental models to determine the magnitude and time course of the effect. Blood 2001;98:3136–3142.
253. Mueller-Eckhardt C, Salama A, Mahn I, Kiefel V, Neuzner J, Graubner M: Lack of efficacy of high-dose intravenous immunoglobulin in autoimmune haemolytic anaemia: A clue to its mechanism. Scand J Haematol 1985;34:394–400.
254. Salama A, Mueller-Eckhardt C, Kiefel V: Effect of intravenous immunoglobulin in immune thrombocytopenia. Lancet 1983;2:193–195.
255. Flores G, Cunningham-Rundles C, Newland AC, Bussel JB: Efficacy of intravenous immunoglobulin in the treatment of autoimmune hemolytic anemia: Results in 73 patients. Am J Hematol 1993;44:237–242.
256. Bussel JB, Cunningham-Rundles C, Abraham C: Intravenous treatment of autoimmune hemolytic anemia with very high dose gammaglobulin. Vox Sang 1986;51:264–269.
257. Ratko TA, Burnett DA, Foulke GE, Matuszewski KA, Sacher RA: Recommendations for off-label use of intravenously administered immunoglobulin preparations. University Hospital Consortium Expert Panel for Off-Label Use of Polyvalent Intravenously Administered Immunoglobulin Preparations. JAMA 1995;273:1865–1870.
258. Ratko TA: Technology Assessment: Intravenous Immunoglobulin Preparations. Oak Brook, IL, University HealthSystem Consortium, 1999.
259. Sacher RA: Intravenous immunoglobulin consensus statement. J Allergy Clin Immunol 2001;108(4 Suppl.):S139–S146.
260. Besa EC: Rapid transient reversal of anemia and long-term effects of maintenance intravenous immunoglobulin for autoimmune hemolytic anemia in patients with lymphoproliferative disorders. Am J Med 1988;84:691–698.
261. Leickly FE, Buckley RH: Successful treatment of autoimmune hemolytic anemia in common variable immunodeficiency with high-dose intravenous gamma globulin. Am J Med 1987;82:159–162.
262. Otheo E, Maldonado MS, Munoz A, Hernandez-Jodra M: High-dose intravenous immunoglobulin as single therapy in a child with autoimmune hemolytic anemia. Pediatr Hematol Oncol 1997;14:487–490.
263. Gonzalez CA: Successful treatment of autoimmune hemolytic anemia with intravenous immunoglobulin in a patient with AIDS. Transplant Proc 1998;30:4151–4152.
264. Vandenberghe P, Zachee P, Verstraete S, Demuynck H, Boogaerts MA, Verhoef GE: Successful control of refractory and life-threatening autoimmune hemolytic anemia with intravenous immunoglobulins in a man with the primary antiphospholipid syndrome. Ann Hematol 1996; 73:253–256.
265. Argiolu F, Diana G, Arnone M, Batzella MG, Piras P, Cao A: High-dose intravenous immunoglobulin in the management of autoimmune hemolytic anemia complicating thalassemia major. Acta Haematol 1990;83:65–68.
266. Salama A, Mahn I, Neuzner J, Graubner M, Mueller-Eckhardt C: IgG therapy in autoimmune haemolytic anaemia of warm type. Blut 1984;48:391–392.
267. Atrah HI, Crawford RJ, Gabra GS, Mitchell R: Successes and failures of intravenous immunoglobulin. Scand J Haematol 1985;34:345–347.
268. American Society of Hospital Pharmacists (ASHP) Commission of Therapeutics: ASHP therapeutic guidelines for intravenous immune globulin. Clin Pharmacol 1992;11: 117–136.
269. Schwartz SA: Clinical use of immune serum globulin as replacement therapy in patients with primary immuno-

deficiency syndromes. In Ballow M (ed): IVIG Therapy Today. Totowa, NJ: Humana Press, 1992:1–12.

270. Sherer Y, Levy Y, Langevitz P, Rauova L, Fabrizzi F, Shoenfeld Y: Adverse effects of intravenous immunoglobulin therapy in 56 patients with autoimmune diseases. Pharmacology 2001; 62:133–137.
271. Sekul EA, Cupler EJ, Dalakas MC: Aseptic meningitis associated with high-dose intravenous immunoglobulin therapy: Frequency and risk factors. Ann Intern Med 1994;121:259–262.
272. Perazella MA, Cayco AV: Acute renal failure and intravenous immune globulin: Sucrose nephropathy in disguise? Am J Ther 1998;5:399–403.
273. Friedman KD, Menitove JE: Preparation and Clinical Use of Plasma and Plasma Fractions. In Beutler E, Lichtman MA, Coller BS, Kipps TJ, Seligsohn U (eds): Williams Hematology. New York: McGraw-Hill, 2001:1917–1934.
274. Epstein JS, Zoon KC: Important drug warning. FDA Dear Doctor Letter. Nov. 13, 1998. Rockville, MD: Center for Biologics Evalulation and Research, Food and Drug Administration.
275. Stahl M, Schifferli JA: The renal risks of high-dose intravenous immunoglobulin treatment. Nephrol Dial Transplant 1998;13:2182–2185.
276. Haskin JA, Warner DJ, Blank DU: Acute renal failure after large doses of intravenous immune globulin. Ann Pharmacother 1999;33:800–803.
277. Gaines A, Varricchio F, Kapit R, Pierce LR, Scott D, Finlayson J: Renal insufficiency and failure associated with immune globulin intravenous therapy-United States (1985–98). Morb Mort Weekly Rpt 1999;48:518–521.
278. Ahsan N: Intravenous immunoglobulin induced-nephropathy: A complication of IVIG therapy. J Nephrol 1998;11:157–161.
279. Laidlaw S, Bainton R, Wilkie M, Makris M: Acute renal failure in acquired haemophilia following the use of high dose intravenous immunoglobulin. Haemophilia 1999;5:270–272.
280. Levy JB, Pusey CD: Nephrotoxicity of intravenous immunoglobulin. QJM 2000;93:751–755.
281. Sati HI, Ahya R, Watson HG: Incidence and associations of acute renal failure complicating high-dose intravenous immunoglobulin therapy. Br J Haematol 2001;113:556–557.
282. Gupta N, Ahmed I, Nissel-Horowitz S, Patel D, Mehrotra B: Intravenous gammglobulin-associated acute renal failure. Am J Hematol 2001;66:151–152.
283. Go RS, Call TG: Deep venous thrombosis of the arm after intravenous immunoglobulin infusion: Case report and literature review of intravenous immunoglobulin-related thrombotic complications. Mayo Clin Proc 2000;75:83–85.
284. Dalakas MC: High-dose intravenous immunoglobulin and serum viscosity: Risk of precipitating thromboembolic events. Neurology 1994;44:223–226.
285. Woodruff RK, Grigg AP, Firkin FC, Smith IL: Fatal thrombotic events during treatment of autoimmune thrombocytopenia with intravenous immunoglobulin in elderly patients. Lancet 1986;2:217–218.
286. Silbert PL, Knezevic WV, Bridge DT: Cerebral infarction complicating intravenous immunoglobulin therapy for polyneuritis cranialis. Neurology 1992;42:257–258.
287. Reinhart WH, Berchtold PE: Effect of high-dose intravenous immunoglobulin therapy on blood rheology. Lancet 1992;339:662–664.
288. Steg RE, Lefkowitz DM: Cerebral infarction following intravenous immunoglobulin therapy for myasthenia gravis. Neurology 1994;44:1180–1181.
289. Brannagan TH, III, Nagle KJ, Lange DJ, Rowland LP: Complications of intravenous immune globulin treatment in neurologic disease. Neurology 1996;47:674–677.
290. Fisman DN, Smilovitch M: Intravenous immunoglobulin, blood viscosity and myocardial infarction. Can J Cardiol 1997;13:775–777.
291. Wolff SN, Fay JW, Herzig RH, et al: High-dose weekly intravenous immunoglobulin to prevent infections in patients undergoing autologous bone marrow transplantation or severe myelosuppressive therapy. A study of the American Bone Marrow Transplant Group. Ann Intern Med 1993;118: 937–942.
292. Klaesson S, Ringden O, Ljungman P, Aschan J, Hagglund H, Winiarski J: Does high-dose intravenous immune globulin treatment after bone marrow transplantation increase mortality in veno-occlusive disease of the liver? Transplantation 1995;60:1225–1230.
293. Rizk A, Gorson KC, Kenney L, Weinstein R: Transfusion-related acute lung injury after the infusion of IVIG. Transfusion 2001;41:264–268.
294. Isbister JP: Therapeutic apheresis. Indian J Pediatr 2001;68:61–67.
295. Grima KM: Therapeutic apheresis in hematological and oncological diseases. J Clin Apheresis 2000;15:28–52.
296. Koo AP: Therapeutic apheresis in autoimmune and rheumatic diseases. J Clin Apheresis 2000;15:18–27.
297. Kiprov DD, Strauss RG, Ciavarella D, Gilcher RO, Kasprisin DO, Klein HG, et al: Management of autoimmune disorders. J Clin Apheresis 1993;8:195–210.
298. McLeod BC, Strauss RG, Ciavarella D, Gilcher RO, Kasprisin DO, Kiprov DD, et al: Management of hematological disorders and cancer. J Clin Apheresis 1993;8:211–230.
299. Branda RF, Moldow CF, McCullough JJ, Jacob HS: Plasma exchange in the treatment of immune disease. Transfusion 1975;15:570–576.
300. Patten E, Reuter FP: Evans' syndrome: Possible benefit from plasma exchange. Transfusion 1980;20:589–593.
301. Rosenfield RE, Jagathambal: Transfusion therapy for autoimmune hemolytic anemia. Semin Hematol 1976;13:311–321.
302. Garelli S, Mosconi L, Valbonesi M, Schieppati G, Navassa G: Plasma exchange for a hemolytic crisis due to autoimmune hemolytic anemia of the IgG warm type. Blut 1980;41:387–391.
303. Bernstein ML, Schneider BK, Naiman JL: Plasma exchange in refractory acute autoimmune hemolytic anemia. J Pediatr 1981;98:774–775.
304. Schroeder JO, Euler HH, Loffler H: Synchronization of plasmapheresis and pulse cyclophosphamide in severe systemic lupus erythematosus. Ann Intern Med 1987;107:344–346.
305. Hughes P, Toogood A: Plasma exchange as a necessary prerequisite for the induction of remission by human immunoglobulin in auto-immune haemolytic anaemia. Acta Haematol 1994;91:166–169.
306. Silberstein LE, Berkman EM: Plasma exchange in autoimmune hemolytic anemia (AIHA). J Clin Apheresis 1983;1:238–242.
307. Brooks BD, Steane EA, Sheehan RG, Frenkel EP: Therapeutic plasma exchange in the immune hemolytic anemias and immunologic thrombocytopenic purpura. Prog Clin Biol Res 1982;106:317–329.
308. Geurs F, Ritter K, Mast A, Van Maele V: Successful plasmapheresis in corticosteroid-resistant hemolysis in infectious mononucleosis: Role of autoantibodies against triosephosphate isomerase. Acta Haematol 1992;88:142–146.
309. Kutti J, Wadenvik H, Safai-Kutti S, Bjorkander J, Hanson LA, Westberg G, et al: Successful treatment of refractory autoimmune haemolytic anaemia by plasmapheresis. Scand J Haematol 1984;32:149–152.
310. Andersen O, Taaning E, Rosenkvist J, Moller NE, Mogensen HH: Autoimmune haemolytic anaemia treated with multiple transfusions, immunosuppressive therapy, plasma exchange, and desferrioxamine. Acta Paediatr Scand 1984;73:145–148.
311. von Keyserlingk H, Meyer-Sabellek W, Arntz R, Haller H: Plasma exchange treatment in autoimmune hemolytic anemia of the warm antibody type with renal failure. Vox Sang 1987;52:298–300.
312. McConnell ME, Atchison JA, Kohaut E, Castleberry RP: Successful use of plasma exchange in a child with refractory immune hemolytic anemia. Am J Pediatr Hematol Oncol 1987;9:158–160.
313. McCarthy LJ, Danielson CF, Fernandez C, Skipworth E, Limiac CA, Prahlow T, et al: Intensive plasma exchange for severe autoimmune hemolytic anemia in a four-month-old infant. J Clin Apheresis 1999;14:190–192.
314. Shehata N, Kouroukis C, Kelton JG: A review of randomized controlled trials using therapeutic apheresis. Transfus Med Rev 2002;16:200–229.
315. Smith JW, Weinstein R, for The AABB Hemapheresis Committee KL: Therapeutic apheresis: A summary of current

indication categories endorsed by the AABB and the American Society for Apheresis. Transfusion 2003;43:820–822.
316. Cash JM, Wilder RL: Treatment-resistant rheumatic disease. Rheum Dis Clin N Am 1995;21:1–170.
317. Lafferty KL, Gazda KS: Costimulation and the regulation of autoimmunity. In Rose NR, Mackay IR (eds): The Autoimmune Diseases. San Diego, CA: Academic Press, 1998:59–74.
318. Bingham SJ, Snowden J, Morgan G, Emery P: High dose immunosuppressive therapy and stem cell transplantation in autoimmune and inflammatory diseases. Int Immunopharmacol 2002;2:399–414.
319. Marmont AM: New horizons in the treatment of autoimmune diseases: Immunoablation and stem cell transplantation. Annu Rev Med 2000;51:115–134.
320. Van Bekkum DW: Autologous stem cell transplantation for treatment of autoimmune diseases. Stem Cells 1999;17:172–178.
321. Moore J, Brooks P: Stem cell transplantation for autoimmune diseases. Springer Semin Immunopathol 2001;23:193–213.
322. Cohen Y, Polliack A, Nagler A: Treatment of refractory autoimmune diseases with ablative immunotherapy using monoclonal antibodies and/or high dose chemotherapy with hematopoietic stem cell support. Curr Pharm Des 2003;9:279–288.
323. Van Bekkum DW: Experimental basis of hematopoietic stem cell transplantation for treatment of autoimmune diseases. J Leukoc Biol 2002;72:609–620.
324. Burt RK, Slavin S, Burns WH, Marmont AM: Induction of tolerance in autoimmune diseases by hematopoietic stem cell transplantation: Getting closer to a cure? Blood 2002;99: 768–784.
325. Morton JL, Siegel BV: Transplantation of autoimmune potential. Development of antinuclear antibodies in H-2 histocompatible recipients of bone marrow from New Zealand Black mice. Proc Natl Acad Sci U S A 1974;71:2162–2166.
326. Ikehara S: Autoimmune diseases as stem cell disorders: Normal stem cell transplant for their treatment [Review]. Int J Mol Med 1998;1:5–16.
327. Ikehara S: Bone marrow transplantation for autoimmune diseases. Acta Haematol 1998;99:116–132.
328. Li H, Kaufman CL, Boggs SS, Johnson PC, Patrene KD, Ildstad ST: Mixed allogeneic chimerism induced by a sublethal approach prevents autoimmune diabetes and reverses insulitis in nonobese diabetic (NOD) mice. J Immunol 1996;156: 380–388.
329. Van Bekkum DW: BMT in experimental autoimmune diseases. Bone Marrow Transplant 1993;11:183–187.
330. Raetz E, Beatty PG, Adams RH: Treatment of severe Evans syndrome with an allogeneic cord blood transplant. Bone Marrow Transplant 1997;20:427–429.
331. De Stefano P, Zecca M, Giorgiani G, Perotti C, Giraldi E, Locatelli F: Resolution of immune haemolytic anaemia with allogeneic bone marrow transplantation after an unsuccessful autograft. Br J Haematol 1999;106:1063–1064.
331a. Oyama Y, Papadopoulos EB, Miranda M, Traynor AE, Burt RK: Allogeneic stem cell transplantation for Evans syndrome. Bone Marrow Transplant 2001;28:903–905.
332. Marmont AM, Gualandi F, Van Lint MT, Bacigalupo A: Refractory Evans' syndrome treated with allogeneic SCT followed by DLI: Demonstration of a graft-versus-autoimmunity effect. Bone Marrow Transplant 2003;31:399–402.
333. Hinterberger W, Hinterberger-Fischer M, Marmont A: Clinically demonstrable anti-autoimmunity mediated by allogeneic immune cells favorably affects outcome after stem cell transplantation in human autoimmune diseases. Bone Marrow Transplant 2002;30:753–759.
334. Burt RK, Traynor AE, Craig R, Marmont AM: The promise of hematopoietic stem cell transplantation for autoimmune diseases. Bone Marrow Transplant 2003;31:521–524.
335. Fassas A: Intense immunosuppression and autologous hematopoietic stem cell transplantation for multiple sclerosis. Haematologica 2003;88:244–245.
336. Openshaw H, Nash RA, McSweeney PA: High-dose immunosuppression and hematopoietic stem cell transplantation in autoimmune disease: Clinical review. Biol Blood Marrow Transplant 2002;8:233–248.
337. Burt RK, Traynor AE: Hematopoietic stem cell transplantation: A new therapy for autoimmune disease. Stem Cells 1999;17:366–372.
338. Huhn RD, Fogarty PF, Nakamura R, et al: High-dose cyclophosphamide with autologous lymphocyte-depleted peripheral blood stem cell (PBSC) support for treatment of refractory chronic autoimmune thrombocytopenia. Blood 2003;101:71–77.
339. Paillard C, Kanold J, Halle P, et al: Two-step immunoablative treatment with autologous peripheral blood CD34(+) cell transplantation in an 8–year-old boy with autoimmune haemolytic anaemia. Br J Haematol 2000;110:900–902.
340. Burt RK, Schroeder J, Rosa R, et al: Autologous hematopoietic stem cell transplantation of patients with severe and refractory systemic lupus erythematosus (SLE): Three year follow-up [abstract]. Blood 2000;96(Suppl. 1):843.
341. Musso M, Porretto F, Crescimanno A, et al: Autologous peripheral blood stem and progenitor (CD34+) cell transplantation for systemic lupus erythematosus complicated by Evans syndrome. Lupus 1998;7:492–494.
342. Snowden JA, Patton WN, O'Donnell JL, Hannah EE, Hart DN: Prolonged remission of longstanding systemic lupus erythematosus after autologous bone marrow transplant for non-Hodgkin's lymphoma. Bone Marrow Transplant 1997;19:1247–1250.
343. Rosler W, Manger B, Repp R, Kalden JR, Gramatzki M: Autologous PBPCT in a patient with lymphoma and Sjogren's syndrome: complete remission of lymphoma without control of the autoimmune disease. Bone Marrow Transplant 1998;22:211–213.
344. Brodsky RA, Sensenbrenner LL, Jones RJ: Complete remission in severe aplastic anemia after high-dose cyclophosphamide without bone marrow transplantation. Blood 1996;87:491–494.
345. Brodsky RA, Petri M, Smith BD, Seifter EJ, Spivak JL, Styler M, et al: Immunoablative high-dose cyclophosphamide without stem-cell rescue for refractory, severe autoimmune disease. Ann Intern Med 1998;129:1031–1035.
346. Brodsky RA, Smith BD: Bone marrow transplantation for autoimmune diseases. Curr Opin Oncol 1999;11:83–86.
347. Nousari HC, Brodsky RA, Jones RJ, Grever MR, Anhalt GJ: Immunoablative high-dose cyclophosphamide without stem cell rescue in paraneoplastic pemphigus: Report of a case and review of this new therapy for severe autoimmune disease. J Am Acad Dermatol 1999;40(5 Pt 1):750–754.
348. Marmont AM: Immunoablation followed or not by hematopoietic stem cells as an intense therapy for severe autoimmune diseases. New perspectives, new problems. Haematologica 2001;86:337–345.
349. Euler HH, Schroeder JO, Harten P, Zeuner RA, Gutschmidt HJ: Treatment-free remission in severe systemic lupus erythematosus following synchronization of plasmapheresis with subsequent pulse cyclophosphamide. Arthritis Rheum 1994;37:1784–1794.
350. Mielcarek M, Sandmaier BM, Maloney DG, Maris M, McSweeney PA, Woolfrey A, et al: Nonmyeloablative hematopoietic cell transplantation: Status quo and future perspectives. J Clin Immunol 2002;22:70–74.
351. Champlin R, Khouri I, Shimoni A, Gajewski J, Kornblau S, Molldrem J, et al: Harnessing graft-versus-malignancy: Nonmyeloablative preparative regimens for allogeneic haematopoietic transplantation, an evolving strategy for adoptive immunotherapy. Br J Haematol 2000;111:18–29.
352. Barrett J, Childs R: Non-myeloablative stem cell transplants. Br J Haematol 2000;111:6–17.
353. Pulsipher MA, Woolfrey A: Nonmyeloablative transplantation in children: Current status and future prospects. Hematol Oncol Clin North Am 2001;15:809–834.
354. Baron F, Beguin Y: Nonmyeloablative allogeneic hematopoietic stem cell transplantation. J Hematother Stem Cell Res 2002;11:243–263.
355. Wilmers MJ, Russell PA: Autoimmune hemolytic anemia in an infant treated by thymectomy. Lancet 1963;2:915.
356. Hancock DM: Autoimmune haemolytic anaemia in an infant treated by thymectomy. Lancet 1963;2:1118.
357. Karaklis AS, Valaes T, Pantelakis SN, Doxiadis SA: Thymectomy in an infant with autoimmune haemollytic anaemia. Lancet 1964;2:778.

358. Oski FA, Abelson NM: Autoimmune hemolytic anemia in an infant: Report of a case treated unsuccessfully with thymectomy. J Pediatr 1965;67:752–758.
359. Hirooka M, Yoshioka K, Ono T, Kubota N, Ikeda S: Autoimmune hemolytic anemia in a child treated with thymectomy. Tohoku J Exp Med 1970;101:227–235.
360. Rennenberg RJ, Pauwels P, Vlasveld LT: A case of thymoma-associated autoimmune haemolytic anaemia. Neth J Med 1997;50:110–114.
361. Albahary C, Homberg JC, Guillaume J, Martin S, Boulangiez JP: Thymoma, myasthenia and auto-immune hemolytic anemia [in French]. Nouv Presse Med 1972;1:1931–1934.
362. Arntzenius AB, Bieger R: Disappearance of autoantibody-induced haemolysis after excision of a malignant thymoma. Neth J Med 1991;38:117–121.
363. Dreyfus B, Aubert P, Patte D, Bolloc'h-Combrisson Le A: Erythroblastopenic chronique decouverte apres une thymectomie. Nouv Rev Fr Hematol 1963;3:765–772.
364. Fischer JT, Lautenschlager J, Pottgen W: Autoimmune haemolytic anaemia following malignant thymoma [in German]. Dtsch Med Wochenschr 1974;99:1867–1869.
365. Halperin IC, Minogue WF, Komninos ZD: Autoimmune hemolytic anemia and myasthenia gravis associated with thymoma. N Engl J Med 1966;275:663–664.
365a. Hennemann HH, Beck T: Autoimmunohaemolytische Anamie nach Bestrahlung eines Thymoma. Dtsch Med Wochenschr 1974;99:1869–1871.
366. Janbon MM, Bertrand L, Bonnet H: Sarcome du thymus avec anemie hemolytique par auto-anticorps. Montpellier Med 1956;49:161–164.
367. Mongan ES, Kern WA Jr, Terry R: Hypogammaglobulinemia with thymoma, hemolytic anemia, and disseminated infection with cytomegalovirus. Ann Intern Med 1966;65:548–554.
368. Pirofsky B: Autoimmune hemolytic anemia and neoplasia of the reticuloendothelium: With a hypothesis concerning etiologic relationships. Ann Intern Med 1968;68:109–121.
369. Ross JF, Finch SC, Street RB, Streider JW: The simultaneous occurrence of benign thymoma and refractory anemia. Blood 1954;9:935.
370. Rubinstein I, Langevitz P, Hirsch R, Berkowicz M, Lieberman Y, Shibi G: Autoimmune hemolytic anemia as the presenting manifestation of malignant thymoma. Acta Haematol 1985; 74:40–42.
371. Taniguchi S, Shibuya T, Morioka E, Okamura T, Okamura S, Inaba S, et al: Demonstration of three distinct immunological disorders on erythropoiesis in a patient with pure red cell aplasia and autoimmune haemolytic anaemia associated with thymoma. Br J Haematol 1988;68:473–477.
372. Tiber C, Casimir M, Nogeire C, Lichtiger B, Conrad FG: Thymoma with red cell aplasia and hemolytic anemia. South Med J 1981;74:1164–1165.
373. Lyckholm LJ, Edmond MB: Images in clinical medicine. Seasonal hemolysis due to cold-agglutinin syndrome. N Engl J Med 1996;334:437.
374. Pisciotta AV: Cold hemagglutination in acute and chronic hemolytic syndromes. Blood 1955;10:295.
375. Firkin BG, Blackwell JB, Johnston GAW: Essential cryoglobulinaemia and acquired haemolytic anaemia due to cold agglutinins. Australian Ann Med 1959;8:151.
376. Schreiber AD, Herskovitz BS, Goldwein M: Low-titer cold-hemagglutinin disease: Mechanism of hemolysis and response to corticosteroids. N Engl J Med 1977;296:1490–1494.
377. Silberstein LE, Berkman EM, Schreiber AD: Cold hemagglutinin disease associated with IgG cold-reactive antibody. Ann Intern Med 1987;106:238–242.
378. Dellagi K, Brouet JC, Schenmetzler C, Praloran V: Chronic hemolytic anemia due to a monoclonal IgG cold agglutinin with anti-Pr specificity. Blood 1981;57:189–191.
379. Nanan R, Scheurlen W, Gerlich M, Huppertz HI: Severe low-titer cold-hemagglutinin disease responsive to steroid pulse therapy. Ann Hematol 1995;71:101–102.
380. Lahav M, Rosenberg I, Wysenbeek AJ: Steroid-responsive idiopathic cold agglutinin disease: A case report. Acta Haematol 1989;81:166–168.
381. Schubothe H: The cold hemagglutinin disease. Semin Hematol 1966;3:27–47.
382. Worlledge SM, Brain MC, Cooper AC, Hobbs JR, Dacie JV: Immmunosuppressive drugs in the treatment of autoimmune haemolytic anaemia. Proc R Soc Med 1968;61:1312–1315.
383. Hippe E, Jensen KB, Olesen H, Lind K, Thomsen PE: Chlorambucil treatment of patients with cold agglutinin syndrome. Blood 1970;35:68–72.
384. Olesen H: Chlorambucil treatment in the cold agglutinin syndrome. Scand J Haematol 1964;1:116.
385. Evans RS, Baxter E, Gilliland BC: Chronic hemolytic anemia due to cold agglutinins: A 20-year history of benign gammopathy with response to chlorambucil. Blood 1973;42:463–470.
386. Ramos RR, Curtis BR, Sadler JE, Eby CS, Chaplin H: Refractory immune hemolytic anemia with a high thermal amplitude, low affinity IgG anti-Pra cold autoantibody. Autoimmunity 1992;12:149–154.
387. Chaplin H Jr: Lymphoma in primary chronic cold hemagglutinin disease treated with chlorambucil. Arch Intern Med 1982;142:2119–2123.
388. Jacobs A: Cold agglutinin hemolysis responding to fludarabine therapy. Am J Hematol 1996;53:279–280.
389. Di Raimondo F, Giustolisi R, Cacciola E, O'Brien S, Kantarjian H, Robertson LB, et al: Autoimmune hemolytic anemia in chronic lymphocytic leukemia patients treated with fludarabine. Leuk Lymphoma 1993;11:63–68.
390. Berentsen S, Tjonnfjord GE, Brudevold R, Gjertsen BT, Langholm R, Lokkevik E, et al: Favourable response to therapy with the anti-CD20 monoclonal antibody rituximab in primary chronic cold agglutinin disease. Br J Haematol 2001;115:79–83.
391. Pulik M, Genet P, Lionnet F, Touahri T: Treatment of primary chronic cold agglutinin disease with rituximab: Maintenance therapy may improve the results. Br J Haematol 2002;117: 998–999.
392. Lee EJ, Kueck B: Rituxan in the treatment of cold agglutinin disease. Blood 1998;92:3490–3491.
393. Bauduer F: Rituximab: A very efficient therapy in cold agglutinins and refractory autoimmune haemolytic anaemia associated with CD20-positive, low-grade non-Hodgkin's lymphoma. Br J Haematol 2001;112:1085–1086.
394. Layios N, Van Den NE, Jost E, Deneys V, Scheiff JM, Ferrant A: Remission of severe cold agglutinin disease after Rituximab therapy. Leukemia 2001;15:187–188.
395. Gharib M, Poynton C: Complete, long-term remission of refractory idiopathic cold haemagglutinin disease after Mabthera. Br J Haematol 2002;117:248–249.
396. Zaja F, Russo D, Fuga G, Michelutti T, Sperotto A, Fanin R, et al: Rituximab in a case of cold agglutinin disease. Br J Haematol 2001;115:232–233.
397. Engelhardt M, Jakob A, Ruter B, Trepel M, Hirsch F, Lubbert M: Severe cold hemagglutinin disease (CHD) successfully treated with rituximab. Blood 2002;100:1922–1923.
398. Silberstein LE, Robertson GA, Harris AC, Moreau L, Besa E, Nowell PC: Etiologic aspects of cold agglutinin disease: Evidence for cytogenetically defined clones of lymphoid cells and the demonstration that an anti-Pr cold autoantibody is derived from a chromosomally aberrant B cell clone. Blood 1986;67:1705–1709.
399. O'Connor BM, Clifford JS, Lawrence WD, Logue GL: Alpha-interferon for severe cold agglutinin disease. Ann Intern Med 1989;111:255–256.
400. Fest T, de Wazieres B, Lamy B, Maskani M, Vuitton D, Dupond JL: Successful response to alpha-interferon 2b in a refractory IgM autoagglutinin-mediated hemolytic anemia. Ann Hematol 1994;69:147–149.
401. Isbister JP, Biggs JC, Penny R: Experience with large volume plasmapheresis in malignant paraproteinaemia and immune disorders. Aust N Z J Med 1978;8:154–164.
402. Wells JV, Fudenberg HH: Paraproteinemias. Dis Mon 1974;1–45.
403. Logue GL, Rosse WF, Gockerman JP: Measurement of the third component of complement bound to red blood cells in patients with the cold agglutinin syndrome. J Clin Invest 1973;52:493.

404. Buskard NA: Plasma exchange and plasmapheresis. Can Med Assoc J 1978;119:681–683.
405. Rodenhuis S, Maas A, Hazenberg CA, Das PC, Nieweg HO: Inefficacy of plasma exchange in cold agglutinin hemolytic anemia—A case study. Vox Sang 1985;49:20–25.
406. Valbonesi M, Guzzini F, Zerbi D, Villa P, Montani F, Angelini G: Successful plasma exchange for a patient with chronic demyelinating polyneuropathy and cold agglutinin disease due to anti-Pra. J Clin Apheresis 1986;3:109–110.
406a. Bell CA, Zwicker H, Sacks HJ: Autoimmune hemolytic anemia: Routine serologic evaluation in a general hospital population. Am J Clin Pathol 1973;60:903–911.
407. von dem Borne AE, Engelfriet CP, Beckers D, Kort-Henkes G, Van Der GM, Van Loghem JJ: Autoimmune haemolytic anaemias. II. Warm haemolysins—Serological and immunochemical investigations and 51Cr studies. Clin Exp Immunol 1969;4:333–343.
408. Evans RS, Bingham M, Turner E: Autoimmune hemolytic disease: Observations of serologic reactions and disease activity. Ann NY Acad Sci 1965;124:422.
409. Evans RS, Turner E, Bingham M, Woods R: Chronic hemolytic anemia due to cold agglutinins. II. The role of C′ in red cell destruction. J Clin Invest 1968;47:691–701.
410. Geffray E, Najman A: Efficacy of danazol in autoimmune hemolytic anemia with cold agglutinins: 4 cases. Presse Med 1992;21:1472–1475.
411. Ramos RR, Curtis BR, Eby CS, Ratkin GA, Chaplin H: Fatal outcome in a patient with autoimmune hemolytic anemia associated with an IgM bithermic anti-ITP. Transfusion 1994;34:427–431.
412. Seldon M, Isbister JP, Raik E, Biggs JC: A fatal case of cold autoimmune hemolytic anemia. Am J Clin Pathol 1980;73: 716–717.
413. Rousey SR, Smith RE: A fatal case of low titer anti-PR cold agglutinin disease. Am J Hematol 1990;35:286–287.
414. Hillen HF, Bakker SJ: Failure of interferon-alpha-2b therapy in chronic cold agglutinin disease. Eur J Haematol 1994;53:242–243.
415. Berentsen S, Tjonnfjord GE, Shammas FV, Bergheim J, Hammerstrom J, Langholm R, et al: No response to cladribine in five patients with chronic cold agglutinin disease. Eur J Haematol 2000;65:88–90.
416. Gottsche B, Salama A, Mueller-Eckhardt C: Donath-Landsteiner autoimmune hemolytic anemia in children: A study of 22 cases. Vox Sang 1990;58:281–286.
417. Banov CH: Paroxysmal cold hemoglobinuria: Apparent remission after splenectomy. JAMA 1960;174:1974.
418. Roy-Burman A, Glader BE: Resolution of severe Donath-Landsteiner autoimmune hemolytic anemia temporally associated with institution of plasmapheresis. Crit Care Med 2002;30:931–934.
418a. Ries CA, Garratty G, Petz LD, Fudenberg HH: Paroxysmal cold hemoglobinuria: Report of a case with an exceptionally high thermal range Donath-Landsteiner antibody. Blood 1971;38:491–499.
419. Mauro FR, Foa R, Cerretti R, Giannarelli D, Coluzzi S, Mandelli F, et al: Autoimmune hemolytic anemia in chronic lymphocytic leukemia: clinical, therapeutic, and prognostic features. Blood 2000;95:2786–2792.
420. Cheson BD, Bennett JM, Rai KR, Grever MR, Kay NE, Schiffer CA, et al: Guidelines for clinical protocols for chronic lymphocytic leukemia: Recommendations of the National Cancer Institute-sponsored working group. Am J Hematol 1988;29:152–163.
421. McCann EL, Shirey RS, Kickler TS, Ness PM: IgM autoagglutinins in warm autoimmune hemolytic anemia: A poor prognostic feature. Acta Haematol 1992;88:120–125.
422. Pisciotta AV, Hirschboeck JS: Therapeutic considerations in chronic lymphocytic leukemia. Arch Intern Med 1957;99: 334–345.
423. Piro LD, Carrera CJ, Beutler E, Carson DA: 2–Chlorodeoxyadenosine: An effective new agent for the treatment of chronic lymphocytic leukemia. Blood 1988;72:1069–1073.
424. Zaucha JM, Halaburda K, Ciepluch H, Hellmann A: 2-Chlorodeoxyadenosine treatment of patients with chronic lymphocytic leukaemia associated with autoimmune haemolysis. Acta Haematol Pol 1994;25:119–127.
425. Coad JE, Matutes E, Catovsky D: Splenectomy in lymphoproliferative disorders: A report on 70 cases and review of the literature. Leuk Lymphoma 1993;10:245–264.
426. Gentile TC, Loughran TP Jr: Resolution of autoimmune hemolytic anemia following splenectomy in CD3+ large granular lymphocyte leukemia. Leuk Lymphoma 1996;23:405–408.
427. Cusack JC Jr, Seymour JF, Lerner S, Keating MJ, Pollock RE: Role of splenectomy in chronic lymphocytic leukemia. J Am Coll Surg 1997;185:237–243.
428. Seymour JF, Cusack JD, Lerner SA, Pollock RE, Keating MJ: Case/control study of the role of splenectomy in chronic lymphocytic leukemia. J Clin Oncol 1997;15:52–60.
429. Neal TF Jr, Tefferi A, Witzig TE, Su J, Phyliky RL, Nagorney DM: Splenectomy in advanced chronic lymphocytic leukemia: a single institution experience with 50 patients. Am J Med 1992;93:435–440.
430. Besa EC: Use of intravenous immunoglobulin in chronic lymphocytic leukemia. Am J Med 1984;76:209–218.
431. Sigler E, Shtalrid M, Goland S, Sthoeger ZM, Berrebi A: Intractable acute autoimmune hemolytic anemia in B-cell chronic lymphocytic leukemia successfully treated with vincristine-loaded platelet infusion. Am J Hematol 1995;50:313–315.
432. Willis F, Marsh JC, Bevan DH, Killick SB, Lucas G, Griffiths R, et al: The effect of treatment with Campath-1H in patients with autoimmune cytopenias. Br J Haematol 2001;114:891–898.
433. Rodon P, Breton P, Courouble G: Treatment of pure red cell aplasia and autoimmune haemolytic anaemia in chronic lymphocytic leukaemia with Campath-1H. Eur J Haematol 2003;70:319–321.
434. Gupta N, Kavuru S, Patel D, Janson D, Driscoll N, Ahmed S, et al: Rituximab-based chemotherapy for steroid-refractory autoimmune hemolytic anemia of chronic lymphocytic leukemia. Leukemia 2002;16:2092–2095.
435. Zaja F, Iacona I, Masolini P, Russo D, Sperotto A, Prosdocimo S, et al: B-cell depletion with rituximab as treatment for immune hemolytic anemia and chronic thrombocytopenia. Haematologica 2002;87:189–195.
436. Kokori SI, Ioannidis JP, Voulgarelis M, Tzioufas AG, Moutsopoulos HM: Autoimmune hemolytic anemia in patients with systemic lupus erythematosus. Am J Med 2000;108:198–204.
437. Voulgarelis M, Kokori SI, Ioannidis JP, Tzioufas AG, Kyriaki D, Moutsopoulos HM: Anaemia in systemic lupus erythematosus: Aetiological profile and the role of erythropoietin. Ann Rheum Dis 2000;59:217–222.
438. Harvey AM, Shulman LE, Tumulty PA, et al: Systemic lupus erythematosus. Review of the literature and clinical analysis of 138 cases. Medicine 1954;33:291–437.
439. Salamon DJ, Ramsey G, Nusbacher J, Yang S, Starzl TE, Israel L: Anti-A production by a group O spleen transplanted to a group A recipient. Vox Sang 1985;48:309–312.
440. Alger M, Alarcon-Segovia D, Rivero SJ: Hemolytic anemia and thrombocytopenic purpura: Two related subsets of systemic lupus erythematosus. J Rheumatol 1977;4:351–357.
441. Ward MM, Pyun E, Studenski S: Mortality risks associated with specific clinical manifestations of systemic lupus erythematosus. Arch Intern Med 1996;156:1337–1344.
442. Alarcon-Segovia D, Deleze M, Oria CV, Sanchez-Guerrero J, Gomez-Pacheco L, Cabiedes J, et al: Antiphospholipid antibodies and the antiphospholipid syndrome in systemic lupus erythematosus. A prospective analysis of 500 consecutive patients. Medicine (Baltimore) 1989;68:353–365.
443. Deleze M, Alarcon-Segovia D, Oria CV, Sanchez-Guerrero J, Fernandez-Dominguez L, Gomez-Pacheco L, et al: Hemocytopenia in systemic lupus erythematosus. Relationship to antiphospholipid antibodies. J Rheumatol 1989;16:926–930.
444. McDonagh JE, Isenberg DA: Development of additional autoimmune diseases in a population of patients with systemic lupus erythematosus. Ann Rheum Dis 2000;59:230–232.
445. Sarles HE, Levin WC: The role of splenectomy in the management of acquired autoimmune hemolytic anemia complicating systemic lupus erythematosus. Amer J Med 1959;26:547.

446. Dubois EL: Systemic lupus erythematosus. M Clin North Am 1952;36:1111.
447. Haserick JR: Modern concepts of systemic lupus erythematosus; a review of 126 cases. J Chronic Dis 1955;1:317.
448. Johnson HM: The effect of splenectomy in acute systemic lupus erythematosus. Arch Dermatol Syph 1953;68:699.
449. Pisciotta AV, Giliberti JJ, Greenwalt TJ, Engstrom WW: Acute hemolytic anemia in disseminated lupus erythematosus. Amer J Clin Path 1951;21:1139.
450. Gruenberg JC, VanSlyck EJ, Abraham JP: Splenectomy in systemic lupus erythematosis. Am Surg 1986;52:366–370.
451. Rivero SJ, Alger M, Alarcon-Segovia D: Splenectomy for hemocytopenia in systemic lupus erythematosus: A controlled appraisal. Arch Intern Med 1979;139:773–776.
452. Drenkard C, Villa AR, Alarcon-Segovia D, Perez-Vazquez ME: Influence of the antiphospholipid syndrome in the survival of patients with systemic lupus erythematosus. J Rheumatol 1994;21:1067–1072.
453. Nossent JC, Swaak AJ: Prevalence and significance of haematological abnormalities in patients with systemic lupus erythematosus. Q J Med 1991;80:605–612.
454. Sthoeger Z, Sthoeger D, Green L, Geltner D: The role of anticardiolipin autoantibodies in the pathogenesis of autoimmune hemolytic anemia in systemic lupus erythematosus. J Rheumatol 1993;20:2058–2061.
455. Xiros N, Binder T, Anger B, Bohlke J, Heimpel H: Idiopathic thrombocytopenic purpura and autoimmune hemolytic anemia in Hodgkin's disease. Eur J Haematol 1988;40:437–441.
456. Eisner E, Ley AB, Mayer K: Coombs'-positive hemolytic anemia in Hodgkin's disease. Ann Intern Med 1967;66:258–273.
457. Levine AM, Thornton P, Forman SJ, et al: Positive Coombs test in Hodgkin's disease: Significance and implications. Blood 1980;55:607–611.
458. Ertem M, Uysal Z, Yavuz G, Gozdasoglu S: Immune thrombocytopenia and hemolytic anemia as a presenting manifestation of Hodgkin disease. Pediatr Hematol Oncol 2000;17:181–185.
459. Shah SJ, Warrier RP, Ode DL, Lele HE, Yu LC: Immune thrombocytopenia and hemolytic anemia associated with Hodgkin disease. J Pediatr Hematol Oncol 1996;18:227–229.
460. Kalmanti M, Polychronopoulou S: Autoimmune hemolytic anemia as an initial symptom in childhood Hodgkin's disease. Pediatr Hematol Oncol 1992;9:393–395.
461. Weitberg AB, Harmon DC: Autoimmune neutropenia, hemolytic anemia, and reticulocytopenia in Hodgkin's disease. Ann Intern Med 1984;100:702–703.
462. Chu J-Y: Autoimmmune hemolytic anemia in childnood Hodgkin's disease. Am J Pediatr Hematol Oncol 1982;4:125–128.
463. Economopoulos T, Stathakis N, Constantinidou M, Papageorgiou E, Anastassiou C, Raptis S: Cold agglutinin disease in non-Hodgkin's lymphoma. Eur J Haematol 1995;55:69–71.
464. Sivakumaran M, Murphy PT, Booker DJ, Wood JK, Stamps R, Sokol RJ: Paroxysmal cold haemoglobinuria caused by non-Hodgkin's lymphoma. Br J Haematol 1999;105:278–279.
465. Sharara AI, Hillsley RE, Wax TD, Rosse WF: Paroxysmal cold hemoglobinuria associated with non-Hodgkin's lymphoma. South Med J 1994;87:397–399.
466. Domingo A, Crespo N, Fernandez dS, Domenech P, Jordan C, Callis M: Hairy cell leukemia and autoimmune hemolytic anemia. Leukemia 1992;6:606–607.
467. Mainwaring CJ, Walewska R, Snowden J, et al: Fatal cold anti-i autoimmune haemolytic anaemia complicating hairy cell leukaemia. Br J Haematol 2000;109:641–643.
468. Cesana C, Brando B, Boiani E, et al: Effective treatment of autoimmune hemolytic anemia and hairy cell leukemia with interferon-alpha. Eur J Haematol 2002;68:120–121.
469. Cohen Y, Polliack A, Zelig O, Goldfarb A: Monotherapy with rituximab induces rapid remission of recurrent cold agglutinin-mediated hemolytic anemia in a patient with indolent lympho-plasmacytic lymphoma. Leuk Lymphoma 2001;42:1405–1408.
470. Mori A, Tamaru J, Sumi H, Kondo H: Beneficial effects of rituximab on primary cold agglutinin disease refractory to conventional therapy. Eur J Haematol 2002;68:243–246.
471. Sokol RJ, Booker DJ, Stamps R: Erythrocyte autoantibodies, autoimmune haemolysis, and carcinoma. J Clin Pathol 1994;47:340–343.
472. Gordon PA, Baylis PH, Bird GW: Tumour-induced autoimmune haemolytic anaemia. Br Med J 1976;1:1569–1570.
473. Horne MK, McAnally TP: Hemolytic anemia with lung carcinoma: Case reports. Milit Med 1978;143:188–189.
474. Carreras Vescio LA, Toblli JE, Rey JA, Assaf ME, De Maria HE, Marletta J: Autoimmune hemolytic anemia associated with an ovarian neoplasm. Medicina (B Aires) 1983;43:415–424.
475. Girelli G, Adorno G, Perrone MP, et al: Kidney carcinoma revealed by autoimmune hemolytic anemia. Haematologica 1988;73:309–311.
476. Adorno G, Girelli G, Perrone MP, et al: A metastatic breast carcinoma presenting as autoimmune hemolytic anemia. Tumori 1991;77:447–448.
477. Hibino S, Stoller RG, Jacobs SA: Autoimmune haemolytic anaemia associated with transitional cell carcinoma. Lancet 1992;340:373.
478. Spira MA, Lynch EC: Autoimmune hemolytic anemia and carcinoma: An unusual association. Am J Med 1979;67:753–758.
479. Bradley GW, Harvey M: Haemolytic anaemia with hypernephroma. Postgrad Med J 1981;57:46–47.
480. Johnson P, Gualtieri RJ, Mohler DN, Carpenter JT: Autoimmune hemolytic anemia associated with a hypernephroma. South Med J 1985;78:1129–1131.
481. Dacie JV: Auto-immune haemolytic anaemia (AIHA): Cold-antibody syndromes III: Haemolytic anaemia following mycoplasma pneumonia. In The Haemolytic Anaemias, 3rd ed. vol. 3, The Auto-Immune Haemolytic Anaemias. New York: Churchill Livingstone, 1992:296–312.
482. Perkin RL, Fox AD, Richards WL, King MH: Acute hemolytic anemia secondary to infectious mononucleosis. Can Med Assoc J 1979;121:1095–1097.
483. Weikert LF, Davis RC: Profound anemia following a respiratory infection. J Tenn Med Assoc 1995;88:270–271.
484. Cherry JD: Anemia and mucocutaneous lesions due to Mycoplasma pneumoniae infections. Clin Infect Dis 1993;17(Suppl. 1):S47–S51.
485. Bartholomew JR, Bell WR, Shirey RS: Cold agglutinin hemolytic anemia: Management with an environmental suit. Ann Intern Med 1987;106:243–244.
485a. Ness PM, Bell WR, Shirey RS: Transfusion medicine illustrated. Novel management of cold agglutinin disease. Transfusion 2003;43:839.
486. Chu CS, Braun SR, Yarbro JW, Hayden MR: Corticosteroid treatment of hemolytic anemia associated with Mycoplasma pneumoniae pneumonia. South Med J 1990;83:1106–1108.
487. Turtzo DF, Ghatak PK: Acute hemolytic anemia with Mycoplasma pneumoniae pneumonia. JAMA 1976;236:1140–1141.
488. Lindstrom FD, Stahl-Furenhed B: Autoimmune haemolytic anaemia complicating Mycoplasma pneumoniae infection. Scand J Infect Dis 1981;13:233–235.
489. Fiala M, Myhre BA, Chinh LT, Territo M, Edgington TS, Kattlove H: Pathogenesis of anemia associated with Mycoplasma pneumoniae. Acta Haematol 1974;51:297–301.
490. Bowman HS, Marsh WL, Schumacher HR, Oyen R, Reihart J: Auto anti-N immunohemolytic anemia in infectious mononucleosis. Am J Clin Pathol 1974;61:465–472.
491. Green N, Goldenberg H: Acute hemolytic anemia and hemoglobinuria complicating infectious mononucleosis. Arch Intern Med 1960;105:108.
492. Keyloun VE, Grace WJ: Acute hemolytic anemia complicating infectious monocucleosis. N Y State J Med 1966;66: 273–275.
493. Tonkin AM, Mond HG, Alford FP, Hurley TH: Severe acute haemolytic anaemia complicating infectious mononucleosis. Med J Aust 1973;2:1048–1050.
494. Dacie JV, Auto-immune haemolytic anaemia (AIHA): Cold-antibody syndromes IV: Haemolytic anaemia following infectious mononucleosis and other viral infections. In The Haemolytic Anaemias, 3rd ed. vol. 3, The Auto-Immune Haemolytic Anaemias. New York: Churchill Livingstone, 1992:313–328.

CHAPTER 12

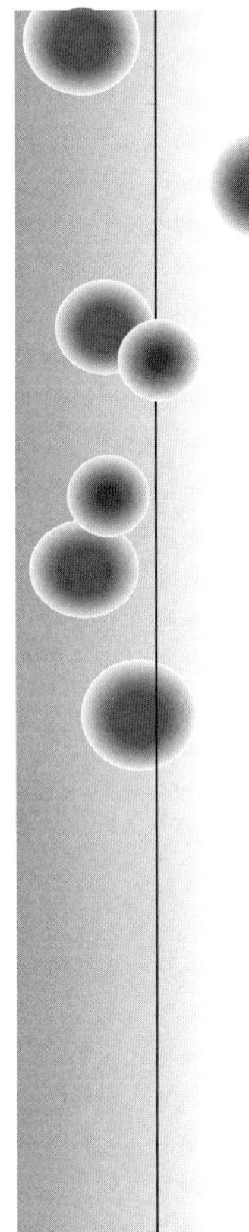

Immune Hemolysis Associated with Transplantation

Immune hemolysis caused by a variety of mechanisms has been noted after transplantation of hematopoietic stem cells or solid organs.[1,2] The evaluation and appropriate mangement of patients at risk requires an understanding of both the manifold causes of hemolysis and the settings in which it can occur.

HEMATOPOIETIC CELL TRANSPLANTATION

The early transplantation literature regarding hematopoietic cell transplantation referred only to bone marrow transplantation (BMT). More recently, there has been increasing use of peripheral blood stem cells (PBSC) or stem cells obtained from umbilical cord blood. Although it is the patient's bone marrow that is reconstituted in each instance, we will maintain the distinctions between BMT, PBSC transplants, and umbilical cord blood transplants where pertinent in this chapter.

Most cases of immune hemolysis associated with hematopoietic cell transplantation are related to the fact that inheritance of blood group antigens is independent of the human leukocyte antigen (HLA) gene complex; consequently, even if the donor and recipient are HLA-matched, their RBCs are likely to be of different phenotypes.[1-5] Of particular significance are those transplants between ABO blood group mismatched donor-recipient pairs.

Major and Minor Blood Group Incompatibility

ABO blood group incompatibility is defined as a "major" incompatibility when the recipient's immune system is capable of producing antibodies against the donor's RBC antigens (e.g., group A donor and group O recipient) and as a "minor" incompatibility when the donor's immune system is capable of producing antibodies against the recipient's RBC antigens (e.g., group O donor and group A recipient). In some instances, both major and minor incompatibilities exist simultaneously—for example, when the donor is group B and the recipient is group A. Similar definitions can also be applied to other blood group systems.

Autoantibodies and Alloantibodies

The terms *autoimmune* and *alloimmune* must be used carefully with regard to antibodies that develop after transplantation. An antibody produced by cells of the donor against RBC antigens of the recipient should be considered an alloantibody, as should antibodies made by the recipient's immune system against RBC antigens of the donor. Donor antidonor or recipient antirecipient antibodies, however, may appropriately be defined as autoantibodies.

MINOR ABO BLOOD GROUP–INCOMPATIBLE HEMATOPOIETIC STEM CELL TRANSPLANTS

The Passenger Lymphocyte Syndrome

A well-recognized syndrome of immune hemolysis after hematopoietic stem cell transplantation has become known as *passenger lymphocyte syndrome*.[1-3,6-17] It occurs in some patients who are transplanted with hematopoietic stem cells from a minor ABO blood group–mismatched donor. Occasionally, mismatches of other blood groups result in similar (although milder) hemolysis. The syndrome has been attributed to proliferation and antibody production by "passenger" lymphocytes, which are infused with the stem cell product. A typical case is illustrated in Figure 12-1, and clinical and laboratory data regarding six patients described by Hows and colleagues[6] are listed in Table 12-1. (In one patient, the passenger lymphocyte syndrome was cause by minor Rh incompatibility.)

Several factors can increase the risk of development of the syndrome: the use of cyclosporine alone in the absence of an antiproliferative agent for graft-vs.-host disease (GVHD) prophylaxis; the use of peripheral blood as a source of the hematopoietic stem cells; the use of a reduced-intensity pretransplant preparative regimen; utilization of a nongenotypically HLA-matched donor and, possibly, use of a female donor.[12,18]

Immune hemolysis generally has its onset near the end of the first week or during the second week after transplantation. In the five patients described by Hows and coworkers,[6] maximum hemolysis was observed on days 10 to 16 after transplantation. Rowley and Braine[10] reported on five patients who showed evidence of hemolysis between days 6 and 10; Haas and colleagues[11] described a patient who developed hemolysis on day 6; and, of the seven patients reported on by Gajewski and coworkers,[12] hemolysis occurred between days 5 and 20 after transplantation.

TABLE 12-1. CLINICAL AND LABORATORY DATA REGARDING SIX PATIENTS WHO HAD BMT FROM A MINOR ABO-INCOMPATIBLE DONOR AND WHO DEVELOPED HEMOLYTIC ANEMIA IN THE POSTTRANSPLANT PERIOD

Case No.	ABO Group and Rh Type: D	R	Details of Hemolysis and RBC Transfusion Requirement
1	O+	A–	Severe intravascular hemolysis; hemoglobinuria; maximum hemolysis day +15; treated with plasma exchange; 9 units RBCs required day +10 to +15
2	O+	A+	Moderate hemolysis, maximum day +16; 6 units RBCs required day +16 to +22
3	O+	B+	Severe hemolysis; hemoglobinuria; maximum day +10; 14 units RBCs required day +10 to +19
4	O+	A+	Moderate hemolysis, maximum day +10; 7 units RBCs required day +9 to +18
5	B+	AB+	Moderate hemolysis; maximum day +12; 6 units RBCs required day +11 to +14
6	A–	A+	Moderate hemolysis, maximum day +13; 5 units RBCs required day +9 to +16

D-Donor; R-Recipient
From Petz LD: Immunohematologic problems unique to bone marrow transplantation. In Garratty G (ed): Red Cell Antigens and Antibodies. Arlington, VA: American Association of Blood Banks, 1986:195–229.

Hemolysis is usually abrupt in onset and can be severe, with a rapidly dropping hemoglobin level, signs of intravascular hemolysis (hemoglobinemia and hemoglobinuria),[6,10-12,19] and renal failure.[10,12,20-22] Less severe cases are characterized by a falling hemoglobin level, increases in serum bilirubin and lactic dehydrogenase (LDH), and decreased serum haptoglobin.

Hemolysis usually persists for 5 to 10 days and then subsides as the patient's residual incompatible RBCs are destroyed and are replaced by transfused

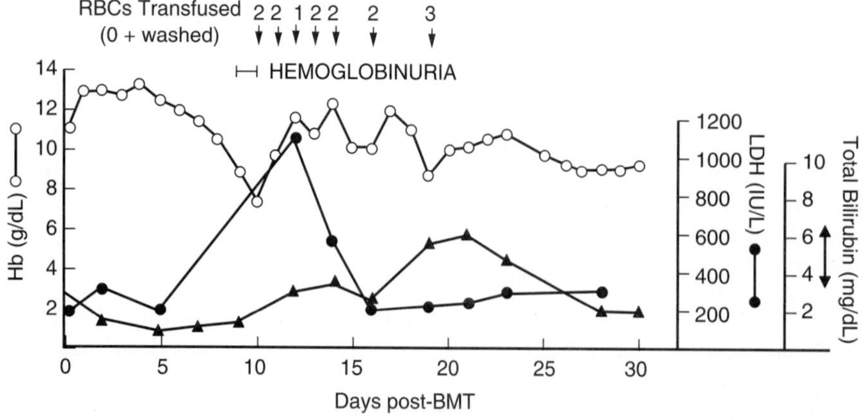

FIGURE 12-1. Minor ABO-mismatched BMT (donor group O, recipient group B). Flow chart shows hematologic and biochemical evidence for hemolysis. Fourteen units of packed group O RBCs were required to maintain the hemoglobin between day 10 and day 19 post-BMT. Note that the hemoglobin, the lactic dehydrogenase, and the total bilirubin were normal for the first 5 days post-BMT. During the hemolytic episode, no incompatible isohemagglutinins were infused; RBCs transfused were washed group O, platelets were group B or washed and resuspended in fresh AB plasma. (From Hows J, Beddow K, Gordon Smith E, et al: Donor-derived red blood cell antibodies and immune hemolysis after allogeneic bone marrow transplantation. Blood 1986;67:177–181.)

group O RBCs and/or by RBCs of donor type produced by cells derived from the engrafted stem cells. Also, antibody production gradually subsides as the passenger lymphocytes that are not engrafted reach the end of their life span.

SEROLOGIC FINDINGS

Table 12-2 displays the results of serological tests for the six patients described by Hows and associates.[6] The direct antibody test (DAT) first became positive on days 4 to 18 after transplanation, and anti-A and/or anti-B were found in eluates from the patients' RBCs and in the patients' sera. In four patients, the DAT was positive with anti-C3 but negative with anti-IgG. Nevertheless, a red cell eluate made from RBCs of two patients with this DAT pattern revealed anti-A.

Of particular interest is that maximum hemolysis occurred in one patient on the 15th day after transplantation, but the DAT did not become positive until day 18. Our subsequent experience has confirmed such findings in that signs of hemolysis might precede one's ability to detect the expected antibody by 1 or 2 days. Similar observations have been reported by Greeno and colleagues,[20] who reported on a patient who developed marked hemolysis on the eighth day after transplanation, although serum anti-A was not detectable until the 10th day. Leo and coworkers[23] emphasized that in their patient, the clinical signs of hemolysis—including a decrease in hemoglobin and a rise in LDH—preceded the detection of the relevant antibody.

Also, Tiplady and associates[16] described a patient who developed signs of hemolysis with a drop in hemoglobin from 10.3 g/dL to 8.3 g/dL on the eighth day after a minor ABO-incompatible peripheral blood stem cell transplant, although no antibody was detectable at that point and the DAT was still negative. On day 9, the hemoglobin fell further to 6.3 g/dL, and although the DAT was now positive, anti-A was not detectable until the next day.

Apparently, significant hemolysis can occur at a time when the amount of anti-A or anti-B is still too small to be detectable by routine serologic tests (also see pages 469–470). Similar findings have been reported after solid organ transplantation.[24]

Measuring anti-A and anti-B titers in the donor before transplantation apparently does not help to predict either which patients will develop passenger lymphocyte syndrome or the severity of hemolysis.[6]

Passenger lymphocyte syndrome is most likely to occur when the donor is group O and the patient group A, a phenomenon which perhaps is related to the fact that IgG anti-A and anti-B are found far more commonly in group O than in group B or A subjects.[25] It is also true that anti-A–sensitized RBCs bind C1q (the earliest reacting component of complement) three to six times more than do anti-B–sensitized RBCs[26] and that an equal level of hemolysis is obtained in vitro only if the fluid phase anti-B is present in concentrations two to four times higher than that of anti-A.[27]

ANTIBODIES OTHER THAN THOSE OF THE ABO BLOOD GROUP SYSTEM PRODUCED BY PASSENGER LYMPHOCYTES

Hows and colleagues[6] evaluated seven D-positive patients receiving marrow from D-negative donors and found that three developed donor-derived anti-D and one of these also developed donor-derived anti-C and anti-E. Only one of the patients had hemolysis. This patient had severe aplastic anemia, was group A, Rh positive, and was transplanted with marrow from a donor who was group A, Rh-negative and whose serum contained anti-D. No antibody was detected in the patient's serum until the 13th day after transplantation, at which time anti-D was found. Moderate hemolysis developed, which reached its maximum on day 13, and the patient required transfusion of 5 units of RBC on days 9 to 16. The antibody titer rose to 256 on day 70; later samples were not

TABLE 12-2. SEROLOGICAL INVESTIGATION OF PATIENTS PRESENTING WITH IMMUNE HEMOLYSIS

Case No.	Maximum Hemolysis Day Post-BMT	ABO Group Rh Type		DAT Positive for	Day Post-BMT DAT First Positive	Antibody in Eluate	Antibody in Serum	Day Post-BMT Serum Antibody Last Detected
		D	R					
1	+15	O+	A–	C3	+18	ND	Anti-A	+38*
2	+16	O+	A+	C3	+15	ND	Anti-A	+24*
3	+10	O+	B+	IgG + C3	+10	Anti-B	Anti-B	+42*
4	+10	O+	A+	C3	+4	Anti-A	Anti-A	+30*
5	+12	B+	AB+	C3	+9	Anti-A	Anti-A	+42*
6	+13	A–	A+	IgG	+13	Anti-D	Anti-D	+70†

DAT, direct antiglobulin test; D, donor; R, recipient; ND, not done.
* Serum antibody not detectable in subsequent follow-up.
† Anti-D titer 256; later samples not tested.
From Hows J, Beddow K, Gordon Smith E, et al: Donor-derived red blood cell antibodies and immune hemolysis after allogeneic bone marrow transplantation. Blood 1986;67:177–181.

tested. The donor-derived anti-D produced in this recipient was, therefore, the result of a secondary immune response to the D antigen by the donor's passenger lymphocytes.

No evidence for donor presensitization to Rh antigens was present, however, in one of the cases reported by Hows and coworkers,[6] in which donor-derived Rh antibodies were produced. This donor was a 15-year-old boy who had not been transfused, suggesting that in this case the production of donor-derived anti-D, -C, and -E after transplantation was due to a primary immune response by the donor lymphocytes. The donor for the third patient, who developed anti-D post-transplant, had no Rh antibodies detectable in her serum, but she had two children who were D positive.

Robertson and associates[28] found anti-Jk^b in the serum and in an eluate of a Jk (b+) recipient 9 days after transplantation of a T-cell depleted marrow from a Jk (b–) donor. No anti-Jk^b was found in the donor before BMT, but she might have been sensitized through pregnancy. The patient did not develop signs of hemolysis.

Ting and colleagues[29] reported production of non-ABO RBC alloantibodies in 12 of 150 patients after BMT. Although none of the antibodies caused hemolysis, the researchers' report is particularly interesting in that it emphasizes the different sources of the antibodies (also see pages 488–490). Passenger lymphocytes were the evident source of antibodies in two patients who developed antibodies within 19 days of transplantation.

Leo and coworkers[23] reported severe hemolysis caused by anti-Jk^a after a PBSC transplant from an HLA-identical sibling donor. The case is of particular interest, as prophylaxis against GVHD consisted of methotrexate (administered on days 5 and 7 after transplantation at a dose of 10 mg/m^2), and cyclosporine (begun on the day before transplantation at a dose of 5 mg/kg). A myeloablative conditioning regimen was used, which included total body irradiation. Hemolysis ensued on the 18th day after transplantation, and the patient was managed with RBC transfusions. The authors pointed out that their case illustrated that clinical signs of hemolysis, such as a decrease in hemoglobin or a rise in LDH, can precede the serologic detection of the responsible antibody.

Young and associates[30] also reported on two patients who developed the passenger lymphocyte syndrome caused by anti-Jk^a. Hemolysis was abrupt in onset and severe, with rapidly dropping hemoglobin, signs of intravascular and extravascular hemolysis, and renal failure. One of the transplants used stem cells from the bone marrow of an unrelated male HLA-matched donor, and the other case was a PBSC transplant from an HLA-matched male sibling. Both transplants used a myeloablative conditioning regimen. They also identified three additional cases in a review of hospital records involving 427 allogeneic stem cell transplants over a 6-year period; antibodies in these three cases were anti-D, -E, and -s. The authors pointed out that cases of non-ABO immune hemolysis frequently involve donors and recipients who have no prior evidence of alloantibodies, thus making it impossible to predict those patients who are at risk.

Franchini and colleagues[31] described a patient who developed anti-D of donor origin and who showed signs of mild hemolytic anemia after a BMT.

LEWIS BLOOD GROUP SYSTEM

A number of authors have pointed out that the Lewis antigens always remain of the recipient type after BMT.[32-35] This finding is consistent with the fact that Lewis antigens are absorbed by RBCs from the plasma and are not synthesized by RBCs or their precursors.[36]

Myser and coworkers[32] described a patient who developed hemolytic anti-Le^a 8 days after BMT. The patient was Le (a-b+) and, at the time of the BMT, a hemolytic anti-Le^a was detected in the Le (a-b-) donor. No hemolysis resulted, but the anti-Le^a interfered with HLA antibody identification in that strong lymphocytotoxic reactions occurred with Le (a+) donors.

SOURCE OF ANTIBODY CAUSING HEMOLYSIS

Detailed serologic studies indicate that the relevant serum antibody is not present in the period immediately after transplantation but rather is first detectable at about the time hemolysis becomes evident.[1-3,5,6] Therefore, passive transfer during infusion of the donor's plasma with the stem cell product cannot account for the presence of the antibody. Also, antibody production and hemolysis generally occur before clinical evidence of engraftment while pancytopenia caused by the pretransplant preparative regimen is present and before immune reconstitution of the patient. Lymphocytes derived from engrafted donor lymphoid cells probably would not be present so soon after transplantation.[8] Instead, the syndrome has been attributed to the production of antibody by rapidly proliferating "passenger" lymphocytes transfused with the donor stem cell product, which are present temporarily until the end of their life spans.

Pertinent data regarding the source of antibody production has come from study of passenger lymphocyte syndrome after solid organ transplantation. Analysis of the immunoglobulin allotypes of the relevant antibodies and comparison with the allotypes of the donor and recipient have documented that the antibodies are produced by antibody-producing cells of donor origin (see page 500).

FREQUENCY OF DONOR-DERIVED ANTIBODY PRODUCTION AND HEMOLYSIS

A retrospective analysis of 21 consecutive cyclosporine-treated BMT patients receiving marrow lacking A, B, or

D antigens that were present in the recipient showed that 15 of 18 patients tested had red cell antibody production against recipient red cell antigens. Despite the frequent presence of donor-derived antibody, however, only 3 of 21 patients (12.5%) developed clinically significant hemolysis.[6] None of the marrow donors had a high titer of anti-A or anti-B, with the highest IgG/IgM titers being 64/128.

Hemolytic anemia was more frequent in a series reported by Rowley and Braine,[10] who found that hemolysis developed in five of seven evaluable minor ABO-mismatched transplants. Hemolysis was severe in several patients—two developing renal failure and one requiring hemodialysis.

Hazlehurst and associates[7] reported that two of nine recipients (22%) of T-cell–depleted minor ABO-incompatible marrow grafts developed hemolysis. Robertson and colleagues[13] reported that two of ten group A patients (20%) receiving T-cell–depleted marrows developed hemolysis, whereas none of five group B patients receiving T-cell–depleted marrows and none of six patients receiving marrows without the removal of T cells (three group A, one group AB, and two group B) developed ABO blood group antibodies or hemolysis. Bensinger and colleagues[37] reported only two episodes of acute hemolysis among 87 patients transplanted with ABO-incompatible marrow.

Young and coworkers[30] identified a total of five patients with hemolysis involving non-ABO red cell alloantibodies among a total of 427 allogeneic hematopoietic stem cell transplants, for an incidence of approximately 1%.

PATIENTS WITH MASSIVE HEMOLYSIS

Of particular concern are the occasional reports of massive hemolysis after minor ABO-incompatible marrow or peripheral blood stem cell allotransplantation[12,14,16,19-22] that lead to renal insufficiency and even fatal multisystem organ failure.[12,20,21,38]

Gajewski and associates[12] described striking hemolysis in seven patients transplanted with minor ABO-incompatible marrow grafts from matched unrelated donors. In four of the patients, the marked hemolysis was accompanied by renal failure severe enough to require hemodialysis. The episodes of hemolysis were typical of the passenger lymphocyte syndrome:

- Hemolysis began 5 to 8 days after transplantation and was manifested by a decreasing hematocrit, elevated bilirubin, elevated LDH, and an increased transfusion requirement.
- Hemolysis persisted for 2 to 12 days.
- A strongly reactive (3+ or 4+) anti-A or anti-B, consistent with donor lymphocyte origin, was found in the serum of each patient.
- No other allo- or autoantibodies were present.
- The DAT was positive during hemolysis in all cases.
- An eluate revealed anti-A or anti-B in three of the four instances in which this was tested.

Three of the patients had massive hemolysis. The course of one of these three patients is illustrated in Figure 12-2.

Transfusion Requirements Exceeding the Recipient's RBC Volume

Transfusion requirements for the three patients with massive hemolysis were far greater than could be accounted for by lysis of the patients' ABO-incompatible RBCs[12] (Table 12-3). The patients' RBC volumes on the fifth day after transplantation ranged from 1592 mL to 2039 mL, whereas the volume of RBCs transfused for each patient was 4680 mL (26 units of RBCs at 180 mL/unit). All of the units of transfused RBCs were group O and were saline washed.

The authors also determined that when the donor and recipient were ABO compatible, the "baseline" RBC transfusion requirement for days 5 to 20 in marrow transplant patients at the same medical center averaged 0.85 times the patient's RBC volume on day 5. This transfusion requirement results from marrow hypoplasia caused by ablative pretransplant radiochemotherapy; in addition, there could be some occult bleeding caused by the hypoproliferative thrombocytopenia. It is also possible that RBC survival is not normal after such high-dose radiochemotherapy, although this has not been measured.

The transfusion requirements for group O RBCs in the three patients with massive hemolysis exceeded the patients' volume of ABO-incompatible RBCs plus the "baseline" transfusion requirement by 908–1735 mL (mean = 1433 mL) (see Table 12-3). Accordingly, even if all of the patients' ABO-incompatible RBCs had been hemolyzed and consideration had been given to the baseline transfusion requirement (as when there is no ABO incompatibility), an average of almost 1500 mL of additional group O RBCs needed to be transfused. As none of the patients demonstrated any signs of bleeding, the inescapable conclusion was that rather large volumes of transfused group O RBCs were hemolyzed in addition to the patients' own RBCs.

Bystander Hemolysis

Because the only RBC antibodies detected in these patients were anti-A and anti-B and yet group O RBCs were also hemolyzed, it appears that hemolysis of antigen-negative RBCs occurred. We refer to this phenomenon as *bystander immune hemolysis*, which we define as immune hemolysis of cells that are intrinsically negative for the antigen against which the relevant antibody is directed.[5,12]

Transplant physicians have been cautious regarding their acceptance of the concept of bystander immune hemolysis, but there has been an increasing number of

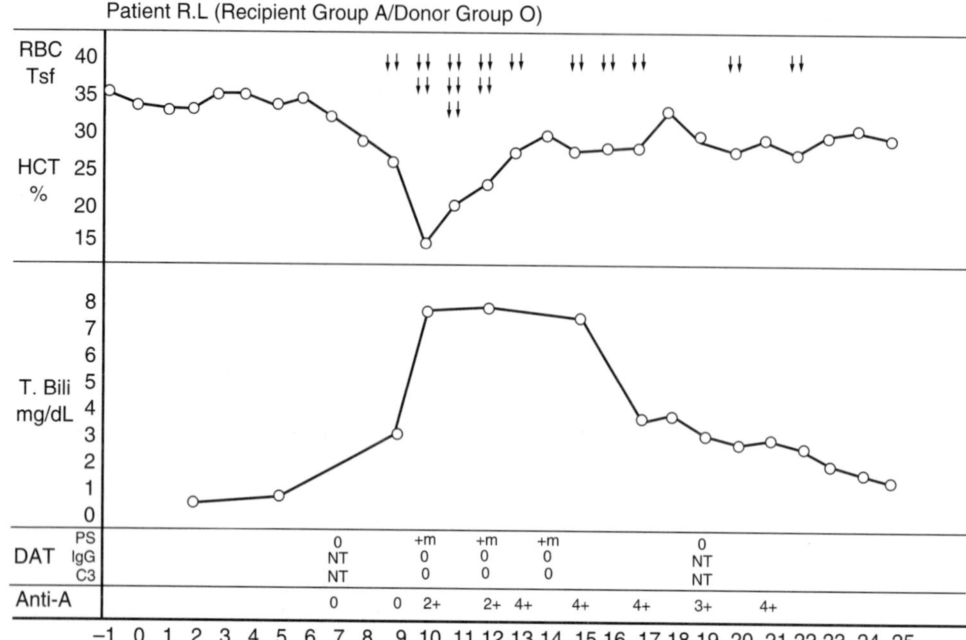

FIGURE 12-2. Flow chart of index group patient not receiving pretransplant exchange transfusion showing transfusion requirements with biochemical and serologic evidence for hemolysis. RBC Tsf, RBC transfusions (*arrows*); DAT, direct antiglobulin reagent (anti-IgG + C3); PS, polyspecific; IgG, anti-IgG reagent; 4+, cells agglutinated in one clump; 3+, cells agglutinated in three to six very large clumps; 2+, cells agglutinated in many medium clumps; 1+, cells agglutinated in numerous tiny clumps, very cloudy background; +m, very tiny agglutinates only seen microscopically; 0, no agglutinates detected; NT, not tested; ↓, transfusion. (From Gajewski JL, Petz LD, Calhoun L, et al: Hemolysis of transfused group O red blood cells in minor ABO-incompatible unrelated-donor bone marrow transplants in patients receiving cyclosporine without posttransplant methotrexate. Blood 1992;79:3076–3085.)

TABLE 12-3. TRANSFUSION REQUIREMENTS OF GROUP O RBCs IN THREE PATIENTS TRANSPLANTED WITH BONE MARROW FROM UNRELATED MINOR ABO-INCOMPATIBLE DONORS

Patient	Patient's RBC Volume Day +5 (mL)	Vol. of RBCs Transfused Day +5 to +20 (mL)	Baseline Transfusion Requirement* Day +5 to +20 (mL)	Excess Transfusion Requirement† Day +5 to +20 (mL)
1	2039	4680	1733	908
2	1592	4680	1353	1735
3	1635	4680	1389	1656

* Baseline transfusion requirement was determined by measuring the transfusion requirements during days +5 to +20 in 61 marrow transplant patients in whom the donor and recipient were ABO identical. This value was 0.85 times the RBC volume on day +5.

† Excess transfusion requirement is defined as the volume of group O RBCs required above the sum of the baseline transfusion requirement and the patient's volume of (ABO incompatible) RBCs on day +5. Thus, even if all of the patient's ABO-incompatible RBCs were hemolyzed and there is, in addition, a baseline transfusion requirement, an average of almost 1.5 liters additional group O RBCs needed to be transfused. Therefore, not only were the patient's ABO-incompatible RBCs hemolyzed, but transfused group O RBCs must have been hemolyzed as well.

From Petz LD: The expanding boundaries of transfusion medicine. In Nance SJ (ed): Clinical and Basic Science Aspects of Immunohematology. Arlington, VA: American Association of Blood Banks, 1991:73–113.

reports of massive hemolysis that is far more extensive than can be explained on the basis of hemolysis of the patient's own RBCs. Accordingly, bystander immune hemolysis has been discussed more frequently in more recent medical literature.[15-17,39]

Bystander immune hemolysis may also occur in a number of other clinical settings, and there are several possible mechanisms.[5] See Chapter 9 for a detailed discussion of this topic and Chapter 14 for a discussion of its possible role in the sickle cell hemolytic transfusion reaction syndrome.

Additional Reports of Severe Hemolysis

Greeno and coworkers[20] reported on a patient who hemolyzed her entire group A RBC population between the 8th and 11th days after transplantation. By day 11, the circulating RBCs were completely group O, but she continued to require transfusion of 2 units of group O RBCs every 2 to 3 days for an additional 10 days, for a total of 16 units of RBCs (about 2800 mL of packed RBCs) (Fig. 12-3). The patient's calculated group A RBC volume on day 7 was only about 1000 mL. The authors pointed out that the mechanism of the hemolysis of the transfused group O RBCs is unknown.

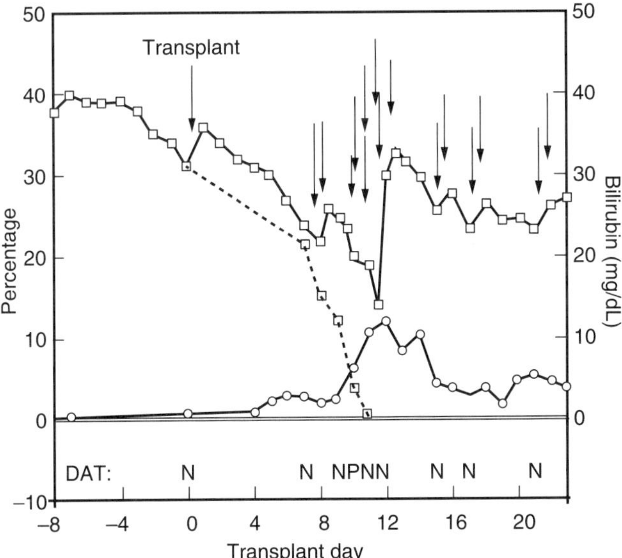

FIGURE 12-3. Shown is the course of the patient's hematocrit (-□-) and total bilirubin (-o-) during her second transplant. The type A hematocrit (---□---) was calculated by multiplying the percentage of A RBCs by the total hematocrit. Each solid arrow represents the transfusion of one unit of RBCs. Along the bottom of the graph are shown the results of the DAT, with N representing negative and P representing positive. (From Greeno EW, Perry EH, Ilstrup SJ, Weisdorf DJ: Exchange transfusion the hard way: Massive hemolysis following transplantation of bone marrow with minor ABO incompatibility. Transfusion 1996;36:71–74.)

Tiplady and colleagues[16] described a 28-year-old man with lymphoblastic lymphoma who received G-CSF mobilized stem cells from his HLA-identical sister. The recipient's blood group was A Rh D positive, and the donor's group was O Rh D positive. The patient received cyclosporine (but not methotrexate) for GVHD prophylaxis. On the eighth day after transplantation, his hemoglobin fell from 10.3 g/dL to 8.3 g/dL, but the DAT was negative and no anti-A was detectable. Three units of group A blood were transfused without complications. On day 9, the hemoglobin fell further to 6.3 g/dL and his DAT became positive (IgG and C3d), but anti-A was not detectable until day 10. From day 9 to day 13, he received 17 units of group O blood (approximately 3 L of RBCs) at a time when his calculated RBC volume was 1 L. By day 26, a further 8 units of blood had been transfused, bringing the total to 28. He had no appreciable blood loss, his bilirubin level remained elevated, and his response to transfusion was short lived. His blood film did not show any evidence of microangiopathic hemolysis. The excessive transfusion requirements led the authors to speculate that the hemolysis of compatible blood was occurring, as only anti-A and anti-B were ever found in the patient's serum. They commented that bystander hemolysis seems to be a very rare, albeit clinically serious complication of hematopoietic stem cell transplantation.

Worel and associates[39] described four patients who developed passenger lymphocyte syndrome, one of whom received 40 units of RBC during the first 30 days after transplantation of a minor ABO-incompatible transplant using peripheral blood stem cells and a nonmyeloablative conditioning regimen. The patient ultimately died of multiorgan failure on day 35. The authors commented that the extent of hemolysis suggested bystander hemolysis in addition to immune hemolysis due to ABO incompatibility.

Herzog and coworkers[40] reported a patient of group A_1 who was transplanted with marrow from a group A_2 donor. On the eighth day after transplantation, coincident with transfusion of 2 units of group A_1 RBC, the patient developed intravascular hemolysis and massive hemoglobinuria. During the next 2 weeks, transfusion of 14 units of group O RBCs was required. The only antibody detectable was anti-A_1. The authors did not comment on the fact that the volume of transfused group O RBCs (about 4000 mL) must have exceeded the volume of the patient's incompatible RBCs (including the transfused group A_1 RBC) that were present at the onset of hemolysis.

Bolan and colleagues[18] reported massive immune hemolysis in three out of ten consecutive patients undergoing HLA-identical, related-donor PBSC transplants with minor ABO incompatibility. Nonablative conditioning had been given to nine of these ten patients, including two patients with hemolysis. Cyclosporine alone was used as prophylaxis against GVHD. Catastrophic hemolysis of 78% of the circulating red cell mass led to anoxic death in the first patient they observed (Fig. 12-4). In their second patient, the authors calculated that hemolysis of more than 80% of the patient's estimated red cell mass had occurred during a 36-hour period. In their third patient, the volume of red cells transfused between days 5 and 11 was equivalent to the patient's entire estimated red cell volume. The patient also required "numerous" additional RBC transfusions, the need for which was attributed to the development of pulmonary hemorrhage on day 13 and thrombotic microangiopathy on day 26. The authors did not seem to accept the notion that transfused group O RBCs were being hemolyzed.

Haas and associates[11] reported on a group A_1 patient who was transplanted with a T-cell–depleted bone marrow from a group O donor. The patient developed a positive DAT, and anti-A_1 was found in the serum. On the sixth day after transplantation, the patient developed life-threatening intravasclar hemolysis, with the hemoglobin dropping from 11.8 g/dL to 3.8 g/dL in 6 hours (Fig. 12-5).

There have been a number of cases of severe hemolysis after PBSC transplantation in addition to those reported by Bolan and coworkers[18] and described previously. Salmon and colleagues[41] reported a 16-year-old boy who underwent an allogeneic PBSC transplant from his mother who was of a different ABO group

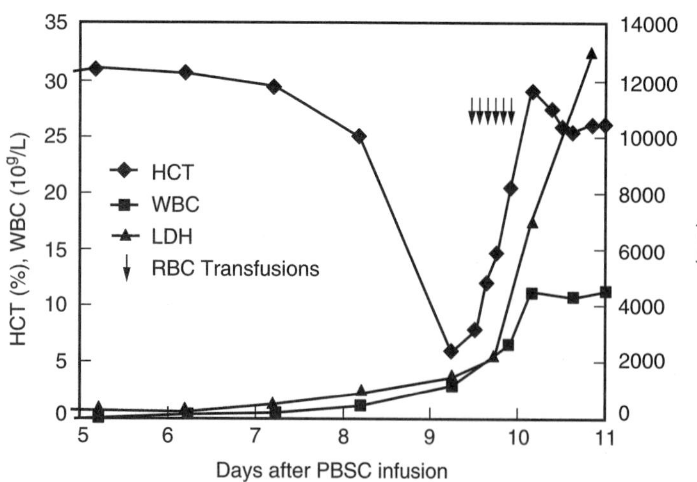

FIGURE 12-4. Course of severe hemolysis in a patient. On days 8 and 9 after transplantation, fever, hemodynamic instability, and renal insufficiency occurred, the hematocrit dropped preciptously, and the LDH doubled. Although the hematocrit responded to transfusions with group O red cells, cardiopulmonary arrest occurred, renal failure ensued, neurological function did not recover, and the patient died on day 16. Serological testing revealed that donor-type anti-A isohemagglutinins were the cause of massive immune hemolysis. (From Bolan CD, Childs RW, Procter JL, Barrett AJ, Leitman SF: Massive immune haemolysis after allogeneic peripheral blood stem cell transplantation with minor ABO incompatibility. Br J Haematol 2001;112:787–795.)

(mother group O, Rh+, patient group A, Rh+). Hemolysis developed abruptly on day 9, and all group A red cells of the recipient were destroyed within 36 hours.

Oziel-Taieb and associates[21] described a group A patient who received a PBSC transplant from a group O donor and developed immune hemolysis starting on day 9. Anti-A was found in the patient's serum and in an eluate from his RBCs. After the onset of hemolysis, the patient was transfused with 10 units of group O RBCs over the next 10 days, but he developed acute renal failure and acute respiratory distress syndrome and died on day 20 from multiorgan failure.

Toren and coworkers[19] described a 12-year-old boy, blood group A, who received an allogeneic PBSC transplant from his HLA-matched sister, blood group O. On day 8, he developed fever, abdominal and bilateral flank pain, and severe intravascular hemolysis with hemoglobinemia and hemoglobinuria and a decrease in his hemoglobin to 5.4 g/dL. The DAT was positive using anti-C3d, and IgM and IgG anti-A antibodies were found in the patient's serum with a titer of 8000. He recovered after being treated with an exchange transfusion of one blood volume, 6 units of packed red cells, fluids, and diuretics.

Laurencet and colleagues[14] described "massive" hemolysis in a 37-year-old man beginning on day 12 after a PBSC transplant with minor ABO incompatibility. Hemolysis was marked, as indicated by the fact that his hematocrit dropped from 30.1% on day 0 to 18.8% on day 12. The patient required transfusion of only 6 units of group O RBCs, however, and he recovered.

The patient reported on by Bornhauser and associates[42] received a G-CSF–mobilized PBSC from an unrelated HLA-matched donor. The blood groups of the patient and donor were bidirectionally incompatible. Signs of "major hemolysis" developed on the fifth day after transplantation, and the patient's hemoglobin reached a nadir of 4.3 g/dL.

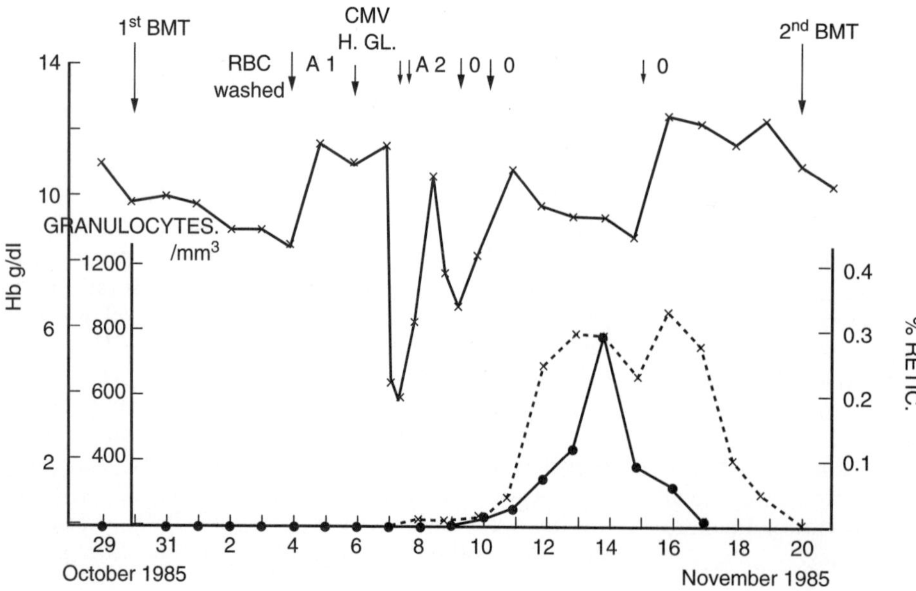

FIGURE 12-5. Hemoglobin (Hb); x—x; reticulocytes: x---x; granulocytes: •—•, of the transplant patient. BMT = bone marrow transplantation; CMV H.Gl. = cytomegalovirus hyperimmune globulin; RBC = red blood cells. (From Haas RJ, Rieber P, Helmig M, Strobel E, Belohradsky BH, Heim MU: Acquired immune haemolysis by anti-A_1 antibody following bone marrow transplantation. Blut 1986;53:401–404.)

Delamaire and coworkers[43] described a patient who had fatal hemolysis after PBSC transplantation.

THE SOURCE OF HEMATOPOIETIC STEM CELLS IN PATIENTS DEVELOPING PASSENGER LYMPHOCYTE SYNDROME

It is possible that the passenger lymphocyte syndrome is more common and more severe among patients who have received PBSC transplants compared with those who have received marrow transplants.[14,15,18,19,21,22,39,41-43] As will be reviewed below regarding the passenger lymphocyte syndrome occurring after solid organ transplants, the incidence and severity of hemolysis in minor ABO-mismatched transplants are related directly to the lymphoid content of the grafted organ.[18,44,45] PBSCs contain a 16-fold increase in CD3+ T lymphocytes and an 11-fold increase in CD19+ B lymphocytes compared with conventional marrow harvests.[46] Also, lymphocytes in PBSC grafts might be specifically primed for antibody production, owing to a switch from a type 1 to a type 2 helper response induced by the administration of granulocyte colony-stimulating factor.[47]

Lapierre and colleagues[48] studied the significance of the hematopoietic stem cell source and concluded that immunohematologic reconstitution differed significantly after granulocyte colony-stimulating factor-mobilized PBSC transplantation compared with bone marrow stem cell transplantation. They suggested that such a difference could contribute to acute hemolysis described after PBSC transplantation.

As of this writing, no instances of passenger lymphocyte syndrome have been reported after umbilical cord blood hematopoietic cell transplants.

SIGNIfiCANCE OF IMMUNE MODULATION AS A CAUSE OF PASSENGER LYMPHOCYTE SYNDROME

The Pretransplant Conditioning Regimen. Two of the three patients reported on by Bolan and associates[18] had received low-intensity nonmyeloablative pretransplant conditioning regimens. Such regimens are being used increasingly in hematopoietic stem cell transplantation. Often, cyclosporine is used as the sole agent for GVHD prophylaxis, and methotrexate or other antiproliferative agents are deliberately avoided with the goal of enhancing immune-mediated donor antitumor effects. Because the conditioning regimen and the anti-GVHD regimen heavily influence engraftment, GVHD, tumor eradication, and the prevention of relapse, altering these regimens for the purposes of prevention of passenger lymphocyte syndrome is not recommended.[18]

Mielcarek and coworkers[49] reported that the passenger lymphocyte syndrome occurred in only two of 40 patients with HLA-matched nonmyeloablative peripheral blood stem cell transplants (23 patients with related donors and 17 with unrelated donors). They commented that the high incidence reported by Bolan and associates[18] could be due to differences in the kind of postgrafting immunosuppression used, as Bolan and associates used cyclosporine only, whereas Mielcrek and coworkers used cyclosporine in combination with the antimetabolite mycophenylate mofetil. The authors commented that the passenger lymphocyte syndrome might occur in a minority of mycophenylate mofetil/cyclosporine-treated nonmyeloablative recipients, whereas it is quite rare among patients treated with methotrexate.

Worel and colleagues[39] reported on four patients who developed severe immune hemolysis after minor ABO-incompatible allogeneic PBSC transplantation. Three of the patients had undergone a nonmyeloablative conditioning regimen. Hemolysis occurred in one of 15 patients (6%) after myeloablative conditioning and in three of ten patients (30%) after dose-reduced conditioning, and only in patients not receiving methotrexate for GVHD prophylaxis. The authors suggested that patients receiving minor or bidirectional ABO-incompatible PBSC grafts in combination with GVHD prophylaxis regimens without methotrexate are at risk of severe hemolysis.

Reduced-intensity pretransplant regimens frequently use fludarabine, which could be an etiologic factor in the development of RBC autoantibodies among patients receiving the drug (see Chapter 8). The role of fludarabine in the development of antibodies in passenger lymphocyte syndrome is uncertain.

T-Cell Depletion. Hazlehurst and associates[7] reported the development of anti-A/B in eight of nine patients transplanted with T-cell–depleted marrow, none of whom had received cyclosporine. The DAT was positive for five patients, and two of these had a fall in hemoglobin of up to 2 g/dL. Also, Haas and coworkers[11] reported one patient and Robertson and colleagues[13] reported two patients who were group A_1, received a T-cell–depleted marrow from a group O donor but did not receive cyclosporine, and developed significant hemolysis due to anti-A or anti-A_1.

Post-transplant Graft-Vs.-Host-Disease Prophylaxis

CYCLOSPORINE/METHOTREXATE

Cyclosporine is a powerful immunosuppressive agent that suppresses lymphocyte proliferative responses to mitogens and alloantigens in a dose-dependent fashion. Primary responses are much more sensitive to the effects of cyclosporine than are secondary responses.[50] T-lymphocyte proliferation is not impaired when presensitized lymphocytes are re-exposed to antigen in the presence of cyclosporine.[6] Although most patients who have developed hemolysis as a result of passenger lymphocyte syndrome have received cyclosporine for immunosuppression, its precise role in facilitating donor-derived antibody production is uncertain.[6]

In all six cases of the passenger lymphocyte syndrome reported by Hows and associates,[6] the patients were treated with cyclosporine for GVHD prophylaxis after BMT. In contrast, a retrospective review of 13 patients in whom methotrexate was used instead of cyclosporine revealed no cases of immune hemolysis due to donor-derived antibody.

As described by Gajewski and coworkers,[12] marked hemolysis occurred among a series of patients receiving minor ABO-incompatible marrow grafts that were not T-cell depleted and that were from unrelated donors. Seven consecutive patients who received received cyclosporine without methotrexate for post-transplant GVHD prophylaxis developed the passenger lymphocyte syndrome with severe hemolysis. In contrast, no hemolysis was observed among similar patients who received both cyclosporine and methotrexate, although weakly positive tests for anti-A or anti-B were found in two of seven patients so treated. The authors suggested that post-transplant immunosuppression with methotrexate might prevent the passenger lymphocyte syndrome from occurring even among patients receiving cyclosporine. Indeed, methotrexate has been shown to be cytotoxic for B lymphocytes and might prevent the antibody production necessary for the passenger lymphocyte syndrome to occur.[51,52] Rowley[15] indicated that special attention must be devoted to the recipient if antiproliferative agents for GVHD prophylaxis (e.g., methotrexate, trimetrexate, and mycophenylate mofetil) are not used as part of the GVHD prophylactic regimen.

With the exception of the patient reported on by Bornhauser and colleagues,[42] cyclosporine without methotrexate was used for post-transplant GVHD prophylaxis for all of the patients described previously who experienced severe hemolysis after PBSC transplants.

Donor-derived antibody, however, has been detected in a number of patients when other means of immune modulation have been used. For example, Bar and associates[53] found donor-derived antibody without hemolysis in three recipients of minor ABO-incompatible marrow transplant patients who received cyclophosphamide rather than cyclosporine immunosuppression. None of these patients received methotrexate, and none developed hemolysis.

TACROLIMUS (FK506)

Greeno and coworkers[20] described a patient who developed no signs of hemolysis after a minor ABO-incompatible BMT after receiving methotrexate, antithymocyte globulin, and prednisone for GVHD prophylaxis. When her leukemia relapsed, however, she underwent a second BMT using marrow from the same donor. Continuous tacrolimus infusion beginning one day before the marrow transplant was the only GVHD prophylaxis given. As described previously, the patient hemolyzed her entire red cell mass between days 8 and 11 after transplantation as a result of anti-A produced by passenger lymphocytes. The authors suggested that tacrolimus could be associated with only modest immunosuppressive activity against donor-derived passenger lymphocytes, but that it might effectively suppress T-cell regulation of B-cell proliferation.

Thus, available data indicate that donor-derived antibody production and hemolysis could occur in association with immune modulation caused by cyclosporine, tacrolimus, or T-cell depletion of the marrow. Additional risk factors might be the use of peripheral blood stem cells, a nonmyeloablative conditioning regimen, use of nongenotypically HLA-matched donors, and the use of female donors.[18]

MANAGEMENT OF PATIENTS RECEIVING HEMATOPOIETIC CELL TRANSPLANTS FROM MINOR ABO-INCOMPATIBLE DONORS

Volume Reduction of Marrow Products to Prevent Hemolytic Transfusion Reaction

Because the volume of a bone marrow product for a transplant recipient can be 700 mL or greater, one must be concerned that the isohemagglutinins in the donor plasma might cause an acute hemolytic transfusion reaction. One option is to measure the anti-A and/or anti-B titer of each marrow donor when there is a minor ABO incompatibility with the intended recipient. If the titer of the relevant ABO antibody is greater than 256, one should consider the advisability of plasma reduction of the marrow product. The decision is reached on the basis of the height of the isohemagglutinin titer, the adequacy of the marrow harvest, and the knowledge that some stem cells will be lost during manipulation of the marrow.

Lasky and colleagues[54] reported that plasma reduction of donor marrow products in five cases resulted in a reduction of the original marrow volume by 54% and a reduction in plasma volume by 71%. The transfused marrow contained a mean of 99.5% of the original nucleated cells present and 203 mL (5 mL/kg) of donor plasma. CFU-C recovery after plasma removal averaged 95.2%.

The degree of volume reduction that would prevent hemolysis by a given antibody is difficult to determine, but some published information is pertinent to this point. Inwood and Zuliani,[55] in reviewing a case of hemolysis resulting from transfusion of a unit of group O packed RBCs to a group A person, determined that the group O unit contained anti-A_1 activity to a titer of 8192. They estimated that the titer of the donor anti-A in the patient's circulation after transfusion was 164. This resulted in intravascular hemolysis and a drop in hemoglobin of 2.4 g/dL.

Studies in bone marrow transplant recipients have indicated that transfusion of ABO-incompatible red cells to patients with isohemagglutinin titers of 16 or lower produced no evident hemolysis.[37] Thus, in calculating the amount of plasma reduction that might be appropriate for a given product, if one reduces the volume of plasma to be transfused so that the post-transfusion isohemagglutinin titer will be lower than 16, it appears likely that serious hemolysis will not occur.

Plasma Reduction of Minor ABO-Incompatible Platelet Products to Prevent Hemolytic Transfusion Reactions

One may reduce the volume of pooled platelet concentrates or plateletpheresis products to minimize risks that are related to the volume of plasma transfused.[56,57] Volume reduction has generally been recommended for prevention of volume overload in infants, for patients in danger of overload from intravenous fluids, patients with acute respiratory distress syndrome, and patients with congestive heart failure.[57] Volume reduction might also be appropriate as a means of diminishing the amount of antibody that would be transfused.

Measuring the isohemagglutinin titers in all minor ABO-incompatible platelet products is impractical and seems unnecessary, however, as episodes of severe hemolysis due to platelet transfusions are rare. Thus, the most practical policy is to try to avoid minor ABO-incompatible platelet transfusions. If only minor incompatible products are available, one must be cognizant of the possible consequences of passively transfused antibody, which can effect compatibility testing and occasionally cause significant hemolysis (see page 494).

An alternative approach for preventing hemolysis is to wash platelets, which removes a large percentage of the plasma. Pineda and associates,[58] however, reported that platelet recovery was decreased significantly in patients receiving washed platelets. The mean platelet recovery was 73% for unwashed platelets, 23% for saline-washed platelets, and 52% for ACD-saline–washed platelets. Platelet survival was not significantly different among patients receiving differently processed platelets, which indicates that a fraction of the platelets remains undamaged and can survive normally.

Pretransplant RBC Exchange Transfusion

One may avoid hemolysis caused by passive transfer of antibody in bone marrow products by performing pretransplant RBC exchange transfusions using RBCs of the donor's type. Because significant hemolysis caused by antibodies in the donor marrow is rare and can be prevented more easily by plasma reduction of the donor marrow product when high-titer antibodies are detected in the donor, it does not seem appropriate to subject patients routinely to such an extensive procedure as exchange transfusion to avoid hemolysis by passive transfer of antibody.

We have performed pretransplant RBC exchange transfusions for a group of patients receiving an ABO-minor mismatched transplants from unrelated donors and who received cyclosporine (but not methotrexate) in the post-transplant period for GVHD prophylaxis.[12] This procedure was performed after observing massive hemolysis in three consecutive such patients. The amount of post-transplant hemolysis among subsequent patients was reduced but not eliminated.

Sniecinski and O'Donnell[59] have recommended prophylactic RBC exchange of the transplant recipient for all patients receiving a minor ABO-incomopatible stem cell product and post-transplant immunosuppression with cyclosporine without concurrent methotrexate. They further recommend that exchanges should be carried out until 70%–80% of the patent's RBC mass is replaced with group O RBCs. In contrast, Bolan and coworkers[18] have concluded that a policy to perform RBC exchanges prophylactically for all subjects at risk seems unwarranted. They determined that after a 10-unit RBC exchange for a patient who weighed 90 kg, more than 40% of the recipient's original RBC mass persisted in circulation after the exchange.

Worel and colleagues[39] also recommend prophylactic RBC exchange, especially for patients who receive a PBSC graft in combination with a GVHD prophylaxis regimen without methotrexate.

Because pretransplant isohemagglutinin titers do not appear to predict the incidence or severity of hemolysis after minor ABO-mismatched transplants,[59] selection of patients to undergo pretransplant exchange transfusion on the basis of these titers would not seem indicated.

Monitoring the Recipient for Development of Passenger Lymphocyte Syndrome

Hemolysis resulting from passenger lymphocyte syndrome usually has its onset between days 3 and 15 after transplantation; therefore, one should routinely monitor all patients receiving a minor ABO-mismatched hematopoietic stem cell transplant for the presence of hemolysis and for donor-derived isohemagglutinins during this period. A note in the medical record can serve to alert the personnel caring for the patient regarding the appropriate procedures and their rationales (Table 12-4). Usually, the syndrome is readily detectable by the presence of signs of hemolysis, a positive DAT, and the relevant antibody

TABLE 12-4. TRANSFUSION MEDICINE SERVICE RECOMMENDATIONS REGARDING ABO MINOR MISMATCHED TRANSPLANTS

This patient has received an ABO minor mismatched transplant (patient type ________ , donor type ________ and is therefore at risk of developing delayed hemolysis from ABO blood group antibody transiently produced by donor "passenger lymphocytes" in the transplanted organ, marrow, or peripheral stem cell product.

"Passenger lymphocyte" hemolysis rarely appears before day 3 after transplantation, usually begins around day 7 to 10, and almost always begins before day 15 if it is going to occur. It can cause a decrease in hemoglobin and hematocrit that can be misconstrued as bleeding. Hemolysis is usually limited in intensity and duration but can be quite serious in some patients.

We will follow the patient from day 3 to day 15 after transplantation for the development of hemolysis, which can impact transfusion need and blood selection. During this time, we recommend the following:

Order daily hemoglobin/hematocrit, LDH, and total/indirect bilirubin.

Beginning on day 3, after transplantation, order a direct antiglobulin test (DAT) three times per week and a reticulocyte count two times per week (solid organ recipients) until day 15.

If there are any questions, please contact the Transfusion Medicine Service.

(usually anti-A or anti-B) in the patient's serum and in a RBC eluate.

We originally had expected that the most sensitive test indicating the possible presence of hemolysis would be the DAT and that serum antibodies would always be readily detectable at the onset of hemolysis. Experience, however, has indicted that in a minority of cases, overt signs of hemolysis in the passenger lymphocyte syndrome might precede the ability to detect the relevant antibodies on the patient's RBCs or in the serum.[16,20,23] Thus, in the proper setting, the diagnosis of passenger lymphocyte syndrome must be accepted provisionally even without confirmatory serologic findings for 24–48 hours. Accordingly, we pay particular attention to signs of hemolysis. The onset of the syndrome is often heralded by an abrupt drop in the patient's hemoglobin and hematocrit associated with a distinct increase in serum bilirubin, especially of the indirect reacting type. Signs of intravascular hemolysis (hemoglobinemia and hemoglobinuria) also can be present.

Bolen and associates[18] found that a positive DAT was found a few days before or at the time of hemolysis in their three patients who developed passenger lymphocyte syndrome. On the other hand, a positive DAT, including strong complement (C3d) coating of RBC, also was detected in some patients who did not develop hemolysis. Also, serum isoagglutinins and RBC eluates with specificity for the relevant ABO antigen occasionally were detected in patients who did not experience hemolysis. The researchers concluded that serological findings—including the intensity of the DAT and the donor isohemagglutinin titer—were not useful for predicting the occurrence of severe hemolysis.

Management of Patients with the Passenger Lymphocyte Syndrome

In most instances, hemolysis caused by the passenger lymphocyte syndrome can be managed by transfusion of compatible RBCs, the empirical use of corticosteroids, avoidance of ABO-incompatible plasma products, and maintenance of adequate renal perfusion. Such supportive care is generally adequate; hemolysis tends to be self-limiting because newly formed red cells produced by the donor marrow generally are not affected by the donor-derived antibody.

In those cases in which massive hemolysis occurs, it is reasonable to consider exchange transfusion, replacing the patient's antigen-positive erythrocytes with group O RBCs. This therapeutic maneuver has been used and perhaps is an effective means of preventing the renal failure that has resulted from hemolysis in some patients.[12] At least equally logical is plasma exchange transfusion, which should decrease the concentration of the causative antibody. Hemolysis severe enough to require exchange transfusion is quite unusual, however.

Selection of Blood Products

In minor ABO-incompatible hematopoietic stem cell transplants, it is generally most practical to transfuse group O red cells. This may be begun at the beginning of the preparative regimen. Although packed RBCs contain isoagglutinins reactive with the patient's RBC, hemolysis caused by transfusion of plasma in packed RBCs is rare (see the foregoing discussion), so the use of washed RBCs is generally unnecessary. (In those unusual cases in which the donor's blood type is group A or B and the recipient's is group AB, the donor's type red cells may be used instead of group O.) (Table 12-5)[60]

Platelets and other plasma-containing products of recipient type are generally used to avoid the transfusion of isohemagglutinins that are reactive against red cells of the patient, even though passive transfusion of isohemagglutinins in plasma products is only infrequently an important contributing factor. When the patient has converted to donor group RBC, ABO-matched platelets would be preferable, as ABO-matched platelets are generally recommended for patients receiving platelet transfusions.[61]

TABLE 12-5. ABO-INCOMPATIBLE BONE MARROW TRANSPLANTATION (FROM PREPARATIVE REGIMEN UNTIL ENGRAFTMENT)

Recipient	Donor	RBCs	Platelets: First Choice	Platelets: Second Choice*	FFP*
Major Incompatible					
O	A	O	A	AB, B, O	A, AB
O	B	O	B	AB, A, O	B, AB
A	AB	A	AB	A, B, O	AB
B	AB	B	AB	B, A, O	AB
O	AB	O	AB	A, B, O	AB
Minor Incompatible					
A	O	O	A	AB, B, O	A, AB
B	O	O	B	AB, A, O	B, AB
AB	O	O	AB	A, B, O	AB
AB	A	A	AB	A, B, O	AB
AB	B	B	AB	B, A, O	AB
Major and Minor Incompatible					
A	B	O	AB	A, B, O	AB
B	A	O	AB	B, A, O	AB

Note: Engraftment occurs when forward and reverse types are of donor and the DAT is negative.
* Avoid high titer ABO antibodies
From Friedberg RC: Transfusion therapy in the patient undergoing hematopoietic stem cell transplantation. Hematol Oncol Clin North Am 1994;8:1105–1116.

PERSISTENCE OF BLOOD GROUP GLYCOSYLTRANSFERASE ACTIVITIES AFTER HEMATOPOIETIC STEM CELL TRANSPLANTATION

The carbohydrate structures of glycoproteins that confer blood group ABO specificities are synthesized by glycosyltransferases, which are determined by genes located in different chromosomal loci. The blood group A- or B-active structures are determined by the incorporation of *N*-acetyl-D-galactosamine or D-galactose onto a common acceptor carbohydrate chain (H substance) by the action of α-3-*N*-acetyl-D-galactosaminyl transferases (A-glycosyltransferase) or α-3-D-galactosyltransferases (B-glycosyltransferase).

Studies of plasma glycosyltransferase activities after bone marrow transplantation have yielded fascinating results. Matsue and coworkers[62] reported that in eight patients transplanted with an ABO-incompatible marrow, the ABO RBC type completely changed from the recipient type to the donor type but that preexistent plasma glycosyltranserase activities of the recipient type persisted in seven of the eight patients. Weak transferase activities of the donor type were observed in all of the patients after marrow grafting. An example of one such patient is illustrated in Figure 12-6.

Yoshida and colleagues[63] reported similar findings in four patients. After BMT, the recipients' A and B enzyme activities changed slightly, and only weak reactivity of donor type was detected. Nevertheless, the blood groups of the patients converted to those of their bone marrow donors in each case (Table 12-6).

RBC Typing Irregularities after ABO Minor Mismatched Hematopoietic Cell Transplants

Maeda and associates[64] studied patients up to 72 weeks after ABO-incompatible marrow transplants. They recognized that isohemagglutinins that one would expect to be produced by the donor marrow after BMT often were not detectable in the patient's serum but, in some patients, were found only on their RBCs. For example, when marrow from a group A donor was used for transplantation of a group B patient, one would expect that, after engraftment and replacement of the patient's group B RBCs with those of the group A marrow donor, one would find anti-B in the patient's serum. Although the expected isohemagglutinin was not found in the serum, the DAT was positive, and anti-B could be eluted from the patient's group A RBCs. Also, weakly positive reactions with anti-B were obtained when testing the patient's RBCs long after engraftment.

The authors considered a number of possible explanations for these findings, including the presence of chronic mixed chimerism. They were unable to demonstrate mixed hematopoietic chimerism in the blood and bone marrow of their patients, however. They suggested that the most likely explanation was that anti-B was produced by the donor marrow and reacted with B antigen adsorbed from the patient's plasma onto RBCs produced by the transplanted marrow cells. Although routine ABO blood grouping after ABO-incompatible marrow transplantation generally indicates conversion to donor type, we have observed weakly positive agglutination reactions a year or more

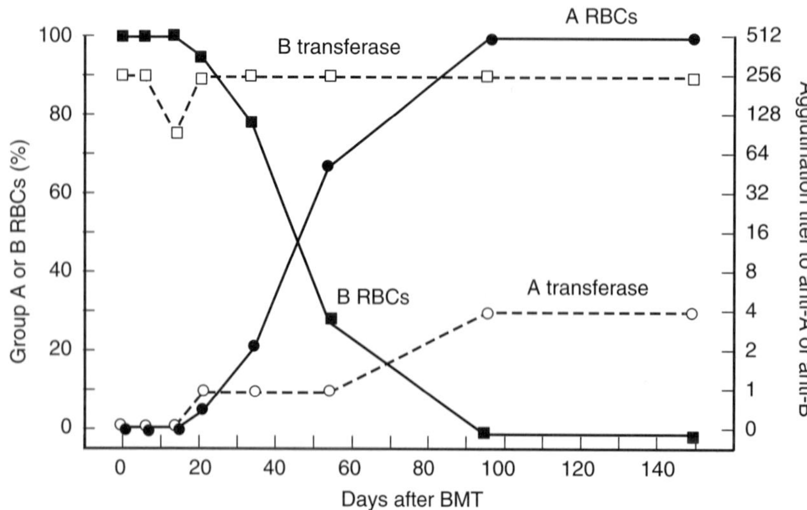

FIGURE 12-6. Blood type and plasma *N*-acetylgalactosaminyltransferase (A-enzyme) activity and galactosyltranferase (B-enzyme) activity before and after bone marrow transplantation. The patient, originally blood group B, received bone marrow from a donor with blood group A. The percentage of RBCs was determined using a microscope by counting agglutinated and nonagglutinated cells, respectively. Transferase activity was assayed after transforming group O RBCs to A or B RBCs by incubation in the presence of the patient's plasma and UDP-N-acetylgalatosamine (for A-tranferase) of UDO-galactose (for B-transferase). The assay was semiquantitated by titration using anti-A or anti-B agglutinin with serial dilutions. (From Matsue K, Yasue S, Matsuda T, et al: Plasma glycosyltransferase activity after ABO-incompatible bone marrow transplantation and development of an inhibitor for glycosyltransferase activity. Exp Hematol 1989;17:827–831.)

after marrow transplantation using anti-A,B sera when testing RBCs from patients who had been group A before transplantation with a group O marrow (Branch DR and Petz LD, unpublished observations).[5]

These findings are consistent with reports of Renton and Hancock,[65] who observed that when group O RBCs are transfused to group A or B recipients, they can acquire small amounts of A or B substance. The uptake of antigen is best demonstrated by using certain group O sera and to a lesser extent with group A and B sera. It can be demonstrated as early as four days after transfusion and reaches a maximum after about 2 weeks (Table 12-7). Also, Crookston and Tilley[66] have reported the adsorption of A antigen by group O RBCs in group A_1 marrow transplant recipients who were transplanted with marrow from group O donors.

To determine whether mixed chimerism or adsorption of plasma antigen is responsible for these reactions, Arndt and coworkers[67] performed flow cytometry on RBCs of people with mixed cell populations, including patients who had been group A and who were transplanted with hematopoietic stem cells from group O donors. They compared these results with flow cytometry patterns obtained when testing mixtures of group O and A RBCs that had a small percentage of group A cells. Their results were consistent with adsorption of group A and B substance (rather than a mixture of group A and O RBCs) as the cause of the weakly positive agglutination reactions found in such post-transplant patients. These findings are discussed further with reference to possible mechanisms of bystander immune hemolysis (see Chapter 9).

TABLE 12-6. BLOOD GROUP AND PLASMA A- AND B-GLYCOSYLTRANSFERASE ACTIVITIES BEFORE AND AFTER BONE MARROW TRANSPLANTATION

Patient Designation	Patient Blood Group		Donor's Blood Group	Patient's Plasma Enzyme Activity*			
	Before BMT	After BMT		Before BMT		After BMT	
				A-Enzyme	B-Enzyme	A-Enzyme	B-Enzyme
UPN 19	A_1	O	O	120	0	55–77	0
UPN 29	O	A_1	A_1	0	0	0–27	0
UPN 35	O	A_1	A_1	0	0	0–10	0
UPN 38	A_1	B	B	90–120	0	48–90	0–5

* Enzyme activity of the patient's plasma was expressed as percentage of mean value of control plasma. Blood group A- and B-enzyme activities are known to differ widely among individuals with phenotype A_1 and B. A-enzyme activity in nine plasma samples with phenotype A_1 ranged from 2.8 to 16.8 (mean value 6.44), and B-enzyme activity in seven plasma samples with phenotype B ranged from 5.0 to 17.5 (mean 10.6), when the activity was expressed as percent of sugar transferred into fucosyllactose under the assay condition.
From Yoshida A, Schmidt GM, Blume KC, Beutler E: Plasma blood group glycosyltransferase activities after bone marrow transplantation. Blood 1980;55:699–701.

TABLE 12-7. AGGLUTINATION OF GROUP O RBCs BY ANTI-A, ANTI-B AND ANTI-A,B AFTER TRANSFUSION TO GROUP A OR B PATIENTS*

Patient	Group	Days after Transfusion	Average Score	
			O Sera	A or B Sera
Mrs. H.D.	A	2	0	0
Mrs. A.S.	B	4	0.2	0
Mrs. D.S.	A	6	0.5	0
Mrs. D.S.	A	13	0.9	0
Mrs. C.O.	A	16	2.1	0.3
Mr. W.C.	B	25	2.1	1.4
Mrs. D.S.	A	29	1.9	1.0
Mrs. D.S.	A	48	1.4	0.3
Mrs. H.D.	A	49	1.5	0
Mr. W.C.	B	76	2.4	0.9

* Following transfusion of group A or B patients with group O RBCs, the patient's RBCs were treated with an excess of high titer anti-A or anti-B, as appropriate, and the unagglutinated RBCs were separated from the agglutinates by a centrifugal method. The free cells were washed and tested with 20 to 30 fresh random group O sera and high-titer group A or B sera. Specificity of the agglutination observed was confirmed by the fact that agglutination was inhibited by A or B secretor saliva but not with nonsecretor saliva or group O secretor saliva. Agglutination was not due to residual A or B cells. The average score was calculated by adding together the scores for all the sera and dividing by the number of sera tested. The average score gives an indication of the amount of antigen that the cells have taken up.
From Renton PH, Hancock JA: Uptake of A and B antigens by transfused group O erythrocytes. Vox Sang 1962;7:33–38.

THE PRESENCE OF ABO ANTIBODIES LONG AFTER MINOR ABO-INCOMPATIBLE HEMATOPOIETIC STEM CELL TRANSPLANTATION

Antibody production by the donor marrow can be present long after hematopoietic stem cell transplantation. For example, Lasky and colleagues[54] reported the presence of ABO antibodies more than 1 year after BMT in three of five recipients of minor ABO-incompatible transplants who survived longer than 5 months after the transplant. The ABO antibodies were first detected at 10 months (anti-A in AB recipient, B donor) and at 21 and 27 months after BMT (anti-A in A recipients, group O donors). Buckner and associates[68] reported that six group A recipients of group O marrow transplants had anti-B (IgG titers of 16–128) more than 1 year after BMT but that none had anti-A. Two other recipients of group O marrow had blood type of group AB, and neither of these had detectable anti-B, but both had weak anti-A. Although A antigen is known to be distributed widely in the tissues, no symptomatology could be ascribed to the presence of the anti-A. Needs and coworkers[33] reported on two group A_2 patients who were engrafted with group O marrow and produced anti-A_1 after 24 months. Robertson and colleagues[13] reported that ABO antibodies were not detected until more than 74 days after transplant in two patients transplanted with marrow from minor ABO-incompatible donors. Gale and associates[34] reported a group O patient who was transplanted with marrow from a group A donor who had IgM anti-B 2 years after BMT.

Lee and coworkers[69] reported that donor-derived ABO antibodies against recipient RBCs were detectable in five out of 36 patients who received minor ABO-incompatible stem cell grafts. The probability of the appearance of ABO antibodies by 1 year after transplant was 17.5%. The ABO antibodies appeared after the disappearance of recipient RBCs except in one patient, in whom there was no clinically detectable hemolysis.

MAJOR ABO BLOOD GROUP INCOMPATIBLE HEMATOPOIETIC STEM CELL TRANSPLANTS

Immune Hemolysis of Red Cells in the Stem Cell Product

Because the volume of RBCs in a bone marrow product could be equal to or greater than that in a unit of RBC, the potential exists for an immediate hemolytic transfusion reaction due to ABO incompatibility. This may be prevented by removal of the RBCs from the donor marrow or by removal of ABO antibodies from the recipient. The latter procedure has sometimes been followed by pretransplant transfusion of incompatible RBCs to adsorb the recipients' hemagglutinins completely.

Delayed Hemolytic Reactions after Transfusion of Incompatible RBCs before Hematopoietic Cell Transplantation

The rebound of ABO antibodies after a transplant procedure is of particular concern for patients who have been transfused with incompatible RBCs in an effort to further reduce the antibody titers by adsorption after plasma exchange. Such transfusions result in the presence of a large volume of incompatible RBCs that are susceptible to hemolysis when the antibody rebound occurs. Indeed, Lasky and colleagues[54] have reported that delayed hemolysis occurred on days 6 to 10 after transplantation in seven of nine patients who received incompatible RBC transfusions before the procedure. In two of these patients, the hemoglobin dropped by 7.9 g/dL and 4.5 g/dL, respectively, over the course of 2 to 3 days. In contrast, none of five patients who had not received donor-type RBCs developed delayed hemolysis. One of the transfused patients, who was group O, had pretransplant anti-A titers of 32/128 (IgM/IgG) and anti-B titers of 64/16. These were reduced to undetectable levels by two-plasma volume plasma exchanges followed by 4 units of incompatible, donor-type RBCs. On day 6 after the transplant procedure, the ABO antibodies reappeared in the patient's serum, signs of acute hemolysis became evident, the DAT was positive for IgG and complement, anti-A and anti-B were eluted from the patient's RBCs, and the hematocrit dropped from 37% to 18%.[70]

Buckner and associates[68] reported on a patient who had been treated with transfusion of incompatible blood before transplantation and in whom a rising anti-A titer after transplantation resulted in acute massive intravascular hemolysis and renal failure. Although this was their only patient in whom hemolysis was a major factor in patient management, unwanted antibody reappeared in the serum of 12 of 14 evaluable patients. Bensinger and coworkers[37] reported on a similar patient who received incompatible RBCs before the transplant procedure and who developed acute hemolysis starting on the third day after transplantation, leading to renal failure that required hemodialysis. These investigators reported that they abandoned as unnecessary the transfusion of incompatible blood for antibody absorption before transplantation.

Hemolysis of RBCs Produced by Newly Engrafted Marrow Caused by Persistence ABO Antibodies

Although ABO antibodies usually become undetectable during the second month after major ABO-incompatible BMT, this is not always the case (Fig. 12-7).[71] Bensinger and colleagues[37] pointed out that IgG antibody was detected for as long as 100 days after a transplant procedure. This suggests the continued production of IgG antibody by plasma cells that survived the pre-BMT cytoreductive therapy, considering that the normal half-life of IgG is 21 days. Other investigators have reported that isohemagglutinins were no longer detectable after 14 days to 4 months after the transplant procedure.[37,54,68,71,72]

Prolonged persistence of ABO antibodies can result in hemolysis of RBCs produced by the newly engrafted marrow. Sniecinski and associates[4] reported that anti-A or anti-B persisted for longer than 120 days after BMT in 9 of 58 evaluable patients receiving a major ABO-incompatible marrow transplant. Five patients developed overt hemolysis at a time when antibodies were still detectable but had decreased to a low titer (≤4). Hemolysis started on days 37 to 105 after BMT (median = +65), persisted for 10–94 days (median = 36 days), and was manifested by a drop in hemoglobin of 1.5–4 g/dL (median = 2.5 g/dL), increases in bilirubin and LDH, and decreases in serum haptoglobin. The five cases of hemolysis occurred among 30 patients who received cyclosporine-prednisone for post-transplant GVHD prophylaxis, and no episodes of hemolysis occurred among 28 patients receiving both methotrexate and prednisone. Before the decrease in the ABO antibody titers to low levels, erythropoiesis was suppressed; after the antibodies decreased to undetectable levels, hemolysis ceased and adequate erythropoiesis developed (Fig. 12-8).

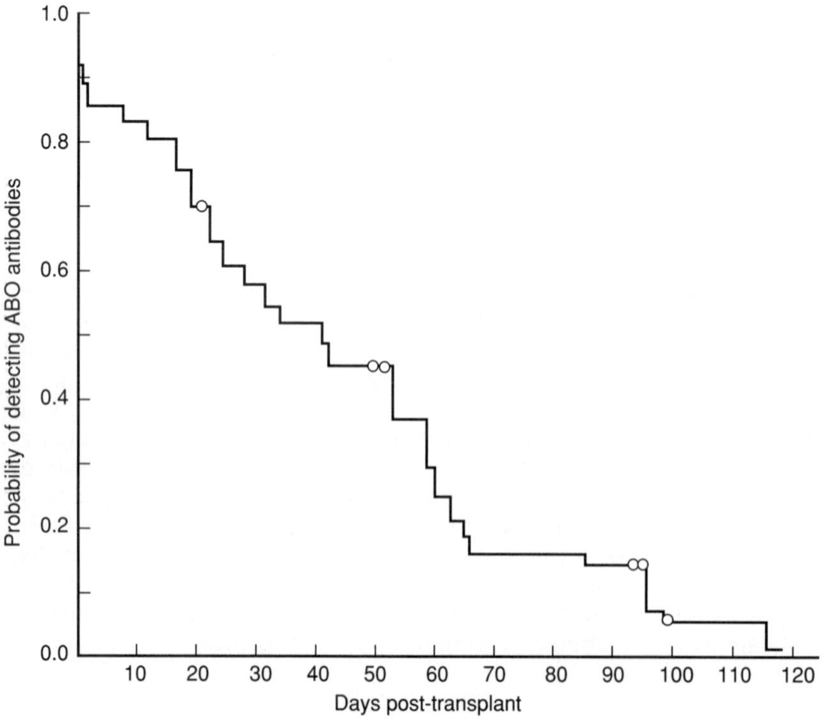

FIGURE 12-7. Probability of detecting host ABO antibodies in 36 major ABO-incompatible marrow receipients at varying times after transplantation. (From Witherspoon RP, Storb R, Ochs HD, et al: Recovery of antibody production in human allogeneic marrow graft recipients: Influence of time posttransplantation, the presence or absence of chronic graft-versus-host disease, and antithymocyte globulin treatment. Blood 1981;58:360–368.)

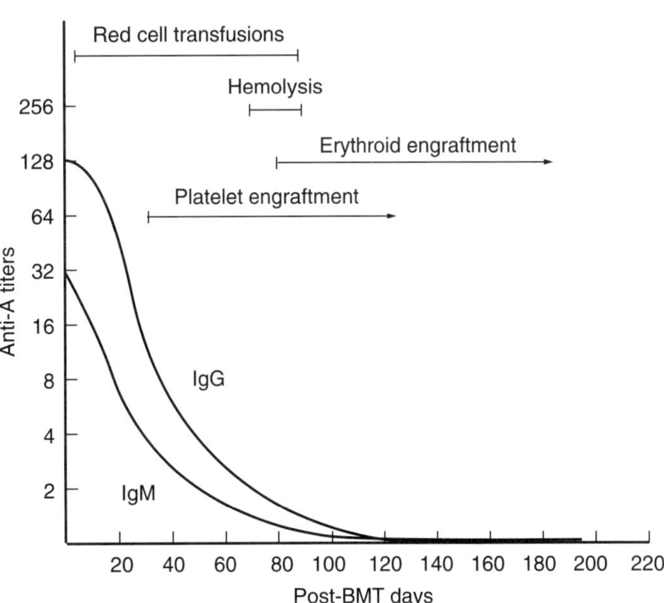

FIGURE 12-8. Post-transplant course in a patient with no RBC production and high ABO antibody titers. Hemolysis occurred when titers were low. Resolution coincided with undetectable antibodies. Findings of hemolysis were present even though donor marrow-derived RBCs were undetectable, suggesting intramedullary hemolysis. *Upper curve* represents immunoglobin G (IgG) ABO antibodies, and *lower curve* represents IgM ABO antibodies. (From Sniecinski IJ, Oien L, Petz LD, et al: Immunohematologic consequences of major ABO-mismatched bone marrow transplantation. Transplantation 1988;45:530–534.)

Lopez and coworkers[73] reported on a major ABO-incompatible BMT patient who developed hemolysis between days 36 and 50 after transplant due to the persistence of recipient isohemagglutinins.

Biggs and colleagues[74] reported hemolysis of newly formed group B RBCs occurring before the 33rd day after transplant in a group O patient transplanted with a group B marrow.

Transient hemolysis caused by immune hemolysis by ABO antibodies of RBCs produced by the newly engrafted marrow seems to be observed infrequently. Neither Gmur and associates[75] nor Bar and coworkers[76] identified episodes of hemolysis in their reports of 15 and 30 evaluable patients, respectively, who were transplanted with major ABO-incompatible marrows.

Suppression of Hematopoiesis by Persistent ABO Antibodies after Major ABO-Incompatible Hematopoietic Cell Transplants

A number of investigators have reported impaired or failed hematopoiesis in some patients with persistent isohemagglutinins after BMT. Figure 12-9 illustrates the findings in a patient with a high titer anti-A at the

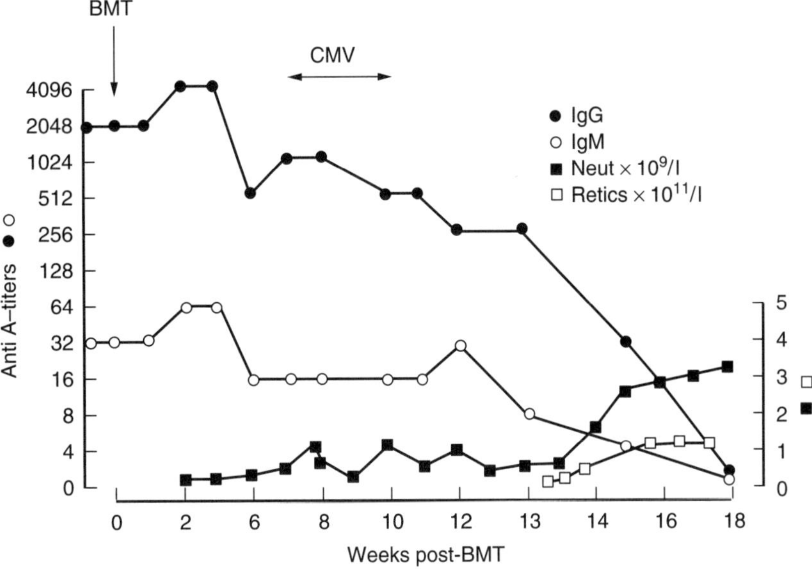

FIGURE 12-9. Serial anti-A titers (reciprocal of dilution) and reticulocyte and neutrophil counts during the weeks after BMT in a group O patient transplanted with marrow from a group A donor. (From Blacklock HA, Gilmore MJ, Prentice HG, et al: ABO-incompatible bone-marrow transplantation: Removal of red blood cells from donor marrow avoiding recipient antibody depletion. Lancet 1982;2:1061–1064.)

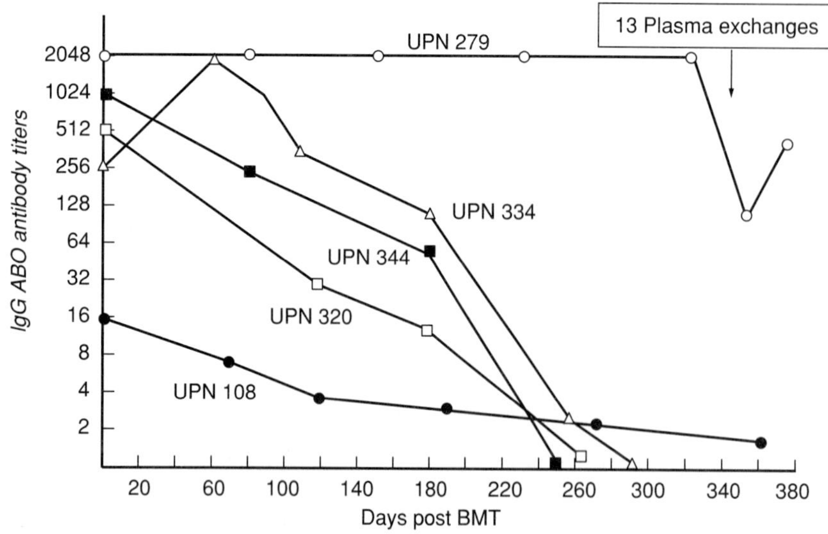

FIGURE 12-10. IgG-ABO antibody titers in five patients whose antibodies persisted for >255 days. (From Sniecinski IJ, Oien L, Petz LD, et al: Immunohematologic consequences of major ABO-mismatched bone marrow transplantation. Transplantation 1988;45:530–534.)

time of transplant, who had detectable antibody until 15 weeks after BMT. She had delayed engraftment of red cells, neutrophils, and platelets (the latter is not illustrated).[77]

Pure Red Cell Aplasia

Much more common than suppression of hematopoiesis is a delay in the production of donor-type RBCs—a temporary development of pure RBC aplasia (PRCA) until the titers of isohemagglutinins reach low levels.[1,4,37,54,59,69,75,76,78-84] This can be explained by the interaction of anti-A or anti-B with donor erythroid precursors expressing the A and/or B antigens.[85-87]

Sniecinski and colleagues[4] reported that, in 9 of 58 evaluable patients who received a major ABO-incompatible BMT from an HLA-matched sibling donor, there was persistence of isohemagglutinins for more than 120 days after BMT. Red cell production was delayed to 40 days or longer in the nine patients and, in five of these, erythropoiesis was markedly delayed to 170 days or longer (Fig. 12-10).

Gmur and associates[75] reported on three patients who developed PRCA lasting from 5 to 8 months. One patient's course is illustrated in Figure 12-11. Bar and coworkers[76] reported that 8 of 30 patients (27%) with major ABO incompatibility had lymphocyte-depleted bone marrow with no detectable donor RBCs for at least 2 months after BMT. In these

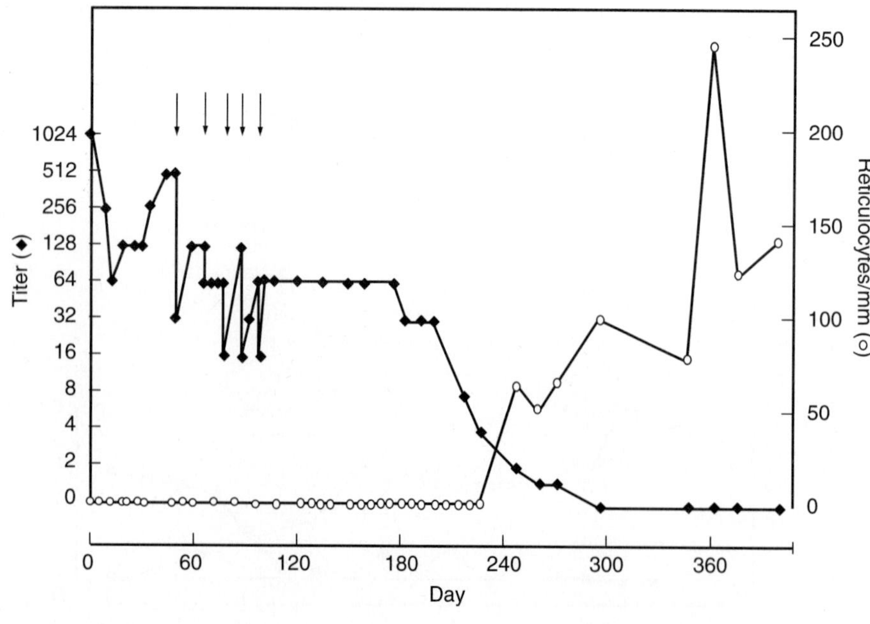

FIGURE 12-11. Course of anti-A agglutinin titer (*squares*) and absolute reticulocytes/mm (*open circles*) after ABO-incompatible BMT in UPN 39. Day 0 is the day of BMT. Arrows indicate plasma exchange. (From Gmur J, Burger J, Schaffner A, et al: Pure red cell aplasia of long duration complicating major ABO-incompatible bone marrow transplantation. Blood 1990;75:290–295.)

patients, there was an early rise in or a persistence of high isohemagglutinin titers (IgG more than IgM), whereas the titers decreased immediately after BMT in patients without delayed erythropoiesis. The median pretransplant IgG isohemagglutinin titer (anti-A or anti-B) was 16 (range, 1–512) in patients without delayed erythropoiesis, in contrast to a median titer of 512 (range, 64–16,000) in patients with a delayed onset of erythropoiesis. The IgM isohemagglutinin titers were the same in both groups. Various reports in the literature do not agree on a correlation between pretransplant ABO titers and the number of days after transplantation before the onset of erythropoiesis.[76]

Lee and colleagues[69] analyzed data for 40 patients with major (and/or minor) ABO incompatibility and reported that recipient-derived ABO antibodies against donor-type RBCs had disappeared by (median) day 89 after the transplant procedure (range, 25–449 days); the probability of ABO antibody disappearance by 1 year after BMT was 97.3%. ABO antibodies against donor-derived RBCs disappeared more rapidly after unrelated donor transplantation (P = 0.006) and in patients with acute GVHD (P = 0.025). Out of 35 patients, 10 (28.6%) evidenced persistent reticulocytopenia for more than 60 days after transplantation.

As with other immunohematologic complications after BMT, the incidence of delayed hematopoiesis appears more common among patients who were treated with cyclosporine for post-transplant GVHD prophylaxis.[4,59,75,76]

PRCA after Reduced-Intensity Nonmyeloablative Conditioning Regimens

Bolan and associates[79] determined PRCA to be present when bone marrow biopsy demonstrated adequate myeloid, lymphoid, and megakaryocyte populations in the setting of absent or nearly absent erythroid precursors and profound peripheral blood reticulocytopenia. The found that PRCA occurred in four of 14 patients (29%) after hematopoietic stem cell transplants using reduced-intensity nonmyeloablative regimens, but in none of 12 patients transplanted using myeloabative conditioning during the same period of time. Donor RBC chimerism (initial detection of donor RBCs in peripheral blood) was delayed markedly after nonmyeloablative regimens (median, 114 days vs. 40 days; P < 0.0001) and correlated strongly with decreasing host anti-donor ABO antibody levels (Figs. 12-12 and 12-13). They pointed out that strategies to further reduce transplant-related toxicity, such as lower-intensity conditioning and more prolonged administration of GVHD prophylaxis, could also be associated with prolonged host ABO antibody production and could result in marked delays in the onset of donor erythropoiesis.

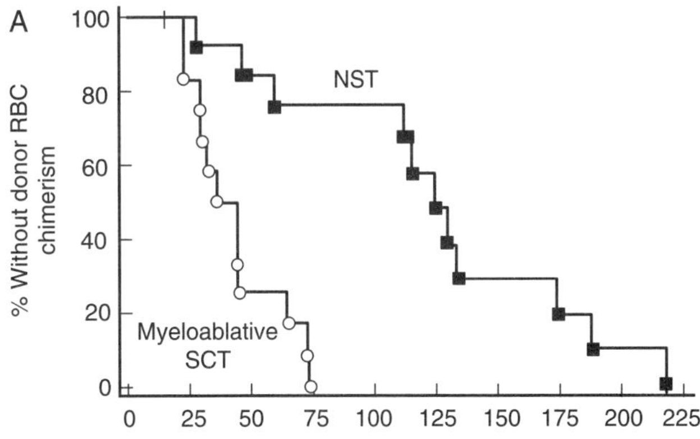

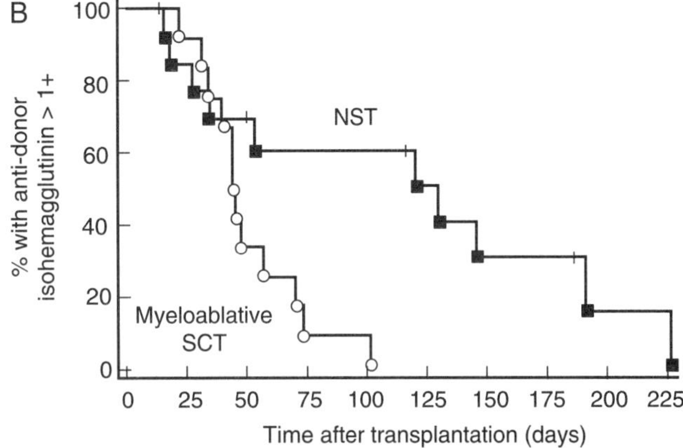

FIGURE 12-12. The onset of donor RBC chimerism and decline in antidonor isohemagglutinin levels after NST compared with myeloablative SCT. The onset of donor RBC chimerism and decline of host antidonor isohemagglutinin to clinically insignificant levels were delayed markedly following major ABO-incompatible NST compared with myeloblative SCT. NST data are represented by solid squares; myeloblative SCT data, by open circles. SCT, stem cell transplant; NST, nonmyeloablative stem cell transplant. (A) Kaplan-Meier plot of the percentage of transplantation. The time until detection of donor RBC chimerism was significantly prolonged following NST vs. myeloblative SCT; P < .0001. (B) Kaplan-Meier plot showing the percentage of patients with persistent host antidonor isohemagglutinins greater that 1+ in strength. Isohemagglutinins decreased significantly faster after myeloblative SCT than after NST; P = .012. (From Bolan CD, Leitman SF, Griffith LM, Wesley RA, Procter JL, Stroncek DF, et al: Delayed donor red cell chimerism and pure red cell aplasia following major ABO-incompatible nonmyeloablative hematopoietic stem cell transplantation. Blood 2001;98:1687–1694.)

Peggs and coworkers[88] reviewed their results with 15 major or bidirectional ABO-incompatible transplants done with nonmyeloalative conditioning regimens. They concluded that the incidence of delayed donor red cell chimerism and PRCA likely differs not only between myeloablative and nonmyeloablative conditioning regimens but also according to the type of nonmyeloablative (or reduced-intensity) conditioning regimen and perhaps also to the degree of B-cell suppression achieved. PRCA after major ABO-incompatible reduced-intensity transplantation has also been reported by Veelken and colleagues.[89]

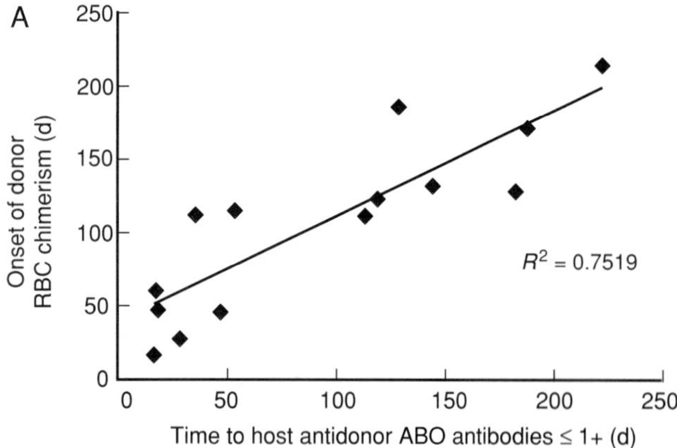

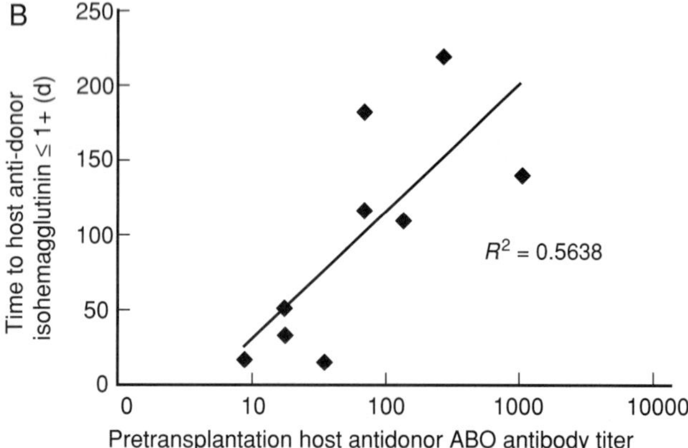

FIGURE 12-13. Correlation of the onset of donor RBC chimerism with a decline in host antidonor ABO antibodies after major ABO-incompatible nonmyeloablative stem cell transplant (NST). The onset of donor RBC chimerism was strongly correlated with a decline in host antidonor ABO antibodies to 1+ or lower, and the time until ABO antibodies decreased to levels 1+ or lower was related to the pretransplantation ABO antibody titer. (A) The onset of donor RBC chimerism after NST strongly correlated with a decline in host isohemagglutinins to clinically insignificant levels (1+ or lower on reverse type; R2 = 0.72, $P < 0.0005$). (B) The time until host antidonor ABO antibodies decreased to levels 1 + or lower correlated with the log value of the pretransplantation ABO antibody titer (R2 = 0.56; $P = 0.02$). (From Bolan CD, Leitman SF, Griffith LM, et al: Delayed donor red cell chimerism and pure red cell aplasia following major ABO-incompatible nonmyeloablative hematopoietic stem cell transplantation. Blood 2001;98:1687–1694.)

MANAGEMENT OF PATIENTS RECEIVING A HEMATOPOIETIC STEM CELL TRANSPLANT FROM A MAJOR ABO-INCOMPATIBLE DONOR

Prevention of Acute Hemolysis

Two general principles are used to prevent acute hemolysis resulting from transfusion of incompatible RBCs at the time of donor marrow infusion. One can either remove RBCs from donor marrow products or remove isohemagglutinins from the patient. In an analogous fashion, one should minimize the RBC content of peripheral blood stem cell products before transplantation or cryopreservation to reduce the amount of hemoglobin transfused with the product.[59]

Red Cell Removal from Donor Marrow

The main objective of removing RBCs from the donor marrow is to remove the majority of RBCs while preserving the hematopoietic progenitors to encourage engraftment. Several manual and automated techniques have been developed to remove RBCs selectively. Some techniques isolate the mononuclear cell-rich component where the cells necessary for engraftment are found, whereas others use the entire buffy coat that contains both mononuclear and polymorphonuclear cells. These techniques have been reviewed by Sniecinski and coworkers.[59]

The major risks of RBC depletion from marrow include stem cell loss during processing and the hazard of infusing small amounts of incompatible RBCs. Dinsmore and associates[90] reported that two patients who received 68 mL and 45 mL of red cells, respectively, developed transient hemoglobinuria without renal impairment. Warkentin and coworkers[91] reported that their marrow products contained 0.4–21.8 mL of red cells but that even the transfusion of these small volumes of red cells resulted in measurable evidence of hemolysis in some patients, although reactions were not severe. Braine and colleagues,[92] whose protocol left 8–38 mL of incompatible erythrocytes in the infusate, reported somewhat more severe reactions, including fever, hypertension, chills, hemoglobinuria, bradycardia, and confusion.

The total volume of RBCs in the marrow product that is infused might determine the frequency of adverse reactions; several authors who reported maximum volumes of residual RBCs of 10 mL or less stated that the infusions caused no clinical symptoms or evidence of hemoysis.[77,93-95] It is also likely that the titer of the patient's ABO antibodies is of significance, although this factor has not been studied extensively in this setting.

Removal of ABO Antibodies from the Patient

The purpose of this approach is to decrease the titer of the potentially offending antibody before marrow infusion. This may be achieved by the use of plasma exchange or plasma immunoadsorption, usually carried out daily over the course of 3 to 4 days before marrow infusion. The goal is to reduce the antibody titers to 16 or less, as transfusion of marrow products to patients with such low titers have been reported to not result in acute hemolytic reactions.[15,37] Supplementation of this procedure by transfusion of incompatible RBCs is not recommended because of the risk of delayed hemolysis caused by antibody rebound in the post-transplant period.

Rowley[15] states that up to 4 days of plasma exchange might be required (1 day for patients with antibody titers of 32–128, two days for titers of 256–512, three days for a titer of 1024, and four days for a titer of 2048). Plasma exchange is unlikely to be adequate for the management of patients with titers greater than 2048; these patients should receive red cell–depleted products.

Disadvantages of methods to remove antibody from the patient are that the procedures are lengthy and need to be carried out during the period immediately before transplantation, when the patient is being conditioned for transplantation with irradiation and chemotherapy.[1,96] Also, the patient is exposed to the risks of transfusion, including allergic reactions and the transmission of infectious diseases. Finally, in a considerable number of patients, the antibody titers rise again after transplantation (Table 12-8).[37,78,96-98]

Prevention of Delayed Erythropoiesis

Some investigators recommend that even if RBCs are removed from the donor marrow product, removal of the patient's isohemagglutinins by plasma exchange should be carried out before transplantation. This recommendation is based on the expectation that recipients who have isohemagglutinins reactive against donor blood group antigens—particularly if they are in high titer—might experience a longer delay in the onset of erythropoiesis than those who have the isohemagglutinins removed. Observations about this point have been in disagreement. Jin and associates[95] found no difference in erythrocyte transfusion requirements between recipients of a red cell–depleted graft and patients who had plasma exchange or immunoadsorption, whereas Lasky and coworkers[54] found that red cell transfusions were required in significantly larger numbers and for a longer time among recipients of red cell–depleted marrow than among patients prepared by plasma exchange.

Blacklock and colleagues[77,85] recommend that recipients with high-titer IgG anti-A, especially when A_1 donors are used, should undergo some form of antibody depletion—perhaps before marrow infusion, but particularly after transplantation—if marrow development is not proceeding. They indicate, however, that donor marrow red cell depletion alone is probably a sufficient measure for the majority of ABO-incompatible transplants, especially among recipients who have low anti-A or anti-B titers.

Patients who have high isohemagglutinin titers before transplantation should be followed with weekly titers after transplantation. A rising titer usually preceeds the onset of delayed erythropoiesis, hemolysis, or both.[59] Plasma exchange or immunoadsorption should then be considered. Lee and associates[69] also reported that 7 of 12 patients who showed a post-transplant increase in titers of isoagglutinins against donor-type RBCs developed delayed erythropoiesis, whereas only 3 of 23 patients who did not show a post-transplant increase in the isoagglutinin titers developed red cell aplasia.

Reviron and coworkers[99,100] suggested that it might be appropriate to remove isohemagglutinins from the patient on day 0 if the titer of antibody is 512 or higher. They did not present data, however, to indicate that outcomes are improved when this strategy is chosen compared with a policy of waiting to perform plasma exchange until after transplantation for patients in whom the isohemagglutinin titers do not diminish spontaneously. They suggest that day 20 after transplantation is an appropriate time to evaluate a patient to determine whether plasma exchange or immunoadsorption should be performed.

TABLE 12-8. SERIAL ANTI-A TITERS FOLLOWING PLASMA EXCHANGES AND INFUSION OF A SUBSTANCE

Time	IgM	IgG
Baseline	2048	512
Postplasma exchange-1 (10 L)	64	32
Post-A-substance	64	32
Preplasma exchange-2	64	32
Postplasma exchange-2 (18 L)	1	2
Transplant	128	64
Day +5	2048	64
Day +12	2048	64
Day +19	512	16
Day +35	0	0
Day +48	0	0

From Hershko C, Gale RP, Ho W, Fitchen J: ABH antigens and bone marrow transplantation. Br J Haematol 1980;44:65–73.

Treatment of Delayed Erythropoiesis

Appropriate management of patients with a delayed onset of erythropoiesis is not clear.[15,79] Treatment successes and failures in PRCA after hematopoietic stem cell transplantation have been described with plasma exchange[4,101–103] and erythropoietin.[73,81,104–106] A patient described by Ohashi and colleagues[104] did not respond to erythropoietin alone, but erythropoiesis began after the addition of methylprednisolone. This development could have been a coincidence, however, as the rise in reticulocytes in this patient was accompanied by a drop in anti-A titer to undetectable levels. Intravenous immune globulin was not found to be beneficial in two case reports; in two other cases, antilymphocyte globulin did result in restoration of erythropoiesis.[82,102]

For most patients, erythroid engraftment occurs spontaneously within 6 months when isohemagglutinin titers decrease to low levels (generally ≤4). Indeed, Benjamin and associates[83] indicated that PRCA rarely requires intervention other than transfusion support. RBC production can be suppressed for more than a year, and in one patient, the onset of erythropoiesis was delayed until 5 years after transplantation,[107] which was long after corticosteroids and multiple plasma exchanges had failed to produce benefit.[4,107] Occasionally, isohemagglutinins might still be present at titers as high as 16 when the red cell aplasia resolves.[4]

Other reports have documented resolution of PRCA after donor lymphocyte infusion.[108,109] Bolan and coworkers[79] reported that erythropoietin was ineffective in all four of their patients, but that discontinuation of cyclosporine appeared to lead to resolution of PRCA. Similarly, Yamaguchi and colleagues[110] described a patient who needed RBC transfusion every week from day 54 after hematopoietic cell transplantation onward. He showed no evidence of GVHD, but with the tapering of cyclosporin after day 123, he developed chronic GVHD around day 145. The patient no longer needed transfusion from day 167, the reticulocyte count began to increase on day 179, and antidonor isohemagglutinin titers became undetectable. They concluded that chronic GVHD induced by tapering of cyclosporin appeared to be related to improvement in the PRCA. A graft-vs.-plasma cell effect is consistent with the data of Lee and associates,[69] cited previously, and of Mielcarek and coworkers.[111]

Treatment of Delayed Hemolysis

Management of this rather uncommon complication of major ABO-incompatible transplants has required only supportive management with transfusion of group O RBCs. Signs of hemolysis of newly formed RBCs can persist for 10–94 days (median = 36 days).

Lopez and colleagues[73] reported on a patient with delayed hemolysis whose treatment included erythropoietin (Fig. 12-14). A 25-year-old male with chronic phase chronic myeloid leukemia (CML) underwent a BMT from his HLA-identical sister. The patient was group O, and the donor was group A. The patient received erythropoietin on days 0 through 36 after transplantation because he was included in a prospective randomized protocol to test the usefulness of erythropoietin in BMT. Anti-A was detected persistently in the patient's serum throughout the post-transplant course until day 175. Between days 36 and 50 after transplantation, his hemoglobin dropped from 12.8 g/dL to 9.7 g/dL. On day 50, his DAT was positive with anti-C3, anti-A was eluted from his RBC, the LDH that had been 381 IU/L on day 36 was now 860 IU/L (normal = <360 IU/L), and the serum haptoglobin value was 0. Administration of erythropoietin was resumed, and reticulocytes rose to as high as 90%. Signs of hemolysis persisted, and the hemoglobin remained stable until after day 78. Thereafter, signs of hemolysis gradually subsided, the hemoglobin improved, and erythropoietin was tapered and then discontinued on day 150. The patient's anti-A titers on day 141 were IgM 8 and IgG 16. In this patient, erythropoietin might have caused release of RBCs by the newly engrafted marrow earlier than would have otherwise occurred in the face of persistent anti-A, thus minimizing the period of red cell aplasia but at the cost of hemolysis, which in this instance caused no adverse consequences.

Selection of Blood Products

From the onset of the preparative regimen, it is advisable to use group O RBCs when transfusion is

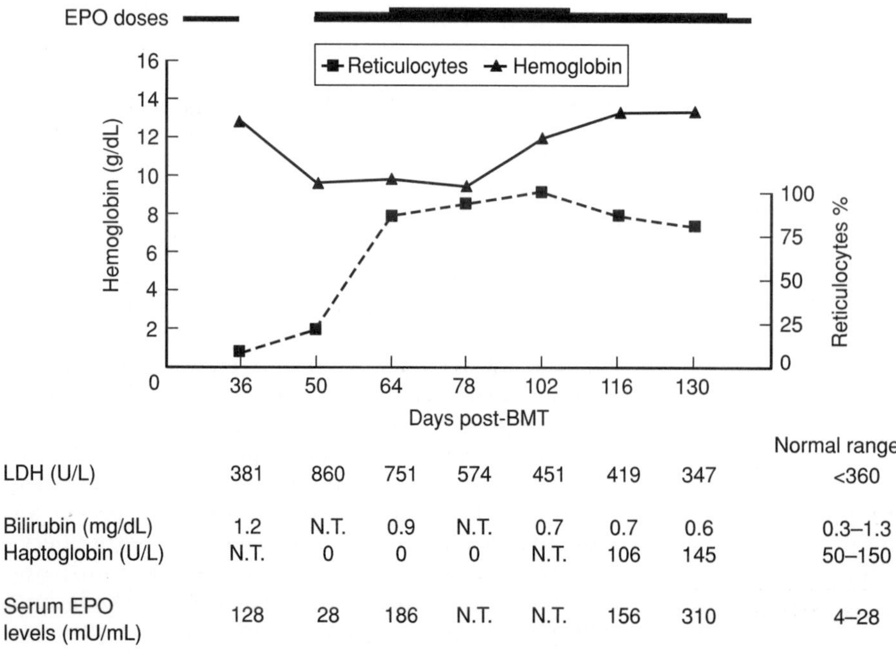

								Normal range
LDH (U/L)	381	860	751	574	451	419	347	<360
Bilirubin (mg/dL)	1.2	N.T.	0.9	N.T.	0.7	0.7	0.6	0.3–1.3
Haptoglobin (U/L)	N.T.	0	0	0	N.T.	106	145	50–150
Serum EPO levels (mU/mL)	128	28	186	N.T.	N.T.	156	310	4–28

FIGURE 12-14. *Top*: Response of hemoglobin and reticulocytes to EPO administration. *Bottom*: Serum EPO levels and parameters of hemolysis before and after EPO therapy. N.T., not tested. (From Lopez J, Steegmann JL, Perez G, et al: Erythopoietin in the treatment of delayed immune hemolysis of a major ABO-incompatible bone marrow transplant. Am J Hematol 1994;45:237.)

necessary, although the recipient's RBC type can be used for group A or B patients in those unusual cases in which the donor is group AB (see Table 12-5). Ultimately, when the patient's hemagglutinins have become undetectable, red cells of the donor's type may be transfused.

Also, it is reasonable to minimize the administration of plasma that contains isohemagglutinins that will react with RBCs of the donor's type. This is best accomplished by providing platelet products that are of the donor's type. If such platelets are not available, volume reduction of the platelets may be performed, although the amount of antibody in the platelet products is usually not a significant factor in causation of hemolysis. The use of washed RBCs or washed platelets as a means of minimizing plasma administration is generally unnecessary.

Other Considerations in Selection of Blood Products

Although the following consideration is not pertinent to the topic of immune hemolysis, one must be aware that all cellular blood products should be γ-irradiated for all hematopoietic stem cell transplant patients beginning with the onset of the preparative regimen. Friedberg[112] also suggests that, for patients who are to have a stem cell transplant, blood products intended for transfusion that might still be circulating at the time of stem cell collection should be γ-irradiated.

One unresolved question concerns the duration of time after transplantation during which irradiated products should be administered. It seems logical to extend their use during the period of posttransplant immune deficiency. This can persist for 1 or 2 years and might be present even longer in patients who have GVHD. A common policy is to irradiate cellular blood products indefinitely in patients who have received a hematopoietic stem cell transplant.[112]

Also, cytomegalovirus (CMV) transmission should be minimized by the use of appropriate CMV-safe products. The indications for CMV-safe products and the choice of products are beyond the scope of this text.

Leukocyte-reduced products are generally given to minimize refractoriness to platelet transfusion. A multi-institutional, randomized, blinded study of alloimmunization to platelets determined that without the use of leukocyte-reduced blood products, 13% of previously untreated patients treated for acute myelogenous leukemia became alloimmunized and refractory to platelet transfusions.[113] With the use of leukocyte-reduced products, 3–4% became alloimmunized and refractory (Fig. 12-15). The study also indicated that patients who had detectable lymphocytotoxic antibodies at entry into the study did not benefit from transfusion of leukocyte-reduced platelets. Finally, platelets obtained by apheresis from single random donors provided no additional benefit compared with pooled platelet concentrates from random donors.

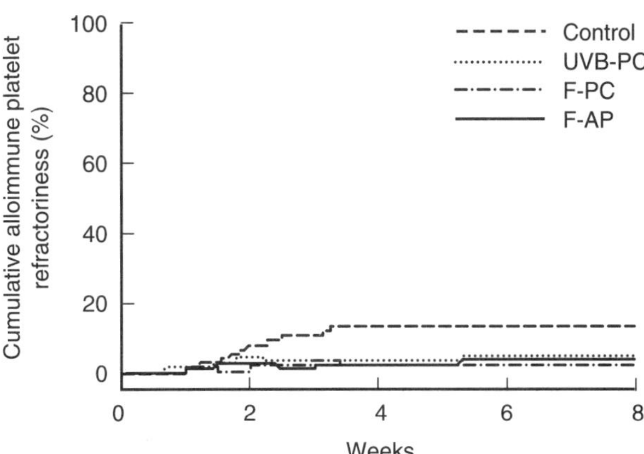

FIGURE 12-15. Development of alloimmune platelet refractoriness in patients who had refractoriness and also were antibody-positive. (From Leukocyte reduction and ultraviolet B irradiation of platelets to prevent alloimmunization and refractoriness to platelet transfusions. The Trial to Reduce Alloimmunization and Refractoriness to Platelets Study Group. N Engl J Med 1997;337:1861–1869.)

THE ROLE OF THE ABO BLOOD GROUP SYSTEM IN GRAFT-VS.-HOST DISEASE, RELAPSE, AND MORTALITY AFTER ALLOGENEIC HEMATOPOIETIC CELL TRANSPLANTATION

Graft-vs.-host disease (GVHD) is most commonly manifested by a generalized maculopapular rash, hepatitis, diarrhea, and a delayed reconstitution of hematopoietic and lymphoid function.[114] GVHD is a pathologic process initiated by engrafted immunocompetent donor T-lymphocytes responding to alloantigens expressed on host cells, particularly cells derived from the lymphohematopoietic system. As the role of ABO incompatibility was being evaluated early in the history of BMT, there was concern that minor ABO blood group incompatibility might be associated with a higher incidence or greater severity of GVHD.

In an early report, Storb and associates[115] stated that their experience did not support the concept that ABO antigens played a role in causing GVHD, as only one of ten patients who received a minor ABO mismatched marrow developed GVHD.

Buckner and coworkers[68] analyzed the results of BMT with regard to the incidence and severity of GVHD among 39 evaluable patients with aplastic anemia or acute leukemia who had minor ABO mismatches with their donors. Only patients who were genotypically HLA-matched at the A, B, and D loci with a sibling donor were included in the analysis. There were 229 evaluable patients with ABO-identical donors available for comparison. Their results suggested no effect of minor ABO incompatibility on the incidence or severity of GVHD.

Hershko and colleagues[98] extended earlier observations[34] and reported a comparison of the incidence of GVHD among 60 patients with ABO-identical or major mismatched grafts with the incidence of GVHD among 15 patients with minor ABO-mismatched marrow transplants. There was no statistically significant difference between the two groups in the incidence of GVHD.

Lasky and associates[54] found no statistical difference in the incidence of GVHD when comparing 13 patients who received a minor ABO-mismatched BMT with 95 patients who received ABO-matched marrow grafts. Other investigators have reached similar conclusions.[77,91,116]

On the other hand, Bacigalupo and coworkers[117] reported an analysis of 174 patients who received a BMT from an HLA-identical sibling for severe aplastic anemia, acute lymphoblastic leukemia, or chronic granulocytic leukemia. Twenty-three transplants were ABO major-mismatched, 27 were ABO minor-mismatched, and 124 were ABO-matched. Double mismatched grafts (A to B and B to A) were excluded from their analysis. They concluded that ABO compatibility clearly was associated with a different risk of grade II–IV acute GVHD (Fig. 12-16). Recipients of ABO minor-mismatched grafts experienced the highest incidence of GVHD, recipients of ABO-identical grafts had an intermediate risk, and patients given an ABO major-mismatched BMT had the lowest incidence. To explain the low incidence of GVHD in ABO major-mismatched BMT, the authors suggested that donor lymphocytes could absorb ABO antigens and then become the target for immune destruction by anti-A/B antibodies, thus contributing to a low incidence of GVHD.

Barone and colleagues[118] retrospectively studied 65 bone marrow transplant patients who had ABO incompatibility (major or minor) and compared the results with a control group whose donors were ABO- and Rh-compatible. They found GVHD in 26 patients (40%) with major ABO incompatibility and in 15 patients (23%) with minor incompatibility. They suggested that GVHD frequency was increased in the group with ABO blood system incompatibility compared with their control group and the data in the literature.

Stussi and associates[119] evaluated the effect of ABO incompatibility on GVHD in 173 consecutive patients receiving allogeneic bone marrow transplants. Univariate analysis suggested a higher incidence of GVHD in minor ABO incompatibility than in ABO identity (14/30, 47% vs. 37/112, 33%; $P = 0.02$). Using logistic regression adjusted for potential confounders, however, the risk of GVHD did not differ significantly between the two groups. In a further report, Stussi and coworkers[120] reported the results of a retrospective two-center analysis of 562 consecutive patients receiving allogeneic bone marrow or peripheral blood stem cell transplantation. The incidence of acute GVHD (grades I–IV) was higher for minor ABO-incompatible transplants compared with transplants involving ABO identity (relative risk [RR], 2.8; 95% confidence interval [CI], 1.3–5.9; $P = 0.009$). This difference was limited to mild GVHD; in moderate-to-severe GVHD (grades II–IV), no significant difference in incidence was found among the groups. Other findings were that RBC engraftment was delayed in major ABO-incompatible transplants and that the relapse rate was not influenced by ABO incompatibility.

Transplant Outcome

Benjamin and colleagues[121] performed a retrospective analysis of a cohort of 292 allogeneic transplant recipients and measured survival in a subgroup of ABO-incompatible bone marrow graft recipients. They found that patients with acute myelogenous leukemia or myelodysplastic syndrome receiving ABO-incompatible non-T-cell–depleted marrow grafts had an 85% greater risk of death within 100 days of transplant (RR, 1.85; 95% CI, 1.33–2.58; $P = 0.003$) than comparable patients receiving ABO-compatible grafts. Both ABO major- and minor-mismatched graft recipients were at risk. The increased mortality rate was not due to an increase in graft failure or acute GVHD; rather, patients died of multiple-organ failure and sepsis, con-

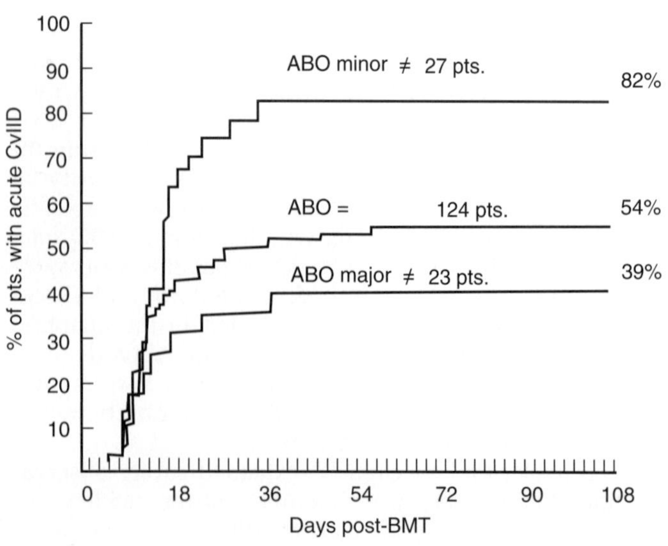

FIGURE 12-16. Occurence of acute GVHD in patients stratified according to donor-recipient ABO compatibility. Recipients of ABO minor-mismatched grafts show a significantly ($P = 0.01$) higher incidence of acute GVHD compared with recipients of ABO-matched and ABO major-mismatched grafts. (From Benjamin RJ, McGurk S, Ralston MS, Churchill WH, Antin JH: ABO incompatibility as an adverse risk factor for survival after allogeneic bone marrow transplantation. Transfusion 1999;39:179–187.)

sistent with regimen-related toxicity. This effect was not seen in a larger group of 112 chronic myelogenous leukemia patients undergoing similar treatment.

In the earlier study by Stussi and associates,[119] the authors found that survival was significantly dependent on ABO-compatibility (P = 0.004). In particular, patients with bidirectional ABO-incompatibility had an excess mortality rate (RR, 7.6; 95% CI, 2.5–23.2; P = 0.0004). They suggested that the role of ABO incompatibility in allogeneic stem cell transplantation should be reevaluated in larger trials. In their subsequent report, they performed a multivariate analysis adjusted for potential confounders and found that survival was significantly associated with ABO incompatibility (P = 0.006).[120] Compared with ABO-identical transplants, bidirectional ABO incompatibility increased the risk of mortality significantly (RR, 2.8; 95% CI 1.5–5.1; P = 0.009), whereas survival rates for patients with minor or major ABO-incompatible transplants were not significantly different from one another.

Similar data were reported by Worel and colleagues[121a] who evaluated 40 patients transplanted after nonmyeloablative conditioning. Eleven patients received a minor or bidirectional ABO-mismatched graft, and eight received a major ABO-mismatched graft. Significantly more patients with ABO mismatched grafts showed transplant-associated complications and died as a result of transplant-related causes.

In contrast, a number of other studies did not find improved relapse-free survival associated with ABO-compatible-vs.-incompatible transplants.[37,54,111,122-125] In particular, Mielcarek and coworkers[111,126] analyzed outcomes of 921 patients with hematologic malignancies transplanted between 1983 and 1998 from HLA-identical–related donors after myeloablative conditioning. In this relatively homogeneous patient population, presence of minor, major, or bidirectional ABO incompatibilities did not affect outcome, and mismatching was not associated with decreased relapse rates or improved survival.

Badros and colleagues[127] performed a retrospective analysis of the effects of ABO incompatibility among multiple myeloma patients who received a nonmyeloablative conditioning regimen. They found that patients with ABO-mismatched transplants had problems with engraftment, including graft rejection, PRCA, and persistence of mixed-lineage chimerism. They suggested that a prospective study to evaluate the effects of ABO mismatch on engraftment in the nonmyeloablative setting was needed.

AUTOIMMUNE HEMOLYTIC ANEMIA AFTER HEMATOPOIETIC STEM CELL TRANSPLANTATION

Another cause of hemolysis after marrow transplantation is autoimmune hemolytic anemia (AIHA). Hemolysis is thought to be due to antibodies produced by the donor's immune system against antigens on red cells of donor origin, thereby qualifying these episodes of hemolytic anemia as AIHA. The source of the autoantibodies has not been documented definitively by immunoglobulin allotyping, however.

Klumpp and associates[128] reported on a patient who developed AIHA 19 months after BMT for chronic myelogenous leukemia using her HLA-identical, ABO-identical brother as the donor. After a rather uneventful clinical course for 18 months, the patient experienced a drop in hematocrit from 30–35% to 21% associated with reticulocytosis (7.8%), mildly elevated serum bilirubin and LDH, and decreased serum haptoglobin. A DAT was positive, and a warm-reacting panspecific IgG and a cold-reacting IgM antibody were demonstrated. The patient also developed leukopenia and thrombocytopenia, and an assay for neutrophil antibody was positive, but platelet antibody could not be demonstrated. Numerous tests for chimerism using chromosome analysis, Southern blot hybridization using a *bcr* probe, and restriction fragment length polymorphism revealed no evidence of residual recipient hematopoiesis or lymphopoiesis. Accordingly, the antibodies were thought to arise as a result of a donor-antidonor reaction.

Bashey and coworkers[129] reported on a 17-year-old male who was transplanted with marrow from his HLA-identical brother; the patient and donor were both group O with Rh phenotype CDce and probable Rh genotype R_1r. After day 170, he developed pancytopenia with hemoglobin at 6.6 g/dL, platelets at 55,000/μL, and WBC count at 1000/μL. Hemolysis was suggested by elevated reticulocyte count (11%), elevated total serum bilirubin (30 μmol/L), and erythroid hyperplasia of the marrow. The DAT was strongly reactive using anti-IgG and anti-C3d sera. The patient's serum contained antibody reacting weakly by lysis and agglutination of papain-treated test cells, and by the IAT using anti-IgG antiglobulin serum. The red cell eluate was strongly reactive in the IAT, and autoantibodies with various specificities within the Rh system were demonstrated in the serum and eluate, including anti-C, D, c, e, and "anti-Rh" (reactive with all cells except Rh-null cells). Granulocyte and platelet antibodies were also present. Efforts to detect residual recipient cells produced negative results using DNA hybridization techniques that are sufficiently sensitive to detect the presence of chimerism when the minority population of cells is present at levels of 1%–5%. Therefore, although production of antibody by a small residual recipient population could not be completely excluded, the authors concluded that that the findings more likely indicated an autoimmune reaction of donor origin to blood cells and their precursors that are also of donor origin. Even a very small percentage of residual host cells can produce readily detectable antibodies, however (see pages 489–490).

Therapy in this case was innovative and produced interesting results. The various components of the pancytopenia showed different responses to therapy in that the hemolysis and the thrombocytopenia responded well to immunosuppressive treatment initially, but the neutropenia did not. Splenectomy produced only a transient rise in neutrophil counts, but total lymphoid irradiation produced a fall in neutrophil antibody levels, with a corresponding amelioration of the neutropenia.

Sokal and colleagues[130] reported the case of an 8-year-old boy with Fanconi's anemia who received a BMT from an unrelated donor. The patient's blood group was O, ccDEe, and the donor's was AB, ccddee. Sustained engraftment was achieved, but the patient developed grade III GVHD, a virus-associated hemophagocytic syndrome, and immune hemolytic anemia. The onset of the immune hemolysis was 6 months after transplantation. The DAT was positive, broadly reactive RBC antibodies were found in the eluate, and anti-c was found in the serum. The authors suggested that the antibodies were probably due to an autoimmune reaction of the graft against its own products, but they recognized that they could not prove the exact origin of the antibodies because both donor and recipient shared the c antigen.

Sokol and associates,[17] in another report, described a 37-year-old male with multiple myeloma who received a BMT from an HLA-matched unrelated donor 8 months after diagnosis. Seven months later, the patient developed warm antibody AIHA (WAIHA), which required treatment with prednisolone and blood transfusions.

Drobyski and coworkers[131] reported on seven adult patients who developed AIHA from a total of 236 patients who received T-cell–depleted marrow grafts (Table 12-9 A,B,C). The onset of AIHA was at a median

TABLE 12-9 AUTOIMMUNE HEMOLYTIC ANEMIA AFTER HEMATOPOIETIC CELL TRANSPLANTATION

A. Treatment of Autoimmune Hemolytic Anemia and Clinical Outcome

UPN	Treatment	Clinical Response	Follow-up after Diagnosis of AIHA (Months)	Clinical Outcome
070	Steroids	NR	2	Death due to candidal sepsis
123	Steroids/immunoglobulins/EPO	CR	57	Off therapy for 3 years
154	Steroids	NR		
	Steroids/splenectomy	NR		
	Steroids/azathioprine	NR	84	Off therapy for 4 years
	Steroids/accessory splenectomy	NR		
	Steroids/cyclosporine	NR		
	Steroids/EPO	CR		
178	Steroids	NR	0.7	Death due to Gram neg. sepsis
295	Steroids/EPO	PR	5	Death due to sepsis, ARDS
	Steroids/splenectomy/EPO	PR		
419	Steroids/immunoglobulin/EPO	PR	41	On low-dose steroids
	Steroids/splenectomy	PR		
434	Steroids Immunoglobulin Prosorba column EPO ATG Danazol/vincristine Plasmapheresis	PR	9	Death due to DIC secondary to AIHA
	Steroids/ATG/cyclophosphamide	PR		

ARDS = acute respiratory distress syndrome; ATG = antithymocyte globulin, DIC = disseminated intravascular coagulation; EPO = erythropoietin; NR = no response; CR = complete response; PR = partial response

B. Clinical Characteristics at Time of Diagnosis of AIHA

UPN	Age/Sex	Disease	Type of Treatment	Onset of AIHA (Months Post-BMT)	History of GVHD (Acute/Chronic)	Concurrent Illness(es)	Immunosuppressive Medications
070	36/M	CML,AP	RM	21	II/extensive	CMV retinitis	Prednisone
123	19/M	Myelodysplasia	RPM	25	I/extensive	Atypical mycobacterial infection	Prednisone, azathioprine
154	18/F	AML, 1 CR	RM	12	II/none	Transverse myelitis, autoimmune thyroiditis, CMV infection	Prednisone
178	46/F	ALL, 1 REL	RM	8	II/none	*Pseudomonas* sepsis	Prednisone
295	21/M	AML, 1 REL	RPM	10	I/limited	None	Prednisone
419	20/M	CML.AP	RPM	7	II/limited	None	Prednisone, cyclosporine
434	27/F	CML.AP	UNR	10	I/limited	None	Cyclosporine

1 CR = first complete remission; 1 REL = first relapse; AP = accelerated phase; RM = related match; RPM = related partial match; UNR = unrelated.

TABLE 12-9. AUTOIMMUNE HEMOLYTIC ANEMIA AFTER HEMATOPOIETIC CELL TRANSPLANTATION, *continued*

C. Laboratory Data at Time of Diagnosis of AIHA

UPN	Hematocrit (%)	DAT			Serum Antibodies
		Polyspecific	IgG	C3	
70	20	4+	3+	3+	Warm autoantibody, allo anti-C
123	15	3+	3+	3+	Warm autoantibody
154	17	4+	4+	0+	Warm autoantibody
178	25	2+	2+	0+	Warm autoantibody, allo anti-E
295	22	3+	4+	3+	Warm autoantibody
419	13	3+	3+	3+	Warm autoantibody
434	28	4+	0+	4+	Cold autoantibody, (anti-I), allo anti-E

From Drobyski WR, Potluri J, Sauer D, Gottschall JL: Autoimmune hemolytic anemia following T cell-depleted allogeneic bone marrow transplantation. Bone Marrow Transplant 1996;17:1093–1099.

of 10 months after transplantation (range 7–25 months) and occurred in 5% of all patients who survived at least 6 months. Six patients had a warm reacting autoantibody, while one patient had a cold-reacting antibody.

In the series reported by Chen and colleagues,[132] nine of 293 patients (3.1%) developed AIHA after marrow transplantation. (Tables 12-10 and 12-11). Three of the nine patients had matched unrelated donors, while the other six had matched sibling donors; some of the marrow products were T-cell depleted. Four patients developed AIHA with cold antibodies, whereas five developed AIHA with warm antibodies. Cold-antibody AIHA had an earlier onset (beginning from 2 to 8 months after transplantation), whereas AIHA associated with warm antibodies developed 6 to 18 months after transplantation. In both series, hemolysis was resistant to treatment and overall prognosis was poor, although no patients died as a direct result of hemolysis but rather from associated problems such as sepsis and GVHD.

Wennerberg and associates[133] reported on a patient who was transplanted with a minor ABO-incompatible marrow. By day 180 after transplantation, her red cell antigen phenotype was essentially donor type, with a conversion from her pretransplant RBC phenotype of A_1, Cde/Cde to that of the donor, which was O, cde/cde. Two years after transplantation, a positive DAT was noted, and shortly thereafter the patient developed WAIHA that required transfusion with group O, Rh-negative RBCs. No specificity of the antibody was noted after autologous and differential allogeneic adsorptions. At that time, RBC mixed chimerism was present, with both group O, Rh-negative and A_1, Rh-positive red cells demonstrable. She was treated with immunosuppressive therapy consisting of corticosteroids, azathioprine, and cyclosporine; she was also treated with intravenous immunoglobulin (IVIG). Mixed-erythrocyte chimerism persisted, and a compensated WAIHA continued for about 1 year but then worsened as immunosuppression was tapered. Shortly thereafter, after differential alloadsorptions to remove the nonspecific red cell autoantibody, anti-S and anti-Fy^b were detected in her serum. One year later, a mimicking anti-C was also demonstrated. She remained on immunosuppressive therapy and underwent splenectomy but continued to have a partially compensated hemolytic anemia. The authors made the interesting observation that RBC antigens that were present on recipient RBCs but absent on donor RBCs

TABLE 12-10. RESULTS OF SEROLOGICAL INVESTIGATION OF NINE PATIENTS WITH AIHA AFTER TRANSPLANTATION

Case	DAT		Antibody Specificity		Blood Group	
	IgG	C3d	Serum	Eluate	Donor	Recipient
1	+	+	NS + anti-e	Nonspecific	B+	A+
2	+	+	Nonspecific	Nonspecific	O+	O+
3	+	+	NS + anti-D	anti-D, E + NS	A+	A+
4	+	+	NS + anti-C, c, e	anti-D, e	O+	O+
5	+	+	Nonspecific	Nonspecific	O+	A+
6	–	+	anti-I	Negative	O+	A+
7	–	+	Nonspecific	ND	O+	O+
8	–	–	anti-Pr	Negative	A–	O–
9	–	+	anti-Pr	Negative	AB+	AB+

Cases 1–5 were warm type and detected at 37°C. Cases 6–9 were cold type and detected by saline methods at 20°C. Patients 2 and 5 also had an allo anti-E (i.e., donor is E-neg). All Rh specificities were enhanced by papainized cells. Patient 6 was lytic at 20°C in saline; patient 7 lysed papainized cells at 20°C; patients 8 and 9 showed no lysis.
ND = not done; NS = nonspecific.
From Chen FE, Owen I, Savage D, et al: Late onset haemolysis and red cell autoimmunisation after allogeneic bone marrow transplant. Bone Marrow Transplant 1996;19:491–495.

TABLE 12-11. CLINICAL COURSE OF THE PATIENTS

		Clinical Association					
Case	**RCAI Type**	**CMV**	**GVHD**	**Relapse**	**Treatment**	**Clinical Outcome**	**Peak Bilirubin (mmol/L)**
1	Warm	+	–	–	Prednisolone Immunoglobulin	Hemolysis resolved Alive and well	27
2	Warm	+	–	+	Prednisolone Immunoglobulin	Resistant hemolysis CML relapse Died from pneumonitis	623
3	Warm	–	–	+	Prednisolone Splenectomy	Hemolysis resolved after splenectomy Alive and well	42
4	Warm	–	–	–	Immunoglobulin Azathioprine Splenectomy Total lymphoid irradiation	Hemolysis eventually resolved but required further donor marrow infusion Alive with no hemolysis	30
5	Warm	–	–	+	Prednisolone Immunoglobulin Splenectomy Vincristine	Also developed ITP Died from multiple thromboembolism	427
6	Cold	–	+	–	Prednisolone Immunoglobulin	Resistant hemolysis Died with GVHD and sepsis	694
7	Cold	+	–	–	Nil	Relapsed with lymphoid blast crisis Subsequently reinduced	27
8	Cold	–	+	–	Nil	No overt hemolysis Resolved	20
9	Cold	+	+	+	Prednisolone	Hemolysis resolved but died from GVHD liver	70

Note that in patient 5, recipient cells were detected 2 months after hemolysis developed but no relapse of CML. In cases 1, 2, and 3, recipient cells were detected 12.2 and 9 months, respectively, before hemolysis. In patient 9, there was transient cytogenetic relapse at the time of hemolysis, both of which resolved after the cyclosporine dose was reduced.

From Chen FE, Owen I, Savage D, et al: Late onset haemolysis and red cell autoimmunisation after allogeneic bone marrow transplant. Bone Marrow Transplant 1996;19:491–495.

included D, C, S, and Fy^b. If the immune-stimulating event was the presence of the minor subpopulation of recipient RBCs, it is interesting that no anti-D or clearly distinguishable alloanti-C was detected, especially as these are considered more immunogenic than are S and Fy^b. The alternative explanation was that the immunizing event was transfusions with group O, Rh-negative RBC, most of which would likely be of the Rh phenotype rr (cde/cde) and would thus not carry the D or C antigens. Whether the RBC autoantibody was produced by cells of the immune system of the donor or recipient was not determined.

Pratt and Kinsey[134] described an 8-year-old boy who developed AIHA 6 months after an allogeneic bone marrow transplant. He required 4 years of immunosuppressive therapy before remission of hemolysis.

Graze and Gale[135] reported evidences of autoimmunity in six patients with chronic GVHD after BMT, including the presence of rheumatoid factor and a positive antinuclear antibody (ANA) test. Four patients developed a positive DAT and clinical evidence of hemolysis, and the authors suggested that AIHA might occasionally complicate chronic GVHD. Insufficient data were provided to document AIHA, however.

Godder and coworkers[136] reported that 18 of 40 patients (45%) developed de novo chronic graft-vs.-host disease (cGVHD) after partially mismatched-related donor BMT. Of those developing cGVHD, five patients (28%) presented with hemolytic anemia on days 112–272 after transplantation (median = 168 days). Four of these patients also had thrombocytopenia (median platelet count = 50,000/μL). Patients with hemolytic anemia were HLA-mismatched with their donors for one antigen (n = 1), two antigens (n = 3), and three antigens (n = 2) and were all sex mismatched. Signs of hemolysis were present, but few serologic findings were reported. Two patients had a positive DAT, and one of these had a positive IAT. In spite of limited evidence of an immune-mediated process, all patients responded to intensive immunosuppressive therapy.

Tamura and colleagues[137] reported a case of cold agglutinin syndrome (CAS) after allogeneic BMT in a 36-year-old male (Fig. 12-17). The cold agglutinin titers of the recipient and the donor before transplant were less than 4 and 4, respectively. Three weeks after transplantation, acrocyanosis developed, and there was evidence of hemolysis with a decrease in hemoglobin level to 5.3 g/dL, undetectable serum haptoglobin, and an increase in both serum indirect bilirubin and

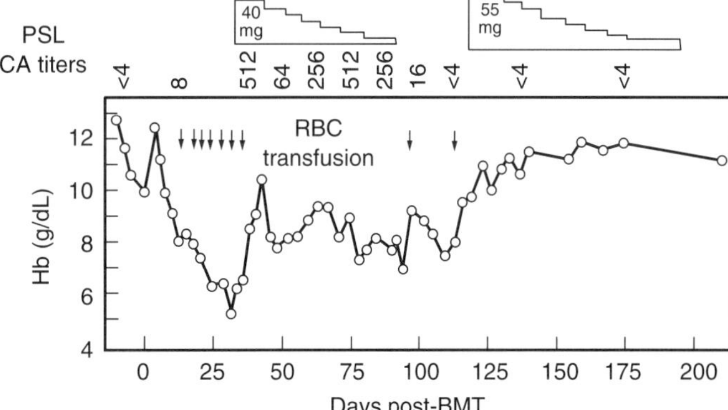

FIGURE 12-17. Clinical course. PSL, predonisolone; CA titers, cold agglutinin titers. (From Tamura T, Kanamori H, Yamazaki E, et al: Cold agglutinin disease following allogeneic bone marrow transplantation. Bone Marrow Transplant 1994;13:321–323.)

LDH. The DAT was positive with anti-C3, the cold agglutinin titer was elevated to 512, and the specificity of the antibody was anti-Pr. Engraftment of donor marrow cells was proven by day 22 using cytogenetic analysis. The patient avoided exposure to cold and was treated with prednisolone. Signs of hemolysis gradually subsided, and on discharge on day 174, the cold agglutinin titer had decreased to less than 4.

Au and associates[138] reported on a 22-year-old woman with CML in second chronic phase who underwent a marrow transplant from a matched unrelated donor. Eleven months after transplantation, she developed an abrupt, painful acrocyanosis up to the thighs and elbows. The peripheral blood film showed extensive RBC agglutination. A cold agglutinin was present to a titer of 8192 at 4°C, with a thermal amplitude up to 30°C. She was treated with high-dose prednisolone, cyclophosphamide, intravenous immunoglobulin, and cessation of cyclosporine. Plasmapheresis was unsuccessful because of extensive extracorporeal agglutination, and exchange transfusion did not reduce the cold agglutinin titer. The patient finally died of infection.

Azuma and coworkers[139] described a 10-year-old male with severe aplastic anemia who was treated with a marrow transplant from his HLA-matched sister. On post-BMT day 67, a diagnosis of CAS was made, and he was treated with plasmapheresis on an emergency basis. Corticosteroids after plasmapheresis had a transient effect. At a second episode of hemolysis 6 months after BMT, immunosuppressive therapy with cyclophosphamide plus corticosteroid was administered successfully without negative effect on engraftment.

Cases of AIHA have been reported after allogeneic marrow transplantation for aplastic anemia,[140] autologous marrow transplantation for recurrent Hodgkin's disease,[141] a mismatched-related allogeneic PBSC transplant for chronic myelogenous leukemia,[142] a partially matched cord blood stem cell transplant for osteopetrosis,[143] and T-cell–depleted haploidentical transplantation for severe combined immunodeficiency.[144] Diagnoses have included Evans's syndrome[141,142,145] and fatal autoimmune pancytopenia.[140]

Dovat and colleagues[145] reported the development of Evans's syndrome after umbilical cord stem cell transplantation of an 8-month-old male with X-linked lymphoproliferative disease. He received multiple courses of IVIG, anti-Rh D immunoglobulin, a pulse of high-dose corticosteroids, and cyclosporine with some improvement of the hemolytic anemia, but no improvement of the thrombocytopenia. Addition of vincristine resulted in long-term resolution of thrombocytopenia and anemia.

Some cases that have been reported as autoimmune hemolysis[11,40] are cases of passenger lymphocyte syndrome, for which the term "autoimmune" is used inappropriately according to the definitions provided earlier in this chapter.

MIXED CHIMERISM AND ITS SIGNIFICANCE IN THE CAUSATION OF RED CELL ANTIBODIES AND IMMUNE HEMOLYSIS AFTER HEMATOPOIETIC CELL TRANSPLANTATION

In Greek mythology, Chimera was a monster with a lion's head, a goat's body, and a serpent's tail (Fig. 2-18). In medical terminology, the term *chimera* is used to designate an organism whose body contains cell populations derived from different individuals of the same or different species, occurring spontaneously or produced artificially.[146] Thus, all successful allogeneic transplants result in the creation of chimeras. When it was recognized that some allogeneic BMT recipients not only had hematopoietic cells of the donor but also retained some of their own hematopoietic system,[147,148] there was a need for a term to distinguish these chimeras from those with complete donor hematopoiesis. The terms generally used are *mixed hematopoietic chimera* or *mixed chimera*, in contrast to *complete chimera* or *donor chimera*.[146,149-151]

Mixed chimerism is detected with increasing frequency as methods for detecting a minor population of cells become more sensitive. Techniques that have been used include cytogenetic markers, red blood cell antigens, immunoglobulin allotypes, HLA typing, persisting RBC antibodies, fluorescence in situ hyrbi-

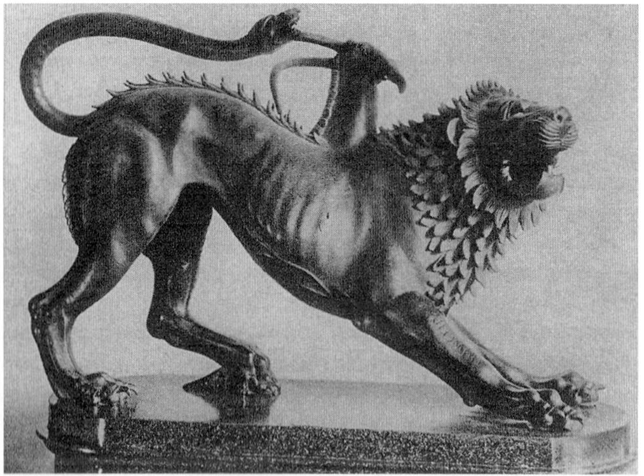

FIGURE 12-18. Chimera, the Greek mythologic creature that, according to one description, was a lion in front, a goat in the middle, and a snake in the back. She devoured many men and animals and was ultimately killed by consent of the gods. In medical science, the term *chimera* is used to designate an organism whose body contains cell populations derived from different individuals of the same or different species, occurring spontaneously or produced artificially. (From Petz LD: Immunohematologic problems unique to bone marrow transplantation. In Garratty G (ed): Red Cell Antigens and Antibodies. Arlington, VA: American Association of Blood Banks, 1986:195–229.)

dization, fluorescence-activated cell sorting (FACS) analysis, in situ hybridization of Y-chromosome,[152] and numerous molecular biology techniques.[150,153] Documenting and characterizing donor and recipient cell populations in the patient after allogeneic BMT was used originally to document engraftment of the donor marrow, but such studies also have the potential to do the following:

1. Better our understanding of mechanisms of graft rejection and marrow failure.
2. Detect the recurrence of leukemia and evaluate whether recurrent leukemia occurs in donor or recipient cells.
3. Determine the clinical significance of mixed chimerism.
4. Provide insights regarding the mechanisms of tolerance and GVHD.
5. Provide information concerning the kinetics of engraftment in various disease states or after different preparative regimens.
6. Determine the origin of cells of the marrow microenvironment.

RED CELL ALLOANTIBODIES OTHER THAN ABO PRODUCED BY ENGRAFTED CELLS OF THE DONOR'S IMMUNE SYSTEM OR BY RESIDUAL CELLS OF THE PATIENT'S IMMUNE SYSTEM AFTER HEMATOPOIETIC STEM CELL TRANSPLANTATION

It is important to appreciate that either complete chimerism or mixed chimerism can exist after hematopoietic stem cell transplantation. Thus, RBC antibodies can be derived from cells of the immune system of the donor, the recipient, or both (Table 12-12). Donor-derived alloantibodies produced as part of the passenger lymphocyte syndrome are thought to be produced by lymphocytes that are transfused with the donor marrow product, proliferate, and produce antibody. The syndrome resolves after the passenger lymphocytes (which are not engrafted) reach the ends of their life spans. Hemolysis has its onset within the first few weeks after BMT and is transient. In contrast, other patients develop donor-derived alloantibodies that are produced by the immune system of the donor long after transplantation, presumably by engrafted cells of the donor's immune system. In still other patients, residual cells of the transplant recipient's immune system produce RBC antibodies.

Alloantibodies Produced by Engrafted Cells of the Donor's Immune System

In seven of the 12 patients reported by Ting and associates[29] who developed non-ABO red cell alloantibodies after BMT, the antibodies were first detected after days 45–330 and seemingly were produced by cells of the engrafted marrow.

Esteve and coworkers[154] reported a 16-year-old boy who was group O, Rh-positive (phenotype ccDEe) and was transplanted with marrow from a group A, Rh-negative donor who had had four pregnancies and whose serum contained anti-D and anti-C. Seven months after transplantation, anti-D was detected in his serum, which was well characterized as being of IgM immunoglobulin class. The antibody persisted for about ten months but disappeared one month after cyclosporine was discontinued as GVHD prophylaxis. The patient did not develop anti-C, possibly due to the lack of an immunizing stimulus, because the patient's RBC did not bear the C antigen. The authors commented that the long follow-up period without appearance of an IgG component suggests a defect in the immunoglobulin isotype switching mechanism.

Heim and colleagues[155] reported a 22-year-old man, blood group O, Rh positive (R_2r), who received bone marrow from his blood group A_1, Rh-negative (rr)

TABLE 12-12. SOURCE OF NON-ABO RED CELL ALLOANTIBODIES FOLLOWING HEMATOPOIETIC CELL TRANSPLANTATION

Donor-Derived
Passenger lymphocyte syndrome
Alloantibodies produced by engrafted cells of the donor's immune system
Recipient-Derived
Alloantibodies produced by residual cells of the patient's immune system

HLA-identical sister for treatment of acute lymphocytic leukemia. Three months after transplantation, the patient was found to be a mixed chimera, with 0.5% of the RBCs still of the host's type. Four months after transplantation, three different Rh antibodies (anti-D, -E, and -G) were detected. It was evident that the engrafted marrow had produced these antibodies, and because the patient had received only Rh-negative RBC transfusions, it appears that he had become immunized to his original red cells.

Lasky and associates[54] reported four Rh-positive patients who received bone marrow from Rh-negative donors. Two developed anti-Rh antibodies 12 and 15 months after BMT, respectively. Both patients received at least four Rh-positive platelet concentrates within the first months after BMT.

Niethammer and coworkers[156] reported a 9-month-old boy who received a BMT from his mother for severe combined immunodeficiency (SCID). The mother was group O, Rh negative (ccdee), and the patient was group O, Rh positive (CcDee). As is not uncommon after BMT for SCID, incomplete chimerism developed, with 100% of the red cells being of the patient's type, while chromosome analysis revealed 4% XX chromosomes and HLA typing revealed that the circulating lymphocytes had the HLA type of the mother. Four months after transplantation, serologic tests revealed anti-D and anti-C and also a weakly positive reaction by indirect antiglobulin test against the mother's RBCs and all other Rh-negative RBCs tested. Hemolysis developed as manifested by erythroid hyperplasia of the marrow and reticulocytosis without an increase in hematocrit. The anti-D and anti-C were most likely produced by the immune system of the donor against antigens on the residual RBCs of the patient. It is difficult to determine what role, if any, the weak, broadly reactive RBC antibody played in the patient's clinical course.

Wennerberg and colleagues[133] reported a patient who became a mixed chimera after allogeneic BMT from an unrelated donor. The patient developed AIHA 3 years after BMT and, 1 year later, alloantibodies of donor origin directed against red cell antigens of the recipient (anti-S and anti-Fy^b).

The distinction between antibody production by passenger lymphocytes that do not engraft and antibody production by engrafted cells of the donor marrow seems clear in many cases on the basis of the time of onset of the antibody and the duration of its production. In some instances, however, the distinction is uncertain, and perhaps both can occur in some patients. For example, Hows and associates[6] described patients who developed Rh antibodies within the first three weeks after BMT that persisted for up to one year.

Ting and coworkers[29] reported on three patients in whom alloantibodies were first observed between days 12 and 18 after transplanation, but neither the donor nor the recipient had the corresponding antigen, so the antibodies could have been donor-derived antibodies produced by passenger lymphocytes or recipient-derived antibodies produced by residual cells of the patient's immune system. Immunization in these cases was probably related to red cell transfusion received after BMT. The source of the antibody was also uncertain in one patient who had a panagglutinin between days 13 and 32.

Alloantibodies Produced by Residual Cells of the Patient's Immune System

Girelli and colleagues[157] reported a group O, Rh-negative female who received an allogeneic bone marrow transplant from an HLA-compatible group O, Rh-positive donor (CcDee). No unexpected antibodies were found in the patient's serum before BMT, and the patient had never been transfused, although she had had two pregnancies with Rh-positive fetuses. On day 5 after transplanation, the RBC phenotype of the patient was CcDee due to persistence of RBCs transfused in the donor marrow product. From day 8 to day 9, the hemoglobin dropped from 9.3 g/dL to 6.1 g/dL, and laboratory evidences of hemolysis were present. On day 11, anti-D was detected in the patient's serum, the red cell phenotype was now ccddee, and the DAT was negative. She was transfused with two units of Rh-negative blood, and signs of hemolysis gradually subsided, only to return on day 21 coincident with evidences of erythropoiesis by the newly engrafted marrow. The RBC phenotype was now CcDee, and anti-D could be eluted from the patient's RBC. Hemolysis gradually subsided, and the anti-D became undetectable in the serum on day 35 but was still detectable on the RBCs until day 46. In this case, the anti-D could only have been produced by the patient's residual immune system. The antibody apparently caused hemolysis of the Rh-positive RBCs that were transfused with the donor marrow product; later, it caused transient hemolysis of Rh-positive RBCs produced by the newly engrafted marrow until the antibody disappeared. The second episode of hemolysis is analogous to that found after some cases of major ABO blood group incompatibility.

Moore and associates[158] reported a 17-year-old boy who was transplanted with marrow from his HLA-identical brother. Both recipient and donor were blood type O, Rh positive. The patient's serum contained anti-Lu^a on day 23, anti-E on day 28, and anti-K on day 31 after transplantation. The antibodies became weaker beginning on day 40, and by day 48, all three were undetectable. The patient had been transfused with 13 units of RBC between 2 and 8 months before transplantation. Retrospectively, the donors of those units were typed for RBC antigens. One was positive for K, and four were positive for E. None was positive for Lu^a. The patient was also exposed to the E and K antigens on transfused RBCs on days 11 and 13 after transplantation, respectively. Cytogenetic studies indicated complete marrow engraftment, and RBC phenotyping

6 months after BMT indicated that the RBCs of donor origin were negative for K, E, and Lu^a antigens. The authors suggested that the antibodies had been produced by residual plasma cells of the patient, possibly as a result of cooperation between elements of residual recipient lymphoid cells and cells of the engrafting donor marrow. Gm allotyping did not help in determining the origin of the antibodies, as both the marrow donor and the recipient had the same allotypes.

In some instances, residual cells of the patient's immune system are presumably responsible for the production of antibodies against antigens on donor RBCs, even though very sensitive techniques fail to detect the residual host cells. In the series reported by Petz and coworkers,[151] RBC antibodies persisting more than 6 months after BMT served as the basis of diagnosing mixed chimerism in seven patients. In two of these patients, immunoglobulin allotyping also indicated mixed chimerism, whereas in the other five patients, immunoglobulin allotyping either was uninformative or was not performed. Anti-A or anti-B antibodies were present in six patients and caused a positive DAT without hemolysis in two patients, a positive DAT with transient hemolytic anemia in one patient, and a delayed onset of erythropoiesis in three patients.

Similar findings were reported by Izumi and colleagues,[159] who described a 26-year-old male who had preexisting alloantibodies to E and c. He received a BMT from a donor whose Rh phenotype was E+, c+. From about one month after the transplant onward, he showed mild hemolysis due to the antibodies. The patient-derived antibodies remained detectable by both DAT and IAT even 20 months after BMT, even though immunomagnetically isolated peripheral circulating B cells were 100% of donor origin. The patient received prednisolone from day 221 onward, and thereafter, the signs of hemolysis disappeared.

von Tol and associates[160] reported that IgG of recipient origin persisted in 15 of 18 informative recipients (83%) until last follow-up (i.e., for several years after BMT) despite the fact that the circulating B cells appeared to be entirely of donor origin at that time. Other investigators have reported similar results.[161,162] Thus, even in this era of sensitive molecular technology, persistence of RBC antibodies and immunoglobulin allotyping, when applicable, appear to be among the most sensitive techniques for indicating the existence of residual cells of the recipient's immune system.

Incidence of Red Cell Antibody Formation after Hematopoietic Cell Transplantation

The incidence of RBC antibody production after BMT appears to be low. Abou-Elella[163] reported that only 4 of 193 patients (2.1%) developed RBC alloantibodies from the date of admission for BMT until the date of hospital discharge (48.5 ± 14.9 days for autologous and 58.7 ± 25.9 days for allogeneic transplants). Three patients each had one RBC antibody, and one patient had two antibodies. The specificities were anti-E (two antibodies), anti-Jk^a, anti-M, and anti-Lu14. The RBC antibody formation rate was 0.1% per unit of RBCs transfused. The authors did not comment on the source of the antibodies. Bar and coworkers[53] reported that none of 230 patients developed unexpected antibodies after BMT.

OTHER IMMUNOHEMATOLOGIC ABNORMALITIES AFTER HEMATOPOIETIC STEM CELL TRANSPLANTATION

Evidences of Autoimmunity after Hematopoietic Stem Cell Transplantation

Immune system imbalance can occur during the reestablishment of immune function and the hematopoietic system after hematopoietic stem cell allografting. The development of humoral and/or cell-mediated immunity directed against smooth muscle, epidermis, mitochondria, cell nuclei, cardiolipin, liver-kidney microsomes, human leukocyte antigens, thyroid antigens, cytoskeletal proteins, and other cellular components has been reported.[9,164-166]

Rouquette-Gally and colleagues[167] studied 53 long-term survivors of allogeneic BMT, 40 of whom had chronic GVHD. They found a high frequency of various autoantibodies, especially considering the young age of their patients (mean age = 20.3 years; range, 4–33). The prevalence of antinuclear, anti–smooth muscle, antimitochondria, anti–liver-kidney microsome, and anti-epidermal antibodies was 62.2%, 49%, 11.3%, 5.6%, and 11.3%, respectively. The screening for anti-DNA, anti-extractable nuclear antigen, anticentromere, and anti-salivary gland duct antibodies was negative. The presence or absence of acute GVHD made no difference in the frequency of autoantibodies. The authors pointed out that although there are clinical features of GVHD that mimic collagen vascular disease, the biological autoimmune profile of GVHD is different.

Immune Thrombocytopenia and Leukopenia after Hematopoietic Cell Transplantation

There are numerous reports of immune cytopenias after hematopoietic stem cell transplantation, and in some of these, the origin (i.e., donor or recipient) of the antibodies has been determined or reasonably inferred. As defined at the beginning of this chapter, antibodies of donor origin against antigens on donor cells, or antibodies of recipient origin against antigens on the recipient's cells, may be considered autoantibodies. In contrast, antibodies produced by cells of host origin against antigens on donor cells should be considered alloantibodies, as should antibodies of donor origin that react with antigens on the recipient's cells. One must keep in mind the difficulty in determining the origin of the antibodies, especially as many of the case reports were published before sensitive techniques were described for detecting the persistence of host cells after transplantation.

Autoimmune Thrombocytopenia

Minchinton and associates[168] described a patient who received an allogeneic BMT from a donor who had an IgM antibody that reacted with his own platelets. The patient had no platelet autoantibodies before grafting, but after transplantation, an IgM platelet antibody was found in the patient's serum that reacted with her circulating platelets and with platelets from the bone marrow donor. After BMT, the peripheral blood neutrophil count was more than 1×10^9/L by the 23rd day, but severe thrombocytopenia persisted until completion of a course of treatment with IVIG, which was started on day 87. It seems reasonable to infer that the donor's autoantibody-producing cells were engrafted by the patient, resulting in a true autoimmune thrombocytopenia (donor vs. donor).

Minchinton and Waters[169] subsequently studied 14 patients who received autologous buffy coat or bone marrow grafts and 32 patients who received allogeneic bone marrow grafts. There was a high incidence (52%) of antibodies to circulating platelets in the early postgraft period. The presence of postgraft antibodies did not predict the development of a cytopenia, however, evidently because of variable in vivo activity of the antibody and the ability of the engrafted bone marrow to compensate for antibody-mediated cell destruction.[170,171] Antibodies demonstrated after autografting were, by definition, autoantibodies. Antibodies in the allografted patients were shown, by immunoglobulin allotyping, to be of marrow donor type and on this basis were thought to be autoantibodies.[169]

Bierling and colleagues[172] described a patient who developed immune thrombocytopenia after allogeneic BMT. The patient's serum contained an IgG antibody that reacted with the patient's platelets (donor origin) and with both of the patient's HLA-identical siblings. The authors suggested that this was an autoimmune thrombocytopenia, apparently concluding that the platelet antibody was produced by engrafted donor cells and reacted with platelets of donor origin.

Benda and associates[173] reported on a patient who developed autoimmune thrombocytopenia after an allogeneic BMT from her HLA-identical sister. An IgG autoantibody was found that bound to the platelet glycoprotein IIb/IIIa, similar to reactions in patients with idiopathic autoimmune thrombocytopenia. In addition, the authors detected an autoantibody to HLA class I proteins.

Other investigators have also reported cases of autoimmune thrombocytopenia after BMT.[9,174-176]

Graft-vs.-Host Disease and Post-transplant Immune Thrombocytopenia

There have been reports that immune thrombocytopenia after BMT could be associated with GVHD. In this setting, autoantibodies rather than alloantibodies have been implicated.

First and coworkers[177] reviewed cases of isolated thrombocytopenia after BMT in 65 fully engrafted patients surviving at least 60 days after transplanation. Nine patients had transient thrombocytopenia with recovery by day 90, whereas 15 patients had chronic thrombocytopenia, in which a normal platelet count was not achieved at any time during the first 4 months after transplantation. The chronic syndrome carried a high mortality and had a high association with both severe (grades 3 to 4) acute GVHD and chronic GVHD. In most cases, bone marrow biopsies demonstrated adequate numbers of platelet precursors, suggesting peripheral platelet destruction or ineffective thrombopoiesis. Platelet antibodies were found in four of eight thrombocytopenic patients tested (one of two transient, three of six chronic). Six patients underwent platelet survival studies (two transient, four chronic), and all showed a markedly decreased platelet half-life (mean of 6 hours compared with normal platelet survival of 6.5 days).

Anasetti and colleagues[178] studied platelet and fibrinogen kinetics and antiplatelet antibodies in 20 patients between 60 and 649 days (median = 90 days) after transplantation (19 allogeneic transplants and one syngeneic transplant). Seventeen patients had isolated thrombocytopenia (<100,000/µL). Platelet survival studies indicated that the major mechanism for thrombocytopenia was increased platelet destruction. Platelet antibodies bound to the patients' platelets were present in five of the 12 patients studied. Patients with platelet antibodies had lower platelet counts and shorter platelet survivals than patients without platelet antibodies. Platelet-bound autoantibodies were present in five of six patients with grade II–IV acute or chronic GVHD but were not present in six patients free of GVHD. The authors concluded that persistent thrombocytopenia after BMT is most often secondary to increased platelet destruction mediated by multiple mechanisms and that platelet autoantibodies are found in patients with acute or chronic GVHD.

Alloimmune Thrombocytopenia—Recipient vs. Donor

Bierling and associates[179] described a patient who had mild, clinically asymptomatic immune thrombocytopenia after allogeneic BMT for CML. A number of studies suggested that all hematopoietic cells were of donor origin. These included cytogenetic studies and molecular analysis of peripheral blood cells, purified B- and T-lymphocyte subpopulations, and bone marrow colonies. Nevertheless, the authors identified anti-HPA-5b (anti-Br^a) of recipient origin that recognized donor platelets. The antibody remained detectable more than 3 years after BMT. Further studies using adsorption-elution techniques demonstrated a small amount of recipient RBCs, and the CML chimeric transcript was detected by the polymerase chain reaction until day 867 after transplantation, indicating persistent mixed chimerism of low level without hematologic relapse. Thus, this case of immune thrombocytopenia was clearly shown to be a result of a recipient-vs.-donor reaction rather than being an autoimmune thrombocytopenia.

Panzer and coworkers[180] described a patient who developed immune thrombocytopenia more than one year after successful allografting for CML. Serologically, the antibody was found to be directed against the donor platelet antigen Pl^{A1}. Determining the phenotypes of the platelets of the patient and his family indicated heterozygosity ($Pl^{A1/A2}$) in the parents and, accordingly, a 25% probability that the patient inherited both Pl^{A2} haplotypes. Further, residual cells of host origin were found in the patient's excised spleen. These findings suggested that this was a recipient-derived immune reaction against the donor's Pl^{A1} platelet antigen rather than an autoimmune reaction.

Szymanski and colleagues[181] also described a patient who had anti-HPA-5b before BMT. It persisted after BMT, indicating that the patient's antibody-producing cells had survived the severe conditioning regimen.

Immune Neutropenia

Immune neutropenia after BMT has been described by a number of investigators.[9,128,171,182,183] Antigranulocyte antibodies can occur in the post-transplant setting and, although often benign, can be the cause of otherwise unexplained neutropenia after autologous or allogeneic BMT.[171] Minchinton and Waters[169] reported that immunoglobulin allotyping on allografted patients indicated that the antibodies were of marrow donor type and were therefore autoantibodies.

Koeppler and Goldman[184] reported on a 32-year-old male who developed isolated neutropenia six months after allogeneic BMT for CML from his HLA-matched brother. The presence of granulocyte-specific IgM and IgG antibodies in the patient's serum indicated an immune-mediated basis for the neutropenia. The patient was in continuous complete remission, suggesting that the antibody was an autoantibody produced by the donor's immune cells. Immunoglobulin allotyping was not performed to document the source of the antibody-producing cells, however.

Stroncek and associates[185] described a 13-year-old girl with large granular lymphocytosis and chronic neutropenia who was treated with granulocyte transfusions before undergoing a transplant with bone marrow from a partially matched, unrelated donor. After the transplant, the patient remained neutropenic, and her serum contained a high-titer antibody against the neutrophil-specific antigen NB1 as well as additional neutrophil antibodies of uncertain specificity present in lower titer. Despite treatment with granulocyte-macrophage colony-stimulating factor, the patient remained neutropenic and died of polymicrobial sepsis and aspergillosis 38 days after transplantation. The authors suggested that the patient probably became alloimmunized as a result of granulocyte transfusions but also pointed out that patients with large granular lymphocytes have a high incidence of autoantibodies, including neutrophil antibodies. Neutrophils from the marrow donor expressed the NB1 antigen, but the authors were unable to phenotype the patient's neutrophils to determine whether the anti-NB1 was an autoantibody or an alloantibody. In contrast to the poor outcome in this case, Warkentin and coworkers[186] reported the successful engraftment (without delayed neutrophil recovery after transplantation) of an NA1-positive bone marrow in a patient with aplastic anemia who had anti-NA1.

Tosi and colleagues[187] described a 26-year-old male with chronic myelogenous leukemia who was the recipient of an HLA-compatible marrow from a matched unrelated donor. Cyclosporine and a short course of methotrexate were administered as GVHD prophylaxis. Good platelet engraftment was observed, but the WBC count remained extremely low, ranging from 0.2 to $0.4 \times 10^9/L$. On day 33 after transplantation, surface-bound neutrophil antibody was detected by immunofluorescence, although the patient's serum was negative when tested with random neutrophils. A repeat test 6 days later was still positive, although with decreased intensity. The granulocytopenia resolved without additional immunosuppressive therapy by day 42, at which time the test for neutrophil antibody was negative. The case represents an example of single-lineage antibody-mediated cytopenia, as neither RBCs nor platelets were affected and their engraftment occurred normally.

THE DIFFERENTIAL DIAGNOSIS OF HEMOLYSIS AFTER HEMATOPOIETIC STEM CELL TRANSPLANTATION

A note of caution is warranted concerning the diagnosis and management of immune hemolysis caused by ABO antibodies after BMT. Hemolysis occurring in the various characteristic clinical settings should quickly lead to a tentative diagnosis, which is then readily confirmed by simple serologic tests. The major pitfalls are that these hemolytic syndromes are rather unusual and often begin abruptly. Accordingly, their sudden and unexpected onset sometimes results in a delay in diagnosis, while more common problems—such as GVHD and veno-occlusive disease of the liver—are inappropriately considered as reasons for elevated bilirubin and anemia. The delay in instituting appropriate therapy to minimize hemolysis can result in unnecessary morbidity, particularly renal insufficiency (Table 12-13).

Minor ABO Blood Group Incompatibility

DIAGNOSIS OF PASSENGER LYMPHOCYTE SYNDROME

Clinical Setting. The diagnosis of passenger lymphocyte syndrome is usually not difficult. Indeed the diagnosis generally should be anticipated because of the characteristic clinical setting. That is, patients are in the early post-transplant period after a hematopoietic stem cell transplant in which there is a minor ABO blood group mismatch between donor and recipient. Additional risk factors are the use of cyclosporine without methotrexate for post-transplant GVHD prophylaxis, the use of stem cells obtained from peripheral blood, and a nonmyeloablative conditioning regimen. Hemolysis characteristically occurs between days 5 and 20 after transplantation. When the onset of hemolysis is delayed beyond several weeks after transplantation, it appears more likely that antibody is being produced by cells of the donor immune system that are engrafted or by residual cells of the patient's immune system. Also, because at least several days are required for proliferation of the transfused lymphocytes, hemolysis during the first few days after BMT is not caused by the passenger lymphocyte syndrome.

The passenger lymphocyte syndrome caused by antibodies of blood group systems other than ABO is rare after hematopoietic stem cell transplantation, although somewhat more common after solid organ transplantation (see page 502).

Laboratory Tests. The causative antibody is usually detectable in the patient's serum and in a RBC eluate throughout the period of time when hemolysis is occurring. One point that deserves emphasis, however, is that signs of hemolysis (e.g., a fall in hemoglobin and hematocrit, elevated bilirubin, and elevated LDH) may occur for a short time (from 1 day to as long as 3 days) before the responsible antibody becomes detectable (see pages 461 and 470). Accordingly, post-transplant follow-up of patients transplanted with a minor mismatched hematopoietic stem cell product should include both laboratory tests to detect hemolysis and serologic studies to detect RBC antibodies.

Antibody in the Donor Marrow Product. Lasky and associates[54] reported on 13 patients who received a marrow transplant from a donor with a minor ABO incompatibility. One patient was managed with exchange transfusion before BMT using RBCs of the donor's type to prevent hemolysis caused by isohemagglutinins in the marrow product. Five patients were managed by centrifuging the bone marrow to remove plasma and thus reduce the amount of antibody. Two of the seven patients who received uncentrifuged bone marrow experienced minimal hemolysis on the first day after transplantation (indirect bilirubin 0.9–1.1 mg/dL). One other patient who received centrifuged marrow developed hemolysis on the sixth post-transplant day, but the delayed onset of hemolysis in this case suggests that it was due to the passenger lymphocyte syndrome rather than to passive transfer of antibody.[1]

TABLE 12-13. THE DIFFERENTIAL DIAGNOSIS OF HEMOLYSIS FOLLOWING HEMATOPOIETIC STEM CELL TRANSPLANTATION

- Minor ABO blood group incompatibility
  - Passenger lymphocyte syndrome
  - Antibody in the donor marrow product
- Major ABO blood group incompatibility
  - Immediate hemolysis (lysis of RBCs in donor stem cell product)
  - Early post-transplant hemolysis (lysis of RBC in donor stem cell product caused by rebound of isohemagglutinins after transplantation in patients treated with plasma exchange prior to transplantation)
  - Delayed hemolysis (lysis of RBCs produced by the newly engrafted marrow caused by residual isohemagglutinins)
- Red cell alloantibodies of blood groups other than ABO
  - Alloantibodies produced by engrafted cells of the donor's immune system
  - Alloantibodies produced by residual cells of the patient's immune system
- Autoimmune hemolytic anemia
- Passive transfer of antibody
  - Plasma transfusion
  - Platelet transfusion
  - Intravenous immunoglobulin
  - Other causes of passive transfer of antibody; packed RBCs, intravenous anti-D, and antilymphocyte globulin
- Drug-induced hemolytic anemia
- Microangiopathic hemolytic anemia
- Miscellaneous additional causes of hemolysis following bone marrow transplantation
  - Infusion of cryopreserved stem cell products
  - Infusion of dimethylsulphoxide (DMSO) and free plasma hemoglobin
- *Clostridium perfringens* septicemia
- Hemolysis associated with hemodialysis

Major Blood Group Incompatibility

IMMEDIATE HEMOLYSIS

Hemolysis at the time of a marrow transplant can, of course, be expected unless the marrow product is depleted of RBCs and/or the serum antibody is removed from the patient by plasma exchange. Even with rather small volumes of residual RBCs, some signs of hemolysis can occur, but this does not result in serious morbidity.

DELAYED HEMOLYSIS

In patients who are treated with pretransplant plasma exchange and transplanted with a marrow that has not been depleted of RBCs, a rebound of the antibody can occur after transplantation causing hemolysis of the RBCs that were transfused with the marrow. Even more serious hemolysis due to rebound of hemagglutinins has been reported in patients who also were transfused with ABO-incompatible RBCs before BMT to absorb isohemagglutinins. Such hemolytic episodes usually occur between days 3 and 10 after transplantation.

Another cause of delayed hemolysis, beginning on day 35 to 105, is most likely a result of destruction of RBCs being produced by the newly engrafted marrow by persistence of isohemagglutinins.

LABORATORY TESTS

Laboratory tests indicative of hemolysis (see Chapter 2) alert one to the diagnosis, which is confirmed readily by the presence of a positive DAT and the expected isohemagglutinins in the patient's serum and in an eluate from the patient's RBCs.

Red Cell Alloantibodies of Blood Groups Other Than ABO

Although ABO blood group antibodies are the most important cause of hemolysis in the post-transplant period, hemolysis also can be caused by alloantibodies of other blood group systems. These episodes of hemolysis occur in less well-defined clinical settings and could be caused by donor-derived or recipient-derived antibodies, as described previously.

Autoimmune Hemolytic Anemia after Hematopoietic Cell Transplantation

Autoimmune hemolytic anemia can occur after hematopoietic stem cell transplantation and is unrelated to the presence or absence of blood group incompatibility between the donor and recipient. This topic is discussed earlier in the chapter, and further information regarding the diagnosis of AIHA is presented in Chapters 2, 5, and 6.

Passive Transfer of Antibody

Human plasma and immunoglobulin derivatives contain alloantibodies to human blood group antigens that can be acquired passively by patients who receive these products. Most commonly of concern in the setting of marrow transplantation are antibodies that might be infused as part of the donor marrow product, platelet transfusions, or IVIG therapy. These antibodies affect cross-matching, antibody screening, and antibody identification testing in addition to potentially causing hemolysis.

The antibodies that are usually responsible for hemolysis are anti-A, anti-B, and anti-D, which are also the antibodies most likely to cause passenger lymphocyte syndrome. Frequently, the clinical setting is valuable in determining the cause of hemolysis because symptoms and signs occur immediately after the passive transfer of antibodies that are capable of causing hemolysis. Because platelet transfusions and IVIG commonly are administered to BMT patients in the post-transplant period, however, hemolysis from passive transfer of antibody can occur during the same time period as the passenger lymphocyte syndrome. Indeed, Kim and coworkers[188] described such a patient, who received a minor ABO-incompatible BMT and was treated with IVIG in the early post-transplant period.

Hemolysis after Platelet Transfusion. Passive transfer of antibody can occur as a result of transfusion of minor ABO-incompatible platelets, as each platelet concentrate obtained from a unit of whole blood contains about 50–70 mL of plasma, and plateletpheresis products can contain about 350 mL of plasma. The use of incompatible platelets is sometimes unavoidable, such as when when inventories are inadequate or when HLA or platelet-specific antibodies are causing refractoriness and the only HLA-matched or cross-matched–compatible platelet donors are ABO incompatible.[189] Cases of severe hemolysis after transfusion of platelets with ABO-incompatible plasma have been reported.[189-201]

Hemolysis occurs when the donors have high titers of antibodies against the recipient's ABO blood group antigens. For example, Pierce and colleagues[193] reported two instances of severe immune hemolysis after transfusion of ABO-incompatible platelet concentrates. One of the reactions resulted in disseminated intravascular coagulation and proved fatal, while the other resulted in hemolysis of an estimated 40% of the patient's RBC mass. They found that the IgG anti-A titer of one donor was 32,000 and the anti-B titer of the other donor was 16,000.

In the case reported by Reis and Coovadia,[195] the plateletpheresis donor's plasma had an anti-B titer of 4096 by indirect antiglobulin testing. In the patient described by Conway and Scott,[192] the donor's saline anti-A titer was 8192, and the titer of dithiothreitol-treated serum was 4096. Transfusion of a plateletpheresis product with a volume of 200 mL resulted in severe hemolysis, disseminated intravascular coagulation, and renal failure requiring dialysis.

The patient reported on by Murphy and associates[189] received two transfusions of plateletpheresis products 25 days apart from the same donor. Stored serum from the donor, taken at the time of the first transfusion, had an anti-A titer of 512 by saline agglutination and a titer of 2048 by indirect antiglobulin test. The patient received 155 mL of plasma with the first platelet product and 448 mL with the second. Hemolysis occurred after both transfusions, and after the second transfusion, the patient's hemoglobin dropped from 11.4 g/dL to 6.0 g/dL in 1 day. She developed renal failure, although dialysis was not required and her renal function returned to normal.

McLeod and coworkers[191] reported on a particularly interesting patient who developed hemolysis after receiving only four platelet concentrates, each containing about 50 mL of plasma. The patient developed serious hemolysis with hemoglobinuria, a drop in hemoglobin from 14.0 g/dL to 8.0 g/dL, and renal insufficiency with a rise in creatinine from 1.6 mg/dL to 6.0 mg/dL. Two of the platelet donors were found by indirect antiglobulin test to have anti-A to a titer of 10,240.

McManigal and Sims[196] described a group AB patient who was transfused with 3380 mL of ABO-incompatible platelet products during a 4-day period. After transfusion of a group O unit of apheresis platelets, she developed classic signs of an intravascular hemolytic transfusion reaction. Although the volume of RBC hemolyzed was apparently small because the hematocrit did not change, the manifestations of the transfusion reaction included chills, flank pain, dyspnea, hemoglobinuria, and life-threatening tachycardia. The authors contacted the United States Food and Drug Administration (FDA) and learned that five deaths caused by ABO-incompatible platelet products had been reported in a 4-year period beginning in 1994.

Incidence of Hemolysis after ABO-Incompatible Platelet Transfusions. In spite of the foregoing case reports, one must keep in mind that hemolysis after ABO-incompatible platelet transfusion is not common. It could become a more common problem as the use of apheresis platelets increases, although this has not been documented.[199] Indeed, Shanwell and colleagues[202] reported that BMT recipients at their institution routinely received single-donor plateletpheresis products from blood group O donors containing about 350 mL of plasma. Over a period of 5 years, about 1000 plateletpheresis products with ABO-incompatible plasma were transfused. Although the researchers noted positive DATs due to passively adsorbed anti-A and/or anti-B from donor plasma, they found no cases of hemolysis. They studied 11 group A patients in detail and found that nine developed a positive DAT and that anti-A could be eluted from their red cells. None developed hemolysis, however. Also, patients of groups A, B, or AB (n = 34) required no more RBC or platelet transfusions than did patients who were group O (n = 47).

More recently, Mair and Benson[200] reported on a group A patient who experienced acute hemolysis, with a drop in hemoglobin from 8.4 g/dL to 5.8 g/dL in 24 hours after a platelet transfusion from a group O donor with a saline anti-A titer of 128. As a result of this reaction, they reviewed their experience and stated that the index case was the only identified episode of hemolysis that occurred after 46,176 platelet transfusions over a 10-year period (October 1986 to October 1986). Given that 21% of all platelets transfused at their medical center are plasma incompatible, the incidence of identified episodes of hemolysis was only one per 9000 incompatible transfusions.

Larsson and associates[199] reported a hemolytic reaction, which was the first that had been recognized at their institution even though more than 6600 single-donor platelet products had been transfused over the previous 9 years.

Although hemolytic reactions to ABO-incompatible platelets are apparently uncommon, they can be serious and even fatal, physicians should therefore be aware of this possibility whenever transfusion of such platelets is necessary.

Immune Hemolysis after Intravenous Immunoglobulin. IVIG is commonly administered to patients after allogeneic BMT, as CMV prophylaxis in seropositive patients and as nonspecific antimicrobial prophylaxis. In addition, the immunomodulatory effect of immunoglobulins on GVHD is the subject of clinical trials and follows the empiric observation that higher immunoglobulin levels are associated with a decreased rate of GVHD.[203]

Positive antiglobulin tests have frequently been reported with the use of IVIG, but usually signs of hemolysis have been absent or minimal.[204-207] A number of reports of significant hemolysis after IVIG administration exist, however.

Patients who have developed hemolysis generally have received rather high doses of IVIG. A common dose for treatment of patients with immune cytopenias is 400 mg/kg daily for 5 days.[208] A female patient described by Copelan and coworkers[208] was treated with 400 mg/kg daily for 10 days; after the sixth day, the DAT became positive, an eluate revealed anti-D, and laboratory evidences of hemolysis were present. During the 10 days of IVIG therapy and the 4 subsequent days, the patient required 6 units of RBCs to maintain her hemoglobin level above 9 g/dL. Another patient received IVIG at a dose of 500 mg/kg for 6 days. The DAT became positive with anti-IgG on the fourth day of therapy, and the eluate showed anti-D and anti-A_1. Hemolysis developed on the sixth day and could have been aggravated by the subsequent transfusion of a single-donor group O, Rh-positive platelet concentrate. Indirect antiglobulin titrations on the IVIG preparations used revealed anti-A (titer 32), anti-B (titers 4 to 8), and anti-D (titers 2 to 4).

Thomas and colleagues[209] reported a case in which a group A_1 patient received 1 g/kg of IVIG on two consecutive days. The following day, signs of hemolysis developed, including the presence of free hemoglobin in his serum and urine. His hemoglobin level dropped from 15 g/dL to 8.7 g/dL, the DAT became positive, an eluate showed anti-A_1, and the IVIG batch used contained anti-A to a titer of 32 against A_1 red cells.

Nicholls and associates[210] reported on a group A, Rh-positive patient who developed signs of hemolysis after the fourth course of IVIG, each course consisting of 400 mg/kg/day for 5 days. Hemolysis recurred during a fifth course of IVIG and was attributed to passively transferred anti-A and anti-D. A second patient also developed hemolysis attributed to passively acquired anti-D and an alloanti-E.

Robertson and coworkers[207] found that 49% of 47 patients who were treated with IVIG after BMT had a positive DAT, and 25.5% had a positive IAT. Antibodies identified in the serums and eluates were anti-A, -B, -D, and -K. Twenty-one lots of IVIG were tested, and all contained anti-A and anti-B; two also contained anti-D, and two others contained anti-K. The observed patterns of anti-D and anti-K reactivity were identical in patients' sera, in red cell eluates, and in the IVIG lots studied. The authors reported "slight hemolysis" in some patients, but no patient developed clinically significant hemolysis.

Kim and colleagues[188] described two BMT recipients who developed hemolysis after IVIG treatment. One of these patients was particularly interesting in that he had received a transplant from a minor ABO-incompatible donor 9 days previous to the IVIG administration. The patient had shaking chills during the IVIG administration; hemoglobinuria occurred 5 hours later and persisted for 4 days. Although IVIG probably precipitated the hemolysis, the passenger lymphocyte syndrome could have been a contributing factor.

Other cases in which overt hemolysis occurred after IVIG administration have been reported by Nakamura and associates,[211] Okubo and coworkers,[212] Brox and colleagues,[213] and Nakagawa and associates.[214]

A number of authors have suggested that steps be taken to minimize the possibility of hemolysis as a result of IVIG administration. Several investigators have suggested that standards should be set for maximum titers of RBC antibodies in IVIG preparations[204,215] and/or that a minor cross-match be performed using the IVIG preparation to be administered.[209,210] Such standards have not been set, however, and currently available literature indicates that ABO antibodies[13,188,208,209,216] and other RBC antibodies[13,208,216] are found commonly in IVIG. Thus, cross-matching would seem to be of limited value, as RBC antibodies would be detected frequently, although commonly at titers that are benign. Determining the titer of red cell alloantibodies in each lot of IVIG would provide more definitive information, although it would be difficult to determine what titers should be considered dangerous. Nevertheless, with further experience, it might be possible to develop guidelines based on titer and dose.

Because experience has indicated that standard doses of IVIG rarely cause immune hemolysis, determinations of red cell antibody titers in IVIG are not performed routinely. Physicians should be aware that hemolysis is a possible outcome, especially with the administration of unusually high doses. Other adverse effects of high-dose IVIG are described in Chapter 11.

Other Causes of Passive Transfer of Antibody: Packed RBC, Intravenous Anti-D, and Antilymphocyte Globulin. Inwood and Zuliani[55] reported a case of intravascular hemolysis after transfusion of packed group O RBCs to a group A patient. The hemoglobin dropped from 6.5 g/dL to 4.4 g/dL, but the patient made an uneventful recovery. The donor's anti-A_1 titer was 8192, and subsequently, it was determined that the donor had participated in a plasmapheresis program in which donors were stimulated for the production of ABO antibodies for subsequent reagent production.[217] The reportability of this case emphasizes the extreme rarity of hemolysis after transfusion of minor ABO-incompatible RBC.[218] Although this possibility must be kept in mind, it is among the least likely causes of hemolysis in transplant recipients.

The administration of intravenous anti-D has proven to be effective in some Rh-positive patients with idiopathic thrombocytopenic purpura (ITP). Transient and slight signs of hemolysis are found frequently, but overt clinical hemolysis has been considered to be unusual.[220,221] A review by Gaines,[222] however, described 15 cases of hemoglobinemia and/or hemoglobinuria that occurred between September 1995 and March 1999. For the 12 patients for whom symptoms were reported, two did not experience any symptoms, while ten had classic findings associated with acute hemolytic transfusion reactions. Information about the duration of hemoglobinuria was available for eight patients. Hemoglobinuria persisted 1 day or less in two patients, 2 days or longer in three patients, 3 days or longer in one patient, 7 days or longer in two patients, and 20 days or longer in one patient. Between May 1999 and October 1999, subsequent to the time period of the review, the FDA received an additional 26 anti-D IVIG adverse event reports of possible or probable hemoglobinemia and/or hemoglobinuria. Three sets of frequency estimates for the development of this complication were calculated (Table 12-14).

Another potential cause of hemolysis is passive transfer of antibody via antilymphocyte globulin, which is used as an immunosuppressant.[17]

Drug-Induced Hemolytic Anemia

Immune reactions to drugs must be considered as a possible cause when transplant patients develop hemolysis. This topic is reviewed in Chapter 8.

Microangiopathic Hemolytic Anemia

The term *microangiopathic hemolytic anemia* was first used by Brain and coworkers[223] to describe the hemolytic anemia associated with fragmented red blood cells that occurred in patients with microvascular disease and that often was associated with thrombocytopenia. These authors suggested that the characteristic RBC morphology, the accelerated RBC destruction, and the thrombocytopenia were secondary consequences of fibrinoid necrosis and hyaline occlusion of arterioles and capillaries in various disease states. Subsequent experimental work and clinical observations have led to the acceptance of these concepts.[224-227]

Microangiopathic hemolytic anemia can occur in association with a large number of clinical conditions:[228–233]

- Disseminated intravascular coagulation
- Acute renal failure
- Radiation nephritis

TABLE 12-14. ESTIMATED FREQUENCY OF HEMOGLOBINEMIA AND/OR HEMOGLOBINURIA FOLLOWING ADMINISTRATION OF ANTI-D IGIV FOR ITP

Source(s) of Data	Reported Patients (*n*)	Total Patients (*n*)	Estimated Incidence Rate (%)	Estimated Reporting Rate (%)	Estimated Incidence
Clinical studies	0	528	0.0	NA	0 in 528
Clinical trial	2	137	1.5	NA	1 in 69
FDA*/IMS	13	14,500*	NA	0.1	1 in 1115

Reported patients experienced hemoglobinemia and/or hemoglobinuria following anti-D IGIV administration during a specified time period. Total patients were treated or estimated to have been treated with anti-D IGIV during a specified time period. NA indicates not applicable.
* Data on file, Office of Biostatistics and Epidemiology, Center for Biologics Evaluation and Research, FDA, Rockville, MD: March 1995–December 1998.
From Gaines AR: Acute onset hemoglobinemia and/or hemoglobinuria and sequelae following Rh(o)(D) immune globulin intravenous administration in immune thrombocytopenic purpura patients. Blood 2000;95:2523–2529.

- Malignant hypertension
- Infections with viral or nonviral agents
- Exposure to a variety of antibiotics
- Severe preeclampsia or eclampsia
- Abruptio placenta
- Adenocarcinomas and other malignant tumors
- Hemangiomas
- Immunologic disorders such as SLE, acute glomerulonephritis, polyarteritis nodosa, Wegener's granulomatosis, and scleroderma

Frequently, the microangiopathic hemolysis in these disorders has occurrred in the context of syndromes known as the hemolytic uremic syndrome (HUS) or thrombotic thrombocytopenic purpura (TTP). In spite of the imposing list of underlying disorders, these syndromes most frequently occur de novo.

Hemolysis associated with fragmented RBCs occurs in patients with cardiovascular abnormalities[234–237] and as a result of prosthetic cardiovascular materials.[237,238] Because there is no microvascular disease, however, these disorders are more appropriately called mechanical, traumatic, or fragmentation hemolysis.[238,239]

THROMBOTIC THROMBOCYTOPENIC PURPURA AND THE HEMOLYTIC-UREMIC SYNDROME AFTER TRANSPLANTATION

The importance of TTP and HUS in transplantation is suggested by the fact that there have been multiple detailed reviews of this topic.[122,240-242]

TTP and HUS were described initially as distinct disorders. At present, some[243] but not all[244] investigators consider TTP and HUS to be different expressions of the same disease process. The precise distinction between the two syndromes remains somewhat arbitrary and controversial.[240,245,246]

The classic pentad of TTP consists of fever, microangiopathic hemolytic anemia, thrombocytopenic purpura, renal insufficiency, and neurologic findings that often fluctuate in both nature and severity.[229,247,248] On the other hand, findings in HUS consist of microangiopathic hemolytic anemia, thrombocytopenia, and renal failure. In recent years, to accelerate the initiation of treatment since the advent of plasma exchange, the diagnosis of TTP-HUS is made on the basis of only the principal features—microangiopathic hemolytic anemia and thrombocytopenia (Table 12-15).[243]

HUS-TTP has been reported to occur after total body irradiation, therapy with a number of chemotherapeutic and immunosuppressive drugs, and among patients who have received a bone marrow or solid organ transplant.

DIFFICULTIES IN DIAGNOSIS IN THE POST-TRANSPLANT SETTING

It often can be difficult to establish a diagnosis of transplant-associated TTP (TA-TTP) in hematopoietic cell transplant patients.[122,242] These patients frequently have multiple potential etiologies for renal dysfunction, fever, and thrombocytopenia, and might display only subtle neurological abnormalities. In addition, the presentation of TA-TTP is highly heterogeneous, ranging from asymptomatic, low-level RBC fragmentation to fulminant disease. The diagnosis of TA-TTP is made most reliably by examination of the peripheral blood film for RBC fragments. Daly and coworkers[122] suggest that an increase in the number of RBC fragments and the biochemical evidence of hemolysis over several observations can make the diagnosis more convincing than finding features compatible with the diagnosis on a single occasion. For this reason, it is essential that blood films be reviewed and reported by experienced staff and that reliable quantitative evaluations or RBC fragmentation be available.

Zomas and colleagues[249] found that mild RBC fragmentation was a common morphologic finding after transplantation but that none of their 58 allograft or 32 autograft patients developed full-blown thrombotic microangiopathy. Indeed, Allford and associates[242] point out that nearly all patients receiving cyclosoporine have some evidence of microangiopathic hemolysis, but the majority do not develop TTP. Furthermore, these authors have observed

TABLE 12-15. EVOLUTION OF DIAGNOSTIC CRITERIA FOR TTP

	Percentage of Patients		
Clinical Sign	**1925–1964**	**1964–1980**	**1982–1989**
Microangiopathic hemolytic anemia	96	98	100
Thrombocytopenia	96	98	100
Neurologic symptoms	92	84	63
Renal disease	88	76	59
Fever	98	59	24

From George JN, El-Harake M: Thrombocytopenia due to enhanced platelet destructon by nonimmunologic mechanisms. In Beutler E, Lichtman MA, Coller BS, Kipps TJ (eds): Williams Hematology. New York: McGraw-Hill Health Professions, 1995:1290–1315.

patients with severe, rapidly fatal post-transplant TTP who had no evidence of hemolysis at the onset of the illness. One group found that LDH was twice the laboratory normal in all 22 patients in their series, so this might be a valuable criterion.[250]

INCIDENCE OF TA-TTP AFTER HEMATOPIETIC STEM CELL TRANSPLANTATION

The exact incidence is difficult to determine due to differences in case definition, reporting bias, and missed diagnoses. Some reported incidence rates have been 0.28%[251] and 4.8%.[250] Other studies support an incidence of 5–15%.[252,253]

Rabinowe and coworkers[254] reported a series of 168 adult patients with hematologic malignancies who underwent autologous or allogeneic bone marrow transplantation and were investigated for the subsequent development of HUS. All patients were conditioned with cyclophosphamide and total body irradiation. Sixteen patients (9.5%) developed clinical and laboratory evidence of HUS between three and 11 months after BMT. Both hemolytic anemia and thrombocytopenia ultimately resolved, but at 18 months after diagnosis, some patients had residual creatinine elevations and persistent hypertension.

Other cases of HUS and TTP have been reported in both children and adults after allogeneic or autologous marrow or peripheral blood stem cell transplantation.[254-266]

RISK FACTORS FOR HUS AND TTP

Risk factors for the development of HUS or TTP after BMT have been analyzed. Irradiation of the kidney (which occurs during total body irradiation) is likely to be involved in the pathogenesis.[267] In fact, the clinical picture of HUS can be indistinguishable from that of radiation nephritis.[268-270] Holler and colleagues[253] reported intravascular hemolysis with RBC fragmentation and de novo thrombocytopenia in 49 of 66 allogeneic marrow graft recipients receiving cyclosporine but none in 11 patients treated with methotrexate for prophylaxis of GVHD. Risk factor analysis revealed a highly significant association of microangiopathy with severity of acute GVHD and the use of cyclosporine. Galli and associates[271] also implicated cyclosporine administration as a cause of HUS in a heart transplant recipient. Hemolysis subsided after treatment with plasma exchange, but rechallenge with cyclosporine caused recurrence of the microangiopathic hemolysis. Tacrolimus (FK506), an alternative immunosuppressive drug that is used in marrow and solid organ transplantation, has also been reported to be associated with HUS and TTP.[272,273]

Paquette and coworkers[263] reviewed clinical data from seven patients diagnosed with severe thrombotic microangiopathy and from 409 patients who underwent BMT during the same time period and survived for at least 100 days afterwards. Univariate analysis revealed an increased risk of thrombotic microangiopathy with the use of an unrelated bone marrow donor ($P = 0.02$), but no significant association with patient age or gender, diagnosis, amount of prior chemotherapy, transplant conditioning regimen, or severity of GVHD. A multivariate exact logistic regression analysis revealed that only the type of GVHD prophylaxis had a significant impact on the risk.

Other reports of HUS after BMT indicated that the patients were heterogeneous with respect to underlying diagnosis, type of BMT (allogeneic or autologous), pretransplant conditioning regimen, presence or absence of GVHD, and use of cyclosporine.[274] Allford and colleagues[242] concluded that the role of cyclosporine in the etiology of TTP remains unclear. Marshall and Sweny[275] reported three cases of HUS after BMT in which none of the patients was treated with cyclosporine, and Chavers and associates[276] reported a case of HUS in a renal transplant recipient who had none of the factors known to contribute to the development of the syndrome. The etiology is likely to be multifactorial.[277,278]

Other reports suggest that patients with TA-TTP are more likely to be female and are significantly older than patients who do not develop the syndrome. Also, grades II–IV acute GVHD and hepatic veno-occlusive disease are associated with an increased risk of TA-TTP.[122]

HUS and TTP have been reported after renal,[276,279–281] liver,[253,272,282,283] and heart[271] transplantation. Schwarz and coworkers[281] reviewed the clinical course of 700 patients with renal transplants and concluded that cyclosporine treatment did not increase the incidence of HUS.

A number of chemotherapeutic agents have been reported to cause HUS or TTP. The most commonly implicated drug is mitomycin, but these syndromes have also been reported in association with carboplatin,[284] gemcitabine,[284] bleomycin, cisplatin, vinca-alkaloids, FK-506, daunorubicin, and methyl-CCNU.[272,273,285-287]

Ticlopidine use has been implicated in numerous cases of TTP.[288,289] Quinine sensitivity is a relatively newly recognized cause of HUS and is unique in that an immune mechanism has been implicated.[290-294]

MANAGEMENT AND PROGNOSIS OF TA-TTP

There is no consensus on what constitutes appropriate therapy for patients with TA-TTP.[122,242] Almost all clinicians stop cyclosporine or tacrolimus, however, and platelet transfusions are avoided if at all possible. Many centers employ plasma exchange, although this strategy is based neither on data nor on logical therapy, as no substance has been identified in the plasma that appears to be associated with disease pathogenesis.[242]

Response rates to plasma exchange have been considerably lower than in classical TTP, and long-term survival rates have been disappointing. Overall, just under half of patients in nine reported case series have achieved a complete or partial remission, but fewer than half of patients who respond to plasma exchange experience prolonged survival.[122] Many of the patients in these reports died of causes other than TA-TTP—most commonly, infection, GVHD, and multisystem organ failure syndrome.

DIFFERENTIATING HUS/TTP FROM IMMUNE HEMOLYSIS IN THE POST-TRANSPLANT SETTING

HUS and TTP are readily distinguished from immune hemolytic syndromes after transplantation. Major points of differentiation are a lack of red cell antibodies in HUS or TTP (with the exception of quinine-dependent antibodies in quinine-induced HUS) and the presence of fragmented RBCs in the peripheral blood film.

The time of onset is often helpful in making a differential diagnosis, as most immune hemolytic syndromes occur earlier after hematopoietic stem cell transplantation than do HUS and TTP, which typically develop at a median time of 5 months after transplantation (range 3 to 7 months).[295] Other reports indicate the median time of onset as 163 days[274] or 61 days.[253] Only occasionally do cases occur within the first month after BMT.[274,277]

HUS caused by mitomycin has its onset at a median time of 1 year from the beginning of treatment.[285] Manifestations of radiation nephritis develop between 6 and 12 months after irradiation.[267]

The time of onset of HUS or TTP after organ transplantation is variable, occurring within the first 1 to 3 weeks after transplantation in some patients[271,279,280,296] and 3 to 16 months after transplantation in others.[272,276,283]

Miscellaneous Additional Causes of Hemolysis after Hematopoietic Stem Cell Transplantation

INFUSION OF CRYOPRESERVED BONE MARROW OR PERIPHERAL BLOOD STEM CELL PRODUCTS; INFUSION OF DIMETHYLSULPHOXIDE (DMSO) AND FREE PLASMA HEMOGLOBIN

Although high concentrations of DMSO cause hemolysis in vitro and in vivo,[297-299] concentrations used in the modern practice of marrow and peripheral blood stem cell transplantation usually produce only mild side effects. These include nausea, chills, fever, hypertension, bradycardia, shortness of breath, and transient substernal chest tightness. Contaminating RBCs that are lysed during the cryopreservation procedure, however, are an obvious cause of hemoglobinemia and hemoglobinuria immediately after administering the stem cell product.

Smith and colleagues[300] reviewed 33 consecutive patients who had received unfractionated cryopreserved autologous bone marrow. Gross hemoglobinuria was noted in all 33 patients, three of whom developed acute renal failure with renal histopathology typical of an acute hemolytic transfusion reaction. Although previous investigators had attributed nephrotoxicity in patients receiving autologous bone marrow to hemolysis caused by DMSO, Smith and associates implicated the hemolysate content of the cryopreserved marrow. Subsequently, they adopted a procedure to remove RBCs from the marrow harvest specimens.

Burger and coworkers[301] reported acute hemoglobinemia and hemoglobinuria after infusion of autologous buffy coat products that contained RBCs and were cryopreserved using DMSO. Although the recipient's free plasma hemoglobin levels after infusion of the products were as high as 932 mg/mL, no overt renal problems resulted. The products contained elevated levels of free hemoglobin due to the presence of lysed RBCs. Accordingly, to minimize RBC contamination, the authors recommended a policy of mononuclear cell separation for patients undergoing autologous marrow transplantation.

Kessinger and colleagues[302] evaluated 100 consecutive autologous peripheral blood stem cell transplants and determined that hemoglobinuria occurred in 92%, elevated serum bilirubin in 43%, and elevated serum creatinine in 15% of patients. Larger volumes of transplanted cells with concomitantly larger doses of DMSO and lysed RBCs were both strongly related to a greater number of side effects of the marrow infusion ($P < 0.0001$). The authors tested a number of procedures to decrease the volume transfused and the number of lysed RBCs in the infusate. All methods eliminated renal toxicity, but several resulted in delayed engraftment. A method involving a repeat centrifugal apheresis of the collected product, harvesting the entire buffy coat and the first 60 mL of discharged cells that have a visible RBC content, eliminated renal toxicity and allowed timely engraftment.

CLOSTRIDIUM PERFRINGENS SEPTICEMIA

Clostridium perfringens is a recognized but rare cause of septicemia and remarkably severe intravascular hemolysis[303-307] and is more likely to occur among immunocompromised patients. Ifthikaruddin and associates[308] reported on a 54-year-old female with acute myeloblastic leukemia who underwent an autologous BMT but failed to engraft. She was followed as an outpatient and was dependent on blood product support. Approximately 4 months after BMT, she was admitted to the hospital with cellulitis of the left inner thigh. On admission, her hemoglobin was 10.6 g/dL. Antibiotics were promptly prescribed, but the patient had signs of septic shock and became unresponsive within hours, during which time hemolysis of her total red cell mass occurred. Just 5 hours after admission, the hemoglobin was 2.3 g/dL, but this value was attributed to free hemoglobin in the plasma because the peripheral blood film failed to show any intact RBCs. The patient also developed disseminated intravascular coagulation and expired on the day of admission. Such massive hemolysis with destruction of essentially all circulating red blood cells strongly suggests a diagnosis of *Clostridium perfringens* septicemia, and this diagnosis was confirmed the following day by the results of blood cultures.

Chaplin[303] reviewed the causes of massive intravascular hemolysis and discussed a patient with "total intravascular hemolysis" caused by *Clostridial perfringens* infection. He reviewed six cases in which the hematocrits were reported to be 0%, 0%, 0.6%, 1%, less than 2%, and less than 5%, respectively. The diagnosis of Clostridial sepsis should be considered at once when gross hemoglobinemia and hemoglobinuria and a rapid fall in hemoglobin level are found, as the immediate institution of appropriate antibiotics and aggressive supportive care could be life saving.

HEMOLYSIS ASSOCIATED WITH HEMODIALYSIS

Occasionally, hemodialysis is indicated for patients who have received a solid organ or marrow transplant. Hemolysis in chronic renal failure is persistent but usually mild.[309] Aggravation of hemolysis can occur in the hemodialysed patient for a number of reasons, however. Acute intravascular hemolysis has been caused by an indwelling hemodialysis catheter.[310] Additional causes are thermal red cell injury such as might be caused by overheated dialysate, osmotic red cell injury caused by hypotonic dialysate, and partial obstruction within the extracorporeal circuit.

IMMUNE HEMOLYSIS ASSOCIATED WITH SOLID ORGAN TRANSPLANTATION

Passenger Lymphocyte Syndrome

The passenger lymphocyte syndrome, with clinical and laboratory findings very similar to those found after BMT, has been reported on numerous occasions after transplantation of kidney,[24,311-324] liver,[325-330] lung,[331-334] heart,[335-337] heart-lung,[334,338,339] spleen,[332] pancreas,[312,340] and pancreas-spleen[341] (Table 12-16).[24,311-324] Ramsey, in a review in 1991,[44] found that among minor ABO-incompatible transplants, 61% of cases involved group O donors and group A recipients, 22% percent involved group O donors and group B recipients, and 17% percent involved group AB patients receiving non-AB organs.

Hemolytic anemia after organ transplantation is more frequently encountered in proportion to the lymphoid mass transplanted.[45,342] Ramsey[44] found that the frequencies of antibodies and hemolysis were lowest in kidney transplant patients (17% and 9%, respectively), intermediate in liver transplant patients (40% and 29%, respectively), and highest in heart-lung transplant patients (both, 70%). Borka and coworkers[24] reported that hemolysis attributed to the passenger lymphocyte syndrome developed in 22 of 237 of their patients (9%) who received a minor incompatible renal transplant. Salerno and colleagues[334] reported that in heart-lung transplantation, the incidence of hemolysis from donor-derived anti-ABO antibodies is as high as 70%.

Triulzi and associates[327] reported that five of nine patients (56%) receiving an ABO minor-mismatched liver transplant developed donor-derived antibody and hemolysis. It is remarkable that the few lymphocytes transplanted with some donor organs are able to proliferate sufficiently to produce adequate quantities of antibody to cause hemolysis of the recipient's RBCs within a week or two after the transplantation. Antibody can be produced even when the donor organs have been perfused copiously with preservative solution and, just before transplantation, with saline.[325,343,344]

IMMUNOGLOBULIN ALLOTYPES OF ANTIBODIES CAUSING THE PASSENGER LYMPHOCYTE SYNDROME

The origin of cells producing immunoglobulins can be investigated by analysis of polymorphic epitopes (allotypes) on the immunoglobulins in instances in which the donor and recipient express different phenotypes.[160] Several groups have confirmed that the

TABLE 12-16. ABO ANTIBODIES FROM SOLID ORGAN TRANSPLANTS: TOTAL REPORTED CASES AND COMBINED FREQUENCIES OF ANTIBODY (Ab) AND HEMOLYSIS (H) IN STUDIED SERIES OF ABO-UNMATCHED ORGANS

Donor-Recipient ABO Blood Groups	Kidney			Liver			Heart-Lung			Heart			Other Cases*	Total Cases
	Cases	%Ab	%H	Cases	%Ab	%H	Cases	%Ab	%H	Cases	%Ab	%H		
Total	46	17	9	45	40	29	7	70	70	2	40	11	6	106
	(33)†	24/144‡	15/165§	(35)	36/90	33/115§	(7)	7/10	7/10	(1)	2/5	1/9§	(3)	(79)
O-A	22	23	8	26	50	44	6	75	75	2	50	14	3	59
	(15)	8/35	4/51	(24)	18/36	16/36	(6)	6/8	6/8	(1)	2/4	1/7	(2)	(48)
O-B	10	9	5	8	40	25	0	0	0	0	0	0	3	21
	(9)	2/22	1/22	(5)	8/20	5/20	—	0/1	0/1	—	0/1	0/1	(1)	(15)
O-AB	2	50	50	4	50	0	1	100	100	—			—	7
	(1)	1/2	1/2	(2)	1/2	0/2	(1)	1/1	1/1					(4)
A-AB	1	6	5	3	50	17	—			0	—	0	—	4
	(1)	1/16	1/20	(2)	3/6	2/12						0/1		(3)
B-AB	3	10	0	2	33	0	—			—			—	5
	(2)	1/10	0/11	(0)	2/6	0/6								(2)
Not given	8			2			—			—			—	10
	(5)			(2)										(7)

* Three pancreas (O-to-B, 1H), two spleen (O-to-A, 2H), and one lung (O-to-A) transplant.
† Number with hemolysis from among those reported; the kidney cases included one kidney-pancreas graft with hemolysis.
‡ Number with Ab or H/total number studied in all series; in the kidney and liver transplants, the total numbers of cases evaluated for the frequencies of Ab and H are greater than the sum of the ABO rows, because several series did not specify ABO groups in all cases.
§ Some patients were evaluated for H but not for Ab; the kidney series included two kidney-pancreas grafts without hemolysis.
From Ramsey G: Red cell antibodies arising from solid organ transplants. Transfusion 1991;31:76–86.

antibodies causing passenger lymphocyte syndrome were produced by donor lymphocytes and not by those of the recipient.[44,323,343-346]

SEROLOGIC FINDINGS

One should be aware that hemolysis is usually abrupt in onset and that serologic abnormalities might not be evident before the onset of hemolysis. Ramsey[44] reported that a positive DAT, serum antibodies, and hemolysis have generally been found at the same time. In our experience, we have been rather disappointed to find that performing DATs and serum antibody studies on patients in the postoperative period are not helpful in predicting the onset of hemolysis. Also, as with hematopoietic stem cell transplantation, hemolysis precedes the ability to detect the relevant antibodies for a day or so in some cases. Triulzi and coworkers[327] reported that hemolysis preceded the first positive DAT in four of five liver transplant recipients who developed passenger lymphocyte syndrome (donors group O, patients group A) by a mean of 1.8 days (range, 0 to 4 days). Similarly, Borka and colleagues[24] reported that antibodies are found after hemolysis has been present for "several days." Accordingly, the most informative laboratory findings are a sudden drop in hemoglobin and hematocrit without evidence of a significant source of bleeding. These findings are associated with an elevation of the serum bilirubin and LDH. The DAT and serum antibody tests, if not immediately positive, will become so during the ensuing days.

The onset of hemolysis is generally between 3 and 24 days, regardless of whether the antibodies are in the ABO or Rh blood group systems. The findings of the DAT in 43 patients with minor ABO-incompatible transplants revealed that 36 patients had IgG on their RBCs, 35 had complement, and 28 had both.[44]

In three kidney and six liver transplant patients, graft anti-A was solely of A_1 specificity. Three of these instances occurred in A_1 patients. The other six occurred in A_2 or A_2B patients. Because hemolysis caused by anti-A_1 is rare,[347] a number of authors have suggested that anti-A could have been absorbed onto RBCs and tissues, with anti-A_1 left circulating as a separate antibody.[44,338] Alternatively, Brecher and associates[347] postulated that anti-A_1 seen after organ transplantation could be the result of cyclosporine-induced altered T-lymphocyte regulation of B cells leading to proliferation of heretofore rarely detected clones of clinically significant anti-A_1–producing B cells.

Hemolysis caused by Rh antibodies has more commonly been reported after solid organ transplantation than after BMT. Specificity has most often been anti-D,[44,317,328,339] but anti-c[316] and anti-e[44,348] also have been noted.

Hareuveni and coworkers[329] reported clinically significant hemolysis associated with the passenger lymphocyte syndrome after liver transplantation caused by anti-Jk^a.

Seltsam and colleagues[349] reported the occurrence of RBC alloimmunization in two of four patients who received different organs from an immunized donor. The donor was a 58-year-old woman who was group O, D+, K-, and Fy(a-). Her serum contained anti-K and anti-Fy^a, and several of her organs were transplanted to different patients. The recipient of her liver developed anti-K, and anti-Fy^a was eluted from her RBCs. A patient who received a pancreas-kidney graft also had RBCs sensitized with anti-Fy^a. The latter patient developed mild hemolysis.

POSSIBLE FACTORS AFFECTING HEMOLYSIS

Patient gender and age did not affect the likelihood of either antibody appearance or hemolysis after minor ABO-incompatible organ transplants.[44] Patients of blood groups A_1 and A_2 had similar frequencies of hemolysis, contrary to the expectation that in group A_2 recipients, the reduced expression of RBC antigen might protect against hemolysis by antibodies from group O organs. The patients' secretor status was also evaluated, as patients who are genetic ABH secretors have more ABH antigen in their plasma than nonsecretors, and the suggestion has been made that soluble ABH antigen could serve to neutralize circulating antibody. This could not be proven on the basis of limited available data, however.

Among patients reviewed by Ramsey,[44] those receiving cyclosporine did not have a significantly higher frequency of antibodies (30%) than those receiving azathioprine (17%). The frequency of hemolysis in patients taking cyclosporine, however, was higher (17% vs. 3%). Subsequently, Povlsen and associates[315] reported two cases of severe but self-limited hemolysis among 34 kidney transplant patients treated with cyclosporine but no cases among 108 patients treated with azathioprine. Borka and coworkers[24] reported that 91% of their 22 renal transplant patients suffering from the passenger lymphocyte syndrome were treated with cyclosporine, in contrast to their entire incompatible group of 237 patients, in whom only 65% were treated with this agent.

Mazarra and colleagues[340] reported on a patient who developed anti-B without hemolysis from day 11 to day 31 after a pancreas transplant, and Lundgren and associates[312] described a patient who developed fulminating hemolysis caused by donor-derived anti-A after a renal allograft. Neither patient received cyclosporine.

Tacrolimus (FK-506) has also been associated with donor-derived antibodies and hemolysis in liver transplant recipients. Bradley and coworkers[350] reported that the DAT was positive in three of five liver transplant patients who had the test performed postoperatively. RBC eluates contained anti-A or anti-B donor-derived RBC antibodies. The donor-derived antibodies appeared a mean of 14 days after transplantation, and one patient developed mild hemolysis requiring a transfusion of 2 units of group O RBCs.

CLINICAL FEATURES

Hemolysis is characteristically acute in onset, and although many cases are mild and self-limited, RBC transfusion is often required. Ramsey[44] reported that the median number of units transfused in 18 renal transplant patients was 6.5 (range of 1 to 18). In seven liver transplant patients, the number of units transfused ranged from 2 to 11 units, and four heart-lung patients received 16–24 units. In some instances, more severe hemolysis has occurred with resultant renal failure requiring dialysis.[282,312,333,346,351]

In contrast to BMT, wherein the patient's RBCs are replaced by those produced by the donor marrow, incompatible red cells continue to be produced by the solid organ transplant recipient. Nevertheless, hemolysis is generally short-lived, evidently because the lymphocytes transferred with the donor organ are able to proliferate only temporarily and are not engrafted permanently. In kidney transplant patients, the final positive DATs were seen 2 to 13 weeks after operation (median, 5), and the last reactive serum specimens were detected at 3 to 23 weeks after transplantation (median, 5.5). In liver transplant patients, the reactive DAT or serum was last detected 10–50 days after surgery (median, 20).[44]

UNUSUAL CASES

Some particularly interesting cases are worth noting. Jacobs and colleagues[352] reported on the simultaneous occurrence of the passenger lymphocyte syndrome and a delayed hemolytic transfusion reaction 16 days after transplantation of an ABO minor mismatched liver. Serologic studies identified a positive DAT and a donor-derived anti-A (i.e., passenger lymphocyte syndrome). In addition, a recipient-derived anti-E was identified in the serum and eluate.

Bracey and Van Buren[353] reported anti-A of donor lymphocyte origin in three group A recipients of organs from the same group O donor. The recipient of the donor's liver developed hemolysis caused by anti-A 10 days after transplantation, and two recipients of the same donor's kidneys developed hemolysis due to anti-A on days 11 and 13, respectively. A similar case was reported by Ramsey and associates,[317] who reported anti-D in two Rh-positive patients receiving renal grafts from an Rh-immunized donor. One patient developed overt hemolysis, whereas evidence of hemolysis was minimal in the other patient.

Bapat[354] reported a patient who had the passenger lymphocyte syndrome caused by anti-A after renal transplantation and in whom thrombocytopenia occurred coincident with the onset of brisk hemolysis and persisted throughout the period of ongoing hemolysis. Platelet-specific antibodies were not detected.

The patient was a 30-year-old male, group A, D positive (Cde/cDE), who received a kidney transplant from a group A, D-positive, E-negative cadaver donor. Forty-eight hours before collection of the kidney, the donor had been transfused with E-positive RBCs. Immunosuppressive therapy, which was started on the day of transplantation, consisted of cyclosporine and prednisone. In the third post-transplant month, the patient was admitted to the hospital because of severe hemolytic anemia with a hemoglobin of 2.6 g/dL, a total bilirubin level of 2.2 mg/dL, and a lactate dehydrogenase level of 1039 IU/L. Serum haptoglobin was below 10 mg/dL, and creatinine was 2.3 mg/dL.

The patient's DAT was positive, and anti-E was detected in the serum and in an eluate from his RBCs. Cyclosporine dosage was reduced, high-dose prednisone therapy was started, and he was transfused with 7 units of group A, E-negative RBCs. Hemolysis gradually resolved. Three months later, the DAT was still positive and anti-E was still present in the patient's serum, but there were no signs of hemolysis. Twelve months after transplantation, the DAT was negative and anti-E could not be detected.

Au and colleagues[330] described a 45-year-old male (group A_1, Rh-positive) who received an orthotopic liver transplant from a male cadaveric donor (group O, Rh-positive). Six units of group A RBCs were transfused in the peritransplant period. On postoperative day 6, the hemoglobin level was normal, but on day 8, the patient developed shock and jaundice accompanied by a dramatic fall in hemoglobin to 3 g/dL. The patient was transfused with 8 units of group O RBCs. The peripheral blood showed numerous spherocytes, the DAT was strongly positive, and anti-A was present to a titer of 512. The donor's titer of anti-A was found to be 2560. Hemolysis persisted for 3 weeks, and 4 more units of group O RBCs were given, after which signs of hemolysis gradually resolved.

DONOR-DERIVED ANTIBODIES PRODUCED LONG AFTER TRANSPLANTATION

Larrea and associates[355] reported a case in which donor-derived anti-E and immune hemolysis was not detected until the third month after transplantation. Accordingly, the antibody was likely produced by cells of the donor that had resulted in microchimerism (see the earlier discussion in this chapter).

Swanson and coworkers[348] reported one patient who had severe hemolytic anemia of 4 months' duration caused by anti-e. Ramsey and colleagues[317] documented the presence of anti-D in two Rh-positive patients for 6 months after each had received a renal transplant from the same Rh-sensitized cadaver donor.

MANAGEMENT OF THE PASSENGER LYMPHOCYTE SYNDROME

Anticipation of the passenger lymphocyte syndrome is important. Unfortunately, the titer of antibody in the donor is not reliable as a means of prediction of

CHAPTER 13

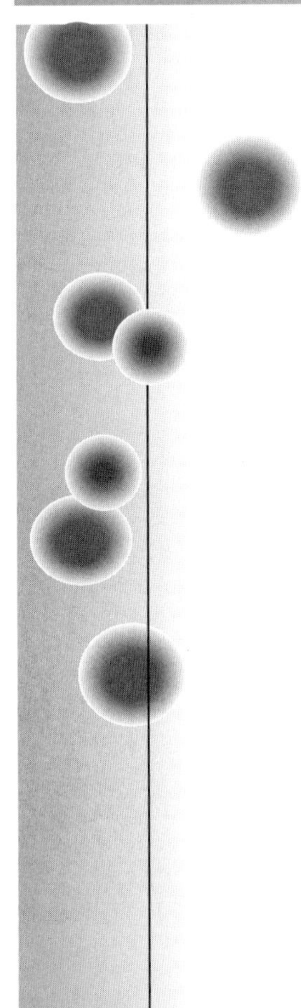

Hemolytic Disease of the Fetus and Newborn

Hemolytic disease of the fetus and newborn (HDFN) is a condition in which fetal or newborn infants' RBCs have a shortened life span due to maternal antibodies. These antibodies cross the placenta and sensitize the fetal RBCs; they are usually IgG alloantibodies but on rare occasions can be IgG maternal autoantibodies. This condition is more commonly called hemolytic disease of the newborn (HDN), but we (and others) prefer the more accurate term, HDFN.[1,2] The hemolytic process varies from severe in utero hemolysis early in pregnancy, resulting in fetal death (often associated with hydrops fetalis), to a mild process that might not be noticeable until a day or more after the baby's birth. Sensitization of the baby's RBCs with maternal antibody does not necessarily lead to HDFN. Many babies are born with a strongly positive direct antiglobulin test (DAT) due to IgG (even Rh antibody) sensitization but have no obvious signs of a hemolytic anemia. This phenomenon has led to some confusion in the literature; in many reports, antibodies are described as being a cause of HDFN because the baby was born with a positive DAT due to a specific maternal antibody, and yet no (or very little) evidence has been presented for the presence of hemolytic anemia. This is particularly the case for ABO HDFN (see the later discussion). Unfortunately, such reports are often perpetuated secondhand by authors quoting the original reference (often without critically reading the original report), or the antibody is added to a list of antibodies purported to cause HDFN. When we refer to HDFN in this chapter, it implies that a hemolytic anemia was present in the fetus and/or the newborn infant, and the antibodies we list as a cause of HDFN are only those for which there is evidence of having caused an immune hemolytic anemia.

The first antibody to be described as a cause of HDFN was anti-D. Until the use of Rh immunoprophylaxis in 1968, anti-D was, by far, the most common antibody to cause HDFN, being responsible for about 98% of all cases.[2,3] Approximately one in 180 of all newborn white infants suffered with HDFN due to anti-D.[2] In 1964, Giblett[3] reported that 93% of antibodies detected in sera of pregnant women were anti-D (or anti-C+D); 6% were of other Rh specificities. In 1967, Polesky[4] reported that 5.7% of pregnant women were alloimmunized; 83% of these involved Rh antibodies, and 1% were associated with specificities other than Rh. In 1969, Queenan and colleagues[5] reported that 3.1% of pregnant women were alloimmunized; 68% of these were associated with anti-D and 1.3% with specificities other than Rh. Since Rh prophylaxis became widespread, the picture has changed, and anti-D is much less common. The comparative incidence of alloantibodies other than anti-D has also been affected by the increased population of pregnant group women who have been transfused; Queenan and colleagues[5] reported that a history of prior transfusion was nine times more frequent among alloimmunized pregnant women. There are a few reports available to illustrate the changing picture after the introduction of Rh prophylaxis. Walker[6] reported that in Michigan (US) in 1969, one in every 175 (0.6%) obstetric patients produced anti-D, but that by 1984 this rate had fallen to 1.7 per 1000 (0.17%) (1.4% of Rh[D] negative women with Rh[D] positive husbands). Over a 12-year period at Walker's hospital, 104 of 55,877 (1/537) deliveries were associated with antibodies of potential clinical significance other than anti-D. Historically, the next most common antibody after anti-D was anti-E (1/1693 or 0.06%), followed by anti-c, -Jk^a, and -K (approximately 1/4000 or 0.3%); these were followed by anti-C, -s, -e, -cE, -Fy^a (approximately 1/14,000 or 0.007%).[6] Kornstad[7] reported that in Norway, the occurrence of new cases of anti-D had fallen from 57.6 cases per 10,000 (0.6%) women in 1967–1969 to 16.5 per 10,000 (0.2%) women during the period 1981–1983. Fifty-eight percent of the new cases of immunization to Rh antigens occurred in Rh(D)-negative women and 42% in Rh(D)-positive women. Rh antibodies other than anti-D accounted for 53% and anti-D for 47% of the "new" antibodies. In an earlier report, Kornstad[8] reported on antibodies that were detected in 148,200 Rh(D)-positive women during a five-year period (1975–1980). These included 99 antibodies with Rh specificities other than anti-D, and 101 antibodies of specificities other than Rh that had the potential to cause HDFN. Anti-E was the most commonly detected antibody in D-positive women, followed by anti-K, -c, -C^w, and -Fy^a. In the same period, 204 D-negative women had anti-D detected in their sera.

Between 12% and 18% of white women are D negative, but a much lower frequency is found in other populations. The D-negative phenotype is rare (1.7%) among Chinese, Japanese, and Southeast Asians and occurs in only 2%–5% of Africans. Some of the Asian D-negative population have a weak D antigen (D_{el}) and do not make anti-D. Thus, HDFN due to anti-D is rare among nonwhites.

ANTIBODIES OF POTENTIAL CLINICAL SIGNIFICANCE PRODUCED DURING PREGNANCY

Antibodies That Cause HDFN

Approximately 3%–6% of pregnant women have antibodies (other than ABO) of potential clinical significance.[2-9] Only antibodies that can cross the placenta cause HDFN; this restricts the cause of clinical problems to IgG antibodies. Table 13-1 shows antibodies, other than ABO, that have been reported to cause HDFN. Although it is clear that obstetric patients are becoming increasingly more commonly immunized to antigens other than D, anti-D is still probably the most common cause of HDFN (i.e., it might not be the most commonly detected antibody, but it still has the greatest potential to destroy fetal RBCs). Although almost any IgG antibody must be considered to have the potential to cause HDFN, very few other than anti-D appear to cause HDFN severe enough to require transfusion. There are many factors that affect the clinical significance of maternal alloantibodies (Table 13-2). Sometimes the respective antigen is not very well developed on the fetal RBCs (Table 13-3); thus, even though a strong IgG antibody is present in the mother's serum, the antibody might cause no HDFN or only a mild case.

Anti-c is usually described as being the next most common cause of severe HDFN after anti-D. Nevertheless, Mollison and coworkers[2] report that only about 30% of babies born with RBCs sensitized with anti-c require exchange transfusion, in contrast to 60% of babies born with anti-D–sensitized red cells. Wenk and associates[10] reported that the frequency of anti-c was 0.52 that of anti-D in their obstetric patients. Of 70 cases with maternal anti-c and c-positive babies, 16 babies (23%) had negative DATs and no evidence of HDFN. Of 46 cases who had HDFN, eight (17%) had mild disease and required no transfusion, 20 (43%) had moderate disease and required transfusion, and 8 (17%) died. Sixty-seven percent of the c-alloimmunized women who delivered babies with HDFN had a history of prior blood transfusion; there was a higher incidence of transfusion in the group of mothers delivering severely affected babies. Although anti-K is probably the most clinically potent antibody after ABO and Rh, it rarely causes HDFN, as only 9% of the white population (i.e., fathers of babies) are K positive. In two studies of 477,000 pregnancies, 0.1% of the women's sera contained anti-K; 78% of these were transfusion-induced.[11,12] As most fathers are K heterozygotes (Kk), fewer than 5% of K-negative mothers will carry a K-positive baby. Table 13-4 shows data from six publications on HDFN associated with anti-K.[13-18]

The pathogenesis of anti-K–related HDFN is often different from Rh disease. It was noted some years ago that babies could be born with severe HDFN due to anti-K and yet have negative DATs and/or low ΔOD values.[19,20] Vaughan and colleagues[21,22] showed that unlike Rh antibodies, anti-K can react with erythroid precursor cells. Thus, one component of the fetal/newborn anemia associated with anti-K could be due to suppressed erythropoiesis; extravascular hemolysis most often is present also.

Hardy and Napier[23] reviewed cases of HDFN in Wales (1948–1978) that were associated with antibodies other than anti-D. Of 557 women with Rh antibodies other than anti-D, 388 delivered babies whose RBCs had the relevant antigen, but only 75% of these had a positive DAT, and only 15% required treatment. There were 128 women with non-Rh antibodies (e.g., anti-K,

TABLE 13-1. BLOOD GROUP ANTIBODIES OTHER THAN ABO REPORTED AS A CAUSE OF HDFN

Blood Group System/Collection	Antibody	Severity of HDFN Most Often Encountered[a,b]
Rh	D	Moderate-severe
	C	Moderate-severe
	E	Moderate-severe
	c	Moderate-severe
	e	Mild-severe
	C^w	Mild-moderate
	C^x	Mild-severe
	E^w	Moderate-severe
	G	Moderate
	Go^a	Severe
	f(ce)	Severe
	Ce	Severe
	Rh:14	Moderate-severe
	Rh:15	Moderate-severe
	Rh:16	Moderate-severe
	Rh:29	Moderate-severe
	Rh:32	Moderate-severe
	Rh:36	Moderate-severe
	Rh:37	Moderate-severe
	Be^a	?
	Evans	?
	Tar	?
	Rh:42	Mild
	Riv	Mild
	Jal	Mild
	Stem	Mild
Kell	K	Mild-severe
	k	Mild-moderate
	Kp^a	Mild
	Kp^b	Mild-severe
	Js^a	Moderate
	Js^b	Mild-severe
	Ku	Mild-severe
	Ul^a	Mild-severe
	K22	Mild-severe
Duffy	Fy^a	Mild-severe
	Fy^b	Moderate
Kidd	Jk^a	Mild-severe
	Jk^b	Mild
	Jk3	Mild
MNSs	M	Mild-severe
	N	Mild
	'N'	Moderate
	S	Severe
	s	Severe
	U	Severe
	Mi^a	Mild-severe
	M^v	Mild
	M^iIII	Severe
	Mit	Mild
	Mt^a	Mild-severe
	V^w	Mild-severe
	Mur	Mild
	Hil	Mild
	Hut	Mild
	En^a	Severe
Globoside	P	Mild
Lutheran	Lu^a	Mild
	Lu^b	Mild
	Lu9	Mild
Diego	Di^a	Mild-severe
	Di^b	Mild-severe
	Wr^a	Mild-severe
	ELO	Mild-severe
Colton	Co^a	Mild-severe
	Co^b	Severe
	Co3	Severe
Gerbich	Ge	Mild-severe
Landsteiner-Weiner	LW	Mild-moderate
High-Frequency Antigens		
Augustine	At^a	Mild
Junior	Jr^a	Mild
Langereis	Lan	Mild-moderate
Vel	Vel	Mild
Low-Frequency Antigens		
Biles	Bi	Mild
Batty	By	Mild
Froese	Fr^a	Mild
Kamhuber	Far(Kam)	Severe
Livesey	Mild	
Gambino	Ga	Mild
Good	Severe	
Heibel	Severe	
Ht^a	Ht^a	Mild
Radin	Rd	Mild
Reid	Re^a	
Zd	Zd	Severe
Jones/Hol	Mild-moderate	
Scianna	Sc2	Moderate
Gonzales	Go^a	Mild
HJK	HJK	Severe
Kg	Kg	Severe
REIT	REIT	Severe

[a] Mild = no transfusions needed; phototherapy usually used
Moderate = transfusion given, but sometimes only after delivery
Severe = fetal death IUT and/or exchange transfusion

[b] Most examples of the antibodies listed, except anti-D, cause no HDFN. Severity relates to cases reported to have evidence of hemolytic anemia; this is sometimes a single case report.

–Fy, –Jk, etc.). These women delivered 35 babies whose RBCs had the appropriate antigen; 91% of these had a positive DAT, but only 6% (one anti-Fy^a and one anti-Kp^a) required treatment. Walker[6] reviewed his experiences over a 12-year period (1972–1983) in which 104 examples of IgG antibodies other than anti-D were encountered; this represented one in 537 deliveries. Approximately 71% of these infants were unaffected by the antibodies; 22% had early onset of jaundice, and 7% had bilirubin levels exceeding 12.9 mg/dL. In only one case (anti-E) was an exchange transfusion required; this was 40 hours after birth and perhaps not related to the anti-E sensitization.

In Manitoba, Canada (population 1 million), the mean annual occurrence of D alloimmunization in pregnant women dropped from 194 in the 5-year period ending October 31, 1967 to 28 in the 6-year period ending October 31, 1988.[11,13] In the same two

TABLE 13-2. FACTORS THAT COULD AFFECT SIGNIfiCANCE OF MATERNAL ALLOANTIBODIES

1. Class and subclass of antibody
2. Strength/quantity of antibody
3. Presence, or strength, of antigen on fetal RBCs (see Table 13-3)
4. Efficiency of placental transfer
5. Efficiency of fetal reticuloendothelial system
6. Competition effect of antigen present in fetal body fluids or fetal tissue
7. Maternal blocking antibodies (capable of blocking fetal macrophage receptors)

TABLE 13-3. PRESENCE AND RELATIVE STRENGTH OF ANTIGENS ON CORD CELLS

Antigen Strength	Blood Group System or Antigen
Well developed at birth	MNSsU
	Rh
	Kell
	Duffy
	Kidd
	Diego
	Dombrock
	Scianna
	Gerbich
	En^{a}
	Yt^{b}
Present at birth but weaker than on adult red cells	ABH
	P
	Lutheran
	Xg^{a}
Very weak or absent at birth	Yt^{a}
	Vel
	Lewis
	I
	Sd^{a}
	Chido

periods, the mean annual occurrence of alloimmunization associated with alloantibodies other than anti-D increased from 14 to 88. It was suggested that this increase was due partially to the increased screening of pregnant D-positive women. This increase was also likely due to an increase in the frequency of blood transfusion. It should be noted that 48% of babies born to mothers with anti-D were affected (i.e., RBCs were sensitized with maternal antibody), but only 51% of these required treatment. If one excludes the one case associated with anti-k, 2.4%–65% of babies born to mothers having antibodies other than anti-D showed any signs of being affected, and only 12%–50% of these required treatment. Table 13-5 shows data, published by Bowman, on the severity of HDFN associated with all antibodies detected in a 26-year period.[11,13] These data represent experiences of 1442 cases of HDFN. Almost half of D-positive babies born to mothers with anti-D did not require therapy. Up to 88% of antigen-positive babies born to mothers with other antibodies (including Rh antibodies other than anti-D) did not require therapy.

The specificity of the antibody should be a good clue to its potential to cause HDFN (see Table 13-1). In some cases (e.g., anti-M), it could be useful to determine the immunoglobulin class (IgG or IgM) of the antibody, which can usually be easily done using 2-mercaptoethanol (2ME) or dithiothreitol (DTT). If the antibody is IgG and has the potential for causing HDFN, knowledge of the father's genotype is another aid to predicting whether the baby is likely to be affected by the antibody. When anti-D is involved, the chances are that the baby's father will be D positive, but it is useful to determine the father's Rh phenotype and hence the possible genotype. This information is also useful if the infant is born affected and the mother wants to plan further pregnancies (i.e., the child of a father homozygous for D will always be D positive, and the outcome of future pregnancies will be similar or worse). Phenotyping the father's RBCs is especially useful when antibodies other than Rh are

TABLE 13-4. HDFN ASSOCIATED WITH ANTI-K

Reference	Period Studied	No. of Anti-K	No. of Mothers Previously Transfused (%)	No. of Affected Babies	No. of Babies Treated or IUFD[b]
13	1977–1983	211	71	7	4
14	1969–1984	127[b]	67	13	9
15	1980–1989	407[c]	88	10	5
16	1944–1990	459	NA	20	8
17	1959–1995	156	63	21	13
18	1984–1996	65	45	18	?11[d]

[a] K+ baby and/or +DAT, with or without HDFN
[b] Intrauterine fetal death (IUFD) or treated with transfusion and/or phototherapy
[c] 0.1% of all pregnancies during this period
[d] Not clear in publication
NA, not available

TABLE 13-5. SEVERITY OF HEMOLYTIC DISEASE IN MANITOBA DURING 26 YEARS[11,13]

Alloantibody	Number of Women	% of Affected Babies*	Not Requiring Treatment
D (13 yrs)	420	48	49
E	350	31	88
c, cE	183	65	62
C, Ce, C^w	108	32	79
K	337	2.4	75
Kp^a	6	33	50
k	1	100	
Fy^a	23	22	80
S	14	57	75

*Affected – any signs suggesting HDFN (e.g., positive DAT because babies' RBCs possess putative antigen)

involved. For instance, anti-K is usually caused by previous transfusions, and there is a good chance that the father and child will be K negative.

Table 13-1 lists antibodies associated with HDFN and the degree of severity reported.

There are many single-case reports in the literature of other antibodies that are said to be associated with HDFN, but no evidence is presented for a hemolytic process; often, the term HDFN is equated with the finding of antibodies in the mother and a baby with a positive DAT. As has been emphasized by Bowman's[11,13] data (see Table 13-5), a positive DAT indicates that the fetal RBCs have become sensitized with antibody, but this does not equate with hemolytic disease.

Predicting the Presence and Severity of HDFN

ANTIBODY SCREENING

Following the discovery that anti-Rh(D) could cause HDFN, it became common practice to screen the sera from all Rh(D)-negative pregnant women for Rh antibodies. Later, when it was found that Rh(D)-positive women could also have babies with HDFN due to Rh antibodies (other than anti-D) and non-Rh antibodies, it was suggested that sera from all pregnant women be screened for antibodies. For some years, the most common practice in the United States has been to screen sera from all women when they first present to the obstetrician. Sera from Rh-negative women are screened again at approximately 28 weeks, and some institutions routinely test pregnant women again at 32–36 weeks. This later screening has received some support from workers in Oxford, England. Bowell and colleagues[24] examined results of screening 70,000 sera from pregnant women. Irregular antibodies were found in 1% of the women, and two thirds of these were found in D-positive women. Seventy percent of the antibodies were detectable in the sample taken at the first visit. Rh-negative women and women with a transfusion history who did not have antibodies detected at the first visit were tested again at 28 weeks; all women were retested at 32–36 weeks. Sampling at 28 weeks alone did not detect all the antibodies developing during pregnancy—fewer than 50% had appeared by this time. Clinically affected infants—in particular those requiring exchange transfusions—were found much more commonly among pregnancies in which antibodies were detected at the first visit (before 26 weeks) than among those in which antibodies developed later; this was found to be true for both anti-D and anti-c.[24,25] Deaths due to anti-D were entirely confined to mothers with antibodies detected at the first visit. Based on their findings, Bowell and colleagues[24] proposed that the practice of screening all mothers before 26 weeks should continue, but only unsensitized Rh-negative and previously transfused mothers should be retested at 28 weeks and at 34–36 weeks; the remaining Rh-positive women need only be retested at 34–36 weeks. It must be emphasized that if this later screening is done, care must be taken not to misinterpret results due to antenatal Rh immunoprophylaxis that could have started at 28 weeks. The proposals suggested by Bowell and colleages[24] are in direct contrast to those of Walker,[6] who suggested (from a cost-benefit point of view) that no screening is necessary for D-positive women. Rothenberg and coworkers[26] found that only six of 9348 (0.06%) D-positive pregnant women developed new antibodies during the third trimester. Heddle and associates[27] found that 58 of 17,568 (0.24%) pregnant women had new antibodies detectable at delivery that were not present during first-trimester testing. In both studies, no significant neonatal problems were encountered due to these new antibodies.

The Scientific Section Coordinating Committee of the American Association of Blood Banks (AABB) has issued guidelines (not AABB standards) for serological testing of pregnant women.[28] Table 13-6 shows their recommendations for prenatal testing.

QUANTITATING THE AMOUNT OF SERUM ANTIBODY

Until the advent of amniocentesis, antibody titers were used routinely in an attempt to predict the severity of HDFN. After the advent of amniocentesis, indirect antiglobulin test (IAT) titers were usually used as a guide to indicate the need to perform amniocentesis. Titers provide only semiquantitative estimates and are not a measure of the total antibody concentration. Titers give only rough estimates of the amount of antibody bound to the target RBCs and do not measure the amount of antibody remaining free in solution at the endpoint of agglutination. Hughes-Jones[29] has shown that the poor correlation between titer and antibody concentration is dependent on the equilibrium constant and heterogeneity index of the

TABLE 13-6. RECOMMENDED PRENATAL TESTING

Testing and Condition	Timing
ABO	
First pregnancy	Initial visit
Subsequent pregnancies	Initial visit
Other	For pretransfusion testing
Rh (test for weak D optional)	
First pregnancy	Initial visit and at 26–28 weeks' gestation
Subsequent pregnancies	Initial visit
Other	For pretransfusion testing
Unexpected Antibodies	
All pregnancies	Initial visit
D– pregnancies	Before Rh Ig therapy (optional)
D+ pregnancies	Third trimester if transfused or history of unexpected antibodies
Other	For pretransfusion testing
Antibody Identification	
Unexpected antibodies present	Upon initial detection
Confirmatory testing	At time of titration
Antibody Titration	
Rh antibodies	Upon initial detection Repeat at 18–20 weeks' gestation Repeat at 2- to 4-week intervals if below critical titer (16–32)
Other potentially significant antibodies	As above, with discussion with obstetrician

From Judd WJ: Practice guidelines for prenatal and perinatal immunotematology, revisited. Transfusion 2001;41:1445–1452.

antibody, the concentration of the RBCs, and the inherent error of the method. Complete reproduction is almost impossible, and only a difference in titer of at least two tubes (more than fourfold), or of a score of 10 (see Chapter 6), should be considered significant. The coefficient of variation with manual titrations is plus or minus 100% or more for intralaboratory replicates and much higher for interlaboratory estimates.[30] Thus, it is perhaps not surprising that titers were not very good at predicting the severity of HDFN. Although an Rh-positive baby born to a mother who has a high titer of anti-D (e.g., >100) is usually affected to some degree, many severely affected babies have been born to mothers with relatively low titers (e.g., 8). Nevertheless, Bowman[11,13] feels that titers have been very useful in his experience of monitoring thousands of cases of HDFN over a period of more than 30 years.

When titers are performed routinely (e.g., at 2- to 4-week intervals after 18 weeks gestation), the technique should be standardized as much as possible (e.g., same test system, same volume of sera/RBCs, RBC phenotype, and preferably the same technologist each time tests are performed), and it is very important that the current serum sample be titrated in parallel with a stored previous sample. A change (i.e., increase) in titer under these conditions yields as much, if not more, valuable information as the absolute value. As mentioned previously, antibody titers are not usually used in current practice to predict the severity of HDFN but rather to indicate the need for amniocentesis and/or other clinical studies. Because of the inaccuracies already mentioned, even the value of this should be questioned. Most hospitals have a titer (e.g., 32) above which they recommend amniocentesis, but they rarely have any data to support the use of this particular value; this has become known as the "critical antibody titer" in the United States. Gall and Miller[31] reported on a retrospective study of Rh-sensitized women over a period of 24 years. Records of 202 obstetric patients representing 280 sensitized pregnancies from a pool of 39,910 deliveries were analyzed. A significant correlation between severity of HDFN and results of amniotic fluid analysis (ΔOD_{450}), cord hematocrit, and bilirubin was noted. Although there was a significant correlation between antibody titer and severity of HDFN, 12 infants had mild to severe HDFN with titers of 16 or less, although it should be pointed out that only three of these babies needed treatment. Gall and Miller[31] suggested that critical antibody titer, as the initiating event to begin amniocentesis, be abandoned. They suggested initiating amniocentesis on any woman who has detectable Rh antibody, regardless of the level. Nevertheless, in the United States, the "critical titer" is still in common use.

In the United Kingdom, it is more common practice to quantitate anti-D in ng or IU/mL using an AutoAnalyzer. Bowell and associates[32,33] found, on examination of the records of 288 pregnancies resulting in D-positive babies, that the chance of producing a severely affected baby rises with increasing maternal anti-D levels. In 140 pregnancies in which the maternal anti-D level remained below 4 IU/mL, only five babies required exchange transfusion, and no baby had a cord hemoglobin below 10 g/dL. On the other hand, of 148 pregnancies in which the anti-D level rose above 4 IU/mL, 99 babies required exchange transfusions, and 25 babies had a cord hemoglobin below 10 g/dL. The researchers concluded that those pregnancies in which anti-D concentrations remained below 4 IU/mL represented a safe group for whom amniocentesis should be avoided. More recently, maternal anti-D concentrations lower than 15 IU/mL were found to be associated with little or no fetal anemia as assessed by fetoscopy.[34] The extent of fetal hemolysis at high concentrations was found to be highly variable. A cutoff value of 10 IU/mL is now generally used in the United Kingdom to indicate the need for invasive tests such as percutaneous umbilical blood sampling (PUBS).[1,2]

PREVIOUS HISTORY OF PREGNANT WOMAN

If an expectant mother has antibodies (e.g., anti-D), it is rare for HDFN to occur in the first pregnancy. Each successive D-positive baby is more likely to suffer with increasingly severe HDFN.[2] If hydrops occurs due to anti-D, there is a 90% chance that the next D-positive fetus will die in utero.[2]

AMNIOTIC FLUID ANALYSIS

As early as 1950, Bevis[35] used amniotic fluid to predict the severity of HDFN. Analysis of a bilirubin pigment in amniotic fluid became popular after publication of a method by Liley[36] in 1961. Amniotic fluid, protected from the light that destroys bilirubin, was centrifuged and filtered. Optical density (OD) measurements above the 350–700 nm range were plotted on semilogarithmic paper using wavelength as the horizontal linear coordinate and OD as the vertical logarithmic coordinate. The plotting readings were corrected, and the deviation from linearity at 450 nm (OD_{450}) was measured. Based on ΔOD_{450} measurements made after 29 weeks in 101 Rh-sensitized pregnancies, Liley[36] divided his readings into three zones. He suggested that fluids that gave ΔOD_{450} measurements in zone 3 were indicative of severe HDFN (e.g., hydrops or fetal death within 7 to 10 days); zone 1 indicated an unaffected or mildly affected baby, and zone 2 measurements were intermediate. It was necessary to relate the ΔOD_{450} values to gestational age. There have been many reports confirming the value of this procedure to monitor the condition of the fetus. For instance, Bowman[37] reported results on 997 pregnant women. He made the following observations:

1. A single ΔOD_{450} reading of 0.400 or higher at any age of gestation is associated with the presence of hydrops fetalis 65% of the time.
2. Occasionally, hydrops might be present at 28 weeks of gestation when the ΔOD_{450} reading is 0.200–0.250.
3. ΔOD_{450} reading at the 80%–85% level in zone 2 can advance to a zone 3 reading and the presence of hydrops within 2 weeks.
4. Rapid increases in ΔOD_{450} and severity of Rh disease can occur. Thus, a reading in low zone 2 at 23 weeks might be followed by a reading in zone 3 2 weeks later, with the presence of an hydropic fetus at the time of the second amniocentesis.
5. On rare occasions, initial ΔOD_{450} readings of 0.200–0.250 at 22–24 weeks' gestation might be associated with an Rh-negative fetus.

Queenan and colleagues[38] pointed out that Liley charts started at 27 weeks' gestation and that projected values before this time were inaccurate. He presented a revised Liley chart (Fig. 13-1), which is now the one commonly used.

In 1996, the American College of Gynecology (ACOG)[39] recommended that amniocentesis or PUBS should be considered if the antibody titer is 32 or

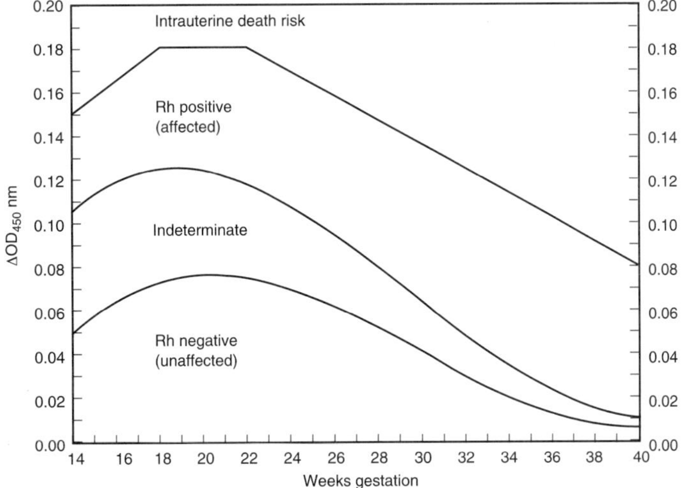

FIGURE 13-1. Amniotic Fluid ΔOD 450 management zones. (From Queenan JT, Tomai TP, Ural SH, et al: Deviation in amniotic fluid optical density at a wavelength of 450 nm in Rh-immunized pregnancies from 14 to 40 weeks gestation: A proposal for clinical management. Am J Obstet Gynecol 1993;168:1370–1376.)

greater. If a patient has had a prior affected pregnancy (neonatal exchange transfusion, early delivery for alloimmunization, or intrauterine transfusion), antibody titers are not necessary because amniocentesis or percutaneous umbilical cord blood sampling will be required. The timing of the initial procedure is determined by past clinical history. It is usually performed at least 4 to 8 weeks earlier than the prior gestational age at which significant morbidity occurred, with some clinicians beginning at 20 weeks or even earlier.

Readings in zone III (the uppermost zone) suggest severe hemolytic disease with a high probability of fetal death within 7 to 10 days. Readings in zone I (the lowest zone) are reassuring, although neonatal exchange transfusion could be necessary occasionally. There are no reliable data concerning the optimal frequency for repeated sampling. In general, amniocentesis is repeated every 1 to 4 weeks if the ΔOD_{450} measurement is in zone II (middle zone) and every 3 to 4 weeks if it has dropped into zone I. The frequency depends on where in zone II the value falls and the pattern established in previous procedures. Declining values are encouraging, although they do not preclude mild hemolytic disease. Stable or rising ΔOD_{450} measurements are causes of concern.[39]

Patients with results in zone I or low zone II can be allowed to proceed to term, at which point labor should be induced. In most cases, patients in the middle of zone II can progress to 36–38 weeks' gestation, at which time delivery should be accomplished, by induction of labor if possible. Depending on gestational age, patients in zone III should either be delivered or should receive intrauterine fetal transfusion. Similar considerations can apply to a rising titer in upper zone II. Delivery is often by cesarean birth because of an unfavorable cervix, but a trial of labor is not contraindicated.[39]

In patients with a poor obstetric history or in whom the initial titer is 16 or greater before 27 weeks, the timing of the initial diagnostic procedure depends on the severity of erythroblastosis in prior pregnancies, on ultrasound findings, and on the degree of titer elevation. In more severely affected cases, many experts currently recommend that fetal blood sampling rather than amniocentesis be used to assess the fetus during the second trimester. This is particularly important if the father is heterozygous for the offending antigen. At the time of the initial blood sampling, the fetal hematocrit and antigen status can be determined. If the fetus is anemic, transfusion is indicated at that time. If the fetus is not anemic and the relevant antigen is found to be present on the fetal blood cells, the timing of future diagnostic procedures will depend on history, serial ultrasound findings, and the hematocrit at the time of the last sample. If the fetus is found to be antigen negative, no further procedures are necessary.[39]

Figure 13-2 shows a management scheme suggested by Moise.[40]

OTHER METHODS FOR ASSESSING AND PREDICTING THE SEVERITY OF HDFN

Ultrasound. The pathophysiology of HDFN predicts that fetal anemia will trigger exaggerated erythropoiesis, resulting in hypertrophy of the placenta and fetal liver or spleen. The placenta will become edematous and the liver parenchyma congested. The obstructive hepatomegaly and hypoproteinemia, together with high-output congestive heart failure, eventually result in fetal abdominal ascites followed by scalp and limb edema, hydrothorax, and pericardial effusion. In its terminal stage, the hydropic fetus could demonstrate cardiomegaly. Some of these changes can be shown using ultrasound. Weiner and coworkers[41] found that ultrasound was slightly more accurate than amniotic fluid analysis in predicting moderate to severe HDFN. In their series of 57 gravidas (including three twin pregnancies), amniotic fluid analysis correctly predicted an affected or healthy neonate in 79% of the cases, with three false-positive predictions. Real-time sonography accurately predicted the clinical course in 86% of the cases, with no false-positive predictions. The authors found that the most useful ultrasound findings were serial measurements of the fetal abdominal circumference and fetal liver size. Others have not found ultrasound to be so valuable.[42,43] Nicolaides and asociates[43] correlated ultrasound findings and the degree of fetal anemia as assessed by fetal blood sampling. Ultrasound was found to be unreliable in predicting fetal anemia in the absence of hydrops.[43] More recently, Doppler ultrasonography, which measures fetal hemodynamics, has been applied.

Fetal Doppler Ultrasonography. Doppler ultrasonography is a noninvasive method of studying fetal hemodynamics.[42] There have been many studies relating Doppler blood velocity evaluations and fetal anemia. The most useful results have resulted from studies of middle cerebral artery time-averaged mean blood velocity. Mari[44] reported the results of a large multicenter study involving 110 alloimmunized pregnancies. They found that moderate and severe fetal anemia could be detected by an increased peak velocity in the middle cerebral artery, with a sensitivity of 100% and a false-positive rate of 12%. Stefos and colleages[45] added confirmatory data. Nevertheless, in 2002 Abdel-Fattah and Soothill[42] reviewed applications of ultrasound (including Doppler) to HDFN and concluded that although the information from the fetal aorta blood velocity measurements resulted in an improvement of the prediction equation, the morphological measurements were of no benefit. They concluded that careful attention to the woman's obstetric history and serial antibody quantitation is equally important to the use of Doppler ultrasonography.

Fetoscopy, Percutaneous Umbilical Blood Sampling (Cordocentesis/Funipuncture), and Chorionic Villus Biopsy. Fetoscopy is a technique in which the second-trimester fetus can be visualized directly and

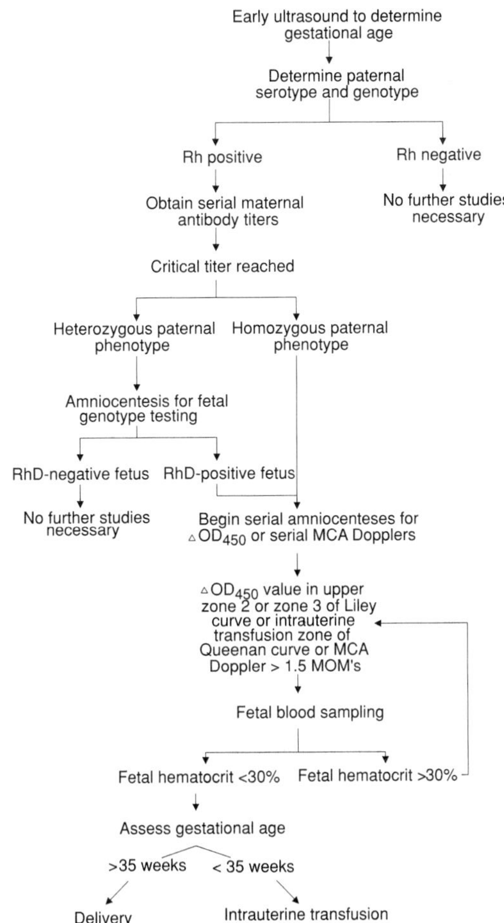

FIGURE 13-2. Flow chart showing a plan for managing the first affected pregnancy. (From Moise KJ Jr: Changing trends in the management of red blood cell alloimmunization in pregnancy. Arch Pathol Lab Med 1994;118:421-428.)

fetal blood (or other tissues) can be sampled through an endoscope introduced transabdominally into the amniotic cavity.[46] The technique is only reliably successful at 16 weeks' gestation and later.[47,48] There is about a 5% mortality rate due to fetoscopy, compared with a 1%–2% mortality rate after midtrimester amniocentesis.[47,48] The fetal blood can be tested for blood type, DAT, hemoglobin, and hematocrit. MacKenzie and coworkers[47,48] suggested that the technique would be of benefit in cases in which the father of the baby is known to be heterozygous for the offending blood group antigen in the following situations:

1. Patients with a history of previous babies having severe HDFN
2. Patients with high-titer anti-D (e.g., in excess of 20 IU/mL) during the first 20 weeks of pregnancy

The authors felt that knowledge that the fetus was blood group incompatible would save considerable time, effort, and expense by obviating the need for further diagnostic tests and exacting methods of treatment. MacKenzie and colleagues[47] gives an example of an Rh-negative woman whose husband was of the probable R_2r (cDE/cde) genotype. The woman had anti-D quantitated at 40 IU/mL at 10 weeks' gestation; fetal blood sampling was not available. The couple, with one living child, were desperate for a second child. They requested repeated plasmapheresis, which was performed on 54 occasions until delivery followed premature rupture of the membranes at 35 weeks' gestation; the baby was Rh-negative and the DAT was negative at birth. In 59 Rh-immunized pregnancies, Nicolaides and colleagues[49] compared the predictive values of the ΔOD_{450} of amniotic fluid and the hemoglobin level of fetal blood obtained by fetal blood sampling. Studies were performed at 18–25 weeks' gestation. The authors found a significant linear correlation between the degree of fetal anemia and ΔOD_{450} of amniotic fluid; however, the values were widely scattered, limiting their predictive value. There was no ΔOD_{450} level that clearly separated severely from mildly affected babies. If the cutoff level was set low enough to include 90% of the severely affected babies (e.g., >0.2 nm), the group would also include 54% of the mildly affected babies. Alternatively, if the cutoff level was set high enough (>0.5 nm), the false-negative rate was 77%. There was an overall linear correlation between fetal hemoglobin and OD_{450}. The normal range of fetal hemoglobin was found not to change within the gestational range of 16–25 weeks. Although the predictive value of the ΔOD_{450} in the third trimester has been said to be 94.5%, the data of Nicolaides and colleagues[49] cast serious doubt on applying the same logic to the second trimester. Of the 31 most severely anemic fetuses (hemoglobin <6 g/dL), which included 14 fetuses with hydrops fetalis, only 10 (32%) would have received intrauterine transfusions at the time of amniocentesis had the "extrapolated" Liley criteria been used.[49] Nicolaides and colleagues[49] conclude by suggesting that although fetal blood sampling could be associated with a marginally greater risk of fetal morbidity than amniocentesis, the only accurate method to assess the severity of fetal anemia in the second trimester is to measure the hemoglobin level of fetal blood. In 1983, Daffos and coworkers[50] reported a new technique for obtaining fetal blood that involved umbilical cord sampling with an ultrasonically guided 20-gauge needle. They later reported a series of 606 fetal blood samplings in 562 pregnancies from 17 to 38 weeks' gestation.[51] Their reported complications were premature delivery (5%), growth retardation (8%), in utero death (1.1%), and spontaneous abortion (0.8%). This PUBS is now more popular than blood sampling using fetoscopy.[52]

Fetoscopy and PUBS have been used to obtain blood for studying the presence and development of blood group antigens on fetal RBCs. These have included ABO and Rh and 30 other blood group antigens.[53,54] Habibi and colleagues[54] confirmed that I, Le^a, and Le^b are not expressed on fetal RBCs and that the expression of A, B, H, P_1, P, Lu^a, and Lu^b antigen is decreased compared with adults. Many antigens, including D, C, c, E, e, K, k, Kp^a, Kp^b, Fy^a, Fy^b, Jk^a, Jk^b, M, N, S, s, Xg^a, Ve^a, and Ge^a, appeared to be fully developed by the second half of gestation. The P antigen was found to be absent from 12% and weakly expressed on 10% of the fetal samples, which were constantly P_1 negative. Some investigators have used a technique known as chorionic villus sampling (CVS) to obtain fetal blood samples during the first trimester of pregnancy. These investigators have studied ABO, Rh, and K antigens on fetal RBCs from CVS between 8 and 12 weeks' gestation.[55-57] They suggest that such studies could be useful in predicting the clinical course of a fetus of an immunized mother, but on the other hand, there is a total pregnancy loss rate of 0.6–0.8% higher than with amniocentesis.[58]

Prenatal Determination of Fetal Blood Group. For many years, the babies' blood group was determined as an educated guess. The process involved serological testing of the mother and father and evaluating the heterozygosity vs. homozygosity of the father by relating to published data of the probability of phenotype results representing a certain genotype. The father's result was reported as a "probable genotype" (Table 13-7). If the father was thought to be homozygous, the baby was assumed to possess the putative antigen. If the father was heterozygous, there was a 50% chance that the baby was antigen positive. With the advent of PUBS, it was possible to obtain RBCs from the fetus to type the fetus using routine serology. It is now possible to determine the Rh(D,c,E), K, Fy^a, and Jk^a status of the fetus accurately, applying molecular techniques to the fetal RBCs, amniocytes, or even the maternal plasma.[59–61] Molecular techniques can also be used to determine the father's true genotype. Although this is the modern approach, readers should be warned that results should be relied on only if they come from laboratories with a trusted knowledge base in the complexity of the Rh system at the DNA level.

In Vitro Predictive Tests Utilizing Functional Cellular Assays. In vitro functional cellular assays, based on the in vivo mechanisms of RBC immune destruction, have been developed and applied to predicting the clinical significance of alloantibodies involved in HDFN and hemolytic transfusion reactions.[62-76] These assays are based on sensitizing RBCs with the putative antibody and adding these sensitized RBCs to monocytes in vitro. The interactions with the monocytes are measured by recording RBC adherence/phagocytosis by a monocyte monolayer assay (MMA), antibody-dependent cellular cytotoxicity (ADCC) using ^{51}Cr-labeled RBCs, or a chemiluminescence test (CL) using luminol. The MMA and CL have been found to be equivalent to performing a 1-hour ^{51}Cr-RBC survival study when evaluating the possibility of transfusing incompatible blood. Application of these assays to predicting severity of HDFN has been more controversial (see the discussion later in this chapter).

In 1995, some international experts reviewed laboratory procedures that were found useful in predicting the severity of HDFN.[65] They were asked: "Is a laboratory procedure used in your country/center to predict the severity of HDFN?" If so:

1. Which assay is used?
2. Why was this assay selected?
3. At which time during pregnancy is the assay performed?
4. How are the results interpreted, and what are the consequences for the management of the case?

If not:

1. How are known cases of maternal alloimmunization managed; that is, how is the status of the fetus controlled?"

The main conclusion from the answers received was that in assessing the clinical significance of maternal

TABLE 13-7. ESTIMATES OF THE LIKELIHOOD OF HOMOZYGOSITY FOR D IN CAUCASIANS

Phenotype	Anti-D	Anti-C	Anti-c	Anti-E	Anti-e	Probable Genotypes*		Likelihood of Homozygosity for D
R_1r	+	+	+	–	+	DCe/dce	R^1r	4.8%
						DCe/Dce	R^1R^0	
R_1R_1	+	+	–	–	+	DCe/DCe	R^1R^1	97.6%
						DCe/dCe	R^1r'	
R_2r	+	–	+	+	+	DcE/dce	R^2r	4.8%
						DcE/Dce	R^2R^0	
R_1R_2	+	+	+	+	+	DCe/DcE	R^1R^2	96.7%
						DCe/dcE	R^1R''	
						dCe/DcE	$r'R^2$	
R_2R_2	+	–	+	+	–	DcE/DcE	R^2R^2	96.6%
						DcE/dcE	R^2r''	

*Rare alternative genotypes have not been shown.

anti-D, functional cellular assays are not used routinely except in the Netherlands. In all other countries, determination of the IAT titer (and in most cases, the determination of the concentration of anti-D using an AutoAnalyzer) are the routine procedures used. If the titer is above a critical level (mostly >16–32) or the anti-D concentration is greater than 4–5 IU, special attention is given to the status of the fetus, and if the concentration is greater than 10–15 IU, the case is usually referred to a center specializing in the management of HDFN. Several answers stressed that an increase in anti-D titer or concentration during pregnancy is of greater significance than the actual titer or concentration. In the Netherlands, the ADCC test with monocytes as effector cells is routinely applied in the Central Laboratory of the Netherlands Red Cross Blood Transfusion Service (now known as the Sanquine Blood Supply Foundation) for the whole country.[65,68] The results of the test determine whether cordocentesis is indicated and whether the case should be referred to a specialized center.[65] In some other countries, a functional assay is used in special cases (e.g., if in a previous pregnancy the severity of the HDFN was much worse than expected from the anti-D titer or concentration, or when there is a rapid increase in anti-D).[68]

It now seems generally accepted, based on the results of several comparative studies, that the ADCC test and the CL test with monocytes as effector cells offer the best predictive value for severity of HDFN, when using functional cellular assays.

Antibody-Dependent Cellular Cytotoxicity. Urbaniak and coworkers[67] used a lymphocyte-driven ADCC assay to predict the severity of HDFN. They sensitized homologous enzyme-treated group O Rh-positive RBCs with maternal antibody and used these as target cells in the ADCC assay, utilizing normal donor lymphocytes as effector cells. They described three cases in which amniotic fluid OD_{450} (Liley low zone in cases one and two and mid-zone in case three) predicted a favorable outcome although maternal anti-D levels predicted a poor outcome (26, 20, and 50 IU/mL, respectively); the ADCC assay results were positive in cases 1 and 3 and negative for case 2. Cases 1 and 3 needed exchange transfusion at birth, whereas case 2 required only "top-up" transfusion. In five cases in which antibody levels were high and OD_{450} predicted the outcome correctly, the ADCC assay was also positive. In two cases in which, despite high anti-D levels, the babies required no treatment, extremely low ADCC assay activity was observed. In one case, the baby was Rh negative and the OD_{450} was high mid-zone, indicating an affected baby; the ADCC assay also gave a false-positive result.

In the Netherlands, an ADCC assay using monocytes rather than lymphocytes is performed in a central laboratory.[65,68] When anti-D is detected for the first time, the ADCC assay is first done during the 32nd week of pregnancy. If anti-D was found in the previous pregnancy, the ADCC test is done for the first time at the 20th week. If the results in a previous pregnancy were predictive of a severe HDFN, the assay is performed between weeks 12 and 14. Based on the analysis of a large number of cases (n = 482), the results of the tests were interpreted as follows:

- ADCC lower than 30%: No hemolysis expected; no amniotic fluid analysis; after week 32, repeat ADCC test every 2 weeks; after week 36, repeat ADCC weekly; before week 32, repeat ADCC test every 3 to 4 weeks.
- ADCC 30%–50%: No hemolysis or moderate hemolysis expected; fetus control by ultrasonography; amniotic fluid analysis, but frequency to depend on the results of the first analysis; after week 32, repeat every 2 weeks; after week 36, repeat ADCC weekly; before week 32, repeat every 3 weeks.
- ADCC greater than 50%: Severe hemolysis expected; patient referred to a center specialized in the management of HDFN.

Oepkes and colleagues[68] compared the ADCC assay with antibody titers and found that the ADCC assay consistently showed a higher predictive value for fetal disease than did the AGT titer.

Monocyte Monolayer Assay. Nance and her Los Angeles colleagues[69,70] compared the efficiency of the MMA with that of titers and amniotic fluid OD_{450}, in predicting the severity of HDFN. Maternal sera were taken at birth or at the time of amniocentesis, from women with antibodies of potential clinical significance in their sera. Cord sera, DAT-positive cord RBCs, and eluates from these RBCs were also tested.[70] The sera and eluates were used to sensitize allogeneic group O RBCs having the reactive antigen (e.g., D). The sensitized RBCs were added to a monocyte monolayer prepared from normal donor· Thirty-one cases with anti-D, 12 cases with other Rh antibodies (six anti-c, two anti-C, one anti-E, two anti-c+E, and one anti-c+s), and seven cases with non-Rh antibodies (two anti-K, one anti-S, one anti-Jk^a, one anti-Jk^b, one anti-Wr^a, and one anti-Di^b) were studied.[70] The babies were divided into five groups. Group 1 (n = 4) were asymptomatic; group 2 (n = 21) had bilirubin levels greater than 5 mg% at 48 hours but required no treatment; group 3 (n = 6) required phototherapy for jaundice; group 4 (n = 6) required IUT or neonatal transfusions; group 5 (n = 4) were fatal cases. The MMA results using maternal sera were better than the others at predicting whether babies would need treatment (groups 3, 4, and 5). As might be expected, the maternal sera gave slightly more false-positive results (e.g., in one case of an Rh-negative infant whose mother's serum contained high-titer anti-D). The antibody titer was better than some other studies have suggested, with an efficiency of 72%–80%; the efficiency of the MMA was 83%, but the predictive value of a negative test was 94% (16 of

17 negative MMAs were associated with a benign clinical course). As the MMA showed a reasonable correlation with the clinical status of the baby at birth, a further study was performed to see how the MMA would compare with amniotic fluid analysis during the pregnancy in predicting severity of HDFN.[70] Parallel studies of amniotic fluid OD_{450} and MMAs were performed on 29 sera from 16 pregnant women with Rh antibodies (nine anti-D, three anti-C+D, two anti-E, one anti-E+D, one anti-c). The predictive value (PV) of positive OD_{450} result (Liley zone mid-2 to -3) was 100%, but the PV of a negative result was only 60%; the efficiency of the OD_{450} was 75%. The PV of a positive MMA was 91% and the PV of a negative MMA was 100%, giving an efficiency of 94%. These results suggested that the MMA would be a very useful test for predicting the severity of HDFN. It was noninvasive and thus did not carry any risks to the mother or baby. Its only disadvantage seemed to be an occasional false-positive result (e.g., when the mother is carrying an Rh-negative baby and has Rh antibodies in her serum). The assay seemed to be a good adjunct to other noninvasive approaches such as ultrasound.

Larson and associates[74] agreed with the findings of Nance and colleagues[70] that the MMA yielded a high PV (a negative PV of 100% and a positive PV of 87.5%). In contrast, Moise and coworkers[75] found there was no difference in MMA results between anemic and nonanemic fetuses. In two later studies by the Los Angeles group, the MMA was found to only have an efficiency of and 66% and 57%, respectively.[62,71] The two latter studies included antibodies other than anti-D and babies who lacked antigens reactive with the maternal antibody; in addition, there were less severely affected babies than in the earlier studies.[62,70] Similar findings were reported by Zupanska and colleagues,[72,73] who at first reported the MMA to be efficient in predicting the severity of HDFN but later found that the assay failed when moderate disease was present.

Chemiluminescence Test. The CL has been compared with ADCC, MMA, and antibody quantitation in predicting the severity of HDFN.[76] The CL appeared to be equivalent to the ADCC assay and more efficient than MMA and antibody quantitation.

IgG Subclass. Most IgG Rh antibodies formed during pregnancy are IgG1 and IgG3. Frankowska and Gorska[77] found that 87.6% of sera from 65 pregnant women contained IgG1 Rh antibodies, 23% contained IgG2 antibodies, 56.9% contained IgG3 antibodies, and 7.7% contained IgG4 antibodies. Most commonly, the sera contained IgG1 alone (33.9%) or IgG1 + IgG3 (32.3%); no sera contained IgG2 and/or IgG4 without IgG1 or IgG3. Ouwehand and associates[78] studied 52 isoimmunized D-negative women; 35% of them produced only IgG1 antibodies, 29% produced only IgG3 anti-D, and 39% produced both IgG1 and IgG3. Parinaud and colleagues[79] found that IgG1 and IgG3 Rh antibodies were equally represented (present in 59% of sera) in 103 isoimmunized women. Nance and coworkers[80] reported on 86 alloimmunized pregnancies (51 anti-D, eight –D,C, six –c, six –E, 2 – cE, two –K, and one each anti-D,E, -D,C,E, -D,C,s, -C, -C^w, -e, -Jk^b, -Wr^a, -Di^b, -U, -Ge) who delivered antigen-positive infants. Seventy-nine percent of the maternal sera contained IgG1 antibodies (31% IgG1 only); 16% contained IgG2 (1% IgG2 only); 62% contained IgG3 (10% IgG3 only); and 12% contained IgG4 (0% contained IgG4 only).

The correlation of IgG subclass and the severity of HDFN is controversial. Schanfield[81] presented a small amount of data that suggested that neonates born with RBCs sensitized with IgG1 Rh antibodies had lower mean cord hemoglobin and higher cord bilirubin levels, with a lower postnatal bilirubin rise, than neonates with IgG3-sensitized RBCs. He suggested that this finding related to the preferential placental transfer of IgG1, which allowed for a longer period of in utero IgG1 sensitization. In contrast, neonates with IgG3 sensitization tended to have higher mean cord hemoglobin and lower cord bilirubin levels, but a higher postnatal rise in bilirubin. This was thought to be due to the shorter in utero exposure to IgG3 but the relative higher efficiency of IgG3 in causing postnatal RBC destruction. Schanfield[81] also suggested that within the IgG1 subclass, G1m(a) antibodies were significantly less effective than G1m(f). Mothers of moderately and severely affected infants showed a striking absence of G1m(a+) IgG1Rh antibodies; the majority of antibodies in this group were G1m(f), G3m(g), or mixtures of IgG1 and IgG3. It was suggested that the differences in transport of subclass-specific antibody across the placenta and their hemolytic potential may account for some of the discrepancies noted between maternal antibody titers and severity of HDFN. For example, a mother with an Rh antibody (titer 2048) that is totally IgG3 might deliver an infant that is not severely affected. The child would probably need therapy postnatally, however. In contrast, an IgG1, G1m(f) antibody of similar titer could cause severe HDFN in utero, leading to a stillborn fetus. Rh IgG1 antibody of lower titer (e.g., 64–128) might be associated with a mildly affected infant at birth, requiring no further treatment. An IgG3 antibody of the same titer, however, might be associated with an infant who is mildly affected at birth but subsequently becomes severely affected. In summary, Schanfield[81] suggested that IgG1 antibodies caused greater destruction in utero followed by a more benign clinical course; in contrast, IgG3 antibodies appeared to cause less destruction in utero but were associated with a much more severe clinical course postnatally. Unfortunately, these data have never been extended, and no one has confirmed the hypothesis thus far.

Frankowska and Gorska[77] could show no correlation between IgG subclass and severity of HDFN. Parinaud and coworkers[79] found that IgG1 Rh antibodies were associated with higher neonatal bilirubinemia than IgG3 antibodies; within the IgG1 group, the G1m(4) allotype was associated with the most severe HDFN. Severe HDFN appeared to be less common when IgG1 and IgG3 were present together; it was suggested that IgG3 might exert a protective effect. Cregut and associates[82] found that IgG3 Rh antibodies were associated with less severe HDFN. In contrast, Taslimi and colleagues[83] found that HDFN occurred only when IgG3 Rh antibodies were present.

Nance and coworkers[80] found that when IgG1 antibodies were present without IgG3 antibodies, 56% of the babies needed treatment (8% phototherapy, 26% transfusion) and 2% had fatal HDFN. When IgG3 was present without IgG1, 47% needed treatment (20% phototherapy, 27% transfusion). When IgG1 and IgG3 were both present, 90% required treatment (21% phototherapy, 63% transfusion), and 5% had fatal HDFN. Several other reports have agreed that IgG1 alone and IgG1 with IgG3 have a higher association with severity of HDFN than IgG3 alone.[84-89]

Lambin and associates[89] found that the median percentages of IgG1 and IgG3 anti-D in maternal sera were 90% and 10%, respectively, whereas on infants' RBCs they were 97% and 3%, respectively. The differences between maternal and infantile percentages were significant ($P < 0.001$). IgG1 and IgG3 anti-D bound to infants' RBCs increased concomitantly with the concentration of IgG1 and IgG3 anti-D in the maternal sera. The severity of HDFN correlated positively with the concentration of IgG1 anti-D in maternal sera, but negatively with the amount of IgG3 anti-D bound to infants' RBCs. In addition, the existence of a high proportion of IgG3 anti-D in maternal serum was associated with a delayed risk of fetal anemia. Thus, the proportion of IgG3 anti-D relative to the total IgG anti-D on infants' RBCs is only one third the proportion present in maternal sera. The study of the correlations between the amount of IgG1 and IgG3 anti-D and the severity of HDFN suggests that IgG1 anti-D was found to be more important than IgG3 anti-D in the pathogenesis of fetal anemia.

Although there is a statistical correlation between severity and IgG subclass, as illustrated in the foregoing discussion, there is so much variation among individual cases (e.g., strong IgG RBC sensitization associated with no hemolysis in one baby and severe hemolysis in another baby), that subclassing has no practical value in predicting the severity of HDFN when testing maternal sera before birth.

RH IMMUNE PROPHYLAXIS

In 1943, Levine[90] pointed out that in matings in which an Rh-negative mother carried an ABO-incompatible fetus, there were significantly fewer cases of Rh HDFN. Later, Race and Sanger[91] speculated that the mechanism of this protection might be that the Rh-positive ABO-incompatible cells of the fetus were rapidly destroyed on entering the mother's circulation and thus were incapable of initiating Rh sensitization. In 1956, Nevanlinna and Vainio[92] examined families in which Rh HDFN had occurred and found that the immunizing pregnancy was always ABO compatible. These and other observations stimulated a group of workers in Liverpool, England, to suggest that perhaps the phenomenon could be mimicked, when the mother and fetus were ABO compatible, by giving an antibody to destroy the Rh-positive fetal RBCs in the maternal circulation.[93] These workers went on to demonstrate, using the Kleihauer-Betke fetal cell staining technique, that the higher the fetal cell score at delivery, the more likely the women were to become immunized.[94] They also tried to give anti-D to Rh-negative volunteers who had been injected with ^{51}Cr-labeled Rh-positive RBCs.[95] Unfortunately, this experiment was a failure, as plasma containing IgM anti-D was used. Fortunately, they were stimulated to repeat the experiment, with plasma containing IgG anti-D,[96] when they heard of work by Stern and coworkers in a Chicago group.[97,98] Stern and coworkers had shown that Rh-negative volunteers failed to make anti-D when they were injected with Rh-positive RBCs coated in vitro with IgG anti-D. In 1961 and 1963, the Liverpool group published the impressive results of their experiments.[95,96,99] Only three of 21 Rh-negative volunteers made anti-D after receiving Rh-positive RBCs if they also received plasma containing IgG anti-D; this was in contrast to the 21 controls who did not receive anti-D, in which group 11 were sensitized to produce anti-D. Independently, another group in the United States was working on the same problem. This group had been stimulated by the early observations of Smith,[100] who, in 1909, had shown that antigen-antibody complexes of diptheria were not immunogenic when the complexes were prepared in antibody excess. Freda and Gorman[101] thought that if an excess of passive antibody (e.g., anti-D) was given to an individual, then subsequent injections of antigen (e.g., O+ red cells) would fail to cause sensitization, the antibody acting as part of the humoral homeostatic mechanism and exerting a negative "feedback" on antibody synthesis. Freda and colleagues[102] carried out a trial in which they injected Rh-negative prisoners in Sing Sing prison with an IgG fraction containing anti-D after the prisoners had received Rh-positive RBCs. This approach was eminently successful. On day 1 of the trial, 27 Rh-negative men received intravenous injections of Rh-positive RBCs (10 mL). Then, 72 hours later, 14 men received intramuscular injections of a sterile hyperimmune anti-Rh gamma globulin preparation (Rh Ig). At 6 months after the procedure, none of the 14 men who received Rh Ig had produced anti-D, but 6 of the 13 controls were immunized. After the success of their experiments, both the British and American groups went ahead with clinical trials. A combined study from British centers and Johns Hopkins Hospital in Baltimore[103] in 1966 and a study by Pollack and associates[104] in 1968, clearly showed the efficiency of Rh Ig in preventing Rh sensitization, with virtually 100% prevention of sensitization being achieved in women who received Rh Ig. One of the main reasons the clinical trials in the United States were so successful with no adverse reactions was the development of a suitable Rh Ig by the Ortho Research Foundation in Raritan, New Jersey. The original preparation was a gamma globulin fraction of pooled sera from a small number of Rh-negative donors who had been hyperimmunized with Rh-positive RBCs. The 16.5% gamma globulin solution was pure IgG (free from IgM) and was sterilized and packaged in 5-mL vials, suitable for intramuscular injections. This product led to the highly standardized successful product RhoGAM, which was licensed by the FDA in 1968.[105] The standard dose for clinical use in the United States is 300 µg, but smaller doses seem to be equally effective and are used in other countries such as England and Australia (100 µg and 125 µg, respectively).[2]

PROBLEMS IN COMPLETELY ERADICATING Rh HDFN

Although Rh Ig was a highly successful approach to eradicating Rh HDFN, it became obvious that failures were occurring. Some of these were due to obvious causes, in that some Rh-negative women were not receiving Rh Ig, and this will probably always occur. Among the group receiving Rh Ig, however, there was still a small number of failures. After about a decade of Rh Ig usage, the failure rate (i.e., an Rh-negative mother making anti-D in a pregnancy subsequent to delivering an Rh-positive baby and receiving Rh Ig), was approximately 1%. The main causes of these failures were shown to be the following:

- Rh-negative women who had aborted[106]
- Rh-negative women who had amniocentesis[106]
- Rh-negative women with a massive fetal maternal hemorrhage (FMH)[106]
- Rh-negative women immunized during pregnancy[93]

These associations led to recommendations that a smaller dose of Rh Ig (e.g., 50 g) be given to all Rh-negative women who abort or undergo amniocentesis. Because the smaller dose effectively suppresses only the response to 2.5 mL of Rh-positive red cells, some workers prefer giving a full dose after amniocentesis, but other workers have suggested that Rh Ig is not necessary after early spontaneous abortion or amniocentesis. The protective effect of Rh Ig is dose dependent. To be able to prevent Rh immunization completely, for every 1 mL of Rh-positive blood (0.5 mL of RBCs), an Rh-negative woman would need to receive 10 µg of Rh Ig. Thus, the 300 µg dose recommended in the United States should prevent immunization when the FMH is less than 30 mL of blood (15 mL of RBCs). An FMH greater than 30 mL produces Rh immunization in about 35% of cases who receive only 300 g of Rh Ig; such cases occur in about 0.2% of pregnancies. Thus, neglecting to screen for a massive FMH will lead to a failure of Rh immunization prevention in less than 0.1% of women at risk.

As early as 1967, Zipursky and Israels[107] noted that the main cause of failure in Rh immunoprophylaxis was sensitization during pregnancy and that the only way to prevent this was antenatal prophylaxis. In a series reported by Bowman and colleagues,[108] Rh immunoprophylaxis was predicted to fail in 1.6% of the Rh-negative women if Rh Ig was given only after delivery. After administration of Rh Ig at 28 and 34 weeks of pregnancy, in addition to a further administration within 72 hours of delivery, the failure rate was only 0.07%. At a conference in 1978, other workers, including those from Europe, the United States, and Canada, showed that of 1078 prior gravidas and multigravidas treated antenatally, only three (0.37%) showed evidence of immunization, compared with 39 of 2550 (1.53%) of women treated only postnatally.[109] Although the data just presented sounds impressive, antenatal prophylaxis remains controversial, especially in some countries.[110-117] Cost-benefit issues are the primary concerns. Some workers in the United Kingdom and the United States have argued that it is not worth the national expense of giving all Rh-negative women Rh Ig antenatally in addition to postnatally; other workers in the same countries have argued for antenatal Rh prophylaxis.[114-117] Mollison[117] makes the point that it is important to make the distinction between the prevention of Rh immunization and the prevention of Rh HDFN. For instance, if a woman is primarily immunized only by her second pregnancy and if she has no further pregnancies, then virtually no harm has been done. Mollison[117] suggests that in these days when most women are content to have just two children, one can make a good argument for giving antenatal prophylaxis during the first pregnancy only. If antenatal Rh Ig is withheld during the following pregnancy despite there being a 1% chance of Rh immunization, routine testing for antibody, premature delivery, and exchange transfusion in the very few cases in which the infant is severely affected, should result in negligible mortality. Mollison[117] makes a final point that antenatal prophylaxis involves waste, not only because it is superfluous in most cases (in which postnatal treatment alone would suffice), but also because in about 40% of cases it is given to women who are carrying Rh-negative infants.

CLINICAL FEATURES OF HDFN

The following features will be those associated with HDFN due to Rh antibodies. HDFN due to ABO antibodies will be dealt with separately later in this chapter. Features of most other IgG alloantibodies, with the possible exception of anti-K (see earlier), will be similar to those of Rh.

HDFN is a result of the fetal RBCs becoming sensitized with IgG antibody. Complement activation rarely occurs and is not thought to be involved in the pathogenesis of the disease (even in ABO HDFN).[2,118,119] The IgG RBCs are removed extravascularly by the mononuclear phagocytic system (MPS); intravascular complement-mediated lysis never occurs (even in ABO HDFN). The fetal MPS is probably capable of destroying sensitized RBCs before the fourth month of pregnancy, as intrauterine death from HDFN has been recorded before the 20th week, although it is uncommon before the 24th week. HDFN varies greatly in severity. It can be associated with a severe hemolytic process leading to intrauterine death. The fetus could die in utero at any time from the 18th week of gestation onward. The incidence of stillbirth associated with Rh-HDFN varies according to the obstetric history of the woman. In first affected infants, the stillbirth rate has been reported as 6%, but in second affected and later infants the rate can be as high as 29%. If a woman has had only a mildly affected infant, her chance of a subsequent stillbirth is probably as low as 2%, but if she has had one previous stillbirth, the risk of subsequent stillbirth is reported to be as high as 70%. In the most severe cases, there is gross enlargement of the liver, spleen, and heart, and sometimes there are also ascites and generalized edema giving rise to the condition known as hydrops fetalis. About 20% of HDFN cases present with fetal hydrops. When born alive, infants with severe HDFN could have cord hemoglobin (Hb) concentrations of 3.5–8 g/dL; the number of nucleated red cells could be as high as 200 × 10^9/L, and the reticulocyte count could be as high as 60%.[2] In such infants, jaundice can develop rapidly. Unless the infant is treated promptly, kernicterus may develop. Kernicterus is a syndrome characterized by signs of damage to the brain. About 70% of infants developing kernicterus die between the second and fifth days of life.[2] At autopsy, these infants are found to have yellow staining of the basal ganglia of the brain. Those that survive have permanent cerebral damage; some infants show deafness as the only sign. There is a close relationship between the peak serum bilirubin concentration and the development of kernicterus. In mature infants, kernicterus rarely develops in association with bilirubin concentrations of less than 18 mg/dL, although in premature infants there is some evidence of kernicterus at lower bilirubin levels. More moderate forms of the disease may present with less anemia and bilirubinemia that respond to transfusions, and these might not necessarily be exchange transfusions.[2]

About 25% of HDFN cases are of moderate severity. Infants with a mild form of HDFN (about 45%–50% of all HDFN cases) might present with little or no jaundice at birth. Mild jaundice and anemia (e.g., slightly more rapid than the normal fall in Hb, remembering that it is normal for the Hb to fall during the first few weeks after birth) might develop after birth, and the baby might need minimal treatment (e.g., phototherapy) or no treatment.[2]

Sometimes a late anemia is associated with HDFN.[2,120] This entity can present as the sudden appearance of anemia in an infant who was born with HDFN at 10–20 days after birth; the anemia is not accompanied by hepatosplenomegaly or jaundice. The anemia seems to be an accentuation of the normal decrease in Hb/Hct that occurs normally at this time. This late anemia can occur in babies who have responded to exchange transfusion at birth or in babies who required little or no treatment at birth. The late anemia is usually only moderately severe and rarely needs treatment with transfusion, but occasionally the anemia can be profound, requiring transfusion.[2] The cause(s) of the late anemia is uncertain and could have multiple origins (e.g., increased RBC destruction due to alloantibodies and/or infection, decreased red cell production due to alloantibodies (e.g., anti-K), erythropoietin deficiency, lack of response to erythropoietin, ineffective erythropoiesis, and/or infection).

Table 13-8 lists some of the clinical problems that can be associated with HDFN.

ASSESSMENT OF SEVERITY OF DISEASE IN THE NEWBORN INFANT

A positive DAT cannot be equated with HDFN. Only about 60% of infants with positive DATs due to Rh(D) sensitization require any form of treatment.[2] There is no direct correlation with the strength of the positive DAT and the severity of HDFN, although the correlation is similar to that discussed in Chapter 4 for AIHA: Most cases of severe HDFN are associated with strongly positive DATs, and most (but not all) babies with weakly positive DATs have mild or no HDFN. Nevertheless, as with AIHA, there are many exceptions to these findings. Hughes-Jones and coworkers[121] measured the amount of red cell-bound IgG Rh antibody on cord RBCs and found 0.4–18 μg/mL. The amount on the RBCs was not highly correlated (correlation coefficient of 0.6) with the infants' cord Hb or bilirubin concentrations. All infants with more than 8 μg/mL of antibody required treatment, but even at a level of 2 μg/mL, six of 14 infants required treatment. Garratty and Nance[122] used flow cytometry to examine the amount of IgG Rh antibody on DAT-positive newborns. Although babies with evidence for

TABLE 13-8. CLINICAL PROBLEMS THAT COULD BE ASSOCIATED WITH SEVERE HDFN

Intrauterine fetal demise
Anemia
Thrombocytopenia
Kernicterus
Coagulation defects (e.g., DIC)
Low serum albumin
Hypoglycemia
Hypocalcemia
Pleural effusion, ascites, hydrops
Respiratory distress syndrome
Birth asphyxia
Preterm delivery

HDFN had higher levels of RBC bound IgG, there was considerable overlap between the clinically affected and nonaffected groups. No clear quantitative hemolytic threshold was obvious. Nance and associates[69,70] also correlated the results of an MMA (using the cord RBCs) with severity of HDFN. Once again, the MMA correlated quite well, but the correlation was not perfect.

Mollison and colleagues[2] reported that the cord blood hemoglobin concentration was the best single criterion of severity; if the logarithm of the hemoglobin concentration was plotted against the probit of the survival rate, a linear relationship was observed. The cord blood bilirubin concentration was of less value on its own, but when taken in conjunction with the cord Hb concentration, it is of great value, especially in assessing dangerously high bilirubin levels. Mollison and colleagues[2] point out that the normal range (mean ± 2 SD) of hemoglobin values in cord blood was approximately 13.6–19.6 g/dL, whereas the range on venous blood drawn in the first 24 hours of life is 14.5–22.5 g/dL. Before Rh prophylaxis, almost 50% of affected infants had cord blood Hb concentrations of 14.5 g/dL or greater, and 30% had values between 3.4 g/dL and 10.4 g/dL. Most infants with cord Hb concentrations within the normal range do not require exchange transfusion.[2] A level of 4 mg/dL or more of cord blood bilirubin (normal range, 0.7–3 mg/dL) or a rapidly rising bilirubin is suggested as an indication for exchange transfusion.[2] If the cord total bilirubin is less than 4–5 mg/dL and rising only slowly, phototherapy might suffice to correct the problem. It should be remembered that the serum bilirubin concentration rises during the first few days of a normal newborn infant's life. This rise is due mainly to the deficiency at birth of glucoronyl transferase, a liver enzyme responsible for conjugating bilirubin with glucuronyl transferase (a liver enzyme responsible for conjugating bilirubin with glucuronic acid) to form a water-soluble compound, bilirubin diglucuronide. This leads to the commonly encountered physiologic jaundice, which is discussed more fully later in the section on ABO HDFN. Bilirubin levels are also affected greatly by prematurity. Hsia and coworkers[123] found that in 12 normal full-term infants, peak bilirubin was on average 7.1 mg/dL and was in all cases less than 13.5 mg/dL. In contrast, the mean bilirubin concentration in 15 premature infants (birthweights below 2250 g) was 11.2 mg/dL, and in five infants the concentration exceeded 15 mg/dL. The amount of albumin present in the plasma also has an effect on bilirubin. Plasma bilirubin is normally bound to albumin, and the risk of damage to the nervous system depends on the amount of bilirubin that is unbound to albumin. Because of this, some workers have recommended infusing albumin to babies with HDFN.[2]

Table 13-9 shows recommendations of the Scientific Coordinating Committee of the AABB for tests at delivery.[28]

AMELIORATION AND TREATMENT OF HDFN

There are many problems to deal with in attempting to salvage a child suffering with HDFN. Table 13-8 shows some of these problems.

Transfusion

In 1950, Allen and associates[124] demonstrated the value of neonatal exchange transfusion in overcoming anemia and preventing kernicterus. In 1954, the same group showed the benefits of preterm delivery; the risk of fetal death due to HDFN was reduced to 25% (from 50%) of the immunized pregnancies.[125] During the last decade, there have been tremendous advances in the care of preterm babies. Most major centers can now claim more than 80% survival rate at 28 weeks' gestation. In 1961, Liley[126] described a technique for intrauterine transfusion (IUT). He transfused fresh Rh-negative blood into the fetal peritoneal cavity, correcting the anemia and allowing the fetus to survive until it was mature enough for preterm delivery. Experiences with this technique have varied. Robertson and colleagues[127] and Palmer and Gordon[128] felt that the value of the technique was questionable, Robertson and colleagues[127] had a fetal mortality rate of 20% due to trauma, and in a further 40% of the stillbirths, death occurred within 48 hours of the IUT. Other centers have reported more success with IUT.[11,13,37,129-135] The reported improved results in the latter reports were undoubtedly due to the expertise gained at these centers and to the use of ultrasound for guiding the needle in the peritoneal cavity. In Winnipeg, Canada, for instance, survival rates increased from 70% in the period 1970–1978 to 92% during the period 1980–1982.[11,13,37] Similarly, the survival rate for hydropic fetuses in the two periods improved from 50% to 75%. Total fetal fatality rates dues to IUT have dropped to less than 5% at centers who perform this procedure regularly.

Because of erratic adsorption, especially in hydropic fetuses, intravascular transfusion has largely replaced the intraperitoneal approach.[39] In an attempt to save two hydropic fetuses, Rodeck and associates[132,133] used fetoscopy to transfuse the fetuses directly into umbilical vessels, at 23 and 25 weeks' gestation, respectively; one baby was delivered at 30 weeks and survived. In 1984, Rodeck and associates[133] reported using the technique on 25 severely affected fetuses (including 15 with hydrops); the neonatal survival rate was 90%. In 1986, Grannum and colleagues[134] performed in utero exchange transfusions on four hydropic fetuses at 24–30 weeks' gestation; three of the four babies survived. Perinatal survival rates for severely affected fetuses after intravascular IUT are now reported in excess of 80%.[13,39]

TABLE 13-9. RECOMMENDED TESTING AT DELIVERY[28]

	Indication
Maternal Blood	
ABO/D	To obtain concordant results of tests on two samples, or if pretransfusion tests requested
Antibody detection	When pretransfusion tests requested
Antibody identification	First detection of alloantibody, D− panel should be used if Rh Ig given during pregnancy
Titration studies	Not indicated
FMH testing	All D− women who deliver a D+ infant
Testing to diagnose HDFN	ABO/D typing and tests for unexpected antibodies if not done during the admission for delivery Test maternal serum against paternal RBCs if there are no unexpected antibodies found by routine reagent screen RBCs and no fetomaternal ABO incompatibility
Cord or Infant Blood	
Infants born to D− women	D status, including test for weak D
Infants born to women with potentially significant antibodies	ABO, D typing, and DAT
No maternal alloimmunization; infant with clinical signs and symptoms of HDFN	ABO/D typing and DAT If fetomaternal ABO incompatibility exists, infant serum should be tested for IgG anti-A and/or -B If no fetal maternal ABO incompatibility exists, maternal serum (see above) or infant eluate should be tested against paternal RBCs

Currently, the decision to perform IUT is usually based on the amniotic fluid OD_{450}, but as discussed previously, other tests (e.g., fetal hemoglobin, MMA) might also be useful in indicating the need for this treatment. The fetal hematocrit at which to initiate transfusion is somewhat arbitrary, but ACOG quotes a hematocrit of 25% as being a reasonable indication.[39] Repeat transfusions are planned for when the fetal hematocrit is predicted to be between 20% and 25%. This may be approximated by assuming a 1% decline per day or by using one of a number of published equations. In fetuses with more severe hemolytic anemia, few fetal RBCs survive the initial transfusion interval, whereas transfused adult RBCs survive for a longer time period. Therefore, the interval between first and second transfusions is usually 7 to 14 days, whereas the interval between subsequent transfusions or birth is 21–28 days.[39]

Indication for neonatal exchange transfusion vary from center to center but generally, if the cord hemoglobin is less than 12g/dL (hematocrit <45%), or if cord unconjugated bilirubin is greater than 75 μmol/L, or if the bilirubin rises at a rate of greater than 10 μmol per hour, most neonatologists would decide to perform an exchange transfusion. The main reason for performing an exchange transfusion is to correct the anemia by removing the baby's sensitized RBCs—which might have a survival time of only 2 to 3 days—and replacing them with donor RBCs with normal survival; removal of bilirubin and antibody are other reasons. Subsequent exchanges are based on the level of unconjugated bilirubin and its rate of increase, but other factors that influence bilirubin transport and the risk of kernicterus must also be taken into account. These include gestational age, low pH, low serum albumin, hypoxia, asphyxia, and infections, all of which predispose to kernicterus at lower bilirubin levels.[134] The blood used for exchange transfusion should preferably be less than 48 hours old and usually partially "packed." Most neonatologists find CPD-A anticoagulated blood acceptable, but some insist on heparinized blood that is less than 12 hours old. The blood should be ABO-compatible with the infant and lack the offending antigen (e.g., D-negative blood is used for an infant suffering from Rh(D)-HDFN). As the blood group of the fetus is usually unknown before the first IUT, fresh group O blood is usually used for the first IUT.

Phototherapy

The irradiation of jaundiced infants with fluorescent lights is currently the most common method for treating hyperbilirubinemia, particularly those with levels below 20 mg%.[136–138] In the United States, about 2.5% of infants receive phototherapy.[137] Some authors have suggested that the technique is overused.[139,140]

Preterm Delivery

Allen[141] and Walker and associates[142] found that approximately 50% of all stillbirths due to HDFN occurred after the 35th week of pregnancy. With the steadily increasing improvement in the case of preterm babies, delivery is now carried out as early as 28–30 weeks' gestation, with some centers claiming a survival rate of greater than 80% after 28 weeks' gestation. Because of the decreasing incidence of HDFN, there is decreasing expertise with IUT. There could be an increasing trend to deliver babies suffering with HDFN as early as 28–30 weeks rather than to risk IUT.

Plasma Exchange

The use of plasma exchange on alloimmunzied mothers to ameliorate HDFN is controversial. The first intensive plasma exchange was carried out on an Rh-immunized woman by Bowman and colleagues[143] in 1968. Since that time, there have been many reports, which were reviewed by Rock[144] in 1984 and by Moise and Whitecarr[145] in 2002. Plasma exchange of three to four liters, up to three or more times a week, might be required for the duration of a pregnancy with an affected fetus. One group claimed that 80% of the mothers showed a reduction in antibody level to at least half the original level when measured by the Auto-Analyzer quantitation method.[146] Some workers[147,148] have suggested that smaller volumes of plasma could be removed. For instance, Rubinstein[147] removed only 250 mL of plasma every week for 20 weeks and decreased antibody levels to 20% of their initial values. Nevertheless, plasma exchange should not be undertaken lightly because the mother is being put to risk as well as the baby; maternal deaths have been reported.[149] Bowman, quoted in Moise and Whitecarr,[145] recommends carrying out plasma exchange starting at 12–14 weeks' gestation if the woman has a homozygous husband, a history of hydropic stillbirths before 30 weeks' gestation, and a quantitative anti-D level greater than 2.5 mg/mL. He believes that plasma exchange is indicated in very severe Rh disease with high levels of anti-D, as these levels can be reduced up to 80%, if only transiently, by intense plasma exchange. For other Rh-immunized women, he feels the procedure is too costly to be justified. Kemp[150] used two-liter exchanges at least twice a week and showed a live birthrate of 66% for 156 patients who had antibody levels greater than 10 IU. If the antibody level cannot be lowered sufficiently by plasma exchange, this author's center transfuses the fetus using fetoscopy as early as 20 weeks' gestation. Robinson and Tovey[151] showed that use of plasma exchange in their treatment regimen changed the live birthrate in 14 women from a predicted value of 38% to an actual value of 75%.

Intravenous Immunoglobulin (IVIG)

IVIG has been used successfully in the antenatal treatment of HDFN.[145,151-157] Moise's group uses a combination of IVIG and plasmapheresis for women who have had a previous fetal loss before 20 weeks' gestation.[145]

Specific Immunoadsorption

Some workers have tried to remove antibody by adsorbing the antibody onto allogenic RBCs containing the reactive antigen and then reinfusing the plasma. Tilz and coworkers[158] were the first to try this with anti-D and Rh(D)-positive RBCs. Robinson[159] reported initial success with a similar technique but subsequently found an increase in antibody titer, presumably due to infusion of contaminating Rh-positive RBCs and/or stroma. Yoshida and associates[160,161] have reported using the procedure successfully to remove IgG anti-M and P from sera of women who had been unsuccessful in delivering live infants in four previous pregnancies, but who after this procedure delivered live babies.

Promethazine Hydrochloride (PMT) Treatment

There have been several reports of the use of PMT to ameliorate the severity of HDFN.[162-166] The largest series was reported by Gusdon,[165] who treated 72 Rh-immunized women (3.7–6.5 mg PMT/Kg/day given orally) for 6 to more than 30 weeks. The total number of perinatal deaths was reduced considerably compared with previous pregnancies, with only three deaths in the treated group; the number of exchange transfusions was significantly lower, with 20 infants requiring 42 exchanges compared with 32 infants needing 82 exchanges in previously affected pregnancies. In contrast, Charles and Blumenthal[166] did not find any ameliorating effects of PMT in 21 Rh-immunized women; the low dosage used in this study has been criticized by others. Scott and coworkers[167] tried combining PMT treatment with plasma exchange; Rock[144] warns that this combination of immuosuppression and plasma exchange could increase the risks of both maternal and neonatal infection during pregnancy.

Erythrocyte Membrane Oral Treatment (EMOT)

In a letter to Lancet in 1979, Bierme and associates[168] reported treating seven Rh-immunized women with daily treatments of stroma prepared from Rh-positive erythrocytes. The stromal extract was taken orally in the form of a capsule. All of these women had previously had stillbirths or intrauterine deaths. While receiving EMOT, their Rh antibodies did not rise in titer, and all six of the Rh-positive babies were born alive at about 35 weeks' gestation. When treatment was stopped after delivery, a rapid rise in Rh antibody titer occurred in three of the women. In 1982, Bierme and colleagues[169] reported on 10 women who had received EMOT over a 9-year period. PMT was given in addition to EMOT in 10 of the 11 pregnancies. The women received 2 g of erythrocyte stromal preparation starting at approximately 10 weeks' gestation. In the group that received EMOT, only 9 of the 11 pregnancies had an Rh incompatibility. In these nine pregnancies, the Rh antibody level remained constant and was always lower than in previous pregnancies. In one case, IUT was performed at 31 weeks' gestation. All nine babies were born alive. The control group showed increases in antibody titer after 30 weeks, and multiple IUTs were necessary.

Other workers have not been so successful with this form of treatment. Barnes and coworkers[170] reported on the use of EMOT in 18 nonsensitized Rh(D)-negative male volunteers injected with Rh-positive RBCs and in six Rh-sensitized women. Sixty-one percent (11/18) of the males who received EMOT (prepared from either Rh-positive or Rh-negative RBCs) before intravenous challenge with Rh-positive RBCs produced detectable antibodies; of these 11, six received Rh-negative EMOT, and five received Rh-positive EMOT. Seventy-two (13/18) of control males who had received no prior EMOT produced Rh antibodies after challenge with Rh-positive RBCs. Three of six presensitized women who received Rh-positive or Rh-negative EMOT for 4 weeks but without intravenous challenge increased their anti-D levels, which peaked at 11–18 weeks; two had received Rh-positive EMOT, and one had received Rh negative EMOT.[170]

HDFN ASSOCIATED WITH ABO ANTIBODIES

In a white population, at least 15% of babies are at risk for HDFN due to ABO antibodies.[2] Group A or B infants born to group O mothers are those at greatest risk, as group O mothers have higher levels of IgG anti-A, -B, -A,B in their plasma compared with group A or B mothers. Although many infants are at risk, and approximately 5% of all births show some sign of ABO HDFN, clinically obvious HDFN is rare.[2] ABO-incompatible infants tend to have lower hemoglobin values and more jaundice (usually slight) than ABO-compatible infants, but the ABO-incompatible infants rarely need treatment of any kind.[2] ABO-incompatible babies often have positive DATs and/or anti-A,B can be eluted from their RBCs, but these findings do not equate with a clinical problem most of the time. The need for exchange transfusion is rare (approximately 1:1000 to 1:5000 of all births).[2] There are suggestions in the literature that ABO HDFN could be more severe in Africans, African-Americans, Chinese, and Arabs.[171-178]

When IgG ABO antibodies cross the placenta, they encounter A and B antigens in the body fluids and on many cells other than RBCs. Fetal RBCs have less A and B sites than adult RBCs, and the carbohydrate chains on the membrane are less branched compared with adult RBCs. IgG ABO antibodies rarely bind complement to the fetal/cord RBCs (i.e., the RBCs react with anti-IgG but not anticomplement antiglobulin sera). All of the RBC destruction is macrophage mediated, similar to Rh HDFN. Severe anemia is uncommon, and hydrops fetalis has been reported in only two or three cases.[2] Hyperbilirubemia leading to kernicterus is the major problem; this usually reaches its peak 24–48 hours after the baby's birth.[2]

Serological Findings in ABO HDFN

MOTHER

Usually, the mother is group O and the baby is A, B, or AB, but sometimes the mother is group A or B.[2] The mother's serum must contain IgG anti-A, anti-B, and/or anti-A,B. The IgG antibody often is of high titer. Voak and Bowley[179] found that 66% and 90% of sera from mothers delivering babies with HDFN due to anti-A and anti-B, respectively, contain IgG antibodies with an IAT titer greater than 256. Brouwers and colleagues[180] found that 100% of sera from group O mothers who previously had delivered a group A or group B baby contained IgG2; 97% of sera contained IgG1, 41% contained IgG4, and 38% contained IgG3 anti-A/B. IgG2 anti-A/B were usually of higher titer than anti-A/B of other subclasses. Although the titer and subclass of the antibodies show some correlation with the presence or severity of HDFN, they are of little practical value, especially in antenatal testing.

INFANT

DAT. There is a large range in the reported incidence of positive DATs associated with ABO HDFN. The low incidence of positive DATs in early reports probably related to the insensitivity of the AGT methods used; more recent data report the incidence as 20%–82%.[181-186] One major problem in relating to the incidence quoted in the literature is the authors' definition of ABO HDFN. Some data relate to positive DATs in infants who are ABO incompatible with their mother, other data relate to infants who have laboratory signs of ABO HDFN, and still other data relate to infants who have evidence of a hemolytic anemia due to anti-A or anti-B. The latter is the definition that should be used, but it is often not clear in the publications. One other way of expressing the data is to apply it to infants who have to be treated for HDFN. Issitt and Anstee[9] reported that infants who have to be treated (transfused) for ABO HDFN always have a positive DAT; this also has been the experience of one of the authors (Garratty, unpublished observations).

There has been much discussion in the literature regarding why the DAT in ABO HDFN is often weakly positive or sometimes negative. Suggestions here ranged from pinocytosis of antigen-antibody complexes, low number of A and B sites in fetal RBCs, and deficiency of branched chains on the fetal RBC membrane.[186-189]

Eluates from Infant's RBCs. One can almost always elute anti-A or anti-B from group A or B infants born to a group O mother, even if the DAT is negative. Because of this, detection of anti-A and anti-B in an eluate has an extremely low predictive value for HDFN. A nonreactive eluate might help exclude ABO antibodies as a cause of the positive DAT and/or jaundice.

Ukita and coworkers[185] showed that 88% and 40% of the IgG anti-A or anti-B eluted from A or B infants born to group O mothers were IgG2 and IgG1, respectively; none were IgG3 or IgG4.

Correlation of Serology with HDFN. It is often difficult to prove that an infant's jaundice is due to ABO HDFN. If the infant is group A or B and the mother is group O, it is usually assumed that the ABO antibodies are to blame, and if a transfusion is needed, group O blood is used.

Dufour and Monaghan[183] found that 252 (38%) of 665 group A and B infants born to group O mothers had laboratory findings compatible with a diagnosis of ABO HDFN (0.8% of ABO-incompatible infants born to group A or B mothers), but only 28 (4%) of the 665 infants (14% of DAT-positive infants) needed treatment (17 phototherapy; seven phototherapy plus exchange transfusion; four exchange transfusion only). Thirty-one percent (208) of the infants were DAT positive; 64% of these infants were jaundiced (26% had bilirubin >12 mg%). Of the DAT-negative (eluate reactive) infants, 21% (38) were jaundiced (8% had bilirubin >12 mg%). It should be noted that 37% of the control group (137 unselected infants) had jaundice (7% had bilirubin >12 mg%).

Desjardins and colleagues[182] reported on 1704 infants born to group O mothers. Of the 680 ABO-incompatible infants, 27 (4%) had clinically significant ABO HDFN. The DAT was positive in 22 (82%) of these infants; in four infants (15%), the DAT was negative, but the eluate was reactive. The group A and B infants had significantly higher bilirubins and lower hemoglobins than the group O infants.

Osborn and coworkers[190] reported on 476 infants born at the University of California, Los Angeles. Forty-seven of the infants (10%, all infants were born to group O mothers), were DAT positive. Of the DAT-positive infants, 92% were found *not* to have clinically significant HDFN and had bilirubin levels indistinguishable from controls (12%–14% of both groups had jaundice). The strength of the DAT was found to be unrelated to the need for phototherapy. The authors emphasized that no laboratory tests predicted HDFN with 100% accuracy and that careful, continuous monitoring of the bilirubin was the only reliable indicator for treatment. The authors developed new, more conservative criteria for treatment of ABO HDFN. The old criteria, when the infants was less than 24 hours old, were that phototherapy was performed if the infant's bilirubin was 5–9 mg%; if the bilirubin was greater than 10 mg%, exchange transfusion was performed instead. When the infant was greater 24 hours old, if the bilirubin was 14–20 mg%, then phototherapy or exchange transfusion, respectively, was performed. Retrospective analysis showed that DAT-positive, ABO-incompatible infants were often treated with phototherapy for 24–48 hours and never developed nonphysiologic jaundice; once treated, bilirubin seldom continued rising, and very few infants ever developed bilirubin levels high enough to warrant exchange transfusion. The criteria were changed to decrease the number of infants treated by lengthening the pretreatment observation period. Phototherapy was performed if the bilirubin was greater than or equal to 10 mg% at less than 12 hours of age; greater than or equal to 12 mg% at less than 18 hours of age; greater than or equal to 14 mg% before 24 hours of age; and greater than 15 mg% after 24 hours of age. Using the new protocol, only 9% of infants needed phototherapy; none needed exchange transfusion. If the old protocol had been used, 82% of the infants would have received phototherapy, and 5% would have had exchange transfusions. The authors commented that exchange transfusion should be used only for severely compromised or asphyxiated infants.[190]

REFERENCES

1. Hadley AG, Soothill P (eds): Alloimmune Disorders of Pregnancy. Cambridge: Cambridge University Press, 2002.
2. Mollison PL, Engelfriet CP, Contreras M: Blood Transfusion in Clinical Medicine, 10th ed. Oxford: Blackwell Scientific, 1997.
3. Giblett ER: Blood group antibodies causing hemolytic disease of the newborn. Clin Obstet Gynecol 1964;7:1044–1055.
4. Polesky HF: Blood group antibodies in prenatal sera. Minn Med 1967;50:601–603.
5. Queenan JT, Smith BD, Haber JM, Jeffrey J, Gadow HC: Irregular antibodies in the obstetric patient. Obstet Gynecol 1969;34:767–770.
6. Walker RH: Relevancy in the selection of serologic tests for the obstetric patient. In Garratty G (ed): Hemolytic Disease of the Newborn. Arlington, VA: American Association of Blood Banks, 1984:173–210.
7. Kornstad L: Occurrence of anti-D and other irregular blood group antibodies in pregnancy. The present situation. In Book of Abstracts, XXI Congress of the International Society of Haematology, XIX Congress of the International Society of Blood Transfusion, 1986:312.
8. Kornstad L: New cases of irregular blood group antibodies other than anti-D in pregnancy. Acta Obstet Gynecol Scand 1983;62:431–436.
9. Issitt PD, Anstee DJ: Applied Blood Group Serology, 4th ed. Durham, NC: Montgomery Scientific Publications, 1998.
10. Wenk RE, Goldstein P, Felix JK: Alloimmunization by hr′(c), hemolytic disease of newborns, and perinatal management. Obstet Gynecol 1986;67:623–626.
11. Bowman JM: Hemolytic disease of the newborn. In Garratty G (ed): Immunobiology of Transfusion Medicine. New York: Dekker, 1994:553–595.
12. Wenk RE, Goldstein P, Felix JK: Kell alloimmunization, hemolytic disease of the newborn, and perinatal management. Obstet Gynecol 1985;66:473–476.
13. Bowman JM: Historical overview: Hemolytic disease of the fetus and newborn. In Kennedy MS, Wilson S, Kelton JG (eds): Perinatal transfusion medicine. Arlington, VA: American Association of Blood Banks, 1990:1–52.
14. Caine ME, Mueller-Heubach E: Kell sensitization in pregnancy. Am J Obstet Gynecol 1986;154:85–90.
15. Mayne KM, Bowell PJ, Pratt GA: The significance of anti-Kell sensitization in pregnancy. Clin Lab Haemat 1990;12:379–385.
16. Bowman JM, Pollock JM, Manning FA, et al: Maternal Kell blood group alloimmunization. Obstet Gynecol 1992;79: 239–244.
17. McKenna DS, Nagaraja HN, O'Shaughnessy R: Management of pregnancies complicated by anti-Kell isoimmunization. Obstet Gynecol 1999;93:667–673.
18. Grant SR, Kilby MD, Meer L, et al: The outcome of pregnancy in Kell alloimmunisation. Br J Obstet Gynaecol 2000;107: 481–485.

19. Berkowitz RL, Beyth Y, Sadovsky E: Death in utero due to Kell sensitization without excessive elevation of the ΔOD_{450} value in amniotic fluid. Obstet Gynecol 1982;60:746–749.
20. Babinszki A, Lapinski RH, Berkowitz RL: Prognostic factors and management in pregnancies complicated with severe Kell alloimmunization: Experiences of the last 13 years. Am J Perinatol 1998;15:695–701.
21. Vaughan JI, Warwick R, Letsky E, et al: Erythropoietic suppression in fetal anemia because of Kell alloimmunization. Am J Obstet Gynecol 1994;171:247–252.
22. Vaughan JI, Manning M, Warwick RM, et al: Inhibition of erythroid progenitor cells by anti-Kell antibodies in fetal alloimmune anemia. N Eng J Med 1998;338:798–803.
23. Hardy J, Napier JAF: Red cell antibodies detected in antenatal tests on rhesus positive women in South and Mid Wales, 1948–1978. Br J Obstet Gynaecol 1981;88:91.
24. Bowell PJ, Allen DL, Entwistle CC: Blood group antibody screening tests during pregnancy. Br J Obstet Gynaecol 1986;93:1038–1043.
25. Bowell PJ, Brown SE, Dike AE, Inskip MJ: The significance of anti-c alloimmunisation in pregnancy. Br J Obstet Gynaecol 1986;93:1044–1048.
26. Rothenberg JM, Weirermiller B, Dirig K, et al: Is a third-trimester antibody screen in Rh+ women necessary? Am J Manag Care 1999;5:1145–1150.
27. Heddle NM, Klama L, Frassetto R, et al: A retrospective study to determine the risk of red cell alloimmunization and transfusion during pregnancy. Transfusion 1993;23:217–220.
28. Judd WJ: Practice guidelines for prenatal and perinatal immunohematology, revisited. Transfusion 2001;41:1445–1452.
29. Hughes-Jones NC: The estimation of the concentration and equilibrium constant of anti-D. Immunology 1967;12: 565–571.
30. Contreras M: Methods for quantitation of anti-D. Plasma Ther Transfus Technol 1984;5:65–71.
31. Gall SA, Miller JM, Jr. Rh isoimmunization: A 24 year experience at Duke University Medical Center. Am J Obstet Gynecol 1981;140:902–908.
32. Bowell P, Wainscoat JS, Peto TEA, Gunson HH: Maternal anti-D concentrations and outcome in rhesus haemolytic disease of the newborn. Br Med J 1982;285:327–329.
33. Bowell PJ, Wainscoat JS, Peto TEA: AutoAnalyzer anti-D measurement and outcome of rhesus-sensitized pregnancies: Serum analysis. Plasma Ther Transfus Technol 1984;5:81–85.
34. Nicolaides KH, Rodeck CH: Maternal serum anti-D antibody concentration and assessment of rhesus isoimmunisation. Br Med J 1992;304:1155–1156.
35. Bevis DCA: Composition of liquor amnii in haemolytic disease of the newborn. Lancet 1950;ii:443.
36. Liley AW: Liquor amnii analysis in management of pregnancy complicated by rhesus immunization. Am J Obstet Gynecol 1961;82:1359.
37. Bowman JM: Management of Rh-isoimmunization. Obstet Gynecol 1978;52:1.
38. Queenan JT, Tomai TP, Ural SH, et al: Deviation in amniotic fluid optical density at a wavelength of 450 nm in Rh-immunized pregnancies from 14 to 40 weeks gestation: A proposal for clinical management. Am J Obstet Gynecol 1993;168:1370–1376.
39. The American College of Obstetricians and Gynecologists. Management of isoimmunization in pregnancy. Washington, DC: American College of Obstetricians and Gynecologists, 1996 (ACOG Technical Bulletin. Number 227:1–7).
40. Moise KJ Jr: Changing trends in the management of red blood cell alloimmunization in pregnancy. Arch Pathol Lab Med 1994;118:421–428.
41. Weiner S, Bolognese RJ, Librizzi RJ: Ultrasound in the evaluation and management of the isoimmunized pregnancy. J Clin Ultrasound 1981;9:315–323.
42. Abdel-Fattah, Soothill P: Assessing the severity of haemolytic disease of the fetus and newborn: Clinical aspects. In Hadley AG, Soothill P, eds. Alloimmune disorders of pregnancy. Cambridge: Cambridge University Press, 2002:153–172.
43. Nicolaides KH, Fontanarosa M, Gabbe SG, et al: Failure of ultrasonographic parameters to predict the severity of fetal anemia in rhesus isoimmunization. Am J Obstet Gynecol 1988;158:920–926.
44. Mari G: Noninvasive diagnosis by Doppler ultrasonography of fetal anemia due to maternal red-cell alloimmunization. N Engl J Med 2000;342:9–14.
45. Stefos T, Cosmi E, Detti L, et al: Correction of fetal anemia on the middle cerebral artery peak systolic velocity. Obstet Gynecol 2002;99:211–215.
46. Rodeck CH, Nicolaides KH: Ultrasound guided invasive procedures in obstetrics. Clinics Obstet Gynecol 1983;10: 515–539.
47. MacKenzie IZ, Guest CM, Bowell PJ: Fetal blood group studies during mid-trimester pregnancy and the management of severe isoimmunization. Prenatal Diagn 1983;3:41–46.
48. MacKenzie IZ: Fetoscopy in the management of hemolytic disease of the newborn. Plasma Ther Transfus Technol 1984;5:33–42.
49. Nicolaides KH, Rodeck CH, Mibashan RS, Kemp JR: Have Liley charts outlived their usefulness? Am J Obstet Gynecol 1986;155:90–94.
50. Daffos F, Capella-Pavlovsky M, Forestier F: A new procedure for fetal blood sampling in utero: Preliminary results of 53 cases. Am J Obstet Gynecol 1983;146:985.
51. Daffos F, Capella-Pavlovsky M, Forestier F: Fetal blood sampling during pregnancy with the use of a needle guided by ultrasound: A study of 606 consecutive cases. Am J Obstet Gynecol 1985;153:655–60.
52. Hobbins JC, Grannum PA, Romero R, Reece EA, Mahoney MJ: Percutaneous umbilical blood sampling. Am J Obstet Gynecol 1985;152:1–6.
53. Philip J, Brandt NJ, Fernandes A, Freiesleben E, Trolle D: ABO and Rh phenotyping of foetal blood obtained by foetoscopy. Clin Genet 1978;14:324–329.
54. Habibi B, Bretagne M, Bretagne Y, Forestier F, Daffos F: Blood group antigens on fetal red cells obtained by umbilical vein puncture under ultrasound guidance: A rapid hemagglutination test to check for contamination with maternal blood. Pediatr Res 1986;20:1082–1084.
55. Gemke RJBJ, Kanhai HHH, Overbeeke MAM, et al: ABO and Rhesus phenotyping of fetal erythrocytes in the first trimester of pregnancy. Brit J Haemat 1986;64:689–697.
56. Kanhai HH, Gravenhorst JB, Gemke RJ, Overbeeke MA, Bernini LF, Beverstock GC: Fetal blood group determination in first trimester pregnancy for the management of severe immunization. Am J Obstet Gynecol 1987;156:120–123.
57. Rodesch F, Lambermount M, Donner C, et al: Chorionic biopsy in management of severe Kell alloimmunization. Am J Obstet Gynecol 1987;156:124–125.
58. Jackson LG, Zachary JM, Fowler SE, et al: A randomized comparison of transcervical and transabdominal chorionic-villus sampling. The U.S. National Institute of Child Health and Human Development Chorionic-Villus Sampling and Amniocentesis Study Group. N Engl J Med 1992;327:594–598.
59. Avent ND: Antenatal genotyping of the blood groups of the fetus. Vox Sang 1998;74(S2):365–374.
60. Avent N: Fetal genotyping. In Hadley AG, Soothill P (eds): Alloimmune Disorders of Pregnancy. Cambridge: Cambridge University Press, 2002:121–139.
61. Allen RW, Ward S, Harris R: Prenatal genotyping for the RhD blood group antigen: Considerations in developing an accurate test. Genet Test 2000;4:377–381.
62. Garratty G: Predicting the clinical significance of red cell antibodies with in vitro cellular assays. Transfus Med Rev 1990; 4:297–312.
63. Engelfriet CP, Ouwehand WH: ADCC and other cellular bioassays for predicting the clinical significance of red cell alloantibodies. In Contreras M (ed): Blood transfusion: The Impact of New Technologies. Baillière's Clinical Haematology. London: Baillière, Tindall, 1990:321–339.
64. Zupanska B: Cellular immunoassays and their use for predicting the clinical significance of antibodies. In Garratty G

(ed): Immunobiology of Transfusion Medicine. New York: Dekker, 1994:465–491.
65. Engelfriet CP, Reesink HW: Laboratory procedures for the prediction of the severity of haemolytic disease of the newborn. Vox Sang 1995;69:61–69.
66. Zupanska B, Lenkiewicz B, Michalewska B, et al: The ability of cellular assays to predict the necessity for cordocenteses in pregnancies at risk of haemolytic disease of the newborn.Vox Sang 2001;80:234–235.
67. Urbaniak SJ, Greiss MA, Crawford RJ, et al: Prediction of the outcome of rhesus haemolytic disease of the newborn. Additional information using an ADCC assay. Vox Sang 1984;46:323–329.
68. Oepkes D, van Kamp IL, Simon MJG, et al: Clinical value of an antibody-dependent cell-mediated cytotoxicity assay in the management of RhD alloimmunization. Am J Obstet Gynecol 2001;184:1015–1020.
69. Nance S, Nelson J, O'Neill P, et al: Correlation of monocyte monolayer assays, maternal antibody titers, and clinical course in hemolytic disease of the newborn (HDFN) [abstract]. Transfusion 1984;24:415.
70. Nance SJ, Nelson J, Horenstein J, et al: Monocyte monolayer assay: An efficient noninvasive technique for predicting the severity of hemolytic disease of the newborn. Am J Clin Pathol 1989;92:89–92.
71. Sacks DA, Nance SJ, Garratty G, et al: Monocyte monolayer assay as a predictor of severity of hemolytic disease of the fetus and newborn. Am J Perinatol 1993;10:428–431.
72. Zupanska B, Brojer E, Richards Y, et al: Serological and immunological characteristics of maternal anti-Rh(D) antibodies in predicting the severity of haemolytic disease of the newborn. Vox Sang 1989;56:247–253.
73. Zupanska B: Cellular immunoassays and their use for predicting the clinical significance of antibodies. In Garratty G (ed): Immunobiology of transfusion medicine. New York: Dekker, 1994:465–491.
74. Larson PJ, Thorp JM Jr, Miller RC, et al: The monocyte monolayer assay: A noninvasive technique for predicting the severity of in utero haemolysis. Am J Perinatol 1995;12: 157–160.
75. Moise KJ, Perkins JT, Sosler SD, et al: The predictive value of maternal serum testing for detection of fetal anaemia in red blood cell alloimmunization. Am J Obstet Gynecol 1995;172: 1003–1009.
76. Hadley AG, Kumpel BM: The role of Rh antibodies in haemolytic disease of the newborn. Bailliere Clin Haematol 1993;6:423–444.
77. Frankowska K, Gorska B: IgG subclasses of anti-Rh antibodies in pregnant women. Arch Immunol et Ther Exper 1978; 26:1095–1100.
78. Ouwehand WH, Engesser L, Huiskes E, et al: Differences in efficacy of IgG1 and IgG3 antibodies in the destruction of red cells. In Ouwehand WH (ed): The activity of IgG1 and IgG3 antibodies in immune mediated destruction of red cells [thesis]. Amsterdam: Rodopi, 1984:44–63.
79. Parinaud J, Blanc M, Grandjean H, et al: IgG subclasses and Gm allotypes of anti-D antibodies during pregnancy: Correlation with the gravity of the fetal disease. Am J Obstet Gynecol 1985;151:1111–1115.
80. Nance S, Arndt P, Nelson J, et al: Correlation of IgG subclass with the severity of hemolytic disease of the newborn [abstract]. Transfusion 1989;29:48S.
81. Schanfield MS: Human immunoglobulin (IgG) subclasses and their biological properties. In Dawson RB (ed): Blood Bank Immunology. Washington, DC: American Association of Blood Banks, 1977:97–112.
82. Cregut R, Pinon F, Brossard Y: Sous-classes d'immunoglobulines anti-Rh(D) et maladie hemolytique du nouveau-ne. Nouv Presse Med 1973;29:1947–1949.
83. Taslimi MM, Sibai BM, Mason JM, et al: Immunoglobulin G subclasses and isoimmunized pregnancy outcome. Am J Obstet Gynecol 1986;154:1327–1332.
84. Nance SJ, Arndt PA, Garratty G: Correlation of IgG subclass with the severity of hemolytic disease of the newborn. Transfusion 1990;30:381–382.
85. Zupanska B, Brojer E, Richards Y, et al: Serological and immunological characteristics of maternal anti-Rh(D) antibodies in predicting the severity of haemolytic disease of the newborn. Vox Sang 1989;56:247–253.
86. Pollock JM, Bowman JM: Anti-Rh(D) IgG subclass and severity of Rh hemolytic disease of the newborn. Vox Sang 1990;59:176–179.
87. Alie-Duran SJ, Dugoujon J-M, Fournie A: Gm typing, IgG subclasses of anti-Rh(D) and severity of hemolytic disease of the newborn. Vox Sang 1992;62:127–128.
88. Iyer YS, Kulkarni SV, Gupte SC: Distribution of IgG subtypes in maternal anti-D sera and their prognostic value in Rh haemolytic disease of the new-born. Acta Haematol 1992;88: 78–81.
89. Lambin P, Debbia M, Puillandre P, et al: Anti-D IgG1 and IgG3 in maternal serum and on the red blood cells of infants suffering from hemolytic disease of the newborn: Relationship with the severity of the disease. Transfusion 2002;42:1537–1546.
90. Levine P: Serological factors as possible causes in spontaneous abortions. J Heredity 1943;34:71–80.
91. Race RR, Sanger R: Blood Groups in Man. Oxford: Blackwell Scientific, 1950:234–236.
92. Nevanlinna HR, Vainio T: The influence of mother-child ABO incompatibility on Rh immunisation. Vox Sang 1956;1:26.
93. Finn R: Erythroblastosis. Lancet 1960;1:526.
94. Finn R, Harper DT, Stallings SA, et al: Transplacental hemorrhage. Transfusion 1963;3:114–124.
95. Finn R, Clarke CA, Donohoe WTA, et al: Experimental studies on the prevention of Rh haemolytic disease. Br Med J 1961;I: 1486–1490.
96. Clarke CA, Donohoe WTA, McConnell RB, et al: Further experimental studies in the prevention of Rh-haemolytic disease. Br Med J 1963;1:979–984.
97. Stern K, Davidsohn I, Masaitis L: Experimental studies on Rh immunization. Am J Clin Pathol 1956;26:833–843.
98. Stern K, Goodman HS, Berger M: Experimental isoimmunization to hemo-antigens in man. J Immunol 1961; 87:189–198.
99. Clarke CA, Donohoe WTA, McConnell RB, et al: Further experimental studies on the prevention of Rh haemolytic disease. Br Med J 1963;I:979–984.
100. Smith T: Active immunity produced by so-called balanced or neutral mixtures of diptheria toxin and antitoxin. J Exp Med 1909;11:241–256.
101. Freda VJ, Gorman JG: Current concepts: Antepartum management of Rh hemolytic disease. Bull Sloane Hosp Women 1962;8:147–158.
102. Freda VJ, Gorman JG, Pollack W: Successful prevention of experimental Rh sensitisation in man with an anti-Rh gammaglobulin antibody preparation. Transfusion 1964;4: 26–32.
103. Combined study. Prevention of Rh haemolytic disease: Results of the clinical trial. A combined study from centres in England and Baltimore. Br Med J 1966;ii:907–914.
104. Pollack W, Gorman JG, Freda VJ, Ascari WQ, Allen AE, Baker WJ: Results of clinical trials of RhoGAM in women. Transfusion 1968;8:151–153.
105. Pollack W, Kochesky RJ: The importance of antibody concentration, binding constant, and heterogeneity in the suppression of immunity to the Rh factor. Int Arch Allergy 1970;38:320–336.
106. Sebring ES, Polesky HF: Fetomaternal hemorrhage: Incidence, risk factors, time of occurrence, and clinical effects. Transfusion 1990;30:344–357.
107. Zipursky A, Israels LG: The pathogenesis and prevention of Rh immunization. Canad Med Assoc J 1967;97:1245.
108. Bowman JM, Chown B, Lewis M, et al: Rh immunization during pregnancy. Antenatal prophylaxis. Canad Med Assoc J 1978;118:623.

109. McMaster Conference on Prevention of Rh Immunization. Vox Sang 1979;36:50–64.
110. Visscher RD, Visscher HC: Do Rh negative women with an early spontaneous abortion need Rh immune prophylaxis? Am J Obstet Gynecol 1972;113:158–162.
111. Bowman JH: The prevention of Rh immunization. Transfus Med Rev 1988;2:129–150.
112. Bowman JH: Controversies in Rh prophylaxis. In Garratty G (ed): Hemolytic disease of the newborn. Arlington, VA: American Association of Blood Banks, 1984:67–85.
113. Urbaniak SJ: Rh(D) haemolytic disease of the newborn: The changing scene. Br Med J 1985;291:4–6.
114. Tovey GH: Should anti-D immunoglobulin be given antenatally? Lancet 1980;ii:466–468.
115. Nusbacher J, Bove JR: Rh immunoprophylaxis: is antepartum therapy desirable? N Eng J Med 1980;303:935–937.
116. Tovey LAD, Taverner JM: A case for the antenatal administration of anti-D immunoglobulin to primigravidae. Lancet 1981;i:878–881.
117. Mollison PL: Some aspects of Rh hemolytic disease and its prevention. In Garratty G (ed): Hemolytic disease of the newborn. Arlington, VA: American Association of Blood Banks, 1984:1–32.
118. Brouwers HAA, Overbeeke MAM, Huiskes E, et al: Complement is not activated in ABO-haemolytic disease of the newborn. Br J Haematol 1988;68:363–366.
119. Vescio LAC, Castro RA: Complement is not activated in ABO-hemolytic disease of the newborn: further support. Vox Sang 1990;58:231.
120. Pochedly C, Palladino N: Etiology of late anemia of hemolytic disease of the newborn. Clin Med 1971;78:30–34.
121. Hughes-Jones NC, Hughes MIJ, Walker W: The amount of anti-D on red cells in haemolytic disease of the newborn. Vox Sang 1967;12:279–285.
122. Garratty G, Nance S: Correlation between in vivo hemolysis and the amount of red cell bound IgG measured by flow cytometry. Transfusion 1990;30:617–621.
123. Hsia DY-Y, Allen FH, Gellis SS, et al: Erythroblastosis fetalis. VIII. Studies of serum bilirubin in relation to kernicterus. N Engl J Med 1952;247:668.
124. Allen FH Jr, Diamond LK, Vaughan VC III: Erythroblastosis fetalis. VI. Prevention of kernicterus. Am J Dis Child 1905;80:779–791.
125. Allen FH Jr, Diamond LK, Jones AR: Erythroblastosis fetalis. IX. The problems of stillbirth. N Eng J Med 1954;251: 453–459.
126. Liley AW: Intrauterine transfusion of foetus in haemolytic disease. Br Med J 1963;ii:1107–1109.
127. Robertson EG, Brown A, Ellis MI, Walker W: Intrauterine transfusion in the management of severe Rhesus isoimmunization. Brit J Obstet Gynecol 1976;83:694–697.
128. Palmer A, Gordon RR: A critical review of intrauterine fetal transfusion. Brit J Obstet Gynecol 1976;83:688–693.
129. Hamilton EG: Intrauterine transfusion. Am J Obstet Gynecol 1977;50:255–260.
130. Frigoletto FD Jr, Umansky I, Birnholz J, et al: Intrauterine fetal transfusion in 365 fetuses during fifteen years. Am J Obstet Gynecol 1981;139:781–790.
131. Buscaglia M, Ferrazzi E, Zuliani G, Caccamo ML, Pardi G: Ultrasound contributions to the management of the severely isoimmunized fetus. J Perinat Med 1986;14:51–58.
132. Rodeck CH, Holman CA, Karnicki J, Kemp JR, Whitmore DN, Austin MA: Direct intravascular fetal blood transfusion by fetoscopy in severe Rhesus isoimmunisation. Lancet 1981;i:625–627.
133. Rodeck CH, Nicolaides KH, Warsof SL, Fysh WJ, Gamsu HR, Kemp JR: The management of severe rhesus isoimmunization by fetoscopic intravascular transfusions. Am J Obstet Gynecol 1984;150:769–774.
134. Grannum PA, Copel JA, Plaxe SC, et al: In utero exchange transfusion by direct intravascular injection in severe erythroblastosis fetalis. N Engl J Med 1986;314:1431–1434.
135. Berkowitz RL, Chitkara U, Goldberg JD, Wilkins I, Chervenak FA: Intravascular transfusion in utero: the percutaneous approach. Am J Obstet Gynecol 1986;154:622–623.
136. Speidel BD: Pediatric management of the severely affected rhesus baby. Plasma Ther Transfus Technol 1984;5:43–46.
137. Brown AK, McDonagh AF: Phototherapy for neonatal hyperbilirubinaemia: Efficiency, mechanism and toxicity. Adv Paediatr 1980;27:341–389.
138. Mathew PM, Wharton BM: Investigation and management of neonatal jaundice: A problem oriented case record. Arch Dis Child 1981;56:949–953.
139. Lewis HM, Campbell RHA, Hambleton G: Use or abuse of phototherapy for physiological jaundice of newborn infants. Lancet 1982;ii:408–410.
140. Hein HA: Why do we keep using phototherapy in healthy newborns? Pediatrics 1984;73:881–882.
141. Allen FH Jr: Induction of labor in the management of erythroblastosis fetalis. Quart Rev Pediat 1957;12:1.
142. Walker W, Murray S, Russell JK: Stillbirth due to haemolytic disease of the newborn. J Obstet Gynaec Br Emp 1957;44:573.
143. Bowman JM, Peddle LJ, Anderson C: Plasmapheresis in severe Rh iso-immunization. Vox Sang 1968;15:272–277.
144. Rock G: Amelioration of Rh disease. In Garratty G (ed): Hemolytic Disease of the Newborn. Arlington, VA: American Association of Blood Banks, 1984:119–143.
145. Moise KJ Jr, Whitecarr PW: Antenatal therapy for haemolytic disease of the fetus and newborn. In Hadley AG, Soothill P (eds): Alloimmune Disorders of Pregnancy. Cambridge: Cambridge University Press, 2002:73–201.
146. Fraser ID, Bennett MO, Bothamley JE, Airth GR: Intensive antenatal plasmapheresis in severe rhesus isoimmunisation. Lancet 1976;1:6–9.
147. Rubinstein P: Repeated small volume plasmapheresis in the management of hemolytic disease of the newborn. In Frigoletto SD, Jewett JF, Konugres AA (eds): Rh Hemolytic Disease, New Strategy for Eradication. Boston: GK Hall and Co, 1981:211–220.
148. Eernisse JG, Gravenhorst JB: 2. Prevention of severe haemolytic disease of the newborn by weekly small-volume plasmapheresis during pregnancy. In Sibinga CTS, Das PC, Forfar JO (eds): Paediatrics and Blood Transfusion. Boston: Martinus Nijhoff, 1982:164–170.
149. Huestis D: Mortality in therapeutic haemapheresis. Lancet 1983;i:1043.
150. Kemp JR: Plasmapheresis: The Lewisham experience. Plas Ther 1984;5:21–22.
151. Robinson AE, Tovey LAD: Intensive plasma exchange in the management of severe Rh disease. Br J Hematol 1980;45: 621–631.
152. Marguiles M, Voto LS, Mathet E: High-dose intravenous IgG for the treatment of severe Rhesus alloimmunization. Vox Sang 1991;61:181–189.
153. Voto LS, Mathet ER, Zapaterio JL, et al: High-dose gammaglobulin (IVIG) followed by intrauterine transfusions (IUT): A new alternative for the treatment of severe fetal hemolytic disease. J Perinat Med 1997;25:85–88.
154. Dooren MC, van Kamp IL, Scherpenisse JW, et al: No beneficial effect of low-dose fetal intravenous gammaglobulin administratin in combination with intravascular transfusions in severe Rh D haemolytic disease. Vox Sang 1994;66:253–257.
155. Rubo J, Albrecht K, Lasch P, et al: High-dose intravenous immune globulin therapy for hyperbilirubinemia caused by Rh hemolytic disease. J Pediatr 1992;121:93–97.
156. Alonso JG, Decaro J, Marrero A, et al: Repeated direct fetal intravascular high-dose immunoglobulin therapy for the treatment of Rh hemolytic disease. J Perinat Med 1994;22:415–419.
157. Gottvall T, Selbing A: Alloimmunization during pregnancy treated with high dose intravenous immunoglobulin. Effects on fetal hemoglobin concentration and anti-D concentrations in the mother and fetus. Acta Obstet Gynecol Scand 1995;74:777–783.

158. Tilz GP, Weiss PAM, Teubl I, Lanzer G, Vollmann H: Succeessful plasma exchange in rhesus incompatibility. Lancet 1977;2:203.
159. Robinson AE: Unsuccessful use of absorbed autologous plasma in Rh incompatible pregnancy. N Eng J Med 1981;305:1346.
160. Yoshida Y, Yoshida H, Tatsumi K, et al: Successful antibody elimination in severe M-incompatible pregnancy. N Eng J Med 1981;305:460–461.
161. Yoshida H, Ito K, Emi N, Kanzaki H, Matsuura S: A new therapeutic antibody removal method using antigen-positive red cells. Vox Sang 1984;47:216–223.
162. Gusdon JP Jr, Witherow C: Possible ameliorating effects of erythroblastosis by promethazine hydrochloride. Am J Obstet Gynecol 1973;117:1101–1108.
163. Rubinstein A, Eidelman AI, Melamed J, Gartner LM, Kandall S, Schulman H: Possible effect of maternal promethazine therapy on neonatal immunologic functions. J Pediatr 1976;89:136–138.
164. Stenchever MA: Promethazine hydrochloride: use in patients with Rh isoimmunization. Am J Obstet Gynecol 1978;130: 665–668.
165. Gusdon JP Jr: The treatment of erythroblastosis with promethazine hydrochloride. J Reprod Med 1981;26:454–458.
166. Charles AG, Blumenthal LS: Promethazine hydrochloride therapy in severely Rh sensitized pregnancies. Obstet Gynecol 1982;60:627–630.
167. Scott JR, Anstall HB, Rote NS, Kochenour NK, Beeson JH: Effect of plasma exchange and immunosuppression on Rh_0(D), viral, and bacterial antibody titers in Rh immunized women. Am J Reprod Immunol 1982;2:46–49.
168. Bierme SJ, Blanc M, Abbal M, Fournie A: Oral Rh treatment for severely immunised mothers. Lancet 1979;i:604–605.
169. Bierme SJ, Blanc M, Fournie A, Abbal M: Desensitization by oral antigen. In Frigoletto FD Jr, Jewett SF, Konugres AA (eds): Rh hemolytic disease: New strategy for eradication. Boston: GK Hall and Co, 1982:247–264.
170. Barnes RMR, Duguid JKM, Roberts FM, et al: Oral administration of erythrocyte membrane antigen does not suppress anti-Rh(D) antibody responses in humans. Clin Exp Immunol 1987;67:220–226.
171. Huntley CC, Lyerly AD, Littlejohn MP, et al: ABO hemolytic disease in Puerto Rico and North Carolina. Pediatrics 1976;57:875–883.
172. Bucher KA, Patterson AM, Elston RC, et al: Racial difference in incidence of ABO hemolytic disease. Am J Public Health 1976;66:854–858.
173. Kirkman HN Jr: Further evidence for a racial difference in frequency of ABO hemolytic disease. J Pediatr 1977;90:717–721.
174. Peevy KJ, Wiseman HJ: ABO hemolytic disease of the newborn: evaluation of management and identification of racial and antigenic factors. Pediatr 1978;61:475–478.
175. Chan-Shu SY, Blair O: ABO hemolytic disease of the newborn. Am J Clin Pathol 1979;71:677–679.
176. Vos GH, Adhikari M, Coovadia HM: A study of ABO incompatibility and neonatal jaundice in Black South African newborn infants. Transfusion 1981;21:744–749.
177. Feng CS, Wan CP, Lau J, et al: Incidence of ABO haemolytic disease of the newborn in a group of Hong Kong babies with severe neonatal jaundice. Paediatr Child Health 1990;26:155–157.
178. Lin M, Broadberry RE: ABO hemolytic disease of the newborn is more severe in Taiwan than in White populations. Vox Sang 1995;68:136.
179. Voak D, Bowley CC: A detailed serological study on the prediction and diagnosis of ABO haemolytic disease of the newborn (ABO HD). Vox Sang 1969;17:321–348.
180. Brouwers HAA, Overbeeke MAM, Gemke RJBJ, et al: Sensitive methods for determining subclasses of IgG anti-A and anti-B in sera of blood–group-O women with a blood-group-A or -B child. Br J Haematol 1987;66:267–270.
181. Orzalesi M, Gloria F, Lucarelli P, et al: ABO system incompatibility: Relationship between direct Coombs test positivity and neonatal jaundice. Pediatr 1973;51:288–289.
182. Desjardins L, Chintu C, Zipursky A: The spectrum of ABO hemolytic disease of the newborn infant. J Pediatr 1979;95: 447–449.
183. Dufour DR, Monaghan WP: ABO hemolytic disease of the newborn. Am J Clin Pathol 1980;73:369–373.
184. Levine DH, Belton H, Meyer P: Newborn screening for ABO hemolytic disease. Clin Pediatr 1985;24:391–394.
185. Ukita M, Takahashi A, Nunotani T, et al: IgG subclasses of anti-A and anti-B antibodies bound to the cord red cells in ABO incompatible pregnancies. Vox Sang 1989;56:181–186.
186. Haberman S, Blanton P, Martin J: Some observations on the ABO antigen sites of the erythrocyte membranes of adults and newborn infants. J Immunol 1967;98:150–160.
187. Voak D, Williams MA: An explanation of the failure of the direct antiglobulin test to detect erythrocyte sensitization in ABO haemolytic disease of the newborn and observations on pinocytosis of IgG anti-A antibodies by infant (cord) red cells. Br J Haematol 1971;20:9–23.
188. Romano EL, Hughes-Jones NC, Mollison PL: Direct antiglobulin reaction in ABO-haemolytic disease of the newborn. Br Med J 1973;1:524–526.
189. Romans DG, Tilley CA, Dorrington KJ: Monogamous bivalency of IgG antibodies. I. Deficiency of branched ABHI-active oligosaccharide chains on red cells of infants causes the weak antiglobulin reactions in hemolytic disease of the newborn due to ABO incompatibility. J Immunol 1980; 124:2807–2811.
190. Osborn LM, Lenarsky C, Oaks RC, et al: Phototherapy in full-term infants with hemolytic disease secondary to ABO incompatibility. Pediatr 1984;74:371–374.

CHAPTER 14

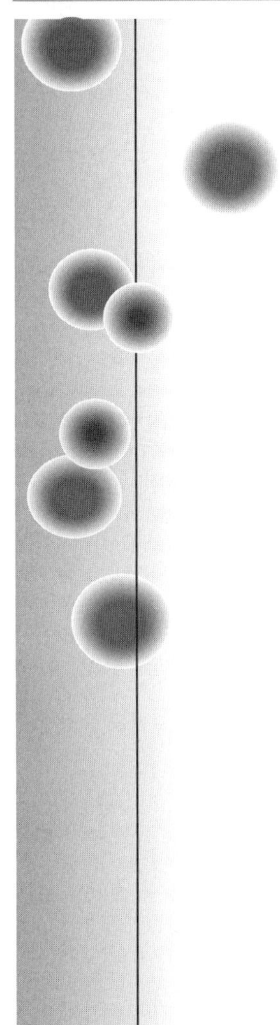

Hemolytic Transfusion Reactions

A hemolytic transfusion reaction (HTR) should be defined as decreased RBC survival following blood transfusion. It is usually the transfused donor RBCs that are destroyed, but on rare occasions, it can be the recipient's RBCs. If this definition is used, then the signs of an HTR could range from obvious signs such as hemoglobinuria/hemoglobinemia and jaundice to a poor post-transfusion increment in hemoglobin and hematocrit. Minimal shortening of RBC survival might not be clinically obvious and shown only by studies such as ^{51}Cr RBC survival tests. An HTR should not be defined by a positive direct antiglobulin test (DAT) alone. Patients can develop a positive DAT without any other signs of HTR; although it is strictly true that such patients have suffered a reaction to the transfused RBCs (i.e., a transfusion reaction) because the RBCs are now sensitized with antibody and/or complement (a "serological" transfusion reaction), the sensitized RBCs often can survive normally. For this reason, a hemolytic transfusion reaction cannot be said to have occurred. Unfortunately, some reports in the literature do not allow one to judge which definition of HTR the authors have used; this is especially true when tables contain many alloantibodies listed together without any clinical data other than a statement that they have caused HTRs.

Hemolytic transfusion reactions can occur in two forms: immediate and delayed. Immediate HTRs (IHTRs) occur during or immediately after the transfusion (i.e., within hours). Delayed HTRs (DHTRs) can occur days or weeks following the transfusion; they usually occur when patients have previously been sensitized to the offending antigen but have no antibody in their plasma at the time of cross-matching or transfusion. On transfusing RBCs containing the offending antigen, a secondary response occurs. This response can occur as early as 24–48 hours after the transfusion but usually takes 5–14 days before it is noticed. The antibody that is produced sensitizes the transfused RBCs having the offending antigen; the patient develops a positive DAT, and the RBCs might or might not have a shortened survival associated with clinical, hematologic, and/or biochemical signs.

INCIDENCE OF ALLOIMMUNIZATION

Antibodies that appear to react (e.g., sensitizing RBCs to react by the antiglobulin test) at 37°C and that are, therefore, of potential clinical significance, have been reported to occur in 1%–3.5% of hospital patients.[1-9] Hoeltge and colleagues[8] reported that 2.9% of 4700 patients had alloantibodies but only 2% were of potential clinical significance. Heddle and coworkers[9] followed 2490 patients given 11,218 red cell transfusions. They found that 2.6% made alloantibodies if they had no antibodies before the transfusion, whereas 3.5% had alloantibodies even before transfusion. If the recipients had at least one antibody before transfusion, then 8.9% made new antibodies. If selected populations (e.g., following massive or multiple transfusions) are examined, the incidence of alloantibodies can be much higher.

Alloimmunization has been reported to occur in 0%–34% (mean of 12.5%, median of 11%) of 3347 random multitransfused patients.[10-16] These patients were transfused for open heart surgery, gastrointestinal bleeds, renal disease, transplants, and hematological conditions. Two reports found that no patients with chronic lymphocytic leukemia made antibodies.[12,13] The highest rate of alloimmunization recorded (34%) was by Lostumbo and associates,[10] who looked for antibodies in a defined time frame (one sample in the second postoperative week and another sample 4–12 months after surgery) and happened to use RBCs that were Lu(a+) for their antibody screen. Their tests included a 22°C phase and a papain test, in addition to an antiglobulin test. They made the unique observation that anti-Lu^a was the most common specificity encountered; the anti-Lu^a appeared earlier than 5 weeks after transfusion and then disappeared. If one subtracts the number of anti-Lu^a and clinically insignificant antibodies in the Lostumbo and colleagues report,[10] the rate of alloimmunization would be 10%, which is similar to that described in other reports.

In six reports, 2714 thalassemias were found to have an alloimmunization rate of 3.7%–23% (mean of 12%, median of 7.7%).[17-23] It has been suggested that the lower rate of immunization among patients with thalassemia compared with patients with sickle cell disease (SCD) (see the discussion later in this chapter) is because patients with thalassemia start transfusions at an earlier age than those with SCD. Michail-Merianou and colleagues[20] showed that thalassemic children who started transfusions at an early age had an alloimmunization rate of 7.7%, compared with a rate of 28% among children who started transfusions later in life. It has also been argued that, compared with SCD patients, the donor blood given to patients with thalassemia is usually from a more genetically similar population.[23,24]

The highest incidence of alloimmunization appears to be associated with SCD and AIHA. In 12 reports, alloimmunization occurred in 8%–35% (mean 25%, median 25%) of 2818 transfused SCD patients.[25-37] Anti-E (21%), -C (14%), and -K (14%) were, by far, the most common antibodies encountered. Anti-Fy^a (7%), -Jk^b (5%), and -S (4%) were the next most common antibodies of possible clinical significance. Lewis system antibodies were also common (11%), but it was unclear from the reports whether they were stimulated by the transfusions or, more probably, were present before transfusion.

It is difficult to calculate the true rate of alloimmunization of multitransfused patients (including patients with SCD), as most of the studies just mentioned calculated their incidence based on antibodies detected after transfusion (without relating to the presence of these antibodies before transfusion) and did not give details of their antibody detection methods. This is particularly relevant to SCD, where Lewis antibodies are often present as naturally occurring antibodies. Other problems are that only a few of the SCD reports segregated patients who had received blood matched for certain antigens from those who received random units. When available, comparison of such data is of great interest. For instance, Wayne and coworkers[35] found an alloimmunization incidence of 17% among patients receiving random units but only 6.4% among those receiving units matched for Rh, K, MNSs, Fy^a, and Fy^b. Tahhan and associates[36] found an incidence of 35% among patients receiving random units but 0% among patients receiving units matched for C, E, K, S, Fy^a, and Fy^b. Most of the reports agree that increasing alloimmunization parallels increasing transfusions. Reisner and colleagues[29] found that the incidence of HTRs was 10% after 50 transfusions, 46% after 100 transfusions, and 57% when 100–199 transfusions were given. Almost all patients who are going to make antibodies make them by the 10th to the 15th transfusion.

The alloimmunization rate among patients with AIHA is high. It has not been so obvious as the high rate reported for SCD, as in AIHA the presence of alloantibodies is often masked by autoantibodies. When adsorption of autoantibodies is carried out, the alloimmunization rate has been reported as 15%–41%. Wallhermfechtel and coworkers,[38] Issitt and associates,[39] and Leger and Garratty[40] performed adsorptions with allogeneic RBCs and found alloantibodies in 15% (19/125), 41% ([14 of 34] and 44% [299 of 674]) of sera, respectively. In studies using adsorptions with autologous RBCs, Issitt and associates,[39] James and colleagues,[41] Laine and Beattie,[42] and Morel and coworkers[43] detected alloantibodies in 27% (11 of 41), 32% (13 of 41), 38% (41 of 109), and 40% (8 of 20) of sera, respectively. Sokol and colleagues[44] detected alloantibodies in 14% (294 of 2149) of their patients, but that series included samples from patients with warm- and cold-reactive autoantibodies and did not distinguish how many patients with warm autoantibodies had alloantibodies. Sokol and colleagues[44] also stated that they issued K–, Rh phenotype-matched blood to decrease the incidence of alloimmunization, so this study cannot be compared directly with the others. Issitt and colleagues[39] found that 69% and 19% of the suspected alloantibodies detected after adsorptions with autologous and allogeneic RBCs, respectively, had autoantbodies that mimicked alloantibodies (see Chapter 7).

As with SCD, a major factor is the number of transfusions the patients have received previously. James and coworkers[41] and Wallhermfechtel and associates[38] found that 75% (3 of 4) and 32% (6 of 19), respectively, of patients who had received more than five transfusions had alloantibodies present. Such a high rate of alloimmunization in patients with warm autoantibodies underscores the need for efficient techniques to evaluate all sera from patients with AIHA for alloantibodies before transfusion (see Chapter 10).

ANTIBODIES HAVING POTENTIAL CLINICAL SIGNIFICANCE

Alloantibodies are of potential clinical significance only if they react at 37°C. Antibodies that react, however strongly, at temperatures below 37°C (e.g., at room temperature) but not at 37°C (e.g., most anti-A_1, -M, -N, -P_1, -Le^a, -Le^b, -I, -HI) will not cause HTRs.[1,45-51] It should be emphasized that if antibodies of any of the specificities mentioned in the previous sentence react at 37°C, then they must be treated as being potentially clinically significant; indeed, some of them have caused HTRs (e.g., anti-M, -P_1, -Le^a), but only when they reacted at 37°C. When an antibody reacts at 37°C, it might or might not be of clinical significance.[1,45,51] Most antibodies should be considered to have potential significance, but some specificities have never been proven to be the cause of an HTR (e.g., anti-Bg, -Chido, -Xg^a); sometimes, blood that is incompatible in vitro at 37°C has been shown to survive normally in vivo.[1,45,51] Antibodies of some specificities are known to cause no RBC destruction in vivo sometimes but on occasion have been shown to cause in vivo destruction (e.g., anti-Lu^b, -Yt^a, -Yt^b, -Ge, -Lan).[44,45] Table 14-1 summarizes the potential clinical significance of some commonly (and less commonly) encountered blood group alloantibodies. The table is a summary of a literature review on antibodies that have been proven to cause hemolytic disease of the newborn (see Chapter 13), HTRs, and in vivo destruction of small amounts (e.g., 1 mL) of ^{51}Cr-labeled RBCs. Increased destruction of these small amounts of ^{51}Cr-labeled RBCs does not always mean that larger volumes (e.g., 500 mL) will have decreased survival.[1,51]

TABLE 14-1. POTENTIAL CLINICAL SIGNIFICANCE OF 37°C-REACTIVE ANTIBODIES

	HDN	HTR	^{51}Cr
Rh	+	+	+
Kell	+	+	+
Duffy	+	+	+
Kidd	+	+	+
SsU	+	+	+
Le^a	0	+	+
Lu^a	(+)	0	0
Lu^b	(+)	+	+
Wr^a	+	+	+
Vel	(+)	+	+
PP_1P^k (Tj^a)	+	+	NA
Holley (Hy)	+	+	NA
Yt^a	0	±	±
Le^b	0	(+)	0
Sd^a	0	(+)	(+)
Xg^a	0	(+)	0
Ch^a	0	0	0
Yk^a	0	0	0

HDN = Antibody has caused hemolytic disease of newborn.
HTR = Antibody has caused hemolytic transfusion reaction.
^{51}Cr = Decreased RBC survival study using RBCs labeled with ^{51}Cr.
\+ = Good evidence indicating potential clinical significance.
(+) = Limited data (e.g., single case report) suggestive of clinical significance (eg, a case of mild HDN in which the mother had anti-Lu^b in her serum, but ABO HDN was not excluded; one case in which anti-Sd^a destroyed RBCs, but this particular donor had a "super" Sd^a antigen).
± = Some examples have been shown to have clinical significance; others have been shown to have no clinical significance.
0 = Evidence (or lack of reports) in the literature suggests that the antibody has no clinical significance.
NA = Data not available.

Table 14-2 shows data extracted from four large series of 37°C-reactive alloantibodies that were detected in hospital patients. The data, reported by Grove-Rasmussen,[3] were from 18 large transfusion centers in the United States, where 1.5 million units of blood were transfused. Anti-D was the most common antibody detected; the next most common specificity was anti-E, followed by anti-K, anti-c, anti-Fy^a, anti-Jk^a, and anti-e. Spielman and Seidl[5] reported on antibodies detected in 55,350 blood recipients in Germany; 443 antibodies were detected (0.8% of all recipients). Tovey[4] reported on 3707 antibodies detected over a 5-year period in England; 3002 were from Rh-negative individuals and contained anti-D with or without anti-C, anti-E, or anti-K. Walker and colleagues[6] reported on 1537 (0.7%) clinically significant antibodies detected in 214,000 patients from two hospitals over a 16-year period.

In the four series, which included 21,499 antibodies detected at 37°C, in blood recipients from three different countries, the findings were as follows: Anti-D was the most common antibody detected (in all four series), followed by anti-C when together with anti-D, and anti-E (approximately the same incidence); then anti-c and anti-Fy^a, followed by anti-Jk^a, anti-e, and, finally, anti-S. These results from data gathered before 1977 might not reflect the impact of Rh prophylaxis. Studies published in the 1990s could reflect the current trend more accurately. In the United States, Hoeltge and coworkers[8] studied alloimmunization in 4700 patients during the period from 1985 to 1993. They found the most common specificities were anti-K (23%), anti-E (18%), anti-D (12%), anti-Le^a (7.3%), anti-C (6.3%), anti-Fy^a (5.7%), anti-c (4.4%), and anti-Jk^a (3%). Heddle and associates[9] (Canada) found that the most common antibodies made by 2490 patients were anti-Jk^a(16.4%), anti-E (16.4%), and anti-K (14.6%).

TABLE 14-2. 37°C-REACTIVE ANTIBODIES DETECTED IN BLOOD TRANSFUSION RECIPIENTS IN FOUR STUDIES FROM THE 1970S*

	Grove-Rasmussen[3]	Tovey[4]	Spielman & Seidl[5]	Walker et al.[6]	Total	Percentage of Total	Order of Frequency
Anti-D	8772	3002	245	778	12,797	61	1
-C (together with D)	2156	28	52	163	2399	11.4	2
-E	1079	231	45	118	1473	7	3
-K (-k)	978	174	41	181	1374	6.5	4
-c	619	154	14	53	840	4	5
-Fy (-Fy^b)	372	72	16	55	515	2.4	6
-Jk^a (-Jk^b)	141	17	12	13	183	0.9	7
-S -s	0	9	0	0	9	0.04	8
Others (e.g., anti-Le^a, -Le^b, -Wr^a, -M, -N, -P$_1$, and unidentified)	1177	0	72	184	1433	6.9	

*See text for comparative rates for the 1990s.

Most Common Antibodies to Cause HTRs

Table 14-3 shows data from three large studies from the 1970s.[3,6,52] The data are based on 280 HTRs (not including ABO) occurring after almost two million transfusions (incidence of one per 7143 transfusions). The most common antibody to cause an HTR was anti-K, followed closely by anti-E. The next most common antibodies were anti-Fy^a, anti-c, and anti-Jk^a. It should be pointed out that the Grove-Rasmussen report[3] was a summary of data from 18 different medical centers. The Mayo Clinic's 10-year study[52-55] also found anti-K to be the most common cause of HTR, but in contrast to the Grove-Rasmussen study,[3] the Mayo researchers found anti-Jk^a to be almost as common a cause of HTR, and they found anti-Fy^a equal to anti-E as the third most common offenders. When DHTRs were examined separately, anti-Jk^a and anti-E were found to be the cause of HTRs more often than anti-K. Anti-Jk^a and anti-E were followed by anti-K and anti-Fy^a, respectively, as causes of DHTR. Unfortunately, it is not clear from the publications how these authors defined a hemolytic transfusion reaction (see the discussion that follows).

INCIDENCE OF HTRs

The reported incidence of HTRs in the transfused population varies considerably in the literature. There are three main reasons for this. First, compatibility techniques have improved. Second, as will be discussed shortly, the incidence varies depending on the criteria that were used to select patients for a particular series of HTRs. The third reason is that the incidence is dependent on the efficiency of the monitoring system. The Mayo Clinic[52-57] published six often-referenced reports relating to their experiences of HTRs, but it should be emphasized that the earlier reports included asymptomatic patients (e.g., patients who developed a positive DAT following transfusion but no clinical symptoms) among those defined as suffering with HTRs. In one of the reports, 13 of 37 patients (35%) described as having HTRs had no clinical symptoms at all.[54] As there was no proven decreased RBC survival in these patients, we would prefer not to include them as HTRs. Nevertheless, the reports from the Mayo Clinic still contain the most substantial hospital experience on HTRs available in the literature. During a 16-year period at the Mayo

TABLE 14-3. ANTIBODIES CAUSING HTRS

	Grove-Rasmussen (1973)[3]	Walker et al. (1977)[6]	Pineda et al. (1978)[52]	Total
Units transfused	1.5 × 10^6	160,000	268,000	2 ×10^6
Number of HTRs	192	41	47	280
K	38	4	10	52
-E	30	10	7	47
-Fy^a	25	3	7	35
-c	25	1	6	32
-D	23	4	4	31
-Jk^a	8	4	9	21
-C (together with -D)	12	0	0	12
-e	4	0	4	8
Other antibodies (e.g., anti-k, -Fyb, -Kp^a, -Js^a, -Le^a, -P$_1$, -M, -C^w)	27	21	5	45

Clinic (1964–1980), 171 cases of HTRs were detected following 649,943 transfusions (one reaction for every 3800 transfusions); if one disregards the asymptomatic cases, the incidence would be approximately one in 5700 transfusions. There were almost twice as many reactions among females compared with males, and an increased frequency of reactions among older patients and among those with conditions requiring large amounts of blood (e.g., acute medical, obstetrical, and surgical situations). A more recent interpretation of the Mayo Clinic data is discussed by Vamvakas and colleagues[56] and Pineda and coworkers.[57]

The first clear report of a DHTR was by Fudenberg and Allen.[58] Since then, many have been reported; usually these have been single reports associated with a particular specificity, but some series of DHTRs have been reported.[52-57] At the Mayo Clinic, DHTRs were reported to occur once in every 3200 transfusions over a 16-year period; there was a great deal of variation in incidence from period to period (e.g., 1:11,650 from 1964 to 1973; 1:4000 from 1974 to 1977; and 1:1500 from 1978 to 1980).[55] Along with the increased incidence of DHTRs since 1974 came a decrease in IHTRs (1:12,000 from 1964 to 1973; 1:21,000 from 1974 to 1977; and 1:17,000 from 1978 to 1980); the overall incidence of IHTRs from 1964 to 1980 was 1:14,000. More recent data from the Mayo Clinic, reviewing two periods (1980–1992 and 1993–1998) and breaking the data into true hemolytic transfusion reactions and serological transfusion reactions (see the discussion later), found an incidence of one DHTR per 5405 and 6715 transfusions, respectively.[56,57] Taswell and colleagues[55] point out that the apparent increase in the incidence of DHTRs at the Mayo Clinic since 1974 was probably due to the following factors:

1. Increased sensitivity of laboratory methods
2. Increased awareness of DHTRs
3. Recognition and inclusion of milder, or entirely asymptomatic, cases (e.g., positive DAT but no clinical symptoms)
4. Improved error recognition and control
5. Increased experience and improved organization (e.g., intravenous service)

These reasons also probably explain why there is a higher incidence of HTRs (especially DHTRs) reported by the Mayo Clinic than from other institutions. For instance, Croucher and associates[59] reported an incidence of only one DHTR for every 22,000 transfusions performed at a Toronto-based hospital; the Mayo Clinic incidence is about three to four times higher.[59] The difference almost certainly does not mean that it is safer to receive blood in Toronto than at the Mayo Clinic, but it does emphasize how much variation exists, even between well-respected workers, in definitions and recognition of a DHTR.

DELAYED HEMOLYTIC TRANSFUSION REACTIONS (DHTRs) VS. DELAYED SEROLOGIC TRANSFUSION REACTIONS (DSTRs)

As mentioned previously, a transfusion reaction can be classified as an HTR only if evidence of hemolysis (i.e., reduced red cell survival) is documented. Ness and colleagues[60] coined the term "delayed serological transfusion reaction" (DSTR) to encompass those reactions in which alloimmunization occurred, leading to a positive DAT following transfusion but without any evidence of hemolytic anemia. They reported 34 cases of DSTR, 70% of which were due to anti-E and/or anti-Jk^a, over a 20-month period. Retrospective review of the medical records found clinical evidence of hemolysis in only six of the 34 (18%) cases; all six were associated with anti-Jk^a. Thus, the incidence of DSTR was one per 151 (0.66%) recipients with post-transfusion samples available for testing, whereas the incidence of DHTR was only one in 854 (0.12%) patients tested. Fifteen of the 34 patients were followed for up to 174 days after the reaction. Twelve of the 15 still demonstrated a positive DAT at 174 days after transfusion. Eluate studies indicated that the persistence of a positive DAT after DSTR or DHTR could involve several immunologic mechanisms, including the development of post-transfusion autoantibodies. Other workers (including those from the Mayo Clinic) have presented transfusion reaction data contrasting DHTRs with DSTRs.[9,56,57,60,61] Table 14-4 shows the results of five studies. It should be noted that Heddle and colleagues[9] used a different definition for DSTR; they included any patient who became alloimmunized after transfusion, without necessarily having a positive DAT. Pineda and colleagues[57] studied two periods (1980–1992 and 1993–1998). The incidence of DHTR/DSTR increased from one in 1899 in the period 1980 through 1992 to one in 1300 in the period 1993 through 1998 ($p < 0.05$). Similarly, DSTRs increased from one in 2990 in the period 1980 through 1992 to one in 1612 in the period 1993 through 1998 ($p < 0.05$). The incidence of DHTR showed a trend toward decrease, from one in 5405 in 1980 through 1992 to one in 6715 in 1993 through 1998. The incidence of Jk^a antibodies increased in 1993 through 1998, while the incidence of other alloantibodies remained stable. These changes were most likely due to a combination of factors, including a decrease in average length of stay and the adoption of the polyethylene glycol (PEG) antibody detection system.[57]

It is obvious from the data that most immune transfusion reactions associated with a positive DAT do not lead to any obvious clinical or laboratory signs of hemolysis. Table 14-5 shows DHTRs or DSTRs, associated with various antibodies, at the Mayo Clinic over a 19-year period.[56,57] Of immune-related transfusion reactions, 65% were DSTR (i.e., positive DAT after

TABLE 14-4. DELAYED HEMOLYTIC TRANSFUSION REACTIONS (DHTRS) VS. DELAYED SEROLOGICAL TRANSFUSION REACTIONS (DSTRS)

	Ness et al.[60]	Pinkerton et al.[61]	Heddle et al.[9]	Vamvakas et al.[56]	Pineda et al.[57]
DHTR					
per unit	1/9094	1/13,680	1/11,328	1/5405[b]	1/9244[c]
per patient	1/854	1/2537	1/2082	NA	NA
DSTR					
per unit	1/1605	1/3040	1/199[a]	1/2990[b]	1/2312[c]
per patient	1/151	1/563	1/37[a]	NA	NA

NA, data not available
[a] Heddle et al. included any patients who made alloantibodies following transfusion, even if the DAT was negative; other investigators used positive DAT, following alloimmunization, to indicate DSTRs.
[b] Mayo Clinic data from 1980–1992.
[c] Mayo Clinic data from 1993–1998.

transfusion but no signs of hemolysis), and 35% were true HTRs. This does not mean that the transfused RBCs in the DSTR group survived normally; none of the studies included RBC survival studies. Nevertheless, the clinical effects were minimal in most cases. The results of these studies also emphasize that the term *HTR* has been applied incorrectly in the past and might still be so in some modern reports; a similar situation applies to the term *hemolytic disease of the newborn*.

In 1984, Salama and Mueller-Eckhardt[62] published an iconoclastic paper suggesting that some of our cherished beliefs concerning the findings associated with DHTRs were incorrect. Some people found these suggestions hard to accept, but in 1990, Ness and colleagues[60] published a study from the United States that confirmed much of what Salama and Mueller-Eckhardt had found.

Salama and Mueller-Eckhardt[62] studied 26 patients with DHTRs. All patients were found to have C3d detectable on their RBCs after the reaction. The RBC-bound C3d, detectable by the DAT, was detected for weeks and even months after the transfusion. RBC-bound IgG was detected by DAT in only 10 of 26 cases (39%), but a radioimmunoassay detected IgG on the RBCs in 16 of 17 patients tested. IgG alloantibodies could be eluted from RBCs of 25 of the 26 patients.

In 1990, Ness and coworkers[60] published results agreeing with the more iconoclastic parts of the article by Salama and Mueller-Eckhardt.[62] Thirty-four transfused patients were studied. All of these patients had serologic evidence (e.g., alloantibodies in the serum and a positive DAT) of a DHTR, but only five (18%) of the 34 patients had clinical evidence of hemolysis. Ness and coworkers[60] suggested that the term *DHTR* be reserved for reactions occurring in patients who show well-defined evidence of hemolysis, whereas the other patients should be described as having DSTR. The incidence of a DHTR was one in 854 patients, and the incidence of a DSTR was one in 151 patients. Results of other studies since then are shown in Table 14-4 and Table 14-5.

Ness and coworkers[60] reported that all 34 patients in their study had a positive DAT. In contrast to Salama and Mueller-Eckhardt,[62] Ness and coworkers[60] detected RBC-bound IgG by the DAT in all patients; 56% also had RBC-bound complement. Alloantibody was eluted from the RBCs of all patients. Fifteen of the 34 patients were followed for up to 194 days after the

TABLE 14-5. DELAYED HEMOLYTIC (DHTR) AND SEROLOGICAL (DSTR) TRANSFUSION REACTIONS AT MAYO CLINIC DURING A 19-YEAR PERIOD (1980–1998)

Specificity	Total Number	DHTR	DSTR*
E	184	47	137
Jk[a]	95	45	50
Fy[a]	62	26	36
K	62	16	46
c	54	18	36
Jk[b]	27	12	15
Fy[b]	12	9	3
C	22	8	14
S	7	4	3
e	12	3	9
C^W	5	3	2
Yt[a]	2	1	1
A_1	2	1	1
Kp[a]	1	1	0
Lu[a]	1	1	0
Lu[b]	1	1	0
D	1	1	0
M	2	0	2
Js[a]	2	0	2
V	2	0	2
G	1	0	1
P_1	1	0	1
Co[b]	1	0	1
Total	559	197 (35%)	362 (65%)

*Alloimmunization with post-transfusion-positive DAT but no obvious hemolytic anemia or clinical signs of a HTR.
From Vamvakas EC, Pineda AA, Reisra R, et al: The differentiation of delayed hemolytic and delayed serologic transfusion reactions: Incidence and predictors of hemolysis. Transfusion 1995;35:26–32 and Pineda AA, Vamvakas EC, Gorden LD, et al: Trends in the incidence of delayed hemolytic and delayed serologic transfusion reactions. Transfusion 1999; 39:1097–1103.

putative transfusion. Twelve of the 15 (80%) still had positive DATs at 194 days after transfusion; at that time, RBC-bound IgG was detectable on the RBCs of 13 of the 15 patients, IgG plus C3 was detected on the RBCs of five patients (33%), and one patient had complement on the RBCs only. Putative alloantibodies were eluted from the RBCs of five (33%) patients 25–168 days after the last transfusion. Panagglutinins (autoantibodies) were eluted from the RBCs of four patients (27%); only specific alloantibodies were found in the sera of these four patients. A mixed-field appearance in the DAT was detected in only six patients (17.7%).

These two reports have changed our expectations of the serology associated with DHTRs.[60,62] The differences from what we previously believed to be typical findings associated with DHTRs, were as follows:

- A mixed-field appearance was not observed commonly in the DAT results.
- A positive DAT was detected for more than 100 days after transfusion in five of seven patients (71%) who were followed up for up to 312 days after transfusion.
- The alloantibody(ies) causing the DHTR could be eluted from the DAT-positive RBCs more than 100 days after transfusion.

The authors emphasized that because so few transfused RBCs would be expected to survive 100 days after transfusion, the alloantibody and complement must be present on autologous RBCs. It was suggested that the syndrome was very similar to post-transfusion purpura (PTP).[62]

HTRs ASSOCIATED WITH SICKLE CELL DISEASE

The literature contains many reports with detailed case histories of HTRs associated with SCD; the incidence of HTRs in SCD is not so well documented.[31,63-81] DHTRs in transfused SCD patients have been reported in four series to have an incidence of 4%, 11%, 17%, and 22%.[29,30,32,64] The incidence of DHTRs in SCD is at least ten times higher than reported for random transfused patients.

Most of the reports of DHTRs in SCD follow the typical pattern of a DHTR, with new alloantibodies (Rh system mainly anti-C and -E [39%], -Jk^b [15%], -Fy^a [10%], and anti-S [7% each], -K, -Fy^b, and -s [3% each]) appearing after 7 to 10 days, obvious signs (laboratory and clinical) of hemolytic anemia, a positive DAT, and decreased survival of the transfused red cells. Many of the reports contain findings that are not typical of DHTR: pain crisis (87%), post-transfusion hemoglobin or hematocrit dropping below pretransfusion levels (83%), hemoglobinuria and/or hemoglobinemia (33%), negative DAT (26%), pulmonary infiltrates (9%), disseminated intravascular coagulation (7%), and new RBC alloantibodies that were not detectable until 72 hours or longer after the DHTR (7%) or that were never detected (20%).[37,70-75] Some patients with SCD and DHTRs develop a life-threatening or fatal anemia (11%) with some, or all, of the unusual findings just described.[37]

The Sickle Cell Hemolytic Transfusion Reaction Syndrome

We, and others, have observed serious and life-threatening signs and symptoms that have occurred in some patients with SCD who have severe HTRs. Petz and colleagues[76] described five such patients, and they felt that there are distinctive features of these hemolytic episodes that justify the designation of a syndrome that they have termed *sickle cell hemolytic transfusion reaction syndrome*. In addition to the usual laboratory manifestations of hemolysis, patients can develop symptoms characteristic of a sickle cell pain crisis, and life-threatening anemia can develop as a result of the hemoglobin and hematocrit falling to levels markedly lower than were present prior to transfusion. Other investigators have reported cases with many similar features, but insufficient emphasis has been given to the constellation of findings that justifies the identification of a distinct syndrome. It is important that the manifestations of this syndrome be recognized, as misinterpretation of the findings could lead to inappropriate management.

Characteristics of Sickle Cell HTR Syndrome

The characteristics of sickle cell HTR syndrome are indicated in Table 14-6, and certain aspects deserve emphasis.

SYMPTOMS OF A SICKLE CELL PAIN CRISIS LEADING TO ERRONEOUS DIAGNOSIS

Symptoms suggestive of a sickle cell pain crisis frequently develop or are intensified during the hemolytic reaction. Indeed, Garratty[37] found that "pain crises" developed in 87% of reported cases of delayed HTRs in patients with SCD. Chaplin and Cassell[80] pointed out the relationship of HTRs to development of pain crises in a remarkably detailed case report. They described a patient with SCD whose multiple episodes of post-transfusion hemolysis were documented with 17 measurements of in vivo RBC survival. A most striking feature of the patient's course was the regular onset of typical painful sickle cell crises coincident with the rapid destruction of large numbers of donor RBCs.

Patients who experience brisk hemolysis often develop fever, chills, flank pain, abdominal pain, chest pain, apprehension, dyspnea, headache, nausea,

TABLE 14-6. COMPONENTS OF THE SICKLE CELL HEMOLYTIC TRANSFUSION REACTION SYNDROME

- Manifestations of an acute or delayed hemolytic transfusion reaction.
- Symptoms suggestive of a sickle cell pain crisis that develop or are intensified during the hemolytic reaction.
- Marked reticulocytopenia (a significant decrease in absolute reticulocyte level compared with the patient's usual value).
- Development of a more severe anemia after transfusion than was previously present. A rapid drop in hemoglobin and hematocrit can occur when hemolysis of donor RBCs is accompanied by suppressed erythropoiesis, as sickle cell RBCs have an intrinsically short survival. In some patients, it is possible that hyperhemolysis of autologous RBCs (bystander immune hemolysis) could play a role in causing the decrease in hemoglobin and hematocrit, although more definitive documentation of this phenomenon is necessary.
- Subsequent transfusions could further exacerbate the anemia, which could become life threatening or even fatal.
- Patients often have multiple RBC alloantibodies and might also have autoantibodies, making it difficult or impossible to find compatible units of RBCs. In other patients, however, no alloantibodies are demonstrable, or patients might have alloantibodies for which antigen-negative RBCs are readily obtainable.
- Serologic studies might not provide an explanation for the hemolytic transfusion reaction. Even RBCs phenotypically matched with multiple patient antigens might be hemolyzed.

From Petz LD, Calhoun L, Shulman IA, et al: The sickle cell hemolytic transfusion reaction syndrome. Transfusion 1997;37:382—392.

vomiting, hemoglobinemia, and hemoglobinuria. Many of these same symptoms can occur as part of a sickle cell "pain crisis." As a result, the diagnosis of an HTR could go unrecognized, and appropriate management could be delayed. Indeed, several groups of investigators have pointed out that many HTRs in sickle cell disease patients are misdiagnosed as typical "vaso-occlusive" or "aplastic" sickle cell crises.[64,65,70] Pain symptoms might simply be part of an HTR, or the HTR might cause symptoms indistinguishable from a true pain crisis.[64-66,70,80,81] In either case, the critical point is that the diagnosis of an HTR could go unrecognized because of the tendency to attribute all signs and symptoms in an acutely ill patient with sickle cell disease to a diagnosis of pain crisis. This is a frequent error, and the delay in making a diagnosis of an HTR contributes significantly to morbidity and to the probability of mortalilty. In this regard, the case described by Reed and colleagues[81] is most dramatic, as the patient's fever and worsening pain after transfusions were attributed to vaso-occlusion, her hemoglobin dropped to 1.4 g/dL, and she expired; the diagnosis of HTR was made postmortem.

THE DEVELOPMENT OF MORE SEVERE ANEMIA THAN WAS PRESENT PRIOR TO TRANSFUSION

One of the most important findings in the sickle cell HTR syndrome is the development of more severe anemia than was present prior to transfusion, as has been indicated in a number of reports.[37,61,65,69,74,75] Indeed, Garratty[37] indicated that in 83% of reported cases of HTRs in SCD, the post-transfusion hemoglobin and hematocrit fell below their pretransfusion levels. The case report visualized in Figure 14-1 (left panel) illustrates this point.

PATIENT 1: A 28-year-old female with SCD was hospitalized with chest, knee, and back pain, diarrhea, and an ankle ulcer. Her blood type was group A, Rh positive. She had a history of multiple previous transfusions, and on admission her serum contained anti-E, -C, -K, and -S red cell alloantibodies. The DAT was negative, LDH was 518 U/L, and total and direct bilirubin levels were 1.3 mg/dL and 0.0 mg/dL, respectively. On hospital day 2, her hematocrit was 13.2%, and she was transfused with 3 units of RBC over the next 5 days, after which her hematocrit rose to 24.7%. All transfused RBCs were negative for E, C, K, and S antigens and were crossmatch compatible.

Her pain symptoms intensified, and on the seventh hospital day, overt signs of a delayed HTR developed, including a drop in hematocrit and increases in total and direct bilirubin to 3.1 mg/dL and 0.2 mg/dL, respectively. On day 9, she received 3 additional units of RBCs, but gross hemoglobinuria developed, and her hematocrit dropped precipitously to 11% on day 12. Two new RBC alloantibodies, anti-Fy^a and -Jk^b, were identified, and the DAT was positive with polyspecific and anti-IgG antiserums. During the next 3 days, the patient received an additional 9 units of blood, all of which were negative for E, C, K, S, Fy^a, and Jk^b antigens and were crossmatch compatible. This resulted in a transient increase in hematocrit to 19%, but the LDH increased to 3580 U/L; the total and direct bilirubin increased to 7.7 mg/dL and 0.6 mg/dL, respectively; reticulocytes reached a nadir of 4.5%; and the hematocrit dropped to 9.3% on day 17. Thus, after transfusion of a total of 15 units of RBCs, her hematocrit had decreased from 13% to 9.3%. Prednisone, 60 mg daily, was begun on day 15, and 2 more units of RBCs were transfused on day 17. Subsequently, signs of hemolysis decreased, and the hematocrit progressively increased. During the hemolytic episode, the patient experienced an increase in pain that began to resolve on about day 17. She was discharged on day 24 with a hematocrit of 22.4%.

Twenty-seven months later, the patient was admitted with symptoms of pain in her chest, knees, and back, and a nonproductive cough and fever (see Fig. 14-1, right panel). The hematocrit was 16.1%; the DAT was negative; total and direct bilirubin were at 2.2 mg/dL and 0.3 mg/dL, respectively; LDH was 386 U/L; and reticulocytes were 10.8%. She was transfused with two units of RBCs that were crossmatch compatible and negative for all six antigens as previously. The hematocrit rose to 25%, and the patient was discharged the next day. She was readmitted 6 days later with persistent pain, however, at which time the hematocrit was 12.7%; total and direct bilirubin were 1.4 mg/dL and 0.2 mg/dL, respectively; and LDH was 509 U/L. The next day, the hematocrit was 10.8% and reticulocytes reached a nadir of 2.8%. Two additional units of RBCs resulted in a hematocrit of 19%, but the patient devel-

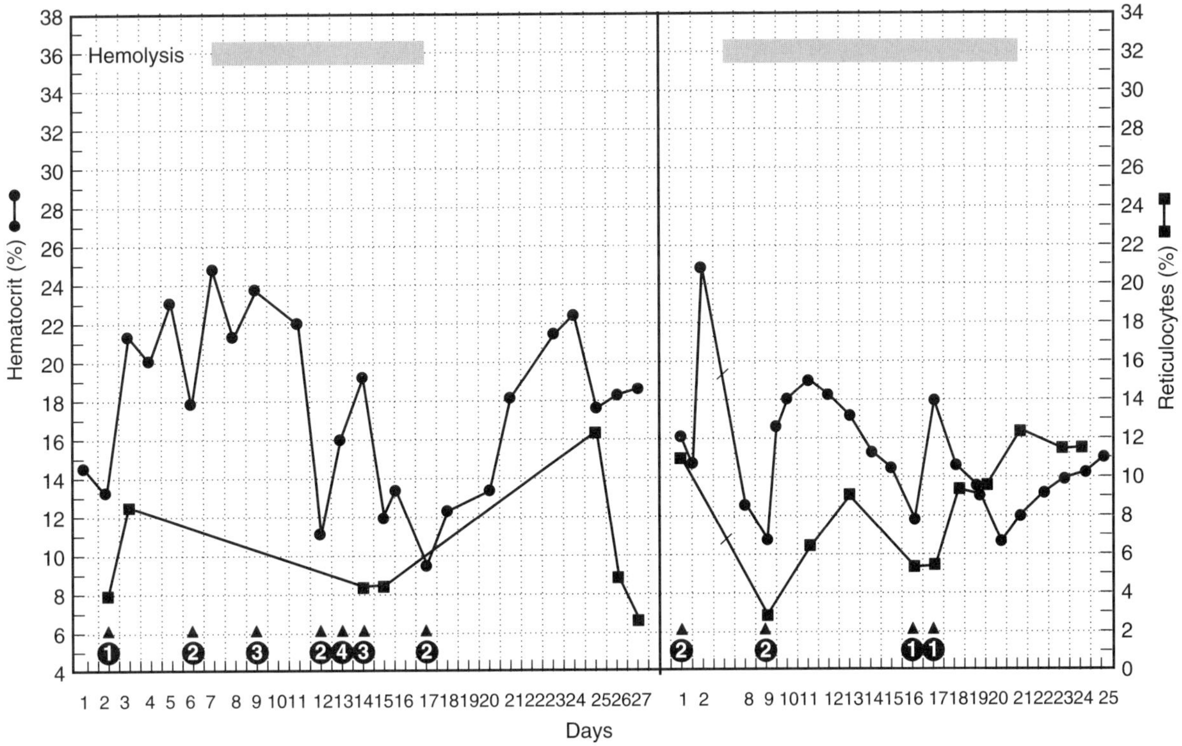

FIGURE 14-1. Clinical course of Patient 1, indicating Hct, uncorrected reiculocyte counts (%), and episodes of hemolysis. Numbers in circles indicate the number of RBCs that were transfused. (From Petz LD, Calhoun L, Shulman IA, et al: The sickle cell hemolytic transfusion reaction syndrome. Transfusion 1997;37:382–392.)

oped dark urine and there was again a progressive fall in hematocrit to 11.8% on day 16. At that time, anti-D was also identified, although it had not been evident previously; a review of previous records from another hospital revealed that the patient was a D mosaic. Two additional units of compatible RBCs resulted in a temporary increase in hematocrit to 17.8%, followed by a progressive fall to 10.5% over the next 3 days, during which time the total and direct bilirubin peaked at 4.5 mg/dL and 0.8 mg/dL and the LDH peaked at 1011 U/L. On day 22, hemoglobin electrophoresis revealed only hemoglobin S, indicating that all donor RBCs had been hemolyzed. Transfusions were discontinued because of the repeated episodes of post-transfusion hemolysis. The patient's hematocrit gradually improved to 15%, and signs of hemolysis and symptoms of pain gradually abated. The patient's DAT remained negative throughout, although flow cytometry on day 23 indicated that the patient's RBCs were weakly coated with IgG. It should be noted that during the first hemolytic episode, her reticulocytes dropped to a nadir of 4.5%, and during the second episode, to 2.8%.

RETICULOCYTOPENIA

Another frequent finding in the sickle cell HTR syndrome, as illustrated in the foregoing case report, is reticulocytopenia, which we have defined as a significant decrease in the absolute reticulocyte level compared with the patient's usual value. Reticulocytosis is a critical mechanism by which patients with SCD partially compensate for their shortened red cell survival. If erythropoiesis is suppressed in patients with a very short RBC survival, a rapid increase in the severity of the anemia will occur. Accordingly, if a patient with SCD has a severe HTR in which transfused RBCs are hemolyzed rapidly and, in addition, the patient's reticulocyte level is significantly depressed, severe and life-threatening anemia could develop.

SEROLOGIC FINDINGS

The sickle cell HTR syndrome most often occurs in patients who have multiple RBC alloantibodies, at times in association with autoantibodies. In some patients, a newly detected RBC alloantibody develops after transfusion as is typical in a DHTR, whereas in other patients, the serologic findings do not provide an explanation for the hemolysis. This could be because no new antibodies become apparent during the DHTR or, in some instances, because no alloantibodies or autoantibodies are demonstrable at any time.

The classic publication by Chaplin and Cassel,[80] cited earlier, described a patient with SCD in whom rapid destruction of transfused RBCs occurred repeatedly despite entirely compatible crossmatch results by a wide variety of serologic methods. Overt hemolysis occurred even after the transfusion of crossmatch–compatible RBCs from two siblings whose blood types were identical to the patient's with respect to numerous RBC antigens. These authors were the first to point out the regular onset of typical sickle pain "crisis" coincident with the rapid destruction of large volumes of donor RBCs.

Diamond and coworkers[64] and Cullis and associates[73] also described patients who had clinical and laboratory findings of a DHTR, although the DAT and antibody screen remained negative.

Although DHTRs in patients with SCD have been reported in which serologic findings do not explain the hemolysis, one must not think of this phenomenon as unique to patients with SCD. Numerous cases of hemolysis of transfused RBCs have been described as occurring in the absence of serologically detectable alloantibodies in patients without SCD.

Additional Reports of Severe HTRs in Patients with SCD

Diamond and colleagues[64] reported DHTRs in three patients with SCD. The patients developed clinical features of painful crises, and the authors pointed out that HTR should be suspected "when patients have recurrent or severe sickle crises after transfusion." Millner and coworkers[65] described ten patients with sickle cell anemia who became acutely ill after blood transfusion. The acute illnesses were attributed to DHTRs although, in two cases, the immunohematologic data were incomplete. Most of the patients developed symptoms characteristic of pain crisis during the hemolysis, and several developed reticulocytopenia and "profound anemia," with the hemoglobin level falling below pretransfusion levels and to values as low as 3.5 g/dL. Two patients died. The authors emphasized that "many of these reactions go unrecognized, being diagnosed as sickle cell crises."

Cullis and associates[73] described one patient who had anti-E, -C, and –Js^b, and who received an exchange transfusion with RBCs negative for these antigens, which increased her hemoglobin from 7.2 g/dL to 9.2 g/dL. At this time, 53% of the hemoglobin was hemoglobin S and 46% hemoglobin A; that is, the hemoglobin S concentration was about 4.9 g/dL. The patient developed severe joint pains, a DHTR ensued, and 6 days later the hemoglobin was only 3.0 g/dL. The authors assumed that the severe anemia was caused by hemolysis of the allogeneic RBCs and "hyperhemolysis" of the patient's RBCs. No follow-up hemoglobin electrophoresis was performed and no reticulocyte counts were reported, however. Suppression of erythropoiesis could have resulted in a drop in the hemoglobin S-containing RBCs from 4.9 g/dL to 3.0 g/dL in 6 days, and all of the allogeneic RBCs could have been hemolyzed. The case is notable in that the patient's DAT remained negative throughout and no previously undetectable RBC alloantibodies could be found on repeated serum samples over the next 8 weeks.

Chaplin and Zarkowsky[82] reported on four patients with SCD who developed severe hemolysis after transfusion. Before transfusion, all four patients had two or more alloantibodies as well as a positive DAT and a RBC autoantibody in the serum. The hemoglobin dropped to levels of 2.8 g/dL to 3.8 g/dL in three patients, and the authors pointed out that these low values occurred during periods of "relative reticulocytopenia." Indeed, the nadir of hemoglobin values were associated with corrected reticulocyte counts (calculated from the authors' data) of 3.52%, 1.1%, and 0.36%. The authors demonstrated autoantibodies in all patients and attributed the accelerated hemolysis to AIHA, which could have been precipitated by alloimmunization associated with transfusion (see Chapter 9). In spite of severe anemia, all patients recovered from the hemolytic episodes, corticosteroids being the mainstay of therapy.

Cummins and colleagues[70] reported two DHTRs in patients with SCD. Both patients developed multiple alloantibodies and an autoantibody, and the nadirs of hemoglobin values during the reactions were 2.6 g/dL and 3.0 g/dL, respectively. Both patients developed pain symptoms while hemolyzing, and the authors emphasized that HTRs in patients with SCD often are mistaken for vaso-occlusive crises.

Solanki and McCurdy[63] reported on five patients with SCD who had DHTRs. Although multiple RBC alloantibodies were ultimately detected in all patients, the responsible antibodies were sometimes undetectable for as long as 72 hours after the reaction. In three patients, painful crises could have been precipitated by the DHTR.

Several additional pertinent reports have appeared only in abstract form and therefore are difficult to evaluate with certainty. Sosler and coworkers[83] described two multiply transfused patients with SCD who developed severe AIHA after transfusion of RBCs lacking the multiple antigens to which they had developed alloantibodies. In both patients, the serologic strength of the autoantibody reactivity increased after transfusion. Hemoglobin levels fell to nadirs of 1.5 g/dL and 4.0 g/dL, respectively. Both patients recovered after prednisone therapy.

Friedman and associates[72] reported on three children with SCD who developed HTRs, with post-transfusion hemoglobin levels falling below pretransfusion levels "despite high reticulocyte counts." (No reticulocyte counts are provided, and it is not clear whether or not the authors are referring to corrected reticulocyte counts.) Serologic evaluations revealed multiple alloantibodies in only one of the patients, and in no case did serologic findings entirely explain the observed hemolysis. One of the patients died, and severe anemia from rapid hemolysis contributed to his death. The authors emphasized that avoidance of further transfusion in these patients is vital, as continued transfusion could be lethal.

King and coworkers[75] described five patients with SCD who experienced a DHTR 7 to 19 days after transfusion. Each patient had received an exchange transfusion of 4 to 5 units of Hb S-negative RBCs in anticipation of elective surgery or for treatment of an acute painful crisis or acute chest syndrome. Three of the patients developed positive DATs after the exchange transfusions, but new RBC alloantibodies were identified that were thought to be responsible for the HTR. Two of the patients had received donor blood matched with the recipient's phenotype for major antigens in the Rh, Kell, Kidd, Duffy, and MNS systems and developed no new allantibodies but nevertheless developed a DHTR.

Syed and colleagues[74] reported the details of DHTRs in four patients with SCD. Three of the patients had been treated with exchange transfusions. Hemoglobin electrophoresis data obtained for one patient during a DHTR showed disappearance of hemoglobin A, and the authors concluded that, in spite of the presence of a warm autoantibody on the patient's RBCs, the hemolysis after transfusion was caused by alloantibodies.

Reed and associates[81] reported a 32-year-old woman with SCD associated with hemoglobin C, who was admitted to the hospital with pain involving the back, chest, and legs. She had been transfused frequently, was 18 weeks pregnant, and had multiple RBC alloantibodies including anti-E, -S, -Jk^b, and Fy3. She was transfused with 1 unit of RBCs, but 1 week later she had worsening pain and her hemoglobin had fallen from 7.7 g/dL to 6.8 g/dL. She was transfused with 2 additional units of RBCs, and 4 days later her hemoglobin fell from 6.0 g/dL to 4.9 g/dL, at which time she quickly became obtunded. Her serum was reddish-brown, the hemoglobin decreased further to 1.4 g/dL, and platelets fell from 131,000/μL to 31,000/μL. No reticulocyte counts were performed. Two group O Rh-negative units, which were not crossmatched, were administered as an emergency, but the patient expired. As indicated previously, her pain was attributed to vaso-occlusion, and the diagnosis of a HTR was made postmortem.

Campbell and coworkers[78] described an 18-year-old woman with SCD who was 37.5 weeks pregnant. Her blood type was group B, Rh-positive, her admission hematocrit was 18%, and she was transfused with 1 unit of group B, Rh-positive RBCs. After delivery of a male infant, her clinical course was complicated by infections, for which she was treated with antibiotics and then discharged. Four days later, however, she presented with intense right femur pain and a hematocrit of 16%. The next day the hemoglobin was 4.2 g/dL, and she was admitted for emergent transfusion and pain management. A decision was made to transfuse phenotypically matched RBCs. No extensively phenotyped group B RBCs were available; instead, group O cells that matched the patient's phenotype were transfused. After receiving approximately 100 mL, however, she experienced chills and an increase in temperature from 36.4°C to 39°C. Serologic studies revealed that the patient had an IgM anti-IH antibody, which reacted with group O RBCs at 30°C and 37°C in both saline and 30% albumin media but did not react in a saline medium with group B cells at 37°C. She was transfused with group B cells, had no adverse reaction, and her post-transfusion hematocrit was 17.2%.

Win and associates[79] reported two cases of severe, life-threatening HTRs in patients with SCD after the transfusion of compatible RBC units. One patient was a 33-year-old woman who was referred for antenatal care for her fourth pregnancy. She had received numerous transfusions in the past. A decision was made to treat her with a gradual exchange transfusion starting at 26 weeks' gestation. The pretransfusion hemoglobin was 7.6 g/dL, the DAT was negative, reticulocytes were 180 × 10^9/L (normal range, 10–100 × 10^9/L), and there were no atypical RBC antibodies. She was transfused with 2 RBC units, and 4 days later she was readmitted with generalized musculoskeletal pain and a 2-day history of passing dark urine. The DAT remained negative, and no RBC alloantibodies were found. In spite of transfusion of an additional unit of RBCs, her hemoglobin fell progressively to a nadir of 4.8 g/dL, and reticulocytes decreased to one tenth their previous value at 18 × 10^9/L. She recovered after treatment with methylprednisolone and IVIG. Analysis of the patient's urine revealed both hemoglobin A and hemoglobin S, which the authors interpreted to mean that both allogeneic and autologous RBC were being destroyed as part of the HTR. No data were provided, however, to indicate that the urine did not contain hemoglobin S regularly as a result of her usual hemolytic state, and the authors pointed out that there is little information on the urinary excretion of free hemoglobin in SCD. Marked reticulocytopenia also occurred in the authors' other patient during an acute episode of hemolysis, and the bone marrow aspirate in both patients revealed erythroid hyperplasia which, in association with reticulocytopenia, indicates ineffective erythropoiesis. The authors speculated that the reticulocytopenia was due to peripheral consumption by hyperactive macrophages.

Tolano and coworkers[84] performed an 11-year retrospective chart review of patients in the pediatric age group with discharge diagnoses of SCD and transfusion reaction. They encountered seven patients (ages 6 to 17 years) who developed nine characteristic episodes of sickle cell HTRs. All patients presented with fever and hemoglobinuria. Symptoms of pain (in the back, abdomen, and/or legs), which initially were ascribed to vaso-occlusive crisis, were present in all but one episode. The hemoglobin decreased from pretransfusion levels in eight of nine episodes, the nadir ranging from 4.0 g/dL to 5.9 g/dL, with a median value of 4.5 g/dL. Of note was the fact that the corrected reticulocyte count at the time of the hemoglobin nadir ranged from 0.2% to 5.6%, with a median value of 1.16%. The DAT was positive in only two of the nine events at presentation. One patient had previous alloantibodies, and four patients developed new identifiable antibodies, which included a warm autoantibody in one patient. The new alloantibodies appeared at the time of the event in two patients but were not detected for one month in a third patient. Severe complications included acute chest syndrome, pancreatitis, congestive heart failure, and acute renal failure. Three patients received additional RBC transfusions that were "completely" phenotypically matched, one patient experienced severe additional hemolysis. The patients responded to treatment with corticosteroids and erythropoietin. For reasons that are not evident, the authors chose to exclude from consideration patients who had acute HTRs, although the syndrome can occur with either acute or delayed HTRs (see Table 14-6).

Similar Hemolytic Transfusion Reaction Syndromes in Patients with Thalassemia

Sirchia and colleagues[85] reported their experience regarding HTRs that occurred in seven patients with β-thalassemia. Their data indicate that findings similar to those described for the sickle cell hemolytic transfusion reaction syndrome might occur in patients with other hemoglobinopathies. Four of the seven patients who developed a HTR had a post-transfusion hemoglobin level that was lower than the pretransfusion value (7.0–3.5; 5.0–4.0; 7.0–5.5; 4.6–3.0), but the authors did not attempt to determine the mechanism of this finding. HTRs occurred in spite of transfusion of RBCs that were compatible as indicated by extensive compatibility test procedures. The serologic findings after transfusion did not clearly explain the cause of the destruction of the transfused RBCs. High-dose steroids were administered to each of the seven patients, and they eventually showed a progressive resolution of the severe anemia manifested during the HTRs.

Grainger and associates[86] reported a 1-year-old girl with newly diagnosed β-thalassemia who developed life-threatening hemolysis after transfusion. The hemoglobin before transfusion was 5.3 g/dL, but 4 weeks after an initial transfusion with red cells matched for Rh and Kell antigens, the hemoglobin had fallen to 3.5 g/dL and she had signs of hemolysis, including gross hemoglobinuria. Serologic findings typical of a delayed HTR were not present, although a weak cold autoantibody reactive up to 18°C was found, and the DAT became positive with C3d on the cells. The hemolysis persisted, and her anemia progressed with subsequent transfusions, even though she was treated with methylprednisilone, IVIG, and splenectomy. One week after splenectomy, her hemoglobin reached a nadir of only 1.9 g/dL. An HLA-identical sibling donor was available, and the patient was prepared for hematopoietic cell transplantation with cyclophosphamide and busulphan over the course of 4 days. During the immunosuppressive transplant conditioning, her hemolysis abated and her DAT became negative.

The findings of Sirchia and colleagues[85] and Grainger and associates[86] are of considerable interest because they indicate that the mechanism of the severe hemolysis which can occur during HTRs in patients with SCD is not related to the presence of hemoglobin S or SCD. Because the finding of a lower hemoglobin level after transfusion than that prior to transfusion has been noted after HTRs in patients with two forms of hereditary hemolytic anemia, one wonders whether a similar occurrence does not sometimes follow HTRs in patients with acquired hemolytic anemias.[87]

The Mechanism Underlying Post-transfusion Fall in Hemoglobin to Values Lower Than Pretransfusion Values

If, following a transfusion, all of the transfused RBCs were hemolzyed, one would expect the hemoglobin to return to the pretransfusion level. In patients who develop the sickle cell HTR syndrome, however, the hemoglobin value after transfusion is significantly lower than that prior to transfusion. Several possible mechanisms, which could be operating concomitantly, have been proposed to explain this remarkable finding.[75,76,88]

"HYPERHEMOLYSIS"

An increased rate of destruction of RBCs in a patient with a chronic hemolytic anemia can be termed *hyperhemolysis*. (Unfortunately, this term is often used simply as a synonym for severe hemolysis, rather than referring to an increased, or hyper-, hemolytic rate.) If an HTR were to cause destruction of all of the transfused RBCs and also result in destruction of the patient's own RBCs, it is evident that the hemoglobin would fall to a level lower than the pretransfusion value. In patients with SCD, the analysis is complicated by the fact that the patient's own RBCs inherently have a markedly short life span. Nevertheless, a number of authors have suggested that hyperhemolysis is frequently the cause of or at least a contributing factor in the development of the marked post-transfusion fall in hematocrit observed in patients with SCD who have an HTR.[37,76,81]

Destruction of the patient's own RBCs during an HTR could occur as a result of "bystander immune hemolysis"—immune lysis of RBCs by antibody directed against an antigen(s) that is not an intrinsic component of the RBC membrane.[86,87] In other words, the hemolysis of transfused RBCs by the patient's alloantibody results in autologous RBCs being hemolyzed as well. This topic is reviewed in detail in the section on bystander immune cytolysis in Chapter 9.

Development of AIHA in Patients with SCD

Another mechanism by which hemolysis of the patient's own RBCs could be destroyed during an HTR is the development of an autoantibody as a result of the transfusion, as reviewed previously in this chapter and in Chapter 9. Indeed, a number of authors have suggested that autoantibodies that developed in association with HTRs in patients with SCD were the cause of hemolysis of the patient's own RBCs.[70,82,83,89] In other reported cases, however, autoantibodies were clearly not present, and for this reason they do not appear to be responsible for the post-transfusion fall in hemoglobin in all cases.[64,65,73,76]

SUPPRESSION OF ERYTHROPOIESIS

In persons whose RBCs have a normal life span, the drop in hemoglobin after an HTR to a value significantly lower than the starting level strongly suggests the destruction of the patient's own RBCs in addition to the transfused RBCs. In patients with SCD or transfusion-dependent thalassemia, however, the patient's own RBCs have a markedly short survival time, thus complicating the analysis. Indeed, when patients with SCD develop suppression of erythropoiesis, such as can be caused by infection, a marked drop in hemoglobin is to be expected because of the short survival of the patients' RBCs. Such an abrupt drop in hemoglobin and hematocrit can be mistaken for hyperhemolysis—a further shortening of the already shortened life span of sickle cells.

Increasing the hematocrit by transfusion also causes suppression of erythropoiesis.[90,91] Accordingly, when there is an unexpectedly low hematocrit after an HTR, it is important to calculate the magnitude of the fall in hematocrit that can be explained on the basis of suppression of erythropoiesis so as to not interpret inappropriately the drop in hematocrit as an indication of hyperhemolysis. The magnitude of a fall in hematocrit that can be explained on the basis of depressed erythropoiesis without hyperhemolysis can be calculated by taking into account the expected loss of RBC volume by senescence while also considering residual RBC production as indicated by hematologic data during this period. We performed these calculations on several patients who developed the sickle cell hemolytic transfusion reaction syndrome.[76]

CALCULATION OF RBC PRODUCTION AND DESTRUCTION THROUGH SENESCENCE

$$\text{Blood volume in mL} = \text{Weight in kg} \times 69\ \text{mL/kg (males) or } 64\ \text{mL/kg (females)}$$

$$\text{RBC volume} = \text{Blood volume (mL)} \times \text{hematocrit}$$

$$\text{Reticulocyte volume} = \text{RBC volume} \times \text{reticulocyte percentage}$$

$$\text{Steady state daily RBC production}/+4\ \text{destruction} = \frac{\text{Reticulocyte volume}}{\text{Life span of reticulocytes (days)}}$$

$$\text{OR} = \frac{\text{(Blood volume) (hematocrit) (reticulocyte percentage)}}{\text{Life span of reticulocytes (days)}}$$

The maturation time of reticulocytes in the peripheral blood is prolonged above the normal of approximately 1 day due to premature delivery of reticulocytes to the circulation in patients with anemias who have marrow stimulation. These reticulocytes, called "shift cells," contain more reticulum than those in the normal subject and require a longer period of time than normal circulating reticulocytes to lose their reticulum. Thus, the index of daily RBC production/destruction must be "corrected" for the life span of reticulocytes in patients with varying degrees of anemia by dividing the reticulocyte volume by the life span of reticulocytes (in days). Based on the data of Hillman and Finch,[92] the following correction factors can be applied: hematocrit 40 to 45, correction 1.0; hematocrit 35 to 40, correction 1.5; hematocrit 25 to 35, correction 2.0; hematocrit lower than 25, correction 2.5. Such corrections do not apply if erythropoiesis is suppressed, as it is, for example, by infection, in which reticulocyte life span is variable.

For example, if steady-state conditions for a 65-kg female include a hematocrit of 22.5% and reticulocytes of 20%, daily RBC production/senescence =

$$\frac{(65\ \text{kg})\ (64\ \text{mL/kg})\ (.225)\ (.20)}{2.5\ \text{days}} = 75\ \text{mL/day}$$

EFFECT OF SUPPRESSION OF ERYTHROPOIESIS IN A PATIENT WITH SICKLE CELL ANEMIA

Petz and associates[76] calculated the amount by which the hematocrit could have fallen on the basis of suppression of erythropoiesis in a patient with sickle cell disease (Fig. 14-2). The volume of RBCs lost by senescence was calculated using data on admission, as these figures provide the best estimate of steady-state conditions. The results of these calculations were consistent with data reported by others for patients with sickle cell anemia in steady-state conditions.[93] In the steady state, RBC production and destruction through senescence are equal.

PATIENT 2: The patient was a 22-year-old male weighing 66 kg, who presented with a hematocrit of 25.9% and a reticulocyte count of 18.1%. Calculation of daily RBC production and senescence using these data are as follows:

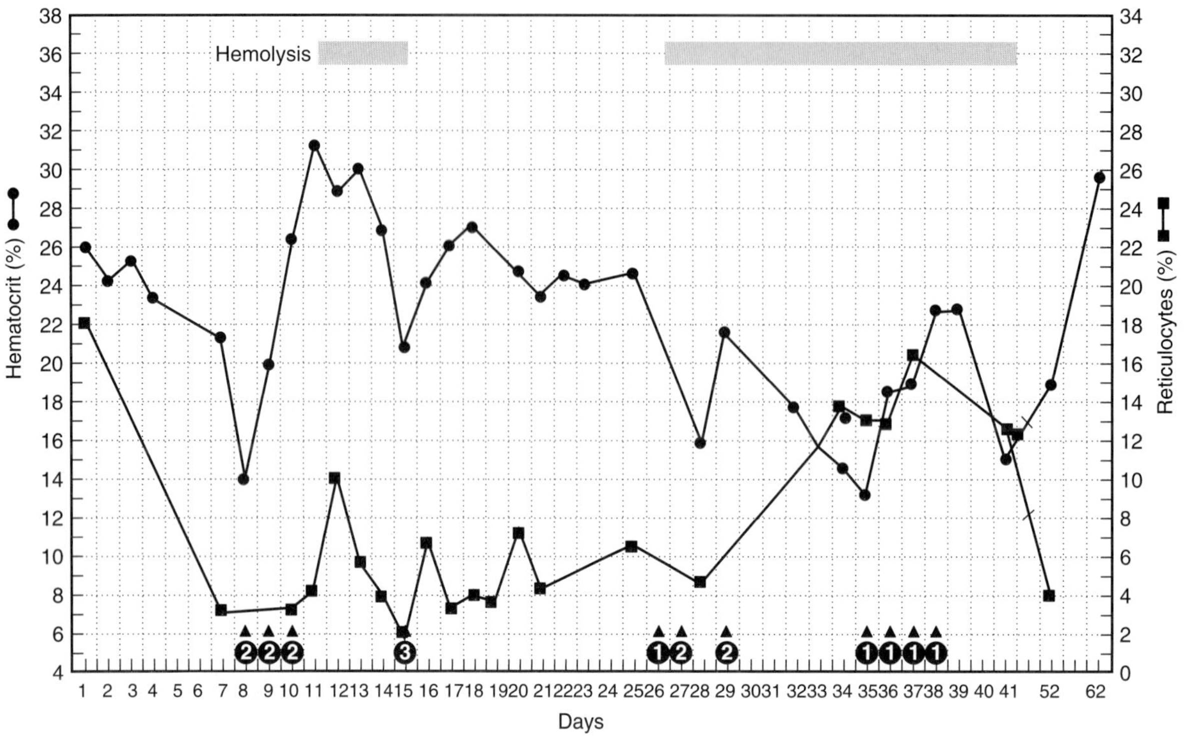

FIGURE 14-2. Clinical course of Patient 2, indicating Hct, uncorrected reticulocyte counts (%), and episodes of hemolysis. Numbers in circles indicates the number of unites of RBCs that were transfused. (From Petz LD, Calhoun L, Shulman IA, et al: The sickle cell hemolytic transfusion reaction syndrome. Transfusion 1997;37:382–392.)

Weight = 66 kg
Period of time = 7 days
Initial hematocrit = 25.9 %
Initial reticulocytes = 18.1%
Initial blood volume = (66 kg) (69 mL/kg) = 4554 mL
Initial red cell volume = (4554 mL) (.259) = 1179 mL

Daily RBC production/senescence

$$= \frac{(4554 \text{ mL}) (.259) (.181)}{2.0 \text{ days}} = 107 \text{ mL/day}$$

By day 8, the hematocrit had fallen to 13.9%. During this time, the patient had an infection manifested by fever, productive cough, purulent sputum, and dyspnea. Suppression of erythropoiesis, presumably a result of infection, was indicated by a drop in the uncorrected reticulocyte count to 3.2% by day 7. The following are the pertinent calculations concerning the mechanism of the patient's marked drop in hematocrit.

For the 7-day period, the volume of RBCs lost through senescence equaled

$$(107 \text{ mL/day}) (7 \text{ days}) = 749 \text{ mL}$$

Therefore, if RBC production dropped to zero and the RBC life span was unchanged throughout this 7-day period, the predicted RBC volume and hematocrit on day 8 would be:

RBC volume = 1179 mL − 749 mL = 430 mL

$$\text{Hematocrit} = \frac{430}{4554} = 9.4\%$$

The measured hematocrit on day 8, however, was 13.9%, indicating an RBC volume on that day of 633 mL (4554 mL × 0.139), which is 203 mL higher than predicted on the basis of zero erythropoiesis. This indicates an average RBC production of 29 mL/day (rather than 0 mL/day).

Production of 29 mL/day is consistent with calculated RBC production during this period of time. A hematocrit and reticulocyte count are available on day 7 and, using these values, calculated RBC production would be 31 mL/day if the life span of reticulocytes was 1 day.

RBC volume day 7 = (4554 mL) (0.213) = 970 mL

$$\text{RBC production} = \frac{(970) (0.032)}{1 \text{ day}} = 31 \text{ mL}$$

If the life span of the patient's reticulocytes was 1.5 days, 2.0 days, or 2.5 days, the corresponding values for RBC production/day would be 20.6 mL, 15.5 mL, and 12.4 mL, respectively.

These calculations indicate that if the patient had been transfused on day 1, and if all allogeneic RBCs had been hemolyzed in an HTR but the life span of autologous RBCs had remained unchanged (that is, if there was no hyperhemolysis), the hematocrit could have fallen alarmingly from 25.9% to 13.9% over a 7-day period simply due to suppression of erythropoiesis.

One may conclude from these calculations that when a patient with SCD develops reticulocytopenia during an HTR, suppression of erythropoiesis is likely to be a significant contributing factor in the development of the marked post-transfusion fall in hematocrit and hemoglobin.

Sickle Cell Crisis as an Explanation for the Post-transfusion Fall in Hemoglobin during an HTR

Some authors suggest that hyperhemolysis is a cardinal manifestation of painful sickle cell episodes.[94] Hematologic studies on sickle cell patients during pain crises do not support such a conclusion, however. Diggs[95] performed daily reticulocyte counts and hemoglobin determinations during 747 episodes of sickle cell pain crisis in 166 subjects. He also measured serum bilirubin and determined the output of fecal urobilinogen. He concluded that a true hemolytic crisis was not observed in any patient with SCD. He observed that in the majority of patients with SCD and secondary viral, bacterial, or protozoal infections and with systemic diseases, there is a decrease in RBC values, and this is primarily the result of defective regeneration rather than of an increase in the hemolytic rate. He concluded, rather emphatically, "The concept of 'hemolytic crisis' in SCD is a myth that should not be perpetuated in the light of present knowledge." In a subsequent report, he restated: "The use of the term 'hemolytic crisis' as a synonym for recurrent painful and febrile crises also is not justified. There is usually no significant decrease in erythrocytes at the time of painful crises compared with asymptomatic intervals."[96]

Further data were published by Naumann and coworkers,[97] who measured plasma hemoglobin during painful crises in patients with SCD. Although they concluded that hyperhemolysis did occur during the first 2 days of crisis, the amounts of plasma hemoglobin detected could be accounted for by the destruction of small volumes of RBCs. Indeed, the highest plasma hemoglobin value observed could have been produced by lysis of only 20 mL of blood, which obviously would have no measurable effect on hemoglobin or hematocrit determinations.

Compelling evidence that sickle cell crisis per se is not an adequate explanation for the remarkable drop in hemoglobin and hematocrit that occur in SCD patients who develop an HTR is provided by the fact that a similar fall in hemoglobin has been reported during HTRs in patients with thalassemia.[85] Suppression of erythropoiesis or development of autoantibodies could occur in either SCD or thalassemia but, of course, sickle cell crisis is not common to both entities.

Management of Patients with Sickle Cell HTR Syndrome

The optimal management of patients with this syndrome is not yet defined.[98] Because continued transfusion could lead to a further fall in the hemoglobin and hematocrit, it is appropriate to discontinue transfusion unless the hemoglobin is so low as to be life threatening. Corticosteroids appear to be helpful when given in doses of 1–2 mg/kg/day of prednisone or equivalent.[76] In addition, IVIG and erythropoietin may be beneficial.[98]

Sirchia and colleagues[85] administered high-dose steroids to each of the seven patients with thalassemia that they reported, and all patients showed a progressive resolution of the severe anemia that developed during HTRs. They cautioned, however, that additional factors could have contributed to the positive outcome in their patients, so that the value of steroid therapy was uncertain.

PATHOPHYSIOLOGY OF HTRs

Most HTRs are associated with destruction of extravascular RBCs. It is rare for any of the antibodies listed in Table 14-3 to activate complement efficiently enough to cause complement-mediated intravascular lysis, but on occasion it has occurred, especially with examples of Kidd antibodies. Complement-mediated intravascular hemolysis is usually associated with HTRs caused by ABO antibodies (anti-A, -B, -H). Although Rh antibodies, however strong, do not activate complement, hemoglobinemia and hemoglobinuria are sometimes found in Rh-mediated HTRs. This is not a sign of complement-mediated intravascular lysis, but rather a consequence of massive extravascular destruction. It could be that such destruction leads to release of hemoglobin into the peripheral circulation because of fragmentation of RBCs during phagocytosis, and possible macrophage-induced cytotoxicity (see Chapter 4). On rare occasions, hemoglobinuria and hemoglobinuria are due directly to blood group antibodies (e.g., Kidd antibodies). Beauregard and Blajchman[99] have reviewed conditions that can mimic HTRs.

To understand what happens in vivo when complement-mediated intravascular lysis occurs (e.g., by ABO antibodies), one has only to understand the classical pathway of complement activation described in Chapter 4. Most other antibodies (e.g., Rh, Kidd, Kell) destroy RBCs by extravascular mechanisms as described in Chapter 4.

Table 14-7 lists the symptoms and Table 14-8 the laboratory findings most commonly associated with HTRs. Figure 14-3 shows the temporal relationship of the laboratory test results to the HTR, and Table 14-9 indicates the volume of lysed RBCs required to produce grossly pink-red plasma. It should be noted that some of the symptoms do not occur if the patient is anesthetized. In the Mayo Clinic series,[52-55] the most common symptoms associated with DHTRs were fever and chills (75% and 34%, respectively). Anemia (usually ≥2 g/dL below previous level), which was seen in 87% of DHTRs, was the leading complication.[53] Oliguria and renal failure were noted in 34% and 13% of patients, respectively.[52-55] If the antibody causing the reaction is capable of activating complement (e.g., ABO), the clinical symptoms could be different from those associated with noncomplement-activating antibody (e.g., Rh). During complement activation, anaphylotoxins (C3a and C5a) are released, which act on smooth muscle and interact with certain cells (e.g., mast cells) to release histamine. These effects play a major role in symptoms such as flushing of the skin, difficulty in breathing, and chest pain, which often are associated with HTRs due to complement-activating antibodies. The most common abnormal laboratory findings were decreased serum haptoglobin (92% of cases); positive (usually weakly or transiently positive) DATs (89% of cases; all negative DATs were associated with ABO immediate HTRs); and elevated serum bilirubin (80% of cases).[52-55] Figure 14-3 shows the temporal relationship of some of these test results.[100]

TABLE 14-7. SYMPTOMS OF DELAYED HEMOLYTIC TRANSFUSION REACTIONS

Symptom	Percentage of Patients Showing These Symptoms
Fever (≥2°F increase)	75
Chills	34
Chest pain	13
Hypotension	13
Nausea	4
Flushing	4
Dyspnea	4
Hemoglobinuria	2

From Pineda AA, Brzica SM, Taswell HF: Hemolytic transfusion reaction. Mayo Clin Proc 1978;53:378; Pineda AA, Taswell HF, Brzica SM: Delayed hemolytic transfusion reaction. Transfusion 1978;18:1; Moore SB, Taswell HF, Pineda AA, et al: Delayed hemolytic transfusion reactions. AM J Clin Pathol 1980;74:94; and Taswell HF, Pineda AA, Moore SB: Hemolytic transfusion reactions: Frequency and clinical and laboratory aspects. In Bell CA (ed): A Seminar on Immune-mediated Cell Destruction. Washington, DC: American Association of Blood Banks, 1981:71.

TABLE 14-8. LABORATORY ABNORMALITIES FOLLOWING HEMOLYTIC TRANSFUSION REACTIONS

	Percentage of Patients Showing These Abnormalities
Low haptoglobin	92
Positive DAT	89[a]
Increased indirect bilirubin	80
Hemoglobin detected in plasma and/or urine	70[b]

[a] All negative DATs were associated with ABO immediate HTRs.
[b] 88% of immediate HTRs and 52% of DHTRs.
From Pineda AA, Brzica SM, Taswell HF: Hemolytic transfusion reaction. Mayo Clin Proc 1978;53:378; Pineda AA, Taswell HF, Brzica SM: Delayed hemolytic transfusion reaction. Transfusion 1978;18:1; Moore SB, Taswell HF, Pineda AA, et al: Delayed hemolytic transfusion reactions. AM J Clin Pathol 1980;74:94; and Taswell HF, Pineda AA, Moore SB: Hemolytic transfusion reactions: Frequency and clinical and laboratory aspects. In Bell CA (ed): A Seminar on Immune-mediated Cell Destruction. Washington, DC: American Association of Blood Banks, 1981:71.

Interrelationships of Mediators of the Inflammatory Response

We have known for some years that some of the clinical signs associated with HTRs are associated with activation of the complement system, (e.g., production of anaphylotoxins [C3a and C5a] and interaction between the complement and coagulation systems). Until recently, it has been a puzzle why similar symptoms could occur with HTRs associated with antibodies that do not activate complement. A number of studies have linked some of these symptoms to a class of biologic mediators known as cytokines.[101-105] Cytokines are hormone-like glycoproteins secreted by a wide variety of cells, including lymphocytes, monocytes, macrophages, fibroblasts, and endothelial cells. Davenport and coworkers[101,102,104,105] showed that several cytokines were produced when ABO- or Rh-incompatible RBCs were added to anti-A/B or anti-D, respectively, in vitro. These cytokines included some interleukins (IL-1, IL-6, IL-8), an interleukin receptor antagonist (IL1ra or IRAP), tumor necrosis factor-alpha (TNF-α), and monocyte chemoattractant protein (MCP-1).

When ABO incompatibility was produced in vitro, Davenport and coworkers[101,102] found that IL-8 was first observed after 2 hours and increased over a 24-hour period. Plasma TNF levels were maximal at 2 hours and declined to control levels by 24 hours. MCP-1 was detected at 24 hours but not at 6 hours. Complement was necessary for optimal production of IL-8 and TNF but was not necessary for MCP-1. Some of the findings have been supported by an in vivo event; Butler and associates[103] studied a patient who was group O and accidentally received a group A unit; TNF levels were found to increase 14-fold after the incompatible transfusion.

When IgG (anti-D)-mediated in vitro incompatibility was studied, Davenport and colleagues[104,105] found that IL-1, IL-6, IL-8, and TNF were produced. The interleukins were detectable in the plasma at 4 to 6 hours and increased up to 24 hours. TNF production peaked at 6 hours. MCP-1 was detectable at 24 hours but not at 6 hours. An interleukin-1 receptor antagonist (IL-1ra) was also produced after IgG-mediated RBC incompatibility. IL-1ra production was evident at

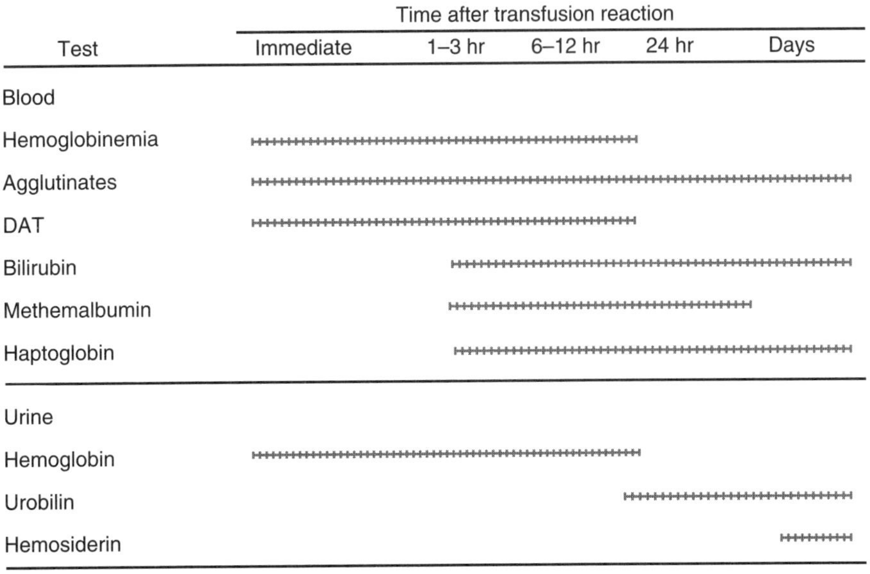

Test	Time after transfusion reaction: Immediate	1–3 hr	6–12 hr	24 hr	Days
Blood					
Hemoglobinemia					
Agglutinates					
DAT					
Bilirubin					
Methemalbumin					
Haptoglobin					
Urine					
Hemoglobin					
Urobilin					
Hemosiderin					

FIGURE 14-3. Temporal results of biochemical and serological tests following a hemolytic transfusion reaction. (From Crookston JH: Transfusion reactions. Am J Med Technol 1968;334:579–588.)

TABLE 14-9. VOLUME OF LYSED RBCs REQUIRED TO PRODUCE GROSSLY PINK-RED PLASMA

Product	Hb Content g	Hb Content mg
100 mL whole blood	15	15,000
100 mL packed RBCs	33	33,000
1 mL packed RBCs	0.33	330
5 mL packed RBCs	1.65	1650

Plasma volume (adult): 3000 mL

$$\frac{1650 \text{ mg Hb}}{3000 \text{ mL plasma}} = 0.55 \text{ mg Hb/mL} \quad \text{or} \quad 55 \text{ mg Hb/100 mL}$$

Barely visible hemolysis	15 mg Hb/100 mL
Plasma definitely pink	45 mg Hb/100 mL
Plasma pink-red	60–100 mg Hb/100 mL

From Masouredis SP, Chaplin H Jr: Transfusion management of autoimmune hemolytic anemia. In Chaplin H Jr (ed): Immune Hemolytic Anemias. New York: Churchill Livingstone, 1985:177.

4 hours and increased progressively over 24 hours. These results suggested that antagonist production might partly account for the variable pathophysiologic events seen in HTRs and AIHA.

Disseminated Intravascular Coagulation Associated with HTRs

Disseminated intravascular coagulation (DIC), characterized by thrombocytopenia, decreased factors I (fibrinogen), V, and VIII and the presence of fibrin degradation products, sometimes occurs as the result of an HTR. Fortunately, it is rare, and it usually occurs only after complement-mediated intravascular red cell destruction, which is usually associated with ABO incompatibility.[1] Abnormal bleeding has been noted many times after transfusion of ABO-incompatible blood.[1] Indeed, blood bankers and anesthetists should be aware that when a patient is undergoing surgery and being transfused, abnormal bleeding and/or hypotension might be the only observable sign of an HTR due to ABO-incompatible blood. The exact relationship between HTRs and DIC is uncertain.

Rare cases of DIC have been described following noncomplement-mediated extravascular RBC destruction; recent data suggest that these could be due to release of cytokines, which, like complement, can interact with the coagulation pathway. Capon and Goldfinger[106] believe that cytokines could play a major role in the coagulation abnormalities after an HTR.

Several reports have suggested that red cell stroma could initiate DIC. Rabiner and Friedman[107] showed that transfusion of autologous lysed dog RBCs led to DIC. Birndorf and colleagues[108] showed that transfusion of sonicated hemoglobin-free stroma into monkeys led to decreased factors I, II, V, and VIII and platelets. Poskitt and coworkers[109] suggested that the ultra structure of red cell stroma resembles endotoxins and that activation of the alternative complement pathway could occur when stroma are present in sufficient quantity.

Renal Failure Associated with HTRs

Mollison and associates[1] reported renal failure as almost always being associated with complement activation during an HTR. Thus, it is usually found in association with acute intravascular lysis, which is usually ABO mediated. Nevertheless, it has been described after DHTRs. Pineda and coworkers[52] found 17% percent of their patients with DHTRs to have associated oliguria and 9% to have renal shutdown, but these patients all had serious underlying disease, and in a later publication from the same institution there were no cases of renal failure in 37 cases of DHTRs.[54] As with DIC, the exact relationship between renal failure and HTR is unclear.

It is unclear from animal experiments whether hemoglobin or RBC stroma is involved in the renal failure. It was first thought that hemoglobin is nephrotoxic, but that is no longer believed to be true, and stroma itself does not seem harmful. Schmidt and Holland[110] transfused large quantities of compatible stroma without any observable reaction, but incompatible (e.g., ABO-incompatible) stroma led to severe reactions (e.g., renal failure).

It is now thought that the renal damage is an indirect result of complement activation. The mechanisms involved could be similar to those seen in renal damage associated with immune complex disease, or those discussed previously for DIC. Anaphylotoxins could cause chemotaxis and subsequent enzyme release from leukocytes, thereby damaging renal tissue, or there could be deposition of fibrin in the renal microcirculation due to activation of the coagulation cascade.

For renal failure after HTRs as for DIC, Capon and Goldfinger[106] believe that cytokines might play an important role.

Treatment of HTRs

Usually, the only treatment necessary is to stop the causative transfusion, investigate its cause, and provide compatible blood for the next transfusion. If the patient develops DIC or renal abnormalities, urgent treatment becomes necessary. Shock and renal failure are the most common causes of death due to HTRs, and as hypotension is an important component of both, this should be treated immediately by maintaining intravascular volume via the immediate infusion of colloids or crystalloids. Diuresis should be induced as soon as possible to increase renal blood flow and to enable detection of renal shutdown. Mannitol (20 g as a 20% solution) was most commonly used for this purpose for years, but more recently, furosemide (80–120 mg intravenously) has exceeded it in popularity. Urine output should be maintained for several hours at a minimum of 0.5 mL/kg/hour.[1] Once oliguria is established, the patient should not be given more water than he or she can excrete (i.e., 500 mL/day). The patient's renal function should be monitored; if blood urea rises less than 20 mg/dL/day, the patient usually responds well to conservative treatment. Greater catabolic rates could suggest that dialysis is necessary. Some workers have suggested that dopamine is useful to combat shock and renal failure and that heparin and even exchange transfusion have been suggested as useful adjuncts to the just-mentioned therapy.[71,72,111-113] Treatment for DIC has been well described in other publications and will not be discussed here, other than to note that immediate rapid infusion of 50–100 mg of aqueous heparin followed by the slow infusion of 250–350 mg of heparin over the course of 24 hours has been recommended.[111-113]

VARIATION IN CLINICAL SYMPTOMS ASSOCIATED WITH ABO-INCOMPATIBLE HTRs

Although ABO incompatibility is by far the most common cause of fatal HTRs, and very small amounts of ABO incompatible blood can cause severe clinical symptoms, the range of symptoms seen among individual patients is extraordinary. Considering how many patients still get transfused with ABO-incompatible blood, it is reassuring to note that only a small percentage of ABO-incompatible transfusions are fatal.[1] In one series of 40 patients receiving ABO-incompatible blood, only four (10%) died.[1] All four patients had been transfused during or immediately after surgery. Severe hypotension and DIC were the main clinical symptoms for all four patients.[1] In two older series describing 12 and 13 patients receiving ABO-incompatible transfusions, none died or experienced renal failure. Six patients received 50 mL of blood or less, but 11 of the 25 patients received 1 or more full units of ABO-incompatible blood. Linden and her colleagues[113a] reported on the outcome of 237 ABO-compatible transfusions in New York State; 47% of the patients had no obvious adverse effects. The five cases that follow show the wide range of clinical symptoms that can occur after ABO-incompatible HTRs in individual patients.

PATIENT 3[114]: A 21-year-old group O male received 3 units of group A blood during surgery for spondylolisthesis. No unusual bleeding was noted; during surgery, pulse, blood pressure, and urine output remained normal. During the first 14 hours after surgery, his temperature rose to 38.3°C but returned to normal the next day. No hemoglobin was visible in the plasma or urine. The DAT was weakly positive. Before transfusion, the anti-A titer was 128; it fell to 4 on the first day after surgery and increased to 4096 at 10 days after surgery. Anti-A hemolysins were not detected until day 10 (titer of 32). Survival of incompatible group A RBCs appeared to be good for 2 days after surgery, then started to disappear over the next 3 days; no A RBCs were detectable at 5 days. The patient did not become jaundiced, the urine was said to be of normal color; bilirubin, BUN, and creatine remained normal from day 1 through day 91 after surgery.

PATIENT 4[115]: A 70-year-old group B male received 3 units of blood postoperatively; 1 unit was later found to be group A. One hour after transfusion, the patient had chills and fever as high as 40°C and experienced a slight fall in blood pressure. The DAT was negative; no hemoglobin was obvious in the plasma. There was no decline in hemoglobin, and bilirubin values were repeatedly normal during the week after the transfusion. The anti-A titer was 8 before transfusion and decreased to 2 after the incompatible transfusion; on day 11, the titer was 128.

PATIENTS 5 AND 6[116]**:** Patients 5 and 6 were group B and group O, respectively; both received ABO-incompatible blood. Patient 3, mistyped as group AB, received 4 units of group AB during surgery and 8 units of AB+ and 18 units of group A blood during the next week. Patient 4 received 2 units of group A during surgery. Both patients had unexpected bleeding thought to be associated with DIC. The ABO incompatibility was not detected in Patients 3 and 4 until the seventh and fifth day, respectively, after surgery. Patient 3 died on day 28 after surgery due to complications resulting from the HTR; Patient 4 died 7 days postoperatively of a myocardial infarction, probably precipitated by the transfusion of 15 units of ABO-incompatible blood.

PATIENT 7[117]**:** A 92-year-old group A, Rh-negative male with diverticulitis was mistyped as group AB because of the use of a particular monoclonal anti-B. The hospital did not detect anti-B in the patient's serum. After a negative antibody screen, blood was issued through an abbreviated cross-match (i.e., immediate-spin crossmatch). The patient was given 3 units of group AB blood and 1 unit of group A blood, and no problems were reported. After the transfusion of a fourth unit of AB blood, the patient had a severe HTR, which resulted in renal failure and death 10 days later. After the transfusion reaction, the patient's pretransfusion RBCs were found to be group A with an acquired B antigen. The monoclonal anti-B used by the hospital was formulated from the ES4 clone, which reacts strongly with even weak acquired B antigens. A sample of the patient's serum taken before the transfusion reaction was later found to contain a weak anti-B, detectable most obviously by the antiglobulin test, which was not performed at the crossmatch stage. The manufacturers of monoclonal anti-B reagents prepared from the ES4 clone have since modified their reagents (i.e., lowered the pH) so that they now detect only the strongest examples of acquired B antigen (similar to other commercial anti-B). This case had several unusual events coming together, but it serves to illustrate that even a very weak ABO antibody (i.e., one not detected by the immediate spin procedure) can cause a problem in a very sick patient.

FATALITIES DUE TO HTRs

Fortunately, fatalities due to HTRs are rare. Schmidt,[118] Myhre,[119] and Honig and Bove[120] examined records of fatalities reported to the FDA for the years 1976–1979 and found an incidence of about 1 fatality per 500,000 transfusions. Honig and Bove[120] found that clerical errors were the major cause of the fatal HTRs; they accounted for 89% of the errors, and in many cases, more than one person was involved. The single most common error was failure to adequately identify the recipient prior to starting the transfusion; this accounted for 46% of the errors. Almost a quarter of the errors were a failure of blood bank technology; for example, four cases (two immediate HTRs and two DHTRs) were associated with compatible crossmatches, and the remaining four cases involved errors of interpretation or judgment. Honig and Bove[120] found that 86.4% of the deaths due to immediate (acute) HTRs were associated with ABO incompatibility; 9% were due to other antibodies (e.g., anti-c, -K, -M plus -P_1, -S plus -c, or -P_1); one death was due to thermal hemolysis in a blood warmer, and in one the cause was unclear. Two deaths were thought to be due to DHTRs (one patient had anti-c and the other anti-c plus anti-E). Evaluation of the reactions due to non-ABO antibodies was difficult, as most of the patients were moribund at the time of transfusion. On analyzing similar records from the FDA, Schmidt[118] felt that many of the deaths reported to the FDA as being due to HTRs were not proven as such, and in his analysis, he eliminated more than half of the cases and included those he felt were proven to be directly attributable to transfusion. In Schmidt's analysis, 100% of the immediate reactions were due to ABO antibodies.[118] Of the 22 fatal immediate reactions due to ABO studied by Schmidt,[118] 17 (77%) were caused by the wrong patient being transfused, five (23%) by an error in test procedure labeling, and none by errors in sample collection. Of 17 patients whose deaths were due to misidentification, 12 deaths (71%) occurred in the operating room or intensive care unit, none occurred in medical wards, and in five cases the location was not reported. Sixteen of the 22 patients who died received 1 or fewer units of blood, six received 2 units, and none received more than 2 units. Nineteen of the 22 patients (82%) were group O and received A or B blood.[118]

In 1990, Sazama[121] reviewed FDA data from 1976 through 1985. During this period, 355 fatalities associated with transfusion were reported, 99 of which were excluded from further review because they were unrelated to transfusion or were caused by transfusion-transmitted infection (e.g., hepatitis or acquired immune deficiency syndrome [AIDS]). Of the remaining 256 reported deaths, 51% resulted from acute hemolysis after the transfusion of ABO-incompatible products. These deaths were due primarily to managerial, not clerical, errors. Other causes of death (in order of frequency of report) included acute pulmonary injury (15%), bacterial contamination of product (10%), delayed hemolysis (10%), damaged product (3%), and graft-versus-host disease (0.4%). Of the deaths due to ABO incompatibility, 85% involved transfusion of A, B, or AB RBCs to a group O recipient. Transfusion of group A RBCs to group O recipients accounted for 30% of all fatalities due to blood transfusion. Nine deaths associated with non-ABO immediate HTRs were attributed to anti-Jk^a, -Jk^a +anti-Jk^b+Jk3, -Fy^a, or -E+K+P_1. Of the 26 fatal DHTRs, anti-c and/or anti-E were implicated in 16 cases (62%). Antibodies in the Kidd system (anti-Jk^a, -Jk^b), Duffy system (anti-Fy^a, -Fy^b, -Fy3), and Kell system (anti-K, -Kp^a) were associated with 10 (39%), 8 (31%), and 7 (27%) of the DHTRs, respectively. As 16 of 26 patients (62%) had more than one antibody specificity present in their sera, it was not clear whether one or more of the specificities were the cause of the fatal HTR.

Mummert and Tourault[122] updated the FDA data gathered up to 1992. They concluded that nearly one third of these fatalities could have been prevented by adherence to proper procedure and reported that transfusion of ABO-incompatible blood cells because of error continues to be the primary cause of preventable death. They identified failures in the following areas:

1. Accurate identification of the patient
2. Recognition of the signs of a transfusion reaction and appropriate action to discontinue the transfusion
3. Verification that equipment in use was functioning properly before and during use
4. Training of employees in adherence to standard operating procedures

The investigators reported that failure to follow standard operating procedures was a significant problem, and they advocated staff education, training, and monitoring for adherence on an ongoing basis. They also reported that failure to identify a reaction in progress contributed to many of the fatalities. They found that most of the errors occurred outside of the blood bank and were largely in violation of existing operating protocols. They advocated facility comprehensive quality assurance programs to identify inappropriate procedures in the facility and to reinforce the purpose and intent of required procedures. They also stressed the importance of the design of systems to prevent and detect errors on an ongoing basis, and the importance of procedures for equipment validation.

REPORTING OF ERRORS AND NEAR MISSES

In New York State, significant incidents involving the collection, processing, or transfusion of blood must be reported. Linden and colleagues[123] reviewed incident reports received over a 22-month period involving transfusion of blood to other than the intended recipient, or release of blood of an incorrect group. Among 1,784,600 transfusions of red cell components, there were 92 cases of erroneous transfusion (1 in 19,000) that met study criteria. There were 54 ABO-incompatible transfusions (1 in 33,000); three of these (1 in 600,000) were fatal. Correction for under-reporting of ABO-compatible errors resulted in an estimate of one per 12,000 as the true risk of transfusion error. National application of New York State data results in an estimate of 800–900 projected red cell-associated errors in the United States annually. The majority of reported errors occurred outside of the blood bank (43% resulted solely from failure to identify the patient and/or unit prior to transfusion, and 11% resulted from phlebotomist error), while the blood bank was responsible for 25% of errors and contributed, with another hospital service, to 17% of the errors. Linden and coworkers[123] considered that the risk of transfusion of ABO-incompatible blood remains significant and that additional precautions to minimize the likelihood of such events should be considered.

In 2000, Linden and Kaplan[124] updated the New York State findings through 1998. Erroneous administration was observed for 1 of 19,000 RBC units administered. Half of these events occurred outside of the blood bank (administration to the wrong recipient, 38%; phlebotomy errors, 13%). Isolated blood bank errors, including testing of the wrong specimen, transcription errors, and issuance of the wrong unit, were responsible for 29% of events. Many events (15%) involved multiple errors; the most common being failure to detect at the bedside that an incorrect unit had been issued.

In 1996, the United Kingdom started a voluntary reporting system of major transfusion complications—the Serious Hazards of Transfusion (SHOT).[125] For the years 1996–1999, 54% of the reports (335 events) concerned the incorrect blood (97 of 335 events involved ABO incompatibility) being given to the wrong patient. There were a total of 28 deaths due to transfusion and nine deaths suspected as being associated with the transfusion. Four deaths were due (and two suspected of being due) to the incorrect components being transfused.[125] Ibojie and Urbaniak[126] performed a retrospective study of transfusion errors in a large Scottish teaching hospital. Seventy-five percent of the errors detected were classified as near misses. The number of patients transfused with the wrong blood was one in 27,007 units supplied. About 50% of the mistransfusion errors occurred at the patient's bedside. The number of near misses was one in 9002. The number of serious errors identified was one per 6752 units issued, or one per 2153 compatibility tests. Fortunately, no fatal HTRs occurred. Callum and colleagues[127] performed a prospective study of near misses using a no-fault medical-event reporting system for transfusion medicine (MERS-TM). Events and near-miss events (total 819) were recorded for a period of 19 months (median number, 51 per month). No serious adverse patient outcome occurred, despite these events, with the transfusion of 17,465 units of RBCs. Sixty-one events (7.4%) were potentially life threatening or could have led to permanent injury (severity level 1). Of most concern were three samples collected from the wrong patient, 13 mislabeled samples, and 22 requests for blood for the wrong patient. Near-miss events were five times more frequent than actual transfusion errors, and 68% of errors were detected before blood was issued. Sixty-one percent of events originated from patient areas, 35% from the blood bank, and 4% from the blood supplier or other hospitals. Repeat collection was required for one in every 94 samples, and one in 346 requests for blood components was incorrect. Education of nurses and alterations to blood bank forms were not by themselves effective in reducing severe errors. An artifactual 50% reduction in the number of errors reported was noted during a 6-month period when two chief members of the event-reporting team were on temporary leave.

Detection, Analysis, Frequency, and Prevention of Errors

Taswell and coworkers[128] reviewed transfusion medicine errors occurring at the Mayo Clinic from 1982 through 1992. They defined an error as any deviation from the standard operating procedure. Twenty-four standard operating procedures were monitored for errors that related to donor processing, testing of donor blood, patient testing, and transfusion. The estimate of the overall error rate and 95% confidence interval fluctuated between 20 and 30 per 10^4 procedures. The transcription error rate declined from 21 to six per 10^4 procedures as a result of changes to systems using computer-generated labels and bar codes.

Several investigators have audited errors occurring from when a unit of blood is first tested in the transfusion service until it is transfused to the patient.[129-131] This approach differs from the reports in the previous section in that these are errors observed by an auditor watching the process, rather than reported errors. It is likely that the audits are nearer to the truth than the reported errors (e.g., FDA data).

Most disturbing data has come from a Belgian study. Baele and associates[129] audited 3485 units of blood transfused to 808 surgical patients. After the units left the blood bank, 165 errors were noted. Fifteen of these errors were defined as major. Seven of 2772 units (0.25%, or one in 400) were transfused to the wrong patient. Luckily, in six instances they provoked no obvious symptoms; in one patient, a few mL of group B blood given to a group O patient caused chills and the transfusion was stopped. It is of concern to note that the episode was noted in the patient's notes, the unit was discarded, and the reaction was not reported to the blood bank.

Shulman and colleagues[130,131] used a multidisciplinary team to address this problem. The team consisted of representatives from the transfusion service, the administration, nursing, medical information services, and quality assessment coordinators from various clinical departments. Acceptable compliance with institutional blood administration policies existed when the following were documented:

1. The intended recipient wore an ID band.
2. Two licensed individuals did each of the following while at the patient's bedside:
   a. They compared the information on the patient's ID band with the information on the blood component labels.
   b. They compared the information on the patient's ID band with the blood component paperwork.
   c. They compared the information on the blood component labels with the blood component paperwork.
3. No deviations from policy were noted for handling of blood components outside of the blood bank, charting of required information, taking of vital signs, use of intravenous solutions, duration of transfusion, or follow-up of possible transfusion reactions.

An initial small audit revealed that variance from the foregoing procedures was observed in three (50%) of six transfusions. The audit data initially demonstrated the following:

1. A systematic failure of transfusionists (mainly nurses, but some physicians and medical students) to identify patients properly before transfusion
2. Sporadic variances in other transfusionists' practices, such as the taking of vital signs and chart documentation

Several factors were found to cause variances from proper blood administration practices, including:

1. Insufficient knowledge due to a deficiency in orientation or training in the procedure
2. Behavioral or performance deficiency due to the lack of acceptance of the procedure, indifference to the procedure, or carelessness
3. System deficits

Even though all nurses are supposed to be orientated and trained in proper blood administration procedures, the audit process demonstrated knowledge deficits. Many nurses failed to perform the pretransfusion clerical cross-check properly because they felt that they knew the patient so well that the clerical checking was unnecessary. These nurses did not realize that a blood bank error could result in issuance of the wrong blood for their patient and that, without the clerical cross-check being done properly, their patient (whom they "knew so well") might get blood that was actually intended for someone else. As transfusionists began to realize that one reason for doing the clerical cross-check was to catch a blood bank error, the hospital blood administration procedures won better acceptance. Furthermore, as each variance from proper blood administration practice was addressed, improvement occurred, and compliance with pretransfusion clerical cross-checking approached 100%. In audits 126 to 175 (50 consecutive transfusions), there was 100% compliance with blood administration policies. Other researchers have reported similar findings.[126,132]

Shulman and Kent[133] studied the incidence of unit placement errors, that is, the placing of RBC units in the wrong section of the refrigerator. In a study of 96,581 units at a large institution, they found an error rate of 0.12% (112 units misplaced, one in 862), with about one third of these potentially leading to ABO-incompatible transfusions if released (an ABO mismatch error rate of 0.04% or 1 in 2610). They noted that placement errors are of concern because a crossmatch cannot always be counted on to detect ABO incompatibility and usually will not detect Rh incompatibility because most Rh-negative patients do not have anti-D. The investigators further noted that placement errors are of great concern when uncrossmatched blood is transfused in emergency situations. Their study showed the importance of frequent verification of unit placement to reduce the chance of an incompatible unit being released by mistake.[133]

Systems for Reducing Incidence of Transfusion of Blood to Wrong Patient

The most commonly used system involves identification of the patient using a wristband. In a College of American Pathologists (CAP) Q-Probe study, Renner and coworkers[134] compared wristband identification errors for 712 hospitals. Phlebotomists checked patient wristbands on 2,463,727 occasions, finding 67,289 errors; in 33,308 instances, patient wristbands were missing entirely. The median total error rate was 2.2%; 10% of participants had error rates of 10.9% or greater. Absent wristbands represented 49.5% of all errors; multiple wristbands with different information, 8.3%; wristbands with incomplete data, 7.5%; wristbands with erroneous data, 8.6%; wristbands with illegible data, 5.7%; and patients wearing wristbands with another patient's identifying information, 0.5%. The monitoring for errors by phlebotomy staff was the most important policy associated with lower error rates. Initial placement of wristbands by nursing staff was the only policy associated with increased error rates. They concluded that wristband identification error rates depend on differences in hospital policy and procedure and should be responsive to quality improvement efforts.[134]

A follow-up study of 204 smaller hospitals compared wristband errors.[135] Phlebotomists examined wristbands on 451,436 occasions and identified 25,800 errors (total error rate, 5.7%). The absence of a wristband accounted for 64.6% of all errors reported; wristbands with missing information, 12.4%; multiple wristbands with different information, 12.1%; wristbands with erroneous information, 6.7%; illegible wristbands, 3.5%; and patients wearing another patient's wristband, 0.7%. Factors found to correlate with lower error rates were the practice of sending written correspondence to the nursing service involved for each error detected, the practice of having nursing staff monitor wristbands on patient transfer, and laboratory accreditation from CAP. Factors found to correlate with higher error rates were the practice of allowing wristbands to be placed on objects that could become separated from the patient (e.g., chart, beds, wall) and the practice of having nurses be responsible for initial wristband placement.[135]

Lau and colleagues[136] designed an improved wristband system. The wristband had the following special features:

- Once attached, it cannot be removed except by cutting.
- It has a pocket containing a transfusion label.
- A unique transfusion barcode is printed simultaneously on each transfusion label and the corresponding wristband by computer technology.
- A transfusion label removed from the wristband after attachment to the patient has a characteristic tear-mark distinguishing it from one removed prior to attachment.

The blood bank accepted only those specimens bearing the tear-marked transfusion labels. All blood units for this patient were labeled with this unique transfusion code together with the patient's details. The nurses counter-checked the transfusion code on the blood units against the transfusion code on the patient's transfusion wristband prior to transfusion. If the blood sample for compatibility testing was drawn from the "wrong" patient, the intended patient either did not carry a wristband or the transfusion codes did not match at all. Pretransfusion compatibility tests were performed on 2189 patient samples using this procedure, which was well accepted by both ward and blood bank staff. Two potential mismatched transfusions were avoided. These two clerical errors would not have been detected because neither patient had previous ABO grouping results.

Other approaches have been suggested. One system consists of a coded locking system so that a blood unit cannot be accessed without matching a three-letter code that can be found only on the patient's wristband. Several authors have reported on the efficiency of this system.[137-139] Jensen and Crosson[140] described a system composed of the following components:

1. A portable bedside scanner that reads barcoded patient and blood unit identification
2. A host computer system that accepts data from the scanner
3. Printed documentation of the transfusion
4. Audit trail monitoring

A commercial variation of this system, which is integrated with an automated blood typing system, has subsequently become available.[141]

Lumadue and colleagues[142] felt that adherence to a strict specimen-labeling policy would be an efficient way to decrease errors leading to HTRs. Incorrectly labeled specimens (rejected samples) were tested for ABO and Rh type, and routine antibody screens were performed. Test results were compared with historic patient data or patient data obtained from subsequently submitted (correctly) labeled specimens. For comparison, all discrepant serologic results from appropriately labeled samples were also recorded. Specimens that failed to meet the criteria for specimen acceptance were 40 times more likely to have a blood grouping discrepancy.

HEMOLYTIC TRANSFUSION REACTIONS DUE TO ANTIBODIES THAT ARE NOT DETECTABLE BY ROUTINE PROCEDURES

Hemolytic transfusion reactions, both immediate and delayed, can occur without antibodies being detected (at the time of the reaction) by routinely used tests.[143-166] These reactions appear to occur among three groups of patients:

1. Patients whose sera do not contain detectable antibody at the time of the reaction but in which detectable antibody appears later
2. Patients whose sera contain antibodies that are not detected by routinely used tests but are detectable by special procedures
3. Patients whose sera appear to contain antibodies that are not detectable by routine procedures or multiple special procedures even after repeated transfusions and reactions

Patients Whose Sera Do Not Contain Detectable Antibody at the Time of the Reaction But in Which Detectable Antibody Appears Later

Although the serology pattern for these patients is similar to classic DHTR, transfused RBCs are destroyed, sometimes rapidly, during the phase when antibody is undetectable. As early as 1957, Fudenberg and Allen[58] described such patients. They performed ^{51}Cr RBC survival studies in three subjects who were known to have anti-s, -S, and -Jk^a, but at the time of the study these were not detectable. The Cr-labeled s+, S+, and Jk(a+) RBCs had half-lives of 55 minutes, 9 hours, and 12 days, respectively. After the study, the anti-s rose to a titer of 1, the anti-S rose to a titer of 8, and the anti-Jk^a was still not detectable. The authors suggested that there might be two main reasons for these findings. The first was that the antibody was present in the serum at the time of the transfusion but the routine techniques were not sensitive enough to detect it. The second suggestion was that there was no antibody in the serum but plenty in the spleen and/or other tissues. The pattern described by Fudenberg and Allen[58] has rarely been described in more recent literature, and it could be that more modern serological procedures detected such antibodies in the pretransfusion sera. The patterns described next seem to be the ones that are observed in contemporary practice.

Patients Whose Sera Contain Antibodies That Are Not Detected by Routinely Used Tests But Are Detectable by Special Procedures

There have been many reports in the literature of patients who had HTRs following transfusion of blood that was compatible by saline, albumin, and routine antiglobulin techniques, but alloantibody was demonstrable by techniques that are not used routinely for cross-matching. In 1978, Snyder and coworkers[143] detected an anti-e that had caused an HTR but was detected only by an automated Polybrene technique. Such antibodies rarely are detectable by routine procedures. In 1982 and 1996, Garratty and associates[144,145] reported on more than 70 patients with HTRs but no detectable antibodies by routine procedures. More than 70% presented with hemoglobinemia and hemoglobinuria. Sera were tested using a manual Polybrene technique, polyethylene glycol (PEG), and ficin-treated RBCs (tube plus capillary), and many were tested with increased amounts of patients' sera, diluted sera, monocyte monolayer assays, and enzyme-linked antiglobulin tests. Twelve of 70 antibodies (18%) (three anti-C, three anti-Jk^a, two anti-S, two anti-e, one anti-E, one anti-Jk^b), that were not detected by routine tests were detected by a Polybrene test; six of these 12 were tested by PEG, and all reacted; three of the 12 reacted by a ficin-capillary technique. Three antibodies (one anti-e, one anti-C, one anti-Vel) became detectable by routine tests after the reaction. Three e– and three C– patients, with antibodies undetectable by any methods, responded poorly to e+ and C+ RBCs but responded well to e– and C– RBCs, respectively (supported by ^{51}Cr RBC survival studies in three cases). Two other patients responded well to RBCs matched for several antigens (C, E, Jk^a, S) that the patients lacked. The most common diagnoses of 67 patients were: leukemia (11 patients: six with chronic lymphocytic leukemia [CLL], five with other leukemias), multiple myeloma (six patients), lymphoma (five patients), cancer (five patients), gastrointestinal bleed (five patients), and sickle cell disease (three patients). One CLL patient who had repeated HTRs with no detectable antibodies was investigated for RBC destruction through an antibody-independent cellular mechanism.[144] The patient's lymphocytes were incubated in vitro with ^{51}Cr-labeled autologous and homologous RBCs in an NK cell cytotoxicity assay. The results were noninformative.

Maynard and associates[146] also found Polybrene useful in detecting clinically significant antibodies not detectable by routine procedures. A patient with macroglobulinemia experienced chills, fever, hemoglobinemia, and hemoglobinuria after the transfusion of one unit of RBCs shown to be compatible by a low-ionic-strength indirect antiglobulin (LIS-IAT) method. Serologic investigation was negative. Intravascular hemolysis occurred with a second "compatible" unit. Serologic tests were again negative by

LIS-IAT and ficin-AG methods but revealed anti-Jk^a by the manual Polybrene technique. Both donors with Jk(a+b–) and ^{51}Cr studies of the second donor's RBCs revealed a $T_{1/2}$ of greater than 30 minutes with marked intravascular hemolysis. RBCs from a C+, c+, Jk(a–) donor that were compatible by LIS-IAT showed a ^{51}Cr $T_{1/2}$ of 100 minutes with slight intravascular lysis. Four transfusions of Jk(a–), C– blood were uneventful, but 5 days later the patient's hemoglobin declined. The following day, anti-E was demonstrable exclusively by the Polybrene test. ^{51}Cr-labeled Jk(a–), C–, E– RBCs had normal 24-hour survival. The patient's hemoglobin rose to 11 g/dL after transfusions of Jk(a–), C–, E– RBCs, and he was discharged.

Others have reported similar findings.[147,148] Although Polybrene appeared to be the most efficient test to detect these unusual antibodies, it might not be the best for routine compatibility test procedures. Lown and Willis[149] tested random antibodies, which were detected by the Polybrene test but negative by IAT, by a monocyte monolayer assay and found that many of these would be predicted to be clinically insignificant.

Patients Whose Sera Appear to Contain Antibodies That Are Not Detectable by Routine Procedures or Multiple Special Procedures Even After Repeated Transfusions and Reactions

As early as 1959, Stewart and Mollison[150] and in 1961, Kissmeyer-Nielsen and colleagues[151] described patients who had HTRs after serologically compatible blood. ^{51}Cr RBC survivals were grossly abnormal. Chaplin and Cassell[80] followed a patient with SCD who had HTRs and no demonstrable alloantibodies for 2 years, and they performed 17 RBC survival studies. Survival of transfused RBCs in this patient varied from a half-life of less than 1 day to a normal survival of 30 days; the 30-day RBC survival was obtained on blood from the patient's sister; therefore, it did appear that the patient had an antibody with a specificity that was not apparent from the RBC survival studies. van Loghem and coworkers[152] also showed rapid destruction of ^{51}Cr-labeled red cells in five patients who had HTRs with no detectable antibody (half-lives varied from 3 hours to 14 days). The authors felt that this phenomenon was not due to circulating antibodies. This conclusion was based on the results of an interesting experiment. They incubated RBCs from a donor (Mrs. G) in the serum of a previous recipient (Mrs. E). Mrs. G's RBCs had been shown previously to be destroyed rapidly in recipient Mrs. E. Following incubation in vitro, the RBCs were labeled with ^{51}Cr and reinjected back into Mrs. G; the RBCs survived normally. This experiment was performed twice: first with serum taken 6 months after the original transfusion of "incompatible" blood and the second time with serum taken 3 weeks after the transfusion; RBC survival was normal both times. This experiment suggested that a factor (e.g., antibody) in Mrs. E's serum was not responsible for the decreased RBC survival observed in the original transfusion or ^{51}Cr studies.

More recently, results of ^{51}Cr RBC survival studies have suggested an antibody with defined blood group specificity as the cause of HTR. Davey and associates[153] described a patient who had HTR with no detectable antibody. The patient had a severe DHTR (hemoglobinemia and hemoglobinuria) 10 days after transfusion of 4 units of blood. No antibodies were detected by multiple serological procedures, either routine or special. Following red cell phenotyping, it was ascertained that the only antigen that the patient lacked and the units possessed was c. ^{51}Cr RBC survival studies showed that c-positive RBCs had 48% survival at 3 hours and less than 1% survival at 24 hours, compared with 93% survival at 3 hours and 80% at 24 hours for c-negative RBCs. Eight c-negative units were transfused with no problems; no anti-c was detectable at the time of transfusion or at 2 months or 6 months after transfusion. Baldwin and colleagues[154] described a similar case. Serological studies using multiple techniques demonstrated only an anti-Bg^a; these studies included both standard procedures and more sensitive experimental techniques. A ^{51}Cr survival study, using RBCs from a random unit compatible in vitro with conventional techniques, showed 72% survival at 1 hour and 7% survival at 24 hours. R_2R_2 (e-negative) RBCs in a second ^{51}Cr survival study showed 90% survival at 1 hour and 92% survival at 6 hours. The patient was transfused with R_2R_2 units, which were tolerated well and survived normally. Extensive serologic testing still demonstrated only an anti-Bg^a. A third ^{51}Cr survival study, 10 months after the first study, with an R_1R_1 (e-positive) sample showed 90% survival at 1 hour and 42% survival at 6 hours. A fourth study, using a larger aliquot of R_2R_2 (e-negative) ^{51}Cr-labeled RBCs, examined over the course of 2 weeks, showed a near-normal 21-day survival of 50%. These ^{51}Cr survival studies, along with normal survival of e-negative units, suggest that this patient destroyed e-positive RBCs despite negative serologic testing.[154]

Garratty and colleagues described two further patients for whom blood was selected on the basis of the patients' phenotypes. Anti-C and anti-e, respectively, were suspected because of proven destruction of RBCs having the appropriate antigen and survival of RBCs lacking the antigen. These antibodies were undetectable by all tests in our lab and those of several specialist labs. RBC survival was studied in one case with ^{51}Cr-labeled RBC and in the other case by differential agglutination. One patient with CLL, who had repeated HTR with no detectable antibodies, was investigated for RBC destruction through a nonantibody-dependent cellular mechanism. Patient's lymphocytes were incubated in vitro with ^{51}Cr-labeled autologous and homologous RBCs (NK cell cytotoxicity assay). The results were noninformative.[144,155]

Harrison and coworkers[156] described an HTR caused by anti-C that was not detectable by any serological procedures, including enzymes, but which was defined by ^{51}Cr studies; the HTR was associated with hemoglobinemia and hemoglobinuria.

Can HLA Antibodies Cause HTRs?

HLA antibodies are usually not considered important with regard to RBC survival. Bg antibodies (anti-HLA-B7, -17, -28) have been shown not to usually destroy reactive RBCs. The antibodies would not be expected to cause many RBC problems because there are very few HLA antigens on mature RBCs. On the other hand, IgG HLA antibodies are known to activate complement efficiently and perhaps, on occasion, they could cause shortened RBC survival. There are some reports in the literature supporting this hypothesis.[157-163] van der Hart and associates[157] performed ^{51}Cr RBC survival studies in a patient with lymphocytotoxic antibodies to HLA-B40, -B13, and -B7, with RBCs from a donor with strong RBC HLA antigens (A2; B7, 40). About 60% of the RBCs were removed, with a T_{50}Cr of about 100 minutes, and the rest with a T_{50}Cr of 20 hours. Nordhagen and Aas[158] studied a patient whose serum reacted with RBCs from HLA-B28–positive donors. A small component (20%) of the incompatible RBCs had a reduced survival (T_{50}Cr of 1.5 days), but the main component had normal survival.

Panzer and colleagues[159] showed that ^{51}Cr-labeled RBCs that were incompatible with HLA antibodies present in the sera of six women had shortened survival in every case, especially when anti-HLA-B7 was involved. In further studies, Panzer and colleagues[160] performed a prospective study to see whether HLA sensitization is associated with increased RBC destruction after HLA-incompatible transfusion; ^{51}Cr-labeled RBC survival and site of sequestration were monitored in nine patients in whom HLA antibodies had developed after RBC transfusion. The donors selected were compatible in ABO- and RBC-specific antigen systems but were mismatched for the HLA antigen in question. Hemolytic transfusion reactions occurred in all four patients who received HLA-B7–incompatible RBCs. A direct radioimmune anti-IgG test became positive, ^{51}Cr RBC survival was very short, and excess sequestration in the spleen was measured. There was a rise in serum lactic dehydrogenase and a fall in haptoglobin. HLA-B7 antibody was detected in the eluate prepared from RBCs collected after transfusion. A similar reaction was found in only one further patient, caused by an HLA-A2 incompatibility. No indications of immune-medicated RBC sequestration were discernable after transfusion of HLA-B7 compatible RBC in one of the patients who had shown a reaction with HLA-B7 incompatible blood, nor in any of the other patients who received HLA-B7–compatible RBCs. The hemolytic transfusion reactions could not be anticipated by conventional cross-match procedures, nor by the measurement of the ^{51}Cr survival 1 hour after transfusion.

Mollison and coworkers[161] criticized the interpretation of the ^{51}Cr survival curves used by Panzer and colleagues.[160] The method used by the latter researchers was meant to be applied to the survival of autologous RBCs, not to potentially incompatible RBCs. When the RBC survival curve has more than one component to the method, it is not applicable. On reinterpreting the data, Mollison and coworkers[161] felt that the ^{51}Cr survival curves published by Panzer and colleagues[160] show that the T_{50}Cr in their cases 3 through 6 was approximately 24–30 days (i.e., probably within normal limits). Cases 1 and 2 showed about 25% destruction of the remaining RBCs in the first 24 hours.

In 1993, Weitekamp and associates[162] reported very convincing data that HLA might sometimes cause HTRs. A woman with gastrointestinal bleeding (one unit RBCs per day), received 13 uncomplicated RBC transfusions in a 2-week period. With the 14th unit of RBCs, she developed shaking chills, nausea, vomiting, and red urine. LDH was 2024 IU/L and haptoglobin less than 5 mg/dL, with a disproportionate decrease in hemoglobin. Similar reactions were seen with 3 of the next 6 units (2 of which were saline washed). Postreaction blood samples were grossly hemolyzed and, despite enhancement, they contained no RBC alloantibodies other than the previously recognized anti-D and -Fy^{b}. The patient's HLA type was A1,26; B44,70. Potent HLA antibodies specific for private A2 and public A2-B17, A2-28, and A2-28-9 were demonstrated by adsorption and elution lymphocytotoxic assays. The patient subsequently received 10 units from HLA compatible donors (6 new) without difficulty. Antibodies reacting 1+ in IAT against HLA-incompatible RBCs were detected 3.5 weeks after hemolysis began. These antibodies reacted with each of the four donors implicated in the transfusion reactions and were negative with RBCs of nine donors (13 units) that were tolerated. HLA typing and AHG white-cell cross-matching showed that all four donors implicated in hemolysis were incompatible with the HLA antibody; whereas the nine donors of tolerated units were HLA compatible. The patient died 2 weeks after total gastrectomy, of surgical complications. This appears to be first reported case of repeated, severe, symptomatic hemolytic reactions after transfusion of HLA-incompatible RBCs. The high titer (128) of the lymphocytotoxic antibody might explain these unusual reactions. The authors suggested that HLA-reactive alloantibodies should be investigated in patients with unexplained hemolytic transfusion reactions.[162] A similar case was described by Benson and associates.[163]

NONHUMORAL MECHANISMS

It is possible that the RBCs are being destroyed by an antibody-independent, cell-mediated mechanism. For instance, NK cells are known to destroy other cells by such a mechanism. Garratty[164] suggested this as a cause of HTRs as early as 1981 but was unable to prove it; an NK cell assay was performed using the donor RBCs and mononuclear cells from a patient with chronic lymphocytic leukemia who had HTRs with no detectable antibodies.[144,164] It is interesting to note that Gilsanz and colleagues[165] have shown in one case that NK cells can cause "DAT-negative" AIHA. Thus, the hypothesis is worth retaining.

HTRs ASSOCIATED WITH PASSIVELY TRANSFUSED ALLOANTIBODIES

The problem of passively acquired alloantibodies is an old one. Because group O blood was first transfused to patients who were not group O, clinicians and immunohematologists have had to deal with the passive transfer of anti-A, anti-B, and anti-A,B to group A, B, or AB recipients. As more plasma products (e.g., platelets, fresh-frozen plasma, coagulation factors) were used for recipients who were sometimes not ABO identical, the problems grew. With the advent of bone marrow transplantation (BMT), the increasing use of intravenous immune gamma globulin (IVIgG), and more recently, the use of intravenous (IV) anti-D (an Rh[D] immune globulin) in Rh-positive recipients, new problems have arisen.[166]

The amount of plasma contained in a unit of RBCs will be influenced by the hematocrit of the donor and how that unit was prepared. (The lowest acceptable hematocrit is 38%; there is no mandated upper value, but the highest normal male hematocrit is around 54%, the hematocrit must be adjusted to take into account the amount of anticoagulant present—63 mL for a 450 mL unit and 70 mL for a 500 mL unit.). Blood centers use a "soft spin" (e.g., 2200 rpm for 7 minutes in a Sorvall RC3 centrifuge) when preparing platelet products from the unit, and a "hard spin" (e.g., 4000 rpm for 6 minutes in a Sorvall RC3 centrifuge) when only plasma is taken off. The resulting hematocrits of the "packed" RBCs before adenine-saline solution (e.g., Adsol, Fenwal Laboratories, Roundlake, IL) is added, are, on average, 81% and 93%, respectively, at the American Red Cross in Los Angeles. Recently, 500 (± 50 mL) units are being collected, in addition to 450 (± 45 mL) units; this, too, will influence the amount of residual plasma. Taking all those factors into account, the amount of plasma remaining in "packed" RBCs can be calculated to be 12–40 mL.[166] As the increasing trend is for blood centers to remove as much plasma as possible from RBC products (e.g., in the Los Angeles Blood Center, two thirds of the "packed" RBCs, before addition of adenine-saline solution, have a hematocrit of about 90%; after adding adenine-saline solution, the hematocrit is 55–65%), the amount of residual plasma is often at the lower end of the range.[166]

TRANSFUSION OF GROUP O BLOOD TO A, B, OR AB RECIPIENTS

When group O blood (even "packed" RBCs) is transfused to group A, B, or AB individuals, anti-A, anti-B, and anti-A,B are almost always transferred. Two major events prevent passively acquired ABO antibodies from causing a clinical problem. First, the antibodies are, of course, diluted in vivo. The average anti-A titer is about 128; thus, if no other factors play a role, a small adult—for instance, a 5-ft, 100-lb woman with a plasma volume of 1200 mL—would need to receive only about 10 mL of plasma to theoretically have detectable antibody.[167,168] In practice, the antibody probably would not be detectable on the patient's RBCs or in the serum because ABH antigens are distributed widely in the recipient, and much of the passively transfused antibody is inhibited by ABH blood group substances present in the recipient's plasma and tissues. Passively acquired ABO antibodies are usually detected in recipients only when the donor antibody is of high titer, and hemolytic transfusion reactions occur only when the plasma contains antibody of exceptionally high titer, when large volumes of plasma are transfused, or when young children or infants receive transfusions.[1,169-171] Mollison and coworkers[1] reviewed early work in which 250 mL of group O plasma was deliberately transfused to group A volunteers. In two studies, the lowest titer of anti-A agglutinins associated with in vivo hemolysis were 512 and 640; 40% and 23%, respectively, of group O donors were found to have anti-A in such titers. Thousands of units of whole blood from "safe" (ABO-antibody titers <200) group O donors were transfused to group A and B recipients in the Korean and Vietnam wars with very few ill effects.[172,173] Schwab and associates[174] performed a 2-year prospective study using group O uncross-matched "packed" RBCs for trauma cases and found no hemolytic transfusion reactions after 880 transfusions.

From a practical point of view, it is usually advised to continue transfusing group O (rather than the patient's own type-specific blood) to a group A or B patient who has had to receive group O blood, until anti-A or -B is no longer detectable (at 37°C or by antiglobulin test) in the patient's serum.[166]

PASSIVE TRANSFER OF RBC ALLOANTIBODIES OTHER THAN ABO

Standard 5.8.3.1 of the 22nd edition of the American Association of Blood Banks (AABB)[175] states that only serum or plasma from donors with a history of transfusion or pregnancy should be tested for unexpected RBC antibodies, but most blood centers find it more convenient to screen all donors. Thus, it is rare for non-ABO alloantibodies to be transferred passively from donor to recipient. As DATs are not performed routinely, RBC-bound autoantibodies can be transferred to the recipient. Such autoantibodies probably have little clinical significance to the recipient if they are causing no problems (i.e., hemolytic anemia) in the donor. Only about 0.2% of blood donors have 37°C-reactive alloantibodies[176]; this frequency is obviously dependent on the techniques used. Even if alloantibodies were present in a unit of blood, they would have to be exceptional antibodies (i.e., of a high enough titer to withstand dilution by recipient plasma) to cause any ill effects in the recipient. High-titer donor alloantibodies can cause positive DATs and perhaps even be detectable in the recipient's plasma, but it is still unlikely that they would cause a significant reaction in the recipient. This statement is supported by the paucity of reports of any such reactions in the literature and is emphasized by the minimal clinical ill effects encountered when D-positive volunteers are transfused (sometimes deliberately) with plasma containing anti-D, anti-C, or anti-K,[177-179] and by the current practice of injecting powerful anti-D into D-positive patients with autoimmune thrombocytopenic purpura.[180]

The literature includes several reports of donor antibodies reacting with another transfused unit ("interdonor incompatibility")[181-187]; most of these were associated with anti-K. The majority of these reactions were mild (e.g., fever, chills, increased bilirubin), but three were quite severe.[182,183,186] Some of the reactions occurred before donor screening was common practice, and two were associated with anti-K that were not detected by an automated enzyme technique.[181,186] It is unknown whether these antibodies would have caused similar reactions if transfused to a K-positive recipient. The association of such reactions with interdonor incompatibility is probably because there would be much more antibody on each K-positive RBC when only 1 unit of RBCs (i.e., the K-positive donor unit) is K positive.

Naczek and colleagues[188] found only minimal serologic and no clinical problems when patients were transfused with RBCs from units containing alloantibodies. They evaluated 42 patients transfused with RBCs from units containing anti-K, anti-D, anti-E, anti-C, anti-C, anti-Fy^a, anti-Jk^a, and anti-A$_1$. Antibodies were detectable in a serum sample from only one recipient; this patient had received 3 units containing anti-E and/or anti-Fy^a. One patient had a positive DAT with anti-D in an eluate from the RBCs. No clinical evidence of hemolysis was observed in any patient.

Combs and coworkers[189] (from Duke University) transfused 253 units of RBCs, from donors who had alloantibodies, to 187 random patients. Only 10% of these recipients had antibody detectable in their serum after transfusion (all detectable antibodies were anti-D or C + D). No HTRs were reported. The antibody-containing units were obtained at a discounted price. The authors concluded that large-scale use of RBC units from donors with alloantibodies is safe and likely to have minimal impact on a busy transfusion service.

PASSIVE TRANSFER OF RBC ALLOANTIBODIES IN PLATELET, GRANULOCYTE, PLASMA, AND COAGULATION PRODUCTS

Platelets and Granulocytes. Any group A, B, or AB patient receiving platelets or granulocytes from donors (who are not group AB) who do not have an identical ABO type could have passively acquired anti-A,B and/or anti-A, and/or anti-B. As discussed previously for transfusion of group O blood, hemolytic anemia rarely ensues, but as larger volumes of plasma are often involved (i.e., apheresis products), there is an increased risk of problems. These problems might involve only a positive DAT due to sensitization of the recipient's RBCs with anti-A or -B. This can confuse the investigator, as eluates are routinely tested against only group O RBCs. Before performing extensive workups (e.g., evaluating drug-dependent antibodies as a cause of a positive DAT), it is always wise to ask whether the patient has received platelets from a donor of different ABO type. On occasions, the passively transfused ABO antibodies cause hemolytic anemia, and on rare occasions this has been fatal.[190-204] Shanwell and colleagues[201] reported that nine of 11 group A recipients developed a positive DAT after receiving platelet concentrates (five had IgG + C3d, and four had only C3d on their RBCs); none of the nine patients showed signs of hemolysis.

Coagulation Factors. Cryoprecipitate, factor VIII, and factor IX products have all caused immune hemolysis in patients.[205-212] The hemolysis was due in all cases to passively transferred ABO antibodies. Mild anemia is common among hemophiliacs, and it has been suggested that immune hemolysis caused by passively acquired antibodies might be a cause of the anemia; Buchanan and associates[211] presented data that did not support this hypothesis. With the advent of more highly purified and recombinant therapeutic coagulation factors, problems with passively transferred ABO antibodies should become even rarer.

LABORATORY INVESTIGATION OF HTRs

The Standards of the AABB[175] suggest that only three tests are mandated to exclude an immune etiology for an HTR. These simple tests are a repeat ABO group, a DAT and visual examination of the recipient's plasma for hemoglobin. The rationale for this is the finding, by the Mayo Clinic, that approximately 90% of recipients have a positive DAT after an HTR.[55,56] The patients who do not have a positive DAT and do have definite signs of a HTR are usually those associated with ABO incompatibility. In ABO incompatibility, all the sensitized RBCs might have been removed from the circulation. In such a case, hemoglobinemia, obvious by visual inspection of the plasma, will always be present. Table 14-9 shows that destruction of 5 mL of RBCs will lead to an obviously pink plasma (especially if compared with pretransfusion plasma), and even destruction of as little as 2 mL of RBCs might be detectable visually.

Many investigators perform more than these three tests. Others might include repeat ABO and Rh typing, antibody screening, and cross-matching. As mentioned earlier, sometimes all the routine serological tests are nonproductive, and if the evidence for an HTR is good, special tests may be performed. These might include different antibody potentiators (e.g., enzymes, PEG, Polybrene), different techniques (gel, solid phase), different antiglobulin sera (anti-C3, -IgA, -IgM), different antibody-antigen ratios (increased volumes of serum), and most important, use of another laboratory (preferably a Reference Laboratory).

REFERENCES

1. Mollison PL, Engelfriet CP, Contreras M: Blood Transfusion in Clinical Medicine, 10th ed. Oxford: Blackwell Scientific, 1997.
2. Grobbelaar BG, Smart E: The incidence of isosensitization following blood transfusion. Transfusion 1967;7:152.
3. Grove-Rasmussen H: Routine compatibility testing. Transfusion 1964;4:200–205.
4. Tovey GH: Preventing the incompatible blood transfusion. Haematologia 1974;8:171–176.
5. Spielmann W, Seidl S: Prevalence of irregular red cell antibodies and their significance in blood transfusion and antenatal care. Vox Sang 1974;26:551–559.
6. Walker RH, Lin D-T, Hartrick MB: Alloimmunization following blood transfusion. Arch Pathol Lab Med 1989;113:254–260.
7. Hewitt PE, Macintyre EA, Devenish A, et al: A prospective study of the incidence of delayed haemolytic transfusion reactions following peri-operative blood transfusion. Br J Haematol 1988;69:541–544.
8. Hoeltge GA, Domen RE, Rybicki LA, Schaffer PA: Multiple red cell transfusions and alloimmunization. Arch Pathol Lab Med 1995;119:42–45.
9. Heddle NM, Soutar RL, O'Hoski PL, et al: A prospective study to determine the frequency and clinical significance of alloimmunization post-transfusion. Br J Haematol 1995;91: 1000–1005.
10. Lostumbo MM, Holland PV, Schmidt PJ: Isoimmunization after multiple transfusions. N Eng J Med 1966;275:141.
11. Perkins HA: Isoantibodies following open heart surgery. In Hollander LP (ed): Proceedings of the 11th Congress International Society for Blood Transfusion, Sydney 1966; Bibl. haemat. No. 29, Part 3. Basel: Karger, 1968:831.
12. Blumberg N, Peck K, Ross K, Avila E: Immune response to chronic red blood cell transfusion. Vox Sang 1983;44:212–217.
13. Ting A, Pun A, Dodds AJ, Atkinson K, Biggs JC: Red cell alloantibodies produced after bone marrow transplantation. Transfusion 1987;17:145–147.
14. Brantley SG, Ramsey G: Red cell alloimmunization in multitransfused HLA-typed patients. Transfusion 1988;28:463–466.
15. Ramsey G, Cornell FW, Hahn LF, et al: Red cell antibody problems in 1000 liver transplants. Transfusion 1989;29:396–400.
16. Fluit CRMG, Kunst VAJM, Drenthe-Schonk AM: Incidence of red cell antibodies after multiple blood transfusions. Transfusion 1990;30:532–535.
17. Economidou J, Constantoulakis M, Augoustaki O, Adinolfi M: Frequency of antibodies to various antigenic determinants in polytransfused patients with homozygous thalassaemia in Greece. Vox Sang 1971;20:252–258.
18. Coles SM, Klein HG, Holland PV: Alloimmunization in two multitransfused patient populations. Transfusion 1981;21:462.
19. Sirchia G, Zanella A, Parravicini A, et al: Red cell alloantibodies in thalassemia major. Transfusion 1985;25:110–112.
20. Michail-Merianou V, Pamphili-Panousopoulou L, Piperi-Lowes L, Pelegrinis E, Karaklis A: Alloimmunization to red cell antigens in thalassemia: Comparative study of usual versus better-match transfusion programmes. Vox Sang 1987;52:95–98.
21. Spanos T, Karageorga M, Ladis V, et al: Red cell alloantibodies in patients with thalassemia. Vox Sang 1990;58:50–55.
22. Prati D: Benefits and complications of regular blood transfusion in patients with beta-thalassaemia major. Vox Sang 2000;79:129–137.
23. Singer ST, Wu V, Mignacca R, et al: Alloimmunization and erythrocyte autoimmunzation in transfusion-dependent thalassemia patients of predominantly Asian descent. Blood 2000;96:3369–3373.
24. Ho H-K, Ha S-Y, Lam C-K, et al: Alloimmunization in Hong Kong southern Chinese transfusion-dependent thalassemia patients. Blood 2001;97:3999–4000.
25. Orlina AR, Unger PJ, Koshy M: Post-transfusion alloimmunization in patients with sickle cell disease. Am J Hematol 1978;5:101–106.
26. Davies SC, McWilliam AC, Hewitt PE, et al: Red cell alloimmunization in sickle cell disease. Br J Haematol 1986; 63:241–245.
27. Sarnaik S, Schornack J, Lusher JM: The incidence of development of irregular red cell antibodies in patients with sickle cell anemia. Transfusion 1986;26:249–252.
28. Ambruso DR, Githens JH, Alcorn R, et al: Experience with donors matched for minor blood group antigens in patients with sickle cell anemia who are receiving chronic transfusion therapy. Transfusion 1987;27:94–98.
29. Reisner EG, Kostyu DD, Phillips G, et al: Alloantibody responses in multiply transfused sickle cell patients. Tissue Antigens 1987;30:161–166.
30. Koshy M, Burd L, Wallace D, et al: Prophylactic red-cell transfusions in pregnant patients with sickle cell disease: A randomized cooperative study. N Eng J Med 1988;319:1447–1452.
31. Cox JV, Steane E, Cunningham G, et al: Risk of alloimmunization and delayed hemolytic transfusion reactions in patients with sickle cell disease. Arch Intern Med 1988;48:2485–2489.
32. Luban NL: Variability in rates of alloimmunization in different groups of children with sickle cell disease: Effect of ethnic background. Am J Pediatr Hematol Oncol 1989;11:314–319.
33. Vichinsky EP, Earles A, Johnson RA, et al: Alloimmunization in sickle cell anemia and transfusion of racially unmatched blood. N Eng J Med 1990;322:1617–1621.
34. Rosse WF, Gallagher D, Kinney TR, et al: Transfusion and alloimmunization in sickle cell disease. Blood 1990;76: 1431–1437.
35. Wayne AS, Kevy SV, Nathan DG: Transfusion management of sickle cell disease. Blood 1993;81:1109–1123.
36. Tahhan HR, Holbrook CT, Braddy LR, et al: Antigen-matched donor blood in the transfusion management of patients with sickle cell disease. Transfusion 1994;34:562–569.
37. Garratty G: Severe reactions associated with transfusion of patients with sickle cell disease. Transfusion 1997;37:357–361.
38. Wallhermfechtel MA, Pohl BA, Chaplin H: Alloimmunization in patients with warm autoantibodies: A retrospective study employing three donor alloabsorptions to aid in antibody detection. Transfusion 1984;24:482–485.
39. Issitt PD, Combs MR, Bumgarner DJ, et al: Studies of antibodies in the sera of patients who have made red cell autoantibodies. Transfusion 1996;36:481–486.
40. Leger RM, Garratty G: Evaluation of methods for detecting alloantibodies underlying warm autoantibodies. Transfusion 1999;39:11–16.
41. James P, Rowe GP, Tozzo GG: Elucidation of alloantibodies in autoimmune haemolytic anaemia. Vox Sang 1988;54:167–171.
42. Laine ML, Beattie KM: Frequency of alloantibodies accompanying autoantibodies. Transfusion 1985;25:545–546.
43. Morel PA, Bergren MO, Frank BA: A simple method for the detection of alloantibody in the presence of warm autoantibody [abstract]. Transfusion 1978;18:388.
44. Sokol RJ, Hewitt S, Booker DJ, et al: Patients with red cell autoantibodies: Selection of blood for transfusion. Clin Lab Haematol 1988;10:257–264.
45. Issitt PD, Anstee DJ: Applied Blood Group Serology, 4th ed. Durham, NC: Montgomery Scientific, 1998:974.
46. Garratty G: Clinical significance of antibodies reacting optimally at 37°C. In Clinically significant and insignificant antibodies. Washington, DC: American Association of Blood Banks, 1979:29–49.
47. Mollison PL: Blood-group antibodies and red-cell destruction. Br Med J 1959;2:1035–1130.